The Latest *Evolution*

Evolve provides online access to free resources designed specifically for you. The resources will provide you with information that enhances the material covered in the book and much more.

Visit the Web address listed below today!

> ▶ **LOGIN:** *http://evolve.elsevier.com/DrugConsult/nurses/*

Evolve Learning Resources for *Mosby's 2005 Drug Consult for Nurses* offer the following features:

- **Continuing Education (CE) Test***
  Earn **4.0 contact hours** of continuing education credit by successfully completing this 26 question multiple-choice test online for a nominal fee. You can use these contact hours for relicensure, recertification, professional development, or personal growth. To request a hard copy of the CE test, contact Gina Clites, Continuing Education Coordinator, Elsevier, 11830 Westline Industrial Drive, St. Louis, MO 63146, 314-453-4810, g.clites@elsevier.com.

- **Quarterly Drug Updates and Alerts**
  Abbreviated monographs on new drugs and updated information on new indications and new dosages for existing drugs. Important information about drugs recently withdrawn from the market, new drug safety information, and other news to help you provide the best possible care.

- **"Do not confuse" Table**
  A complete listing of drug names that sound alike and are often confused.

- **Less Commonly Used Drugs**
  Find vital information about drugs used less often in everyday practice.

*Mosby Continuing Education and Training (CET) is accredited as a provider for continuing education in nursing by the American Nurses Credentialing Center's Commission on Accreditation (ANCC-COA). This approval is reciprocal in all states for all specialty organizations that recognize the ANCC approval process.

Think outside the book... *evolve*.

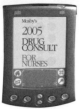

ERRATA NOTICE

Location of error: p. 1248, two thirds of the page down under the "Prophylaxis of transplant rejection" heading

Currently reads: "IV infusion *Children (without preexisting liver or renal dysfunction).* 0.05-1.5 mg/kg/day."

Should read: "IV infusion *Children (without preexisting liver or renal dysfunction).* 0.03-0.15 mg/kg/day."

Mosby's
2005
DRUG CONSULT
FOR NURSES

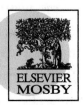

ELSEVIER
MOSBY

ELSEVIER
MOSBY

11830 Westline Industrial Drive
St. Louis, Missouri 63146

Mosby's 2005 Drug Consult for Nurses   **ISBN 0-323-02847-0**
Copyright © 2005, Mosby, Inc. All rights reserved.

NOTICE

Pharmacology is an ever-changing field. Standard safety precautions must
be followed, but as new research and clinical experience broaden our
knowledge, changes in treatment and drug therapy may become necessary
or appropriate. Readers are advised to check the most current product
information provided by the manufacturer of each drug to be administered
to verify the recommended dose, the method, and duration of administration, and contraindications. It is the responsibility of the licensed prescriber,
relying on experience and knowledge of the patient, to determine dosages
and the best treatment for each individual patient. Neither the publisher nor
the author assumes any liability for any injury and/or damage to persons
or property arising from this publication.

International Standard Book Number 0-323-02847-0

Vice President, Publishing Director: Sally Schrefer
Executive Publisher: Barbara Nelson Cullen
Executive Editor: Cindy Tryniszewski, MSN, RN
Managing Editor: Robin Levin Richman
Editorial Consultants: Gina Hopf, Nancy Priff
Editorial Assistant: Shaheen Kadri
Publishing Services Manager: Melissa Lastarria
Designer: Amy Buxton

Printed in the United States of America

Last digit is the print number: 9   8   7   6   5   4   3   2   1

SPECIAL CONTRIBUTORS

Barbara B. Hodgson, RN, OCN
Cancer Institute
St. Joseph's Hospital
Tampa, Florida

Robert J. Kizior, BS, RPh
Education Coordinator
Department of Pharmacy
Alexian Brothers Medical
    Center
Elk Grove Village, Illinois

CONTRIBUTORS

Maryann Foley, RN, BSN
Clinical Consultant
Flourtown, Pennsylvania

Doris Greggs-McQuilkin, RN, BSN, MA
President
Academy of Medical-Surgical Nurses
Washington, D.C.

Esperanza Villanueva Joyce, EdD, RN
Dean and Professor
Our Lady of the Lake College
Baton Rouge, Louisiana

Eileen S. Robinson, RN, MSN
Continuing Education Consultant
Chadds Ford, Pennsylvania

Evelyn Salerno, BS, PharmD, RPh
Consultant Pharmacist
Editor
Mosby's/Saunders ePharmacology Update
Formerly affiliated with School of Nursing
Florida International University
Clinical Assistant Professor
Nova-Southeastern College of Pharmacy
Miami, Florida

Colleen Seeber-Combs, RN, MSN
Clinical Consultant
Philadelphia, Pennsylvania

ADVISORY BOARD

REVIEWERS

Cathy R. Boone, RN
Torrance Memorial Medical
  Center
Pacific Hospital of
  Long Beach, California
Long Beach, California

Joyce Christmann, RN
Wildwood, Missouri

**Andrea Gargaro, RN, BSN,
MA, Ed**
Professor Emeritus, Nursing
Harbor College
Harbor City, California

Bridget K. Harrell, RN
St. Joseph Hospital
Kirkwood, Missouri

**Kathleen J. Haydon, RN, MS,
BC CRRN**
Rancho Los Amigos National
  Rehabilitation Center
Downey, California

Eleanor Hudson, RN
Fountain Valley Regional
  Hospital
Fountain Valley, California

Karen Elizabeth Johnson, RN
Private Consultant
Huntington Beach, California

**Christiana Lassen, RN, MS,
BC, CRRN**
Rancho Los Amigos National
  Rehabilitation Center
Downey, California

Dana McCoy, RN
College Hospital Cerritos
Cerritos, California

Winifred U. Meehan, RN
Retired
St. Louis, Missouri

**Kathleen Montgomery-Krethel,
RN**
Odyssey Health Care Hospice
St. Louis, Missouri

Patricia Neudecker, RN
Lutheran Senior Services
St. Louis, Missouri

**Teresa Tockstein, RN, ACLS,
BCLS, PALS**
Little Company of Mary
  San Pedro Hospital
San Pedro, California

FOREWORD

Nurses are the front-line care providers for patients in all settings, ranging from hospitals to long-term care facilities, transitional care units, and even patients' homes. So as a nurse, your actions—including drug administration—directly affect patient outcomes. In today's fast-paced, high-tech world, drug administration errors pose a constant threat and are a leading cause of morbidity, mortality, and litigation. To help prevent life-threatening errors, you need a drug reference that gives you the vital information you need in the most useful way possible. *Mosby's 2005 Drug Consult for Nurses* provides you with a resource to help you provide optimal patient care related to drug therapy.

This portable drug handbook is completely new. Of course, it includes all the essential information you need to administer thousands of generic and trade drugs, but it does *more*. Because it's organized by therapeutic class and lists drugs alphabetically by generic name in each class, it allows you to scan related drugs easily and compare factors that may affect their use in certain patients.

Mosby's 2005 Drug Consult for Nurses is written by the well-respected nurse and pharmacist authors of the *Saunders Nursing Drug Handbook*, Barbara B. Hodgson, RN, OCN, and Robert J. Kizior, BS, RPh. Their reputation for authoritative, clinically relevant drug information—in collaboration with our panel of expert nurse and pharmacist advisors—ensures that this new reference meets the highest standards for reliability and accuracy.

Whether you're a student, novice, or seasoned nurse, you'll find that the book's convenient organization and accurate, comprehensive drug information make it an essential tool on the job, one that you'll use every day.

WHAT MAKES THIS BOOK SPECIAL
Besides providing detailed information in each drug entry, *Mosby's 2005 Drug Consult for Nurses* offers many special features designed to help make drug administration easier, faster, and flawless.

KEY FEATURES
Organization by therapeutic class. By grouping drug entries within therapeutic classes, the book helps you identify drugs by clinical application and compare information about alternate drugs used for the same purpose. Each class includes an overview with key information about the drugs' therapeutic uses and mechanisms of action.

Practice-oriented nursing considerations. In every drug entry, this reference provides extensive, practice-oriented nursing considerations, putting essential drug facts directly into the context of your care.

Vital lifespan considerations. Throughout its pages, the book highlights key points related to drug therapy in pregnant, breast-feeding, pediatric, and geriatric patients.

Herbal medicine section. This portion of the book includes full-length entries for the most commonly used herbs.

Handy compatibility charts. For everyday reference, the book features an IV Compatibility Chart that folds out for easy use and is bound into the book to prevent accidental loss.

Comprehensive appendices. In ready-reference format, the appendices give you easy access to additional vital drug-related information, such as an English-Spanish Drug Translator to help you provide drug therapy and teaching to Spanish-speaking patients.

UNIQUE FEATURES

Insightful illustrations. Nearly two dozen, detailed, two-color illustrations help enhance your understanding of the mechanism or site of action for selected drugs and drug classes.

Prioritized side effects. Each drug entry ranks side effects by frequency of occurrence from most common to least common. It also includes the percentage of frequency, when known. This information helps you focus your care by knowing which effects to monitor more closely.

Highlights on serious reactions. In each drug entry, the book calls attention to dangerous or life-threatening reactions so you can identify them easily and act on them promptly.

Alert icons. The pages use an *Alert* icon to spotlight critical nursing considerations that require your special attention.

Continuing education option. As a bonus with the book, the online continuing education (CE) test at http://evolve.elsevier.com/ DrugConsult/nurses/ offers an opportunity to earn CE contact hours, which you can use for relicensure, certification, or professional advancement.*

---

*Mosby Continuing Education and Training (CET) is accredited as a provider of continuing education in nursing by the American Nurses Credentialing Center's Commission on Accreditation (ANCC-COA). This approval is reciprocal in all states and for all specialty organizations that recognize the ANCC approval process.

Free updates. The companion web site, http://evolve.elsevier.com/DrugConsult/nurses/, provides free late-breaking drug information, to keep you up to date on new drugs and indications, recent warnings, withdrawals from the market, and more.

HOW TO USE THIS BOOK

Mosby's 2005 Drug Consult for Nurses is divided into major sections, such as central nervous system agents, which are then divided into chapters of drugs in the same therapeutic classification, such as antianxiety agents. Each chapter introduction explains the drugs' general uses and actions (often with illustrations), lists generic drugs in the class, and identifies combination products by trade name with generic components and their strengths.

Within each chapter, detailed entries provide all the information you need about the generic drugs in the class. In every drug entry, you'll find:

Generic name, pronunciation, and trade names. Each generic drug name is listed alphabetically—and spelled phonetically—for quick identification.

Do not confuse with. This unique feature identifies generic and trade names that resemble the featured drug to help you avoid drug errors.

Category and schedule. This section lists the drug's pregnancy risk category and, when appropriate, its controlled substance schedule or over-the-counter (OTC) status.

Mechanism of action. Expanding on the chapter overview information, this section clearly and concisely details the drug's mechanism of action and therapeutic effects.

Pharmacokinetics. Under this heading, a quick-reference chart outlines the drug's route, onset, peak, and duration, when known. It's followed by a discussion of the drug's absorption, distribution, metabolism, excretion, and half-life.

Availability. This section identifies the forms that the drug comes in, for example, in tablets, sustained-release capsules, or an injectable solution. Plus, it lists the available doses and concentrations.

Indications and dosages. Here, you'll find the approved indications and routes, along with the dosage information for all age groups, including adults, elderly patients, children, neonates, and those with pre-existing conditions such as liver or kidney disease.

Unlabeled uses. This section brings you up to date on the unlabeled uses commonly seen in practice.

Contraindications. In this section, conditions that prohibit the use of the drug are listed.

Interactions. For drugs, herbal supplements, and food, this section supplies vital information about interactions with the topic drug.

Diagnostic test effects. Under this heading, you'll see a brief description of the drug's effects of laboratory and diagnostic test results, such as liver enzyme levels and electrocardiogram tracings.

IV incompatibilities and IV compatibilities. These twin sections let you know which IV drugs can't and can be given with the featured drug, whether by IV push or Y-site or IV piggyback administration.

Side effects. Unlike other handbooks that mix common, deadly effects with rare, minor ones in a long, undifferentiated list, this book ranks side effects by frequency of occurrence as expected, frequent, occasional, and rare. This section also includes the percentage of occurrence, when known.

Serious reactions. Because serious reactions are life-threatening responses that require prompt intervention, this section highlights them, apart from other side effects, for easy identification.

Nursing considerations. Using a practice-oriented format, this section presents nursing considerations in five main categories:

- *Baseline assessment* tells what to assess before giving the first dose of a drug.
- *Lifespan considerations* contains age-specific recommendations as well as information related to pregnancy and breast-feeding.
- *Precautions* alerts you to specific conditions or circumstances that call for caution when administering the drug.
- *Administration and handling* features the do's and don'ts of drug administration, with guidelines for PO, IV, IM, and other forms of the drug. It gives clear-cut instructions about how to store, prepare, and administer the drug.
- *Intervention and evaluation* describes ongoing interventions and ways to monitor the drug's therapeutic and adverse effects.
- *Patient teaching* explains exactly what to teach your patients to help them achieve the maximum therapeutic response to drugs while minimizing possible adverse effects.

We think you'll agree that *Mosby's 2005 Drug Consult for Nurses* is an indispensable tool for delivering the best possible patient care. We know you'll love the way this unique, comprehensive reference book is organized to help you focus on the drugs used in your daily practice. Whether you keep it in your lab coat pocket, on the drug cart, or at the nurse's station, you'll surely turn to it again and again for drug information you can trust.

Doris Greggs-McQuilkin, RN, BSN, MA
President
Academy of Medical-Surgical Nurses
Washington, D.C.

Evelyn Salerno, BS, PharmD, RPh
Consultant Pharmacist
Editor
Mosby's/Saunders ePharmacology Update
Formerly affiliated with
School of Nursing
Florida International University
Clinical Assistant Professor
Nova-Southeastern College of Pharmacy
Miami, Florida

ACKNOWLEDGMENTS

A technical book of this magnitude requires the dedicated commitment of many persons. Each of us appreciates the other's enduring commitment to excellence, completeness, and accuracy in compiling the information for this book. Our partnership and friendship has bridged many years and many personal challenges, and it has endured and grown with each publication. We give special thanks to Gina Hopf for her tireless efforts to develop and facilitate the format that you will see within. It has been our pleasure to work with Gina on several projects, and she continues to be an invaluable partner in our work. It has been our pleasure working with Cindy Tryniszewski, who also gave so much of her time and effort turning this project into a reality. We offer grateful acknowledgment to the editorial staff at Elsevier–who have encouraged our best efforts and who have contributed valuable ideas for content, format, and presentation. Our thanks also go to the staff at Graphic World Publishing Services for their efforts in presenting this work in an attractive and easy-to-use manner. Thanks go as well to our family and friends—personal and professional—who listen to and critique our bright ideas, make suggestions that make our work better, and provide support and encouragement at every turn.

Robert (Bob) Kizior and Barbara Hodgson

TABLE OF CONTENTS

DRUG MONOGRAPHS
Anti-Infective Agents

Antineoplastic Agents

Cardiovascular Agents

Central Nervous System Agents

Gastrointestinal Agents

Hematologic Agents

Hormonal Agents

Immunomodulating Agents

Natural Medicines

Nutritional and Electrolyte Agents

Renal and Genitourinary Agents

Respiratory Agents

APPENDIXES

INDEXES

DRUGS BY DISORDER

Generic names appear first, followed by brand names in parentheses.

Allergy
Beclomethasone (Beclovent, Vanceril)
Betamethasone (Celestone)
Budesonide (Pulmicort, Rhinocort)
Clemastine (Tavist)
Desloratadine (Clarinex)
Dexamethasone (Decadron)
Dimenhydrinate (Dramamine)
Diphenhydramine (Benadryl)
Epinephrine (Adrenalin)
Fexofenadine (Allegra)
Flunisolide (AeroBid, Nasalide)
Fluticasone (Flovent)
Hydrocortisone (Solu-Cortef)
Loratadine (Claritin)
Prednisolone (Prelone)
Prednisone (Deltasone)
Promethazine (Phenergan)
Triamcinolone (Kenalog)

Alzheimer's disease
Donepezil (Aricept)
Galantamine (Reminyl)
Memantine (Namenda)
Rivastigmine (Exelon)
Tacrine (Cognex)

Angina
Amlodipine (Norvasc)
Atenolol (Tenormin)
Diltiazem (Cardizem, Dilacor)
Isosorbide (Imdur, Isordil)
Metoprolol (Lopressor)
Nadolol (Corgard)
Nicardipine (Cardene)
Nifedipine (Adalat, Procardia)
Nitroglycerin
Propranolol (Inderal)
Timolol (Blocadron)
Verapamil (Calan, Isoptin)

Anxiety
Alprazolam (Xanax)
Buspirone (BuSpar)
Diazepam (Valium)
Doxepin (Sinequan)
Hydroxyzine (Atarax, Vistaril)
Lorazepam (Ativan)
Oxazepam (Serax)

Arrhythmias
Acebutolol (Sectral)
Adenosine (Adenocard)
Amiodarone (Cordarone, Pacerone)
Digoxin (Lanoxin)
Diltiazem (Cardizem, Dilacor)
Disopyramide (Norpace)
Dofetilide (Tikosyn)
Esmolol (Brevibloc)
Ibutilide (Corvert)
Lidocaine
Mexiletine (Mexitil)
Moricizine (Ethmozine)
Phenytoin (Dilantin)
Procainamide (Pronestyl, Procan)
Propafenone (Rythmol)
Propranolol (Inderal)
Quinidine
Sotalol (Betapace)
Tocainide (Tonocard)
Verapamil (Calan, Isoptin)

Arthritis, rheumatoid
Adalimumab (Humira)
Anakinra (Kineret)
Aspirin
Auranofin (Ridaura)
Aurothioglucose (Solganal)
Azathioprine (Imuran)
Betamethasone (Celestone)
Capsaicin (Zostrix)
Celecoxib (Celebrex)

Cyclosporine (Sandimmune)
Diclofenac (Cataflam, Voltaren)
Diflunisal (Dolobid)
Etanercept (Enbrel)
Hydroxychloroquine (Plaquenil)
Infliximab (Remicade)
Leflunomide (Arava)
Methotrexate
Prednisone (Deltasone)
Rofecoxib (Vioxx)
Valdecoxib (Bextra)

Asthma
Albuterol (Proventil, Ventolin)
Aminophylline (Theophylline)
Beclomethasone (Beclovent, Vanceril)
Budesonide (Pulmicort)
Cromolyn (Crolom, Intal)
Dexamethasone (Decadron)
Epinephrine (Adrenalin)
Flunisolide (AeroBid)
Fluticasone (Flovent)
Formoterol (Foradil)
Hydrocortisone (Solu-Cortef)
Ipratropium (Atrovent)
Levalbuterol (Xopenex)
Metaproterenol (Alupent)
Methylprednisolone (Solu-Medrol)
Montelukast (Singulair)
Nedocromil (Tilade)
Prednisolone (Prelone)
Prednisone (Deltasone)
Salmeterol (Serevent)
Terbutaline (Brethine)
Theophylline (SloBid)
Zafirlukast (Accolate)

Attention deficit hyperactivity disorder (ADHD)
Atomoxetine (Strattera)
Desipramine (Norpramin)
Dexmethylphenidate (Focalin)
Dextroamphetamine (Dexedrine)
Imipramine (Tofranil)
Methylphenidate (Ritalin)
Pemoline (Cylert)

Benign prostatic hypertrophy (BPH)
Alfuzosin (UroXatral)
Doxazosin (Cardura)
Finasteride (Proscar)
Tamsulosin (Flomax)
Terazosin (Hytrin)

Bronchospasm
Albuterol (Proventil, Ventolin)
Epinephrine (Adrenalin)
Levalbuterol (Xopenex)
Metaproterenol (Alupent)
Salmeterol (Serevent)
Terbutaline (Brethine)
Theophylline (SloBid)

Cancer
Abarelix (Plenaxis)
Aldesleukin (Proleukin)
Alemtuzumab (Campath)
Anastrozole (Arimidex)
Arsenic trioxide (Trisenox)
Asparaginase (Elspar)
BCG (Tice BCG, TheraCys)
Bexarotene (Targretin)
Bicalutamide (Casodex)
Bleomycin (Blenoxane)
Bortezumib (Velcade)
Busulfan (Myleran)
Capecitabine (Xeloda)
Carboplatin (Paraplatin)
Carmustine (BiCNU)
Chlorambucil (Leukeran)
Cisplatin (Platinol)
Cyclophosphamide (Cytoxan)
Cytarabine (Cytosar, Ara-C)
Dacarbazine (DTIC)
Daunorubicin (Cerubidine, DaunoXome)
Docetaxel (Taxotere)
Doxorubicin (Adriamycin, Doxil)
Epirubicin (Ellence)
Estramustine (Emcyt)
Etoposide (VePesid)
Fludarabine (Fludara)
Fluorouracil
Flutamide (Eulexin)

Fulvestrant (Faslodex)
Gefitnib (Iressa)
Gemcitabine (Gemzar)
Gemtuzumab (Mylotarg)
Goserelin (Zoladex)
Hydroxyurea (Hydrea)
Idarubicin (Idamycin)
Ifosfamide (Ifex)
Imatinib (Gleevec)
Interferon alfa-2a (Roferon A)
Interferon alfa-2b (Intron A)
Irinotecan (Camptosar)
Letrozole (Femara)
Leuprolide (Lupron)
Lomustine (CeeNU)
Megestrol (Megace)
Melphalan (Alkeran)
Mercaptopurine (Purinethol)
Methotrexate
Mitomycin (Mutamycin)
Mitotane (Lysodren)
Mitoxantrone (Novantrone)
Nilutamide (Nilandron)
Oxaliplatin (Eloxatin)
Paclitaxel (Taxol)
Plicamycin (Mithracin)
Procarbazine (Matulane)
Rituximab (Rituxan)
Tamoxifen (Nolvadex)
Temozolomide (Temodar)
Teniposide (Vumon)
Thiotepa (Thioplex)
Topotecan (Hycamtin)
Toremifene (Fareston)
Tositumomab (Bexxar)
Trastuzumab (Herceptin)
Valrubicin (Valstar)
Vinblastine (Velban)
Vincristine (Oncovin)
Vinorelbine (Navelbine)

Cerebrovascular accident (CVA)
Aspirin
Clopidogrel (Plavix)
Heparin
Nimodipine (Nimotop)
Ticlopidine (Ticlid)
Warfarin (Coumadin)

Chronic obstructive pulmonary disease (COPD)
Albuterol (Proventil, Ventolin)
Aminophylline (Theophylline)
Budesonide (Pulmicort)
Epinephrine (Adrenalin)
Formoterol (Foradil)
Levalbuterol (Xopenex)
Metaproterenol (Alupent)
Salmeterol (Serevent)
Theophylline (SloBid)

Congestive heart failure (CHF)
Amlodipine (Norvasc)
Bumetanide (Bumex)
Captopril (Capoten)
Carvedilol (Coreg)
Digoxin (Lanoxin)
Dobutamine (Dobutrex)
Dopamine (Intropin)
Enalapril (Vasotec)
Eprosartan (Teveten)
Fosinopril (Monopril)
Furosemide (Lasix)
Hydralazine (Apresoline)
Isosorbide (Isordil)
Lisinopril (Prinivil, Zestril)
Losartan (Cozaar)
Metoprolol (Lopressor)
Milrinone (Primacor)
Moexipril (Univasc)
Nitroglycerin
Nitroprusside (Nipride)
Quinapril (Accupril)
Ramipril (Altace)

Constipation
Bisacodyl (Dulcolax)
Docusate (Colace)
Lactulose (Kristalose)
Methylcellulose (Citrucel)
Milk of magnesia (MOM)
Psyllium (Metamucil)
Senna (Senokot)

Crohn's disease
Cyclosporine (Neoral)
Hydrocortisone (Cortenema)

Infliximab (Remicade)
Mesalamine (Asacol, Pentasa)
Olsalazine (Dipentum)
Sulfasalazine (Azulfidine)

Deep vein thrombosis (DVT)
Dalteparin (Fragmin)
Enoxaparin (Lovenox)
Heparin
Tinzaparin (Innohep)
Warfarin (Coumadin)

Depression
Amitriptyline (Elavil, Endep)
Bupropion (Wellbutrin)
Citalopram (Celexa)
Clomipramine (Anafranil)
Desipramine (Norpramin)
Doxepin (Sinequan)
Escitalopram (Lexapro)
Fluoxetine (Prozac)
Imipramine (Tofranil)
Mirtazapine (Remeron)
Nefazodone (Serzone)
Nortriptyline (Aventyl, Pamelor)
Paroxetine (Paxil)
Phenelzine (Nardil)
Sertraline (Zoloft)
Tranylcypromine (Parnate)
Trazodone (Desyrel)
Venlafaxine (Effexor)

Diabetes mellitus
Acarbose (Precose)
Glimepiride (Amaryl)
Glipizide (Glucotrol)
Glyburide (Micronase)
Insulin
Metformin (Glucophage)
Miglitol (Glyset)
Nateglinide (Starlix)
Pioglitazone (Actos)
Repaglinide (Prandin)
Rosiglitazone (Avandia)

Diarrhea
Bismuth subsalicylate
   (Pepto-Bismol)
Diphenoxylate and atropine
   (Lomotil)
Loperamide (Imodium)
Octreotide (Sandostatin)

Duodenal/gastric ulcer
Cimetidine (Tagamet)
Esomeprazole (Nexium)
Famotidine (Pepcid)
Lansoprazole (Prevacid)
Nizatidine (Axid)
Omeprazole (Prilosec)
Pantoprazole (Protonix)
Rabeprazole (Aciphex)
Ranitidine (Zantac)
Sucralfate (Carafate)

Edema
Amiloride (Midamor)
Bumetanide (Bumex)
Chlorthalidone (Hygroton)
Furosemide (Lasix)
Hydrochlorothiazide
   (HydroDIURIL)
Indapamide (Lozol)
Metolazone (Zaroxolyn)
Spironolactone (Aldactone)
Torsemide (Demadex)
Triamterene (Dyrenium)

Epilepsy
Carbamazepine (Tegretol)
Clonazepam (Klonopin)
Clorazepate (Tranxene)
Diazepam (Valium)
Fosphenytoin (Cerebyx)
Gabapentin (Neurontin)
Lamotrigine (Lamictal)
Levetiracetam (Keppra)
Lorazepam (Ativan)
Oxcarbazepine (Trileptal)
Phenobarbital
Phenytoin (Dilantin)
Primidone (Mysoline)
Tiagabine (Gabitril)
Topiramate (Topamax)
Valproic acid (Depakene, Depakote)
Zonisamide (Zonegran)

Esophageal reflux, esophagitis
Cimetidine (Tagamet)
Esomeprazole (Nexium)
Famotidine (Pepcid)
Lansoprazole (Prevacid)
Nizatidine (Axid)
Omeprazole (Prilosec)
Pantoprazole (Protonix)
Rabeprazole (Aciphex)
Ranitidine (Zantac)

Fever
Acetaminophen (Tylenol)
Aspirin
Ibuprofen (Advil, Motrin)
Indomethacin (Indocin)
Naproxen (Anaprox, Naprosyn)

Gastritis
Cimetidine (Tagamet)
Famotidine (Pepcid)
Nizatidine (Axid)
Ranitidine (Zantac)

Gastroesophageal reflux disease (GERD)
Cimetidine (Tagamet)
Esomeprazole (Nexium)
Famotidine (Pepcid)
Lansoprazole (Prevacid)
Metoclopramide (Reglan)
Nizatidine (Axid)
Omeprazole (Prilosec)
Pantoprazole (Protonix)
Rabeprazole (Aciphex)
Ranitidine (Zantac)

Glaucoma
Acetazolamide (Diamox)
Apraclonidine (Iopidine)
Betaxolol (Betoptic)
Bimatoprost (Lumigan)
Brimonidine (Alphagan)
Brinzolamide (Azopt)
Carbachol
Carteolol (Ocupress)
Dipivefrin (Propine)
Dorzolamide (Trusopt)
Echothiophate iodide (Phospholine)

Latanoprost (Xalatan)
Levobunolol (Betagan)
Metipranolol (OptiPranolol)
Pilocarpine (Isopto Carpine)
Timolol (Timoptic)
Travoprost (Travatan)
Unoprostone (Rescula)

Gout
Allopurinol (Zyloprim)
Colchicine
Indomethacin (Indocin)
Naproxen (Anaprox, Naprosyn)
Probenecid (Benemid)
Sulindac (Clinoril)

Human immunodeficiency virus (HIV)
Abacavir (Ziagen)
Amprenavir (Agenerase)
Atazanavir (Reyataz)
Delavirdine (Rescriptor)
Didanosine (Videx)
Efavirenz (Sustiva)
Emtricitabine (Emtriva)
Enfuvirtide (Fuzeon)
Indinavir (Crixivan)
Lamivudine (Epivir)
Lopinavir/ritonavir (Kaletra)
Nelfinavir (Viracept)
Nevirapine (Viramune)
Ritonavir (Norvir)
Saquinavir (Fortovase, Invirase)
Stavudine (Zerit)
Tenofovir (Viread)
Zalcitabine (Hivid)
Zidovudine (AZT, Retrovir)

Hypercholesterolemia
Atorvastatin (Lipitor)
Cholestyramine (Questran)
Colesevelam (Welchol)
Ezetimibe (Zetia)
Fenofibrate (Tricor)
Fluvastatin (Lescol)
Gemfibrozil (Lopid)
Lovastatin (Mevacor)
Niacin (Niaspan)
Pravastatin (Pravachol)

Rosuvastatin (Crestor)
Simvastatin (Zocor)

Hyperphosphatemia
Aluminum salts
Calcium slats
Sevelamer (Renagel)

Hypertension
Amiloride (Midamor)
Amlodipine (Norvasc)
Atenolol (Tenormin)
Benazepril (Lotensin)
Bisoprolol (Zebeta)
Candesartan (Atacand)
Captopril (Capoten)
Clonidine (Catapres)
Diltiazem (Cardizem, Dilacor)
Doxazosin (Cardura)
Enalapril (Vasotec)
Eplerenone (Inspra)
Eprosartan (Teveten)
Felodipine (Plendil)
Fosinopril (Monopril)
Hydralazine (Apresoline)
Hydrochlorothiazide
   (HydroDIURIL)
Indapamide (Lozol)
Irbesartan (Avapro)
Isradipine (DynaCirc)
Labetalol (Normodyne, Trandate)
Lisinopril (Prinivil, Zestril)
Losartan (Cozaar)
Methyldopa (Aldomet)
Metolazone (Diulo, Zaroxolyn)
Metoprolol (Lopressor)
Minoxidil (Loniten)
Moexipril (Univasc)
Nadolol (Corgard)
Nicardipine (Cardene)
Nifedipine (Adalat, Procardia)
Nitroglycerin
Nitroprusside (Nipride)
Olmesartan (Benicar)
Perindopril (Aceon)
Prazosin (Minipress)
Propranolol (Inderal)
Quinapril (Accupril)
Ramipril (Altace)

Spironolactone (Aldactone)
Telmisartan (Micardis)
Terazosin (Hytrin)
Timolol (Blocadren)
Trandolapril (Mavik)
Valsartan (Dovan)
Verapamil (Calan, Isoptin)

Hypertriglyceridemia
Atorvastatin (Lipitor)
Fenofibrate (Tricor)
Fluvastatin (Lescol)
Gemfibrozil (Lopid)
Lovastatin (Mevacor)
Niacin (Niaspan)
Pravastatin (Pravachol)
Rosuvastatin (Crestor)
Simvastatin (Zocor)

Hyperuricemia
Allopurinol (Zyloprim)
Colchicine
Probenecid (Benemid)

Hypotension
Norepinephrine (Levophed)
Phenylephrine (AK-Dilate)

Hypothyroidism
Levothyroxine (Levoxyl, Synthroid)
Liothyronine (Cytomel)

**Idiopathic thrombocytopenic
   purpura (ITP)**
Azathioprine (Imuran)
Cyclophosphamide (Cytoxan)
Dexamethasone (Decadron)
Prednisone
Vincristine (Oncovin)

Infection
Amikacin (Amikin)
Amoxicillin (Trimox)
Amoxicillin/clavulanic acid
   (Augmentin)
Ampicillin (Principen)
Ampicillin/sulbactam (Unasyn)
Azithromycin (Zithromax)
Cefaclor (Ceclor)

Cefadroxil (Duricef)
Cefazolin (Ancef)
Cefdinir (Omnicef)
Cefepime (Maxipime)
Cefotaxime (Claforan)
Cefotetan (Cefotan)
Cefoxitin (Mefoxin)
Cefpodoxime (Vantin)
Cefprozil (Cefzil)
Ceftazidime (Fortaz)
Ceftizoxime (Cefizox)
Ceftriaxone (Rocephin)
Cefuroxime (Ceftin, Zinacef)
Cephalexin (Keflex)
Ciprofloxacin (Cipro)
Clarithromycin (Biaxin)
Dirithromycin (Dynabac)
Erythromycin (E-Mycin)
Gatifloxacin (Tequin)
Gemifloxacin (Factive)
Gentamicin (Garamycin)
Levofloxacin (Levaquin)
Lomefloxacin (Maxaquin)
Loracarbef (Lorabid)
Moxifloxacin (Avelox)
Norfloxacin (Noroxin)
Ofloxacin (Floxin)
Oxacillin
Penicillin G (Pfizerpen)
Penicillin V (Pen-Vee K)
Piperacillin/tazobactam (Zosyn)
Ticarcillin/clavulanate (Timentin)
Tobramycin (Nebcin)
Vancomycin (Vancocin)

Insomnia
Diphenhydramine (Benadryl)
Flurazepam (Dalmane)
Temazepam (Restoril)
Triazolam (Halcion)
Zaleplon (Sonata)
Zolpidem (Ambien)

Migraine headaches
Almotriptan (Axert)
Amitriptyline (Elavil)
Dihydroergotamine (Migranal)
Eletriptan (Relpax)
Ergotamine (Ergomar)

Frovatriptan (Frovan)
Naratriptan (Amerge)
Propranolol (Inderal)
Rizatriptan (Maxalt)
Sumatriptan (Imitrex)
Zolmitriptan (Zomig)

Multiple sclerosis
Glatiramer (Copaxone)
Interferon beta-1a (Avonex, Rebif)
Interferon beta-1b (Betaseron)
Mitoxantrone (Novantrone)

Myocardial infarction
Alteplase (Activase)
Aspirin
Atenolol (Tenormin)
Captopril (Capoten)
Clopidogrel (Plavix)
Dalteparin (Fragmin)
Diltiazem (Cardizem, Dilacor)
Enalapril (Vasotec)
Enoxaparin (Lovenox)
Heparin
Lidocaine
Lisinopril (Prinivil, Zestril)
Metoprolol (Lopressor)
Morphine
Nitroglycerin
Propranolol (Inderal)
Quinapril (Accupril)
Ramipril (Altace)
Reteplase (Retavase)
Streptokinase
Timolol (Blocadren)
Verapamil (Calan, Isoptin)
Warfarin (Coumadin)

Nausea
Aprepitant (Emend)
Chlorpromazine (Thorazine)
Dexamethasone (Decadron)
Dimenhydrinate (Dramamine)
Dolasetron (Anzemet)
Dronabinol (Marinol)
Granisetron (Kytril)
Hydroxyzine (Vistaril)
Lorazepam (Ativan)
Meclizine (Antivert)

Metoclopramide (Reglan)
Ondansetron (Zofran)
Palonosetron (Aloxi)
Prochlorperazine (Compazine)
Promethazine (Phenergan)
Trimethobenzamide (Tigan)

Obsessive-compulsive disorder
Citalopram (Celexa)
Clomipramine (Anafranil)
Fluoxetine (Prozac)
Fluvoxamine (Luvox)
Paroxetine (Paxil)
Sertraline (Zoloft)

Osteoporosis
Alendronate (Fosamax)
Calcitonin
Calcium salts
Conjugated estrogens (Premarin)
Estradiol (Estrace)
Raloxifene (Evista)
Risedronate (Actonel)
Teriparatide (Forteo)
Vitamin D (Calcitriol)

Paget's disease
Alendronate (Fosamax)
Calcitonin
Etidronate (Didronel)
Pamidronate (Aredia)
Risedronate (Actonel)
Tiludronate (Skelid)

Pain, mild to moderate
Acetaminophen (Tylenol)
Aspirin
Celecoxib (Celebrex)
Codeine
Diclofenac (Voltaren)
Diflunisal (Dolobid)
Etodolac (Lodine)
Flurbiprofen (Ansaid)
Ibuprofen (Motrin)
Ketorolac (Toradol)
Naproxen (Naprosyn)
Propoxyphene (Darvon)
Salsalate (Disalcid)
Tramadol (Ultram)

Pain, moderate to severe
Butorphanol (Stadol)
Fentanyl (Duragesic)
Hydromorphone (Dilaudid)
Meperidine (Demerol)
Methadone (Dolophine)
Morphine (MS Contin)
Nalbuphine (Nubain)
Oxycodone (OxyFast)

Panic attack disorder
Alprazolam (Xanax)
Clonazepam (Klonopin)
Paroxetine (Paxil)
Sertraline (Zoloft)

Parkinsonism
Amantadine (Symmetrel)
Bromocriptine (Parlodel)
Carbidopa/levodopa (Sinemet)
Diphenhydramine (Benadryl)
Entacapone (Comtan)
Pergolide (Permax)
Pramipexole (Mirapex)
Ropinirole (Requip)
Selegiline (Eldepryl)
Tolcapone (Tasmar)

Peptic ulcer disease
Cimetidine (Tagamet)
Esomeprazole (Nexium)
Famotidine (Pepcid)
Lansoprazole (Prevacid)
Nizatidine (Axid)
Omeprazole (Prilosec)
Pantoprazole (Protonix)
Rabeprazole (Aciphex)
Ranitidine (Zantac)
Sucralfate (Carafate)

Pneumonia
Amoxicillin (Trimox)
Amoxicillin/clavulanate
  (Augmentin)
Ampicillin (Principen)
Azithromycin (Zithromax)
Cefaclor (Ceclor)
Cefpodoxime (Vantin)
Ceftriaxone (Rocephin)

Cefuroxime (Zinacef)
Clarithromycin (Biaxin)
Co-trimoxazole (Bactrim,
 Septra)
Dirithromycin (Dynabac)
Erythromycin (E-Mycin)
Gentamicin (Garamycin)
Loracarbef (Lorabid)
Piperacillin/tazobactam (Zosyn)
Tobramycin (Nebcin)
Vancomycin (Vancocin)

Pneumonia, *Pneumocystis carinii*
Atovaquone (Mepron)
Clindamycin (Cleocin)
Co-trimoxazole (Bactrim, Septra)
Pentamidine (Pentam)
Trimethoprim (Trimpex)
Trimetrexate (Neutrexin)

Prostatic hyperplasia, benign
Alfuzon (UroXatral)
Doxazosin (Cardura)
Finasteride (Proscar)
Tamsulosin (Flomax)
Terazosin (Hytrin)

Pruritus
Amcinonide (Cyclocort)
Cetirizine (Zyrtec)
Clemastine (Tavist)
Clobetasol (Temovate)
Desonide (Tridesilon)
Desoximetasone (Topicort)
Desloratadine (Clarinex)
Diphenhydramine (Benadryl)
Fluocinolone (Synalar)
Fluocinonide (Lidex)
Halobetasol (Ultravate)
Hydrocortisone (Cort-Dome,
 Hytone)
Hydroxyzine (Atarax, Vistaril)
Prednisolone (Prelone)
Prednisone (Deltasone)
Promethazine (Phenergan)

Psychosis
Aripiprazole (Abilify)
Chlorpromazine (Thorazine)

Clozapine (Clozaril)
Haloperidol (Haldol)
Lithium (Lithobid)
Olanzapine (Zyprexa)
Quetiapine (Seroquel)
Risperidone (Risperdal)
Thioridazine (Mellaril)
Thiothixene (Navane)
Ziprasidone (Geodon)

**Reflux esophagitis
 (GERD)**
Cimetidine (Tagamet)
Esomeprazole (Nexium)
Famotidine (Pepcid)
Lansoprazole (Prevacid)
Metoclopramide (Reglan)
Nizatidine (Axid)
Omeprazole (Prilosec)
Pantoprazole (Protonix)
Rabeprazole (Aciphex)
Ranitidine (Zantac)

**Respiratory distress syndrome
 (RDS)**
Beractant (Survanta)
Calfactant (Infasurf)
Poractant alfa (Curosurf)

Schizophrenia
Aripiprazole (Abilify)
Chlorpromazine (Thorazine)
Clozapine (Clozaril)
Haloperidol (Haldol)
Olanzapine (Zyprexa)
Quetiapine (Seroquel)
Risperidone (Risperdal)
Thioridazine (Mellaril)
Thiothixene (Navane)
Ziprasidone (Geodon)

Smoking cessation
Bupropion (Wellbutrin)
Clonidine (Catapres)
Nicotine (Nicoderm, Nicotrol)

Thrombosis
Dalteparin (Fragmin)
Enoxaparin (Lovenox)
Heparin
Tinzaparin (Innohep)
Warfarin (Coumadin)

Thyroid disorders
Levothyroxine (Levoxyl, Synthroid)
Liothyronine (Cytomel)

Transient ischemic attack
Aspirin
Clopidogrel (Plavix)
Ticlopidine (Ticlid)
Warfarin (Coumadin)

Tremor
Atenolol (Tenormin)
Chlordiazepoxide (Librium)
Diazepam (Valium)
Lorazepam (Ativan)
Metoprolol (Lopressor)
Nadolol (Corgard)
Propranolol (Inderal)

Tuberculosis
Ethambutol (Myambutol)
Isoniazid (INH)
Pyrazinamide
Rifabutin (Mycobutin)
Rifampin (Rifadin)
Rifapentine (Priftin)
Streptomycin

Urticaria
Cetirizine (Zyrtec)
Cimetidine (Tagamet)

Clemastine (Tavist)
Diphenhydramine (Benadryl)
Hydroxyzine (Atarax,
   Vistaril)
Loratadine (Claritin)
Promethazine (Phenergan)
Ranitidine (Zantac)

Vertigo
Dimenhydrinate (Dramamine)
Diphenhydramine (Benadryl)
Meclizine (Antivert)
Scopolamine (Trans-Derm Scop)

Vomiting
Aprepiant (Emend)
Chlorpromazine (Thorazine)
Dexamethasone (Decadron)
Dimenhydrinate (Dramamine)
Dolasetron (Anzemet)
Dronabinol (Marinol)
Granisetron (Kytril)
Hydroxyzine (Vistaril)
Lorazepam (Ativan)
Meclizine (Antivert)
Metoclopramide (Reglan)
Ondansetron (Zofran)
Palonosetron (aloxi)
Prochlorperazine (Compazine)
Promethazine (Phenergan)
Trimethobenzamide (Tigan)

Zollinger-Ellison syndrome
Aluminum salts
Cimetidine (Tagamet)
Esomeprazole (Nexium)
Famotidine (Pepcid)
Lansoprazole (Prevacid)
Omeprazole (Prilosec)
Pantoprazole (Protonix)
Rabeprazole (Aciphex)
Ranitidine (Zantac)

1 Aminoglycosides

amikacin sulfate
gentamicin sulfate
kanamycin sulfate
neomycin sulfate
streptomycin sulfate
tobramycin sulfate

Uses: Aminoglycosides are used to treat serious infections when other, less toxic agents aren't effective, are contraindicated, or require adjunctive therapy (such as penicillins or cephalosporins). Aminoglycosides primarily treat infections caused by gram-negative microorganisms, such as *Proteus mirabilis, Klebsiella pneumoniae, Pseudomonas aeruginosa, Escherichia coli, Serratia marcescens,* and *Enterobacter* species. They're inactive against most gram-positive microorganisms. These agents aren't well absorbed systemically from the gastrointestinal (GI) tract and must be administered parenterally for systemic infections. Oral agents are given to suppress intestinal bacteria.

Action: Aminoglycosides are transported across bacterial cell membranes and are bactericidal. These drugs irreversibly bind to specific receptor proteins on bacterial ribosomes, thereby interfering with protein synthesis, preventing cell reproduction, and eventually causing cell death. (See illustration, *Sites and Mechanisms of Action: Anti-infective Agents,* page 2.)

COMBINATION PRODUCTS

NEOSPORIN GU IRRIGANT: neomycin/polymyxin B (an anti-infective) 40 mg/200,000 units/ml.

NEOSPORIN OINTMENT, TRIPLE ANTIBIOTIC: neomycin/polymyxin B (an anti-infective)/bacitracin (an anti-infective) 3.5 mg/5,000 units/400 units/g; 3.5 mg/10,000 units/400 units/g.

TOBRADEX: tobramycin/dexamethasone (a steroid) 0.3%/0.1% per ml or per g.

amikacin sulfate
am-ih-**kay**-sin
(Amikin)
Do not confuse with Amicar.

CATEGORY AND SCHEDULE
Pregnancy Risk Category: C

MECHANISM OF ACTION
An aminoglycoside antibiotic agent that irreversibly binds to protein on bacterial ribosomes. *Therapeutic Effect:* Interferes with protein synthesis of susceptible microorganisms.

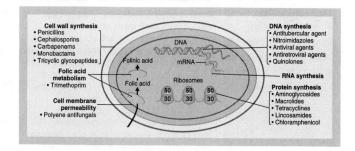

Sites and Mechanisms of Action: Anti-infective Agents

The goal of anti-infective therapy is to kill or inhibit the growth of microorganisms, such as bacteria, viruses, and fungi. To achieve this goal, anti-infective agents must reach their targets, which usually occurs through absorption and distribution by the circulatory system. When the target is reached, a drug can kill or suppress microorganisms by:

- Inhibiting cell wall synthesis or activating enzymes that disrupt the cell wall, which leads to cellular weakening, lysis, and death. Penicillins (ampicillin), cephalosporins (cefazolin), carbapenems (imipenem), monobactams (aztreonam), and tricyclic glycopeptides (vancomycin) act in this way.
- Altering cell membrane permeability through direct action on the cell wall, which allows intracellular substances to leak out and destabilizes the cell. Polyene antifungals (amphotericin) work by this mechanism.
- Altering protein synthesis by binding to bacterial ribosomes (50/30) or affecting ribosomal function, which leads to cell death or slowed growth respectively. Aminoglycosides (gentamicin), macrolides (erythromycin), tetracyclines (doxycycline), lincosamides (clindamycin), and the miscellaneous anti-infective chloramphenicol use the action.
- Inhibiting deoxyribonucleic acid (DNA) or ribonucleic acid (RNA), including messenger RNA (mRNA), synthesis by binding to nucleic acids or interacting with enzymes required for their synthesis. Antitubercular agents (rifampin), nitroimidazoles (metronidazole), antiviral agents (acyclovir), antiretroviral agents (stavudine), and quinolones (ciprofloxacin) act like this.
- Inhibiting the metabolism of folic acid and folinic acid or other cellular components that are essential for bacterial cell growth. The miscellaneous anti-infective trimethoprim employs this mechanism of action.

PHARMACOKINETICS

Rapid, complete absorption after intramuscular (IM) administration. Protein binding: 0%–10%. Widely distributed (does not cross blood-brain barrier, low concentrations in cerebrospinal fluid [CSF]). Excreted unchanged in urine. Removed by hemodialysis. **Half-life:** 2–4 hrs (increased in reduced renal function, neonates; decreased in cystic fibrosis, burn or febrile patients).

AVAILABILITY

Injection: 50 mg/ml, 250 mg/ml.

INDICATIONS AND DOSAGES
▸ **Uncomplicated urinary tract infections**
IM/IV
Adults, Elderly. 250 mg q12h.
▸ **Moderate to severe infections**
IM/IV
Adults, Elderly, Children. 15 mg/kg/day in divided doses q8–12h. Do not exceed 15 mg/kg or 1.5 g/day.
Neonates. Loading dose: 10 mg/kg, then 7.5 mg/kg q12h.
▸ **Dosage in Renal Impairment**
Dosage and frequency is modified based on degree of renal impairment and serum concentration of the drug. After a loading dose of 5–7.5 mg/kg, the maintenance dose and frequency is based on serum creatinine or creatinine clearance.

CONTRAINDICATIONS
Sensitivity to amikacin or any component

INTERACTIONS
Drug
Nephrotoxic medications, other aminoglycosides, ototoxic-producing medications: May increase risk of amikacin toxicity. May increase effects of neuromuscular blocking agents.
Herbal
None known.
Food
None known.

DIAGNOSTIC TEST EFFECTS
May increase serum bilirubin, BUN, serum creatinine, LDH concentrations, SGOT (AST), SGPT (ALT). May decrease serum calcium, magnesium, potassium, and sodium concentrations. Therapeutic blood serum level: Peak: 20–30 mcg/ml; toxic serum level: greater than 30 mcg/ml; Trough: 1–9 mcg/ml; toxic serum level: greater than 10 mcg/ml.

IV INCOMPATIBILITIES
Amphotericin, ampicillin, cefazolin (Ancef), heparin, propofol (Diprivan)

IV COMPATIBILITIES
Amiodarone (Cordarone), aztreonam (Azactam), calcium gluconate, cefepime (Maxipime), cimetidine (Tagamet), ciprofloxacin (Cipro), clindamycin (Cleocin), diltiazem (Cardizem), enalapril (Vasotec), esmolol (BreviBloc), fluconazole (Diflucan), furosemide (Lasix), levofloxacin (Levaquin), lorazepam (Ativan), magnesium sulfate, midazolam (Versed), morphine, ondansetron (Zofran), potassium chloride, ranitidine (Zantac), vancomycin

SIDE EFFECTS
Frequent
Pain, induration at IM injection site, phlebitis, thrombophlebitis with IV administration
Occasional
Hypersensitivity reactions manifested as rash, fever, urticaria, pruritus
Rare
Neuromuscular blockade manifested as difficulty breathing, drowsiness, weakness

SERIOUS REACTIONS
• Nephrotoxicity as evidenced by increased thirst, decreased appetite, nausea, vomiting, increased BUN and serum creatinine, and decreased creatinine clearance; neurotoxicity manifested as muscle twitching, visual disturbances, seizures, and tingling; and ototoxicity as evidenced by tinnitus, dizziness, or loss of hearing may occur.

NURSING CONSIDERATIONS

Baseline Assessment
- Determine the patient's history of allergies, especially to aminoglycosides and sulfite.
- Expect to correct dehydration before beginning aminoglycoside therapy.
- Establish the patient's baseline hearing acuity before beginning therapy.
- Expect to obtain a specimen for culture and sensitivity testing before giving the first dose. Therapy may begin before test results are known.

Lifespan Considerations
- Be aware that amikacin readily crosses the placenta and small amounts are distributed in breast milk. Amikacin may produce fetal nephrotoxicity.
- Be aware that neonates and premature infants may be more susceptible to amikacin toxicity due to immature renal function.
- In the elderly, age-related renal impairment presents a higher risk of amikacin toxicity.
- In the elderly there is an increased risk of hearing loss.

Precautions
- Use cautiously in patients with 8th cranial nerve impairment (vestibulocochlear nerve), decreased renal function, myasthenia gravis, and Parkinson's disease.

Administration and Handling
◀ALERT▶ Space amikacin doses evenly around the clock. The drug dosage is based on the patient's ideal body weight. Peak, trough blood serum levels are determined periodically to maintain desired serum concentrations to minimize the risk of amikacin toxicity. Therapeutic blood serum level: Peak: 20 to 30 mcg/ml; toxic serum level: greater than 30 mcg/ml; Trough: 1 to 9 mcg/ml; toxic serum level: greater than 10 mcg/ml.

IM
- Give deep IM injections slowly to minimize patient discomfort. Injections administered into the gluteus maximus are less painful than injections into the lateral aspect of the thigh.

IV
- Store vials at room temperature.
- Solutions appear clear but may become pale yellow. The pale yellow color does not affect the drug's potency. Discard if precipitate forms or dark discoloration occurs.
- Intermittent IV infusion (piggyback) is stable for 24 hours at room temperature.
- Dilute each 500 mg with 100 ml 0.9% NaCl or D_5W.
- Infuse over 30 to 60 minutes for adults and older children. Infuse over 60 to 120 minutes for infants and young children.

Intervention and Evaluation
- Monitor the patient's intake and output to maintain hydration.
- Expect to monitor urinalysis results to detect casts, red blood cells, white blood cells, and a decrease in specific gravity, and the results of peak and trough amikacin serum levels.
- Be alert to ototoxic and neurotoxic symptoms.
- Check the IM injection site for pain and induration.
- Evaluate the IV site for phlebitis as evidenced by heat, pain, and red streaking over the vein.
- Assess the patient's skin for a rash.
- Assess the patient for superinfection, particularly changes in the oral mucosa, diarrhea, and genital or anal pruritus.
- In patients with neuromuscular

disorders, assess the respiratory response carefully.

Patient Teaching
• Explain to the patient the importance of receiving the full course of amikacin treatment.
• Warn the patient that IM injection may cause discomfort.
• Instruct the patient to notify the physician in the event of any hearing, visual, balance, or urinary problems that occur, even if they start after therapy is completed.
• Caution the patient not to take any other medications without first notifying the physician.
• Advise the patient that lab tests are an essential part of therapy.

gentamicin sulfate
jen-tah-**my**-sin
(Alcomicin[CAN],
Cidomycin[CAN], Garamycin,
Genoptic, Gentacidin)

CATEGORY AND SCHEDULE
Pregnancy Risk Category: C

MECHANISM OF ACTION
An aminoglycoside that irreversibly binds to the protein of bacterial ribosomes. *Therapeutic Effect:* Interferes in protein synthesis of susceptible microorganisms. Bactericidal.

PHARMACOKINETICS
Rapid, complete absorption after intramuscular (IM) administration. Protein binding: less than 30%. Widely distributed. Does not cross the blood-brain barrier and appears in low concentrations in cerebrospinal fluid [CSF]. Excreted unchanged in urine. Removed by hemodialysis. **Half-life:** 2–4 hrs (half-life is increased with impaired renal function as is found in neonates; half-life is decreased in cystic fibrosis, burn or febrile patients).

AVAILABILITY
Injection: 10 mg/ml, 40 mg/ml, 2 mg/ml (Intrathecal).
Ophthalmic Solution: 3 mg/ml.
Ophthalmic Ointment: 3 mg/g.
Cream: 0.5%.
Ointment: 0.1%.

INDICATIONS AND DOSAGES
▸ **Treatment of acute pelvic, bone, complicated urinary tract, intra-abdominal, joint, respiratory tract, and skin/skin structure infections, burns, septicemia, meningitis and for postoperative patients**
IM/IV
Adults, Elderly. Usual dosage 3–6 mg/kg/day in divided doses q8h or 4–6.6 mg/kg once a day.
Children 5–12 yrs. Usual dosage 2–2.5 mg/kg/dose q8h.
Children younger than 5 yrs. Usual dosage 2.5 mg/kg/dose q8h.
Neonates. Usual dosage 2.5–3.5 mg/kg/dose q8–12h.
▸ **Hemodialysis**
IM/IV
Adults, Elderly. 0.5–0.7 mg/kg/dose postdialysis.
Children. 1.25–1.75 mg/kg/dose postdialysis.
▸ **Intrathecal**
Adults. 4–8 mg/day.
Children 3 mos–12 yrs. 1–2 mg/day.
Neonates. 1 mg/day.
▸ **Superficial eye infections**
Ophthalmic Ointment
Adults, Elderly. Usual dosage, thin strip to conjunctiva 2–3 times a day.
Ophthalmic Solution
Adults, Elderly, Children. Usual dosage 1–2 drops q2–4h up to 2 drops q hour.

▸ **Superficial skin infections**
Topical
Adults, Elderly. Usual dosage.
Apply 3–4 times a day.

UNLABELED USES
Topical: Prophylaxis of minor
bacterial skin infections, treatment
of dermal ulcer

CONTRAINDICATIONS
Hypersensitivity to gentamicin or
other aminoglycosides (cross-
sensitivity). Sulfite sensitivity may
result in anaphylaxis, especially in
asthmatics.

INTERACTIONS
Drug
*Other aminoglycosides, nephrotoxic
or ototoxic-producing medications:*
May increase risk of gentamicin
toxicity.
Neuromuscular blocking agents:
May increase effects of neuromus-
cular blocking agents.
Herbal
None known.
Food
None known.

DIAGNOSTIC TEST EFFECTS
May increase serum creatinine,
serum bilirubin, BUN, serum LDH
concentrations, SGOT (AST), and
SGPT (ALT) levels. May decrease
serum calcium, magnesium, potassium, and sodium concentrations.
Therapeutic peak serum level is
6–10 mcg/ml and trough is 0.5–2
mcg/ml. Toxic peak serum level is
greater than 10 mcg/ml and trough
is greater than 2 mcg/ml.

IV INCOMPATIBILITIES
Allopurinol (Aloprim), amphotericin
B complex (Abelcet, AmBisome,
Amphotec), furosemide (Lasix),
heparin, hetastarch (Hespan), idaru-
bicin (Idamycin), indomethacin
(Indocin), propofol (Diprivan)

IV COMPATIBILITIES
Amiodarone (Cordarone), diltiazem
(Cardizem), enalapril (Vasotec),
filgrastim (Neupogen), hydromorphone (Dilaudid), insulin, lorazepam
(Ativan), magnesium sulfate, midazolam (Versed), morphine, multivitamins

SIDE EFFECTS
Occasional
IM: Pain, induration at IM injection
site
IV: Phlebitis, thrombophlebitis with
IV administration; hypersensitivity
reactions such as fever, pruritus,
rash, and urticaria
Ophthalmic: Burning, tearing,
itching, blurred vision
Topical: Redness, itching
Rare
Alopecia, hypertension, weakness

SERIOUS REACTIONS
• Nephrotoxicity, as evidenced
by increased BUN and serum
creatinine and decreased creatinine
clearance, may be reversible if the
drug is stopped at the first sign of
symptoms.
• Irreversible ototoxicity manifested
as tinnitus, dizziness, ringing or
roaring in the ears, and impaired
hearing, and neurotoxicity as evidenced by headache, dizziness,
lethargy, tremors, and visual disturbances occur occasionally. The risk
of irreversible ototoxicity and neurotoxicity is greater with higher
dosages, prolonged therapy, or if the
solution is applied directly to the
mucosa.
• Superinfections, particularly with
fungi, may result from bacterial
imbalance via any route of administration.

• Ophthalmic application may cause paresthesia of conjunctiva or mydriasis.

NURSING CONSIDERATIONS
Baseline Assessment
• Expect to correct dehydration before beginning parenteral therapy.
• Establish the patient's baseline hearing acuity.
◀ALERT▶ Determine if the patient has a history of allergies, especially to aminoglycosides and sulfites, as well as parabens for topical and ophthalmic routes before giving drug.
Lifespan Considerations
• Be aware that gentamicin readily crosses the placenta and that it is unknown if gentamicin is distributed in breast milk.
• Use cautiously in neonates as their immature renal function increases gentamicin half-life and risk of toxicity.
• In the elderly, age-related renal impairment may require dosage adjustment.
Precautions
◀ALERT▶ Cumulative effects may occur with concurrent systemic administration and topical application to large areas.
• Use cautiously in elderly and neonate patients because of age-related renal insufficiency or immaturity.
• Use cautiously in patients with neuromuscular disorders as there is a potential for respiratory depression.
• Use cautiously in patients with prior hearing loss, renal impairment or vertigo.
Administration and Handling
◀ALERT▶ Space parenteral doses evenly around the clock. Gentamicin dosage is based on ideal body weight. As ordered, monitor serum peak and trough levels periodically to maintain the desired serum con-

centrations and to minimize the risk of toxicity. Be aware that the recommended peak serum level is 6 to 10 mcg/ml and trough level is 0.5 to 2 mcg/ml. Also, the toxic peak serum level is greater than 10 mcg/ml and the trough is greater than 2 mcg/ml.
IM
• To minimize discomfort, give deep IM injection slowly.
• To minimize injection site pain, administer the IM injection in the gluteus maximus rather than lateral aspect of thigh.
IV
• Store vials at room temperature.
• The solution normally appears clear or slightly yellow.
• Intermittent IV infusion or IV piggyback solution is stable for 24 hours at room temperature.
• Discard the IV solution if precipitate forms.
• Dilute with 50 to 200 ml D_5W or 0.9% NaCl. The amount of diluent for infants and children depends on individual needs.
• Infuse over 30 to 60 minutes for adults and older children. Infuse over 60 to 120 minutes for infants and young children.
Intrathecal
• Use only 2 mg/ml intrathecal preparation without preservative.
• Mix with 10% estimated CSF volume or NaCl.
• Use intrathecal forms immediately after preparation. Discard unused portion.
• Give over 3 to 5 minutes.
Ophthalmic
• Place a gloved finger on the patient's lower eyelid and pull it out until a pocket is formed between the eye and lower lid.
• Hold the dropper above the pocket and place the correct number of drops (or ¼ to ½ inch of ointment)

into the pocket. Close the eye gently.
• For ophthalmic solution apply digital pressure to the lacrimal sac for 1 to 2 minutes to minimize drainage into the nose and throat, thereby reducing the risk of systemic effects.
• For ophthalmic ointment close the patient's eye for 1 to 2 minutes. Instruct the patient to roll the eyeball to increase the contact area of the drug to the eye.
• Remove excess solution or ointment around eye with tissue.

Intervention and Evaluation
• Monitor the patient's intake and output and urinalysis results as appropriate. Urge the patient to drink fluids to maintain adequate hydration. Monitor the urinalysis results for casts, red blood cells (RBCs) and white blood cells (WBCs) or a decrease in specific gravity.
• Be alert to ototoxic and neurotoxic signs and symptoms.
• Check the IM injection site for induration.
• Evaluate the IV infusion site for signs and symptoms of phlebitis such as heat, pain, and red streaking over the vein.
• Assess the patient's skin for rash. If giving gentamicin for ophthalmic use, monitor the patient's eye for burning, itching, redness, and tearing. If giving gentamicin for topical use, monitor the patient for signs of itching and redness.
• Be alert for signs and symptoms of superinfection, particularly changes in the oral mucosa, diarrhea, and genital or anal pruritus.
• When treating those with neuromuscular disorders, assess the patient's respiratory response carefully.

• Be aware that the therapeutic peak serum level is 6 to 10 mcg/ml and the trough is 0.5 to 2 mcg/ml. Also, know that the toxic peak serum level is greater than 10 mcg/ml and the trough is greater than 2 mcg/ml.

Patient Teaching
• Explain to the patient that discomfort may occur with IM injection.
• Advise the patient that blurred vision or tearing may occur briefly after each ophthalmic dose.
• Instruct the patient receiving topical gentamicin to cleanse the area gently before applying the ointment.
• Warn the patient to notify the physician of any balance, hearing, urinary, or vision problems that develop, even after gentamicin therapy is completed.
• Warn the patient taking ophthalmic gentamicin to notify the physician if irritation, redness, or tearing continues.
• Warn the patient taking topical gentamicin to notify the physician if itching or redness occurs.

kanamycin sulfate
can-ah-**my**-sin
(Kantrex)

CATEGORY AND SCHEDULE
Pregnancy Risk Category:
Unavailable for irrigating solution.

MECHANISM OF ACTION
An aminoglycoside antibiotic that irreversibly binds to protein on bacterial ribosomes. *Therapeutic Effect:* Interferes in protein synthesis of susceptible microorganisms.

AVAILABILITY
Injection: 1 g/3 ml.

INDICATIONS AND DOSAGES
▸ **Wound and surgical site irrigation**
Adults, Elderly. 0.25% solution to
irrigate pleural space, ventricular or
abscess cavities, wounds, or surgical
sites.

CONTRAINDICATIONS
Hypersensitivity to aminoglycosides, kanamycin

INTERACTIONS
Drug
None significant.
Herbal
None significant.
Food
None significant.

DIAGNOSTIC TEST EFFECTS
None known.

SIDE EFFECTS
Occasional
Hypersensitivity reactions: fever,
pruritus, rash, urticaria
Rare
Headache

SERIOUS REACTIONS
• None known.

NURSING CONSIDERATIONS
Baseline Assessment
• Assess the patient for hypersensitivity to aminoglycosides or kanamycin
Lifespan Considerations
• There are no age-related precautions noted in children or the elderly.

neomycin sulfate
nee-oh-**my**-sin
(Mycifradin, Myciguent,
Neosulf[AUS])

CATEGORY AND SCHEDULE
Pregnancy Risk Category: C
OTC (topical ointment 0.5%
only)

MECHANISM OF ACTION
An aminoglycoside antibiotic that
binds to bacterial microorganisms.
Therapeutic Effect: Interferes with
bacterial protein synthesis.

AVAILABILITY
Topical ointment (OTC): 0.5%.
Tablets (Rx): 500 mg.

INDICATIONS AND DOSAGES
▸ **Preop bowel antisepsis**
PO
Adults, Elderly. 1 g each hr for
4 doses; then 1 g q4h for 5 doses
or 1 g at 1 p.m., 2 p.m., 10 p.m.
(with erythromycin) on day before
surgery.
Children. 90 mg/kg/day in divided
doses q4h for 2 days or 25 mg/kg
at 1 p.m., 2 p.m., 10 p.m. on day
before surgery.
▸ **Liver encephalopathy**
PO
Adults, Elderly. 4–12 g/day in
divided doses q4–6h.
Children. 2.5–7 g/m^2/day in divided
doses q4–6h.
▸ **Diarrhea caused by *Eserichia coli***
PO
Adults, Elderly. 3 g/day in divided
doses q6h.
Children. 50 mg/kg/day in divided
doses q6h.
▸ **Minor skin infections**
Topical
Adults, Elderly, Children. Usual

dosage, apply to affected area 1–3 times a day.

CONTRAINDICATIONS
Hypersensitivity to aminoglycosides

INTERACTIONS
Drug
Other aminoglycosides, other nephrotoxic or ototoxic medications: If significant systemic absorption occurs, neomycin may increase nephrotoxicity and ototoxicity of these drugs.
Herbal
None known.
Food
None known.

DIAGNOSTIC TEST EFFECTS
None known.

SIDE EFFECTS
Frequent
Systemic: Nausea, vomiting, diarrhea, irritation of mouth or rectal area
Topical: Itching, redness, swelling, rash
Rare
Systemic: Malabsorption syndrome, neuromuscular blockade as evidenced by difficulty breathing, drowsiness, or weakness

SERIOUS REACTIONS
• Nephrotoxicity, as evidenced by increased BUN and serum creatinine and decreased creatinine clearance, may be reversible if the drug is stopped at the first sign of nephrotoxic symptoms.
• Irreversible ototoxicity manifested as tinnitus, dizziness, ringing or roaring in the ears, and impaired hearing, and neurotoxicity as evidenced by headache, dizziness, lethargy, tremors, and visual disturbances, occur occasionally.

• Severe respiratory depression and anaphylaxis occur rarely.
• Superinfections, particularly fungal infections, may occur.

NURSING CONSIDERATIONS
Baseline Assessment
• Expect to correct dehydration before beginning aminoglycoside therapy.
• Establish the patient's baseline hearing acuity before beginning therapy.
Precautions
• Use cautiously in the elderly, infants, and patients with renal insufficiency or immaturity, neuromuscular disorders, history of hearing loss, renal impairment, or vertigo.
Intervention and Evaluation
• Assess the patient for signs and symptoms of ototoxicity and neurotoxicity.
• Evaluate the patient for signs and symptoms of a hypersensitivity reaction. With topical application a hypersensitivity reaction may appear as rash, redness, or itching.
• Watch the patient for signs and symptoms of superinfection, particularly changes in the oral mucosa, diarrhea, or genital or anal pruritus.
Patient Teaching
• Advise the patient to continue the antibiotic for the full length of treatment and to evenly space doses around the clock.
• Instruct patients receiving topical neomycin to cleanse the affected area gently before applying the drug.
• Warn patients receiving topical neomycin to notify the physician if any itching or redness occurs.
• Warn the patient to notify the

physician if he or she experiences dizziness, impaired hearing, or ringing in the ears.

streptomycin
strep-toe-**mye**-sin

CATEGORY AND SCHEDULE
Pregnancy Risk Category: D

MECHANISM OF ACTION
An aminoglycoside that binds directly to the 30S ribosomal subunits causing faulty peptide sequence to form in the protein chain. *Therapeutic effect:* Inhibits bacterial protein synthesis.

AVAILABILITY
Injection: 1 g.

INDICATIONS AND DOSAGES
▸ **Tuberculosis**
IM
Adults. 15 mg/kg/day. Maximum: 1 g.
Elderly: 10 mg/kg/day. Maximum: 750 mg/day.
Children. 20–40 mg/kg/day. Maximum: 1 g.
▸ **Dosage in renal impairment:**

Creatinine Clearance	Dosage Interval
10–50 ml/min	every 24–72 hrs
less than 10 ml/min	every 72–96 hrs

CONTRAINDICATIONS
Pregnancy

INTERACTIONS
Drug
Amphotericin, loop diuretics: May increase the nephrotoxicity of streptomycin.

Neuromuscular blocking agents: May increase the effects of streptomycin.
Herbal
None known.
Food
None known.

DIAGNOSTIC TEST EFFECTS
None known.

SIDE EFFECTS
Occasional
Hypotension, drowsiness, headache, drug fever, paresthesia, skin rash, nausea, vomiting, anemia, arthralgia, weakness, tremor

SERIOUS REACTIONS
• Symptoms of ototoxicity, nephrotoxicity, and neuromuscular toxicity may occur.

NURSING CONSIDERATIONS
Baseline Assessment
• Determine if the patient is hypersensitive to aminoglycosides, pregnant, or being treated for other medical conditions such as myasthenia gravis and parkinsonism.
Precautions
• Use cautiously in patients with hearing loss, neuromuscular disorders, pre-existing vertigo, renal impairment, and tinnitus.
Administration and Handling
IM/IV
• Give IM injection deeply into a large muscle mass.
• May be given IV over 30 to 60 minutes.
Intervention and Evaluation
• Monitor the patient's hearing, renal function, and serum concentrations of streptomycin.
Patient Teaching
• Warn the patient to notify the physician if he or she experiences

any unusual symptoms of hearing loss, dizziness, fullness in the ears, or roaring noises.

tobramycin sulfate
tow-bra-**my**-sin
(Nebcin, Tobi, Tobrex)

CATEGORY AND SCHEDULE
Pregnancy Risk Category: C.
(B, Ophthalmic form)

MECHANISM OF ACTION
An aminoglycoside antibiotic that irreversibly binds to protein on bacterial ribosomes. *Therapeutic Effect:* Interferes in protein synthesis of susceptible microorganisms.

PHARMACOKINETICS
Rapid, complete absorption after IM administration. Protein binding: less than 30%. Widely distributed but does not cross the blood-brain barrier and is in low concentrations in cerebrospinal fluid (CSF). Excreted unchanged in urine. Removed by hemodialysis. **Half-life:** 2–4 hrs. Half-life is increased with impaired renal function and in neonates. Half-life is decreased in cystic fibrosis, febrile, or burn patients.

AVAILABILITY
Injection: 10 mg/ml, 40 mg/ml.
Powder for Injection: 1.2 g.
Ophthalmic Solution: 0.3%.
Ophthalmic Ointment: 3 mg/g.
Inhalation Solution: 300 mg/5 ml.

INDICATIONS AND DOSAGES
▸ **Skin/skin structure, bone, joint, respiratory tract infections, postoperative, burn, intra-abdominal infections, complicated urinary tract infections, septicemia, meningitis**
IM/IV
Adults, Elderly. 3–6 mg/kg/day in 3 divided doses. May use 4–6.6 mg/kg once a day.
▸ **Superficial eye infections, including blepharitis, conjunctivitis, keratitis, corneal ulcers**
Ointment
Adults, Elderly. Usual dosage, a thin strip to conjunctiva q8–12h (q3–4h for severe infections).
Solution
Adults, Elderly. Usual dosage, 1–2 drops q4h (2 drops every hour for severe infections) to the affected eye.
▸ **Bronchopulmonary infections in patients with cystic fibrosis**
Inhalation
Adults. Usual dosage, 60–80 mg twice a day for 28 days, then off for 28 days.
Children. 40–80 mg 2–3 times/day.
▸ **Dosage in Renal Impairment**
Dosage and frequency are modified based on degree of renal impairment and the serum concentration of the drug. After a loading dose of 1–2 mg/kg, the maintenance dose and frequency are based on serum creatinine levels and creatinine clearance.

CONTRAINDICATIONS
Hypersensitivity to aminoglycosides (cross-sensitivity)

INTERACTIONS
Drug
Other aminoglycosides, nephrotoxic and ototoxic-producing medications: May increase the risk of tobramycin toxicity.
Neuromuscular blocking agents: May increase the effects of neuromuscular blocking agents.

Herbal
None known.
Food
None known.

DIAGNOSTIC TEST EFFECTS

May increase serum bilirubin, BUN, serum creatinine, serum LDH concentrations, SGOT (AST), and SGPT (ALT) levels. May decrease serum calcium, magnesium, potassium, and sodium concentrations. Therapeutic blood level: Peak is 5–20 mcg/ml; trough is 0.5–2 mcg/ml. Toxic blood level: Peak is greater than 20 mcg/ml; trough is greater than 2 mcg/ml.

IV INCOMPATIBILITIES

Amphotericin B complex (Abelcet, AmBisome, Amphotec), heparin, hetastarch (Hespan), indomethacin (Indocin), propofol (Diprivan), sargramostim (Leukine, Prokine)

IV COMPATIBILITIES

Amiodarone (Cordarone), calcium gluconate, diltiazem (Cardizem), furosemide (Lasix), hydromorphone (Dilaudid), insulin, magnesium sulfate, midazolam (Versed), morphine, theophylline

SIDE EFFECTS

Occasional
IM: Pain, induration at IM injection site
IV: Phlebitis, thrombophlebitis
Topical: Hypersensitivity reaction such as fever, pruritus, rash, and urticaria
Ophthalmic: Tearing, itching, redness, swelling of eyelid
Rare
Hypotension, nausea, vomiting

SERIOUS REACTIONS

• Nephrotoxicity, as evidenced by increased BUN and serum creatinine and decreased creatinine clearance, may be reversible if the drug is stopped at the first sign of nephrotoxic symptoms.
• Irreversible ototoxicity, manifested as tinnitus, dizziness, ringing or roaring in ears, impaired hearing and neurotoxicity, as evidenced by headache, dizziness, lethargy, tremors, and visual disturbances, occur occasionally. The risk of irreversible neurotoxicity and ototoxicity is greater with higher dosages, prolonged therapy, or if the solution is applied directly to the mucosa.
• Superinfections, particularly with fungi, may result from bacterial imbalance with any route of administration.
• Anaphylaxis may occur.

NURSING CONSIDERATIONS

Baseline Assessment

• Expect to correct dehydration before beginning parenteral therapy.
◀ ALERT ▶ Determine the patient's history of allergies, especially to aminoglycosides, sulfites, and parabens (for topical and ophthalmic routes) before giving the drug. Establish a baseline for the patient's hearing acuity.

Lifespan Considerations

• Be aware that tobramycin readily crosses the placenta and is distributed in breast milk.
• Be aware that tobramycin may cause fetal nephrotoxicity. The ophthalmic form should not be used in breastfeeding mothers and only when specifically indicated in pregnancy.
• Be aware that immature renal function in neonates and premature infants may increase the risk of toxicity.
• In the elderly, age-related renal

impairment may increase the risk of toxicity. Dosage adjustment is recommended.

Precautions

• Use cautiously in patients who also use neuromuscular blocking agents or who have impaired renal function or preexisting auditory or vestibular impairment.

Administration and Handling

◀ALERT▶ Be sure to carefully coordinate the drawing of peak and trough blood levels with the drug's administration times.

◀ALERT▶ Evenly space parenteral doses around the clock. Be aware that dosages are based on ideal body weight. Monitor blood peak and trough levels to ensure that the desired blood concentrations are maintained and to minimize the risk of toxicity.

IM

• To minimize injection site discomfort, give deep IM injection slowly. Also, to reduce pain, administer the injection into the gluteus maximus rather than the lateral aspect of the thigh.

IV

• Store vials at room temperature.

• Solutions may be discolored by light or air, but discoloration does not affect drug potency.

• Dilute with 50 to 200 ml D_5W or 0.9% NaCl. The amount of diluent for infant and children dosages depends on individual needs.

• Infuse over 20 to 60 minutes.

Ophthalmic

• Place a gloved finger on the patient's lower eyelid and pull it out until a pocket is formed between the eye and lower lid.

• Hold the dropper above the pocket and place the correct number of drops (or ¼–½ inch of ointment) into the pocket. Have patient close the eye gently.

• To administer ophthalmic solution, apply digital pressure to the lacrimal sac for 1 to 2 minutes to minimize drainage into the patient's nose and throat, thereby reducing the risk of systemic effects.

• To administer ophthalmic ointment, close the patient's eye for 1 to 2 minutes. Have the patient roll the eyeball to increase the contact area of the drug to the eye.

• Remove excess solution or ointment around the eye with tissue.

Intervention and Evaluation

• Monitor the patient's intake and output and urinalysis results, as appropriate. To maintain adequate hydration, encourage the patient to drink fluids. Monitor urinalysis results for casts, red blood cells (RBCs), and white blood cells (WBCs) or a decrease in specific gravity.

• Expect to monitor the results of peak and trough blood tests. Keep in mind that the therapeutic peak blood level is 5 to 20 mcg/ml and trough is 0.5 to 2 mcg/ml. Also, know that the toxic peak blood level is greater than 20 mcg/ml and trough is greater than 2 mcg/ml.

◀ALERT▶ Assess the patient for ototoxic and neurotoxic symptoms.

• Evaluate the IV site for signs and symptoms of phlebitis such as heat, pain, and red streaking over the vein.

• Assess the patient's skin for rash.

• Be alert for signs and symptoms of superinfection, particularly changes in the oral mucosa, diarrhea, or genital or anal pruritus.

• When treating patients with neuromuscular disorders, assess the patient's respiratory response frequently.

• Assess patients receiving ophthalmic tobramycin for itching, redness, swelling, and tearing.

Patient Teaching

• Warn the patient to notify the physician if any balance, hearing, urinary, or vision problems develop, even after therapy is completed.

• Advise patients receiving ophthalmic tobramycin that blurred vision and tearing may occur briefly after application.

• Warn patients receiving ophthalmic tobramycin to notify the physician if irritation, redness, or tearing continues.

2 Antifungal Agents

amphotericin B
caspofungin acetate
fluconazole
griseofulvin
itraconazole
ketoconazole
nystatin
terbinafine
  hydrochloride
voriconazole

Uses: Antifungal agents are used to treat systemic and superficial fungal infections. They're effective against opportunistic and nonopportunistic *systemic* fungal infections. Opportunistic infections, which include candidiasis, aspergillosis, and cryptococcosis, occur primarily in debilitated or immunocompromised patients. Nonopportunistic infections, which include blastomycosis, histoplasmosis, and coccidioidomycosis, are less common.

Antifungal agents are especially effective against *superficial* fungal infections caused by *Candida* species and dermatophytes (ringworm). Candidiasis usually affects the mucus membranes and moist skin areas; in chronic infection, organisms may invade the scalp, skin, and nails. Dermatophytosis typically affects only the skin, hair, and nails.

Action: The three types of antifungal agents act in different ways. *Polyene antifungals,* such as amphotericin and nystatin, bind to sterols in fungal cell walls, forming pores or channels that increase cell wall permeability and allow the leakage of small molecules. *Imidazole antifungals,* such as ketoconazole, inhibit cytochrome P-450 in fungal cells, which impairs ergosterol synthesis and fungal growth. *Antimetabolite antifungals,* such as flucytosine, disrupt the synthesis of deoxyribonucleic acid (DNA) and ribonucleic acid (RNA) in fungal cells. (See illustration, *Sites and Mechanism of Action: Antifungal Agents*, page 17.)

COMBINATION PRODUCTS

MYCOLOG: nystatin/triamcinolone (a steroid) 100,000 units/0.1%.
MYCO-TRIACET: nystatin/triamcinolone (a steroid) 100,000 units/0.1%.

amphotericin B
am-foe-**tear**-ih-sin
(Abelcet, AmBisome, Amphotec, Fungizone)

CATEGORY AND SCHEDULE
Pregnancy Risk Category: B

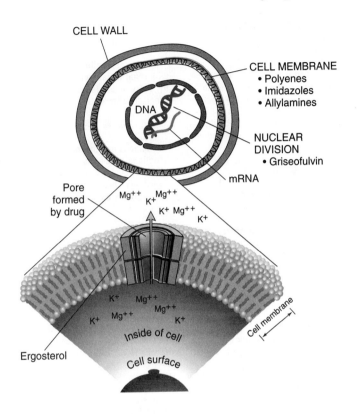

CELL WALL

CELL MEMBRANE
• Polyenes
• Imidazoles
• Allylamines

DNA

NUCLEAR DIVISION
• Griseofulvin

mRNA

Pore formed by drug

Mg^{++} K^+ Mg^{++}
K^+ Mg^{++}
K^+

K^+ Mg^{++}
K^+ Mg^{++} Mg^{++}
K^+
Inside of cell

Cell membrane

Ergosterol

Cell surface

Sites and Mechanism of Action: Antifungal Agents

Antifungal agents primarily affect fungi at one of two sites: the cell membrane or the cell nucleus. Most of these agents, such as polyene, imidazole, and allylamine antifungals, act on the fungal cell membrane. Polyene antifungals, such as amphotericin B, bind to ergosterol and increase cell membrane permeability. Imidazole antifungals, such as fluconazole and ketoconazole, interfere with ergosterol synthesis by inhibiting the cytochrome P_{450} enzyme system, altering the cell membrane, and inhibiting fungal growth. Allylamine antifungals, such as terbinafine, inhibit the enzyme squaline epoxidase, which disrupts ergosterol production—and cell membrane integrity. When cell membrane permeability increases, cellular components, including potassium (K^+) and magnesium (Mg^{++}), leak out. Loss of these cellular components leads to cell death.

Another antifungal agent, griseofulvin directly affects the fungal nucleus, interfering with mitosis. By binding to structures in the mitotic spindle, it prevents cells from dividing, which eventually leads to their death.

MECHANISM OF ACTION

This antifungal and antiprotozoal is generally fungistatic but may become fungicidal with high dosages or very susceptible microorganisms. This drug binds to sterols in the fungal cell membrane. *Therapeutic Effect:* Increases fungal cell-membrane permeability, allowing loss of potassium, and other cellular components.

PHARMACOKINETICS

Protein binding: 90%. Widely distributed. Metabolic fate unknown. Cleared by nonrenal pathways. Minimal removal by hemodialysis. Amphotec and Abelcet are not dialyzable. **Half-life:** 24 hrs (half-life increased in neonates, children). Amphotec half-life is 26–28 hrs. Abelcet half-life is 7.2 days. AmBisome half-life is 100–153 hrs.

AVAILABILITY

Injection: 50 mg, 50 mg (Fungizone), 100 mg (Amphotec), 50 mg (AmBisone).
Suspension for Injection: 5 mg/ml (Amphotericin B lipid complex, Abelcet).
Cream, Lotion, Ointment: 3%

INDICATIONS AND DOSAGES

▶ **Invasive fungal infections unresponsive or intolerant to Fungizone (Abelcet)**
IV Infusion
Adults, Children. 5 mg/kg at rate of 2.5 mg/kg/hr.
▶ **Empiric treatment for fungal infection in patients with febrile neutropenia; for aspergillus, candida, or cryptococcus infections unresponsive to Fungizone; or for patients with renal impairment or toxicity from Fungizone (AmBisome)**
IV Infusion
Adults, Children. 3–5 mg/kg over 1 hr.
▶ **Invasive aspergillus in patients with renal impairment, renal toxicity, or treatment failure with Fungizone.(Amphotec)**
IV Infusion
Adults, Children. 3–4 mg/kg over 2–4 hrs.
▶ **Cutaneous and mucocutaneous infections caused by *Candida albicans,* such as paronychia, oral thrush, perlche, diaper rash, and intertriginous candidiasis (Topical)**
Adults, Elderly, Children. Apply liberally to the affected area and rub in 2–4 times/day.
▶ **Cryptococcosis; blastomycosis; systemic candidiasis; disseminated forms of moniliasis, coccidioidomycosis, and histoplasmosis; zygomycosis; sporotrichosis; and aspergillosis (Fungizone)**
IV Infusion
Adults, Elderly. Dosage based on pt tolerance, severity of infection. Initially, 1-mg test dose is given over 20–30 min. If test dose is tolerated, 5-mg dose may be given the same day. Subsequently, increases of 5 mg/dose are made q12–24h until desired daily dose is reached. Alternatively, if test dose is tolerated, a dose of 0.25 mg/kg is given same day; increased to 0.5 mg/kg the second day. Dose increased until desired daily dose reached. Total daily dose: 1 mg/kg/day up to 1.5 mg/kg every other day. Do not exceed maximum total daily dose of 1.5 mg/kg.
Children. Test dose: 0.1 mg/kg/dose (maximum 1 mg) infused over 20–60 min. If tolerated, then initial dose: 0.4 mg/kg same day; Dose may be increased in 0.25 mg/kg

increments. Maintenance dose: 0.25–1 mg/kg/day.

CONTRAINDICATIONS

Hypersensitivity to amphotericin B, sulfite

INTERACTIONS
Drug
Bone marrow depressants: May increase risk for anemia.
Digoxin: May increase risk of digoxin toxicity from hypokalemia.
Nephrotoxic medications: May increase risk of nephrotoxicity.
Steroids: May cause severe hypokalemia.
Herbal
None known.
Food
None known.

DIAGNOSTIC TEST EFFECTS

May increase BUN, serum alkaline phosphatase, serum creatinine, SGOT (AST), and SGPT (ALT) levels. May decrease serum calcium, magnesium, and potassium levels.

IV INCOMPATIBILITIES

Abelcet/Amphotec/AmBisome: Do not mix with any other drug, diluent, or solution. Fungizone: Allopurinol (Aloprim), amifostine (Ethyol), aztreonam (Azactam), calcium gluconate, cefepime (Maxipime), cimetidine (Tagamet), ciprofloxacin (Cipro), docetaxel (Taxotere), dopamine (Intropin), doxorubicin (Adriamycin), enalapril (Vasotec), etoposide (VP-16), filgrastim (Neupogen), fluconazole (Diflucan), fludarabine (Fludara), foscarnet (Foscavir), gemcitabine (Gemzar), magnesium sulfate, meropenem (Merrem IV), ondansetron (Zofran), paclitaxel (Taxol), piperacillin/tazobactam (Zosyn), potassium chloride,

propofol (Diprivan), vinorelbine (Navelbine)

IV COMPATIBILITIES

None known; do not mix with other medications or electrolytes.

SIDE EFFECTS

Frequent (greater than 10%)
Abelcet: Chills, fever, increased serum creatinine, multiple organ failure
AmBisome: Hypokalemia, hypomagnesemia, hyperglycemia, hypocalcemia, edema, abdominal pain, back pain, chills, chest pain, hypotension, diarrhea, nausea, vomiting, headache, fever, rigors, insomnia, dyspnea, epistaxis, increased liver/renal function test results
Amphotec: Chills, fever, hypotension, tachycardia, increased creatinine, hypokalemia, bilirubinemia
Fungizone: Fever, chills, headache, anemia, hypokalemia, hypomagnesemia, anorexia, malaise, generalized pain, nephrotoxicity
Topical: Local irritation, dry skin
Rare
Topical: Skin rash

SERIOUS REACTIONS

• Cardiovascular toxicity as evidenced by hypotension and ventricular fibrillation and anaphylaxis occur rarely.
• Vision and hearing alterations, seizures, liver failure, coagulation defects, multiple organ failure, and sepsis may be noted.

NURSING CONSIDERATIONS
Baseline Assessment
• Determine the patient's history of allergies, especially to amphotericin B and sulfites, before giving the drug.
• Be aware that other nephrotoxic

medications should be avoided, if possible.
- Check for or obtain orders for drugs to reduce the risk or severity of adverse reactions during IV therapy. Antiemetics, antihistamines, antipyretics, or small doses of corticosteroids may be given before or during amphotericin administration to help control adverse reactions.

Lifespan Considerations
- Be aware that amphotericin B crosses the placenta and that it is unknown if amphotericin B is distributed in breast milk.
- Be aware that the safety and efficacy of amphotericin B have not been established in children. Therefore, expect to use the smallest dose necessary to achieve optimal results.
- There are no age-related precautions noted in the elderly.

Precautions
- Use cautiously in patients with renal impairment and in combination with antineoplastic therapy. Drug is prescribed only for progressive, potentially fatal fungal infection.
- Keep in mind that conventional amphotericin, Fungizone, is more nephrotoxic than the alternative formulations of amphotericin B, including Albecet, AmBisonme, and Amphotec.

Administration and Handling
IV
- Observe strict aseptic technique because no bacteriostatic agent or preservative is present in the diluent.
- Refrigerate Abelcet as unreconstituted solution. Albecet reconstituted solution is stable for 48 hours if refrigerated and 6 hours at room temperature.
- Refrigerate AmBisome as unre-

constituted solution. AmBisone reconstituted solution of 4 mg/ml is stable for 24 hours. AmBisone reconstituted solution concentration of 1–2 mg/ml is stable for 6 hours.
- Store Amphotec as unreconstituted solution at room temperature. Amphotec reconstituted solution is stable for 24 hours.
- Refrigerate Fungizone as unreconstituted solution. Fungizone reconstituted solution is stable for 24 hours at room temperature or 7 days if refrigerated. Diluted solution less than or equal to 0.1 mg/ml should be used promptly. Do not use the solution if it is cloudy or contains a precipitate.
- Shake Abelcet 20-ml (100-mg) vial gently until contents are dissolved. Withdraw required Abelcet dose using a 5-micron filter needle supplied by manufacturer.
- Inject Abelcet dose into D_5W; 4 ml D_5W is required for each 1 ml (5 mg) to final concentration of 1 mg/ml. Reduce dose by half for pediatric, fluid-restricted patients (2 mg/ml).
- Reconstitute each 50-mg AmBisome vial with 12 ml Sterile Water for Injection to provide concentration of 4 mg/ml.
- Shake AmBisome vial vigorously for 30 seconds. Then, withdraw the required AmBisone dose and empty the syringe contents through a 5-micron filter into an infusion of D_5W to provide final concentration of 1 to 2 mg/ml.
- Add 10 ml Sterile Water for Injection to each 50-mg Amphotec vial to provide a concentration of 5 mg/ml. Shake the Amphotec vial gently.
- Further dilute Amphotec vial only with D_5W using specific amount recommended by manufacturer to

provide concentration of 0.16 to
0.83 mg/ml.
• Rapidly inject 10 ml Sterile Water
for Injection to each 50-mg Fungizone vial to provide concentration
of 5 mg/ml. Immediately shake
Fungizone vial until the solution
is clear.
• Further dilute each 1 mg Fungizone in at least 10 ml D₅W to provide a concentration of 0.1 mg/ml.
• Be aware that the potential for
thrombophlebitis may be less with
the use of pediatric scalp vein
needles or by adding dilute heparin
solution, as prescribed.
• Infuse conventional amphotericin,
Fungizone, over 2 to 6 hours by
slow IV infusion.
• Infuse Abelcet over 2 hours by
slow IV infusion. Shake the contents if the infusion is greater than
2 hours.
• Infuse Amphotec over 2 to 4
hours by slow IV infusion.
• Infuse AmBisome over 1 to 2
hours by slow IV infusion.

Intervention and Evaluation
• Monitor the patient's blood pressure (B/P), pulse, respirations, and
temperature twice every 15 minutes,
then every 30 minutes for the initial
4 hours of the infusion to assess for
adverse reactions. Adverse reactions
include abdominal pain, anorexia,
chills, fever, nausea, shaking, and
vomiting. If signs and symptoms of
adverse reactions occur, slow the
infusion and give prescribed drugs
to provide symptomatic relief. For a
severe reaction or for patients without orders for symptomatic relief,
stop the infusion and notify the
physician.
• Evaluate the IV site for signs
of phlebitis as evidenced by heat,
pain, and red streaking over the
vein.
• Monitor the patient's intake and

output and renal function test results
to assess for nephrotoxicity.
• Check the patient's serum potassium and magnesium levels, as well
as hematologic and liver function
test results.
• Assess the patient's skin for
burning, irritation, or itching.

Patient Teaching
• Explain to the patient that prolonged amphotericin B therapy over
weeks or months is usually necessary to achieve therapeutic effect.
• Tell the patient that the fever
reaction may decrease with continued therapy.
• Advise the patient that muscle
weakness may be noted during
therapy from hypokalemia.
• Teach patient to thoroughly rub in
the topical cream or lotion because
this may prevent staining of the
skin or nails. Assure the patient that
soap and water or dry cleaning will
remove fabric stains caused by
topical applications.
• Warn the patient not to use other
preparations or occlusive coverings
without consulting the physician.
• Urge the patient to keep affected
areas clean, dry, to wear light clothing, and to separate out personal
items with direct contact to the
affected area.

caspofungin acetate
cas-poe-**fun**-gin
(Cancidas)

CATEGORY AND SCHEDULE
Pregnancy Risk Category: C

MECHANISM OF ACTION
An antifungal that inhibits the
synthesis of glucan, a vital component of fungal cell formation,

thereby damaging the fungal cell membrane. *Therapeutic Effect:* Fungistatic.

PHARMACOKINETICS

Distributed in tissue. Extensively bound to albumin. Protein binding: 97%. Slowly metabolized in liver to active metabolite. Primarily excreted in urine and to a lesser extent in feces. Not removed by hemodialysis. **Half-life:** 40–50 hrs.

AVAILABILITY

Powder for Injection: 50-mg, 70-mg vials.

INDICATIONS AND DOSAGES

▶ **Aspergillosis**
IV
Adults, Elderly. Give single 70-mg loading dose on day 1, followed by 50 mg a day thereafter. Patients with moderate liver insufficiency, daily dose reduced to 35 mg.

CONTRAINDICATIONS

None known.

INTERACTIONS

Drug
Carbamazepine, cyclosporine, dexamethasone, efavirenz, nelfinavir, nevirapine, phenytoin, or rifampin: May increase blood concentration of caspofungin.
Tacrolimus: May decrease the effect of tacrolimus.
Herbal
None known.
Food
None known.

DIAGNOSTIC TEST EFFECTS

May increase serum alkaline phosphatase, serum bilirubin, serum creatinine, LDH concentrations, prothrombin time, SGOT (AST), SGPT (ALT), serum uric acid, urine pH, urine protein, urine red blood cells (RBCs), and urine white blood cells (WBCs). May decrease Hgb, Hct, platelet count, serum albumin, serum bicarbonate, serum protein, and serum potassium.

IV INCOMPATIBILITIES

Do not mix with any other medication or use dextrose as a diluent.

SIDE EFFECTS

Frequent (26%)
Fever
Occasional (11%–4%)
Headache, nausea, phlebitis
Rare (3% or less)
Paresthesia, vomiting, diarrhea, abdominal pain, myalgia, chills, tremor, insomnia

SERIOUS REACTIONS

• Hypersensitivity reactions characterized by rash, facial swelling, pruritus, and a sensation of warmth occur.

NURSING CONSIDERATIONS

Baseline Assessment
• Obtain the patient's baseline temperature, liver function test results, and history of allergies before giving the drug.
Lifespan Considerations
• Be aware that caspofungin crosses the placental barrier, may be embryotoxic, and is distributed in breast milk.
• Be aware that the safety and efficacy of caspofungin have not been established in children
• In the elderly, age-related moderate renal impairment may require dosage adjustment.
Precautions
• Use cautiously in patients with liver function impairment.

Administration and Handling
IV
• Refrigerate but warm it to room temperature before preparing it with the diluent.
• The reconstituted solution, before prepared as the patient infusion solution, may be stored at room temperature for 1 hour before infusion.
• The final infusion solution can be stored at room temperature for 24 hours.
• Discard the solution if it contains particulate or is discolored.
• For a 50- to 70-mg loading dose, add 10.5 ml 0.9% NaCl to the vial. Transfer 10 ml of the reconstituted solution to 250 ml 0.9% NaCl.
• For 35-mg dose in patients with moderate liver insufficiency, add 10.5 ml 0.9% NaCl to the vial. Transfer 10 ml of reconstituted solution to 100 or 250 ml 0.9% NaCl for 50- to 70-mg a day dose. For moderate liver insufficiency, transfer 7 ml to 100 or 250 ml 0.9% NaCl.
• Infuse over 60 minutes.

Intervention and Evaluation
• Assess the patient for signs and symptoms of liver dysfunction.
• Expect to monitor liver enzyme test results in patients with preexisting liver dysfunction.

Patient Teaching
• Advise the patient to notify the physician if he or she develops increased shortness of breath, itching, facial swelling, or a rash.
• Urge the patient to report pain, burning, or swelling at the IV infusion site.

fluconazole
flu-**con**-ah-zole
(Apo-Fluconazole[CAN], Diflucan)
Do not confuse with diclofenac.

CATEGORY AND SCHEDULE
Pregnancy Risk Category: C

MECHANISM OF ACTION
A fungistatic antifungal that interferes with cytochrome, an enzyme necessary for ergosterol formation. *Therapeutic Effect:* Directly damages fungal membrane, altering membrane function.

PHARMACOKINETICS
Well absorbed from gastrointestinal (GI) tract. Widely distributed, including cerebrospinal fluid (CSF). Protein binding: 11%. Partially metabolized in liver. Primarily excreted unchanged in urine. Partially removed by hemodialysis. **Half-life:** 20–30 hrs (half-life is increased with impaired renal function).

AVAILABILITY
Tablets: 50 mg, 100 mg, 150 mg, 200 mg.
Powder for Oral Suspension: 10 mg/ml, 40 mg/ml.
Injection: 2 mg/ml (in 100- or 200-ml containers).

INDICATIONS AND DOSAGES
▶ **Oropharyngeal Candidiasis**
PO/IV
Adults, Elderly. Initially, 200 mg once, then 100 mg/day for at least 14 days.
Children. Initially, 6 mg/kg/day once, then 3 mg/kg/day.
▶ **Esophageal Candidiasis**
PO/IV
Adults, Elderly. 200 mg once, then 100 mg/day (up to 400 mg/day) for

21 days and at least 14 days following resolution of symptoms.
Children. 6 mg/kg/day once, then 3 mg/kg/day (up to 12 mg/kg/day).
▶ **Vaginal Candidiasis**
PO
Adults. 150 mg once.
▶ **Candidiasis Prevention**
PO
Adults. 400 mg/day.
▶ **Systemic Candidiasis**
PO/IV
Adults, Elderly. Initially, 400 mg once, then 200 mg/day (up to 400 mg/day) for at least 28 days and at least 14 days following resolution of symptoms.
Children. 6–12 mg/kg/day.
▶ **Cryptococcal Meningitis**
PO/IV
Adults, Elderly. Initially, 400 mg once, then 200 mg/day (up to 800 mg/day). Continue for 10–12 wks after CSF becomes negative (200 mg/day for suppression of relapse in patients with AIDS).
Children. 12 mg/kg/day once, then 6–12 mg/kg/day; 6 mg/kg/day for suppression.
▶ **Onychomycosis**
PO
Adults. 150 mg weekly.
▶ **Dosage in Renal Impairment**
After loading dose of 400 mg, the daily dosage is based on creatinine clearance:

Creatinine Clearance (ml/min)	% of Recommended Dose
greater than 50	100
21–50	50
11–20	25
Dialysis	Dose after dialysis

UNLABELED USES
Treatment of coccidioidomycosis, cryptococcosis, fungal pneumonia, onychomycosis, ringworm of the hand, septicemia

CONTRAINDICATIONS
None known.

INTERACTIONS
Drug
Cyclosporine: High fluconazole doses increase cyclosporine blood concentration.
Oral hypoglycemics: May increase blood concentration and effects of oral hypoglycemics.
Phenytoin, warfarin: May decrease the metabolism of these drugs.
Rifampin: May increase fluconazole metabolism.
Herbal
None known.
Food
None known.

DIAGNOSTIC TEST EFFECTS
May increase serum alkaline phosphatase, serum bilirubin, SGOT (AST), and SGPT (ALT) levels.

IV INCOMPATIBILITIES
Amphotericin (Fungizone), amphotericin B complex (Abelcet, Amphotec, AmBisome), ampicillin (Polycillin), calcium gluconate, cefotaxime (Claforan), ceftazidime (Fortaz), ceftriaxone (Rocephin), cefuroxime (Zinacef), chloramphenicol (Chloromycetin), clindamycin (Cleocin), diazepam (Valium), digoxin (Lanoxin), erythromycin (Erythrocin), furosemide (Lasix), haloperidol (Haldol), hydroxyzine (Vistaril), imipenem/cilastatin (Primaxin), sulfamethoxazole-trimethoprim (Bactrim)

IV COMPATIBILITIES
Diltiazem (Cardizem), dobutamine (Dobutrex), dopamine (Intropin), heparin, lorazepam (Ativan),

midazolam (Versed), propofol
(Diprivan)

SIDE EFFECTS
Occasional (4%–1%)
Hypersensitivity reaction including
chills, fever, pruritus, and rash;
dizziness, drowsiness, headache,
constipation, diarrhea, nausea,
vomiting, abdominal pain

SERIOUS REACTIONS
• Exfoliative skin disorders, serious
liver effects, and blood dyscrasias
such as eosinophilia, thrombocytopenia, anemia, and leukopenia have
been reported rarely.

NURSING CONSIDERATIONS
Baseline Assessment
• Expect to obtain baseline tests for
complete blood count, liver function, and serum potassium.
Lifespan Considerations
• Be aware that it is unknown if
fluconazole is excreted in breast
milk.
• There are no age-related precautions noted in children.
• In the elderly, age-related renal
impairment may require dosage
adjustment.
Precautions
• Use cautiously in patients
with liver or renal impairment,
hypersensitivity to other triazoles,
such as itraconazole or terconazole,
or hypersensitivity to imidazoles,
such as butoconazole and ketoconazole.
Administration and Handling
PO
• Give without regard to meals.
• Be aware that PO and IV therapy
are equally effective and that IV
therapy is for patients intolerant
of the drug or unable to take it
orally.

IV
• Store at room temperature.
• Do not remove from outer wrap
until ready to use.
• Squeeze inner bag to check for
leaks.
• Do not use parenteral form if the
solution is cloudy, a precipitate
forms, the seal is not intact, or it is
discolored.
• Do not add another medication to
the solution.
• Do not exceed maximum flow rate
200 mg/hour.
Intervention and Evaluation
• Assess the patient for signs
and symptoms of a hypersensitivity reaction, including chills or
fever.
• Expect to monitor the patient's
complete blood count (CBC), liver
and renal function test results,
platelet count, and serum potassium
levels.
• Warn the patient to report any
itching or rash promptly.
• Monitor the patient's temperature
daily.
• Assess the patient's daily pattern
of bowel activity and stool consistency.
• Evaluate the patient for dizziness and provide assistance as
needed.
Patient Teaching
• Caution the patient not to drive or
use machinery until his or her
response to the drug is established.
• Warn the patient to notify the
physician if he or she develops
dark urine, pale stool, rash with
or without itching, or yellow skin
or eyes.
• Teach patients with oropharyngeal
infections about good oral hygiene.
• Advise the patient to consult the
physician before taking any other
medications.

griseofulvin

griz-ee-oh-**full**-vin
(Fulvicin P/G, Fulvicin U/F,
Grifulvin V, Gris-PEG,
Grisovin[AUS])

CATEGORY AND SCHEDULE

Pregnancy Risk Category: C

MECHANISM OF ACTION

An antifungal that inhibits fungal
cell mitosis by disrupting mitotic
spindle structure. *Therapeutic
Effect:* Fungistatic.

AVAILABILITY

Tablets (microsize): 250 mg,
500 mg.
Tablets (ultramicrosize): 125 mg,
250 mg, 330 mg.
Oral Suspension: 125 mg/5 ml.

INDICATIONS AND DOSAGES

▶ **Treatment of tineas (ringworm):
t. capitis, t. corporis, t. cruris,
t. pedis, t. unguium**
Microsize Tablets
Adults. Usual dosage 500–1,000 mg
as single or divided doses.
Children. Usual dosage 10–20
mg/kg/day.
Ultramicrosize Tablets
Adults. Usual dosage 330–750
mg/day as single or divided
doses.
Children older than 2 yrs. 5–10
mg/kg/day.

CONTRAINDICATIONS

Porphyria, hepatocellular failure

INTERACTIONS

Drug
Oral contraceptives, warfarin: May
decrease the effects of these drugs.
Herbal
None known.

Food
None known.

DIAGNOSTIC TEST EFFECTS

None known.

SIDE EFFECTS

Occasional
Hypersensitivity reaction, such as
pruritus, rash, and urticaria; headache, nausea, diarrhea, excessive
thirst, flatulence, oral thrush, dizziness, insomnia
Rare
Paresthesia of hands or feet,
proteinuria, photosensitivity
reaction

SERIOUS REACTIONS

• Granulocytopenia occurs rarely.

NURSING CONSIDERATIONS

Baseline Assessment
• Determine the patient's history of
allergies, especially to griseofulvin
and penicillins, before giving the
drug.
Precautions
• Use cautiously in patients with
hypersensitivity to penicillins or in
those who are exposed to sun or
ultraviolet light because photosensitivity may develop.
Intervention and Evaluation
◀ALERT▶ The duration of treatment
depends on the site of infection.
• Evaluate the patient's skin for
rash and therapeutic response to the
drug.
• Assess the patient's daily pattern
of bowel activity and stool consistency.
◀ALERT▶ Monitor the patient's
granulocyte count as appropriate. If
the patient develops granulocytopenia, notify the physician and expect
to discontinue the drug.
• In patients experiencing headache,

establish and document the head-ache's location, onset and type.
• Assess the patient for dizziness.

Patient Teaching
• Explain to the patient that prolonged therapy over weeks or months is usually necessary.
• Advise the patient not to miss a dose and to continue therapy as long as is ordered.
• Warn the patient to avoid consuming alcohol as this may produce flushing or tachycardia.
• Advise the patient that griseofulvin may cause a photosensitivity reaction, so he or she should avoid exposure to sunlight.
• Urge the patient to maintain good hygiene to help prevent superinfection.
• Encourage the patient to separate personal items that come in direct contact with affected areas.
• Teach the patient to keep affected areas dry and to wear light clothing for ventilation.
• Advise the patient to take griseofulvin with foods high in fat, such as milk or ice cream, to reduce GI upset and assist in drug absorption.

---

itraconazole
eye-tra-**con**-ah-zoll
(Sporanox)
Do not confuse with Suprax.

CATEGORY AND SCHEDULE
Pregnancy Risk Category: C

MECHANISM OF ACTION
An antifungal that inhibits the synthesis of ergosterol, a vital component of fungal cell formation, thereby damaging the fungal cell membrane. *Therapeutic Effect:* Fungistatic.

PHARMACOKINETICS
Moderately absorbed from the gastrointestinal (GI) tract. Absorption is increased if the drug is taken with food. Protein binding: 99%. Widely distributed, primarily in the fatty tissue, liver, and kidney. Metabolized in liver to active metabolite. Primarily excreted in urine. Not removed by hemodialysis. **Half-life:** 21 hrs; metabolite, 12 hrs.

AVAILABILITY
Capsules: 100 mg.
Oral Solution: 10 mg/ml.
Injection: 10 mg/ml, 25-ml amp.

INDICATIONS AND DOSAGES
▶ **Blastomycosis, histoplasmosis**
IV
Adults, Elderly. 200 mg 2 times/day for 4 doses then 200 mg once a day.
PO
Adults, Elderly. Initially, 200 mg once a day. May increase to maximum of 400 mg/day in 2 divided doses.
▶ **Aspergillosis**
IV
Adults, Elderly. 200 mg 2 times/day for 4 doses then 200 mg once a day.
PO
Adults, Elderly. 600 mg/day in 3 divided doses for 3–4 days, then 200–400 mg/day in 2 divided doses.
▶ **Esophageal Candidiasis**
PO
Adults, Elderly. Swish 10 ml in the mouth for several seconds then swallow. Maximum dose: 200 mg/day.
▶ **Oropharyngeal Candidiasis**
PO
Adults, Elderly. Swish 10 ml in the mouth for several seconds then swallow.

UNLABELED USES
Suppression of histoplasmosis; treatment of disseminated sporotrichosis, fungal pneumonia and septicemia, ringworm of the hand

CONTRAINDICATIONS
Hypersensitivity to itraconazole, fluconazole, ketoconazole, miconazole

INTERACTIONS
Drug
Antacids, didanosine, H_2 antagonists: May decrease itraconazole absorption.
Buspirone, cyclosporine, digoxin, lovastatin, simvastatin: May increase blood concentrations of these drugs.
Oral anticoagulants: May increase the effect of oral anticoagulants.
Phenytoin, rifampin: May decrease itraconazole blood concentrations.
Herbal
None known.
Food
Grapefruit juice: May alter itraconazole absorption.

DIAGNOSTIC TEST EFFECTS
May increase serum LDH concentrations, serum alkaline phosphatase, serum bilirubin, SGOT (AST), and SGPT (ALT) levels. May decrease serum potassium.

IV INCOMPATIBILITIES
◀ALERT▶ Dilution compatibility with other than 0.9% NaCl unknown. Do not mix with D_5W or lactated Ringer's. Do not give any medication in same bag of itraconazole or through same IV line. Not for IV bolus administration. Do not mix with any other medication.

SIDE EFFECTS
Frequent (11%–9%)
Nausea, rash
Occasional (5%–3%)
Vomiting, headache, diarrhea, hypertension, peripheral edema, fatigue, fever
Rare (2% or less)
Abdominal pain, dizziness, anorexia, pruritus

SERIOUS REACTIONS
• Hepatitis as evidenced by anorexia, abdominal pain, unusual tiredness or weakness, jaundice, and dark urine occurs rarely.

NURSING CONSIDERATIONS
Baseline Assessment
• Obtain the patient's baseline temperature, check the liver function test results, as appropriate, and determine if the patient has a history of allergies before giving the drug.
Lifespan Considerations
• Be aware that itraconazole is distributed in breast milk.
• Be aware that the safety and efficacy of itraconazole have not been established in children.
• In the elderly, age-related renal impairment may require dosage adjustment.
Precautions
• Use cautiously in patients with achlorhydria, hepatitis, HIV-infection, hypochlorhydria, or impaired liver function.
Administration and Handling
◀ALERT▶ Doses larger than 200 mg should be given in 2 divided doses.
PO
• Give capsules with food to increase absorption.
• Give solution on an empty stomach.

IV
• Store at room temperature. Do not freeze.
• Use only components provided by the manufacturer.
• Do not dilute with any other diluent.
• Add full contents of amp (250 mg/10 ml) to infusion bag provided (50 ml 0.9% NaCl) and mix gently.
• Infuse over 60 minutes using the extension line and infusion set provided.
• After administration, flush infusion set with 15 to 20 ml 0.9% NaCl over 30 seconds to 15 minutes and discard entire infusion line.

Intervention and Evaluation
• Assess the patient for signs and symptoms of liver dysfunction.
• Expect to monitor the liver enzyme test results in patients with preexisting liver dysfunction.

Patient Teaching
• Instruct the patient to take itraconazole capsules with food and itraconazole solution on an empty stomach.
• Advise the patient that therapy will continue for at least 3 months and until lab tests and the patient's overall condition indicate that the infection is controlled.
• Warn the patient to report any anorexia, dark urine, nausea, pale stool, unusual fatigue, yellow skin, or vomiting to the physician.
• Caution the patient to avoid grapefruit and grapefruit juice as they may alter itraconazole absorption.

ketoconazole
keet-oh-**con**-ah-zol
(Apo-Ketocomazole[CAN], Nizoral, Nizoral AD, Sebizole[AUS])
Do not confuse with Nasarel.

CATEGORY AND SCHEDULE
Pregnancy Risk Category: C
OTC (1% shampoo only)

MECHANISM OF ACTION
An imidazole derivative that changes the permeability of the fungal cell wall. *Therapeutic Effect:* Inhibits fungal biosynthesis of triglycerides, phospholipids. Fungistatic.

AVAILABILITY
Tablets: 200 mg.
Cream: 2%.
Shampoo: 2%, 1% (OTC).

INDICATIONS AND DOSAGES
▸ **Treatment of histoplasmosis, blastomycosis, candidiasis, chronic mucocutaneous candidiasis, coccidioidomycosis, paracoccidioidomycosis, chromomycosis, seborrheic dermatitis, tineas (ringworm): t. corporis, t. capitis, t. manus, t. cruris, t. pedis, t. unguium (onychomycosis), oral thrush, candiduria**
PO
Adults, Elderly. 200–400 mg/day.
Children. 3.3–6.6 mg/kg/day.
Maximum: 800 mg/day in 2 divided doses.
Topical
Adults, Elderly. Apply 1–2 times/day to affected area for 2–4 wks.
Dandruff Shampoo
Adults, Elderly. 2 times/wk for 4 wks, allowing at least 3 days between shampooing. Intermittent use to maintain control.

UNLABELED USES
Systemic: Treatment of fungal pneumonia, prostate cancer, septicemia

CONTRAINDICATIONS
None known.

INTERACTIONS
Drug
Alcohol, hepatotoxic medications: May increase hepatotoxicity of ketoconazole.
Antacids, anticholinergics, H_2 antagonists, omeprazole: May decrease ketoconazole absorption.
Cyclosporine, lovastatin, simvastatin: May increase blood concentration and risk of toxicity of these drugs.
Isoniazid, rifampin: May decrease blood ketoconazole concentration.
Herbal
Echinacea: May have additive hepatotoxic effects.
Food
None known.

DIAGNOSTIC TEST EFFECTS
May increase serum alkaline phosphatase, serum bilirubin, SGOT (AST), and SGPT (ALT) levels. May decrease serum corticosteroid and testosterone concentrations.

SIDE EFFECTS
Occasional (10%–3%)
Nausea, vomiting
Rare (less than 2%)
Abdominal pain, diarrhea, headache, dizziness, photophobia, pruritus
Topical: itching, burning, irritation

SERIOUS REACTIONS
• Hematologic toxicity as evidenced by thrombocytopenia, hemolytic anemia, and leukopenia occurs occasionally.
• Hepatotoxicity may occur within first week to several months of therapy.
• Anaphylaxis occurs rarely.

NURSING CONSIDERATIONS
Baseline Assessment
• Confirm that a culture or histologic test was done for accurate diagnosis; therapy may begin before results are known.
Precautions
• Use cautiously in patients with liver impairment.
Administration and Handling
PO
• Give with food to minimize gastrointestinal (GI) irritation.
• Tablets may be crushed.
• Ketoconazole requires acidity; give antacids, anticholinergics, H_2 blockers, and omeprazole at least 2 hours after dosing.
Shampoo
• Apply to wet hair, massage for 1 minute, rinse thoroughly, reapply for 3 minutes, then rinse.
Topical
• Apply and rub gently into the affected and surrounding area.
Intervention and Evaluation
• Expect to monitor the patient's liver function test results. Be alert for signs and symptoms of hepatotoxicity, including anorexia, dark urine, fatigue, nausea, pale stools, and vomiting, that are unrelieved by giving the medication with food.
• Monitor the patient's complete blood count (CBC) for evidence of hematologic toxicity.
• Assess the patient's daily pattern of bowel activity and stool consistency.
• Assess the patient for dizziness, provide assistance as needed, and institute safety precautions.

• Evaluate the patient's skin for itching, rash, and urticaria.
• If the patient is receiving topical ketoconazole, check the patient's skin for local burning, itching, and irritation.

Patient Teaching
• Explain to the patient that prolonged therapy over weeks or months is usually necessary.
• Instruct the patient not to miss a dose and to continue therapy as long as directed.
• Advise the patient to avoid alcohol to avoid potential liver toxicity.
• Warn the patient to avoid tasks that require mental alertness or motor skills until his or her response to the drug is established.
• Encourage the patient to take antacids or antiulcer medications at least 2 hours after taking ketoconazole.
• Warn the patient to notify the physician if he or she develops dark urine, increased irritation in topical use, onset of other new symptoms, pale stool, or yellow skin or eyes.
• Teach the patient receiving topical ketoconazole to avoid drug contact with the eyes, keep the skin clean and dry, rub the drug well into affected areas, and wear light clothing for ventilation.
• Encourage the patient to separate personal items that come in direct contact with the affected area.
• Instruct the patient to use the ketoconazole shampoo initially twice weekly for 4 weeks with at least 3 days between shampooing. Also explain that further shampooing will be based upon the patient's response to the initial treatment.

nystatin
nigh-**stat**-in
(Mycostatin, Nilstat, Nyaderm, Nystop)
Do not confuse with Nitrostat.

CATEGORY AND SCHEDULE
Pregnancy Risk Category: C

MECHANISM OF ACTION
An antifungal that binds to sterols in fungal cell membranes, increasing permeability, permitting loss of potassium, and other cell components. *Therapeutic Effect:* Fungistatic.

PHARMACOKINETICS
PO: Poorly absorbed from the gastrointestinal (GI) tract. Eliminated unchanged in feces. Topical: Not absorbed systemically from intact skin.

AVAILABILITY
Tablets: 500,000 units.
Oral Suspension: 100,000 units/ml.
Troches: 200,000 units.
Vaginal Tablets: 100,000 units.
Cream: 100,000 units/g.
Ointment: 100,000 units/g.
Powder: 100,000 units/g.

INDICATIONS AND DOSAGES
▸ **Intestinal candidiasis**
PO
Adults, Elderly. 500,000–1,000,000 units 3 times a day.
Children. 500,000 units 4 times a day.
▸ **Oral candidiasis**
PO
Adults, Elderly, Children. Oral suspension: 400,000–600,000 units 4 times a day. Troches: 200,000–400,000 units 4–5 times a day up to 14 days.

Infants. 100,000–200,000 units 4 times a day.

▸ **Vulvovaginal candidiasis**
Intravaginal
Adults, Elderly. 1 tablet high in vagina 1–2 times a day for 14 days.

▸ **Topical fungal infections**
Topical
Adults, Elderly. Apply to affected area 2–4 times a day.

UNLABELED USES

Prophylaxis and treatment of, oro-pharyngeal candidiasis, tinea barbae, tinea capitis

CONTRAINDICATIONS

None known.

INTERACTIONS

Drug
None known.
Herbal
None known.
Food
None known.

DIAGNOSTIC TEST EFFECTS

None known.

SIDE EFFECTS

Occasional
PO: None known
Topical: Skin irritation
Vaginal: Vaginal irritation

SERIOUS REACTIONS

• High dosage with oral form may produce nausea, vomiting, diarrhea, an GI distress.

NURSING CONSIDERATIONS

Baseline Assessment
• Confirm that cultures or histo-logic tests were done for accu-rate diagnosis before giving the drug.

Lifespan Considerations
• Be aware that it is unknown if nystatin is distributed in breast milk.
• During pregnancy, vaginal appli-cators may be contraindicated, requiring manual insertion of tablets.
• There are no age-related precau-tions noted for suspension or topical use in children.
• Be aware that lozenges are not recommended for use in children 5 years old or younger.
• There are no age-related precau-tions noted in the elderly.

Precautions
• None known.

Administration and Handling
PO
• Have the patient dissolve lozenges (troches) slowly and completely in the mouth for optimal therapeutic effect. Lozenges should not be chewed or swallowed whole.
• Shake suspension well before administration.
• Instruct the patient to place and hold the suspension in the mouth or swish throughout the mouth as long as possible before swallowing.

Intervention and Evaluation
• Assess the patient for increased irritation with topical application or increased vaginal discharge with vaginal application.

Patient Teaching
• Advise the patient not to miss a dose and to complete the full length of treatment.
• Explain that vaginal use should be continued during menses.
• Teach the patient to insert the vaginal form high into the vagina.
• Advise the patient receiving the vaginal form to check with the physician regarding douching and sexual intercourse.
• Warn the patient that the topical

form must not come in contact with the eyes.

• Explain that nystatin cream or powder should be used sparingly on erythematous areas.

• Teach the patient to rub the topical form well into affected areas, to keep affected areas clean and dry, and to wear light clothing for ventilation.

• Encourage the patient to separate personal items that come in contact with affected areas.

• Warn the patient to notify the physician if diarrhea, nausea, stomach pain, or vomiting develops.

terbinafine hydrochloride
tur-**bin**-ah-feen
(Lamisil, Lamisil Derma Gel)
Do not confuse with Lamictal, terbutaline.

CATEGORY AND SCHEDULE
Pregnancy Risk Category: B

MECHANISM OF ACTION
An antifungal that inhibits the enzyme squalene epoxidase, thereby interfering with biosynthesis in fungi. *Therapeutic Effect:* Results in fungal cell death.

AVAILABILITY
Tablets: 250 mg.
Cream: 1%.
Topical Solution: 1%.

INDICATIONS AND DOSAGES
▶ **Tinea pedis**
Topical
Adults, Elderly, Children 12 yrs and older. Apply 2 times a day until signs and symptoms significantly improve.

▶ **Tinea cruris, Tinea corporis**
Topical
Adults, Elderly, Children 12 yrs and older. Apply 1–2 times a day until signs and symptoms significantly improve.
▶ **Onychomycosis**
PO
Adults, Elderly, Children 12 yrs and older. 250 mg/day for 6 wks (fingernails), 12 wks (toenails).
▶ **Tinea versicolor**
Topical (solution)
Adults, Elderly. Apply to the affected area 2 times/day for 7 days.
▶ **Systemic mycosis**
PO
Adults, Elderly. 250-500 mg/day for up to 16 mos.

CONTRAINDICATIONS
Oral: Preexisting liver disease or renal impairment (creatinine clearance of 50 ml/min or less) and in children younger than 12 years of age.

INTERACTIONS
Drug
Alcohol, other hepatotoxic medications: May increase risk of hepatotoxicity.
Liver enzyme inducers, including rifampin: May increase terbinafine clearance.
Liver enzyme inhibitors, including cimetidine: May decrease terbinafine clearance.
Herbal
None known.
Food
None known.

DIAGNOSTIC TEST EFFECTS
May increase SGOT (AST) and SGPT (ALT) levels.

SIDE EFFECTS
Frequent (13%)
Oral: Headache

Occasional (6%–3%)
Oral: Diarrhea, rash, dyspepsia, pruritus, taste disturbance, nausea
Rare
Oral: Abdominal pain, flatulence, urticaria, visual disturbance
Topical: Irritation, burning, itching, dryness

SERIOUS REACTIONS
• Hepatobiliary dysfunction, including cholestatic hepatitis, serious skin reactions, and severe neutropenia occur rarely.
• Ocular lens and retinal changes have been noted.

NURSING CONSIDERATIONS
Baseline Assessment
• As appropriate, monitor liver function in patients receiving treatment for longer than 6 weeks.
Precautions
• None known
Intervention and Evaluation
◀ALERT▶ Topical therapy may be used for a minimum of 1 week and is not to exceed 4 weeks.
• Assess the patient for signs of a therapeutic response.
• Discontinue the medication and notify the physician if a local reaction occurs. Signs and symptoms of a local reaction include blistering, burning, irritation, itching, oozing, redness, and swelling.
Patient Teaching
• Teach the patient to keep affected areas clean and dry and to wear light clothing to promote ventilation.
• Encourage the patient to separate personal items that come in contact with affected areas.
• Warn the patient to avoid topical cream contact with eyes, mouth, nose, or other mucous membranes.

• Instruct the patient to rub the topical form well into the affected and surrounding area. Reinforce that the treated area should not be covered with an occlusive dressing.
• Warn the patient to notify the physician if diarrhea or skin irritation occurs.

voriconazole
voor-ih-**con**-ah-zole
(Vfend)

CATEGORY AND SCHEDULE
Pregnancy Risk Category: D

MECHANISM OF ACTION
A triazole derivative that inhibits the synthesis of ergosterol, a vital component of fungal cell wall formation. *Therapeutic Effect:* Damages fungal cell wall membrane.

PHARMACOKINETICS
Rapidly, completely absorbed after PO administration. Widely distributed. Protein binding: 98%. Metabolized in the liver. Primarily excreted as metabolite in the urine. **Half-life:** 6 hrs.

AVAILABILITY
Tablets: 50 mg, 200 mg.
Powder for Injection: 200 mg.

INDICATIONS AND DOSAGES
▸ **Antifungal**
IV
Adults, Elderly. Initially, 6 mg/kg q12h for 2 doses, then 4 mg/kg q12h.
PO
Adults, Elderly, weighing 40 kg and more. Initially, 400 mg q12h for 2 doses, then 200 mg q12h.

Adults, Elderly, weighing less than 40 kg. Initially, 200 mg q12h times 2 doses, then 100 mg q12h.

CONTRAINDICATIONS
Coadministration of carbamazepine, ergot alkaloids, pimozide or quinidine (may cause QT prolongation or torsades de pointes), rifabutin, rifampin, sirolimus

INTERACTIONS
Drug
Cyclosporine, omeprazole, phenytoin, rifabutin, sirolimus, tacrilimus, warfarin: May increase concentrations of these drugs.
Phenytoin, rifabutin, rifampin: May decrease voriconazole concentration.
Herbal
None known.
Food
None known.

DIAGNOSTIC TEST EFFECTS
May increase serum alkaline phosphatase and SGPT (ALT) levels.

IV INCOMPATIBILITIES
Do not mix with any other medications.

SIDE EFFECTS
Frequent (20%–5%)
Abnormal vision, fever, nausea, rash, vomiting
Occasional (5%–2%)
Headache, chills, hallucinations, photophobia, tachycardia, hypertension

SERIOUS REACTIONS
• Liver toxicity occurs rarely.

NURSING CONSIDERATIONS
Baseline Assessment
• Expect to obtain baseline liver function and renal function test results before giving the drug.
Lifespan Considerations
• Be aware that voriconazole may cause fetal harm.
• Be aware that the safety and efficacy of voriconazole have not established in children younger than 12 years.
○ There are no age-related precautions noted in the elderly.
Precautions
• Use cautiously in patients with hypersensitivity to other antifungal agents or impaired renal or liver function.
Administration and Handling
PO
• Give 1 hour before or 1 hour after a meal.
IV
• Store powder for injection at room temperature.
• Use reconstituted solution immediately.
• Do not use reconstituted solution after 24 hours when refrigerated.
• Reconstitute 200-mg vial with 19 ml Sterile Water for Injection to provide a concentration of 10 mg/ml. Further dilute with 0.9% NaCl or D_5W to provide a concentration of 5 mg/ml or less.
• Infuse over 1 to 2 hours at a concentration of 5 mg/ml or less.
Intervention and Evaluation
• Expect to monitor the patient's liver and renal function test results.
• Evaluate and monitor the patient's visual function, including color perception, visual acuity, and visual field, for drug therapy lasting longer than 28 days.
Patient Teaching
• Instruct the patient to take voriconazole at least 1 hour before or 1 hour after a meal.

• Warn the patient to avoid driving at night because voriconazole may cause visual changes, such as blurred vision or photophobia.

• Caution the patient to avoid performing hazardous tasks if changes in vision occur.

• Encourage the patient to avoid direct sunlight.

• Caution the patient to avoid becoming pregnant while taking voriconazole and explain that the drug may have detrimental effects on the fetus. Also, teach the patient the importance of using effective contraception.

3 Antiretroviral Agents

abacavir
amprenavir
atazanavir sulfate
delavirdine mesylate
didanosine
efavirenz
emtricitabine
enfuvirtide
fosamprenavir
indinavir
lamivudine
lopinavir-ritonavir
nelfinavir
nevirapine
ritonavir
saquinavir
stavudine (dT4)
tenofovir
zalcitabine
zidovudine

Uses: Antiretroviral agents are used to treat human immunodeficiency virus (HIV) infection. HIV treatment aims to greatly reduce the viral load, which allows the CD4 cell count to remain at a level that's adequate to fight infections. Antiretroviral therapy typically includes more than one antiretroviral agent, each with a different mechanism of action. By attacking the virus through different mechanisms of action, the risk of resistance is reduced.

Action: The five classes of antiretroviral agents act in different ways. *Nucleoside reverse transcriptase inhibitors (NRTIs)*, such as stavudine and zalcitabine, compete with natural substrates for formation of proviral deoxyribonucleic acid (DNA) by reverse transcriptase inhibiting viral replication. *Fusion inhibitors*, such as enfuvirtide, inhibit fusion of viral and cellular membranes. *Nucleotide reverse transcriptase inhibitors (NtRTIs)*, such as tenofovir, inhibit reverse transcriptase by competing with the natural substrate deoxyadenosine triphosphate and by DNA chain termination. *Nonnucleoside reverse transcriptase inhibitors (NNRTIs)*, such as delavirdine and efavirenz, directly bind to reverse transcriptase and block ribonucleic acid (RNA)-dependent and DNA-dependent DNA polymerase activities by disrupting the enzyme's catalytic site. *Protease inhibitors (PIs)*, such as indinavir and nelfinavir, bind to the active site of HIV-1 protease and therefore prevent the binding of the enzyme protease. This action prevents protease from processing HIV polyproteins, which renders the structural proteins and enzymes of HIV unable to function. Therefore, the virus remains immature and noninfectious. (See illustration, *Mechanisms and Sites of Action: Antiretroviral Agents*, page 38.)

COMBINATION PRODUCTS
COMBIVIR: lamivudine/zidovudine (an antiretroviral) 150 mg/300 mg.

TRIZIVIR: abacavir/lamivudine (an antiretroviral)/zidovudine (an antiretroviral) 300 mg/150 mg/300 mg.

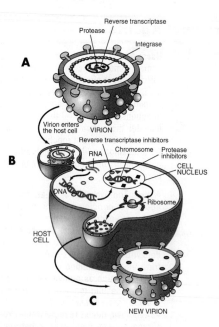

Mechanisms and Sites of Action: Antiretroviral Agents

To understand how antiretroviral agents work, you need to know how viruses reproduce. First, the infectious viral particle or virion (A) enters the host cell. The virion attaches to the cell's surface and then inserts itself into the host cell (B). Once inside, the virion uncoats, and the enzyme reverse transcriptase makes two copies of the viral ribonucleic acid (RNA): one copy is identical; the other is a mirror image. These two copies merge to form double-stranded viral deoxyribonucleic acid (DNA). This newly formed viral DNA enters the host cell's nucleus, where it inserts itself into the host cell's DNA with the help of the enzyme integrase. Then viral DNA reprograms the host cell to produce additional viral RNA, which begins the process of forming new viruses. Specifically, messenger RNA (mRNA) instructs ribosomal RNA (rRNA) to produce a new chain of proteins and enzymes that are used to form new viruses. Protease, another enzyme, cuts the chains of proteins, creating individual proteins. These individual proteins combine with new RNA to create new virions, which bud and are then released from the host cell (C).

Antiretroviral agents target specific enzymes during viral reproduction. Many of them work to inhibit reverse transcriptase. Nucleoside reverse transcriptase inhibitors, such as stavudine, interfere with the action of reverse transcriptase by mimicking naturally occurring nucleosides. Nucleotide reverse transcriptase inhibitors, such as tenofovir, block reverse transcriptase by competing with the natural substrate deoxyadenosine triphosphate and by causing DNA chain termination. Nonnucleoside reverse transcriptase inhibitors, such as delavirdine, work by directly binding to reverse transcriptase. All of these actions block the conversion of single-stranded viral RNA into double-stranded DNA. As a result, no viral DNA is available to insert itself into the host cell's DNA. Protease inhibitors, such as indinavir, bind to and interfere with the action of protease. By blocking protease, the new chain of proteins formed by rRNA can't be cut into individual proteins to make new viruses.

abacavir
ah-bah-**kay**-veer
(Ziagen)

CATEGORY AND SCHEDULE
Pregnancy Risk Category: C

MECHANISM OF ACTION
This antiretroviral agent inhibits the activity of HIV-1 reverse transcriptase by competing with natural substrate dGTP and by its incorporation into viral DNA. *Therapeutic Effect:* Inhibits viral DNA growth.

PHARMACOKINETICS
Rapidly, extensively absorbed following PO administration. Protein binding: 50%. Widely distributed, including cerebrospinal fluid (CSF) and erythrocytes. Metabolized in liver to inactive metabolites. Primarily excreted in urine. Unknown if removed by hemodialysis. **Half-life:** 1.5 hrs.

AVAILABILITY
Tablets: 300 mg.
Oral Solution: 20 mg/ml.

INDICATIONS AND DOSAGES
▶ **HIV (in combination)**
PO
Adults. 300 mg 2 times/day.
Children (3 mos–16 yrs). 8 mg/kg 2 times/day. Maximum: 300 mg 2 times/day.

CONTRAINDICATIONS
Hypersensitivity to any component

INTERACTIONS
Drug
Alcohol: May increase abacavir blood concentration and half-life.

Herbal
St. John's wort: May decrease abacavir blood concentration and effect.
Food
None known.

DIAGNOSTIC TEST EFFECTS
May increase blood glucose, GGT, SGOT (AST), SGPT (ALT), and triglycerides.

SIDE EFFECTS
Adult
Frequent
Nausea (47%), nausea with vomiting (16%), diarrhea (12%), decreased appetite (11%)
Occasional
Insomnia (7%)
Children
Frequent
Nausea with vomiting (39%), fever (19%), headache, diarrhea (16%), rash (11%)
Occasional
Decreased appetite (9%)

SERIOUS REACTIONS
• Hypersensitivity reaction (may be life-threatening) signs and symptoms include fever, rash, fatigue, intractable nausea and vomiting, severe diarrhea, abdominal pain, cough, pharyngitis, and dyspnea.
• Life-threatening hypotension may occur.
• Lactic acidosis and severe hepatomegaly may occur.

NURSING CONSIDERATIONS
Baseline Assessment
• Determine if the patient is pregnant.
• Expect to obtain baseline laboratory testing, especially liver function tests, before beginning therapy and at periodic intervals during therapy.

• Offer emotional support to the patient.

Lifespan Considerations

• Be aware that it is unknown whether abacavir is excreted in breast milk. Patients taking abacavir should not breast-feed because this may increase the potential for adverse effects in the infant as well as the risk of HIV transmission.

• Abacavir may be used safely in children ages 3 months to 13 years.

• Be aware that there is no information on the safety and efficacy of the drug in the elderly.

Precautions

• Use cautiously in patients with impaired liver function.

Administration and Handling

PO

• May give without regard to food.

• Oral solution may be refrigerated. Do not freeze.

Intervention and Evaluation

• Assess the patient for nausea and vomiting.

• Determine the patient's pattern of bowel activity and stool consistency.

• Assess the patient's eating pattern.

• Monitor the patient for weight loss.

• Monitor lab values carefully, particularly liver function.

Patient Teaching

• Explain to the patient that he or she should not take any medications, including over-the-counter (OTC) drugs, without consulting the physician.

• Encourage the patient to ingest small, frequent meals to help offset anorexia and nausea.

• Instruct the patient that abacavir is not a cure for HIV infection, nor does it reduce the risk of transmission to others.

amprenavir
am-**prenn**-ah-veer
(Agenerase)

CATEGORY AND SCHEDULE
Pregnancy Risk Category: C

MECHANISM OF ACTION
This antiviral inhibits HIV-1 protease by binding to the active site of HIV-1 protease, preventing processing of viral precursors and forming immature noninfectious viral particles. *Therapeutic Effect:* Produces impairment of HIV viral replication and proliferation.

PHARMACOKINETICS
Rapidly absorbed after PO administration. Protein binding: 90%. Metabolized in the liver. Primarily excreted in feces. **Half-life:** 7.1–10.6 hrs.

AVAILABILITY
Capsules: 50 mg, 150 mg.
Oral Solution: 15 mg/ml.

INDICATIONS AND DOSAGES
▸ **HIV-1 infection**
PO
Adults, Children 13–16 yrs (capsules). 1,200 mg 2 times/day.
Children 4–12 yrs, 13–16 yrs weighing less than 50 kg. 20 mg/kg 2 times/day or 15 mg/kg 3 times/day. Maximum: 2,400 mg/day.
Children 4–12, 13–16 yrs weighing less than 50 kg (oral solution). 22.5 mg/kg/day (1.5 ml/kg) 2 times/day or 17 mg/kg/day (1.1 ml/kg) 3 times/day. Maximum: 2,800 mg/day.

▶ **Dosage in liver impairment**

Child-Pugh Score	Capsules	Oral Solution
5–8	450 mg bid	513 mg bid
9–12	300 mg bid	342 mg bid

CONTRAINDICATIONS
None known

INTERACTIONS
Drug
Amiodarone, bepridil, ergotamine, lidocaine, midazolam, oral contraceptives, quinidine, triazolam, tricyclic antidepressants: May interfere with the metabolism of these drugs.
Antacids, didanosine: May decrease amprenavir absorption.
Carbamazepine, phenobarbital, phenytoin, rifampin: May decrease amprenavir blood concentration.
Clozapine, HMG-CoA reductase inhibitors, including statins, warfarin: May increase the blood concentration of these drugs.
Herbal
St. John's wort: May decrease amprenavir blood concentration.
Food
High-fat meals: May decrease amprenavir absorption.

DIAGNOSTIC TEST EFFECTS
May increase blood cholesterol, glucose, and triglyceride levels.

SIDE EFFECTS
Frequent
Diarrhea or loose stools (56%), nausea (38%), oral paresthesia (30%), rash (25%), vomiting (20%)
Occasional
Rash (18%), peripheral paresthesia (12%), depression (4%)

SERIOUS REACTIONS
• Severe hypersensitivity reactions or Stevens-Johnson syndrome as evidenced by blisters, peeling of the skin, loosening of skin and mucous membranes, and fever may occur.

NURSING CONSIDERATIONS
Baseline Assessment
• Expect to obtain baseline laboratory testing before beginning therapy and at periodic intervals during therapy.
• Offer the patient emotional support.
Lifespan Considerations
• Be aware that it is unknown if amprenavir crosses the placenta or is distributed in breast milk.
• Be aware that the safety and efficacy of amprenavir have not established in children younger than 4 years.
• In the elderly, age-related liver impairment may require decreased dosage.
Precautions
• Use cautiously in patients with diabetes mellitus, hemophilia, hypersensitivity to sulfa drugs, liver function impairment, or vitamin K deficiency from anticoagulant malabsorption.
Administration and Handling
PO
• May give without regard to food.
Intervention and Evaluation
• Observe the patient for any nausea or vomiting.
• Determine the patient's pattern of bowel activity and stool consistency.
• Evaluate the patient's eating pattern and monitor the patient for weight loss.
• Examine the patient for tingling or numbness of the peripheral extremities and skin rash.

Patient Teaching
• Urge the patient to avoid high-fat meals because they may decrease drug absorption.
• Encourage the patient to consume small, frequent meals to help offset anorexia and nausea.
• Advise the patient that amprenavir is not a cure for HIV infection, nor does it reduce risk of transmission to others.

atazanavir sulfate
ah-tah-**zan**-ah-veer
(Reyataz)

CATEGORY AND SCHEDULE
Pregnancy Risk Category: B

MECHANISM OF ACTION
An antiretroviral that acts as an HIV-1 protease inhibitor, selectively prevents the processing of viral polyproteins found in HIV-1 infected cells. *Therapeutic Effect:* Prevents formation of the mature HIV viral cell.

PHARMACOKINETICS
Rapidly absorbed following oral administration. Protein binding: 86%. Extensively metabolized in the liver. Primarily excreted in urine with a lesser extent in the feces. **Half-life:** 5–8 hrs.

AVAILABILITY
Capsules: 100 mg, 150 mg, 200 mg.

INDICATIONS AND DOSAGES
▶ **HIV-1 infection**
PO
Adults, Elderly. 400 mg (2 capsules) once a day given with food.

▶ **Concurrent therapy with efavirenz**
PO
Adults, Elderly. 300 mg atazanavir and 100 mg ritonavir and 600 mg efavirenz given as a single daily dose with food.
▶ **Concurrent therapy with didanosine**
PO
Adults, Elderly. Give atazanavir with food 2 hours before or 1 hour following didanosine.
▶ **Mild to moderate liver function impairment:**
PO
Adults, Elderly. 300 mg once a day given with food.

CONTRAINDICATIONS
Concurrent use with ergot derivatives, midazolam, pimozide, triazolam, severe liver insufficiency

INTERACTIONS
Drug
Antacids, H₂ receptor antagonists, proton pump inhibitors, rifampin: Decreases atazanavir plasma concentrations.
Atorvastatin, calcium channel blockers, immunosuppressants, irinotecan, lovastatin, sildenafil, simvastatin, tricyclic antidepressants: May result in increased atazanavir plasma concentrations.
Herbal
St. John's wort: May decrease atazanavir blood concentration.
Food
High fat meals: May decrease the absorption of atazanavir.

DIAGNOSTIC TEST EFFECTS
May increase serum amylase, bilirubin, lipase, SGOT (AST), and SGPT (ALT) levels. May decrease blood Hgb and neutrophil and platelet counts. May alter LDL cholesterol, triglycerides.

SIDE EFFECTS
Frequent (16%–14%)
Nausea, headache
Occasional (9%–4%)
Rash, vomiting, depression, diarrhea, abdominal pain, fever
Rare (3% or less)
Dizziness, insomnia, cough, fatigue, back pain

SERIOUS REACTIONS
• Severe hypersensitivity reaction, such as angioedema and chest pain, and jaundice may occur.

NURSING CONSIDERATIONS
Baseline Assessment
• Obtain the patient's baseline laboratory testing, including a complete blood count (CBC) and liver function tests before beginning atazanavir therapy and at periodic intervals during therapy.
• Offer the patient emotional support.
Lifespan Considerations
• Be aware that it is unknown if atazanavir crosses the placenta or distributed in breast milk.
• Be aware that hyperbilirubinemia, kernicterus, and lactic acidosis syndrome have been reported in pregnant and breast-feeding women.
• Be aware that the safety and efficacy of atazanavir have not been established in children younger than 3 months of age.
• In the elderly, age-related liver impairment may require dose reduction.
Precautions
• Use extremely cautiously in patients with liver impairment.
• Use cautiously in elderly patients and patients with diabetes mellitus, impaired renal function, and pre-existing conduction system disease, including first-degree atrioventricular (AV) block or second- or third-degree AV block.
Administration and Handling
PO
• Give atazanavir with food.
Intervention and Evaluation
• Evaluate the patient's eating pattern.
• Assess the patient for nausea and vomiting.
• Assess the patient's daily pattern of bowel activity and stool consistency.
• Examine the patient's skin for rash.
• Determine if the patient experiences headache.
• Monitor the patient for the onset of depression.
Patient Teaching
• Teach the patient to take atazanavir with food. Explain that eating small, frequent meals may offset atazavir's side effects of nausea and vomiting.
• Instruct the patient that atazanavir is not a cure for HIV infection, nor does it reduce risk of transmission to others.

delavirdine mesylate
dell-ah-**veer**-deen
(Rescriptor)

CATEGORY AND SCHEDULE
Pregnancy Risk Category: C

MECHANISM OF ACTION
A nonnucleoside reverse transcriptase inhibitor that inhibits catalytic reaction of HIV reverse transcriptase that is independent of nucleoside binding. *Therapeutic Effect:* Interrupts HIV replication, slows progression of HIV infection.

PHARMACOKINETICS

Rapidly absorbed after PO administration. Primarily distributed in blood plasma. Protein binding: 98%. Metabolized in the liver. Eliminated in feces and urine. **Half-life:** 2–11 hrs.

AVAILABILITY

Tablets: 100 mg, 200 mg.

INDICATIONS AND DOSAGES

▸ **HIV infection**
PO
Adults. 400 mg 3 times a day on an empty stomach.

CONTRAINDICATIONS

None known.

INTERACTIONS

Drug
Benzodiazepines, calcium channel blockers: May cause life-threatening adverse effects.
Carbamazepine, phenobarbital, phenytoin: May decrease delavirdine blood concentration.
H_2 blockers: May decrease delavirdine absorption.
Rifampin: May decrease delavirdine blood concentrations.
Herbal
None known.
Food
None known.

DIAGNOSTIC TEST EFFECTS

May increase SGOT (AST) and SGPT (ALT) levels. May decrease neutrophil count.

SIDE EFFECTS

Frequent (18%)
Rash, pruritus
Occasional (greater than 2%)
Headache, nausea, diarrhea, fatigue, anorexia

SERIOUS REACTIONS

• None known.

NURSING CONSIDERATIONS

Baseline Assessment
• Expect to obtain the patient's baseline laboratory testing, especially liver function tests, before giving the first dose and at periodic intervals during therapy.
• Offer the patient emotional support.
Lifespan Considerations
• Be aware that it is unknown if delavirdine crosses the placenta or is distributed in breast milk.
• Be aware that the safety and efficacy of delavirdine have not been established in children younger than 16 years and in the elderly.
Precautions
• Use cautiously in patients with liver impairment.
Administration and Handling
PO
• May disperse in water before consumption.
• May give with or without food.
• Patients with achlorhydria should take delavirdine with orange juice or cranberry juice.
Intervention and Evaluation
• Assess the patient's skin for evidence of rash.
• Evaluate the patient for nausea.
• Determine the patient's daily pattern of bowel activity and stool consistency.
• Assess the patient's eating pattern and monitor for weight loss.
• Expect to monitor lab values carefully, particularly liver function.
Patient Teaching
• Advise the patient not to take any medications, including over-the-

counter (OTC) drugs, without notifying the physician.
• Instruct the patient that small, frequent meals may offset anorexia, nausea.
• Explain to the patient that delavirdine is not a cure for HIV infection, nor does it reduce risk of transmission to others.

didanosine
dye-**dan**-oh-sin
(Videx, Videx-EC)

CATEGORY AND SCHEDULE
Pregnancy Risk Category: B

MECHANISM OF ACTION
A purine nucleoside analogue that is intracellularly converted into a triphosphate, interfering with RNA-directed DNA polymerase (reverse transcriptase). *Therapeutic Effect:* Virustatic, inhibiting replication of retroviruses, including HIV.

PHARMACOKINETICS
Variably absorbed from the gastrointestinal (GI) tract. Protein binding: less than 5%. Rapidly metabolized intracellularly to active form. Primarily excreted in urine. Partially (20%) removed by hemodialysis. **Half-life:** 1.5 hrs; metabolite: 8–24 hrs.

AVAILABILITY
Tablets (chewable): 25 mg, 50 mg, 100 mg, 150 mg, 200 mg.
Capsules (delayed-release): 125 mg, 200 mg, 250 mg, 400 mg.
Powder for Oral Solution (single-dose packet): 100 mg.
Pediatric Solution: 10 mg/ml.

INDICATIONS AND DOSAGES
▸ **HIV infection**
Adults, children 13 yrs and older, weighing 60 kg or more.
200 mg q12h or 400 mg once a day.
Oral solution
Adults, children 13 yrs and older, weighing 60 kg or more.
250 mg q12h.
Delayed-release capsules
Adults, children 13 yrs and older, weighing 60 kg or more.
400 mg once a day.
Adults, children 13 yrs and older, weighing less than 60 kg. 125 mg q12h or 250 mg once a day.
Oral solution
Adults, children 13 yrs and older, weighing less than 60 kg. 167 mg q12h.
Delayed-release capsules
Adults, children 13 yrs and older, weighing less than 60 kg. 250 mg once a day
Children 3 mos to less than 13 yrs. 180–300 mg/m^2/day in divided doses q12h.
Children younger than 3 mos. 50 mg/m^2/day in divided doses q12h.
▸ **Dosage in renal impairment**
Patients weighing less than 60 kg:

CrCl	Tablets	Oral Solution	Delayed-Release Capsules
30–59 ml/min	75 mg 2 times a day	100 mg 2 times a day	125 mg once a day
10–29 ml/min	100 mg once a day	100 mg once a day	125 mg once a day
less than 10 ml/min	75 mg once a day	100 mg once a day	N/A

CrCl = creatinine clearance

Patients weighing 60 kg or more:

CrCl	Tablets	Oral Solution	Delayed-Release Capsules
30–59 ml/ min	100 mg 2 times a day	100 mg 2 times a day	200 mg once a day
10–29 ml/ min	150 mg once a day	167 mg once a day	125 mg once a day
less than 10 ml/ min	100 mg once a day	100 mg once a day	125 mg once a day

CrCl = creatinine clearance

CONTRAINDICATIONS
Hypersensitivity to drug or any component of preparation

INTERACTIONS
Drug
Dapsone, flouroquinolones, itraconazole, ketoconazole, tetracyclines: May decrease absorption of these drugs.
Medications producing pancreatitis or peripheral neuropathy: May increase risk of pancreatitis, peripheral neuropathy with these drugs.
Stavudine: May increase risk of fatal lactic acidosis in pregnancy.
Herbal
None known.
Food
Decreases absorption of didanosine.

DIAGNOSTIC TEST EFFECTS
May increase serum alkaline phosphatase, amylase, bilirubin, lipase, triglycerides, and uric acid levels and SGOT (AST) and SGPT (ALT) levels. May decrease serum potassium levels.

SIDE EFFECTS
Frequent
Adults (greater than 10%)
Diarrhea, neuropathy, chills and fever
Children (greater than 25%)
Chills, fever, decreased appetite, pain, malaise, nausea, diarrhea, vomiting, abdominal pain, headache, nervousness, cough, rhinitis, dyspnea, asthenia, rash, itching
Occasional
Adults (9%–2%)
Rash, itching, headache, abdominal pain, nausea, vomiting, pneumonia, myopathy, decreased appetite, dry mouth, dyspnea
Children (25%–10%)
Failure to thrive, decreased weight, stomatitis, oral thrush, ecchymosis, arthritis, myalgia, insomnia, epistaxis, pharyngitis

SERIOUS REACTIONS
• Pneumonia and opportunistic infection occur occasionally.
• Peripheral neuropathy and potentially fatal pancreatitis are the major toxicities.

NURSING CONSIDERATIONS
Baseline Assessment
• Expect to obtain the patient's baseline values for complete blood count (CBC), renal and liver function tests, vital signs, and weight.
Lifespan Considerations
• Be aware that didanosine should be used during pregnancy only if clearly needed and that breast-feeding should be discontinued during didanosine therapy.
• Be aware that didanosine is well tolerated in children older than 3 months.
• In the elderly, age-related renal impairment may require dosage adjustment.
Precautions
• Use cautiously in patients with alcoholism, elevated triglycerides,

renal or liver dysfunction, or T-cell counts less than 100 cells/mm^3.

• Use didanosine with extreme caution in patients with a history of pancreatitis.

• Use cautiously in patients on phenylketonuria and sodium-restricted diets because didanosine contains phenylalanine and sodium.

Administration and Handling

PO

• Store at room temperature.

• Tablets dispersed in water are stable for 1 hour at room temperature; after reconstitution of buffered powder, oral solution is stable for 4 hours at room temperature.

• Pediatric powder for oral solution following reconstitution, as directed, is stable for 30 days refrigerated.

• Give 1 hour before or 2 hours after meals because food decreases the rate and extent of didanosine absorption.

• Thoroughly crush and disperse chewable tablets in at least 30 ml water before having the patient swallow. Stir the mixture well (up to 2 to 3 minutes) and have the patient immediately swallow it.

• Reconstitute buffered powder for oral solution before giving it by pouring the contents of the packet into 4 oz of water; stir until completely dissolved (up to 2 to 3 minutes). Don't mix with fruit juice or other acidic liquid because didanosine is unstable with an acidic pH.

• Add 100 to 200 ml water to 2 or 4 g of the unbuffered pediatric powder, respectively, to provide a concentration of 20 mg/ml. Immediately mix with an equal amount of an antacid to provide a concentration of 10 mg/ml. Shake thoroughly before removing each dose.

• Have the patient swallow enteric-coated capsules whole take them on an empty stomach.

Intervention and Evaluation

◀ ALERT ▶ Contact the physician if the patient experiences abdominal pain, elevated serum amylase or triglycerides, nausea, and vomiting before administering the medication because these symptoms may indicate pancreatitis.

• Assess the patient for signs and symptoms peripheral neuropathy, including burning feet, "restless leg syndrome" (unable to find comfortable position for legs and feet), and lack of coordination.

• Monitor the consistency and frequency of the patient's stools.

• Check the patient's skin for eruptions and rash.

• As appropriate, monitor the patient's blood chemistry values and complete blood count (CBC).

• Assess the patient for signs and symptoms of opportunistic infections, including cough or other respiratory symptoms, fever, or oral mucosa changes.

• Check the patient's weight at least twice a week.

• Assess the patient for visual or hearing difficulty and provide protection from light if photophobia develops.

Patient Teaching

• Advise the patient to avoid the intake of alcohol.

• Warn the patient to notify the physician if he or she experiences nausea, numbness, persistent severe abdominal pain, or vomiting.

• Teach the patient to shake the oral suspension well before using it, to keep it refrigerated, and to discard the solution after 30 days and obtain a new supply.

efavirenz
eh-fah-**vir**-enz
(Stocrin[AUS], Sustiva)

CATEGORY AND SCHEDULE
Pregnancy Risk Category: C

MECHANISM OF ACTION
A nonnucleoside reverse transcriptase inhibitor that inhibits the activity of HIV reverse transcriptase (RT) of HIV-1. *Therapeutic Effect:* Interrupts HIV replication, slowing progression of HIV infection.

PHARMACOKINETICS
Rapidly absorbed after PO administration. Protein binding: 99%. Metabolized to major isoenzymes in liver. Eliminated in urine and feces. **Half-life:** 40–55 hrs.

AVAILABILITY
Capsules: 50 mg, 100 mg, 200 mg.
Tablets: 600 mg.

INDICATIONS AND DOSAGES
▸ **HIV infection**
PO
Adults, Elderly. 600 mg once a day in combination with other antiretroviral agents at bedtime.
Children 3 yrs and older weighing 40 kg and more. 600 mg once a day.
Children older than 3 yrs weighing 32.5 kg–less than 40 kg. 400 mg once a day.
Children older than 3 yrs weighing 25 kg–less than 32.5 kg. 350 mg once a day.
Children older than 3 yrs weighing 20 kg–less than 25 kg. 300 mg once a day.
Children older than 3 yrs weighing 15 kg–less than 20 kg. 250 mg once a day.
Children older than 3 yrs weighing
between 10 kg–less than 15 kg. 200 mg once a day.

CONTRAINDICATIONS
Concurrent administration with ergot derivatives, midazolam, or triazolam; a history of hypersensitivity to efavirenz; monotherapy

INTERACTIONS
Drug
Alcohol, psychoactive drugs: May produce additive central nervous system (CNS) effects.
Clarithromycin: Decreases clarithromycin plasma levels.
Ergot derivatives, midazolam, triazolam: May cause serious or life-threatening events, such as arrhythmias, prolonged sedation, or respiratory depression.
Indinavir, saquinavir: Decreases the plasma concentrations of these drugs.
Nelfinavir, ritonavir: Increases the plasma concentrations of these drugs.
Phenobarbital, rifabutin, rifampin: Lowers efavirenz plasma concentration.
Warfarin: Alters warfarin plasma concentrations.
Herbal
None known.
Food
None known.

DIAGNOSTIC TEST EFFECTS
May produce false-positive urine test results for cannabinoid and increase liver enzyme, total cholesterol, SGOT (AST), SGPT (ALT), and serum triglyceride levels.

SIDE EFFECTS
Frequent (52%)
Mild to severe symptoms: Dizziness, vivid dreams, insomnia, confusion, impaired concentration, amnesia, agitation, depersonalization, hallucinations, euphoria

Occasional

Mild to moderate degree maculo-papular rash (27%); nausea, fatigue, headache, diarrhea, fever, cough (less than 26%)

SERIOUS REACTIONS

• None known.

NURSING CONSIDERATIONS

Baseline Assessment

• Offer emotional support to the patient and family.

• Expect to obtain the baseline SGOT (AST) and SGPT (ALT) levels in patients with a history of hepatitis B or C before giving the drug.

• Expect to obtain the patient's baseline serum cholesterol and triglycerides levels before giving the drug and at regular intervals during therapy.

• Obtain the patient's history of all prescription and nonprescription medications before giving the drug because efavirenz interacts with several drugs.

Lifespan Considerations

• Be aware that breast-feeding is not recommended for patients on efavirenz.

• Be aware that the safety and efficacy of efavirenz have not been established in children younger than 3 years.

• In children, there may be an increased incidence of rash.

• There are no age-related precautions noted in the elderly.

Precautions

• Use cautiously in patients with a history of liver impairment, mental illness, or substance abuse.

Administration and Handling

PO

• Give without regard to meals.

• High-fat meals may increase

drug absorption and should be avoided.

• For adult and elderly patients, administer the drug at bedtime during the first 2 to 4 weeks because of the increased risk of temporary CNS side effects.

Intervention and Evaluation

• Monitor the patient for signs and symptoms of adverse CNS psychologic side effects, such as abnormal dreams, dizziness, impaired concentration, insomnia, severe acute depression, including suicidal ideation or attempts, and somnolence. Be aware that insomnia may begin during the first or second day of therapy and generally resolves in 2 to 4 weeks.

• Assess the patient for evidence of a rash, a common side effect.

• As appropriate, monitor the patient's liver enzyme studies for abnormalities.

• Assess the patient for diarrhea, headache, and nausea.

Patient Teaching

• Advise the patient to avoid high-fat meals during therapy.

• Warn the patient to notify the physician immediately if a rash appears.

• Explain to the patient that CNS psychologic symptoms occur in more than half of patients and may cause delusions, depression, dizziness, and impaired concentration. Advise the patient to notify the physician if these continue or become problematic.

• Advise the patient to take the medication every day as prescribed. Warn the patient not to alter the dose or discontinue the medication without first notifying the physician.

• Warn the patient to avoid tasks that require mental alertness or motor skills until his or her response to the drug is established.

• Explain that efavirenz is not a cure for HIV infection, nor does it reduce risk of transmission to others.

emtricitabine
em-trih-**sit**-ah-bean
(Emtriva)

CATEGORY AND SCHEDULE
Pregnancy Risk Category: B

MECHANISM OF ACTION
An antiretroviral agent that inhibits HIV-1 reverse transcriptase by incorporating into viral DNA, resulting in chain termination. *Therapeutic Effect:* Slows HIV replication, reducing progression of HIV infection.

PHARMACOKINETICS
Rapidly and extensively absorbed from the gastrointestinal (GI) tract. Primarily excreted in urine (86%) with a lesser amount excreted in feces (14%). 30% removed by hemodialysis. Unknown if removed by peritoneal dialysis. **Half-life:** 10 hrs.

AVAILABILITY
Capsules: 200 mg.

INDICATIONS AND DOSAGES
▶ **HIV infection**
PO
Adults, Elderly. 200 mg once a day.

▶ **Dosage in renal impairment**

Creatinine Clearance	Dosage
30–49 ml/min	200 mg q48h
15–29 ml/min	200 mg q72h
less than 15 ml/min, hemodialysis patients	200 mg q96h

CONTRAINDICATIONS
None known

INTERACTIONS
Drug
None known.
Herbal
None known.
Food
None known.

DIAGNOSTIC TEST EFFECTS
May elevate serum amylase, lipase, SGPT (ALT), SGOT (AST), and triglyceride levels. May alter blood glucose levels.

SIDE EFFECTS
Frequent (23%–13%)
Headache, rhinitis, rash, diarrhea, nausea
Occasional (14%–4%)
Cough, vomiting, abdominal pain, insomnia, depression, paresthesia, dizziness, peripheral neuropathy, dyspepsia, including heartburn and epigastric distress, myalgia
Rare (3%–2%)
Arthralgia, abnormal dreams

SERIOUS REACTIONS
• Lactic acidosis and hepatomegaly with steatosis, or excess fat in liver, occur rarely and may be severe.

NURSING CONSIDERATIONS
Baseline Assessment
• Expect to obtain the patient's baseline laboratory testing,

especially liver function tests and triglycerides before beginning emtricitabine therapy, and at periodic intervals during therapy.

• Offer the patient emotional support.

Lifespan Considerations

• Be aware that breast-feeding is not recommended for this patient population.

• Be aware that the safety and efficacy of this drug have not been established in children.

• In the elderly, age-related decreased renal function may require dosage adjustment.

Precautions

• Use cautiously in patients with impaired liver or renal function.

Administration and Handling

PO

• Give emtricitabine without regard to food.

Intervention and Evaluation

• Assess the patient's daily pattern of bowel activity and stool consistency.

• Evaluate the patient for nausea and pruritus or itching.

• Examine the patient's skin for rash and urticaria.

• Monitor the patient's clinical chemistry tests for marked laboratory abnormalities.

Patient Teaching

• Explain to the patient that emtricitabine use may cause the redistribution of body fat.

• Tell the patient to continue emtricitabine therapy for the full length of treatment.

• Instruct the patient that emtricitabine is not a cure for HIV infection, nor does it reduce risk of transmission to others. Explain to the patient that he or she may continue to acquire illnesses associated with advanced HIV infection. Also stress to the patient that emtricitabine use does not preclude the need to continue practices to prevent transmission of HIV.

enfuvirtide
en-**few**-vir-tide
(Fuzeon)

CATEGORY AND SCHEDULE
Pregnancy Risk Category: B

MECHANISM OF ACTION
A fusion inhibitor that interferes with the entry of HIV-1 into CD4+ cells by inhibiting fusion of viral and cellular membranes. *Therapeutic Effect:* Slows HIV replication, reducing progression of HIV infection.

PHARMACOKINETICS
Comparable absorption when injected into subcutaneous tissue of abdomen, arm, or thigh. Protein binding: 92%. Undergoes catabolism to amino acids. **Half-life:** 3.8 hrs.

AVAILABILITY
Powder for Injection: 108 mg (approximately 90 mg/ml when reconstituted) vials.

INDICATIONS AND DOSAGES
▸ **HIV infection**
Subcutaneous
Adults, Elderly. 90 mg (1 ml) twice a day.
Children 6–16 yrs. 2 mg/kg twice a day up to a maximum dose of 90 mg twice a day.

Pediatric dosing guidelines

Weight: kg (lbs)	Dose: mg (ml)
11–15.5 (24–34)	27 (0.3)
15.6–20 (more than 34–44)	36 (0.4)
20.1–24.5 (more than 44–54)	45 (0.5)
24.6–29 (more than 54–64)	54 (0.6)
29.1–33.5 (more than 64–74)	63 (0.7)
33.6–38 (more than 74–84)	72 (0.8)
38.1–42.5 (more than 84–94)	81 (0.9)
more than 42.5 (more than 94)	90 (1)

CONTRAINDICATIONS
None known.

INTERACTIONS
Drug
None known.
Herbal
None known.
Food
None known.

DIAGNOSTIC TEST EFFECTS
May elevate blood glucose, serum amylase, serum creatine phosphokinase, serum lipase, serum triglycerides, SGOT (AST) and SGPT (ALT) levels. May decrease blood hemoglobin levels and white blood cell (WBC) counts.

SIDE EFFECTS
Expected (98%)
Local injection site reactions (pain, discomfort, induration, erythema, nodules, cysts, pruritus, ecchymosis)
Frequent (26%–16%)
Diarrhea, nausea, fatigue
Occasional (11%–4%)
Insomnia, peripheral neuropathy, depression, cough, weight or appetite decrease, sinusitis, anxiety, asthenia (loss of energy, strength), myalgia, cold sores
Rare (3%–2%)
Constipation, influenza, upper abdominal pain, anorexia, conjunctivitis

SERIOUS REACTIONS
• Enfuvirtide use may potentiate bacterial pneumonia development.
• Hypersensitivity (rash, fever, chills, rigors, hypotension), thrombocytopenia, neutropenia, and renal insufficiency or failure may occur rarely.

NURSING CONSIDERATIONS

Baseline Assessment
• Expect to obtain baseline laboratory testing, especially liver function tests and serum triglyceride levels, before beginning enfuvirtide therapy and at periodic intervals during therapy.
• Offer the patient emotional support.

Lifespan Considerations
• Breast-feeding is not recommended in this patient population due to the possibility of HIV transmission.
• Be aware that the safety and efficacy of enfuvirtide have not been established in children younger than 6 years of age.
• There are no age-related precautions noted in the elderly.

Administration and Handling
• Store at room temperature. Refrigerate reconstituted solution; use within 24 hours.
• Bring reconstituted solution to room temperature before injection.
• Reconstitute with 1.1 ml Sterile Water for Injection. Visually inspect vial for particulate matter. Solution normally appears clear, colorless. Discard unused portion.
• Administer subcutaneously into the upper abdomen, anterior thigh, or arm. Administer each injection at a different site that the preceding injection site.

Intervention and Evaluation
• Assess the patient's skin for hypersensitivity reaction and local injection site reaction.
• Observe the patient for evidence of fatigue or nausea.
• Evaluate the patient's sleep patterns.
• Monitor the patient for signs and symptoms of depression and insomnia.
• Monitor the patient's blood chemistry test results for marked abnormalities.

Patient Teaching
• Warn the patient that an increased rate of bacterial pneumonia has occurred in patients taking enfuvirtide and to seek medical attention if cough with fever, rapid breathing, or shortness of breath occurs.
• Advise the patient to continue taking enfuvirtide for the full length of treatment.
• Instruct the patient that enfuvirtide is not a cure for HIV infection, nor does it reduce the risk of transmission to others. Explain to the patient that he or she still needs to continue practices to prevent transmission of HIV.

fosamprenavir calcium
foss-am-**pren**-ah-vur
(Lexiva)

CATEGORY AND SCHEDULE
Pregnancy Risk Category: C

MECHANISM OF ACTION
An antiretroviral that is rapidly converted to amprenavir which inhibits HIV-1 protease by binding to active site of HIV-1 protease, preventing processing of viral precursors and forming immature noninfectious viral particles. *Therapeutic Effect:* Produces impairment of HIV viral replication and proliferation.

AVAILABILITY
Tablets: 700 mg, equivalent to 600 mg amprenavir

INDICATIONS AND DOSAGES
▸ **Therapy-naive patients**
PO
Adults, Elderly. 1,400 mg 2 times/day. When given with ritonavir, 1,400 mg once a day or 700 mg 2 times/day.
▸ **Protease inhibitor-experienced patients**
PO
Adults, Elderly. 700 mg fosamprenavir twice a day plus 100 mg ritonavir twice a day.
▸ **Concurrent therapy with efavirenz**
PO
Adults, Elderly. In patients receiving fosamprenavir plus ritonavir once a day in combination with efavirenz, the recommended dose of ritonavir is 300 mg a day.
▸ **Mild to moderate liver function impairment**
PO
Adults, Elderly. 700 mg twice a day.

CONTRAINDICATIONS
Concurrent use with amprenavir, dihydroergotamine, ergonovine, ergotamine, methylergonovine, pimozide, midazolam, or triazolam. If fosamprenavir is given currently with ritonavir, then flecainide and propafenone are also contraindicated.

INTERACTIONS
Drug
Amiodarone, bepridil, ergotamine, lidocaine, oral contraceptives,

midazolam, quinidine, triazolam, tricyclic antidepressants: May interfere with the metabolism of the aforementioned drugs.
Antacids, didanosine: May decrease the absorption of fosamprenavir.
Carbamazepine, phenobarbital, phenytoin, rifampin: May decrease fosamprenavir blood concentration.
Clozapine, HMG-CoA reductase inhibitors (statins), warfarin: May increase blood concentrations of the aforementioned drugs.

Herbal
St. John's wort: May decrease fosamprenavir blood concentration.

Food
None known.

DIAGNOSTIC TEST EFFECTS
May increase blood glucose levels, serum lipase, SGPT (ALT), SGOT (AST), and serum triglyceride levels.

SIDE EFFECTS
Frequent (39%–35%)
Nausea, rash, diarrhea
Occasional (19%–8%)
Headache, vomiting, fatigue, depression
Rare (7%–2%)
Pruritus, abdominal pain, oral paresthesia

SERIOUS REACTIONS
• Severe or life-threatening skin reactions occur rarely (less than 1%).

NURSING CONSIDERATIONS
Baseline Assessment
• Expect to obtain baseline lab values, including blood glucose levels, serum lipase, SGPT (ALT), SGOT (AST), and serum triglyceride levels.
• Find out which other drugs the patient is taking, including ritonavir. Makes sure the patient is not also taking amprenavir, because it is chemically similar to fosamprenavir.

Precautions
• Use extremely cautiously in patients with liver impairment.
• Use cautiously in elderly patients and patients with diabetes mellitus, impaired renal function, and known sulfonamide allergy.

Administration and Handling
PO
• Do not chew, crush, or break film-coated tablets.
• May give without regard to food.

Patient Teaching
• Tell the patient to report any side effects, including nausea rash and diarrhea.
• Instruct the patient that fosamprenavir is not a cure for HIV infection, nor does it reduce risk of transmission to others.

indinavir
in-**din**-oh-vir
(Crixivan)
Do not confuse with Denavir.

CATEGORY AND SCHEDULE
Pregnancy Risk Category: C

MECHANISM OF ACTION
A protease inhibitor that suppresses HIV protease, an enzyme necessary for splitting viral polyprotein precursors into mature and infectious virus particles. *Therapeutic Effect:* Resultant effect interrupts HIV replication, forms immature noninfectious viral particles.

PHARMACOKINETICS
Rapidly absorbed after PO administration. Protein binding: 60%. Me-

tabolized in liver. Primarily excreted in urine. Unknown if removed by hemodialysis. **Half-life:** 1.8 hrs (half-life is increased with impaired liver function).

AVAILABILITY
Capsules: 100 mg, 200 mg, 333 mg, 400 mg.

INDICATIONS AND DOSAGES
▶ **HIV infection**
PO
Adults. 800 mg (two 400-mg capsules) q8h.
▶ **HIV infection with liver insufficiency**
PO
Adults. 600 mg q8h.

UNLABELED USES
Prophylaxis following occupational exposure to HIV

CONTRAINDICATIONS
Hypersensitivity to indinavir; nephrolithiasis

INTERACTIONS
Drug
Midazolam, triazolam: Concurrent administration of indinavir with these drugs raises the risk of developing arrhythmias and prolonged sedation.
Herbal
St. John's wort: May decrease indinavir blood concentration and effect.
Food
Avoid meals high in fat, calories, and protein.
Grapefruit: May decrease indinavir blood concentration and effect.

DIAGNOSTIC TEST EFFECTS
May increase serum bilirubin (occurs in 10% of patients), SGOT (AST), and SGPT (ALT) levels.

SIDE EFFECTS
Frequent
Nausea (12%), abdominal pain (9%), headache (6%), diarrhea (5%)
Occasional
Vomiting, asthenia, fatigue (4%); insomnia; accumulation of fat in waist, abdomen, or back of neck
Rare
Abnormal taste sensation, heartburn, symptomatic urinary tract disease, transient kidney dysfunction

SERIOUS REACTIONS
• Nephrolithiasis (flank pain with or without hematuria) occurs in 4% of patients.

NURSING CONSIDERATIONS
Baseline Assessment
• Offer emotional support to the patient.
• Establish the patient's baseline lab values.
• Monitor the patient's renal function before and during therapy, and in particular, evaluate the results of the serum creatinine and urinalysis tests.
Lifespan Considerations
• Be aware that it is unknown if indinavir is excreted in breast milk. Breast-feeding is not recommended in this patient population because of the possibility of HIV transmission.
• Be aware that the safety and efficacy of this drug have not been established in children.
• There is no information on the effects of this drug's use in the elderly.
Precautions
• Use cautiously in patients with renal or liver function impairment.
Administration and Handling
PO
• Store drug at room temperature, keep it in the original bottle, and

protect it from moisture. Keep in mind that indinavir capsules are sensitive to moisture.

• For optimal drug absorption, give indinavir with water only and without food 1 hour before or 2 hours after a meal. Give indinavir with coffee, juice, skim milk, tea, or water with a light meal (e.g. dry toast with jelly).

• Do not give indinavir with meals high in fat, calories, and protein.

• If indinavir and didanosine are given concurrently, give the drugs at least 1 hour apart on an empty stomach.

Intervention and Evaluation

• To maintain adequate hydration, have the patient drink 48 oz (1.5 L) of liquid over each 24-hour period during therapy.

◀**ALERT**▶ Monitor the patient for signs and symptoms of nephrolithiasis as evidenced by flank pain and hematuria, and notify the physician if symptoms occur. If nephrolithiasis occurs, expect therapy to be interrupted for 1 to 3 days.

• Assess the patient's pattern of daily bowel activity and stool consistency.

• Evaluate the patient for abdominal discomfort or headache.

• Expect to monitor the patient's serum amylase, bilirubin, blood glucose, complete blood count (CBC), CD4 cell count, cholesterol, lipase, liver function tests, and triglyceride levels.

Patient Teaching

• Advise the patient that indinavir is not a cure for HIV, and the condition may progress despite treatment.

• Explain to the patient that if a dose is missed, to take the next dose at the regularly scheduled time, not to double the dose.

• Teach the patient that indinavir is

best taken with water only and without food for optimal drug absorption 1 hour before or 2 hours after a meal. Explain that indinavir may be taken with coffee, juice, skim milk, tea, or water with a light meal.

• Tell the patient that St. John's wort and grapefruit or grapefruit juice will lower indinavir levels. Urge the patient to avoid them during treatment.

lamivudine
lah-**mih**-view-deen
(Heptovir[CAN], Epivir,
Zeffix[AUS])
Do not confuse with lamotrigine.

CATEGORY AND SCHEDULE
Pregnancy Risk Category: C

MECHANISM OF ACTION
An antiviral that inhibits HIV reverse transcriptase via viral DNA chain termination. Also inhibits RNA- and DNA-dependent DNA polymerase, an enzyme necessary for viral HIV replication. *Therapeutic Effect:* Slows HIV replication, reduces progression of HIV infection.

PHARMACOKINETICS
Rapidly, completely absorbed from the gastrointestinal (GI) tract. Protein binding: less than 36%. Widely distributed (crosses the blood-brain barrier). Primarily excreted unchanged in urine. Not removed by hemodialysis or peritoneal dialysis. **Half-life:** 11–15 hrs (intracellular); serum (adults) 2–11 hrs, (children) 1.7–2 hrs. Half-life is increased with impaired renal function.

AVAILABILITY
Tablets: 100 mg, 150 mg, 300 mg.
Oral Solution: 5 mg/ml, 10 mg/ml.

INDICATIONS AND DOSAGES
▸ **HIV infection**
PO
Adults, Children 12–16 yrs, weighing more than 50 kg (more than 100 lbs). 150 mg twice a day or 300 mg once a day.
Adults weighing less than 50 kg. 2 mg/kg twice a day.
Children 3 mos–11 yrs. 4 mg/kg twice a day (up to 150 mg/dose).
▸ **Chronic hepatitis B**
PO
Adults, Children 17 yrs or older. 100 mg daily.
Children younger than 17 yrs. 3 mg/kg/day. Maximum: 100 mg/day.
▸ **Dosage in renal impairment**
Dosage and frequency are modified based on creatinine clearance.

Creatinine Clearance (ml/min)	Dosage
50 or greater	150 mg twice a day
30–49	150 mg once a day
15–29	150 mg first dose, then 100 mg once a day
5–14	150 mg first dose, then 50 mg once a day
less than 5	50 mg first dose, then 25 mg once a day

UNLABELED USES
Prophylaxis in health care workers at risk of acquiring HIV after occupational exposure to virus

CONTRAINDICATIONS
None known

INTERACTIONS
Drug
Trimethoprim-sulfamethoxazole: Increases lamivudine blood concentration.

Herbal
St. John's wort: May decrease lamivudine blood concentration and effect.
Food
None known.

DIAGNOSTIC TEST EFFECTS
May increase blood Hgb values, neutrophil count, and serum amylase, SGOT (AST), and SGPT (ALT) levels.

SIDE EFFECTS
Frequent
Headache (35%), nausea (33%), malaise and fatigue (27%), nasal disturbances (20%), diarrhea, cough (18%), musculoskeletal pain, neuropathy (12%), insomnia (11%), anorexia, dizziness, fever or chills (10%)
Occasional
Depression (9%); myalgia (8%); abdominal cramps (6%); dyspepsia, arthralgia (5%)

SERIOUS REACTIONS
• Pancreatitis occurs in 13% of pediatric patients.
• Anemia, neutropenia, and thrombocytopenia occur rarely.

NURSING CONSIDERATIONS
Baseline Assessment
• Before starting drug therapy, check the patient's baseline lab values, especially renal function.
Lifespan Considerations
• Be aware that lamivudine crosses the placenta and it is unknown if lamivudine is distributed in breast milk. Breast-feeding is not recommended in this patient population because of the possibility of HIV transmission.
• Be aware that the safety and efficacy of this drug have not been

established in children younger than 3 months.
• In the elderly, age-related renal impairment may require dosage adjustment.

Precautions
• Use cautiously in patients with impaired renal function, a history of pancreatitis, or a history of peripheral neuropathy.
• Use cautiously in young children.

Administration and Handling
PO
• Give without regard to meals.

Intervention and Evaluation
• Expect to monitor the patient's serum amylase, BUN, and serum creatinine levels.
• Evaluate the patient for altered sleep patterns, cough, dizziness, headache, and nausea.
• Assess the patient's pattern of daily bowel activity and stool consistency.
• Modify the patient's diet or administer a laxative, if ordered, as needed.
• If pancreatitis in a pediatric patient occurs, help the patient to sit up or flex at the waist to relieve abdominal pain aggravated by movement.

Patient Teaching
• Advise the patient to continue taking lamivudine for the full length of treatment and to evenly space drug doses around the clock.
• Explain to the patient that lamivudine is not a cure for HIV and that he or she may continue to experience illnesses, including opportunistic infections.
• Advise the parents of pediatric patients to closely monitor the patient for symptoms of pancreatitis, manifested as clammy skin, hypotension, nausea, severe and steady abdominal pain often radiating to the back, and vomiting accompanying abdominal pain.
• Warn the patient not to engage in activities that require mental acuity if he or she is experiencing dizziness.

lopinavir/ritonavir
low-**pin**-ah-veer/rih-**ton**-ah-veer (Kaletra)
Do not confuse with Keppra.

CATEGORY AND SCHEDULE
Pregnancy Risk Category: C

MECHANISM OF ACTION
A protease inhibitor combination. Lopinavir acts on protease enzyme late in the HIV replication process and inhibits its activity. *Therapeutic Effect:* Formation of immature, noninfectious viral particles. Ritonavir inhibits the metabolism of lopinavir. *Therapeutic Effect:* Increases plasma concentrations of lopinavir.

PHARMACOKINETICS
Readily absorbed after PO administration (increased when taken with food). Protein binding: 98%–99%. Metabolized in liver. Primarily eliminated in feces. Not removed by hemodialysis. **Half-life:** 5–6 hrs.

AVAILABILITY
Capsules: 133.3 mg lopinavir/ 33.3 mg ritonavir.
Oral Solution: 80 mg lopinavir/ 20 mg ritonavir per ml.

INDICATIONS AND DOSAGES
▸ **HIV infection**
PO
Adults. 400/100 mg of lopinavir/ ritonavir (3 capsules or 5 ml) twice

a day. Increase to 533/133 mg (4 capsules or 6.5 ml) when taken with efavirenz or nevirapine.
Children weighing 15–50 kg.
11 mg/kg 2 times/day.
Children weighing 7 kg to less than 15 kg and not taking efavirenz or nevirapine. 12 mg/kg 2 times/day.
Children weighing 15–40 kg.
10 mg/kg 2 times/day.
Children weighing 7 kg to less than 15 kg and taking efavirenz or nevirapine. 13 mg/kg 2 times/day.

CONTRAINDICATIONS
Hypersensitivity to lopinavir or ritonavir; concomitant use of ergot derivatives (causes peripheral ischemia of extremities and vasospasm), flecainide, midazolam, pimozide, propafenone (increases the risk of serous cardiac arrhythmias), and triazolam (increases sedation or respiratory depression)

INTERACTIONS
Drug
Atorvastatin: May increase lopinavir/ritonavir blood concentration and risk of myopathy with this drug.
Atovaquone, methadone, oral contraceptives: May decrease blood concentration and effects of these drugs.
Carbamazepine, corticosteroids, efavirenz, nevirapine, phenobarbital, phenytoin, rifampin: May decrease lopinavir/ritonavir blood concentration and effect.
Clarithromycin, felodipine, immunosuppressants, nicardipine, nifedipine, rifabutin: May increase the blood concentration and effects of these drugs.
Herbal
St. John's wort: May decrease lopinavir/ritonavir blood concentration and effect.

Food
None known.

DIAGNOSTIC TEST EFFECTS
May increase blood glucose, GGT, serum uric acid, SGOT (AST), SGPT (ALT), total cholesterol, and triglyceride levels.

SIDE EFFECTS
Frequent (14%)
Diarrhea, mild to moderate severity
Occasional (6%–2%)
Nausea, asthenia (loss of strength, energy), abdominal pain, headache, vomiting
Rare (less than 2%)
Insomnia, rash

SERIOUS REACTIONS
• Anemia, leukopenia, lymphadenopathy, deep vein thrombosis, Cushing's syndrome, pancreatitis, and hemorrhagic colitis occur rarely.

NURSING CONSIDERATIONS
Baseline Assessment
• Expect to establish the patient's baseline values for complete blood count (CBC), renal and liver function tests, and weight.
Lifespan Considerations
• Be aware that it is unknown if lopinavir/ritonavir is excreted in breast milk. Breast-feeding is not recommended in this patient population because of the possibility of HIV transmission.
• Be aware that the safety and efficacy of lopinavir/ritonavir have not been established in children younger than 6 months.
• In the elderly, age-related cardiac function, renal, or liver impairment requires caution.

Precautions
• Use cautiously in patients with hepatitis B or C or impaired liver function.
◀ **ALERT** ▶ High-doses of itraconazole or ketoconazole are not recommended in patients taking lopinavir/rotinavir. Lopinavir/ritonavir oral solution contains alcohol and should not be given to patients receiving metronizole because this combination may cause a disulfiram-type reaction.
Administration and Handling
PO
• Refrigerate until dispensed and avoid exposure to excessive heat.
• If stored at room temperature, use within 2 months.
• Give with food.
Intervention and Evaluation
• Assess the patient's pattern of daily bowel activity and stool consistency.
• Evaluate the patient for signs and symptoms of opportunistic infections as evidenced by cough, onset of fever, oral mucosa changes, or other respiratory symptoms.
• Check the patient's weight at least twice a week.
• Evaluate the patient for nausea and vomiting.
• Monitor the patient for signs and symptoms of pancreatitis as evidenced by abdominal pain, nausea, and vomiting.
• Monitor the patient's blood glucose, CBC with differential, CD4 count cell count, serum cholesterol, HIV RNA levels (viral load), serum electrolytes, and liver function tests.
Patient Teaching
• Teach the patient how to properly take the medication.
• Encourage the patient to eat small, frequent meals to offset nausea or vomiting.

• Explain to the patient that lopinavir/ritonavir is not a cure for HIV infection, nor does it reduce risk of transmission to others.

nelfinavir
nell-**fine**-ah-veer
(Viracept)

CATEGORY AND SCHEDULE
Pregnancy Risk Category: B

MECHANISM OF ACTION
Inhibits the activity of HIV-1 protease, the enzyme necessary for the formation of infectious HIV. *Therapeutic Effect:* Formation of immature noninfectious viral particles rather than HIV replication.

PHARMACOKINETICS
Well absorbed after PO administration. Protein binding: greater than 98%. Absorption increased with food. Metabolized by the liver. Highly bound to plasma proteins. Eliminated primarily in feces. Unknown if removed by hemodialysis. **Half-life:** 3.5–5 hrs.

AVAILABILITY
Tablets: 250 mg, 625 mg.
Powder: 50 mg/g.

INDICATIONS AND DOSAGES
▶ **HIV infection**
PO
Adults. 750 mg (three 250-mg tablets) 3 times/day, or 1,250 mg 2 times/day in combination with nucleoside analogues (enhances antiviral activity).
Children 2–13 yrs. 20–30 mg/kg/dose, 3 times a day. Maximum: 750 mg q8h.

CONTRAINDICATIONS

Concurrent administration with midazolam, rifampin, or triazolam

INTERACTIONS
Drug

Alcohol, psychoactive drugs: May produce additive central nervous system (CNS) effects.

Anticonvulsants, rifabutin, rifampin: Lower nelfinavir plasma concentration.

Indinavir, saquinavir: Increases plasma concentration of these drugs.

Oral contraceptives: Decreases the effects of these drugs.

Ritonavir: Increases nelfinavir plasma concentration.

Herbal

St. John's wort: May decrease nelfinavir plasma concentration and effect.

Food

Increases nelfinavir plasma concentration.

DIAGNOSTIC TEST EFFECTS

May decrease Hgb values, neutrophils, and white blood cells (WBCs). May increase serum creatine kinase, SGOT (AST), and SGPT (ALT) levels.

SIDE EFFECTS

Frequent (20%)
Diarrhea
Occasional (7%–3%)
Nausea, rash
Rare (2%–1%)
Flatulence, asthenia

SERIOUS REACTIONS

• None known.

NURSING CONSIDERATIONS

Baseline Assessment
• Expect to check the patient's hematology and liver function tests to establish an accurate baseline before beginning drug therapy.

Lifespan Considerations
• Be aware that it is unknown if nelfinavir is distributed in breast milk.
• There are no age-related precautions noted in children over 2 years old.
• There is no information on the effects of this drug's use in the elderly.

Precautions
• Use cautiously in patients with liver function impairment.

Administration and Handling
PO
• Give with food, a light meal or snack.
• Mix oral powder with a small amount of dietary supplement, formula, milk, soy formula, soy milk, or water. The entire contents must be consumed in order to ingest a full dose.
• Do not mix with acidic food such as apple juice, applesauce, or orange juice, or with water in its original container.

Intervention and Evaluation
• Assess the patient's pattern of daily bowel activity and stool consistency.
• Monitor the patient's liver enzyme studies for abnormalities.
◄ALERT► Monitor the patient for signs and symptoms of opportunistic infections as evidenced by chills, cough, fever, and myalgia.

Patient Teaching
• Instruct the patient to take nelfinavir with food to optimize the drug's absorption.
• Advise the patient to take the medication every day as prescribed and to evenly space drug doses around the clock.
• Caution the patient not to alter the dose or discontinue the medication without first notifying the physician.

• Explain to the patient that this medication is not a cure for HIV infection nor does it reduce the risk of transmitting HIV to others, and that he or she may continue to experience illnesses associated with advanced HIV infection, including opportunistic infections.

nevirapine
neh-**vear**-ah-peen
(Viramune)

CATEGORY AND SCHEDULE
Pregnancy Risk Category: C

MECHANISM OF ACTION
A nonnucleoside reverse transcriptase inhibitor that binds directly to virus type 1 (HIV-1) reverse transcriptase (RT), blocking RNA and DNA-dependent DNA polymerase activity by changing the shape of the RT enzyme. *Therapeutic Effect:* Slows HIV replication, reducing progression of HIV infection.

PHARMACOKINETICS
Readily absorbed after PO administration. Protein binding: 60%. Widely distributed. Extensively metabolized in liver; primarily excreted in urine. **Half-life:** 45 hrs (single dose); 25–30 hrs (multiple doses).

AVAILABILITY
Tablets: 200 mg.
Oral Suspension: 50 mg/5 ml.

INDICATIONS AND DOSAGES
▸ **HIV infection**
PO
Adults. 200 mg a day for 14 days reduces the risk of rash.
Maintenance: 200 mg twice a day

in combination with nucleoside analogue antiretroviral agents.
Children 2 mos–8 yrs. 4 mg/kg once a day for 14 days; then 7 mg/kg 2 times/day.
Children older than 8 yrs. 4 mg/kg once a day for 14 days; then 4 mg/kg 2 times/day. Maximum: 400 mg/day.

UNLABELED USES
Reduces the risk of transmitting HIV from infected mother to newborn

CONTRAINDICATIONS
None known

INTERACTIONS
Drug
Ketoconazole, oral contraceptives, protease inhibitors: May decrease the plasma concentrations of these drugs.
Rifabutin, rifampin: May decrease nevirapine blood concentration.
Herbal
St. John's wort: May decrease nevirapine blood concentration and effects.
Food
None known.

DIAGNOSTIC TEST EFFECTS
May significantly increase serum bilirubin, GGT, SGOT (AST), and SGPT (ALT) levels. May significantly decrease Hgb level and neutrophil and platelet count.

SIDE EFFECTS
Frequent (8%–3%)
Rash, fever, headache, nausea
Occasional (3%–1%)
Stomatitis, a burning or erythema of the oral mucosa, mucosal ulceration, dysphagia
Rare (less than 1%)

Paresthesia, myalgia, abdominal pain

SERIOUS REACTIONS
• The rash may become severe and life-threatening.
• Hepatitis occurs rarely.

NURSING CONSIDERATIONS
Baseline Assessment
• Check the patient's baseline diagnostic test results and laboratory values, especially liver function tests, before starting therapy and at intervals during therapy.
• Obtain the patient's medication history, especially regarding the use of oral contraceptives.
Lifespan Considerations
• Be aware that nevirapine crosses the placenta and is distributed in breast milk. Breast-feeding is not recommended in this patient population because of the possibility of HIV transmission.
• Granulocytopenia occurs more frequently in children.
• There is no information on the effects of this drug's use in the elderly.
Precautions
• Use cautiously in patients with elevated SGOT (AST) or SGPT (ALT) levels, a history of chronic hepatitis (B or C), or renal or liver dysfunction.
Administration and Handling
◀ALERT▶ Be aware that nevirapine is always prescribed in combination with at least one additional antiretroviral agent because a resistant HIV virus appears rapidly when nevirapine is given as monotherapy.
PO
• Give without regard to meals.
Intervention and Evaluation
• Closely monitor the patient for evidence of rash, which usually appears on the extremities, face, or trunk, within the first 6 weeks of drug therapy.
• Evaluate the patient for rash accompanied by blistering, conjunctivitis, fever, general malaise, muscle or joint aches, oral lesions, and swelling.
Patient Teaching
• Instruct the patient that if nevirapine therapy is missed for more than 7 days, to restart therapy by using one 200-mg tablet each day for the first 14 days, followed by one 200-mg tablet twice a day.
• Advise the patient to continue nevirapine therapy for the full length of treatment and to evenly space drug doses around the clock.
• Explain to the patient that nevirapine is not a cure for HIV infection, nor does it reduce the risk of transmission to others.
• Warn the patient that if he or she experiences a rash, to notify the physician before continuing therapy.

ritonavir
rih-**tone**-ah-vir
(Norvir)
Do not confuse with Retrovir.

CATEGORY AND SCHEDULE
Pregnancy Risk Category: B

MECHANISM OF ACTION
Inhibits HIV-1 and HIV-2 proteases, rendering the enzymes incapable of processing the polypeptide precursor that leads to production of immature HIV particles. *Therapeutic Effect:* Slows HIV replication, reducing progression of HIV infection.

PHARMACOKINETICS

Well absorbed after PO administration (extent of absorption increased with food). Protein binding: 98%–99%. Extensively metabolized by liver to active metabolite. Primarily eliminated in feces. Unknown if removed by hemodialysis. **Half-life:** 2.7–5 hrs.

AVAILABILITY

Soft Gelatin Capsules: 100 mg.
Oral Solution: 80 mg/ml.

INDICATIONS AND DOSAGES
▸ **HIV infection**
PO
Adults, Children 12 yrs or older: 600 mg 2 times/day. If nausea becomes apparent upon initiation of 600 mg twice a day, give 300 mg twice a day for 1 day, 400 mg twice a day for 2 days, 500 mg twice a day for 1 day, then 600 mg twice a day thereafter.
Children younger than 12 yrs. Initially, 250 mg/m^2/dose 2 times/day. Increase by 50 mg/m^2/dose up to 400 mg/m^2/dose. Maximum: 600 mg/dose 2 times/day.

CONTRAINDICATIONS

Due to the potential for serious or life-threatening drug interactions, the following medications should not be given concomitantly with ritonavir: amiodarone, astemizole, bepridil, bupropion, cisapride, clozapine, encainide, flecainide, meperidine, piroxicam, propafenone, propoxyphene, quinidine, rifabutin, terfenadine (increases risk of arrhythmias, hematologic abnormalities, seizures). Alprazolam, clorazepate, diazepam, estazolam, flurazepam, midazolam, triazolam, and zolpidem may produce extreme sedation and respiratory depression.

INTERACTIONS
Drug
Desipramine, fluoxetine, other antidepressants: May increase the blood concentration of these drugs.
Disulfiram or drugs causing disulfiram-like reaction, such as metronidazole: May produce disulfiram-like reaction if taken with these drugs.
Enzyme inducers, including carbamazepine, dexamethasone, nevirapine, phenobarbital, phenytoin, rifabutin, rifampin: May increase ritonavir metabolism and decrease the ritonavir's efficacy.
Oral contraceptives, theophylline: May decrease the effectiveness of these drugs.
Herbal
St. John's wort: May decrease ritonavir blood concentration and effect.
Food
None known.

DIAGNOSTIC TEST EFFECTS

May alter serum CPK, GGT, triglyceride, and uric acid and SGOT (AST), and SGPT (ALT) levels, and creatinine clearance.

SIDE EFFECTS

Frequent
Gastrointestinal (GI) disturbances (abdominal pain, anorexia, diarrhea, nausea, and vomiting), neurologic disturbances (circumoral and peripheral paresthesias, especially around the feet, hands, or lips, change in sense of taste), headache, dizziness, fatigue, weakness
Occasional
Allergic reaction, flu syndrome, hypotension

SERIOUS REACTIONS

• None known.

NURSING CONSIDERATIONS

Baseline Assessment
• Patients beginning combination therapy with ritonavir and nucleosides may promote GI tolerance by first beginning ritonavir alone and then by adding nucleosides before completing 2 weeks of ritonavir monotherapy.
• Check the patient's baseline laboratory test results, if ordered, especially liver function tests and serum triglycerides, before beginning ritonavir therapy and at periodic intervals during therapy.
• Offer the patient emotional support.

Lifespan Considerations
• Be aware that breast-feeding is not recommended in this patient population because of the possibility of HIV transmission.
• There are no age-related precautions noted in children older than 2 years.
• There is no known effects of this drug's use in the elderly.

Precautions
• Use cautiously in patients with impaired hepatic function.

Administration and Handling
PO
• Store capsules or solution in the refrigerator.
• Protect the drug from light.
• Refrigerate the oral solution unless it is used within 30 days and stored below 77°F.
• May give without regard to meals, but preferably give with food.
• May improve the taste of the oral solution by mixing it with Advera, chocolate milk, or Ensure within 1 hour of dosing.

Intervention and Evaluation
• Closely monitor the patient for signs and symptoms of GI disturbances or neurologic abnormalities, particularly paresthesias.

• Monitor the patient's blood glucose, CD4 cell count, liver function tests, and plasma levels of HIV RNA.

Patient Teaching
• Advise the patient to continue therapy for the full length of treatment and to evenly space drug doses around the clock.
• Explain to the patient that ritonavir is not a cure for HIV infection, nor does it reduce risk of transmission to others. Also explain that he or she may continue to develop illnesses associated with advanced HIV infection.
• Instruct the patient that, if possible, he or she should take ritonavir with food.
• Suggest to the patient that he or she mask the taste of the solution by mixing it with Advera, chocolate milk, or Ensure.
• Warn the patient to notify the physician if he or she experiences abdominal pain, frequent urination, increased thirst, nausea or vomiting.

saquinavir
sah-**quin**-ah-vir
(Fortovase, Invirase)
Do not confuse with Sinequan.

CATEGORY AND SCHEDULE
Pregnancy Risk Category: B

MECHANISM OF ACTION
Inhibits HIV protease, rendering the enzyme incapable of processing the polyprotein precursor to generate functional proteins in HIV-infected cells. *Therapeutic Effect:* Slows HIV replication, reducing progression of HIV infection.

PHARMACOKINETICS
Poorly absorbed after PO adminis-tration (high-calorie and high-fat meal increases absorption). Protein binding: 99%. Metabolized in liver to inactive metabolite. Primarily eliminated in feces. Unknown if removed by hemodialysis. **Half-life:** 13 hrs.

AVAILABILITY
Capsules (Invirase): 200 mg.
Capsules (gelatin) (Fortovase): 200 mg.

INDICATIONS AND DOSAGES
▶ **HIV infection in combination with other antiretroviral agents**
PO
Adults, Elderly. Fortovase: 1,200 mg 3 times/day. Invirase: Three 200-mg capsules given 3 times a day within 2 hrs after a full meal. Do not give less than 600 mg/day (does not produce antiviral activity). Recommended daily doses of other antiretroviral agents are zalcitabine (ddC) 0.75 mg 3 times a day or zidovudine (AZT) 200 mg 3 times a day.

CONTRAINDICATIONS
Clinically significant hypersensitiv-ity to drug; concurrent use with ergot medications, lovastatin, mida-zolam, simvastatin, and triazolam

INTERACTIONS
Drug
Calcium channel blockers, clinda-mycin, dapsone, quinidine, triazolam: May increase the plasma concentrations of these drugs.
Carbamazepine, dexamethasone, phenobarbital, phenytoin, rifampin: May reduce saquinavir plasma concentration.
Ketoconazole: Increases saquinavir plasma concentration.

Herbal
Garlic, St. John's wort: May de-crease saquinavir plasma concentra-tions and effect.
Food
Grapefruit juice: May increase saquinavir plasma concentration.

DIAGNOSTIC TEST EFFECTS
May alter serum CPK levels, ele-vate serum transaminase levels, and lower blood glucose levels.

SIDE EFFECTS
Occasional
Diarrhea, abdominal discomfort and pain, nausea, photosensitivity, buc-cal mucosa ulceration
Rare
Confusion, ataxia, weakness, head-ache, rash

SERIOUS REACTIONS
• None known.

NURSING CONSIDERATIONS
Baseline Assessment
• Check the patient's baseline labo-ratory and diagnostic test results, especially liver function test results, if ordered, before beginning saquinavir therapy and at periodic intervals during therapy.
• Offer emotional support to the patient.
• Expect to obtain the patient's medication history.
Lifespan Considerations
• Breast-feeding is not recom-mended in this patient population because of the possibility of HIV transmission.
• Be aware that the safety and efficacy of saquinavir have not been established in children.
• There is no information on the effects of this drug's use in the elderly.

Precautions
• Use cautiously in patients with diabetes mellitus or liver impairment.

Administration and Handling
PO
• Give within 2 hours after a full meal. Keep in mind that if saquinavir is taken on an empty stomach, the drug may not produce antiviral activity.

Intervention and Evaluation
• Monitor the patient's liver function tests, CD4 cell count, blood glucose, HIV RNA levels, and serum triglyceride levels.
• Closely monitor the patient for signs and symptoms of gastrointestinal (GI) discomfort.
• Assess the patient's pattern of daily bowel activity and stool consistency.
• Inspect the patient's mouth for signs of mucosal ulceration.
• Monitor the patient's blood chemistry test results for marked abnormalities.
• If serious or severe toxicities occur, withhold the drug and notify the physician.

Patient Teaching
• Warn the patient to notify the physician if he or she experiences nausea, numbness, persistent abdominal pain, tingling, or vomiting.
• Encourage the patient to avoid exposure to artificial light sources and sunlight.
• Advise the patient to continue therapy for the full length of treatment and to evenly space drug doses around the clock.
• Explain to the patient that saquinavir is not a cure for HIV infection, nor does it reduce the risk of transmission to others. Also explain that he or she may continue to develop illnesses associated with advanced HIV infection.

• Instruct the patient to take saquinavir within 2 hours after a full meal.
• Warn the patient to avoid grapefruit products while taking saquinavir.

stavudine (d4T)
stay-view-deen
(Zerit)

CATEGORY AND SCHEDULE
Pregnancy Risk Category: C

MECHANISM OF ACTION
Inhibits HIV reverse transcriptase via viral DNA chain termination. Also inhibits RNA- and DNA-dependent DNA polymerase, an enzyme necessary for viral HIV replication. *Therapeutic Effect:* Slows HIV replication, reducing progression of HIV infection.

PHARMACOKINETICS
Rapidly, completely absorbed after PO administration. Undergoes minimal metabolism. Excreted in urine. **Half-life:** 1.5 hrs (half-life is increased with impaired renal function).

AVAILABILITY
Capsules: 15 mg, 20 mg, 30 mg, 40 mg.
Oral Solution: 1 mg/ml.

INDICATIONS AND DOSAGES
▸ **HIV infection**
PO
Adults weighing 60 kg and more.
40 mg twice a day.
Adults weighing less than 60 kg.
30 mg twice a day.
▸ **HIV infection with recent history and complete resolution of symp-**

toms of peripheral neuropathy or elevations in serum concentrations of hepatic transaminases
Adults weighing 60 kg and more.
20 mg twice a day.
Adults weighing less than 60 kg.
15 mg twice a day.
Children weighing more than 30 kg.
20 mg twice a day.
Children weighing less than 30 kg.
2 mg/kg/day.
▸ **Dosage in renal impairment**
Dosage and frequency are modified based on creatinine clearance and patient weight.

Creatinine Clearance (ml/min)	Weight 60 kg or more	Weight less than 60 kg
greater than 50	40 mg q12h	30 mg q12h
26–50	20 mg q12h	15 mg q12h
10–25	20 mg q24h	15 mg q24h

CONTRAINDICATIONS
None known

INTERACTIONS
Drug
None known.
Herbal
None known.
Food
None known.

DIAGNOSTIC TEST EFFECTS
Commonly increases SGOT (AST) and SGPT (ALT) levels. May decrease blood neutrophil count.

SIDE EFFECTS
Frequent
Headache (55%), diarrhea (50%), chills and fever (38%), nausea or vomiting, myalgia (35%), rash (33%), asthenia (loss of strength, energy) (28%), insomnia, abdominal pain (26%), anxiety (22%), arthralgia (18%), back pain (20%), sweating (19%), malaise (17%), depression (14%)
Occasional
Anorexia, weight loss, nervousness, dizziness, conjunctivitis, dyspepsia, dyspnea
Rare
Constipation, vasodilation, confusion, migraine, urticaria, abnormal vision

SERIOUS REACTIONS
• Peripheral neuropathy, characterized by numbness, tingling, or pain in the hands and feet occurs frequently (15%–21%).
• Ulcerative stomatitis (erythema or ulcers of oral mucosa, glossitis, and gingivitis), pneumonia, and benign skin neoplasms occur occasionally.
• Pancreatitis and lactic acidosis occur rarely.

NURSING CONSIDERATIONS

Baseline Assessment
• Check patient's baseline laboratory test results, if ordered, especially liver function test results, before beginning stavudine therapy and at periodic intervals during therapy.
• Offer the patient emotional support.
• Determine the patient's history of peripheral neuropathy.
Lifespan Considerations
• Breast-feeding is not recommended in this patient population because of the possibility of HIV transmission.
• There are no age-related precautions noted in children.
• There is no information on the effects of this drug's use in the elderly.

Precautions
• Use cautiously in patients with a history of peripheral neuropathy or liver or renal impairment.
Administration and Handling
PO
• Give without regard to meals.
Intervention and Evaluation
• Monitor the patient for signs and symptoms of peripheral neuropathy, which is characterized by numbness, pain, or tingling in the feet or hands. Be aware that peripheral neuropathy symptoms resolve promptly if stavudine therapy is discontinued. Also, know that symptoms may worsen temporarily after the drug is withdrawn. If symptoms resolve completely, expect to resume drug therapy at a reduced dosage.
• Assess the patient for dizziness, headache, muscle or joint aches, myalgia, nausea, and vomiting.
• Monitor the patient for evidence of a rash and signs of chills or a fever.
• Determine the patient's pattern of daily bowel activity and stool consistency.
• Assess the patient for a change in sleep pattern.
• Assess the patient's eating pattern and monitor the patient for weight loss.
• Examine the patient's eyes for signs of conjunctivitis.
• Monitor the patient's CD4 cell count, complete blood count (CBC), Hgb and HIV RNA levels, and renal and liver function test results.
Patient Teaching
• Advise the patient to continue stavudine therapy for the full length of treatment and to evenly space doses around the clock.
• Caution the patient not to take any medications, including over-the-counter (OTC) drugs, without first notifying the physician.

• Explain to the patient that stavudine is not a cure for HIV infection, nor does it reduce risk of transmission to others, and that he or she may continue to develop illnesses, including opportunistic infections.
• Warn the patient to report abdominal discomfort, burning, dyspnea, fatigue, nausea, numbness, pain, tingling, vomiting, and weakness to the physician.

tenofovir
ten-**oh**-fah-vir
(Viread)

CATEGORY AND SCHEDULE
Pregnancy Risk Category: B

MECHANISM OF ACTION
A nucleotide analogue that inhibits HIV viral reverse transcriptase by being incorporated into the viral DNA and then by causing DNA chain termination. *Therapeutic Effect:* Slows HIV replication, reduces HIV RNA levels (viral load).

AVAILABILITY
Tablets: 300 mg.

INDICATIONS AND DOSAGES
▸ **HIV infection**
PO
Adults, Elderly, Children 18 yrs and older. 300 mg once a day.

CONTRAINDICATIONS
None known

INTERACTIONS
Drug
Didanosine: May increase didanosine concentrations.

Indinavir, lamivudine, lopinavir, ritonavir: May decrease the blood concentrations of these drugs.

Herbal

None known.

Food

High-fat food: Increases tenofovir bioavailability.

DIAGNOSTIC TEST EFFECTS

May elevate serum transaminase levels. May alter serum CPK, creatinine clearance, GGT, serum uric acid, SGOT (AST), SGPT (ALT), and triglyceride levels.

SIDE EFFECTS

Occasional

Gastrointestinal (GI) disturbances such as diarrhea, flatulence, nausea, and vomiting

SERIOUS REACTIONS

• Lactic acidosis and hepatomegaly with steatosis (excess fat in liver) occur rarely, but may be severe.

NURSING CONSIDERATIONS

Baseline Assessment

• Check patient's baseline laboratory test results, if ordered, especially liver function test results and serum triglyceride levels before beginning tenofovir therapy and at periodic intervals during therapy.

• Offer the patient emotional support.

Precautions

• Use cautiously in patients with impaired liver or renal function.

Administration and Handling

PO

• Give with food.

Intervention and Evaluation

• Closely monitor the patient for signs and symptoms of GI discomfort.

• Assess the patient's pattern of

daily bowel activity and stool consistency.

• Monitor the patient's CD4 cell count, complete blood count (CBC), Hgb levels, HIV RNA plasma levels, liver function test results, and reticulocyte count.

Patient Teaching

• Advise the patient to continue drug therapy for the full length of treatment.

• Explain to the patient that tenofovir is not a cure for HIV infection, nor does it reduce risk of transmission to others. Explain that he or she may continue to develop illnesses associated with advanced HIV infection.

• Instruct the patient to take tenofovir with a meal to increase the drug's absorption.

• Warn the patient to notify the physician if he or she experiences nausea, persistent abdominal pain, or vomiting.

zalcitabine

zal-**site**-ah-bean

(Hivid)

CATEGORY AND SCHEDULE

Pregnancy Risk Category: C

MECHANISM OF ACTION

A nucleoside reverse transcriptase inhibitor that is intracellularly converted to active metabolite. Inhibits viral DNA synthesis. *Therapeutic Effect:* Prevents replication of HIV-1.

PHARMACOKINETICS

Readily absorbed from the gastrointestinal (GI) tract. Food decreases the drug's absorption. Protein binding: less than 4%. Undergoes phosphorylation intracellularly to the active metabolite. Primarily excreted in urine. Removed by hemodialysis. **Half-life:** 1–3 hrs; metabolite: 2.6–10 hrs (half-life is increased with impaired renal function).

AVAILABILITY
Tablets: 0.375 mg, 0.75 mg.

INDICATIONS AND DOSAGES
▶ **HIV infection**
PO
Adults, Children 13 yrs and older. 0.75 mg q8h (may be given with zidovudine).
Children younger than 13 yrs. 0.01 mg/kg q8h. Range: 0.005–0.01 mg/kg q8h.
▶ **Dosage in renal impairment**
Based on creatinine clearance.

Creatinine Clearance	Dose
10–40 ml/min	0.75 mg q12h
less than 10 ml/min	0.75 mg q24h

CONTRAINDICATIONS
Patients with moderate or severe peripheral neuropathy

INTERACTIONS
Drug
Medications associated with peripheral neuropathy, including cisplatin, disulfiram, phenytoin, vincristine: May increase the risk of neuropathy. *Medications causing pancreatitis, including IV pentamidine:* May increase the risk of pancreatitis.
Herbal
None known.
Food
None known.

DIAGNOSTIC TEST EFFECTS
May increase serum alkaline phosphatase, amylase, bilirubin, lipase, SGOT (AST), SGPT (ALT), and triglyceride levels. May decrease serum calcium, magnesium, and phosphates. May alter blood glucose and sodium levels.

SIDE EFFECTS
Frequent (28%–11%)
Peripheral neuropathy, fever, fatigue, headache, rash
Occasional (10%–5%)
Diarrhea, abdominal pain, oral ulcers, cough, pruritus, myalgia, weight loss, nausea, vomiting
Rare (4%–1%)
Fatigue, nasal discharge, dysphagia, depression, night sweats, confusion

SERIOUS REACTIONS
• Peripheral neuropathy occurs commonly (17%–31%) and is characterized by numbness, tingling, burning, and pain of the lower extremities. This situation may be followed by sharp, shooting pain and progress to a severe, continuous, burning pain that may be irreversible if the drug is not discontinued in time.
• Pancreatitis, leukopenia, neutropenia, eosinophilia, and thrombocytopenia occur rarely.

NURSING CONSIDERATIONS
Baseline Assessment
• Offer emotional support to the patient and the patient's family.
• Expect to monitor the patient's complete blood count (CBC), serum amylase, and serum triglyceride levels before and during therapy.
Lifespan Considerations
• Be aware that it is unknown if zalcitabine crosses the placenta or is distributed in breast milk. Breast-feeding is not recommended in this patient population because of the possibility of HIV transmission.
• There are no age-related precautions in children younger than 6 months.

• In children, dosages are not established.
• In the elderly, age-related renal impairment may require dosage adjustment.

Precautions

◀ALERT▶ Use extremely cautiously in patients with preexisting neuropathy and low CD4 cell counts because of an increased risk of developing peripheral neuropathy.
• Use cautiously in patients with a history of alcohol abuse, diabetes, liver disease, peripheral neuropathy, renal impairment, or weight loss.

Administration and Handling

PO
• Zalcitabine is best taken on an empty stomach because food decreases drug absorption.
• May take with food to decrease GI distress.
• Space doses evenly around the clock.

Intervention and Evaluation

• Withhold the drug and notify the physician immediately if signs and symptoms of peripheral neuropathy develop, including burning, numbness, shooting, or tingling pains of the extremities and loss of the ankle reflex or vibratory sense.
◀ALERT▶ Although rare, assess the patient for impending, potentially fatal pancreatitis as evidenced by abdominal pain, increasing serum amylase levels, rising triglyceride levels, nausea, and vomiting. If the patient develops any of these signs or symptoms, particularly abdominal pain, withhold the drug and immediately notify the physician.
• Assess the patient for signs and symptoms of a therapeutic response to drug therapy, including decreased fatigue, increased energy, and weight gain.
• Evaluate the patient's complete blood count (CBC) for evidence of blood dyscrasias.

Patient Teaching

• Explain to the patient that zalcitabine is not a cure for HIV, nor does it reduce transmission of the disease, and that he or she may continue to contract opportunistic illnesses associated with advanced HIV infection.
• Warn the patient to notify the physician if he or she experiences any signs or symptoms of pancreatitis or peripheral neuropathy.
• Caution women of childbearing age to avoid pregnancy. Teach female patients of childbearing age about contraception use.

zidovudine
zye-**dough**-view-deen
(Apo-Zidovudine[CAN], AZT, Novo-AZT[CAN], Retrovir)
Do not confuse with Combivent or ritonavir.

CATEGORY AND SCHEDULE
Pregnancy Risk Category: C

MECHANISM OF ACTION
A nucleoside reverse transcriptase inhibitor that interferes with viral RNA-dependent DNA polymerase, an enzyme necessary for viral HIV replication. *Therapeutic Effect:* Slows HIV replication, reducing progression of HIV infection.

PHARMACOKINETICS
Rapidly, completely absorbed from the gastrointestinal (GI) tract. Protein binding: 25%–38%. Undergoes first-pass metabolism in liver. Widely distributed. Crosses blood-brain barrier, cerebrospinal fluid (CSF). Primarily excreted in urine. Minimal

removal by hemodialysis. **Half-life:** 0.8–1.2 hrs (half-life is increased with impaired renal function).

AVAILABILITY
Capsules: 100 mg.
Tablets: 300 mg.
Syrup: 50 mg/5 ml.
Injection: 10 mg/ml.

INDICATIONS AND DOSAGES
▶ **HIV infection**
IV
Adults, Elderly, Children older than 12 yrs. 1–2 mg/kg/dose q4h.
Children 12 yrs and younger. 120 mg/m²/dose q6h.
Neonates. 1.5 mg/kg/dose q6h.
PO
Adults, Elderly, Children older than 12 yrs. 200 mg q8h or 300 mg q12h.
Children 12 yrs and younger. 160 mg/m²/dose q8h. Range: 90–180 mg/m²/dose q6–8h.
Neonates. 2 mg/kg/dose q6h.

UNLABELED USES
Prophylaxis in patients at risk of acquiring HIV after occupational exposure

CONTRAINDICATIONS
Life-threatening allergies to zidovudine or components of preparation

INTERACTIONS
Drug
Bone marrow depressants, ganciclovir: May increase myelosuppression.
Clarithromycin: May decrease zidovudine blood concentration.
Probenecid: May increase zidovudine blood concentrations and the risk of zidovudine toxicity.
Herbal
None known.

Food
None known.

DIAGNOSTIC TEST EFFECTS
May increase mean corpuscular volume.

IV INCOMPATIBILITIES
None known

IV COMPATIBILITIES
Dexamethasone (Decadron), dobutamine (Dobutrex), dopamine (Intropin), heparin, lorazepam (Ativan), morphine, potassium chloride

SIDE EFFECTS
Expected (46%–42%)
Nausea, headache
Frequent (20%–16%)
GI pain, asthenia (loss of energy, strength), rash, fever
Occasional (12%–8%)
Diarrhea, anorexia, malaise, myalgia, somnolence
Rare (6%–5%)
Dizziness, paresthesia, vomiting, insomnia, dyspnea, altered taste

SERIOUS REACTIONS
• Anemia, occurring most commonly after 4–6 weeks of therapy, and granulocytopenia, particularly significant in those who have low levels before therapy begins, occur rarely.
• Neurotoxicity as evidenced by ataxia, fatigue, lethargy, and nystagmus, as well as seizures may occur.

NURSING CONSIDERATIONS
Baseline Assessment
• Be aware that the patient should not receive drugs that are cytotoxic, myelosuppressive, or nephro-

toxic, because these drugs may increase the risk of zidovudine toxicity.

* Expect to obtain patient specimens for viral diagnostic tests before starting therapy. Therapy may begin before results are obtained.
* Check the patient's hematology reports to establish an accurate baseline.

Lifespan Considerations

* Be aware that it is unknown if zidovudine crosses the placenta or is distributed in breast milk.
* Be aware that it is unknown if fetal harm or effects on fertility can occur from use of this drug.
* There are no age-related precautions noted in children.
* There is no information on the effects of this drug's use in the elderly.

Precautions

* Use cautiously in patients with bone marrow compromise, decreased liver blood flow, and renal and liver dysfunction.

Administration and Handling

PO
* Keep capsules in a cool, dry place. Protect from light.
* Food or milk does not affect GI absorption of zidovudine.
* Space doses evenly around the clock.
* The patient should be in an upright position when giving the medication to prevent esophageal ulceration.

IV
* After dilution, IV solution is stable for 24 hours at room temperature; 48 hours if refrigerated.
* Use within 8 hours if stored at room temperature; 24 hours if refrigerated.

* Do not use if particulate matter is present or discoloration occurs.
* Must dilute before administration. Remove calculated dose from vial and add to D_5W to provide a concentration no greater than 4 mg/ml.
* Infuse over 1 hour.

Intervention and Evaluation

* Monitor the patient's CD4 cell count, complete blood count (CBC), Hgb levels, HIV RNA plasma levels, mean corpuscular volume (MCV), and reticulocyte count.
* Assess the patient for bleeding, dizziness, headache, and insomnia.
* Assess the patient's pattern of daily bowel activity and stool consistency.
* Evaluate the patient's skin for acne or rash.
* Assess the patient for signs and symptoms of opportunistic infections, such as chills, cough, fever, and myalgia.
* Monitor the patient's intake and output, as well as his or her renal and liver function test results.

Patient Teaching

* Advise the patient that zidovudine doses should be evenly spaced around the clock and that blood tests are an essential part of therapy because of the bleeding potential.
* Explain to the patient that zidovudine does not cure HIV or AIDS, but acts to reduce symptoms and slow or arrest disease progression.
* Caution the patient not to take any medications without the physician's prior approval.
* Warn the patient to report bleeding from gums, nose, or rectum to the physician immediately.

- Suggest to the patient that dental work be done before therapy or after blood counts return to normal, which is often weeks after therapy has stopped.
- Warn the patient to notify the physician if he or she experiences difficulty breathing, headache, inability to sleep, muscle weakness, rash, signs of infection, or unusual bleeding.

4 Antitubercular Agents

ethambutol
isoniazid
pyrazinamide
rifabutin
rifampin
rifapentine

Uses: Antitubercular agents are used to treat tuberculosis, an infectious disease usually caused by *Mycobacterium tuberculosis* or *Mycobacterium bovis*. Treatment, which aims to eliminate symptoms and prevent relapse, typically consists of combination drug therapy. By using more than one drug, the risk of drug resistance is minimized. Treatment may require three or more drugs and may continue for 6 to 24 months.

Action: First-line agents act in different ways, combining the greatest efficacy with an acceptable degree of toxicity. For example, *ethambutol* blocks enzymes in mycobacteria, preventing cell wall synthesis. *Isoniazid* inhibits the synthesis of mycolic acids, which are important to mycobacterial cell walls. *Pyrazinamide* affects enzymes involved in mycolic acid synthesis. *Rifabutin, rifampin,* and *rifapentine* inhibit deoxyribonucleic acid (DNA)-dependent ribonucleic acid (RNA) polymerase in mycobacteria. (See illustration, *Sites and Mechanisms of Action: Anti-infective Agents,* page 2.)

COMBINATION PRODUCTS
RIFAMATE: isoniazid/rifampin (an antitubercular) 150 mg/300 mg.
RIFATER: isoniazid/pyrazinamide (an antitubercular)/rifampin (an antitubercular) 50 mg/300 mg/120 mg.

ethambutol
eth-**am**-byoo-toll
(Etibi[CAN], Myambutol)
Do not confuse with Nembutal.

CATEGORY AND SCHEDULE
Pregnancy Risk Category: B

MECHANISM OF ACTION
An isonicotinic acid derivative that interferes with RNA synthesis.

Therapeutic Effect: Suppresses mycobacterial multiplication.

PHARMACOKINETICS
Rapidly, well absorbed from the gastrointestinal (GI) tract. Widely distributed. Protein binding: 20%–30%. Metabolized in liver. Primarily excreted in urine. Removed by hemodialysis. **Half-life:** 3–4 hrs (half-life is increased with impaired renal function).

AVAILABILITY
Tablets: 100 mg, 400 mg.

INDICATIONS AND DOSAGES
▸ **Tuberculosis**
PO
Adults, Elderly, Children. 15–25 mg/kg/day as a single dose or

50 mg/kg 2 times/wk. Maximum:
2.5 g/dose.
▸ **Nontuberculosis mycobacterium**
PO
Adults, Elderly, Children. 15 mg/
kg/day. Maximum: 1 g/day.
▸ **Dosage in renal impairment**

Creatinine Clearance	Dosage Interval
10–50 ml/min	q24–36h
less than 10 ml/min	q48h

UNLABELED USES

Treatment of atypical mycobacterial infections

CONTRAINDICATIONS

Optic neuritis

INTERACTIONS

Drug
Neurotoxic medications: May increase the risk of neurotoxicity.
Herbal
None known.
Food
None known.

DIAGNOSTIC TEST EFFECTS

May increase serum uric acid levels.

SIDE EFFECTS

Occasional
Acute gouty arthritis (as evidenced by chills, pain, swelling of joints with hot skin), confusion, abdominal pain, nausea, vomiting, anorexia, headache
Rare
Rash, fever, blurred vision, eye pain, red-green color blindness

SERIOUS REACTIONS

• Optic neuritis (occurs more often with high ethambutol dosage or long-term ethambutol therapy),

peripheral neuritis, and thrombocytopenia, and anaphylactoid reaction occur rarely.

NURSING CONSIDERATIONS

Baseline Assessment
• Evaluate the patient's initial complete blood count (CBC) and renal and liver function test results.
Lifespan Considerations
• Be aware that ethambutol crosses the placenta and is excreted in breast milk.
• Be aware that the safety and efficacy of ethambutol have not been established in children younger than 13 years of age.
• In the elderly, age-related renal impairment may require dosage adjustment.
Precautions
• Use cautiously in patients with cataracts, diabetic retinopathy, gout, recurrent ocular inflammatory conditions, and renal dysfunction.
• Ethambutol use is not recommended for children younger than 13 years of age.
Administration and Handling
PO
• Give with food to decrease GI upset.
Intervention and Evaluation
• Assess the patient for the first signs of vision changes, including altered color perception and decreased visual acuity. If vision changes occur, discontinue the drug and notify the physician immediately.
• Give ethambutol to the patient with food if GI distress occurs.
• Monitor the patient's serum uric acid levels. Also, assess the patient for signs and symptoms of gout, including hot, painful, or swollen joints, especially in the ankle, big toe, or knee.
• Assess the patient for signs and

symptoms of peripheral neuritis as evidenced by burning, numbness, or tingling of the extremities. Notify the physician if peripheral neuritis occurs.

Patient Teaching

• Advise the patient not to skip drug doses and to take ethambutol for the full length of therapy, which may be months or years.

• Warn the patient to notify the physician immediately of any visual problems. Explain to the patient that visual effects are generally reversible after ethambutol is discontinued, and that in rare cases visual problems may take up to a year to disappear or may become permanent.

• Warn the patient to promptly report burning, numbness, or tingling of the feet or hands, and pain and swelling of joints.

---

isoniazid
eye-sew-**nye**-ah-zid
(INH, Isotamine[CAN], Nydrazid, PMS Isoniazid[CAN])

CATEGORY AND SCHEDULE
Pregnancy Risk Category: C

MECHANISM OF ACTION
An isonicotinic acid derivative that inhibits mycolic acid synthesis. Active only during bacterial cell division. *Therapeutic Effect:* Causes disruption of bacterial cell wall and loss of acid-fast properties in susceptible mycobacteria. Bactericidal.

PHARMACOKINETICS
Readily absorbed from the gastrointestinal (GI) tract. Protein binding: 10%–15%. Widely distributed (including cerebrospinal fluid [CSF]). Metabolized in liver. Primarily

excreted in urine. Removed by hemodialysis. **Half-life:** 0.5–5 hrs.

AVAILABILITY
Tablets: 100 mg, 300 mg.
Syrup: 50 mg/5 ml.
Injection: 100 mg/ml.

INDICATIONS AND DOSAGES
▸ **To treat tuberculosis**
PO/IM
Adults, Elderly. 5 mg/kg/day (Maximum 300 mg/day) as a single dose.
Children. 10–15 mg/kg/day (Maximum 300 mg/day) as a single dose.
▸ **To prevent tuberculosis**
PO/IM
Adults, Elderly. 300 mg/day as a single dose.
Children. 10 mg/kg/day (maximum 300 mg/day) as a single dose.

CONTRAINDICATIONS
Acute liver disease, history of hypersensitivity reactions or liver injury with previous isoniazid therapy

INTERACTIONS
Drug
Alcohol: May increase hepatotoxicity and isoniazid metabolism.
Carbamazepine, phenytoin: May increase the toxicity of these drugs.
Disulfiram: May increase central nervous system (CNS) effects.
Hepatotoxic medications: May increase hepatotoxicity.
Ketoconazole: May decrease blood concentration of this drug.
Herbal
None known.
Food
None known.

DIAGNOSTIC TEST EFFECTS
May increase serum bilirubin, SGOT (AST), and SGPT (ALT) levels.

SIDE EFFECTS
Frequent
Nausea, vomiting, diarrhea, abdominal pain
Rare
Pain at injection site, hypersensitivity reaction

SERIOUS REACTIONS
• Neurotoxicity, as evidenced by clumsiness or unsteadiness and numbness, tingling, burning, or pain in the hands and feet, optic neuritis, and liver toxicity occur rarely.

NURSING CONSIDERATIONS

Baseline Assessment
◀ALERT▶ Determine the patient's history of hypersensitivity reactions or liver injury from isoniazid, as well as his or her sensitivity to nicotinic acid or chemically related medications before starting drug therapy.
• Before beginning therapy, be sure that appropriate specimens are obtained from the patient for culture and sensitivity testing.
• Evaluate the patient's initial liver function test results.

Lifespan Considerations
• Be aware that prophylactic use of isoniazid is usually postponed until after childbirth.
• Be aware that isoniazid crosses the placenta and is distributed in breast milk.
• There are no age-related precautions noted in children.
• The elderly are more susceptible to developing hepatitis.

Precautions
• Use cautiously in patients who are alcoholics or have chronic liver disease or severe renal impairment because these patients may be cross sensitive to nicotinic acid or other chemically related medications.

Administration and Handling
PO
• Give 1 hour before or 2 hours after meals. May give with food to decrease GI upset, but this will delay isoniazid absorption.
• Administer at least 1 hour before antacids, especially those containing aluminum.

Intervention and Evaluation
◀ALERT▶ Monitor the patient's liver function test results. Also, assess the patient for signs and symptoms of hepatitis as evidenced by anorexia, dark urine, fatigue, jaundice, nausea, vomiting, and weakness. If you suspect hepatitis, withhold the drug and notify the physician promptly.
• Assess the patient for burning, numbness, and tingling of the extremities. Be aware that patients at risk for neuropathy, such as alcoholics, those with chronic liver disease, diabetics, the elderly, and malnourished individuals, may receive pyridoxine prophylactically.
• Be alert for signs and symptoms of hypersensitivity reaction, including fever and skin eruptions.

Patient Teaching
• Advise the patient not to skip doses and to continue taking isoniazid for the full length of therapy (6 to 24 months).
• Instruct the patient to take the drug preferably 1 hour before or 2 hours after meals. Explain that the medication may be taken with food if GI upset occurs.
• Urge the patient to avoid consuming alcohol during treatment.
• Caution the patient not to take any other medications without first notifying the physician, including antacids. Explain to the patient that he or she must take isoniazid at least 1 hour before taking an antacid.
• Warn the patient to avoid foods

containing tyramine, including aged cheeses, sauerkraut, smoked fish, and tuna because these foods may cause a reaction such as headache, a hot or clammy feeling, lightheadedness, pounding heartbeat, and red or itching skin. Warn the patient to notify the physician if any of these reactions occur. Also, provide the patient with a list of tyramine-containing foods.

• Warn the patient to notify the physician of any new symptoms, immediately for dark urine, fatigue, nausea, numbness or tingling of the feet or hands, vision difficulties, vomiting, and yellowing of the skin and eyes.

pyrazinamide
peer-a-**zin**-a-mide
(Pyrazinamide, Tebrazid[CAN], Zinamide[AUS])

CATEGORY AND SCHEDULE
Pregnancy Risk Category: C

MECHANISM OF ACTION
An antitubercular whose exact mechanism is unknown. *Therapeutic Effect:* Pyrazinamide is either bacteriostatic or bactericidal, depending on its concentration at the infection site and the susceptibility of infecting bacteria.

AVAILABILITY
Tablets: 500 mg.

INDICATIONS AND DOSAGES
▸ **Tuberculosis**
PO
Adults. 15–30 mg/kg/day in 1–4 doses. Maximum: 2 g/day.
Children. 20–40 mg/kg/day in 1 or 2 doses. Maximum: 2 g/day.

CONTRAINDICATIONS
Severe liver dysfunction

INTERACTIONS
Drug
Allopurinol, colchicine, probenecid, sulfinpyrazone: May decrease the effects of these drugs.
Herbal
None known.
Food
None known.

DIAGNOSTIC TEST EFFECTS
May increase SGOT (AST) and SGPT (ALT) levels and serum uric acid concentrations.

SIDE EFFECTS
Frequent
Arthralgia, myalgia (usually mild and self-limiting)
Rare
Hypersensitivity (rash, pruritus, urticaria), photosensitivity

SERIOUS REACTIONS
• Hepatotoxicity, thrombocytopenia, and anemia occur rarely.

NURSING CONSIDERATIONS
Baseline Assessment
• Determine the patient's hypersensitivity to ethionamide, isoniazid, niacin, and pyrazinamide.
• Ensure the collection of patient specimens for culture and sensitivity tests before beginning drug therapy.
• Evaluate the results of the patient's initial complete blood count (CBC), liver function tests, and serum uric acid levels.
Precautions
• Use cautiously in patients with diabetes mellitus, a history of gout, and renal impairment.

• Use cautiously in patients with a possible cross-sensitivity to ethionamide, isoniazid, and niacin.
• Be aware that the safety and efficacy of pyrazinamide have not been established in children.

Intervention and Evaluation

• Monitor the patient's liver function test results and be alert for liver reactions such as anorexia, fever, jaundice, liver tenderness, malaise, nausea, and vomiting. If any liver reactions occur, stop the drug and notify the physician promptly.
• Check the patient's serum uric acid levels and assess for signs and symptoms of gout, such as hot, painful, swollen joints, especially the ankle, big toe, or knee.
• Evaluate the patient's blood glucose levels, especially in patients with diabetes mellitus, because pyrazinamide administration may make diabetic management difficult.
• Assess the patient's skin for rash or skin eruptions.
• Monitor the patient's CBC for anemia and development of thrombocytopenia.

Patient Teaching

• Advise the patient not to skip drug doses and to complete the full length of therapy, which may be months or years.
• Explain to the patient that follow-up physician office visits and lab tests are essential parts of treatment.
• Instruct the patient to take pyrazinamide with food to reduce GI upset.
• Encourage the patient to avoid overexposure to sun or ultraviolet light to prevent photosensitivity reactions.
• Warn the patient to immediately notify the physician of any new symptoms, especially fever, hot, painful, swollen joints; unusual tiredness, or yellow eyes or skin.

rifabutin
rye-fah-**byew**-tin
(Mycobutin)
Do not confuse with rifampin.

CATEGORY AND SCHEDULE
Pregnancy Risk Category: B

MECHANISM OF ACTION
An antitubercular that inhibits DNA-dependent RNA polymerase, an enzyme in susceptible strains of *E. coli* and *Bacillus subtilis*. *Therapeutic Effect:* Prevents *Mycobacterium avium* complex (MAC) disease.

PHARMACOKINETICS
Readily absorbed from the gastrointestinal (GI) tract. High-fat meals slow absorption. Protein binding: 85%. Widely distributed. Crosses blood-brain barrier. Extensive intracellular tissue uptake. Metabolized in liver to active metabolite. Excreted in urine; eliminated in feces. Unknown if removed by hemodialysis. **Half-life:** 16–69 hrs.

AVAILABILITY
Capsules: 150 mg.

INDICATIONS AND DOSAGES
▸ **Prophylaxis (first episode M. avium complex [MAC])**
PO
Adults, Elderly. 300 mg as a single or in 2 divided doses.
▸ **Prophylaxis (recurrent MAC)**
PO
Adults, Elderly. 300 mg/day (in combination)

▸ **Dosage in renal impairment**
Creatinine Clearance less
than 30 ml/min, reduce dose
by 50%.

CONTRAINDICATIONS
Active tuberculosis, hypersensitivity
to other rifamycins, including
rifampin

INTERACTIONS
Drug
Oral contraceptives: May decrease
the effects of these drugs.
Zidovudine: May decrease blood
concentration of zidovudine, but
does not affect the inhibition of
HIV by zidovudine.
Herbal
None known.
Food
None known.

DIAGNOSTIC TEST EFFECTS
May increase serum alkaline phosphatase, SGOT (AST), and SGPT
(ALT) levels. May cause anemia,
leukopenia, neutropenia, or thrombocytopenia.

SIDE EFFECTS
Frequent (30%)
Red-orange or red-brown discoloration of urine, feces, saliva, skin,
sputum, sweat, or tears
Occasional (11%–3%)
Rash, nausea, abdominal pain,
diarrhea, dyspepsia (heartburn,
indigestion, epigastric pain), belching, headache, altered taste, uveitis,
corneal deposits
Rare (2% or less)
Anorexia, flatulence, fever, myalgia,
vomiting, insomnia

SERIOUS REACTIONS
• Hepatitis and thrombocytopenia
occur rarely.

NURSING CONSIDERATIONS
Baseline Assessment
• Expect the patient to undergo
a biopsy of suspicious nodes, if
present. Also, expect to obtain
blood or sputum cultures and a
chest x-ray to rule out active tuberculosis.
• If ordered, obtain the patient's
baseline complete blood count
(CBC) and liver function test
results.
Lifespan Considerations
• Be aware that it is unknown if
rifabutin crosses the placenta or is
excreted in breast milk.
• There are no age-related precautions noted in children or the
elderly.
Precautions
• Use cautiously in patients with
liver or renal impairment.
• The safety of this drug for use in
children is not established.
Administration and Handling
PO
• Give without regard to food. Give
with food if GI irritation occurs.
• May mix with applesauce if the
patient is unable to swallow capsules whole.
Intervention and Evaluation
• Monitor the patient's CBC and
platelet count and Hgb, Hct, and
liver function test results.
• Avoid giving the patient IM injections, taking the patient's rectal
temperature, and any other trauma
that may induce bleeding.
• Check the patient's body temperature and notify the physician of
flu-like syndrome, GI intolerance,
or rash.
Patient Teaching
• Inform the patient that his or her
feces, perspiration, saliva, skin,
sputum, tears, and urine may be
discolored brown-orange during

drug therapy. Also warn the patient that soft contact lenses may be permanently discolored.
• Caution the patient that rifabutin may decrease the effectiveness of oral contraceptives. Teach the patient about alternative methods of contraception.
• Warn the patient to avoid crowds and those with known infection.
• Warn the patient to notify the physician if he or she experiences dark urine, flu-like symptoms, nausea, unusual bleeding or bruising, any visual disturbances, or vomiting.

rifampin
rif-**am**-pin
(Rifadin, Rimactane, Rimycin[aus], Rofact[can])
Do not confuse with rifabutin, Rifamate, rifapentine, or Ritalin.

CATEGORY AND SCHEDULE
Pregnancy Risk Category: C

MECHANISM OF ACTION
This antitubercular interferes with bacterial RNA synthesis by binding to DNA-dependent RNA polymerase, preventing attachment of the enzyme to DNA, and thereby blocking RNA transcription. *Therapeutic Effect:* Bactericidal activity occurs in susceptible microorganisms.

PHARMACOKINETICS
Well absorbed from the gastrointestinal (GI) tract (food delays absorption). Protein binding: 80%. Widely distributed. Metabolized in liver to active metabolite. Primarily eliminated via biliary system. Not removed by hemodialysis. **Half-life:** 3–5 hrs (increased in liver impairment).

AVAILABILITY
Capsules: 150 mg, 300 mg.
Powder for Injection: 600 mg.

INDICATIONS AND DOSAGES
▸ **Tuberculosis**
IV/PO
Adults, Elderly. 10 mg/kg/day. Maximum: 600 mg/day.
Children. 10–20 mg/kg/day in divided doses q12–24h.
▸ **Meningococcal prophylaxis**
IV/PO
Adults, Elderly. 600 mg q12h for 2 days.
Children. 20 mg/kg/day in divided doses q12–24h. Maximum: 600 mg/dose.
Infants younger than 1 mo. 10 mg/kg/day in divided doses q12h for 2 days.
▸ **Staphylococcal infections**
IV/PO
Adults, Elderly. 600 mg once a day.
Children. 15 mg/kg/day in divided doses q12h.
▸ **Synergy for *S. aureas* infections**
PO
Adults, Elderly. 300–600 mg 2 times/day (in combination).
Neonates. 5–20 mg/kg/day in divided doses q12h (in combination).
▸ ***H influenza* prophylaxis**
PO
Adults, Elderly. 600 mg/day for 4 days.
Children 1 mo and older. 20 mg/kg/day in divided doses q12h for 5–10 days.
Children younger than 1 mo. 10 mg/kg/day in divided doses q12h for 2 days.

UNLABELED USES
Prophylaxis of *H. influenzae* type b infection; treatment of atypical

mycobacterial infection, serious infections caused by *Staphylococcus* species

CONTRAINDICATIONS
Concomitant therapy with amprenavir, hypersensitivity to rifampin or any rifamycins

INTERACTIONS
Drug
Alcohol, liver toxic medications: May increase risk of liver toxicity.
Aminophylline, theophylline: May increase creatinine clearance of these drugs.
Chloramphenicol, digoxin, disopyramide, fluconazole, methadone, mexiletine, oral anticoagulants, oral hypoglycemics, phenytoin, quinidine, tocainide, verapamil: May decrease the effects of these drugs.
Herbal
None known.
Food
None known.

DIAGNOSTIC TEST EFFECTS
May increase serum alkaline phosphatase, bilirubin, and uric acid, as well as SGOT (AST) and SGPT (ALT) levels.

IV INCOMPATIBILITIES
Diltiazem (Cardizem)

SIDE EFFECTS
Expected
Red-orange or red-brown discoloration of feces, saliva, skin, sputum, sweat, tears, or urine
Occasional (5%–2%)
Hypersensitivity reaction, such as flushing, pruritus, or rash
Rare (2%–1%)
Diarrhea, dyspepsia, nausea, fungal overgrowth as evidenced by sore mouth or tongue

SERIOUS REACTIONS
• Liver toxicity (risk is increased when rifampin is taken with isoniazid), hepatitis, blood dyscrasias, Stevens-Johnson syndrome, and antibiotic-associated colitis occur rarely.

NURSING CONSIDERATIONS
Baseline Assessment
• Determine the patient's hypersensitivity to rifampin and rifamycins before beginning drug therapy.
• Ensure the collection of patient specimens for culture and sensitivity tests before beginning drug therapy.
• Evaluate the patient's initial complete blood count (CBC) and liver function test results.
Precautions
• Use cautiously in patients with active alcoholism, a history of alcohol abuse, or liver dysfunction.
Lifespan Considerations
• Be aware that rifampin crosses the placenta and is distributed in breast milk.
• There are no age-related precautions noted in children or the elderly.
Administration and Handling
PO
• Preferably give rifampin 1 hour before or 2 hours after meals with 8 oz of water. Rifampin may be given with food to decrease GI upset; but this will delay the drug's absorption.
• For those patients unable to swallow capsules, rifampin's contents may be mixed with applesauce or jelly.
• Give rifampin at least 1 hour before administering antacids, especially antacids containing aluminum.

IV

◀**ALERT**▶ Administer rifampin by IV infusion only. Avoid IM and subcutaneous administration.

• Reconstituted vial is stable for 24 hours.

• Once the reconstituted vial is further diluted, it is stable for 4 hours in D_5W or 24 hours in 0.9% NaCl.

• Reconstitute 600-mg vial with 10 ml Sterile Water for Injection to provide a concentration of 60 mg/ml.

• Withdraw the desired dose and further dilute with 500 ml D_5W.

• Evaluate the patient periodically for extravasation as evidenced by local inflammation and irritation.

• Infuse over 3 hours (may dilute with 100 ml D_5W and infuse over 30 minutes).

Intervention and Evaluation

• Assess the patient's IV site at least hourly during infusion. At the first sign of extravasation, restart the IV at another site.

• Monitor the patient's liver function test results and assess the patient for signs and symptoms of hepatitis as evidenced by anorexia, fatigue, nausea, jaundice, vomiting, and weakness. If any signs or symptoms of hepatitis occur, withhold rifampin and inform the physician immediately.

• Report hypersensitivity reactions such as flu-like syndromes and skin eruptions promptly.

• Assess the patient's pattern of daily bowel activity and stool consistency.

• Monitor CBC results for blood dyscrasias and observe the patient for bleeding, bruising, infection manifested as a fever or sore throat, and unusual tiredness and weakness.

Patient Teaching

• Instruct the patient to take rifampin on an empty stomach with 8 oz of water 1 hour before or 2 hours after a meal. If GI upset occurs, tell the patient that he or she can take rifampin with food.

• Warn the patient to avoid consuming alcohol while taking this drug.

• Explain to the patient that he or she should not take any other medications, including antacids, while taking rifampin without first consulting the physician. Teach the patient to take rifampin at least 1 hour before taking an antacid.

• Inform the patient that his or her feces, sputum, sweat, tears, or urine may become red-orange colored and that soft contact lenses may be permanently stained.

• Warn the patient to notify the physician of any new symptoms and to notify the physician immediately if he or she experiences fatigue, fever, flu, nausea, unusual bleeding or bruising, vomiting, weakness, or yellow eyes and skin.

• Caution women taking oral contraceptives to check with the physician. Explain that the reliability of oral contraceptives may be affected by rifampin. Teach the female patient about barrier contraception.

rifapentine
rif-ah-**pen**-teen
(Priftin)

CATEGORY AND SCHEDULE
Pregnancy Risk Category: C

MECHANISM OF ACTION
An antitubercular that inhibits DNA-dependent RNA polymerase in *Mycobacterium tuberculosis*.

Interferes with bacterial RNA synthesis, preventing attachment of enzyme to DNA, thereby blocking RNA transcription. *Therapeutic Effect:* Bactericidal activity.

AVAILABILITY
Tablets: 150 mg.

INDICATIONS AND DOSAGES
▸ **Tuberculosis**
PO
Adults, Elderly. Intensive phase: 600 mg 2 times/wk for 2 mos (interval between doses no less than 3 days). Continuation phase: 600 mg weekly for 4 mos.

CONTRAINDICATIONS
None known

INTERACTIONS
Drug
None known.
Herbal
None known.
Food
None known.

DIAGNOSTIC TEST EFFECTS
None known.

SIDE EFFECTS
Rare (less than 4%)
Red-orange or red-brown discoloration of feces, saliva, skin, sputum, sweat, tears or urine, arthralgia, pain, nausea, vomiting, headache, dyspepsia (epigastric pain, heartburn, indigestion), hypertension, dizziness, diarrhea

SERIOUS REACTIONS
• Hyperuricemia, neutropenia, proteinuria, and hematuria occur rarely.

NURSING CONSIDERATIONS
Baseline Assessment
• Evaluate the patient's initial complete blood count (CBC) and liver function test results.
Precautions
• Use cautiously in alcoholic patients and patients with liver function impairment.
Administration and Handling
◀ALERT▶ Be aware that rifapentine is used only in combination with another antituberculosis agent.
Intervention and Evaluation
• Monitor the patient's liver function test results.
• Assess the patient's pattern of daily bowel activity and stool consistency.
• Evaluate the patient for diarrhea, gastrointestinal (GI) upset, nausea, or vomiting.
Patient Teaching
• Inform the patient that his or her feces, sputum, sweat, tears, and urine may become red-orange or red-brown colored and that soft contact lenses may be permanently stained.
• Caution women taking oral contraceptives to check with the physician. Explain that the reliability of oral contraceptives may be affected by rifapentine. Teach the female patient about barrier contraception.
• Warn the patient to notify the physician if he or she experiences dark urine, decreased appetite, fever, nausea, pain or swelling of the joints, vomiting, or yellow skin and eyes.

acyclovir
adefovir dipivoxil
amantadine
  hydrochloride
cidofovir
famciclovir
fomivirsen
foscarnet sodium
ganciclovir sodium
oseltamivir
ribavirin
rimantadine
  hydrochloride
valacyclovir
valganciclovir
  hydrochloride
zanamivir

Uses: Antiviral agents are used to treat cytomegalovirus (CMV) retinitis in patients with acquired immunodeficiency syndrome (AIDS), acute herpes zoster infection (shingles), recurrent genital herpes infection, chickenpox, influenza A viral illness, and mucosal and cutaneous infections with herpes simplex virus.

Action: To be effective, antiviral agents must inhibit virus-specific nucleic acid and protein synthesis. They may act by interfering with viral deoxyribonucleic acid (DNA) synthesis and viral replication, inactivating viral DNA polymerases, incorporating into and halting the growth of viral DNA chains, preventing the release of viral nucleic acid into host cells, or blocking viral penetration into cells. (See illustration, *Sites and Mechanisms of Action: Anti-infective Agents,* page 2.)

COMBINATION PRODUCTS

REBETRON: ribavirin/interferon alfa-2b (an immunologic agent) Packaged as ribavirin (Rebetol) 200 mg capsules together with recombinant interferon alfa-2b (Intron A) injection as 3 million international units per 0.5 ml or 3 million international units per 0.2 ml.

acyclovir

aye-**sigh**-klo-veer
(Aciclovir-BC IV[AUS],
Acihexal[AUS], Acyclo-V[AUS],
Avirax[CAN], Lovir[AUS], Zovirax,
Zyclir[AUS])
Do not confuse with Zostrix.

CATEGORY AND SCHEDULE

Pregnancy Risk Category: B

MECHANISM OF ACTION

A synthetic nucleoside that converts to acyclovir triphosphate, becoming part of the DNA chain. *Therapeutic Effect:* Interferes with DNA synthesis and viral replication. Virustatic.

PHARMACOKINETICS

Poorly absorbed from the gastrointestinal (GI) tract; minimal absorption following topical application. Protein binding: 9%–36%. Widely distributed. Partially metabolized in liver. Excreted primarily in urine. Removed by hemodialysis. **Half-life:** 2.5 hrs (increased in impaired renal function).

AVAILABILITY

Tablets: 400 mg, 800 mg.
Capsules: 200 mg.
Oral Suspension: 200 mg/5 ml.
Powder for Injection: 500 mg, 1,000 mg.

Ointment: 5%/50 mg.
Cream: 5%.

INDICATIONS AND DOSAGES
▶ **Herpes simplex**
IV
Adults, Elderly, Children older than 12 yrs. 5 mg/kg/dose q8h for 5–10 days.
▶ **Genital herpes**
PO
Adults, Elderly, Children older than 12 yrs. 200 mg q4h (5 times/day) for 10 days (initial episode) or 5 days (recurrent episode).
▶ **Varicella zoster (chickenpox)**
IV
Adults, Elderly, Children older than 12 yrs. 10 mg/kg/dose q8h for 7 days.
PO
Adults, Elderly. 600–800 mg/dose q4h (5 times/day) for 7–10 days or 1000 mg q6h for 5 days.
Children. 10–20 mg/kg/dose (Maximum: 800 mg) 4 times/day for 5 days.
▶ **Herpes zoster (shingles)**
IV
Adults, Children. 10 mg/kg/dose q8h.
Elderly. 7.5 mg/kg/dose
PO
Adults. 800 mg q4h (5 times/day) for 7–10 days.
Children. 250–600 mg/m^2/dose 4–5 times/day for 7–10 days.
Topical
Adults, Elderly. 3–6 times/day for 7 days.
▶ **Dosage in renal impairment**
Dosage and frequency are modified based on severity of infection and degree of renal impairment.
PO
Creatinine clearance of less than or equal to 10 ml/1.73 m^2: 200 mg q12h.

IV

Creatinine Clearance (ml/min)	Dosage Percent	Dosage Interval
greater than 50	100	8 hrs
25–50	100	12 hrs
10–25	100	24 hrs
less than 10	50	24 hrs

UNLABELED USES
Herpes simplex ocular infections, infectious mononucleosis

CONTRAINDICATIONS
Acyclovir reconstituted with bacteriostatic water containing benzyl alcohol should not be used in neonates

INTERACTIONS
Drug
Nephrotoxic medications (e.g., aminoglycosides): May increase nephrotoxicity of acyclovir.
Probenecid: May increase half-life of acyclovir.
Herbal
None known.
Food
None known.

DIAGNOSTIC TEST EFFECTS
May increase BUN, serum creatinine concentrations.

IV INCOMPATIBILITIES
Aztreonam (Azactam), cefepime (Maxipime), diltiazem (Cardizem), dobutamine (Dobutrex), dopamine (Intropin), levofloxacin (Levaquin), meropenem (Merrem IV), ondansetron (Zofran), piperacillin-tazobactam (Zosyn)

IV COMPATIBILITIES
Allopurinol (Alloprim), amikacin (Amikin), ampicillin, cefazolin

(Ancef), cefotaxime (Claforan), ceftazidime (Fortaz), ceftriaxone (Rocephin), cimetidine (Tagamet), clindamycin (Cleocin), famotidine (Pepcid), fluconazole (Diflucan), gentamicin, heparin, hydromorphone (Dilaudid), imipenem (Primaxin), lorazepam (Ativan), magnesium sulfate, methylprednisolone (SoluMedrol), metoclopramide (Reglan), metronidazole (Flagyl), morphine, multivitamins, potassium chloride, propofol (Diprivan), ranitidine (Zantac), trimethoprim-sulfamethoxazole (Bactrim, Septa), vancomycin

SIDE EFFECTS
Frequent
Parenteral (9%–7%): Phlebitis or inflammation at IV site, nausea, vomiting
Topical (28%): Burning, stinging
Occasional
Parenteral (3%): Itching, rash, hives
Oral (12%–6%): Malaise, nausea, headache
Topical (4%): Itching
Rare
Parenteral (2%–1%): Confusion, hallucinations, seizures, tremors
Topical (less than 1%): Skin rash
Oral (3%–1%): Vomiting, rash, diarrhea, headache

SERIOUS REACTIONS
• Rapid parenteral administration, excessively high doses, or fluid and electrolyte imbalance may produce renal failure exhibited by such signs and symptoms as abdominal pain, decreased urination, decreased appetite, increased thirst, nausea, and vomiting.
• Toxicity not reported with oral or topical use.

NURSING CONSIDERATIONS
Baseline Assessment
• Determine if the patient has a history of allergies, particularly to acyclovir.
• Assess herpes simplex lesions before treatment to compare baseline with treatment effect.
Lifespan Considerations
• Acyclovir crosses the placenta and is distributed in breast milk.
• Be aware that safety and efficacy have not been established in children less than 2 years of age or less than 1 year of age for IV use.
• In the elderly, age-related renal impairment may require dosage adjustment.
Precautions
• Use cautiously in patients with concurrent use of nephrotoxic agents, dehydration, fluid and electrolyte imbalance, neurologic abnormalities or renal or hepatic impairment.
Administration and Handling
PO
• May give without regard to food.
• Do not crush or break capsules.
• Store capsules at room temperature.
Topical
• Avoid eye contact.
• Use finger cot or rubber glove to prevent autoinoculation.
IV
• Store vials at room temperature. Solutions of 50 mg/ml will remain stable for 12 hours at room temperature; may form precipitate when refrigerated. Potency not affected by precipitate and redissolution.
• IV infusion (piggyback) stable for 24 hours at room temperature. Yellow discoloration does not affect potency.
• Add 10 ml sterile water for injec-

tion to each 500-mg vial (50 mg/ml). Do not use bacteriostatic water for injection containing benzyl alcohol or parabens because this will cause a precipitate to form.
• Shake well until solution is clear.
• Further dilute with at least 100 ml D5W or 0.9% NaCl. Final concentration should be less than or equal to 7 mg/ml.
• Infuse over at least 1 hour because renal tubular damage may occur with too rapid administration.
• Maintain adequate hydration during infusion and for two hours following IV administration.

Intervention and Evaluation
• Assess IV site for signs and symptoms of phlebitis, including heat, pain, or red streaking over the vein.
• Evaluate cutaneous lesions for signs of effective drug treatment.
• Ensure adequate ventilation.
• Be sure to maintain appropriate isolation precautions in patients with chickenpox and disseminated herpes zoster.
• Provide analgesics and comfort measures, especially to the elderly.
• Encourage the patient to drink water.

Patient Teaching
• Encourage the patient to drink adequate fluids.
• Advise the patient to avoid touching lesions with fingers to prevent spreading infection to new sites.
• Urge the genital herpes patient to continue therapy for the full length of treatment and to evenly space doses around the clock.
• Instruct the patient to use a finger cot or rubber glove to apply topical ointment.
• Caution the patient to avoid sexual intercourse while visible lesions are present to prevent infecting his or her partner.

• Warn the patient that acyclovir does not cure herpes.
• Encourage the female patient to have a pap smear at least annually because of the increased risk of cervix cancer of cervix in women with genital herpes.

adefovir dipivoxil
(add-eh-**foe**-vur)
Hepsera
CATEGORY AND SCHEDULE
Pregnancy Risk Category: C

MECHANISM OF ACTION
An antiviral that inhibits the enzyme DNA polymerase, causing DNA chain termination after its incorporation into viral DNA. *Therapeutic Effect:* Prevents DNA cell replication.

PHARMACOKINETICS
Following oral administration, binds to proteins. Excreted in the urine. **Half-life:** 7 hrs (half-life is increased with impaired renal function).

AVAILABILITY
Tablets: 10 mg.

INDICATIONS AND DOSAGES
▸ **Chronic hepatitis B in patients with normal renal function**
PO
Adults, Elderly. 10 mg once a day.
▸ **Chronic hepatitis B in patients with impaired renal function**
Adults, Elderly with creatinine clearance 50 ml/min or more. 10 mg q24h.
Adults, Elderly with creatinine clearance 20–49 ml/min. 10 mg q48h.

Adults, Elderly with creatinine clearance 10–19 ml/min. 10 mg q72h.
Adults, Elderly on hemodialysis. 10 mg every 7 days following dialysis.

CONTRAINDICATIONS
None known.

INTERACTIONS
Drug
Ibuprofen: Increases adefovir plasma concentration.
Herbal
None known.
Food
None known.

DIAGNOSTIC TEST EFFECTS
May increase serum amylase, serum creatinine, SGOT (AST), and SGPT (ALT) levels.

SIDE EFFECTS
Frequent (13%)
Asthenia (loss of energy, strength)
Occasional (9%–4%)
Headache, abdominal pain, nausea, flatulence
Rare (3%)
Diarrhea, dyspepsia (epigastric discomfort, heartburn)

SERIOUS REACTIONS
• Nephrotoxicity characterized by an increase in serum creatinine and decrease in serum phosphorus is a treatment-limiting toxicity of adefovir therapy.
• Lactic acidosis and severe hepatomegaly may occur rarely, particularly in female patients.

NURSING CONSIDERATIONS
Baseline Assessment
• As ordered, obtain baseline renal function laboratory values before therapy begins and routinely thereafter.

• Expect to adjust adefovir dosage in those patients with pre-existing renal insufficiency.
• Expect to obtain a blood specimen for HIV antibody testing before therapy begins because unrecognized or untreated HIV infection may result in an emergence of HIV resistance.
Precautions
• Use cautiously in patients with impaired renal function and known risk factors for liver disease.
• Use cautiously in elderly patients.
Administration and Handling
PO
• Give adefovir without regard to food.
Intervention and Evaluation
• Monitor the patient's intake and output and serum creatinine levels.
• Closely monitor the patient for serious reactions, especially in those patients taking other medications that are excreted by the kidneys or with other drugs known to affect renal function.
Patient Teaching
• Encourage patient to have follow-up laboratory testing done. Explain that these tests will help monitor the patient's kidney function, liver function, and hepatitis B virus levels.
◄ALERT► Warn the patient to immediately notify the physician if he or she experiences unusual muscle pain, stomach pain with nausea and vomiting, cold feeling in arms and legs, and dizziness. Explain that these signs and symptoms may signal the onset of lactic acidosis.
◄ALERT► Warn the patient to continue to take adefovir as prescribed or he or she will be at risk for developing a worse or very serious hepatitis if the drug is stopped.

• Advise patient to immediately notify physician for yellow skin color or yellowing of the whites of the eyes or other unusual signs or symptoms. Explain that these may indicate serious liver problems.
• Instruct patient to use reliable methods of contraception.

amantadine hydrochloride
ah-**man**-tih-deen
(Endantadine [CAN], PMS-Amantadine[CAN], Symmetrel)

CATEGORY AND SCHEDULE
Pregnancy Risk Category: C

MECHANISM OF ACTION
A dopaminergic agonist that blocks the uncoating of influenza A virus, preventing penetration into the host, and inhibiting M2 protein in the assembly of progeny virions. Amantadine locks the reuptake of dopamine into presynaptic neurons and causes direct stimulation of postsynaptic receptors. *Therapeutic Effect:* Antiviral, antiparkinson activity.

PHARMACOKINETICS
Rapidly, completely absorbed from gastrointestinal (GI) tract. Protein binding: 67%. Widely distributed. Primarily excreted in urine. Minimally removed by hemodialysis. **Half-life:** 11–15 hrs (half-life increased in elderly, decreased in impaired renal function).

AVAILABILITY
Liquid: 50 mg/5 ml.
Syrup: 50 mg/5 ml.
Tablets: 100 mg.

INDICATIONS AND DOSAGES
▸ **Prophylaxis, symptomatic treatment of respiratory illness due to influenza A virus**
PO
Elderly. 100 mg/day.
Children older than 12 yrs. 200 mg/day.
Children 9–12 yrs. 100 mg 2 times/day.
Children 1–8 yrs. 5 mg/kg/day (up to 150 mg/day).
▸ **Parkinson's disease, extrapyramidal symptoms**
PO
Adults, Elderly. 100 mg 2 times/day. May increase up to 300 mg/day in divided doses.
▸ **Dosage in renal impairment**
Dosage and frequency are modified based on creatinine clearance (Ccr).

Creatinine Clearance	Dosage
30–50 ml/min	200 mg first day; 100 mg/day thereafter
15–29 ml/min	200 mg first day; 100 mg on alternate days
less than 15 ml/min	200 mg every 7 days

UNLABELED USES
Treatment of attention-deficit hyperactivity disorder (ADHD) and of fatigue associated with multiple sclerosis

CONTRAINDICATIONS
None known.

INTERACTIONS
Drug
Anticholinergics, antihistamines, phenothiazine, tricyclic antidepressants: May increase anticholinergic effects of amantadine.
Hydrochlorothiazide, triamterene: May increase amantadine blood concentration and risk for toxicity.

Herbal
None known.
Food
None known.

DIAGNOSTIC TEST EFFECTS
None known.

SIDE EFFECTS
Frequent (10%–5%)
Nausea, dizziness, poor concentration, insomnia, nervousness
Occasional (5%–1%)
Orthostatic hypotension, anorexia, headache, livedo reticularis evidenced by reddish blue, netlike blotching of skin, blurred vision, urinary retention, dry mouth or nose
Rare
Vomiting, depression, irritation or swelling of eyes, rash

SERIOUS REACTIONS
• Congestive heart failure (CHF), leukopenia, and neutropenia occur rarely.
• Hyperexcitability, convulsions, and ventricular arrhythmias may occur.

NURSING CONSIDERATIONS
Baseline Assessment
• When treating infections caused by influenza A virus, expect to obtain specimens for viral diagnostic tests before giving first dose. Therapy may begin before test results are known.
Lifespan Considerations
• Be aware that it is unknown if amantadine crosses the placenta or is distributed in breast milk.
• There are no age-related precautions noted in children less than 1 year of age.
• The elderly may exhibit increased sensitivity to amantadine's anticholinergic effects.

• In the elderly, age-related decreased renal function may require dosage adjustment.
Precautions
• Use cautiously in patients with cerebrovascular disease, CHF, history of seizures, liver disease, orthostatic hypotension, peripheral edema, recurrent eczema-toid dermatitis, renal dysfunction, and those receiving CNS stimulants.
Administration and Handling
PO
◀ALERT▶ Give as a single or in 2 divided doses.
• May give without regard to food.
• Administer night-time dose several hours before bedtime to prevent insomnia.
Intervention and Evaluation
• Expect to monitor the patient's intake and output and renal function tests, if ordered.
• Check for peripheral edema. Assess the patient's skin for blotching or rash.
• Evaluate the patient's food tolerance and episodes of nausea or vomiting.
• Assess the patient for dizziness.
• For patients with Parkinson's disease, assess for clinical reversal of symptoms as evidenced by an improvement of the masklike facial expression, muscular rigidity, shuffling gait, and tremor of the head and hands at rest.
Patient Teaching
• Advise the patient to continue therapy for the full length of treatment and to evenly space drug doses around the clock.
• Explain to the patient that he or she should not take any medications, including over-the-counter (OTC) drugs, without first consulting the physician.

* Warn the patient to avoid alcoholic beverages.
* Caution the patient not to drive, use machinery, or engage in other activities that require mental acuity if he or she is experiencing dizziness or blurred vision.
* Teach the patient to get up slowly from a sitting or lying position.
* Stress to the patient that he or she notify the physician of new symptoms, especially any blurred vision, dizziness, nausea or vomiting, and skin blotching or rash.
* Tell the patient to take the night-time dose several hours before bedtime to prevent insomnia.

cidofovir
sid-**dough**-foe-vir
(Vistide)

CATEGORY AND SCHEDULE
Pregnancy Risk Category: C

MECHANISM OF ACTION
An anti-infective that suppresses cytomegalovirus (CMV) replication. *Therapeutic Effect:* Inhibits viral DNA synthesis. Incorporation of cidofovir in growing viral DNA chain results in reduction in rate of viral DNA synthesis.

PHARMACOKINETICS
Protein binding: less than 6%. Excreted primarily unchanged in urine. Effect of hemodialysis unknown. Elimination **half-life:** 1.4–3.8 hrs.

AVAILABILITY
Injection: 75 mg/ml (5-ml amp).

INDICATIONS AND DOSAGES
▶ **In combination with probenecid CMV retinitis in patients with AIDS**
IV infusion
Adults. (Induction) Usual dosage 5 mg/kg at constant rate over 1 hr once weekly for 2 consecutive wks. Give 2 g of PO probenecid 3 hrs before cidofovir dose, and then give 1 g 2 and again at 8 hrs after completion of the 1-hr cidofovir infusion (total of 4 g). 1 liter 0.9% NaCl given over 1–2 hrs immediately before cidofovir infusion. If tolerated, a second liter may be given at start or immediately after cidofovir infusion and infused over 1–3 hrs. Maintenance: 5 mg/kg cidofovir at constant rate over 1 hr once every 2 wks.
▶ **Dosage in renal impairment**
Dosages are based on creatinine clearance.

Creatinine Clearance	Induction Dose	Maintenance Dose
41–55 ml/min	2 mg/kg	2 mg/kg
30–40 ml/min	1.5 mg/kg	1.5 mg/kg
20–29 ml/min	1 mg/kg	1 mg/kg
19 ml/min or less	0.5 mg/kg	0.5 mg/kg

UNLABELED USES
Antiviral with activity against acyclovir-resistant herpes simplex virus (HSV) or varicella zoster virus (VZV), adenovirus, foscarnet-resistant CMV, and ganciclovir-resistant CMV

CONTRAINDICATIONS
Direct intraocular injection, history of clinically severe hypersensitivity to probenecid or other sulfa-containing medication, hypersensitivity to cidofovir, renal function impairment (serum

creatinine greater than 1.5 mg/dl or creatinine clearance 55 ml/min or less or urine protein greater than 100 mg/dl)

INTERACTIONS
Drug
Nephrotoxic medications, including aminoglycosides, amphotericin B, foscarnet, IV pentamidine: Avoid concurrent cidofovir administration with these drugs because of the increased risk of nephrotoxicity.
Herbal
None known.
Food
None known.

DIAGNOSTIC TEST EFFECTS
May decrease neutrophil count, and serum bicarbonate, phosphate, and uric acid levels. May elevate serum creatinine levels.

IV INCOMPATIBILITIES
No information available via Y-site administration.

SIDE EFFECTS
Frequent
Nausea, vomiting (65%), fever (57%), asthenia (46%), rash (30%), diarrhea (27%), headache (27%), alopecia (25%), chills (24%), anorexia (22%), dyspnea (22%), abdominal pain (17%)

SERIOUS REACTIONS
• Proteinuria (80%), nephrotoxicity (53%), neutropenia (31%), serum creatinine elevations (29%), infection (24%), anemia (20%), ocular hypotony (12%) (a decrease in intraocular pressure), and pneumonia (9%) occur. Concurrent probenecid use may produce a hypersensitivity reaction including rash, fever, chills, and anaphylaxis.
• Acute renal failure occurs rarely.

NURSING CONSIDERATIONS
Baseline Assessment
• For those patients also taking zidovudine (AZT), expect to temporarily discontinue zidovudine administration or decrease zidovudine dose by 50% on days of cidofovir infusion. Be aware that concurrent probenecid use reduces the metabolic clearance of zidovudine.
• Closely monitor the patient's renal function through serum creatinine levels and urinalysis during therapy.
Lifespan Considerations
• Be aware that cidofovir is embryotoxic and results in reduced fetal body weight in animals.
• Be aware that it is unknown if cidofovir is excreted in breast milk. Do not administer to breast-feeding patients. Breast-feeding is not recommended in this patient population because of the possibility of HIV transmission.
• Be aware that the safety and efficacy of cidofovir have not been established in children.
• In the elderly, age-related renal impairment may require dosage adjustment.
Precautions
• Use cautiously in patients with preexisting diabetes.
Administration and Handling
◀ALERT▶ Do not exceed the recommended dosage, frequency, or infusion rate.
IV
• Store cidofovir at controlled room temperature (68° to 77°F).
• Refrigerate admixtures for no more than 24 hours. Allow refrigerated admixtures to warm to room temperature before use.
• Dilute in 100 ml 0.9% NaCl and infuse over 1 hour.
• Prepare to administer IV hydration with 0.9% NaCl and probenecid

with each cidofovir infusion to minimize the risk of nephrotoxicity.
• Have the patient eat food before each dose of probenecid to help reduce nausea and vomiting. As prescribed, administer an antiemetic to reduce the risk of nausea.

Intervention and Evaluation
• Monitor the patient's serum creatinine, urine protein, and white blood cell (WBC) count before giving each dose.
• Monitor the patient for signs and symptoms of proteinuria, which may be early indicator of dose-dependent nephrotoxicity.
• Periodically evaluate the patient's visual acuity and ocular symptoms.
• Obtain an order for an antiemetic and administer to the patient as needed.

Patient Teaching
• Advise the patient of the importance of obtaining regular follow-up ophthalmologic exams.
• Caution female patients of child-bearing age to use effective contraception during and for 1 month after cidofovir treatment. Explain that pregnancy should be avoided as cidofovir is embryotoxic.
• Warn male patients to practice barrier contraceptive methods during and for 3 months after treatment.
• Advise the patient that she cannot breast-feed while taking cidofovir.
• Explain to the patient that he or she must complete full course of probenecid with each cidofovir dose.

famciclovir
fam-**sigh**-klo-vir
(Famvir)

CATEGORY AND SCHEDULE
Pregnancy Risk Category: B

MECHANISM OF ACTION
A synthetic nucleoside that inhibits viral DNA synthesis. *Therapeutic Effect:* Suppresses herpes simplex virus and varicella-zoster virus replication.

PHARMACOKINETICS
Rapidly, extensively absorbed after PO administration. Protein binding: 20%–25%. Rapidly metabolized to penciclovir by enzymes in gut wall, liver, and plasma. Eliminated unchanged in urine. Removed by hemodialysis.
Half-life: 2 hrs.

AVAILABILITY
Tablets: 125 mg, 250 mg, 500 mg.

INDICATIONS AND DOSAGES
▸ **Herpes zoster**
PO
Adults. 500 mg q8h for 7 days.
▸ **Recurrent genital herpes**
PO
Adults. 125 mg twice a day for 5 days.
▸ **Suppression of recurrent genital herpes**
PO
Adults. 250 mg twice a day for up to 1 yr.
▸ **Recurrent herpes simplex**
PO
Adults. 500 mg twice a day for 7 days.
▸ **Dosage in renal impairment**
Dosages are based on creatinine clearance (ml/min):

Creatinine Clearance	Herpes Zoster	Genital Herpes
40–59	500 mg q12h	125 mg q12h
20–39	500 mg q24h	125 mg q24h
less than 20	250 mg q24h	125 mg q24h

▶ **Hemodialysis Patients**
PO
Adults. 250 mg (herpes zoster) or
125 mg (genital herpes) after each
dialysis treatment.

CONTRAINDICATIONS
None known

INTERACTIONS
Drug
None known.
Herbal
None known.
Food
None known.

DIAGNOSTIC TEST EFFECTS
None known.

SIDE EFFECTS
Frequent
Headache (23%), nausea (12%)
Occasional (10%–2%)
Dizziness, somnolence, numbness of
feet, diarrhea, vomiting, constipa-
tion, decreased appetite, fatigue,
fever, pharyngitis, sinusitis, pruritus
Rare (less than 2%)
Inability to sleep, abdominal pain,
dyspepsia, flatulence, back pain,
arthralgia

SERIOUS REACTIONS
• None known.

NURSING CONSIDERATIONS

Lifespan Considerations
• Be aware that famciclovir causes
an increase in mammary adenocarcinoma in animals.
• Be aware that it is unknown if
famciclovir is excreted in breast
milk.
• Be aware that the safety and
efficacy of famciclovir have not
been established in children.

• In the elderly, age-related renal
function impairment may require
dosage adjustment.
Precautions
• Use cautiously in patients
with liver or renal function impairment.
Administration and Handling
PO
• Give without regard to
meals.
Intervention and Evaluation
• Evaluate the patient for cutaneous
lesions.
• Assess the patient for signs
and symptoms of neurologic effects including dizziness and headache.
• Provide the patient with analgesics, if ordered, and comfort
measures. Be aware that famciclovir administration is especially exhausting to elderly
patients.
Patient Teaching
• Advise the patient to take the
famciclovir for the full length of
treatment.
• In genital herpes patients, advise
the patient to evenly space doses
around the clock.
• Encourage the patient to drink
adequate fluids.
• Teach the patient to keep his or
her fingernails short and hands
clean.
• Caution the patient not to touch
lesions with his or her fingers to
avoid spreading infection to new
sites.
• Warn the patient to avoid sexual
intercourse during the duration of
lesions to prevent infecting his or
her partner.
• Tell the patient to notify
the physician if his or her lesions do not improve or if they
recur.

fomivirsen
foam-ih-**verse**-inn
(Vitravene)

CATEGORY AND SCHEDULE
Pregnancy Risk Category: C

MECHANISM OF ACTION
An antiviral that binds to mRNA, which blocks replication of cytomegalovirus. *Therapeutic Effect:* Inhibits synthesis of viral proteins.

AVAILABILITY
Intravitreal Injection: 6.6 mg/ml.

INDICATIONS AND DOSAGES
▶ **Cytomegalovirus (CMV) retinitis**
Intravitreal injection
Adults. 330 mcg (0.05 ml) every other week for 2 doses, then 330 mcg q4wks.

CONTRAINDICATIONS
None significant.

INTERACTIONS
Drug
None significant.
Herbal
None significant.
Food
None significant.

DIAGNOSTIC TEST EFFECTS
May alter liver function tests and serum alkaline phosphatase. May decrease blood Hgb levels and neutrophils and platelet counts.

SIDE EFFECTS
Frequent (10%–5%)
Fever, headache, nausea, diarrhea, vomiting, abdominal pain, anemia, uveitis, abnormal vision
Occasional (5%–2%)
Chest pain, confusion, dizziness, depression, neuropathy, anorexia, decreased weight, pancreatitis, dyspnea, cough

SERIOUS REACTIONS
• Thrombocytopenia may occur.

NURSING CONSIDERATIONS
Precautions
• Be aware that fomivirsen use should be avoided in patients who have received cidofovir within 2 to 4 weeks of fomivirsen therapy.
• Use cautiously in patients with increased intraocular pressure.
Intervention and Evaluation
• After fomivirsen injection, expect the physician to evaluate the patient's light perception, optic nerve head perfusion, and intraocular pressure.
• Monitor the patient for signs and symptoms of extraocular CMV infection, including pneumonitis and colitis. Also, assess for signs and symptoms of CMV infection in the untreated eye if only one eye is undergoing treatment.
Patient Teaching
• Instruct the patient that fomivirsen only treats and does not cure CMV retinitis of the eye. Explain to the patient that regular eye exams and follow-up care will be required.

foscarnet sodium
fos-**car**-net
(Foscavir)

CATEGORY AND SCHEDULE
Pregnancy Risk Category: C

MECHANISM OF ACTION
An antiviral that selectively inhibits binding sites on virus-specific DNA

polymerases and reverse transcriptases. *Therapeutic Effect:* Inhibits replication of herpes virus.

PHARMACOKINETICS

Sequestered into bone, cartilage. Protein binding: 14%–17%. Primarily excreted unchanged in urine. Removed by hemodialysis. **Half-life:** 3.3–6.8 hrs (half-life is increased with impaired renal function).

AVAILABILITY

Injection: 24 mg/ml.

INDICATIONS AND DOSAGES
▸ **Cytomegalovirus (CMV) retinitis**
IV
Adults, Elderly. Initially, 60 mg/kg q8h (may dose as 100 mg q12h) for 2–3 wks. Maintenance: 90–120 mg/kg/day as a single IV infusion.
▸ **Herpes simplex**
IV
Adults. 40 mg/kg q8–12h for 2–3 wks or until healed.
▸ **Dosage in renal impairment**
Dosages are individualized according to the patient's creatinine clearance. Refer to the dosing guide provided by the manufacturer.

CONTRAINDICATIONS

None known

INTERACTIONS
Drug
Nephrotoxic medications: May increase the risk of renal toxicity. *Pentamidine (IV):* May cause reversible hypocalcemia, hypomagnesemia, and nephrotoxicity. *Zidovudine (AZT):* May increase anemia.
Herbal
None known.
Food
None known.

DIAGNOSTIC TEST EFFECTS

May increase serum alkaline phosphatase, bilirubin, and creatinine, as well as SGOT (AST) and SGPT (ALT) levels. May decrease serum magnesium and potassium levels. May alter serum calcium and phosphate concentrations.

IV INCOMPATIBILITIES

Acyclovir (Zovirax), amphotericin (Fungizone), diazepam (Valium), digoxin (Lanoxin), diphenhydramine (Benadryl), dobutamine (Dobutrex), droperidol (Inapsine), ganciclovir (Cytovene), haloperidol (Haldol), leucovorin, midazolam (Versed), pentamidine (Pentam IV), prochlorperazine (Compazine), trimethoprim-sulfamethoxazole (Bactrim), vancomycin (Vancocin)

IV COMPATIBILITIES

Dopamine (Intropin), heparin, hydromorphone (Dilaudid), lorazepam (Ativan), morphine, potassium chloride

SIDE EFFECTS
Frequent
Fever (65%); nausea (47%); vomiting, diarrhea (30%)
Occasional (5% or greater)
Anorexia, pain and inflammation at injection site, fever, rigors, malaise, hypertension or hypotension, headache, paresthesia, dizziness, rash, diaphoresis nausea, vomiting, abdominal pain
Rare (5%–1%)
Back or chest pain, edema, hypertension or hypotension, flushing, pruritus, constipation, dry mouth

SERIOUS REACTIONS
• Renal impairment is a major toxicity that occurs to some extent in most patients.
• Seizures and mineral or electrolyte

imbalances may occur and be life-threatening.

NURSING CONSIDERATIONS

Baseline Assessment
• Expect to obtain the patient's baseline complete blood count (CBC) values, mineral and electrolyte levels, renal function, and vital signs.
• Know that the risk of renal impairment is reduced by ensuring sufficient fluid intake to promote diuresis before and during dosing.

Lifespan Considerations
• Be aware that it is unknown if foscarnet is distributed in breast milk.
• Be aware that the safety and efficacy of foscarnet have not been established in children.
• In the elderly, age-related renal impairment may require dosage adjustment.

Precautions
• Use cautiously in patients with altered serum calcium or other serum electrolyte levels, a history of renal impairment, or cardiac or neurologic abnormalities.

Administration and Handling
IV
• Store parenteral vials at room temperature.
• After dilution, foscarnet is stable for 24 hours at room temperature.
• Do not use if foscarnet solution is discolored or contains particulate material.
• Use the standard 24 mg/ml solution without diluting it when a central venous catheter is used for infusion; the 24 mg/ml solution *must* be diluted to 12 mg/ml when you're giving the drug through a peripheral vein catheter. Use only D_5W or 0.9% NaCl solution for injection for dilution.

• Because foscarnet dosage is calculated on body weight, remove the unneeded quantity before the start of infusion to avoid overdosage. Use an IV infusion pump to administer foscarnet and prevent accidental overdose.
• Use aseptic technique and administer the solution within 24 hours of the first entry into the sealed bottle.
◄ ALERT ► Do not give foscarnet as an IV injection or by rapid infusion because these routes increase the drug's toxicity. Administer foscarnet by IV infusion at a rate not faster than 1 hour for doses up to 60 mg/kg and 2 hours for doses greater than 60 mg/kg.
• To minimize the risk of phlebitis and toxicity, use central venous lines or veins with an adequate blood flow to permit rapid dilution and dissemination of foscarnet.

Intervention and Evaluation
• Monitor the patient's blood Hct and Hgb levels, renal function test results, and serum calcium, creatinine, magnesium, phosphorus, and potassium levels. Also monitor the results of ophthalmic exams, as appropriate.
• Assess the patient for signs and symptoms of electrolyte imbalances, especially hypocalcemia as evidenced by numbness or paresthesia of the extremities and peri-oral tingling, and hypokalemia manifested as irritability, muscle cramps, numbness or tingling of the extremities, and weakness.
• Evaluate the patient for signs and symptoms of anemia, bleeding, superinfections, and tremors. Institute safety measures for potential seizures.

Patient Teaching
• Warn the patient to report numbness in the extremities, paresthesias,

or peri-oral tingling, during or after infusion as this may indicate electrolyte abnormalities.
• Warn the patient to report tremors promptly because the drug may cause seizures.

ganciclovir sodium
gan-**sye**-klo-vir
(Cymevene[AUS], Cytovene, Vitrasert)
Do not confuse with Cytosar.

CATEGORY AND SCHEDULE
Pregnancy Risk Category: C

MECHANISM OF ACTION
This synthetic nucleoside is converted intracellularly, competes with viral DNA polymerases, and directly incorporates into growing viral DNA chains. *Therapeutic Effect:* Interferes with DNA synthesis and viral replication.

PHARMACOKINETICS
Widely distributed. Protein binding: 1%–2%. Undergoes minimal metabolism. Primarily excreted unchanged in urine. Removed by hemodialysis.
Half-life: 2.5–3.6 hrs (half-life is increased with impaired renal function).

AVAILABILITY
Capsules: 250 mg, 500 mg.
Powder for Injection: 500 mg.
Implant: 4.5 mg.

INDICATIONS AND DOSAGES
▸ **Cytomegalovirus retinitis**
IV
Adults, Children older than 3 mos.
10 mg/kg/day in divided doses q12h for 14–21 days, then 5 mg/kg/day as a single daily dose.
▸ **Prevention of cytomegalovirus (CMV) in transplant patients**
IV
Adults, Children. 10 mg/kg/day in divided doses q12h for 7–14 days, then 5 mg/kg/day as a single daily dose.
▸ **Other CMV infections**
IV
Adults. Initially, 10 mg/kg/day in divided doses q12h for 14–21 days, then 5 mg/kg/day as a single daily dose. Maintenance: 1,000 mg 3 times/day or 500 mg q3h (6 times/day).
Children. Initially, 10 mg/kg/day in divided doses q12h for 14–21 days, then 5 mg/kg/day as a single daily dose. Maintenance: 30 mg/kg/dose q8h.
▸ **Intravitreal implant**
Adults. 1 implant q6–9mos plus ganciclovir orally.
Children older than 9 yrs. 1 implant q6–9mos plus ganciclovir orally (30 mg/dose q8h).
▸ **Adult dosage in renal impairment**

CrCl	IV Indications	IV Maintenance	Oral
50–69 ml/min	2.5 mg/kg q12h	2.5 mg/kg q24h	1,500 mg/day
25–49 ml/min	2.5 mg/kg q24h	1.25 mg/kg q24h	1,000 mg/day
10–24 ml/min	1.25 mg/kg q24h	0.625 mg/kg q24h	500 mg/day
10–24 ml/min	1.25 mg/kg 3 times/wk	0.625 mg/kg 3 times/wk	500 mg 3 times/wk

CrCl = creatinine clearance

UNLABELED USES

Treatment of other CMV infections, such as gastroenteritis, hepatitis, pneumonitis

CONTRAINDICATIONS

Absolute neutrophil count less than 500/mm^3, platelet count less than 25,000/mm^3, hypersensitivity to acyclovir or ganciclovir. Not for use in nonimmunocompromised persons or those with congenital or neonatal CMV disease.

INTERACTIONS

Drug

Bone marrow depressants: May increase bone marrow depression.
Imipenem-cilastatin: May increase the risk of seizures.
Zidovudine (AZT): May increase the risk of liver toxicity.

Herbal

None known.

Food

None known.

DIAGNOSTIC TEST EFFECTS

May increase serum alkaline phosphatase and bilirubin, as well as SGOT (AST) and SGPT (ALT) levels.

IV INCOMPATIBILITIES

Aldesleukin (Proleukin), amifostine (Ethyol), aztreonam (Azactam), cefepime (Maxipime), cytarabine (ARA-C), doxorubicin (Adriamycin), fludarabine (Fludara), foscarnet (Foscavir), gemcitabine (Gemzar), ondansetron (Zofran), piperacillin/tazobactam (Zosyn), sargramostim (Leukine), vinorelbine (Navelbine)

IV COMPATIBILITIES

Amphotericin, enalapril (Vasotec), filgrastim (Neupogen), fluconazole (Diflucan), propofol (Diprivan)

SIDE EFFECTS

Frequent
Diarrhea (41%), fever (40%), nausea (25%), abdominal pain (17%), vomiting (13%)
Occasional (11%–6%)
Diaphoresis, infection, paresthesia, flatulence, pruritus
Rare (4%–2%)
Headache, stomatitis, dyspepsia, vomiting, phlebitis

SERIOUS REACTIONS

• Hematologic toxicity occurs commonly: leukopenia (29%–41%) and anemia (19%–25%).
• Intraocular insertion produces visual acuity loss, vitreous hemorrhage, and retinal detachment occasionally.
• Gastrointestinal (GI) hemorrhage occurs rarely.

NURSING CONSIDERATIONS

Baseline Assessment

• Evaluate the patient's hematologic baseline.
• Obtain specimens (blood, feces, throat culture, urine) from the patient for culture and sensitivity testing, as ordered, before giving the drug. Keep in mind that test results are needed to support the differential diagnosis and rule out retinal infection as the result of hematogenous dissemination.

Lifespan Considerations

• Be aware that ganciclovir should not be used during pregnancy and breast-feeding should be discontinued during ganciclovir use. Breast-feeding may be resumed no sooner than 72 hours after the last dose of ganciclovir.
• Be aware that effective contraception should be used during ganciclovir therapy.
• Be aware that the safety and

efficacy of ganciclovir have not been established in children younger than 12 years of age.

• In the elderly, age-related renal impairment may require dosage adjustment.

Precautions

• Use cautiously in pediatric patients. The long-term safety of this drug has not been determined because of the potential for long-term adverse reproductive and carcinogenic effects.

• Use cautiously in patients with impaired renal function, neutropenia, and thrombocytopenia.

Administration and Handling

PO

• Give ganciclovir with food.

IV

• Store vials at room temperature. Do not refrigerate.

• Reconstituted solution in vial is stable for 12 hours at room temperature.

• After dilution, refrigerate and use within 24 hours.

• Discard the solution if precipitate forms or discoloration occurs.

• Avoid inhaling the solution. Also avoid solution exposure to the eyes, mucous membranes, or skin. Use latex gloves and safety glasses during preparation and handling of ganciclovir solution. If the solution comes in contact with mucous membranes or the skin, wash the affected area thoroughly with soap and water; rinse eyes thoroughly with plain water.

• Reconstitute 500-mg vial with 10 ml Sterile Water for Injection to provide a concentration of 50 mg/ml; do not use Bacteriostatic Water which contains parabens, and is therefore incompatible with ganciclovir.

• Further dilute with 100 ml D_5W, 0.9% NaCl, lactated Ringer's, or any combination thereof to provide a concentration of 5 mg/ml.

◀ALERT▶ Do not give by IV push or rapid IV infusion because these routes increase the risk of ganciclovir toxicity. Administer only by IV infusion over 1 hour.

• Protect the patient from infiltration because the high pH of this drug causes severe tissue irritation.

• Use large veins to permit rapid dilution and dissemination of ganciclovir and to minimize the risk of phlebitis Keep in mind that central venous ports tunneled under subcutaneous tissue may reduce catheter-associated infection.

Intervention and Evaluation

• Monitor the patient's intake and output and ensure the patient is adequately hydrated. (minimum 1,500 ml/24 hours).

• Diligently evaluate the patient's hematology reports for decreased platelets, neutropenia, and thrombocytopenia.

• Evaluate the patient for altered vision, complications, and therapeutic improvement.

• Assess the patient for signs and symptoms of infiltration, phlebitis, pruritus and rash.

Patient Teaching

• Instruct the patient that ganciclovir provides suppression, but is not a cure for CMV retinitis.

• Explain to the patient that frequent blood tests and eye exams are necessary during therapy because of toxic nature of drug.

• Stress to the patient that it is essential to report any new symptom promptly to the physician.

• Tell male patients that ganciclovir may temporarily or permanently inhibit sperm production.

• Tell female patients that ganciclovir use may suppress fertility.

• Urge patients to use barrier contraception during ganciclovir administration and for 90 days after therapy because of mutagenic potential.

oseltamivir
oh-sell-**tam**-ih-veer
(Tamiflu)

CATEGORY AND SCHEDULE
Pregnancy Risk Category: C

MECHANISM OF ACTION
A selective inhibitor of influenza virus neuraminidase, an enzyme essential for viral replication. Acts against both influenza A and B viruses. *Therapeutic Effect:* Suppresses spread of infection within respiratory system and reduces duration of clinical symptoms.

PHARMACOKINETICS
Readily absorbed. Protein binding: 3%. Extensively converted to active drug in the liver. Primarily excreted in urine. **Half-life:** 6–10 hrs.

AVAILABILITY
Capsules: 75 mg.
Oral Suspension: 12 mg/ml.

INDICATIONS AND DOSAGES
▸ **Influenza**
PO
Adults, Elderly. 75 mg 2 times/day for 5 days.
Children weighing more than 40 kg. 75 mg twice a day.
Children weighing 23–40 kg. 60 mg twice a day.
Children weighing 15–23 kg. 45 mg twice a day.
Children weighing less than 15 kg. 30 mg twice a day.

▸ **Prophylaxis against influenza**
PO
Adults, Elderly. 75 mg once a day.
▸ **Dosage in renal impairment**
PO
Adults, Elderly. 75 mg once a day for at least 7 days up to 6 wks.

CONTRAINDICATIONS
None known

INTERACTIONS
Drug
None known.
Herbal
None known.
Food
None known.

DIAGNOSTIC TEST EFFECTS
None known.

SIDE EFFECTS
Frequent (greater than 5%)
Nausea, vomiting, diarrhea
Occasional (5%–1%)
Abdominal pain, bronchitis, dizziness, headache, cough, insomnia, fatigue, vertigo

SERIOUS REACTIONS
• Colitis, pneumonia, and pyrexia occur rarely.

NURSING CONSIDERATIONS
Lifespan Considerations
• Be aware that it is unknown if oseltamivir is excreted in breast milk.
• Be aware that the safety and efficacy of this drug have not been established in children younger than 1 year of age.
• There are no age-related precautions noted in the elderly.
Precautions
• Use cautiously in patients with renal function impairment.

Administration and Handling
PO
• Give oseltamivir without regard to food.
Intervention and Evaluation
• Monitor the patient's renal function.
• In diabetic patients, monitor blood glucose levels.
Patient Teaching
• Instruct the patient to begin taking oseltamivir as soon as possible from first appearance of flu symptoms.
• Warn the patient to avoid contact with those who are at high risk for influenza.
• Advise the patient that oseltamivir is not a substitute for a flu shot.

ribavirin
rye-bah-**vi**-rin
(Copegus, Rebetol, Virazole)
Do not confuse with riboflavin.

CATEGORY AND SCHEDULE
Pregnancy Risk Category: X

MECHANISM OF ACTION
A synthetic nucleoside that inhibits replication of RNA and DNA viruses. Inhibits influenza virus RNA polymerase activity and interferes with expression of messenger RNA. *Therapeutic Effect:* Inhibits viral protein synthesis.

AVAILABILITY
Powder for Reconstitution (Aerosol): 6 g/100 ml.
Capsules: 200 mg.
Tablets: 200 mg.

INDICATIONS AND DOSAGES
▶ **Severe lower respiratory tract infection caused by respiratory syncytial virus (RSV)**

Inhalation
Children, Infants. Use with Viratek small-particle aerosol generator at a concentration of 20 mg/ml (6 g reconstituted with 300 ml sterile water) 12–18 hrs/day for 3 days or up to 7 days.
▶ **Chronic hepatitis C**
PO (capsule in combination with interferon alfa-2b)
Adults, Elderly. 1000–1200 mg/day in 2 divided doses.
PO (capsule in combination with peginterferon alfa-2b)
Adults, Elderly. 800 mg/day in 2 divided doses.
PO (tablets in combination with peginterferon alfa-2b)
Adults, Elderly. 800–1200 mg/day in 2 divided doses.

UNLABELED USES
Treatment of influenza A or B and west Nile virus

CONTRAINDICATIONS
Pregnancy, women of childbearing age who will not use contraception reliably

INTERACTIONS
Drug
Didanosine: May increase the risk of pancreatitis and peripheral neuropathy. May decrease the effects of this drug.
Nucleoside analogues, including adefovir, didanosine, lamivudine, stavudine, zalcitabine, zidovudine: May increase the risk of lactic acidosis.
Herbal
None known.
Food
None known.

DIAGNOSTIC TEST EFFECTS
None known.

SIDE EFFECTS

Frequent (greater than 10%)
Dizziness, headache, fatigue, fever, insomnia, irritability, depression, emotional lability, impaired concentration, alopecia, rash, pruritus, nausea, anorexia, dyspepsia, vomiting, decreased hemoglobin, hemolysis, arthralgia, musculoskeletal pain, dyspnea, sinusitis, flu-like symptoms
Occasional (1%–10%)
Nervousness, altered taste, weakness

SERIOUS REACTIONS

• Cardiac arrest, apnea and ventilator dependence, bacterial pneumonia, pneumonia, and pneumothorax occur rarely.
• If ribavirin therapy exceeds 7 days, anemia may occur.

NURSING CONSIDERATIONS

Baseline Assessment

• Expect to obtain respiratory tract secretions for diagnostic testing before giving the first dose of ribavirin or at least during the first 24 hours of therapy.
• Assess the patient's respiratory status and establish a baseline.
• In patients taking oral ribavirin, expect to obtain the patient's complete blood count (CBC) with differential and to pretreat and test the female patient of childbearing age monthly for pregnancy.

Precautions

• Use inhaled ribavirin cautiously in patients with asthma and chronic obstructive pulmonary disease (COPD).
• Use inhaled ribavirin cautiously in patients requiring mechanical ventilation.
• Use oral ribavirin cautiously in elderly patients and patients with cardiac or pulmonary disease.

• Use oral ribavirin cautiously in patients with a history of psychiatric disorders.

Administration and Handling

Inhalation

◀ALERT▶ Ribavirin may be given via nasal or oral inhalation.
• Solution normally appears clear and colorless and is stable for 24 hours at room temperature. Discard solution for nebulization after 24 hours. Discard solution if discolored or cloudy.
• Add 50 to 100 ml Sterile Water for Injection or inhalation to 6-g vial.
• Transfer to a flask, serving as reservoir for aerosol generator.
• Further dilute to final volume of 300 ml, giving a solution concentration of 20 mg/ml.
• Use only aerosol generator available from manufacturer of drug.
• Do not give at the same time with other drug solutions for nebulization.
• Discard reservoir solution when fluid levels are low and at least every 24 hours.
◀ALERT▶ Be aware that there is controversy over the safety of administering ribavirin to ventilator-dependent patients; only experienced personnel should administer the drug.

Oral

• Capsules may be taken without regard to food.
• Tablets should be given with food.

Intervention and Evaluation

• Monitor the patient's intake and output and fluid balance carefully.
• Check the patient's hematology reports for anemia due to reticulocytosis when therapy exceeds 7 days.
• For ventilator-assisted patients, watch for "rainout" in tubing and empty frequently.
• Be alert to impaired ventilation

and gas exchange due to drug precipitate.
• Periodically assess the patient's lung sounds and assess the patient's skin for rash.
• Monitor the patient's blood pressure and respirations.

Patient Teaching
• Instruct patient to immediately report any difficulty breathing or itching, redness, or swelling of the eyes.
• Educate female patients about prevention of pregnancy and the need for regular pregnancy testing.
• Educate male patients about protection of female partners from pregnancy.

rimantadine hydrochloride
rye-**man**-tah-deen
(Flumadine)
Do not confuse with flunisolide, flutamide, or ranitidine.

CATEGORY AND SCHEDULE
Pregnancy Risk Category: C

MECHANISM OF ACTION
An antiviral that appears to exert an inhibitory effect early in viral replication cycle. May inhibit uncoating of virus. *Therapeutic Effect:* Prevents replication of influenza A virus.

AVAILABILITY
Tablets: 100 mg.
Syrup: 50 mg/5 ml.

INDICATIONS AND DOSAGES
▸ **Prophylaxis against influenza A virus**
PO
Adults, Elderly, Children 10 yrs and older. 100 mg 2 times/day for at least 10 days after known exposure (usually 6–8 weeks).
Children younger than 10 yrs. 5 mg/kg once a day. Maximum: 150 mg.
▸ **Severe liver or renal impairment**
Elderly nursing home patients. 100 mg/day.
▸ **Treatment of influenza A virus**
PO
Adults, Elderly. 100 mg 2 times/day for 7 days.
▸ **Severe liver or renal impairment**
Elderly nursing home patients. 100 mg/day for 7 days.

CONTRAINDICATIONS
Hypersensitivity to amantadine or rimantadine

INTERACTIONS
Drug
Acetaminophen, aspirin: May decrease rimantadine blood concentration.
Anticholinergics, central nervous system (CNS) stimulants: May increase side effects of rimantadine.
Cimetidine: May increase rimantadine blood concentration.
Herbal
None known.
Food
None known.

DIAGNOSTIC TEST EFFECTS
None known.

SIDE EFFECTS
Occasional (3%–2%)
Insomnia, nausea, nervousness, impaired concentration, dizziness
Rare (less than 2%)
Vomiting, anorexia, dry mouth, abdominal pain, asthenia (loss of energy, strength), fatigue

SERIOUS REACTIONS
• None known.

NURSING CONSIDERATIONS

Precautions
• Use cautiously in patients with history of recurrent eczematoid dermatitis, liver disease, renal impairment, seizures, and uncontrolled psychosis.
• Use cautiously in patients who also receive CNS stimulants.

Administration and Handling
PO
• Give rimantadine without regard to food.

Intervention and Evaluation
• Assess the patient for nervousness and evaluate the patient's sleep pattern for insomnia.
• Provide assistance to the patient if he or she experiences dizziness.

Patient Teaching
• Stress to the patient that he or she should avoid contact with those who are at high risk for developing influenza A (rimantadine-resistant virus may be shed during therapy).
• Warn the patient not to drive or perform tasks that require mental alertness if he or she experiences decreased concentration or dizziness.
• Caution the patient against taking acetaminophen, aspirin, or compounds containing these drugs.
• Advise the patient that rimantadine may cause dry mouth.

valacyclovir
val-ah-**sigh**-klo-veer
(Valtrex)

CATEGORY AND SCHEDULE
Pregnancy Risk Category: B

MECHANISM OF ACTION
An antiviral that is converted to acyclovir triphosphate, becoming part of viral DNA chain. Virustatic.

Therapeutic Effect: Interferes with DNA synthesis and viral replication of herpes simplex and varicella zoster virus.

PHARMACOKINETICS
Rapidly absorbed after PO administration. Protein binding: 13%–18%. Rapidly converted by hydrolysis to active compound, acyclovir. Widely distributed to tissues and body fluids (including cerebrospinal fluid [CSF]). Primarily eliminated in urine. Removed by hemodialysis. **Half-life:** 2.5–3.3 hrs (half-life is increased with impaired renal function).

AVAILABILITY
Tablets: 500 mg, 1,000 mg.

INDICATIONS AND DOSAGES
▶ **Herpes zoster (shingles)**
PO
Adults, Elderly. 1 g 3 times a day for 7 days.
▶ **Recurrent genital herpes**
PO
Adults, Elderly. 500 mg twice a day for 3 days.
▶ **Cold sores**
PO
Adults, Elderly. 2 g twice a day for 1 day.
▶ **Prevention of herpes**
PO
Adults, Elderly. 500–1,000 mg/day.
▶ **Initial treatment of genital herpes**
PO
Adults, Elderly. 1 g twice a day for 10 days.
▶ **Dosage in renal impairment**

Creatinine Clearance (ml/min)	Herpes Zoster	Genital Herpes
50 or higher	1 g q8h	500 mg q12h
30–49	1 g q12h	500 mg q12h
10–29	1 g q24h	500 mg q24h
less than 10	500 mg q24h	500 mg q24h

UNLABELED USES
Reduce heterosexual transmission of genital herpes

CONTRAINDICATIONS
Hypersensitivity or intolerance to acyclovir, components of formulation, or valacyclovir

INTERACTIONS
Drug
Cimetidine, probenecid: May increase acyclovir blood concentration.
Herbal
None known.
Food
None known.

DIAGNOSTIC TEST EFFECTS
None known.

SIDE EFFECTS
Frequent
Herpes zoster (17%–10%): Nausea, headache
Genital herpes (17%): Headache
Occasional
Herpes zoster (7%–3%): Vomiting, diarrhea, constipation (50 yrs or older), asthenia, dizziness (50 yrs or older)
Genital herpes (8%–3%): Nausea, diarrhea, dizziness
Rare
Herpes zoster (3%–1%): Abdominal pain, anorexia
Genital herpes (3%–1%): Asthenia, abdominal pain

SERIOUS REACTIONS
• None known.

NURSING CONSIDERATIONS
Baseline Assessment
• Determine the patient's history of allergies, particularly to acyclovir and valacyclovir, before beginning drug therapy.
• Expect to obtain tissue cultures from herpes simplex and herpes zoster patients before giving the first dose of valacyclovir. Therapy may proceed before test results are known.
• Assess the patient's medical history, especially in those with advanced HIV infection, bone marrow or renal transplantation, and impaired liver or renal function.
Lifespan Considerations
• Be aware that valacyclovir may cross the placenta and be distributed in breast milk.
• The safety and efficacy of this drug have not been established in children.
• In the elderly, age-related renal impairment may require dosage adjustment.
Precautions
• Use cautiously in patients with advanced HIV infection, bone marrow or renal transplantation, concurrent use of nephrotoxic agents, dehydration, fluid or electrolyte imbalance, neurologic abnormalities, and renal or liver impairment.
Administration and Handling
◀ALERT▶ Be aware that therapy should be initiated at the first sign of shingles and that valacyclovir is most effective within 48 hours of the onset of zoster rash.
PO
• Give valacyclovir without regard to meals.
• Do not crush or break tablets.
Intervention and Evaluation
• Evaluate the patient for cutaneous lesions.

• Monitor the patient's complete blood count (CBC), liver or renal function tests, and urinalysis.
• Manage herpes zoster patients with strict isolation, according to the institution's policies and procedures.
• For herpes zoster patients, provide analgesics, if ordered, and comfort measures. Know that herpes zoster is especially exhausting for the elderly.
• Provide the patient with adequate fluids.
• Keep the patient's fingernails short and hands clean.

Patient Teaching
• Encourage the patient to drink adequate fluids.
• Stress to the patient that he or she should not touch lesions with fingers to avoid spreading infection to new sites.
• Advise genital herpes patients to continue therapy for the full length of treatment and to evenly space doses around the clock.
• Warn genital herpes patients to avoid sexual intercourse during the duration of lesions to prevent infecting partner.
• Instruct the patient that valacyclovir does not cure herpes.
• Warn the patient to notify the physician if lesions do not improve or recur.
• Explain to the female genital herpes patient that pap smears should be done at least annually due to increased risk of cervical cancer in women with genital herpes.
• Teach the patient to initiate valacyclovir treatment at the first sign of a recurrent episode of genital herpes or herpes zoster. Explain to the patient that early treatment, that is,

within first 24 to 48 hours, is imperative for therapeutic results.

valganciclovir hydrochloride
val-gan-**sye**-klo-vir
(Valcyte)

CATEGORY AND SCHEDULE
Pregnancy Risk Category: C

MECHANISM OF ACTION
A synthetic nucleoside that is converted intracellularly; competes with viral DNA esterases and incorporates directly into growing viral DNA chains. *Therapeutic Effect:* Interferes with DNA synthesis and viral replication.

PHARMACOKINETICS
Well absorbed and rapidly converted to ganciclovir by intestinal and hepatic enzymes. Widely distributed. Slowly metabolized intracellularly. Primarily excreted unchanged in urine. Removed by hemodialysis. **Half-life:** 18 hrs (half-life is increased with impaired renal function).

AVAILABILITY
Tablets: 450 mg.

INDICATIONS AND DOSAGES
▶ **Cytomegalovirus (CMV) retinitis (in patients with normal renal function)**
PO
Adults. Initially, 900 mg (two 450-mg tablets) twice a day for 21 days with food. Maintenance: 900 mg once a day with food.

▶ **Dosage in renal impairment**

Creatinine Clearance	Induction Dosage	Mainte-nance Dosage
60 ml/min or more	900 mg twice/day	900 mg once/day
40–59 ml/min	450 mg twice/day	450 mg once/day
25–39 ml/min	450 mg once/day	450 mg q2 days
10–24 ml/min	450 mg q2 days	450 mg twice weekly

CONTRAINDICATIONS
Hypersensitivity to acyclovir or ganciclovir

INTERACTIONS
Drug
Amphotericin B, cyclosporine: Concurrent use of these drugs may produce nephrotoxicity.
Bone marrow depressants: May increase bone marrow depression.
Imipenem-cilastatin: May increase the risk of seizures.
Probenecid: Reduces renal clearance of valganciclovir.
Zidovudine (AZT): May increase the risk of hematologic toxicity.
Herbal
None known.
Food
Food maximizes drug bioavailability.

DIAGNOSTIC TEST EFFECTS
May decrease blood Hct, Hgb levels, and platelet count, serum creatinine, and white blood cell count (WBC).

SIDE EFFECTS
Frequent (16%–9%)
Diarrhea, neutropenia, headache
Occasional (8%–3%)
Nausea, anemia, thrombocytopenia

Rare (less than 3%)
Insomnia, paresthesia, vomiting, abdominal pain, pyrexia

SERIOUS REACTIONS
• Hematologic toxicity (mainly neutropenia), anemia, and thrombocytopenia may occur.
• Retinal detachment occurs rarely.
• Overdose may result in renal toxicity.
• May decrease sperm production and fertility.

NURSING CONSIDERATIONS
Baseline Assessment
• Evaluate the patient's blood chemistry, hematologic baselines, and serum creatinine levels.
Lifespan Considerations
• Effective contraception should be used during therapy because of the drug's mutagenic potential.
• Valganciclovir should not be used during pregnancy because of the drug's mutagenic potential.
• Female patients taking valganciclovir should avoid breast-feeding. Breast-feeding may be resumed no sooner than 72 hours after the last dose of valganciclovir.
• Be aware that the safety and efficacy of this drug have not been established in children younger than 12 years of age.
• In the elderly, age-related renal impairment may require dosage adjustment.
Precautions
• Use extremely cautiously in children because of long-term carcinogenicity and risk of reproductive toxicity.
• Use cautiously in elderly patients who are at a greater risk of renal impairment.
• Use cautiously in patients with a history of cytopenic reactions to

other drugs, preexisting cytopenias, and renal impairment.

Administration and Handling

PO

• Do not break or crush tablets (potentially carcinogenic).

• Avoid contact with skin. Wash skin with soap and water if contact occurs.

• Give valganciclovir with food.

Intervention and Evaluation

• Monitor the patient's intake and output and ensure the patient maintains adequate hydration (minimum 1,500 ml/24 hours).

• Diligently evaluate complete blood count (CBC) for decreased blood Hct and Hgb, platelet, and WBC levels.

• Evaluate the patient's complications, therapeutic improvement, and vision.

Patient Teaching

• Instruct the patient that valganciclovir provides suppression, not a cure, of CMV retinitis.

• Stress to the patient that frequent blood tests are necessary during therapy because of the toxic nature of drug.

• As advised by the physician, explain to the patient that he or she should have an ophthalmologic exam every 4 to 6 weeks during treatment.

• Warn the patient to report any new symptoms promptly to the physician.

• Explain to the male patient that valganciclovir may temporarily or permanently inhibit sperm production. Explain to the female patient that valganciclovir may temporarily or permanently suppress fertility. Teach patients to use barrier contraception during and for 90 days after therapy because of the drug's mutagenic potential.

zanamivir
zah-**nam**-ih-vur
(Relenza)

CATEGORY AND SCHEDULE
Pregnancy Risk Category: B

MECHANISM OF ACTION

An antiviral that appears to inhibit the influenza virus enzyme neuraminidase, which is essential for viral replication. *Therapeutic Effect:* Prevents viral release from infected cells.

AVAILABILITY

Blisters of powder for inhalation: 5 mg.

INDICATIONS AND DOSAGES

▶ **Treatment of influenza virus**
Inhalation
Adults, Elderly, Children 7 yrs and older. 2 inhalations (one 5-mg blister per inhalation for a total dose of 10 mg) twice a day (approximately 12 hrs apart) for 5 days.

▶ **Prevention of influenza virus**
Inhalation
Adults, Elderly. 2 inhalations once a day for the duration of the exposure period.

CONTRAINDICATIONS

None known

INTERACTIONS

Drug
None known.
Herbal
None known.
Food
None known.

DIAGNOSTIC TEST EFFECTS

May increase serum CPK and liver enzymes.

SIDE EFFECTS
Occasional (3%–2%)
Diarrhea, sinusitis, nausea, bronchitis, cough, dizziness, headache
Rare (less than 1.5%)
Malaise, fatigue, fever, abdominal pain, myalgia, arthralgia, urticaria

SERIOUS REACTIONS
• Neutropenia may occur.
• Bronchospasm may occur in those with history of chronic obstructive pulmonary disease (COPD) or bronchial asthma.

NURSING CONSIDERATIONS
Baseline Assessment
• Be aware that patients requiring an inhaled bronchodilator at the same time as zanamivir should receive the bronchodilator before zanamivir.
Precautions
• Use cautiously in patients with asthma and COPD.
Administration and Handling
• Inhalation
• Using the Diskhaler device provided, instruct the patient to exhale completely; then, holding the mouthpiece 1 inch away from the patient's lips, instruct the patient to inhale and hold his or her breath as long as possible before exhaling.
• Have the patient rinse his or her mouth with water immediately after inhalation to prevent mouth and throat dryness.
• Store at room temperature.
Intervention and Evaluation
• Provide assistance to the patient if he or she experiences dizziness.
• Assess the patient's pattern of daily bowel activity and stool consistency.
Patient Teaching
• Instruct the patient on how to use the delivery device.
• Stress to the patient that he or she avoid contact with those who are at high risk for influenza.
• Advise the patient to continue treatment for the full 5-day course and to evenly space doses around the clock.
• Teach patients with respiratory disease to be sure an inhaled bronchodilator is always readily available.

6 Carbapenems

ertapenem
imipenem/cilastatin
   sodium
meropenem

Uses: Carbapenems are used to treat a wide variety of infections caused by aerobic and anaerobic organisms, including *Streptococci, Enterococci, Staphylococci, Pseudomonas* species, and *Acinetobacter* species, and *Bacteroides fragilis.* They have a broader spectrum of activity than most other beta-lactam antibiotics.

Action: Carbapenems bind to penicillin-binding proteins, disrupting bacterial cell wall synthesis. Through this action, they're bactericidal. (See illustration, *Sites and Mechanisms of Action: Anti-infective Agents,* page 2.)

ertapenem
er-tah-**pen**-em
(Invanz)

CATEGORY AND SCHEDULE
Pregnancy Risk Category: B

MECHANISM OF ACTION
A carbapenem that penetrates the bacterial cell wall of microorganisms, inhibiting cell wall synthesis. *Therapeutic Effect:* Produces bacterial cell death.

PHARMACOKINETICS
Almost completely absorbed after IM administration. Protein binding: 85%–95%. Widely distributed. Primarily excreted in urine with smaller amount eliminated in feces. Removed by hemodialysis. **Half-life:** 4 hrs.

AVAILABILITY
Lyophilized Powder: 1-g vial.

INDICATIONS AND DOSAGES
▶ **Infection**
IM
Adults, Elderly. 1 g given once a day for up to 7 days.
IV
Adults, Elderly. 1 g given once a day for up to 14 days.
▶ **Dosage in renal impairment**
IM/IV
Adults, Elderly with creatinine clearance less than 30 ml/min. 500 mg once a day.

CONTRAINDICATIONS
History of hypersensitivity to beta-lactams (imipenem-cilastin, meropenem); hypersensitivity to local anesthetics of amide type (IM)

INTERACTIONS
Drug
Probenecid: Reduces renal excretion of ertapenem (do not use concurrently).
Herbal
None known.
Food
None known.

DIAGNOSTIC TEST EFFECTS

May increase serum alkaline phosphatase, SGOT (AST), and SGPT (ALT) levels. May decrease blood Hct, Hgb, platelet count, and potassium levels.

IV INCOMPATIBILITIES

Do not mix or confuse with any other medications. Do not use diluents or IV solutions containing dextrose.

IV COMPATIBILITIES

Compatible with Water for Injection, 0.9% NaCl

SIDE EFFECTS

Frequent (10%–6%)
Diarrhea, nausea, headache
Occasional (5%–2%)
Altered mental status, insomnia, rash, abdominal pain, constipation, vomiting, edema or swelling, fever
Rare (less than 2%)
Dizziness, cough, oral candidiasis, anxiety, tachycardia, phlebitis at IV site

SERIOUS REACTIONS

• Antibiotic-associated colitis and other superinfections may occur.
• Anaphylactic reactions in those concurrently receiving beta-lactams have occurred.
• Seizures may occur in those with central nervous system (CNS) disorders, including patients with brain lesions or a history of seizures, and in patients with bacterial meningitis or severely impaired renal function.

NURSING CONSIDERATIONS

Baseline Assessment
◀ALERT▶ Determine the patient's history of allergies, particularly to beta-lactams, cephalosporins, and penicillins before beginning drug therapy.
• Determine the patient's history of seizures.

Lifespan Considerations
• Be aware that ertapenem is distributed in breast milk.
• Be aware that the safety and efficacy of ertapenem have not been established in children younger than 18 years.
• In the elderly, advanced renal insufficiency and end-stage renal insufficiency may require dosage adjustment.

Precautions
• Use cautiously in patients with CNS disorders (particularly with brain lesions or history of seizures), a hypersensitivity to cephalosporins, penicillins, or other allergens, and impaired renal function.

Administration and Handling
IM
• Reconstitute with 3.2 ml 1% lidocaine HCl injection (without epinephrine).
• Shake vial thoroughly.
• Give deep IM injections slowly to minimize patient discomfort. To further minimize discomfort, administer IM injections into the gluteus maximus instead of the lateral aspect of the thigh.
• Administer suspension within 1 hour after preparation.
IV
• Solution normally appears colorless to yellow (variation in color does not affect potency).
• Discard if solution contains precipitate.
• Reconstituted solution is stable for 6 hours at room temperature, 24 hours if refrigerated.
• Dilute 1-g vial with 10 ml, 0.9% NaCl or Bacteriostatic Water for Injection.
• Shake well to dissolve.

• Further dilute with 50 ml 0.9% NaCl.
• Give by intermittent IV infusion (piggyback). Do not give IV push.
• Infuse over 20 to 30 minutes.

Intervention and Evaluation
• Assess the patient's pattern of daily bowel activity and stool consistency.
• Evaluate the patient for hydration status, nausea, and vomiting.
• Check the patient's IV injection site for inflammation.
• Assess the patient's skin for rash.
• Evaluate the patient's mental status.
• Observe the patient for signs of possible seizures and tremors.
• Assess the patient' s sleep pattern for evidence of insomnia.

Patient Teaching
• Warn the patient to notify the physician if he or she experiences diarrhea, rash, seizures, tremors, or any other new symptoms.

imipenem/cilastatin sodium
im-ih-**peh**-nem/sill-as-**tah**-tin
(Primaxin)

CATEGORY AND SCHEDULE
Pregnancy Risk Category: C

MECHANISM OF ACTION
A fixed-combination carbapenem. Imipenem binds to bacterial cell membrane. *Therapeutic Effect:* Inhibits cell wall synthesis. Bactericidal. Cilastatin competitively inhibits the enzyme dehydropeptidase. *Therapeutic Effect:* Prevents renal metabolism of imipenem.

PHARMACOKINETICS
Readily absorbed after IM administration. Widely distributed. Protein binding: 13%–21%. Metabolized in kidney. Primarily excreted in urine. Removed by hemodialysis. **Half-life:** 1 hr (half-life is increased in those with impaired renal function).

AVAILABILITY
IM Injection: 500 mg, 750 mg.
IV Injection: 250 mg, 500 mg.

INDICATIONS AND DOSAGES
▶ **Serious respiratory tract, skin and skin-structure, gynecologic, bone, joint, intra-abdominal, nosocomial, and urinary tract infections; endocarditis; polymicrobic infections; and septicemia**
IV
Adults, Elderly. 2–4 g/day in divided doses q6h.
▶ **Mild to moderate respiratory tract, skin and skin-structure, gynecologic, bone, joint, intra-abdominal, and urinary tract infections; endocarditis; polymicrobic infections; and septicemia**
IV
Adults, Elderly. 1–2 g/day in divided doses q6–8h.
Children 3 mos and older–12 yrs. 60–100 mg/kg/day in divided doses q6h. Maximum: 4 g/day.
Children 1–less than 3 mos. 100 mg/kg/day in divided doses q6h.
Children younger than 1 mo. 20–25 mg/kg/dose q8–24h.
IM
Adults, Elderly. 500–750 mg q12h.
▶ **Dosage in renal impairment**
Dosage and frequency are modified based on creatinine clearance and the severity of infection.

Creatinine Clearance	Dosage
31–70 ml/min	500 mg q8h
21–30 ml/min	500 mg q12h
5–20 ml/min	250 mg q12h

CONTRAINDICATIONS
None known

INTERACTIONS
Drug
None known.
Herbal
None known.
Food
None known.

DIAGNOSTIC TEST EFFECTS
May increase BUN, serum alkaline phosphatase, bilirubin, creatinine, LDH, SGOT (AST), and SGPT (ALT) levels. May decrease blood Hct and Hgb.

IV INCOMPATIBILITIES
Allopurinol (Aloprim), amphotericin B complex (Abelcet, AmBisome, Amphotec), fluconazole (Diflucan)

IV COMPATIBILITIES
Diltiazem (Cardizem), insulin, propofol (Diprivan)

SIDE EFFECTS
Occasional (3%–2%)
Diarrhea, nausea, vomiting
Rare (2%–1%)
Rash

SERIOUS REACTIONS
• Antibiotic-associated colitis and other superinfections may occur.
• Anaphylactic reactions in those concurrently receiving beta-lactams have occurred.

NURSING CONSIDERATIONS
Baseline Assessment
◀ALERT▶ Determine the patient's history of allergies, particularly to beta-lactams, cephalosporins, and penicillins before beginning drug therapy.

• Determine the patient's history of seizures.
Lifespan Considerations
• Be aware that imipenem crosses the placenta and is distributed in amniotic fluid, breast milk, and cord blood.
• This drug may be used safely in children younger than 12 years.
• In the elderly, age-related renal function impairment may require dosage adjustment.
Precautions
• Use cautiously in patients with a history of seizures, renal impairment, and sensitivity to penicillins.
Administration and Handling
IM
• Prepare with 1% lidocaine without epinephrine, as prescribed; 500-mg vial with 2 ml, 750-mg vial with 3 ml lidocaine HCl.
• Administer suspension within 1 hour of preparation.
• Don't mix the suspension with any other medications.
• Give deep IM injections slowly into a large muscle to minimize patient discomfort. To further minimize discomfort, administer IM injections into the gluteus maximus instead of the lateral aspect of the thigh. Be sure to aspirate with the syringe before injecting the drug to decrease risk of injection into a blood vessel.
IV
• Solution normally appears colorless to yellow; discard if solution turns brown.
• IV infusion (piggyback) is stable for 4 hours at room temperature, 24 hours if refrigerated.
• Discard if precipitate forms.
• Dilute each 250- or 500-mg vial with 100 ml D_5W; 0.9% NaCl.
• Give by intermittent IV infusion (piggyback). Do not give IV push.

• Infuse over 20 to 30 minutes (1-g dose longer than 40 to 60 minutes).
• Observe the patient during the first 30 minutes of the infusion for possible hypersensitivity reaction.

Intervention and Evaluation

• Monitor the patient's hematologic, liver, and renal function tests.
• Evaluate the patient for phlebitis as evidenced by heat, pain, and red streaking over vein.
• Evaluate that patient for pain at the IV injection site.
• Assess the patient for gastrointestinal (GI) discomfort, nausea, and vomiting.
• Assess the patient's pattern of daily bowel activity and stool consistency.
• Assess the patient's skin for rash.
• Observe the patient for possible seizures and tremors.

Patient Teaching

• Warn the patient to immediately notify the physician if he or she experiences severe diarrhea and to avoid taking antidiarrheals until directed to do so by the physician.
• Explain to the patient that he or she should notify the physician of the onset of troublesome or serious adverse reactions, including infusion site pain, redness, or swelling, nausea or vomiting, or skin rash or itching.

meropenem
murr-**oh**-pen-em
(Merrem IV)

CATEGORY AND SCHEDULE
Pregnancy Risk Category: B

MECHANISM OF ACTION
A carbapenem that binds to penicillin-binding proteins. *Therapeutic Effect:* Inhibits bacterial cell wall synthesis. Bactericidal.

PHARMACOKINETICS
After IV administration, widely distributed into tissues and body fluids, including cerebrospinal fluid (CSF). Protein binding: 2%. Primarily excreted unchanged in urine. Removed by hemodialysis. **Half-life:** 1 hr.

AVAILABILITY
Powder for Injection: 500 mg, 1 g.

INDICATIONS AND DOSAGES
▸ **Mild to moderate infections**
IV
Adults, Elderly. 0.5–1 g q8h.
Children 3 mos and older. 20 mg/kg/dose q8h.
Children younger than 3 mos. 20 mg/kg/dose q8–12h.
▸ **Meningitis**
IV
Adults, Elderly, Children weighing 50 kg or more. 2 g q8h.
Children 3 mos and older, weighing less than 50 kg. 40 mg/kg q8h. Maximum: 2 g/dose.
▸ **Dosage in renal impairment**
Reduce dosage in patients with creatinine clearance less than 50 ml/min.

Creatinine Clearance	Dosage	Interval
26–49 ml/min	Recommended dose (1,000 mg)	q12h
10–25 ml/min	½ recommended dose	q12h
less than 10 ml/min	½ recommended dose	q24h

UNLABELED USES
Lowers respiratory tract infections, febrile neutropenia, gynecologic and obstetric infections, sepsis

CONTRAINDICATIONS
None known

INTERACTIONS
Drug
Probenecid: Inhibits renal excretion of meropenem (do not use concurrently).
Herbal
None known.
Food
None known.

DIAGNOSTIC TEST EFFECTS
May increase BUN, serum alkaline phosphatase, serum bilirubin, serum creatinine, serum LDH, SGOT (AST), and SGPT (ALT) levels. May decrease blood Hct and, Hgb, and serum potassium levels.

IV INCOMPATIBILITIES
Acyclovir (Zovirax), amphotericin B (Fungizone), diazepam (Valium), doxycycline (Vibramycin), metronidazole (Flagyl), ondansetron (Zofran)

IV COMPATIBILITIES
Dobutamine (Dobutrex), dopamine (Intropin), heparin, magnesium

SIDE EFFECTS
Frequent (5%–3%)
Diarrhea, nausea, vomiting, headache, inflammation at injection site
Occasional (2%)
Oral moniliasis, rash, pruritus
Rare (less than 2%)
Constipation, glossitis

SERIOUS REACTIONS
• Antibiotic-associated colitis and other superinfections may occur.
• Anaphylactic reactions in those concurrently receiving beta lactams have occurred.
• Seizures may occur in those with bacterial meningitis, central nervous system (CNS) disorders (including brain lesions and a history of seizures), and impaired renal function.

NURSING CONSIDERATIONS
Baseline Assessment
• Determine the patient's history of seizures.
Lifespan Considerations
• Be aware that it is unknown if meropenem is distributed in breast milk.
• Be aware that the safety and efficacy of meropenem have not been established in children younger than 3 months.
• In the elderly, age-related renal impairment may require dosage adjustment.
Precautions
• Use cautiously in patients with CNS disorders (particularly a history of seizures), hypersensitivity to cephalosporins, penicillins, or other allergens, and renal function impairment.
Administration and Handling
◄ALERT► Space drug doses evenly around the clock.
IV
• Store vials at room temperature.
• After reconstitution with 0.9% NaCl, solution is stable for 2 hours at room temperature, 18 hours if refrigerated (with D_5W, stable for 1 hour at room temperature, 8 hours if refrigerated).
• Reconstitute each 500 mg with 10 ml Sterile Water for Injection to provide a concentration of 50 mg/ml.
• Shake to dissolve until clear.
• May further dilute with 100 ml 0.9% NaCl or D_5W.
• May give by IV push or IV intermittent infusion (piggyback).
• If administering as IV intermittent

infusion (piggyback), give over
15 to 30 minutes; if administered
by IV push (5 to 20 ml), give over
3 to 5 minutes.

Intervention and Evaluation

• Assess the patient's pattern of
daily bowel activity and stool consistency.

• Evaluate the patient for hydration
status, nausea, and vomiting.

• Check the patient's IV injection
site for inflammation.

• Assess the patient's skin for rash.

• Monitor the patient's electrolytes
(especially potassium), intake and
output, and renal function test
results.

• Observe the patient's mental status
and be alert to possible seizure or
tremor development.

• Assess the patient's blood pressure
(B/P) and temperature twice a day,
more often if necessary.

Patient Teaching

• Warn the patient to immediately
notify the physician if he or she
experiences severe diarrhea and to
avoid taking antidiarrheals until
directed to do so by the physician.

• Explain to the patient that he or
she should notify the physician of
the onset of troublesome or serious
adverse reactions, including infusion
site pain, redness, or swelling,
nausea or vomiting, or skin rash or
itching.

cefaclor
cefadroxil
cefazolin sodium
cefdinir
cefditoren
cefepime
cefotaxime sodium
cefotetan disodium
cefoxitin sodium
cefpodoxime proxetil
cefprozil
ceftazidime
ceftibuten
ceftizoxime sodium
ceftriaxone sodium
cefuroxime axetil,
  cefuroxime sodium
cephalexin
loracarbef

Uses: Cephalosporins are used to treat a number of diseases, including respiratory diseases, skin and soft tissue infections, bone and joint infections, and genitourinary (GU) infections. These broad-spectrum antibiotics also are used prophylactically in some surgical procedures. First-generation cephalosporins have good activity against gram-positive organisms and moderate activity against gram-negative organisms, including *Escherichia coli, Klebsiella pneumoniae,* and *Proteus mirabilis.* Second-generation cephalosporins have increased activity against gram-negative organisms. Third-generation cephalosporins are less active against gram-positive organisms but more active against the Enterobacteriaceae with some activity against *Pseudomonas aeruginosa.* Fourth-generation cephalosporins have good activity against gram-positive organisms, such as *Staphylococcus aureus,* and gram-negative organisms, such as *P. aeruginosa.*

Action: Cephalosporins inhibit bacterial cell wall synthesis or activate enzymes that disrupt the cell wall, causing a weakening in the cell wall, cell lysis, and cell death. (See illustration, *Sites and Mechanisms of Action: Anti-infective Agents,* page 2.) Cephalosporins may be bacteriostatic or bactericidal and are most effective against rapidly dividing cells.

cefaclor
sef-ah-klor
(Apo-Cefaclor[CAN], Ceclor, Ceclor CD, Cefkor[AUS], Cefkor CD[AUS], Keflor[AUS])

CATEGORY AND SCHEDULE
Pregnancy Risk Category: B

MECHANISM OF ACTION
A second-generation cephalosporin that binds to bacterial cell membranes. *Therapeutic Effect:* Inhibits synthesis of bacterial cell wall. Bactericidal.

PHARMACOKINETICS
Well absorbed from the gastrointestinal (GI) tract. Protein binding: 25%. Widely distributed. Primarily excreted unchanged in urine. Moderately removed by hemodialysis. **Half-life:** 0.6–0.9 hrs (half-life is increased with impaired renal function).

AVAILABILITY
Capsules: 250 mg, 500 mg.
Tablets (extended-release):
375 mg, 500 mg.
Oral Suspension: 125 mg/5 ml,
187 mg/5 ml, 250 mg/5 ml,
375 mg/5 ml.

INDICATIONS AND DOSAGES
▶ **Mild to moderate infections**
PO
Adults, Elderly. 250 mg q8h.
Children older than 1 mo.
20 mg/kg/day in divided
doses q8h.
▶ **Severe infections**
PO
Adults, Elderly. 500 mg q8h.
Maximum: 4 g/day.
Children older than 1 mo. 40 mg/
kg/day in divided doses q8h.
Maximum: 2 g/day.
PO (extended-release tablets)
Adults, Children older than 16 yrs.
375–500 mg q12h.
▶ **Otitis media**
PO
Children older than 1 mo. 40 mg/
kg/day in divided doses q8h.
Maximum: 1 g/day.
▶ **Dosage in renal impairment**
Reduced dosage may be necessary
in those with creatinine clearance
less than 40 ml/min.

CONTRAINDICATIONS
History of anaphylactic reaction to
penicillins or hypersensitivity to
cephalosporins

INTERACTIONS
Drug
Probenecid: May increase cefaclor
blood concentration.
Herbal
None known.
Food
None known.

DIAGNOSTIC TEST EFFECTS
Positive direct or indirect Coombs'
test. May increase BUN, serum
alkaline phosphatase, bilirubin,
creatinine, and LDH, and
SGOT (AST), and SGPT (ALT)
levels.

SIDE EFFECTS
Frequent
Oral candidiasis (sore mouth or
tongue), mild diarrhea, mild abdominal cramping, vaginal candidiasis
(discharge, itching)
Occasional
Nausea, serum sickness reaction
(fever, joint pain)
Serum sickness reaction usually
occurs after the second course of
therapy and resolves after the drug
is discontinued.
Rare
Allergic reaction as evidenced by
pruritus, rash, and urticaria

SERIOUS REACTIONS
• Antibiotic-associated colitis manifested as severe abdominal pain and
tenderness, fever, and watery and
severe diarrhea, and other superinfections, may result from altered
bacterial balance.
• Nephrotoxicity may occur, especially in patients with preexisting
renal disease.
• Severe hypersensitivity reaction
including severe pruritus, angioedema, bronchospasm, and anaphylaxis, particularly in patients with a
history of allergies, especially to
penicillin, may occur.

◼NURSING CONSIDERATIONS

Baseline Assessment
◀ALERT▶ Determine the patient's
history of allergies, particularly
cephalosporins and penicillins,
before beginning drug therapy.

Lifespan Considerations
• Be aware that cefaclor readily crosses the placenta and is distributed in breast milk.
• There are no age-related precautions noted in children older than 1 month.
• In the elderly, age-related renal impairment may require dosage adjustment.

Precautions
• Use cautiously in patients with a history of GI disease (especially antibiotic-associated colitis or ulcerative colitis), and renal impairment.
• Use cautiously in patients concurrently using nephrotoxic medications.

Administration and Handling
PO
• After reconstitution, oral solution is stable for 14 days if refrigerated.
• Shake oral suspension well before using.
• Give without regard to meals; if GI upset occurs, give with food or milk.
• Do not cut, crush, or chew extended-release tablets.

Intervention and Evaluation
• Assess the patient's mouth for white patches on the mucous membranes and tongue.
• Assess the patient's pattern of daily bowel activity and stool consistency. Although mild GI effects may be tolerable, an increase in their severity may indicate the onset of antibiotic-associated colitis.
• Monitor the patient's intake and output and renal function reports for nephrotoxicity.
• Be alert for signs and symptoms of superinfection including abdominal pain, moderate to severe diarrhea, severe anal or genital pruritus, and severe mouth soreness.

Patient Teaching
• Advise the patient to continue therapy for the full length of treatment and to evenly space doses around the clock.
• Explain to the patient that cefaclor may cause GI upset. Instruct the patient to take the drug with food or milk if GI upset occurs.
• Teach the patient to refrigerate cefaclor oral suspension.

cefadroxil
sef-ah-**drocks**-ill
(Duricef)

CATEGORY AND SCHEDULE
Pregnancy Risk Category: B

MECHANISM OF ACTION
A first-generation cephalosporin that binds to bacterial cell membranes. *Therapeutic Effect:* Inhibits synthesis of bacterial cell wall. Bactericidal.

PHARMACOKINETICS
Well absorbed from the gastrointestinal (GI) tract. Protein binding: 15%–20%. Widely distributed. Primarily excreted unchanged in urine. Removed by hemodialysis. **Half-life:** 1.2–1.5 hrs (half-life is increased with impaired renal function).

AVAILABILITY
Capsules: 500 mg.
Tablets: 1,000 mg.
Oral Suspension: 250 mg/5 ml, 500 mg/5 ml.

INDICATIONS AND DOSAGES
▸ **Urinary tract infections**
PO
Adults, Elderly. 1–2 g/day in 1–2 divided doses.

▸ **Skin/skin-structure infections, group A beta-hemolytic streptococcal pharyngitis, tonsillitis**
PO
Adults, Elderly. 1–2 g in 2 divided doses.
Children. 30 mg/kg/day in 2 divided doses. Maximum: 2 g/day.
▸ **Dosage in renal impairment**
Dosage and frequency are based on the degree of renal impairment and the severity of infection. After initial 1-g dose:

Creatinine Clearance	Dosage Interval
25–50 ml/min	500 mg q12h
10–25 ml/min	500 mg q24h
0–10 ml/min	500 mg q36h

CONTRAINDICATIONS
Anaphylactic reaction to penicillins, history of hypersensitivity to cephalosporins

INTERACTIONS
Drug
Probenecid: Increases cefadroxil blood concentration.
Herbal
None known.
Food
None known.

DIAGNOSTIC TEST EFFECTS
Positive direct or indirect Coombs' test. May increase BUN, serum alkaline phosphatase, bilirubin, creatinine, and LDH, and SGOT (AST), and SGPT (ALT) levels.

SIDE EFFECTS
Frequent
Oral candidiasis (sore mouth or tongue), mild diarrhea, mild abdominal cramping, vaginal candidiasis (discharge, itching)

Occasional
Nausea, unusual bruising or bleeding, serum sickness reaction (fever, joint pain)
Serum sickness reaction usually occurs following the second course of therapy and resolves after the drug is discontinued.
Rare
Allergic reaction (rash, pruritus, urticaria), thrombophlebitis (pain, redness, swelling at injection site)

SERIOUS REACTIONS
• Antibiotic-associated colitis as evidenced by severe abdominal pain and tenderness, fever, and watery and severe diarrhea, and other superinfections may result from altered bacterial balance.
• Nephrotoxicity may occur, especially in patients with preexisting renal disease.
• Severe hypersensitivity reaction including severe pruritus, angioedema, bronchospasm, and anaphylaxis, particularly in patients with history of allergies, especially penicillin, may occur.

NURSING CONSIDERATIONS
Baseline Assessment
◀ALERT▶ Determine the patient's history of allergies, particularly to cephalosporins and penicillins before beginning drug therapy.
Precautions
• Use cautiously in patients with a history of allergies or GI disease (especially antibiotic-associated colitis or ulcerative colitis) and renal impairment.
• Use cautiously in patients concurrently using nephrotoxic medications.
Lifespan Considerations
• Be aware that cefadroxil readily crosses the placenta and is distributed in breast milk.

• There are no age-related precautions noted in children.
• In the elderly, age-related decreased renal function may require dosage adjustment.

Administration and Handling
PO
• After reconstitution, oral solution is stable for 14 days if refrigerated.
• Shake oral suspension well before using.
• Give without regard to meals; if GI upset occurs, give with food or milk.

Intervention and Evaluation
• Assess the patient's mouth for white patches on the mucous membranes and tongue.
• Assess the patient's pattern of daily bowel activity and stool consistency. Although mild GI effects may be tolerable, an increase in their severity may indicate onset of antibiotic-associated colitis.
• Monitor the patient's intake and output and renal function reports for nephrotoxicity.
• Be alert for signs and symptoms of superinfection as evidenced by abdominal pain, anal or genital pruritus, moderate to severe diarrhea, moniliasis, and sore mouth or tongue.

Patient Teaching
• Advise the patient to continue therapy for the full length of treatment and to evenly space doses around the clock.
• Explain that cefadroxil may cause GI upset. Instruct the patient to take the drug with food or milk if GI upset occurs.
• Teach the patient to refrigerate cefadroxil oral suspension.

cefazolin sodium
cef-ah-**zoe**-lin
(Ancef, Kefzol)
Do not confuse with cefprozil or Cefzil.

CATEGORY AND SCHEDULE
Pregnancy Risk Category: B

MECHANISM OF ACTION
A first-generation cephalosporin that binds to bacterial cell membranes. *Therapeutic Effect:* Inhibits synthesis of bacterial cell wall. Bactericidal.

PHARMACOKINETICS
Widely distributed. Protein binding: 85%. Primarily excreted unchanged in urine. Moderately removed by hemodialysis. **Half-life:** 1.4–1.8 hrs (half-life is increased with impaired renal function).

AVAILABILITY
Injection: 500 mg, 1 g.
Ready-to-Hang Infusion: 1 g/50 ml, 2 g/100 ml.

INDICATIONS AND DOSAGES
▶ **Uncomplicated urinary tract infection (UTI)**
IM/IV
Adults, Elderly. 1 g q12h.
▶ **Mild to moderate infections**
IM/IV
Adults, Elderly. 250–500 mg q8–12h.
▶ **Severe infections**
IM/IV
Adults, Elderly. 0.5–1 g q6–8h.
▶ **Life-threatening infections**
IM/IV
Adults, Elderly. 1–1.5 g q6h.
Maximum: 12 g/day.
▶ **Perioperative prophylaxis**
IM/IV
Adults, Elderly. 1 g 30–60 min

before surgery, 0.5–1 g during surgery, and q6–8h for up to 24 hrs postoperatively.

▶ **Usual pediatric dosage**
Neonates 7 days and younger: 40 mg/kg/day in divided doses q12h.
Neonates older than 7 days. 40–60 mg/kg/day in divided doses q8–12h.
Children. 50–100 mg/kg/day in divided doses q8h.

▶ **Dosage in renal impairment**

Creatinine Clearance	Dosing Interval
10–30 ml/min	q12h
less than 10 ml/min	q24h

CONTRAINDICATIONS
Anaphylactic reaction to penicillins, history of hypersensitivity to cephalosporins

INTERACTIONS
Drug
Probenecid: Increases cefazolin blood concentration.
Herbal
None known.
Food
None known.

DIAGNOSTIC TEST EFFECTS
Positive direct or indirect Coombs' test. May increase BUN, serum alkaline phosphatase, bilirubin, creatinine, and LDH, and SGOT (AST), and SGPT (ALT) levels.

IV INCOMPATIBILITIES
Amikacin (Amikin), amiodarone (Cordarone), hydromorphone (Dilaudid)

IV COMPATIBILITIES
Calcium gluconate, diltiazem (Cardizem), famotidine (Pepcid), heparin, insulin (regular), lidocaine, magnesium sulfate, midazolam (Versed), morphine, multivitamins, potassium chloride, propofol (Diprivan), vecuronium (Norcuron)

SIDE EFFECTS
Frequent
Discomfort with IM administration, oral candidiasis (sore mouth or tongue), mild diarrhea, mild abdominal cramping, vaginal candidiasis (discharge, itching)
Occasional
Nausea, serum sickness reaction (fever, joint pain)
Serum sickness reaction usually occurs after the second course of therapy and resolves after the drug is discontinued.
Rare
Allergic reaction (rash, pruritus, urticaria), thrombophlebitis (pain, redness, swelling at injection site)

SERIOUS REACTIONS
• Antibiotic-associated colitis manifested as severe abdominal pain and tenderness, fever, and watery and severe diarrhea, and other superinfections may result from altered bacterial balance.
• Nephrotoxicity may occur, especially in patients with preexisting renal disease.
• Severe hypersensitivity reaction including severe pruritus, angioedema, bronchospasm, and anaphylaxis, particularly in patients with a history of allergies, especially to penicillin, may occur.

NURSING CONSIDERATIONS
Baseline Assessment
◀ **ALERT** ▶ Determine the patient's history of allergies, particularly cephalosporins and penicillins, before beginning drug therapy.

Lifespan Considerations
• Be aware that cefazolin readily crosses the placenta and is distributed in breast milk.
• There are no age-related precautions noted in children.
• In the elderly, age-related renal impairment may require dosage adjustment.

Precautions
• Use cautiously in patients with a history GI disease (especially antibiotic-associated colitis or ulcerative colitis), and renal impairment.
• Use cautiously in patients concurrently using nephrotoxic medications.

Administration and Handling
IM
• To minimize discomfort, give IM injection deep and slowly. To minimize injection site discomfort, give the IM injection in the gluteus maximus rather than lateral aspect of thigh.

IV
• Solution normally appears light yellow to yellow.
• IV infusion (piggyback) is stable for 24 hours at room temperature and 96 hours if refrigerated.
• Discard solution if precipitate forms.
• Reconstitute each 1 g with at least 10 ml Sterile Water for Injection.
• May further dilute in 50 to 100 ml D_5W or 0.9% NaCl to decrease the incidence of thrombophlebitis.
• For IV push, administer over 3 to 5 minutes.
• For intermittent IV infusion (piggyback), infuse over 20 to 30 minutes.

Intervention and Evaluation
• Evaluate the patient's IM site for induration and tenderness.
• Assess the patient's mouth for white patches on the mucous membranes or tongue.
• Assess the patient's pattern of daily bowel activity and stool consistency carefully. Although mild GI effects may be tolerable, an increase in their severity may indicate the onset of antibiotic-associated colitis.
• Monitor the patient's intake and output and renal function reports for nephrotoxicity.
• Be alert for signs and symptoms of superinfection including abdominal pain, moderate to severe diarrhea, severe anal or genital pruritus, and severe mouth soreness.

Patient Teaching
• Explain to the patient that discomfort may occur with IM injection.
• Advise the patient to continue the antibiotic therapy for the full length of treatment and to evenly space drug doses around the clock.

cefdinir
cef-din-ur
(Omnicef)

CATEGORY AND SCHEDULE
Pregnancy Risk Category: B

MECHANISM OF ACTION
A third-generation cephalosporin that binds to bacterial cell membranes. *Therapeutic Effect:* Inhibits synthesis of bacterial cell wall. Bactericidal.

PHARMACOKINETICS
Moderately absorbed from the gastrointestinal (GI) tract. Protein binding: 60%–70%. Widely distributed. Not appreciably metabolized. Primarily excreted unchanged in urine. Minimally removed by hemodialysis. **Half-life:** 1–2 hrs (half-life is increased in those with impaired renal function).

AVAILABILITY
Capsules: 300 mg.
Oral Suspension: 125 mg/5 ml.

INDICATIONS AND DOSAGES
▶ **Community-acquired pneumonia**
PO
Adults, Elderly, Children 13 yrs and older. 300 mg q12h for 10 days.
▶ **Acute exacerbation of chronic bronchitis**
PO
Adults, Elderly. 300 mg q12h for 5 days.
▶ **Acute maxillary sinusitis**
PO
Adults, Elderly, Children 13 yrs and older. 300 mg q12h or 600 mg q24h for 10 days.
Children 6 mos–12 yrs. 7 mg/kg q12h or 14 mg/kg q24h for 10 days.
▶ **Pharyngitis or tonsillitis**
PO
Adults, Elderly, Children 13 yrs and older. 300 mg q12h for 5–10 days or 600 mg q24h for 10 days.
Children 6 mos–12 yrs. 7 mg/kg q12h for 5–10 days or 14 mg/kg q24h for 10 days.
▶ **Uncomplicated skin/skin-structure infections**
PO
Adults, Elderly, Children 13 yrs and older. 300 mg q12h for 10 days.
Children 6 mos–12 yrs. 7 mg/kg q12h for 10 days.
▶ **Acute bacterial otitis media**
PO
Children 6 mos–12 yrs. 7 mg/kg q12h or 14 mg/kg q24h for 10 days.
▶ **Oral suspension**
Infants weighing less than 20 lbs. 2.5 ml (tsp) q12h or 5 ml (1 tsp) q24h.
Children weighing 20–40 lbs. 5 ml (1 tsp) q12h or 10 ml (2 tsp) q24h.
Children weighing 41–60 lbs. 7.5

ml (1 tsp) q12h or 15 ml (3 tsp) q24h.
Children weighing 61–80 lbs. 10 ml (2 tsp) q12h or 20 ml (4 tsp) q24h.
Children weighing 81–95 lbs. 12.5 ml (2.5 tsp) q12h or 25 ml (5 tsp) q24h.
▶ **Dosage in renal impairment**
Creatinine clearance less than 30 ml/min: 300 mg/day as single daily dose.
Hemodialysis patients: 300 mg or 7 mg/kg dose every other day.

CONTRAINDICATIONS
Hypersensitivity to cephalosporins

INTERACTIONS
Drug
Antacids: Decrease cefdinir blood concentration.
Probenecid: Increases cefdinir blood concentration.
Herbal
None known.
Food
None known.

DIAGNOSTIC TEST EFFECTS
May produce a false-positive reaction for ketones in urine. May increase serum alkaline phosphatase, bilirubin, and LDH, and SGOT (ALT), and SGPT (AST) levels.

SIDE EFFECTS
Frequent
Oral candidiasis (sore mouth or tongue), mild diarrhea, mild abdominal cramping, vaginal candidiasis (discharge, itching)
Occasional
Nausea, serum sickness reaction (fever, joint pain)
Serum sickness reaction usually occurs after the second course of therapy and resolves after the drug is discontinued.

Rare
Allergic reaction (rash, pruritus,
urticaria)

SERIOUS REACTIONS
• Antibiotic-associated colitis manifested as severe abdominal pain and
tenderness, fever, and watery and
severe diarrhea, and other superinfections may result from altered
bacterial balance.
• Nephrotoxicity may occur, especially in patients with preexisting
renal disease.
• Severe hypersensitivity reaction
including severe pruritus, angioedema, bronchospasm, and anaphylaxis, particularly in patients with a
history of allergies, especially to
penicillins, may occur.

NURSING CONSIDERATIONS
Baseline Assessment
◀ALERT▶ Determine the patient's
hypersensitivity to cefdinir and
other cephalosporins and penicillins
before beginning drug therapy.
Lifespan Considerations
• Be aware that cefdinir crosses the
placenta but is not detected in
breast milk.
• Be aware that infants and newborns may have lower renal clearance of cefdinir.
• In the elderly, age-related decreases in renal function may require decreased cefdinir dosage or
increased dosing interval.
Precautions
• Use cautiously in patients with
hypersensitivity to penicillins or
other drugs, a history of GI disease
(e.g., colitis), impaired liver function, and renal impairment.
Administration and Handling
PO
• Give without regard to meals.
• To reconstitute oral suspension,

for the 60-ml bottle, add 39 ml
water; for the 120-ml bottle, add
65 ml water.
• Shake oral suspension well before
administering.
• Store mixed suspension at room
temperature. Discard unused portion
after 10 days.
Intervention and Evaluation
• Assess the patient's pattern of
daily bowel activity and stool consistency. Although mild GI effects
may be tolerable, an increasing in
their severity may indicate the onset
of antibiotic-associated colitis.
• Be alert for signs and symptoms
of superinfection including anal or
genital pruritus, changes or ulceration of the oral mucosa, moderate to
severe diarrhea, and new or increased fever.
• Monitor the patient's hematology
reports.
Patient Teaching
• Instruct the patient to take antacids 2 hours prior to or following
taking this medication.
• Advise the patient to continue
therapy for the full length of treatment and to evenly space doses
around the clock.
• Warn the patient to notify the
nurse or physician of any persistent
diarrhea.

cefditoren
sef-dih-**tore**-inn
(Spectracef)

CATEGORY AND SCHEDULE
Pregnancy Risk Category: B

MECHANISM OF ACTION
A third generation cephalosporin
that binds to bacterial cell membranes. *Therapeutic effect:* Inhibits

synthesis of bacterial cell wall. Bactericidal.

AVAILABILITY
Tablets: 200 mg.

INDICATIONS AND DOSAGES
▶ **Pharyngitis or tonsillitis, uncomplicated skin and skin-structure infections**
PO
Adults, elderly, children older than 11 yrs. 200 mg 2 times/day for 10 days.
▶ **Acute bacterial exacerbation of chronic bronchitis**
PO
Adults, elderly, children older than 11 yrs. 400 mg 2 times/day for 10 days.
▶ **Dosage in renal impairment**

Creatinine Clearance	Dosage
30–49 ml/min	200 mg 2 times/day
less than 30 ml/min	200 mg once a day

CONTRAINDICATIONS
History of anaphylactic reaction to penicillins or hypersensitivity to cephalosporins, carnitine deficiency

INTERACTIONS
Drug
Antacids containing magnesium and aluminum, H_2 receptor antagonists: May reduce absorption of cefditoren.
Probenecid: Increases absorption of cefditoren.
Herbal
None known.
Food
None known.

DIAGNOSTIC TEST EFFECTS
None known.

SIDE EFFECTS
Frequent
Diarrhea, nausea, headache, abdominal pain, vaginal moniliasis, dyspepsia, vomiting

SERIOUS REACTIONS
• Antibiotic associated colitis manifested as severe abdominal pain and tenderness, fever, watery and severe diarrhea, may occur.
• Severe hypersensitivity reaction manifested as severe pruritus, angioedema, bronchospasm, and anaphylaxis, particularly in patients with a history of allergies, may occur.

NURSING CONSIDERATIONS
Baseline Assessment
◀ ALERT ▶ Determine if the patient is hypersensitive cephalosporins, penicillins, other drugs.
Precautions
• Use cautiously in patients with a history of allergies and renal impairment.
Administration and Handling
PO
• Give with meals to enhance drug absorption.
Intervention and Evaluation
• Examine the patient's mouth for white patches on mucous membranes and tongue.
• Assess the patient's pattern of daily bowel activity and stool consistency.
• Monitor the patient's intake and output and renal function reports.
Patient Teaching
• Advise the patient to continue cefditoren for the full length of treatment.
• Caution the patient against skipping drug doses.
• Explain to the patient that cefdi-

toren is best taken with food to increase the absorption of the drug.

cefepime
sef-eh-**peem**
(Maxipime)

CATEGORY AND SCHEDULE
Pregnancy Risk Category: B

MECHANISM OF ACTION
A fourth-generation cephalosporin that binds to bacterial cell membranes. *Therapeutic Effect:* Inhibits synthesis of bacterial cell wall. Bactericidal.

PHARMACOKINETICS
Well absorbed after IM administration. Protein binding: 20%. Widely distributed. Primarily excreted unchanged in urine. Removed by hemodialysis. **Half-life:** 2–2.3 hrs (half-life is increased with impaired renal function, and in the elderly).

AVAILABILITY
Powder for Injection: 500 mg, 1 g, 2 g.

INDICATIONS AND DOSAGES
▸ **Pneumonia, bronchitis, skin and skin-structure infections, intra-abdominal infections, bacteremia, septicemia, complicated intra-abdominal infections (with metronidazole)**
IM/IV
Adults. Usual dosage 1–2 g q12h.
▸ **Urinary tract infections (UTIs)**
IM/IV
Adults, Elderly. 500 mg q12h.
▸ **Empiric therapy for febrile neutropenia**
IV
Adults. 2 g q8h.
▸ **Usual pediatric dosage**
Children 2 mos–16 yrs. Usual dosage 50 mg/kg q8–12h. Do not exceed maximum adult dose.
▸ **Dosage in renal impairment**
Dosage and frequency are based on the degree of renal impairment (creatinine clearance) and the severity of infection.

Creatinine Clearance	Dose
30–60 ml/min	0.5–2 g q24h
11–29 ml/min	0.5–1 g q24h
10 ml/min or less	0.25–0.5 g q24h

CONTRAINDICATIONS
Anaphylactic reaction to penicillins, history of hypersensitivity to cephalosporins

INTERACTIONS
Drug
Probenecid: May increase cefepime blood concentration.
Herbal
None known.
Food
None known.

DIAGNOSTIC TEST EFFECTS
Positive direct or indirect Coombs' test may occur. May increase serum alkaline phosphatase, bilirubin, and LDH, and SGOT (AST), and SGPT (ALT) levels.

IV INCOMPATIBILITIES
Acyclovir (Zovirax), amphotericin (Fungizone), cimetidine (Tagamet), ciprofloxacin (Cipro), cisplatin (Platinol), dacarbazine (DTIC),

daunorubicin (Cerubidine), diazepam (Valium), diphenhydramine (Benadryl), dobutamine (Dobutrex), dopamine (Intropin), doxorubicin (Adriamycin), etoposide (VePesid), droperidol (Inapsine), famotidine (Pepcid), ganciclovir (Cytovene), haloperidol (Haldol), magnesium, magnesium sulfate, mannitol, meperidine (Demerol), metoclopramide (Reglan), morphine, ofloxacin (Floxin), ondansetron (Zofran), vancomycin (Vancocin)

IV COMPATIBILITIES

Bumetanide (Bumex), calcium gluconate, furosemide (Lasix), hydromorphone (Dilaudid), lorazepam (Ativan), propofol (Diprivan)

SIDE EFFECTS

Frequent
Discomfort with IM administration, oral candidiasis (sore mouth or tongue), mild diarrhea, mild abdominal cramping, vaginal candidiasis (discharge, itching)
Occasional
Nausea, serum sickness reaction (fever, joint pain)
Serum sickness reaction usually occurs after the second course of therapy and resolves after the drug is discontinued.
Rare
Allergic reaction (rash, pruritus, urticaria), thrombophlebitis (pain, redness, swelling at injection site)

SERIOUS REACTIONS

• Antibiotic-associated colitis manifested as severe abdominal pain and tenderness, fever, and watery and severe diarrhea, and other superinfections may result from altered bacterial balance.
• Nephrotoxicity may occur, especially in patients with preexisting renal disease.

• Severe hypersensitivity reaction including severe pruritus, angioedema, bronchospasm, and anaphylaxis, particularly in patients with a history of allergies, especially to penicillins, may occur.

NURSING CONSIDERATIONS

Baseline Assessment
◀ALERT▶ Determine the patient's history of allergies, particularly to cephalosporins and penicillins, before beginning drug therapy.
Lifespan Considerations
• Be aware that it is unknown if cefepime is distributed in breast milk.
• There are no age-related precautions noted in children older than 2 months.
• In the elderly, age-related decreased renal function may require reduced cefepime dosage or increased dosing interval.
Precautions
• Use cautiously in patients with renal impairment.
Administration and Handling
IM
• Add 1.3 ml Sterile Water for Injection, 0.9% NaCl, or D_5W to 500-mg vial (2.4 ml for 1-g and 2-g vials).
• To minimize the pain experienced by the patient, give IM injection slowly and deeply into a large muscle mass (e.g., upper gluteus maximus) instead of the lateral aspect of the thigh.
IV
• Solution is stable for 24 hours at room temperature or 7 days if refrigerated.
• Add 5 ml to 500-mg vial (10 ml for 1-g and 2-g vials).
• Further dilute with 50 to 100 ml 0.9% NaCl, or D_5W.

• For IV push, administer over 3 to 5 minutes.
• For intermittent IV infusion (piggyback), infuse over 30 minutes.

Intervention and Evaluation
• Evaluate the patient's IM site for induration and tenderness.
• Check the patient's mouth for white patches on the mucous membranes and tongue.
• Assess the patient's pattern of daily bowel activity and stool consistency. Although mild GI effects may be tolerable, an increasing in their severity may indicate the onset of antibiotic-associated colitis.
• Monitor the patient's intake and output and renal function reports for nephrotoxicity.
• Be alert for signs and symptoms of superinfection including abdominal pain, moderate to severe diarrhea, severe anal or genital pruritus, and severe mouth soreness.

Patient Teaching
• Explain to the patient that discomfort may occur with IM injection.
• Advise the patient to continue the antibiotic therapy for the full length of treatment and to evenly space drug doses around the clock.

cefotaxime sodium
seh-fo-**tax**-eem
(Claforan)
Do not confuse with cefoxitin, ceftizoxime, or cefuroxime.

CATEGORY AND SCHEDULE
Pregnancy Risk Category: B

MECHANISM OF ACTION
A third-generation cephalosporin that binds to bacterial cell membranes. *Therapeutic Effect:* Inhibits synthesis of bacterial cell wall. Bactericidal.

PHARMACOKINETICS
Widely distributed, including cerebrospinal fluid (CSF). Protein binding: 30%–50%. Partially metabolized in liver to active metabolite. Primarily excreted in urine. Moderately removed by hemodialysis.
Half-life: 1 hr (half-life is increased with impaired renal function).

AVAILABILITY
Powder for Injection: 500 mg, 1 g, 2 g.

INDICATIONS AND DOSAGES
▸ **Uncomplicated infections**
IM/IV
Adults, Elderly. 1 g q12h.
▸ **Mild to moderate infections**
IM/IV
Adults, Elderly. 1–2 g q8h.
▸ **Severe infections**
IM/IV
Adults, Elderly. 2 g q6–8h.
▸ **Life-threatening infections**
IM/IV
Adults, Elderly. 2 g q4h.
Children: 2 g q4h. Maximum: 12 g/day.
▸ **Uncomplicated gonorrhea**
IM
Adults. 1 g one time.
▸ **Perioperative prophylaxis**
IM/IV
Adults, Elderly. 1 g 30–90 min before surgery.
▸ **Cesarean section**
IV
Adults. 1 g as soon as umbilical cord is clamped, then 1 g 6 and 12 hrs after first dose.
▸ **Usual pediatric dosage**
Children 1 mo–12 yrs weighing less than 50 kg. 100–200 mg/kg/day in divided doses q6–8h.
Children weighing 50 kg or more. 1–2 g q6–8h.

▶ **Dosage in renal impairment**
Creatinine clearance less than 20
ml/min: Give half dose at usual
dosing intervals.

UNLABELED USES
Treatment of Lyme disease

CONTRAINDICATIONS
Anaphylactic reaction to penicillins,
history of hypersensitivity to cephalosporins

INTERACTIONS
Drug
Probenecid: May increase cefo-
taxime blood concentration.
Herbal
None known.
Food
None known.

DIAGNOSTIC TEST EFFECTS
Positive direct or indirect Coombs'
test. May increase liver function
tests.

IV INCOMPATIBILITIES
Allopurinol (Aloprim), filgrastim
(Neupogen), fluconazole (Diflucan),
hetastarch (Hespan), pentamidine
(Pentam IV), vancomycin
(Vancocin)

IV COMPATIBILITIES
Diltiazem (Cardizem), famotidine
(Pepcid), hydromorphone (Dilaudid), lorazepam (Ativan), magnesium sulfate, midazolam (Versed),
morphine, propofol (Diprivan)

SIDE EFFECTS
Frequent
Discomfort with IM administration,
oral candidiasis (sore mouth or
tongue), mild diarrhea, mild abdominal cramping, vaginal candidiasis
(discharge, itching)

Occasional
Nausea, serum sickness reaction
(fever, joint pain)
Serum sickness reaction usually
occurs after the second course of
therapy and resolves after the drug
is discontinued.
Rare
Allergic reaction (rash, pruritus,
urticaria), thrombophlebitis (pain,
redness, swelling at injection site)

SERIOUS REACTIONS
• Antibiotic-associated colitis manifested as severe abdominal pain and
tenderness, fever, and watery and
severe diarrhea, and other superinfections may result from altered
bacterial balance.
• Nephrotoxicity may occur, especially in patients with preexisting
renal disease.
• Severe hypersensitivity reaction
including severe pruritus, angioedema, bronchospasm, and anaphylaxis, particularly in patients with a
history of allergies, especially to
penicillins, may occur.

NURSING CONSIDERATIONS
Baseline Assessment
◀ALERT▶ Determine the patient's
history of allergies, particularly to
cephalosporins and penicillins
before beginning drug therapy.
Lifespan Considerations
• Be aware that cefotaxime readily
crosses the placenta and is distributed in breast milk.
• There are no age-related precautions noted in children.
• In the elderly, age-related renal
impairment may require dosage
adjustment.
Precautions
• Use cautiously in patients concurrently using nephrotoxic medications.

- Use cautiously in patients with a history of gastrointestinal (GI) disease (especially antibiotic-associated colitis and ulcerative colitis).
- Use cautiously in patients with renal impairment with a creatinine clearance less than 20 ml/min.

Administration and Handling

◀ALERT▶ Space drug doses evenly around the clock.

IM

- Reconstitute with Sterile Water for Injection or Bacteriostatic Water for Injection.
- Add 2, 3, or 5 ml to 500-mg, 1-g, or 2-g vial, respectively, providing a concentration of 230 mg, 300 mg, or 330 mg/ml, respectively.
- To minimize discomfort, give IM injection deeply and slowly into the gluteus maximus rather than lateral aspect of thigh.
- For 2-g IM dose, give at 2 separate sites.

IV

- Solution normally appears light yellow to amber. IV infusion (piggyback) may darken in color (does not indicate loss of potency).
- IV infusion (piggyback) is stable for 24 hours at room temperature, 5 days if refrigerated.
- Discard the solution if precipitate forms.
- Reconstitute with 10 ml Sterile Water for Injection to provide a concentration of 50 mg, 95 mg, or 180 mg/ml for 500-mg, 1-g, or 2-g vials, respectively.
- May further dilute with 50 to 100 ml 0.9% NaCl or D_5W.
- For IV push, administer over 3 to 5 minutes.
- For intermittent IV infusion (piggyback), infuse over 20 to 30 minutes.

Intervention and Evaluation

- Evaluate the patient's IM injection sites for induration and tenderness.

- Assess the patient's mouth for white patches on the mucous membranes and tongue.
- Assess the patient's pattern of daily bowel activity and stool consistency. Although mild GI effects may be tolerable, an increase in their severity may indicate the onset of antibiotic-associated colitis.
- Monitor the patient's intake and output and renal function reports for nephrotoxicity.
- Be alert for signs and symptoms of superinfection including abdominal pain, moderate to severe diarrhea, severe anal or genital pruritus, and severe mouth soreness.

Patient Teaching

- Explain to the patient that discomfort may occur with IM injection.
- Advise the patient to continue the antibiotic therapy for the full length of treatment and to evenly space drug doses around the clock.

cefotetan disodium

seh-fo-**teh**-tan
(Cefotan)
Do not confuse with cefoxitin or Ceftin.

CATEGORY AND SCHEDULE

Pregnancy Risk Category: B

MECHANISM OF ACTION

A second-generation cephalosporin that binds to bacterial cell membranes. *Therapeutic Effect:* Inhibits synthesis of bacterial cell wall. Bactericidal.

PHARMACOKINETICS

Widely distributed. Protein binding: 78%–91%. Primarily excreted unchanged in urine. Minimally removed by hemodialysis. **Half-life:** 3–4.6 hrs (half-life is increased with impaired renal function).

AVAILABILITY
Powder for Injection: 1 g, 2 g.

INDICATIONS AND DOSAGES
▸ **Urinary tract infections (UTIs)**
IM/IV
Adults, Elderly. 1–2 g in divided doses q12–24h.
▸ **Mild to moderate infections**
IM/IV
Adults, Elderly. 1–2 g q12h.
▸ **Severe infections**
IM/IV
Adults, Elderly. 2 g q12h.
▸ **Life-threatening infections**
IM/IV
Adults, Elderly. 3 g q12h.
▸ **Perioperative prophylaxis**
IV
Adults, Elderly. 1–2 g 30–60 min before surgery.
▸ **Cesarean section**
IV
Adults. 1–2 g as soon as umbilical cord is clamped.
▸ **Usual pediatric dosage**
Children. 40–80 mg/kg/day in divided doses q12h. Maximum: 6 g/day.
▸ **Dosage in renal impairment**
Dosage and frequency are modified on the basis of creatinine clearance and the severity of infection.

Creatinine Clearance	Dosage Interval
10–30 ml/min	Usual dose q24h
less than 10 ml/min	Usual dose q48h

CONTRAINDICATIONS
Anaphylactic reaction to penicillins, history of hypersensitivity to cephalosporins

INTERACTIONS
Drug
Alcohol: A disulfiram reaction (facial flushing, headache, nausea, sweating, tachycardia) may occur when alcohol is ingested during cefotetan therapy.
Anticoagulants, heparin, thrombolytics: May increase the risk of bleeding with these drugs.
Herbal
None known.
Food
None known.

DIAGNOSTIC TEST EFFECTS
Positive direct or indirect Coombs' test may occur. Drug interferes with crossmatching procedures and hematologic tests. Prothrombin times may be prolonged. May increase BUN, serum alkaline phosphatase, serum creatinine, SGOT (AST), and SGPT (ALT) levels.

IV INCOMPATIBILITIES
Vancomycin (Vancocin)

IV COMPATIBILITIES
Diltiazem (Cardizem), famotidine (Pepcid), heparin, insulin (regular), morphine, propofol (Diprivan)

SIDE EFFECTS
Frequent
Discomfort with IM administration, oral candidiasis (sore mouth or tongue), mild diarrhea, mild abdominal cramping, vaginal candidiasis (discharge, itching)
Occasional
Nausea, unusual bleeding or bruising, serum sickness reaction (fever, joint pain)
Serum sickness reaction usually occurs after the second course of therapy and resolves after the drug is discontinued.

Rare
Allergic reaction (rash, pruritus, urticaria), thrombophlebitis (pain, redness, swelling at injection site)

SERIOUS REACTIONS

• Antibiotic-associated colitis manifested as severe abdominal pain and tenderness, fever, and watery and severe diarrhea, and other superinfections may result from altered bacterial balance.
• Nephrotoxicity may occur, especially in patients with preexisting renal disease.
• Severe hypersensitivity reaction including severe pruritus, angioedema, bronchospasm, and anaphylaxis, particularly in patients with a history of allergies, especially to penicillins, may occur.

NURSING CONSIDERATIONS

Baseline Assessment
◀ ALERT ▶ Determine the patient's history of allergies, particularly to cephalosporins and penicillins before beginning drug therapy.
Lifespan Considerations
• Be aware that cefotetan readily crosses the placenta and is distributed in breast milk.
• The safety and efficacy of this drug have not been established in children.
• In the elderly, age-related renal impairment may require dosage adjustment.
Precautions
• Use cautiously in patients with a history GI disease (especially antibiotic-associated colitis or ulcerative colitis), and renal impairment.
• Use cautiously in patients concurrently using nephrotoxic medications.

Administration and Handling
◀ ALERT ▶ Give by IM injection, IV push, or intermittent IV infusion (piggyback) only.
IM
• Add 2, 3 ml Sterile Water for Injection or other appropriate diluent to 1 g, 2 g providing a concentration of 400 mg/ml or 500 mg/ml, respectively.
• To minimize injection site discomfort, give the IM injection deeply and slowly into the gluteus maximus rather than the lateral aspect of thigh.
IV
• Solution normally appears colorless to light yellow.
• Color change to deep yellow does not indicate loss of potency.
• IV infusion (piggyback) is stable for 24 hours at room temperature, 96 hours if refrigerated.
• Discard solution if precipitate forms.
• Reconstitute each 1 g with 10 ml Sterile Water for Injection to provide a concentration of 95 mg/ml.
• May further dilute with 50 to 100 ml 0.9% NaCl or D_5W.
• For IV push, administer over 3 to 5 minutes.
• For intermittent IV infusion (piggyback), infuse over 20 to 30 minutes.
Intervention and Evaluation
• Evaluate the patient's IV site for signs and symptoms of phlebitis as evidenced by heat, pain, and red streaking over the vein.
• Evaluate the patient's IM injection sites for induration and tenderness.
• Assess the patient's mouth for white patches on the mucous membranes and tongue.
• Assess the patient's pattern of daily bowel activity and stool

consistency. Although mild GI effects may be tolerable, an increase in their severity may indicate the onset of antibiotic-associated colitis.
• Monitor the patient's intake and output and renal function reports for nephrotoxicity.
• Be alert for signs and symptoms of superinfection including abdominal pain, moderate to severe diarrhea, severe anal or genital pruritus, and severe mouth soreness.
Patient Teaching
• Explain to the patient that discomfort may occur with IM injection.
• Advise the patient to continue the antibiotic therapy for the full length of treatment and to evenly space drug doses around the clock.
• Warn the patient to avoid consuming alcohol and alcohol-containing preparations, such as cough syrups, salad dressings, and sauces, during treatment and for 72 hours after the last dose of cefotetan.

cefoxitin sodium
seh-**fox**-ih-tin
(Mefoxin)
Do not confuse with cefotaxime, cefotetan, or Cytoxan.

CATEGORY AND SCHEDULE
Pregnancy Risk Category: B

MECHANISM OF ACTION
A second-generation cephalosporin that binds to bacterial cell membranes. *Therapeutic Effect:* Inhibits synthesis of bacterial cell wall. Bactericidal.

AVAILABILITY
Powder for Injection: 1 g, 2 g.

INDICATIONS AND DOSAGES
▶ **Mild to moderate infections**
IM/IV
Adults, Elderly. 1–2 g q6–8h.
▶ **Severe infections**
IM/IV
Adults, Elderly. 1 g q4h or 2 g q6–8h up to 2 g q4h.
▶ **Uncomplicated gonorrhea**
IM
Adults. 2 g one time with 1 g probenecid.
▶ **Perioperative prophylaxis**
IM/IV
Adults, Elderly. 2 g 30–60 min before surgery and q6h up to 24 hrs postop.
Children older than 3 mos. 30–40 mg/kg 30–60 min before surgery and q6h postop for no more than 24 hrs.
▶ **Cesarean section**
IV
Adults. 2 g as soon as umbilical cord is clamped, then 2 g 4 and 8 hrs after first dose, then q6h for no more than 24 hrs.
▶ **Usual pediatric dosage**
Children older than 3 mos. 80–160 mg/kg/day in 4–6 divided doses. Maximum: 12 g/day.
Neonates. 90–100 mg/kg/day in divided doses q6–8h.
▶ **Dosage in renal impairment**
After loading dose of 1–2 g, dosage and frequency are modified on the basis of creatinine clearance and the severity of infection.

Creatinine Clearance	Dosage
30–50 ml/min	1–2 g q8–12h
10–29 ml/min	1–2 g q12–24h
5–9 ml/min	500 mg–1 g q12–24h
less than 5 ml/min	500 mg–1 g q24–48h

CONTRAINDICATIONS
Anaphylactic reaction to penicillins, history of hypersensitivity to cephalosporins

INTERACTIONS
Drug
Probenecid: Increases serum concentrations of cefoxitin.
Herbal
None known.
Food
None known.

DIAGNOSTIC TEST EFFECTS
Positive direct or indirect Coombs' test may occur (interferes with crossmatching procedures, hematologic tests). May increase BUN, serum alkaline phosphatase, serum creatinine, SGOT (AST), and SGPT (ALT) levels.

IV INCOMPATIBILITIES
Filgrastim (Neupogen), pentamidine (Pentam IV), vancomycin (Vancocin)

IV COMPATIBILITIES
Diltiazem (Cardizem), famotidine (Pepcid), heparin, hydromorphone (Dilaudid), magnesium sulfate, morphine, multivitamins, propofol (Diprivan)

SIDE EFFECTS
Frequent
Discomfort with IM administration, oral candidiasis (sore mouth or tongue), mild diarrhea, mild abdominal cramping, vaginal candidiasis (discharge, itching)
Occasional
Nausea, serum sickness reaction (fever, joint pain). Serum sickness reaction usually occurs after the second course of therapy and resolves after the drug is discontinued.
Rare
Allergic reaction (pruritus, rash, urticaria), thrombophlebitis (pain, redness, swelling at injection site)

SERIOUS REACTIONS
• Antibiotic-associated colitis manifested as severe abdominal pain and tenderness, fever, and watery and severe diarrhea, and other superinfections may result from altered bacterial balance.
• Nephrotoxicity may occur, especially in patients with preexisting renal disease.
• Severe hypersensitivity reaction including severe pruritus, angioedema, bronchospasm, and anaphylaxis, particularly in those with history of allergies, especially to penicillins, may occur.

NURSING CONSIDERATIONS
Baseline Assessment
◀ALERT▶ Determine the patient's history of allergies, particularly to cephalosporins and penicillins before beginning drug therapy.
Precautions
• Use cautiously in patients with a history of gastrointestinal (GI) disease, especially antibiotic-associated colitis or ulcerative colitis, and renal impairment.
• Use cautiously in patients concurrently using nephrotoxic medications.
Administration and Handling
◀ALERT▶ Give by IM, intermittent IV infusion (piggyback), or IV push.
◀ALERT▶ Space doses evenly around the clock.
IM
• Reconstitute each 1 g with 2 ml Sterile Water for Injection or lidocaine to provide concentration of 400 mg/ml.
• Give deep IM injections slowly to minimize patient discomfort. To further minimize discomfort, administer IM injections into the gluteus

maximus instead of the lateral aspect of the thigh.
IV
• Solution normally appears colorless to light amber but may darken (does not indicate loss of potency).
• IV infusion (piggyback) is stable for 24 hours at room temperature, 48 hours if refrigerated.
• Discard if precipitate forms.
• Reconstitute each 1 g with 10 ml Sterile Water for Injection to provide concentration of 95 mg/ml.
• May further dilute with 50 to 100 ml 0.9% Sterile Water for Injection, NaCl, or D_5W.
• For IV push, administer over 3 to 5 minutes.
• For intermittent IV infusion (piggyback), infuse over 15 to 30 minutes.

Intervention and Evaluation
• Evaluate the patient's IV site for phlebitis as evidenced by heat, pain, and red streaking over the vein.
• Assess the patient's IM injection sites for induration and tenderness.
• Assess the patient's mouth for white patches on the mucous membranes and tongue.
• Assess the patient's pattern of daily bowel activity and stool consistency. Mild GI effects may be tolerable, but increasing severity may indicate the onset of antibiotic-associated colitis.
• Monitor the patient's intake and output and renal function reports for signs of nephrotoxicity.
• Be alert for signs and symptoms of superinfection including abdominal pain, moderate to severe diarrhea, severe anal or genital pruritus, and severe mouth soreness.

Patient Teaching
• Explain to the patient that discomfort may occur with IM injection.
• Advise the patient to continue the antibiotic therapy for the full length

of treatment and to evenly space drug doses around the clock.

cefpodoxime proxetil
sef-poe-**docks**-em
(Vantin)
Do not confuse with Ventolin.

CATEGORY AND SCHEDULE
Pregnancy Risk Category: B

MECHANISM OF ACTION
A third-generation cephalosporin that binds to bacterial cell membranes. *Therapeutic Effect:* Inhibits synthesis of bacterial cell wall. Bactericidal.

PHARMACOKINETICS
Well absorbed from the gastrointestinal (GI) tract (food increases absorption). Protein binding: 21%–40%. Widely distributed. Primarily excreted unchanged in urine. Partially removed by hemodialysis. **Half-life:** 2.3 hrs (half-life is increased in the elderly and those with impaired renal function).

AVAILABILITY
Tablets: 100 mg, 200 mg.
Oral Suspension: 50 mg/5 ml, 100 mg/5 ml.

INDICATIONS AND DOSAGES
▸ **Chronic bronchitis, pneumonia**
PO
Adults, Elderly, Children older than 13 yrs. 200 mg q12h for 10–14 days.
▸ **Gonorrhea, rectal gonococcal infection (female patients only)**
PO
Adults, Children older than 13 yrs. 200 mg as single dose.

▶ **Skin and skin-structure infections**
PO
Adults, Elderly, Children older than 13 yrs. 400 mg q12h for 7–14 days.
▶ **Pharyngitis, tonsillitis**
PO
Adults, Elderly, Children older than 13 yrs. 100 mg q12h for 5–10 days.
Children 6 mos–13 yrs. 5 mg/kg q12h for 5–10 days. Maximum: 100 mg/dose.
▶ **Acute maxillary sinusitis**
PO
Adults, Children older than 13 yrs. 200 mg twice a day for 10 days.
Children 2 mos–13 yrs. 5 mg/kg q12h for 10 days. Maximum: 400 mg/day.
▶ **Urinary tract infection**
PO
Adults, Elderly, Children older than 13 yrs. 100 mg q12h for 7 days.
▶ **Acute otitis media**
PO
Children 6 mos–13 yrs. 5 mg/kg q12h for 5 days. Maximum: 400 mg/dose.
▶ **Dosage in renal impairment**
Dosage and frequency are based on the degree of renal impairment and creatinine clearance. Creatinine clearance less than 30 ml/min: dose q24h.
Patients on hemodialysis: 3 times/wk after dialysis.

CONTRAINDICATIONS
History of anaphylactic reaction to penicillins, hypersensitivity to cephalosporins

INTERACTIONS
Drug
Antacids, H_2 antagonists: May decrease cefpodoxime absorption.
Probenecid: May increase cefpodoxime blood concentration.
Herbal
None known.
Food
None known.

DIAGNOSTIC TEST EFFECTS
Positive direct or indirect Coombs' test. May increase BUN, serum alkaline phosphatase, serum bilirubin, serum creatinine, serum LDH, SGOT (AST), and SGPT (ALT) levels.

SIDE EFFECTS
Frequent
Oral candidiasis (sore mouth or tongue), mild diarrhea, mild abdominal cramping, vaginal candidiasis (discharge, itching)
Occasional
Nausea, serum sickness reaction (fever, joint pain)
Serum sickness reaction usually occurs after the second course of therapy and resolves after the drug is discontinued.
Rare
Allergic reaction (pruritus, rash, urticaria)

SERIOUS REACTIONS
• Antibiotic-associated colitis manifested as severe abdominal pain and tenderness, fever, and watery and severe diarrhea, and other superinfections may result from altered bacterial balance.
• Nephrotoxicity may occur, especially in patients with preexisting renal disease.
• Severe hypersensitivity reaction including severe pruritus, angioedema, bronchospasm, and anaphylaxis, particularly in patients with a history of allergies, especially to penicillins, may occur.

NURSING CONSIDERATIONS

Baseline Assessment
◀ALERT▶ Determine the patient's history of allergies, particularly cephalosporins and penicillins before beginning drug therapy.

Lifespan Considerations
• Be aware that cefpodoxime readily crosses the placenta and is distributed in breast milk.
• Be aware that the safety and efficacy of cefpodixime have not been established in children younger than 6 months.
• In the elderly, age-related renal impairment may require dosage adjustment.

Precautions
• Use cautiously in patients with a history of allergies or GI disease, especially antibiotic-associated colitis or ulcerative colitis, and renal impairment.
• Use cautiously in patients concurrently using nephrotoxic medications.

Administration and Handling
PO
• Administer with food to enhance drug absorption.
• After reconstitution, oral suspension is stable for 14 days if refrigerated.

Intervention and Evaluation
• Assess the patient's mouth for white patches on the mucous membranes and tongue.
• Assess the patient's pattern of daily bowel activity and stool consistency. Mild GI effects may be tolerable, but increasing severity may indicate the onset of antibiotic-associated colitis.
• Monitor the patient's intake and output and renal function reports for signs of nephrotoxicity.
• Be alert for signs and symptoms of superinfection including abdominal pain, moderate to severe diarrhea, severe anal or genital pruritus, and severe mouth soreness.

Patient Teaching
• Advise the patient to continue cefpodoxime therapy for the full length of treatment and to evenly space drug doses around the clock.
• Instruct the patient to refrigerate the oral suspension, to shake the oral suspension well before using, and to take the oral suspension with food.

cefprozil
sef-**proz**-ill
(Cefzil)
Do not confuse with Cefazolin or Ceftin.

CATEGORY AND SCHEDULE
Pregnancy Risk Category: B

MECHANISM OF ACTION
A second-generation cephalosporin that binds to bacterial cell membranes. *Therapeutic Effect:* Inhibits synthesis of bacterial cell wall. Bactericidal.

PHARMACOKINETICS
Well absorbed from the gastrointestinal (GI) tract. Protein binding: 36%–45%. Widely distributed. Primarily excreted unchanged in urine. Moderately removed by hemodialysis. **Half-life:** 1.3 hrs (half-life is increased in those with impaired renal function).

AVAILABILITY
Tablets: 250 mg, 500 mg.
Oral Suspension: 125 mg/5 ml, 250 mg/5 ml.

INDICATIONS AND DOSAGES

▸ **Pharyngitis, tonsillitis**

PO

Adults, Elderly. 500 mg q24h for 10 days.

Children 2–12 yrs. 7.5 mg/kg q12h for 10 days.

▸ **Acute bacterial exacerbation of chronic bronchitis, secondary bacterial infection of acute bronchitis**

PO

Adults, Elderly. 500 mg q12h for 10 days.

▸ **Skin and skin-structure infections**

PO

Adults, Elderly. 250–500 mg q12h for 10 days.

Children. 20 mg/kg q24h.

▸ **Acute sinusitis**

PO

Adults, Elderly. 250–500 mg q12h.

Children 6 mos–12 yrs. 7.5–15 mg/kg q12h.

▸ **Otitis media**

PO

Children 6 mos–12 yrs. 15 mg/kg q12h for 10 days. Maximum: 1 g/day.

▸ **Dosage in renal impairment**

Dosage and frequency are based on the degree of renal impairment and creatinine clearance. Creatinine clearance less than 30 ml/min: 50% dosage at usual interval.

CONTRAINDICATIONS

History of anaphylactic reaction to penicillins, hypersensitivity to cephalosporins

INTERACTIONS

Drug

Probenecid: Increases serum concentrations of cefprozil.

Herbal

None known.

Food

None known.

DIAGNOSTIC TEST EFFECTS

Positive direct or indirect Coombs' test may occur (interferes with crossmatching procedures, hematologic tests). May increase liver function test results.

SIDE EFFECTS

Frequent

Oral candidiasis (sore mouth or tongue), mild diarrhea, mild abdominal cramping, vaginal candidiasis (discharge, itching)

Occasional

Nausea, serum sickness reaction (fever, joint pain)

Serum sickness reaction usually occurs after the second course of therapy and resolves after the drug is discontinued.

Rare

Allergic reaction (pruritus, rash, urticaria)

SERIOUS REACTIONS

• Antibiotic-associated colitis manifested as severe abdominal pain and tenderness, fever, and watery and severe diarrhea, and other superinfections may result from altered bacterial balance.

• Nephrotoxicity may occur, especially in patients with preexisting renal disease.

• Severe hypersensitivity reaction including severe pruritus, angioedema, bronchospasm, and anaphylaxis, particularly in patients with a history of allergies, especially to penicillins, may occur.

NURSING CONSIDERATIONS

Baseline Assessment

◂ **ALERT** ▸ Determine the patient's history of allergies, particularly cephalosporins and penicillins before beginning drug therapy.

Lifespan Considerations
• Be aware that cefprozil readily crosses the placenta and is distributed in breast milk.
• Be aware that the safety and efficacy of cefprozil have not been established in children younger than 6 months.
• In the elderly, age-related renal impairment may require dosage adjustment.

Precautions
• Use cautiously in patients with a history of GI disease, especially antibiotic-associated colitis or ulcerative colitis, and renal impairment.
• Use cautiously in patients concurrently using nephrotoxic medications.

Administration and Handling
PO
• After reconstitution, oral suspension is stable for 14 days if refrigerated.
• Shake oral suspension well before using.
• Give without regard to meals; if GI upset occurs, give with food or milk.

Intervention and Evaluation
• Assess the patient's mouth for white patches on the mucous membranes and tongue.
• Assess the patient's pattern of daily bowel activity and stool consistency. Mild GI effects may be tolerable, but increasing severity may indicate the onset of antibiotic-associated colitis.
• Monitor the patient's intake and output and renal function reports for signs of nephrotoxicity.
• Be alert for signs and symptoms of superinfection including abdominal pain, moderate to severe diarrhea, severe anal or genital pruritus, and severe mouth soreness.

Patient Teaching
• Advise the patient to continue cefprozil therapy for the full length of treatment and to evenly space drug doses around the clock.
• Explain to the patient that cefprozil may cause GI upset. Instruct the patient to take the drug with food or milk if GI upset occurs.

ceftazidime
sef-**taz**-ih-deem
(Ceptaz, Fortaz, Fortum[AUS], Tazicef, Tazidime)
Do not confuse with ceftizoxime.

CATEGORY AND SCHEDULE
Pregnancy Risk Category: B

MECHANISM OF ACTION
A third-generation cephalosporin that binds to bacterial cell membranes. *Therapeutic Effect:* Inhibits synthesis of bacterial cell wall. Bactericidal.

PHARMACOKINETICS
Widely distributed (including cerebrospinal fluid [CSF]). Protein binding: 5%–17%. Primarily excreted unchanged in urine. Removed by hemodialysis. **Half-life:** 2 hrs (half-life is increased in those with impaired renal function).

AVAILABILITY
Powder for Injection: 500 mg, 1 g, 2 g.

INDICATIONS AND DOSAGES
▸ **Urinary tract infections**
IM/IV
Adults. 250–500 mg q8–12h.
▸ **Mild to moderate infections**
IM/IV
Adults. 1 g q8–12h.

▸ **Uncomplicated pneumonia, skin and skin-structure infections**
IM/IV
Adults. 0.5–1 g q8h.
▸ **Bone and joint infection**
IM/IV
Adults. 2 g q12h.
▸ **Meningitis, serious gynecologic, intra-abdominal infections**
IM/IV
Adults. 2 g q8h.
▸ **Pseudomonal pulmonary infections in patients with cystic fibrosis**
IV
Adults. 30–50 mg/kg q8h.
Maximum: 6 g/day.
▸ **Usual elderly dosage**
Elderly (normal renal function).
500 mg–1 g q12h.
▸ **Usual pediatric dosage**
Children 1 mo–12 yrs. 100–150 mg/kg/day in divided doses q8h.
Maximum: 6 g/day.
Neonates 0–4 wks. 100–150 mg/kg/day in divided doses q8–12h.
▸ **Dosage in renal impairment**
After initial 1-g dose, dosage and frequency are modified on the basis of creatinine clearance and the severity of infection.

Creatinine Clearance (ml/min)	Dosage Interval
30–50	q12h
10–30	q24h
less than 10	q24–48h

CONTRAINDICATIONS
History of anaphylactic reaction to penicillins, hypersensitivity to cephalosporins

INTERACTIONS
Drug
None known.
Herbal
None known.
Food
None known.

DIAGNOSTIC TEST EFFECTS
Positive direct or indirect Coombs' test (interferes with crossmatching procedures, hematologic tests). May increase BUN, serum alkaline phosphatase, serum creatinine, serum LDH, SGOT (AST), and SGPT (ALT) levels.

IV INCOMPATIBILITIES
Amphotericin B complex (AmBisome, Amphotec, Abelcet), doxorubicin liposome (Doxil), fluconazole (Diflucan), idarubicin (Idamycin), midazolam (Versed), pentamidine (Pentam IV), vancomycin (Vancocin)

IV COMPATIBILITIES
Diltiazem (Cardizem), famotidine (Pepcid), heparin, hydromorphone (Dilaudid), morphine, propofol (Diprivan)

SIDE EFFECTS
Frequent
Discomfort with IM administration, oral candidiasis (sore mouth or tongue), mild diarrhea, mild abdominal cramping, vaginal candidiasis (discharge, itching)
Occasional
Nausea, serum sickness reaction (fever, joint pain)
Serum sickness reaction usually occurs after the second course of therapy and resolves after the drug is discontinued.
Rare
Allergic reaction (pruritus, rash, urticaria), thrombophlebitis (pain, redness, swelling at injection site)

SERIOUS REACTIONS
• Antibiotic-associated colitis manifested as severe abdominal pain and tenderness, fever, and watery and severe diarrhea, and other superin-

fections may result from altered bacterial balance.

• Nephrotoxicity may occur, especially in patients with preexisting renal disease.

• Severe hypersensitivity reaction including severe pruritus, angioedema, bronchospasm, and anaphylaxis, particularly in patients with a history of allergies, especially to penicillins, may occur.

NURSING CONSIDERATIONS

Baseline Assessment
◀ALERT▶ Determine the patient's history of allergies, particularly cephalosporins and penicillins before beginning drug therapy.

Lifespan Considerations
• Be aware that ceftazidime readily crosses the placenta and is distributed in breast milk.

• There are no age-related precautions noted in children.

• In the elderly, age-related renal impairment may require dosage adjustment.

Precautions
• Use cautiously in patients with a history of gastrointestinal (GI) disease, especially antibiotic-associated colitis or ulcerative colitis, and renal impairment.

• Use cautiously in patients concurrently using nephrotoxic medications.

Administration and Handling
◀ALERT▶ Give by IM injection, direct IV injection, or intermittent IV infusion (piggyback).

IM
• For reconstitution, add 1.5 ml Sterile Water for Injection or lidocaine 1% to 500 mg, if prescribed, or 3 ml to 1-g vial to provide a concentration of 280 mg/ml.

• Give deep IM injections slowly to minimize patient discomfort. To further minimize discomfort, administer IM injections into the gluteus maximus instead of the lateral aspect of the thigh.

IV
• Solution normally appears light yellow to amber, tends to darken (color change does not indicate loss of potency).

• IV infusion (piggyback) stable for 18 hours at room temperature, 7 days if refrigerated.

• Discard if precipitate forms.

• Add 10 ml Sterile Water for Injection to each 1 g to provide concentration of 90 mg/ml.

• May further dilute with 50 to 100 ml 0.9% NaCl, D_5W, or other compatible diluent.

• For IV push, administer over 3 to 5 minutes.

• For intermittent IV infusion (piggyback), infuse over 15 to 30 minutes.

Intervention and Evaluation
• Evaluate the patient's IV site for phlebitis as evidenced by heat, pain, and red streaking over the vein.

• Assess the patient's IM injection site for induration and tenderness.

• Assess the patient's mouth for white patches on the mucous membranes or tongue.

• Assess the patient's pattern of daily bowel activity and stool consistency. Mild GI effects may be tolerable, but increasing severity may indicate the onset of antibiotic-associated colitis.

• Monitor the patient's intake and output and renal function reports for signs of nephrotoxicity.

• Be alert for signs and symptoms of superinfection including abdominal pain, moderate to severe diarrhea, severe anal or genital pruritus, and severe mouth soreness.

Patient Teaching
• Explain to the patient that discomfort may occur with IM injection.
• Advise the patient to continue ceftazidime therapy for the full length of treatment and explain that doses will be evenly spaced around the clock.

ceftibuten
sef-tih-**byew**-ten
(Cedax)

CATEGORY AND SCHEDULE
Pregnancy Risk Category: B

MECHANISM OF ACTION
A third-generation cephalosporin that binds to bacterial cell membranes. *Therapeutic Effect:* Inhibits bacterial cell wall synthesis. Bactericidal.

AVAILABILITY
Capsules: 400 mg.
Oral Suspension: 90 mg/5 ml.

INDICATIONS AND DOSAGES
▸ **Chronic bronchitis, acute bacterial otitis media, pharyngitis, tonsillitis**
PO
Adults, Elderly, Children 12 yrs and older. 400 mg/day as single daily dose for 10 days.
Children younger than 12 yrs. 9 mg/kg/day as single daily dose for 10 days. Maximum: 400 mg/day.
▸ **Dosage in renal impairment**
Based on creatinine clearance.

Creatinine Clearance	Dosage
greater than 50 ml/min	400 mg or 9 mg/kg q24h
30–49 ml/min	200 mg or 4.5 mg/kg q24h
less than 30 ml/min	100 mg or 2.25 mg/kg q24h

CONTRAINDICATIONS
Hypersensitivity to cephalosporins

INTERACTIONS
Drug
Aminoglycosides: Increased risk of nephrotoxicity with concurrent use of drugs in this class.
Probenecid: Increases serum levels of cephalosporins.
Herbal
None known.
Food
None known.

DIAGNOSTIC TEST EFFECTS
Positive direct or indirect Coombs' test. May increase BUN, serum alkaline phosphatase, serum bilirubin, serum creatinine, serum LDH, SGOT (AST), and SGPT (ALT) levels.

SIDE EFFECTS
Frequent
Oral candidiasis (sore mouth or tongue), mild diarrhea, mild abdominal cramping, vaginal candidiasis (discharge, itching)
Occasional
Nausea, serum sickness reaction (fever, joint pain)
Serum sickness reaction usually occurs after the second course of therapy and resolves after the drug is discontinued.
Rare
Allergic reaction (rash, pruritus, urticaria)

SERIOUS REACTIONS
• Antibiotic-associated colitis manifested as severe abdominal pain and tenderness, fever, and watery and severe diarrhea, and other superinfections may result from altered bacterial balance.
• Nephrotoxicity may occur, especially in patients with preexisting renal disease.
• Severe hypersensitivity reaction including severe pruritus, angioedema, bronchospasm, and anaphylaxis, particularly in patients with a history of allergies, especially to penicillins, may occur.

NURSING CONSIDERATIONS
Baseline Assessment
◀ALERT▶ Determine the patient's history of allergies, particularly cephalosporins and penicillins before beginning drug therapy.
Precautions
• Use cautiously in patients with a history of allergies or gastrointestinal (GI) disease (especially antibiotic-associated colitis or ulcerative colitis), hypersensitivity to penicillins or other drugs, and renal impairment.
Administration and Handling
◀ALERT▶ Use this drug's oral suspension to treat otitis media to achieve higher peak blood levels.
Intervention and Evaluation
• Assess the patient's mouth for white patches on the mucous membranes and tongue.
• Assess the patient's pattern of daily bowel activity and stool consistency. Mild GI effects may be tolerable, but increasing severity may indicate the onset of antibiotic-associated colitis.
• Monitor the patient's intake and output and renal function reports for signs of nephrotoxicity.
• Be alert for signs and symptoms

of superinfection including abdominal pain, moderate to severe diarrhea, severe anal or genital pruritus, and severe mouth soreness.
Patient Teaching
• Advise the patient to continue ceftibuten therapy for the full length of treatment and to evenly space drug doses around the clock.
• Explain to the patient that ceftibuten may cause GI upset. Instruct the patient to take the drug with food or milk if GI upset occurs.

ceftizoxime sodium
cef-tih-**zox**-eem
(Cefizox)
Do not confuse with cefotaxime or ceftazidime.

CATEGORY AND SCHEDULE
Pregnancy Risk Category: B

MECHANISM OF ACTION
A third-generation cephalosporin that binds to bacterial cell membranes. *Therapeutic Effect:* Inhibits synthesis of bacterial cell wall. Bactericidal.

PHARMACOKINETICS
Widely distributed (including cerebrospinal fluid [CSF]). Protein binding: 30%. Primarily excreted unchanged in urine. Moderately removed by hemodialysis. **Half-life:** 1.7 hrs (half-life is increased in those with impaired renal function).

AVAILABILITY
Powder for Injection: 1 g, 2 g.

INDICATIONS AND DOSAGES
▶ **Uncomplicated urinary tract infections (UTIs)**
IM/IV
Adults, Elderly. 500 mg q12h.

▸ Mild to moderate to severe infections of the biliary, respiratory, and genitourinary (GU) tracts; skin, bone and intra-abdominal infections; meningitis; septicemia
IM/IV
Adults, Elderly. 1–2 g q8–12h.
▸ Pelvic inflammatory disease (PID)
IV
Adults. 2 g q4–8h.
▸ Life-threatening infections of the biliary, respiratory, and GU tracts; skin, bone and intra-abdominal infections; meningitis; septicemia
IV
Adults, Elderly. 3–4 g q8h, up to 2 g q4h.
▸ Uncomplicated gonorrhea
IM
Adults. 1 g one time.
▸ Usual pediatric dosage
Children older than 6 mos: 50 mg/kg q6–8h. Maximum: 12 g/day.
▸ Dosage in renal impairment
After loading dose of 0.5–1 g, dosage and frequency are modified on the basis of creatinine clearance and the severity of infection.

Creatinine Clearance	Dosage Interval
50–80 ml/min	q8–12h
10–50 ml/min	q36–48h
less than 10 ml/min	q48–72h

CONTRAINDICATIONS
History of anaphylactic reaction to penicillins, hypersensitivity to cephalosporins

INTERACTIONS
Drug
Probenecid: Increases serum concentration of ceftizoxime.
Herbal
None known.
Food
None known.

DIAGNOSTIC TEST EFFECTS
Positive direct or indirect Coombs' test may occur. May increase BUN, serum alkaline serum phosphatase, serum creatinine, SGOT (AST), and SGPT (ALT) levels.

IV INCOMPATIBILITIES
Filgrastim (Neupogen)

IV COMPATIBILITIES
Hydromorphone (Dilaudid), morphine, propofol (Diprivan)

SIDE EFFECTS
Frequent
Discomfort with IM administration, oral candidiasis (sore mouth or tongue), mild diarrhea, mild abdominal cramping, vaginal candidiasis (discharge, itching)
Occasional
Nausea, serum sickness reaction (fever, joint pain)
Serum sickness reaction usually occurs after the second course of therapy and resolves after the drug is discontinued.
Rare
Allergic reaction (rash, pruritus, urticaria), thrombophlebitis (pain, redness, swelling at injection site)

SERIOUS REACTIONS
• Antibiotic-associated colitis manifested as severe abdominal pain and tenderness, fever, and watery and severe diarrhea, and other superinfections may result from altered bacterial balance.
• Nephrotoxicity may occur, especially in patients with preexisting renal disease.
• Severe hypersensitivity reaction including severe pruritus, angioedema, bronchospasm, and anaphylaxis, particularly in patients with a history of allergies, especially to penicillins, may occur.

NURSING CONSIDERATIONS

Baseline Assessment
◀ALERT▶ Determine the patient's history of allergies, particularly cephalosporins and penicillins before beginning drug therapy.

Lifespan Considerations
• Be aware that ceftizoxime readily crosses the placenta and is distributed in breast milk.
• Be aware that ceftizoxime use in children is associated with transient elevations of serum creatine kinase, blood eosinophil count, SGOT (AST), and SGPT (ALT) levels.
• In the elderly, age-related renal impairment may require dosage adjustment.

Precautions
• Use cautiously in patients with a history of gastrointestinal (GI) disease, especially antibiotic-associated colitis or ulcerative colitis, and liver or renal impairment.

Administration and Handling
IM
• Add 1.5 ml Sterile Water for Injection to each 0.5 g to provide concentration of 270 mg/ml.
• Give deep IM injections slowly to minimize patient discomfort.
• When giving 2-g dose, divide dose and give in different large muscle masses.

IV
• Solutions normally appears clear to pale yellow. Color change from yellow to amber does not indicate loss of potency.
• IV infusion (piggyback) is stable for 24 hours at room temperature, 96 hours if refrigerated.
• Discard if precipitate forms.
• Add 5 ml Sterile Water for Injection to each 0.5 g to provide concentration of 95 mg/ml.

• May further dilute with 50 to 100 ml 0.9% NaCl, D_5W, or other compatible fluid.
• For IV push, administer over 3 to 5 minutes.
• For intermittent IV infusion (piggyback), infuse over 15 to 30 minutes.

Intervention and Evaluation
• Assess the patient's mouth for white patches on the mucous membranes and tongue.
• Assess the patient's pattern of daily bowel activity and stool consistency. Mild GI effects may be tolerable, but increasing severity may indicate the onset of antibiotic-associated colitis.
• Monitor the patient's intake and output and renal function reports for signs of nephrotoxicity.
• Be alert for signs and symptoms of superinfection including abdominal pain, moderate to severe diarrhea, severe anal or genital pruritus, and severe mouth soreness.

Patient Teaching
• Advise the patient to continue ceftizoxime therapy for the full length of treatment and explain that the doses will be evenly spaced around the clock.
• Explain to the patient that discomfort may occur with IM injection.

ceftriaxone sodium
cef-try-**ax**-zone
(Rocephin)

CATEGORY AND SCHEDULE
Pregnancy Risk Category: B

MECHANISM OF ACTION
A third-generation cephalosporin that binds to bacterial cell membranes. *Therapeutic Effect:* Inhibits

synthesis of bacterial cell wall. Bactericidal.

PHARMACOKINETICS
Widely distributed (including cerebrospinal fluid [CSF]). Protein binding: 83%–96%. Primarily excreted unchanged in urine. Not removed by hemodialysis. **Half-life:** 4.3–4.6 hrs IV; 5.8–8.7 hrs IM (half-life is increased in those with impaired renal function).

AVAILABILITY
Powder for Injection: 250 mg, 500 mg, 1 g, 2 g.

INDICATIONS AND DOSAGES
▸ **Mild to moderate respiratory and genitourinary (GU) tract, bone, intra-abdominal, and biliary tract infections and septicemia**
IM/IV
Adults, Elderly. 1–2 g given as single dose or 2 divided doses.
▸ **Serious respiratory and GU tract, bone, intra-abdominal, and biliary tract infections and septicemia**
IM/IV
Adults, Elderly. Up to 4 g/day in 2 divided doses.
Children. 50–75 mg/kg/day in divided doses q12h. Maximum: 2 g/day.
▸ **Skin and skin-structure infections**
IM/IV
Children. 50–75 mg/kg/day as single or 2 divided doses. Maximum: 2 g/day.
▸ **Meningitis**
IV
Children. Initially, 75 mg/kg, then 100 mg/kg/day as single or in divided doses q12h. Maximum: 4 g/day.
▸ **Lyme disease**
IV
Adults, Elderly. 2–4 g a day for 10–14 days.

▸ **Acute bacterial otitis media**
IM
Children. 50 mg/kg a day for 3 days as single dose. Maximum: 1 g/day.
▸ **Perioperative prophylaxis**
IM/IV
Adults, Elderly. 1 g 0.5–2 hrs before surgery.
▸ **Uncomplicated gonorrhea**
IM
Adults. 250 mg one time plus doxycycline.
▸ **Dosage in renal impairment**
Dosage modification is usually unnecessary but should be monitored in those with both renal and liver impairment or severe renal impairment.

CONTRAINDICATIONS
History of anaphylactic reaction to penicillins, hypersensitivity to cephalosporins

INTERACTIONS
Drug
None known.
Herbal
None known.
Food
None known.

DIAGNOSTIC TEST EFFECTS
Positive direct or indirect Coombs' test may occur (interferes with crossmatching procedures, hematologic tests). May increase BUN, serum alkaline phosphatase, bilirubin, creatinine, SGOT (AST), and SGPT (ALT) levels.

IV INCOMPATIBILITIES
Aminophylline, amphotericin B complex (AmBisome, Amphotec, Abelcet), filgrastim (Neupogen), fluconazole (Diflucan), labetalol (Normodyne), pentamidine (Pentam IV), vancomycin (Vancocin)

IV COMPATIBILITIES

Diltiazem (Cardizem), heparin, lidocaine, morphine, propofol (Diprivan)

SIDE EFFECTS

Frequent

Discomfort with IM administration, oral candidiasis (sore mouth or tongue), mild diarrhea, mild abdominal cramping, vaginal candidiasis (discharge, itching)

Occasional

Nausea, serum sickness reaction (fever, joint pain)

Serum sickness reaction usually occurs after the second course of therapy and resolves after the drug is discontinued.

Rare

Allergic reaction (rash, pruritus, urticaria), thrombophlebitis (pain, redness, swelling at injection site)

SERIOUS REACTIONS

• Antibiotic-associated colitis manifested as severe abdominal pain and tenderness, fever, and watery and severe diarrhea, and other superinfections may result from altered bacterial balance.

• Nephrotoxicity may occur, especially in patients with preexisting renal disease.

• Severe hypersensitivity reaction including severe pruritus, angioedema, bronchospasm, and anaphylaxis, particularly in patients with a history of allergies, especially to penicillins, may occur.

NURSING CONSIDERATIONS

Baseline Assessment

◄ALERT► Determine the patient's history of allergies, particularly cephalosporins and penicillins before beginning drug therapy.

Lifespan Considerations

• Be aware that ceftriaxone readily crosses the placenta and is distributed in breast milk.

• Be aware that ceftriaxone use in children may displace serum bilirubin from serum albumin.

• Use ceftriaxone with caution in neonates, who may become hyperbilirubinemic.

• In the elderly, age-related renal impairment may require dosage adjustment.

Precautions

• Use cautiously in patients with a history of allergies or gastrointestinal (GI) disease, especially antibiotic-associated colitis or ulcerative colitis, and liver or renal impairment.

• Use cautiously in patients concurrently using nephrotoxic medications.

Administration and Handling

IM

• Add 0.9 ml Sterile Water for Injection, 0.9% NaCl, D_5W, Bacteriostatic Water and 0.9% Benzyl Alcohol or lidocaine to each 250 mg to provide concentration of 250 mg/ml.

• Give deep IM injections slowly to minimize patient discomfort. To further minimize discomfort, administer IM injections into the gluteus maximus instead of the lateral aspect of the thigh.

IV

• Solution normally appears light yellow to amber.

• IV infusion (piggyback) is stable for 3 days at room temperature, 10 days if refrigerated.

• Discard if precipitate forms.

• Add 2.4 ml Sterile Water for Injection to each 250 mg to provide concentration of 100 mg/ml.

• May further dilute with 50 to 100 ml 0.9% NaCl, D_5W.

• For intermittent IV infusion (piggyback), infuse over 15 to 30 minutes for adults, 10 to 30 minutes in children, neonates.

• Alternate IV sites and use large veins to reduce the potential for phlebitis development.

Intervention and Evaluation

• Assess the patient's mouth for white patches on the mucous membranes and tongue.

• Assess the patient's pattern of daily bowel activity and stool consistency. Mild GI effects may be tolerable, but increasing severity may indicate the onset of antibiotic-associated colitis.

• Monitor the patient's intake and output and renal function reports for nephrotoxicity.

• Be alert for signs and symptoms of superinfection including abdominal pain, moderate to severe diarrhea, severe anal or genital pruritus, and severe mouth soreness.

Patient Teaching

• Advise the patient to continue ceftriaxone therapy for the full length of treatment and explain that doses will be evenly spaced around the clock.

• Explain to the patient that discomfort may occur with IM injection.

---

cefuroxime axetil
sef-yur-**ox**-ime
(Ceftin, Zinnat[AUS])
Do not confuse with cefotaxime or Cefzil.

cefuroxime sodium
(Kefurox, Zinacef)

CATEGORY AND SCHEDULE
Pregnancy Risk Category: B

MECHANISM OF ACTION

A second-generation cephalosporin that binds to bacterial cell membranes. *Therapeutic Effect:* Inhibits synthesis of bacterial cell wall. Bactericidal.

PHARMACOKINETICS

Rapidly absorbed from the gastrointestinal (GI) tract. Protein binding: 33%–50%. Widely distributed (including cerebrospinal fluid [CSF]). Primarily excreted unchanged in urine. Moderately removed by hemodialysis. **Half-life:** 1.3 hrs (half-life is increased in those with impaired renal function).

AVAILABILITY

Tablets: 250 mg, 500 mg.
Oral Suspension: 125 mg/5 ml, 250 mg/5 ml.
Powder for Injection: 750 mg, 1.5 g.

INDICATIONS AND DOSAGES

▸ **Ampicillin-resistant influenza; bacterial meningitis; early Lyme disease; genitourinary tract, gynecologic, skin, and bone infections; septicemia; gonorrhea, and other gonococcal infections**
IM/IV
Adults, Elderly. 750 mg to 1.5 g q8h.
Children. 75–100 mg/kg/day divided q8h. Maximum: 8 g/day.
Neonates. 50–100 mg/kg/day divided q12h.
PO
Adults, Elderly. 125–500 mg 2 times/day depending on the infection.
▸ **Pharyngitis, tonsillitis**
PO
Children 3 mos–12 yrs. Tablets: 125 mg q12h. Suspension: 20 mg/kg/day in 2 divided doses.

▶ **Acute otitis media, acute bacterial maxillary sinusitis, impetigo**
PO
Children 3 mos–12 yrs. Tablets: 250 mg q12h. Suspension: 30 mg/kg/day in 2 divided doses.
▶ **Bacterial meningitis**
IV
Children 3 mos–12 yrs. 200–240 mg/kg/day in divided doses q6–8h.
▶ **Perioperative prophylaxis**
IV
Adults, Elderly. 1.5 g 30–60 min before surgery and 750 mg q8h postop.
▶ **Usual neonate dosage**
IM/IV
Neonates. 20–100 mg/kg/day in divided doses q12h.
▶ **Dosage in renal impairment**
Adult dosage is modified on the basis of creatinine clearance and the severity of infection.

Creatinine Clearance	Dosage Interval
10–20 ml/min	q12h
less than 10 ml/min	q24h

CONTRAINDICATIONS
History of anaphylactic reaction to penicillins, hypersensitivity to cephalosporins

INTERACTIONS
Drug
Probenecid: Increases serum concentration of cefuroxime.
Herbal
None known.
Food
None known.

DIAGNOSTIC TEST EFFECTS
Positive direct or indirect Coombs' test may occur (interferes with crossmatching procedures, hematologic tests). May increase serum alkaline phosphatase, serum bilirubin, serum LDH, SGOT (AST), and SGPT (ALT) levels.

IV INCOMPATIBILITIES
Filgrastim (Neupogen), fluconazole (Diflucan), midazolam (Versed), vancomycin (Vancocin)

IV COMPATIBILITIES
Diltiazem (Cardizem), hydromorphone(Dilaudid), morphine, propofol (Diprivan)

SIDE EFFECTS
Frequent
Discomfort with IM administration, oral candidiasis (sore mouth or tongue), mild diarrhea, mild abdominal cramping, vaginal candidiasis (discharge, itching)
Occasional
Nausea, serum sickness reaction (fever, joint pain)
Serum sickness reaction usually occurs after the second course of therapy and resolves after the drug is discontinued.
Rare
Allergic reaction (rash, pruritus, urticaria), thrombophlebitis (pain, redness, swelling at injection site)

SERIOUS REACTIONS
• Antibiotic-associated colitis manifested as severe abdominal pain and tenderness, fever, and watery and severe diarrhea, and other superinfections may result from altered bacterial balance.
• Nephrotoxicity may occur, especially in patients with preexisting renal disease.
• Severe hypersensitivity reaction including severe pruritus, angioedema, bronchospasm, and anaphylaxis, particularly in patients with a history of allergies, especially to penicillins, may occur.

NURSING CONSIDERATIONS

Baseline Assessment

◀ALERT▶ Determine the patient's history of allergies, particularly cephalosporins and penicillins, before beginning drug therapy.

Lifespan Considerations

• Be aware that cefuroxime readily crosses the placenta and is distributed in breast milk.

• There are no age-related precautions noted in children.

• In the elderly, age-related renal impairment may require dosage adjustment.

Precautions

• Use cautiously in patients with a history of GI disease, especially antibiotic-associated colitis or ulcerative colitis, and renal impairment.

• Use cautiously in patients concurrently using nephrotoxic medications.

Administration and Handling

PO

• Give without regard to meals. If GI upset occurs, give with food or milk.

• Avoid crushing tablets due to bitter taste.

• Suspension must be given with food.

IM

• Give deep IM injections slowly to minimize patient discomfort. To further minimize discomfort, administer IM injections into the gluteus maximus instead of the lateral aspect of the thigh.

IV

• Solution normally appears light yellow to amber; may darken, but color change does not indicate loss of potency

• IV infusion (piggyback) is stable for 24 hours at room temperature, 7 days if refrigerated.

• Discard if precipitate forms.

• Reconstitute 750 mg in 8 ml (1.5 g in 14 ml) Sterile Water for Injection to provide a concentration of 100 mg/ml.

• For intermittent IV infusion (piggyback), further dilute with 50 to 100 ml 0.9% NaCl or D_5W.

• For IV push, administer over 3 to 5 minutes.

• For intermittent IV infusion (piggyback), infuse over 15 to 60 minutes.

Intervention and Evaluation

• Assess the patient's mouth for white patches on the mucous membranes and tongue.

• Assess the patient's pattern of daily bowel activity and stool consistency. Mild GI effects may be tolerable, but increasing severity may indicate the onset of antibiotic-associated colitis.

• Monitor the patient's intake and output and renal function reports for signs of nephrotoxicity.

• Be alert for signs and symptoms of superinfection including abdominal pain, moderate to severe diarrhea, severe anal or genital pruritus, and severe mouth soreness.

Patient Teaching

• Advise the patient to continue cefuroxime therapy for the full length of treatment and to evenly space drug doses around the clock.

• Explain to the patient that cefuroxime may cause GI upset. Instruct the patient to take the drug with food or milk if GI upset occurs.

• Explain to the patient that discomfort may occur with IM injection.

cephalexin
cef-ah-**lex**-in
(Apo-Cephalex[CAN],
Ceporex[AUS], Ibilex[AUS], Keflex,
Keftab, Novolexin[CAN])

CATEGORY AND SCHEDULE
Pregnancy Risk Category: B

MECHANISM OF ACTION
A first-generation cephalosporin that
binds to bacterial cell membranes.
Therapeutic Effect: Inhibits synthesis
of bacterial cell wall. Bactericidal.

PHARMACOKINETICS
Rapidly absorbed from the gastrointestinal (GI) tract. Protein binding:
10%–15%. Widely distributed.
Primarily excreted unchanged in
urine. Moderately removed by
hemodialysis. **Half-life:** 0.9–1.2 hrs
(half-life is increased in those with
impaired renal function).

AVAILABILITY
Capsules: 250 mg, 500 mg.
Tablets: 250 mg, 500 mg, 1 g.
Oral Suspension: 125 mg/5 ml,
250 mg/5 ml.
Tablets for Oral Suspension: 125
mg, 250 mg.

INDICATIONS AND DOSAGES
▸ **Bone infections; prophylaxis of
rheumatic fever, follow-up to par-
enteral therapy**
PO
Adults, Elderly. 250–500 mg q6h up
to 4 g/day.
▸ **Streptococcal pharyngitis, skin
and skin-structure infections, un-
complicated cystitis**
PO
Adults, Elderly. 500 mg q12h.
▸ **Usual pediatric dosage**
Children. 25–100 mg/kg/day in
2–4 divided doses.

▸ **Otitis media**
PO
Children. 75–100 mg/kg/day in
4 divided doses.
▸ **Dosage in renal impairment**
After usual initial dose, dosage and
frequency are modified on the basis
of creatinine clearance and the
severity of infection.

Creatinine Clearance	Dosage Interval
10–40 ml/min	q8–12h
less than 10 ml/min	q12–24h

CONTRAINDICATIONS
History of anaphylactic reaction to
penicillins, hypersensitivity to
cephalosporins

INTERACTIONS
Drug
Probenecid: Increases serum con-
centration of cephalexin.
Herbal
None known.
Food
None known.

DIAGNOSTIC TEST EFFECTS
Positive direct or indirect Coombs'
test may occur (interferes with
crossmatching procedures, hematologic tests). May increase serum
alkaline phosphatase, SGOT (AST),
and SGPT (ALT) levels.

SIDE EFFECTS
Frequent
Oral candidiasis (sore mouth or
tongue), mild diarrhea, mild abdominal cramping, vaginal candidiasis
(discharge, itching)
Occasional
Nausea, serum sickness reaction
(fever, joint pain)
Serum sickness reaction usually
occurs after the second course of

therapy and resolves after the drug is discontinued.

Rare

Allergic reaction (rash, pruritus, urticaria)

SERIOUS REACTIONS

• Antibiotic-associated colitis manifested as severe abdominal pain and tenderness, fever, and watery and severe diarrhea, and other superinfections may result from altered bacterial balance.

• Nephrotoxicity may occur, especially in patients with preexisting renal disease.

• Severe hypersensitivity reaction including severe pruritus, angioedema, bronchospasm, and anaphylaxis, particularly in patients with a history of allergies, especially to penicillin, may occur.

NURSING CONSIDERATIONS

Baseline Assessment

◀ALERT▶ Determine the patient's history of allergies, particularly cephalosporins and penicillins, before beginning drug therapy.

Lifespan Considerations

• Be aware that cephalexin readily crosses the placenta and is distributed in breast milk.

• There are no age-related precautions noted in children.

• In the elderly, age-related renal impairment may require dosage adjustment.

Precautions

• Use cautiously in patients with a history of GI disease, especially antibiotic-associated colitis or ulcerative colitis, and renal impairment.

• Use cautiously in patients concurrently using nephrotoxic medications.

Administration and Handling

◀ALERT▶ Space drug doses evenly around the clock.

PO

• After reconstitution, oral suspension is stable for 14 days if refrigerated.

• Shake oral suspension well before using.

• Give without regard to meals. If GI upset occurs, give with food or milk.

Intervention and Evaluation

• Assess the patient's mouth for white patches on the mucous membranes and tongue.

• Assess the patient's pattern of daily bowel activity and stool consistency. Mild GI effects may be tolerable, but increasing severity may indicate the onset of antibiotic-associated colitis.

• Monitor the patient's intake and output and renal function reports for signs of nephrotoxicity.

• Be alert for signs and symptoms of superinfection including abdominal pain, moderate to severe diarrhea, severe anal or genital pruritus, and severe mouth soreness.

Patient Teaching

• Advise the patient to continue cephalexin therapy for the full length of treatment and to evenly space drug doses around the clock.

• Explain to the patient that cephalexin may cause GI upset. Instruct the patient to take the drug with food or milk if GI upset occurs.

• Teach the patient to refrigerate cephalexin's oral suspension.

loracarbef

laur-ah-**car**-bef
(Lorabid)
Do not confuse with Lortab.

CATEGORY AND SCHEDULE

Pregnancy Risk Category: B

MECHANISM OF ACTION

A cephalosporin that acts as a bactericidal by binding to bacterial cell membranes. *Therapeutic Effect:* Inhibits bacterial cell wall synthesis.

AVAILABILITY

Capsules: 200 mg, 400 mg.
Powder for PO Suspension: 100 mg/5 ml, 200 mg/5 ml.

INDICATIONS AND DOSAGES

▸ **Bronchitis**
PO
Adults, Elderly, Children older than 12 yrs. 200–400 mg q12h for 7 days.

▸ **Pharyngitis**
PO
Adults, Elderly, Children older than 12 yrs. 200 mg q12h for 10 days.
Children 6 mos–12 yrs. 7.5 mg/kg q12h for 10 days.

▸ **Pneumonia**
PO
Adults, Elderly, Children older than 12 yrs. 400 mg q12h for 14 days.

▸ **Sinusitis**
PO
Adults, Elderly, Children older than 12 yrs. 400 mg q12h for 10 days.
Children 6 mos–12 yrs. 15 mg/kg q12h for 10 days.

▸ **Skin, soft tissue infections**
PO
Adults, Elderly, Children older than 12 yrs. 200 mg q12h for 7 days.
Children 6 mos–12 yrs. 7.5 mg/kg q12h for 7 days.

▸ **Urinary tract infections (UTIs)**
PO
Adults, Elderly, Children 6 mos–12 yrs. 200–400 mg q12h for 7–14 days.

▸ **Otitis media**
PO
Children 6 mos–12 yrs. 15 mg/kg q12h for 10 days.

CONTRAINDICATIONS

History of anaphylactic reaction to penicillins, hypersensitivity to cephalosporins

INTERACTIONS

Drug
Probenecid: Increases serum concentrations and half-life of loracarbef.
Herbal
None known.
Food
None known.

DIAGNOSTIC TEST EFFECTS

May increase BUN, serum alkaline phosphatase, serum creatinine, SGOT (AST), and SGPT (ALT) levels. May decrease blood leukocyte and platelet counts.

SIDE EFFECTS

Frequent
Abdominal pain, anorexia, nausea, vomiting, diarrhea
Occasional
Skin rash, itching
Rare
Dizziness, headache, vaginitis

SERIOUS REACTIONS

• Antibiotic-associated colitis and other superinfections may result from altered bacterial balance.
• Hypersensitivity reactions (ranging from rash, urticaria, and fever to anaphylaxis) occur in less than 5% of patients. Generally, hypersensitivity reactions develop in those patients with a history of allergies, especially to penicillins.

NURSING CONSIDERATIONS

Baseline Assessment
◀ **ALERT** ▶ Determine the patient's history of allergies, particularly cephalosporins and penicillins before beginning drug therapy.

Precautions
• Use cautiously in patients with a history of colitis or renal impairment.

Administration and Handling
PO
• Give 1 hour before or 2 hours after meals.
• After reconstitution, powder for suspension may be kept at room temperature for 14 days.
• Discard unused portion after 14 days.
• Shake oral suspension well before using.

Intervention and Evaluation
• Assess the patient for nausea or vomiting.
• Assess the patient's pattern of daily bowel activity and stool consistency.
• Evaluate the patient's skin for rash, especially in the diaper area in children.
• Monitor the patient's intake and output, renal function reports, and urinalysis results for signs of nephrotoxicity.
• Be alert for signs and symptoms of superinfection including abdominal pain, anal or genital pruritus, moderate to severe diarrhea, moniliasis, and sore mouth or tongue.

Patient Teaching
• Advise the patient to continue loracarbef therapy for the full length of treatment and to evenly space drug doses around the clock, giving the drug 1 hour before or 2 hours after a meal.

8 Macrolides

azithromycin
clarithromycin
dirithromycin
erythromycin

Uses: Macrolides are used to treat pharyngitis, tonsillitis, sinusitis, chronic bronchitis, pneumonia, and uncomplicated skin and skin structure infections.

Action: Macrolides can be bacteriostatic or bactericidal and act primarily against gram-positive microorganisms and gram-negative cocci by reversibly binding to the P site of the 50S ribosomal subunit of susceptible organisms This action inhibits ribonucleic acid (RNA)-dependent protein synthesis and causes bacterial cell death. (See illustration, *Sites and Mechanisms of Action: Anti-infective Agents,* page 2.) Azithromycin and clarithromycin appear to be more potent than erythromycin.

COMBINATION PRODUCTS

ERYZOLE: erythromycin/sulfisoxazole (a sulfonamide) 200 mg/600 mg per 5 ml.
PEDIAZOLE: erythromycin/sulfisoxazole (a sulfonamide) 200 mg/600 mg per 5 ml.

azithromycin

aye-**zith**-row-my-sin
(Zithromax)
Do not confuse with erythromycin.

CATEGORY AND SCHEDULE
Pregnancy Risk Category: B

MECHANISM OF ACTION
A macrolide antibiotic that binds to ribosomal receptor sites of susceptible organisms. *Therapeutic Effect:* Inhibits RNA-dependent protein synthesis.

PHARMACOKINETICS
Rapidly absorbed from the gastrointestinal (GI) tract. Protein binding: 7%–50%. Widely distributed. Eliminated primarily unchanged via biliary excretion. **Half-life:** 68 hrs.

AVAILABILITY
Tablets: 250 mg, 500 mg, 600 mg.
Injection: 500 mg.
Oral Suspension: 100 mg/5 ml, 200 mg/5 ml.

INDICATIONS AND DOSAGES
▶ **Respiratory tract infections**
PO
Adults, Elderly. 500 mg once, then 250 mg each day for 4 days.
▶ **Acute bacterial exacerbations of chronic obstructive pulmonary disease (COPD)**
PO
Adults. 500 mg/day for 3 days.
▶ **Skin/skin-structure infections**
PO
Adults, Elderly. 500 mg once, then 250 mg each day for 4 days.
▶ **Otitis media**
PO
Children older than 6 mos. 10 mg/kg once (maximum 500 mg) then 5 mg/kg/day for 4 days (maximum 250 mg).

▸ **Pharyngitis, tonsillitis**
PO
Children 2 yrs and older. 12 mg/kg/
day (maximum 500 mg) for 5 days.
▸ **Treatment of *Mycobacterium
avium* complex (MAC)**
PO
Adults, Elderly. 500 mg/day in
combination.
Children. 5 mg/kg/day (maximum
250 mg) in combination.
▸ **MAC prevention**
PO
Adults, Elderly. 1200 mg/wk alone
or with rifabutin.
Children. 5 mg/kg/day (maximum
250 mg) or 20 mg/kg/wk (maxi-
mum 1200 mg) alone or with
rifabutin.
▸ **Usual pediatric dosage**
Children older than 6 mos.
10 mg/kg once (maximum: 500 mg)
then 5 mg/kg/day for 4 days
(maximum 250 mg).

UNLABELED USES
Chlamydial infections, gonococcal
pharyngitis, uncomplicated gonococcal infections of cervix, urethra,
and rectum

CONTRAINDICATIONS
Hypersensitivity to azithromycin,
erythromycins, or any macrolide
antibiotic

INTERACTIONS
Drug
*Aluminum or magnesium-
containing antacids:* May decrease azithromycin blood concentration. Give azithromycin
1 hour before or 2 hours after
antacids.
*Carbamazepine, cyclosporine,
theophylline, warfarin*: May increase the serum concentrations
of these drugs.

Herbal
None known.
Food
None known.

DIAGNOSTIC TEST EFFECTS
May increase serum CPK, SGOT
(AST), and SGPT (ALT) levels.

IV INCOMPATIBILITIES
Information is not available.

IV COMPATIBILITIES
None known; do not mix with other
medications.

SIDE EFFECTS
Occasional
Nausea, vomiting, diarrhea, abdomi-
nal pain
Rare
Headache, dizziness, allergic reaction

SERIOUS REACTIONS
• Superinfections, especially
antibiotic-associated colitis as evidenced by abdominal cramps, severe, watery diarrhea, and fever, may
result from altered bacterial balance.
• Acute interstitial nephritis occurs
rarely.

NURSING CONSIDERATIONS
Baseline Assessment
• Determine the patient's history of
hepatitis or allergies to azithromycin
and erythromycin.
Lifespan Considerations
• Be aware that it is unknown if
azithromycin is distributed in breast
milk.
• Be aware that the safety and
efficacy of azithromycin have not
been established in children less
than 16 years old for IV use and
less than 6 months old for oral use.
• In those elderly with normal renal
function, no age-related precautions
are noted.

Precautions
• Use cautiously in patients with liver or renal dysfunction.

Administration and Handling
PO
• May give tablets without regard to food.
• Store the suspension at room temperature. The suspension is stable for 10 days after reconstitution.
• Do not administer oral suspension with food. Give at least 1 hour before or 2 hours after meals.
IV
• Store vials at room temperature.
• Following reconstitution, the solution is stable for 24 hours at room temperature or 7 days if refrigerated.
• Reconstitute each 500-mg vial with 4.8 ml Sterile Water for Injection to provide concentration of 100 mg/ml.
• Shake well to ensure dissolution.
• Further dilute with 250 or 500 ml 0.9% NaCl or D_5W to provide final concentration of 2 mg with 250 ml diluent or 1 mg/ml with 500 ml diluent.
• Infuse over 60 minutes.

Intervention and Evaluation
• Assess the patient for gastrointestinal (GI) discomfort, nausea, or vomiting.
• Assess the patient's pattern of daily bowel activity and stool consistency.
• Monitor the patient's liver function test results.
• Assess the patient for signs and symptoms of hepatotoxicity manifested as abdominal pain, fever, GI disturbances, and malaise.
• Evaluate the patient for signs and symptoms of superinfection including genital or anal pruritus, sore mouth or tongue, and moderate to severe diarrhea.

Patient Teaching
• Advise the patient to continue therapy for the full length of treatment and to evenly space drug doses around the clock.
• Teach patients to take oral medication with 8 oz of water at least 1 hour before or 2 hours after consuming any food or beverages.

clarithromycin
clair-**rith**-row-my-sin
(Biaxin, Biaxin XL, Klacid[AUS])

CATEGORY AND SCHEDULE
Pregnancy Risk Category: C

MECHANISM OF ACTION
A macrolide that is bacteriostatic and binds to ribosomal receptor sites. May be bactericidal with high dosage or very susceptible microorganisms. *Therapeutic Effect:* Inhibits protein synthesis of bacterial cell wall.

PHARMACOKINETICS
Well absorbed from the gastrointestinal (GI) tract. Protein binding: 65%–75%. Widely distributed. Metabolized in liver to active metabolite. Primarily excreted in urine. Not removed by hemodialysis. **Half-life:** 3–7 hrs; metabolite: 5–7 hrs (half-life is increased in those with impaired renal function).

AVAILABILITY
Tablets: 250 mg, 500 mg.
Tablets (extended-release): 500 mg.
Oral Suspension: 125 mg/5 ml.

INDICATIONS AND DOSAGES
▶ **Usual adult and elderly dosage**
PO
Adults, Elderly. Immediate-release: 250–500 mg q12h for 7–14 days. Extended-release: Two 500-mg tablets a day for 7–14 days.

▸ **Acute otitis media**
Children. 15 mg/kg/day in
2 divided doses for 10 days.
▸ **Respiratory, skin, and skin-structure infections**
PO
Children. 15 mg/kg/day in
2 divided doses for 7–14 days.
▸ **Dosage in renal impairment**
Creatinine clearance less than 30
ml/min: Reduce dose by 50% and
administer once or twice a day.

CONTRAINDICATIONS
Hypersensitivity to clarithromycin,
erythromycins, any macrolide anti-biotic

INTERACTIONS
Drug
Carbamazepine, digoxin, theo-phylline: May increase blood con-centration and toxicity of these
drugs.
Rifampin: May decrease clarithro-mycin blood concentration.
Warfarin: May increase warfarin
effects.
Zidovudine: May decrease blood
concentration of zidovudine.
Herbal
None known.
Food
None known.

DIAGNOSTIC TEST EFFECTS
May rarely increase BUN, SGOT
(AST), and SGPT (ALT) levels.

SIDE EFFECTS
Occasional (6%–3%)
Diarrhea, nausea, altered taste,
abdominal pain
Rare (2%–1%)
Headache, dyspepsia

SERIOUS REACTIONS
• Antibiotic-associated colitis as
evidenced by severe abdominal pain

and tenderness, fever, and watery
and severe diarrhea, and other
superinfections may result from
altered bacterial balance.
• Hepatotoxicity and thrombocyto-penia occur rarely.

NURSING CONSIDERATIONS

Baseline Assessment
◀ **ALERT** ▶ Determine the patient's
allergies, especially to clarithromy-cin and erythromycins, and history
of hepatitis before beginning drug
therapy.
Lifespan Considerations
• Be aware that it is unknown if
clarithromycin is distributed in
breast milk.
• Be aware that the safety and
efficacy of this drug have not been
established in children younger than
6 months.
• In the elderly, age-related renal
impairment may require dosage
adjustment.
Precautions
• Use cautiously in patients with
liver and renal dysfunction and in
elderly patients with severe renal
impairment.
Administration and Handling
PO
• Give without regard to food.
• Do not crush or break tablets.
Intervention and Evaluation
• Assess the patient's pattern of
daily bowel activity and stool con-sistency. Mild gastrointestinal (GI)
effects may be tolerable, but in-creasing severity may indicate the
onset of antibiotic-associated colitis.
• Be alert for signs and symptoms
of superinfection, including abdomi-nal pain, anal or genital pruritus,
moderate to severe diarrhea, and
mouth soreness.
Patient Teaching
• Advise the patient to continue
clarithromycin therapy for the full

length of treatment and to evenly space drug doses around the clock.
* Instruct the patient to take this medication with 8 oz of water. Explain that the drug may be taken without regard to food.

dirithromycin
dih-**rith**-row-my-sin
(Dynabac)
Do not confuse with Dynacin or DynaCirc.

CATEGORY AND SCHEDULE
Pregnancy Risk Category: C

MECHANISM OF ACTION
A macrolide that binds to ribosomal receptor sites of susceptible organisms. *Therapeutic Effect:* Inhibits bacterial protein synthesis.

PHARMACOKINETICS
Rapidly absorbed from the gastrointestinal (GI) tract. Widely distributed into tissues and within cells. Protein binding: 15%–30%. Eliminated primarily unchanged via biliary excretion. Not removed by hemodialysis. **Half-life:** 30–44 hrs.

AVAILABILITY
Tablets (enteric-coated): 250 mg.

INDICATIONS AND DOSAGES
▶ **Pharyngitis, tonsillitis**
PO
Adults, Elderly, Children 12 yrs and older. 500 mg once a day for 10 days.
▶ **Acute bronchitis, chronic bronchitis**
PO
Adults, Elderly, Children 12 yrs and older. 500 mg once a day for 7 days.

▶ **Community-acquired pneumonia**
PO
Adults, Elderly, Children 12 yrs and older. 500 mg once a day for 14 days.
▶ **Skin and skin-structure infections**
PO
Adults, Elderly, Children 12 yrs and older. 500 mg once a day for 7 days.

CONTRAINDICATIONS
Hypersensitivity to dirithromycin, erythromycins, any macrolide antibiotic

INTERACTIONS
Drug
Aluminum- and magnesium-containing antacids: May decrease dirithromycin blood concentration (give 1 hr before or 2 hrs after antacid). *H_2 antagonists:* Increases dirithromycin absorption.
Herbal
None known.
Food
None known.

DIAGNOSTIC TEST EFFECTS
May increase serum CPK, blood eosinophil count, blood neutrophil count, platelet count, and serum potassium levels.

SIDE EFFECTS
Frequent (10%–8%)
Abdominal pain, headache, nausea, diarrhea
Occasional (3%–2%)
Vomiting, dyspepsia, dizziness, nonspecific pain, asthenia
Rare (less than 2%)
Increased cough, flatulence, rash, dyspnea, pruritus and urticaria, insomnia

SERIOUS REACTIONS
* Superinfections, especially antibiotic-associated colitis as evi-

denced by abdominal cramps, watery and severe diarrhea, and fever, may result from altered bacterial balance.

NURSING CONSIDERATIONS

Baseline Assessment
◀ALERT▶ Determine the patient's history of allergies to dirithromycin and erythromycins before beginning drug therapy.

Lifespan Considerations
• Be aware that it is unknown if dirithromycin is distributed in breast milk.
• Be aware that the safety and efficacy of dirithromycin have not been established in children younger than 12 years of age.
• There are no age-related precautions noted in the elderly.

Precautions
• Use cautiously in patients with liver or renal dysfunction.

Administration and Handling
PO
• Administer to the patient with food or within 1 hour after a meal because food increases absorption.
• Have the patient swallow the tablets whole. Don't crush or cut or have the patient chew the tablets.

Intervention and Evaluation
• Monitor the patient's white blood cell count (WBC) for signs of infection improvement.
• Evaluate the patient for diarrhea, gastrointestinal (GI) discomfort, headache, and nausea.
• Assess the patient's pattern of daily bowel activity and stool consistency.
• Evaluate the patient for signs and symptoms of superinfection including anal or genital pruritus, moderate to severe diarrhea, and sore mouth or tongue.

Patient Teaching
• Advise the patient to continue dirithromycin therapy for the full length of treatment.
• Instruct the patient to take dirithromycin with food or within 1 hour after a meal.
• Teach the patient not to take the drug with aluminum or magnesium-containing antacids. Explain to the patient that these antacids will lower dirithromycin's blood concentration.

erythromycin
eh-rith-row-**my**-sin
(Akne-Mycin, Apo-Erythro Base[CAN], EES, Eryacne[AUS], Erybid[CAN], Eryc, Eryc LD[AUS], EryDerm, EryPed, Ery-Tab, Erythrocin, Erythromid[CAN], PCE)

CATEGORY AND SCHEDULE
Pregnancy Risk Category: B

MECHANISM OF ACTION
A macrolide that is bacteriostatic and penetrates bacterial cell membranes and reversibly binds to bacterial ribosomes. *Therapeutic Effect:* Inhibits bacterial protein synthesis.

PHARMACOKINETICS
Variably absorbed from the gastrointestinal (GI) tract (affected by dosage form used). Widely distributed. Protein binding: 70%–90%. Metabolized in liver. Primarily eliminated in feces via bile. Not removed by hemodialysis.
Half-life: 1.4–2 hrs (half-life is increased in those with impaired renal function).

AVAILABILITY
Powder for Injection: 500 mg, 1 g.
Tablets (Base): 250 mg, 333 mg,
500 mg.
Tablets (delayed-release [Base]):
333 mg.
Capsules (delayed-release): 250 mg.
Tablets (Estolate): 500 mg.
Capsules (Estolate): 250 mg.
Oral Suspension (Estolate):
125 mg/5 ml, 250 mg/5 ml.
Tablets (chewable [Ethylsuccinate]):
200 mg.
Tablets (Ethylsuccinate): 400 mg.
Oral Suspension (Ethylsuccinate):
200 mg/5 ml, 400 mg/5 ml.
Oral Drops (Ethylsuccinate):
100 mg/2.5 ml.
Tablets (Stearate): 250 mg, 500 mg.
Ophthalmic Ointment (Stearate): 5%.
Topical Solution (Stearate): 1.5%, 2%.
Topical Gel (Stearate): 2%.
Topical Ointment (Stearate): 2%.

INDICATIONS AND DOSAGES
▶ **Respiratory infections, otitis media, pertussis, diphtheria (adjunctive therapy), Legionnaires' disease, intestinal amebiasis**
IV
Adults, Elderly, Children. 15–20
mg/kg/day in divided doses.
Maximum: 4 g/day.
PO
Adults, Elderly. 250 mg q6h; 500
mg q12h; or 333 mg q8h. Increase
up to 4 g/day.
Children. 30–50 mg/kg/day in
divided doses up to 60–100 mg/kg/
day for severe infections.
Neonates. 20–40 mg/kg/day in
divided doses q6–12h.
▶ **Preop intestinal antisepsis**
PO
Adults, Elderly. Give 1 g at 1 pm,
2 pm, and 11 pm on day before
surgery (with neomycin).
Children. 20 mg/kg; same regimen
as above.

▶ **Acne vulgaris**
Topical
Adults. Apply thin layer to the
affected area 2 times/day.
▶ **Gonococcal ophthalmia neonatorum**
Ophthalmic
Neonates. 0.5–2 cm no later than
1 hr after delivery.

UNLABELED USES
Systemic: Treatment of acne vulgaris, chancroid, *Campylobacter* enteritis, gastroparesis, Lyme disease
Topical: Treatment of minor bacterial skin infections
Ophthalmic: Treatment of blepharitis, conjunctivitis, keratitis, chlamydial trachoma

CONTRAINDICATIONS
Do not administer the fixed-combination, Pediazole, to infants younger than 2 months.
History of hepatitis due to erythromycins, hypersensitivity to erythromycins, preexisting liver disease

INTERACTIONS
Drug
Buspirone, cyclosporine, felodipine, lovastatin, simvastatin: May increase the blood concentration and toxicity of these drugs.
Carbamazepine: May inhibit the metabolism of carbamazepine.
Chloramphenicol, clindamycin: May decrease the effects of chloramphenicol and clindamycin.
Hepatotoxic medications: May increase the risk of liver toxicity.
Theophylline: May increase the risk of theophylline toxicity.
Warfarin: May increase the effects of this drug.
Herbal
None known.

Food
None known.

DIAGNOSTIC TEST EFFECTS
May increase serum alkaline phosphatase, serum bilirubin, SGOT (AST), and SGPT (ALT) levels.

IV INCOMPATIBILITIES
Fluconazole (Diflucan)

IV COMPATIBILITIES
Aminophylline, amiodarone (Cordarone), diltiazem (Cardizem), heparin, hydromorphone (Dilaudid), lidocaine, lorazepam (Ativan), magnesium sulfate, midazolam (Versed), morphine, multivitamins, potassium chloride

SIDE EFFECTS
Frequent
IV: Abdominal cramping or discomfort, phlebitis or thrombophlebitis
Topical: Dry skin (50%)
Occasional
Nausea, vomiting, diarrhea, rash, urticaria
Rare
Ophthalmic: Sensitivity reaction with increased irritation, burning, itching, inflammation
Topical: Urticaria

SERIOUS REACTIONS
• Superinfections, especially antibiotic-associated colitis as evidenced by genital and anal pruritus, sore mouth or tongue, and moderate to severe diarrhea, and reversible cholestatic hepatitis may occur.
• High dosages in patients with renal impairment may lead to reversible hearing loss.
• Anaphylaxis occurs rarely.

NURSING CONSIDERATIONS
Baseline Assessment
◀ALERT▶ Determine the patient's history of allergies, particularly to erythromycins, and hepatitis before beginning drug therapy.
Lifespan Considerations
• Be aware that erythromycin crosses the placenta and is distributed in breast milk.
• Be aware that erythromycin estolate may increase liver function enzymes in pregnant women.
• There are no age-related precautions noted in children or the elderly.
• Be aware that high dosages in patients with decreased liver or renal function increase the risk of hearing loss.
Precautions
• Use cautiously in patients with liver dysfunction.
• Consider the precautions of sulfonamides if erythromycin is used in combination therapy Pediazole).
• IV erythromycin may cause tachycardia and prolonged QT interval.
Administration and Handling
PO
• Store capsules, tablets at room temperature.
• Oral suspension is stable for 14 days at room temperature.
• Administer erythromycin base, stearate 1 hour before or 2 hours following food. Erythromycin estolate, ethylsuccinate may be given without regard to meals, but optimal absorption occurs when given on empty stomach.
• Give with 8 oz water.
• If the patient has difficulty swallowing, sprinkle capsule contents on teaspoon of applesauce and follow with water.
• Be sure the patient doesn't swallow chewable tablets whole.

IV
• Store parenteral form at room temperature.
• Initial reconstituted solution in vial is stable for 2 weeks refrigerated or 24 hours at room temperature.
• Diluted IV solutions are stable for 8 hours at room temperature, 24 hours if refrigerated.
• Discard if precipitate forms.
• Reconstitute each 500 mg with 10 ml Sterile Water for Injection without preservative to provide a concentration of 50 mg/ml.
• Further dilute with 100 to 250 ml D_5W or 0.9% NaCl.
• For intermittent IV infusion (piggyback), infuse over 20 to 60 minutes.
• For continuous infusion, infuse over 6 to 24 hours.
Ophthalmic:
• Place a gloved finger on the patient's lower eyelid and pull the lower eyelid out until a pocket is formed between eye and lower lid. Place ¼–½ inch ointment into pocket.
• Have the patient close the eye gently for 1 to 2 minutes and roll the eyeball to increase the contact area of drug to eye.
• Remove excess ointment around the eye with tissue.
Intervention and Evaluation
• Assess the patient's pattern of daily bowel activity and stool consistency.
• Assess the patient' s skin for rash.
• Evaluate the patient for signs and symptoms of liver toxicity, including abdominal pain, fever, gastrointestinal (GI) disturbances, and malaise.

• Evaluate the patient for signs and symptoms of superinfection.
• Check the patient's injection site for signs and symptoms of phlebitis as evidenced by heat, pain, and red streaking over the vein.
• Monitor the patient for signs of high dose hearing loss.
Patient Teaching
• Advise the patient to continue erythromycin therapy for the full length of treatment and to evenly space drug doses around the clock.
• Instruct the patient to take the oral form of erythromycin with 8 oz water 1 hour before or 2 hours after food or beverage. Teach the patient not to swallow chewable tablets whole.
• Warn patients receiving the ophthalmic form of erythromycin to notify the physician if they experience burning, inflammation, and itching.
• Advise patients receiving the topical form of erythromycin to notify the physician if they experience burning, excessive dryness, and itching.
• Explain to the patient that acne improvement may not occur for 1 to 2 months and that the maximum benefit of the drug may take 3 months to appear. Also inform the patient that erythromycin therapy may last months or years.
• Warn patients taking erythromycin for acne vulgaris to use caution if using other topical acne preparations containing abrasive or peeling agents, abrasive or medicated soaps, and cosmetics containing alcohol (e.g., astringents, aftershave lotion).

9 Penicillins

amoxicillin
amoxicillin/
  clavulanate
  potassium
ampicillin sodium
ampicillin/sulbactam
  sodium
oxacillin
penicillin G
  benzathine
penicillin G potassium
penicillin V potassium
piperacillin sodium/
  tazobactam sodium
ticarcillin disodium/
  clavulanate
  potassium

Uses: Penicillins may be used to treat a large number of infections, including pneumonia and other respiratory diseases, urinary tract infections, septicemia, meningitis, intra-abdominal infections, gonorrhea, syphilis, and bone and joint infections.

These agents are classified by antimicrobial spectrum:

Natural penicillins, such as penicillin G benzathine and penicillin V potassium, are very active against gram-positive cocci, but ineffective against most strains of *Staphylococcus aureus* because the drugs are inactivated by the enzyme penicillinase, which is produced by these organisms.

Penicillinase-resistant penicillins, such as oxacillin, are effective against penicillinase-producing *S. aureus* but are less effective against gram-positive cocci than the natural penicillins.

Broad-spectrum penicillins, such as amoxicillin and ampicillin sodium, are effective against gram-positive cocci and some gram-negative bacteria, such as *Haemophilus influenzae, Escherichia coli,* and *Proteus mirabilis.*

Extended-spectrum penicillins, such as piperacillin sodium-tazobactam sodium and ticarcillin disodium-clavulanate potassium, are effective against *Pseudomonas aeruginosa, Enterobacter* species, *Proteus* species, *Klebsiella* species, and some other gram-negative organisms.

Action: Penicillins inhibit cell wall synthesis or activate enzymes that disrupt bacterial cell walls, weakening the walls and causing cell lysis and death. They may be bacteriostatic or bactericidal and are most effective against bacteria undergoing active growth and division. (See illustration: *Mechanisms of Action: Penicillins,* page 170.)

COMBINATION PRODUCTS
BICILLIN CR: penicillin G benzathine/ penicillin procaine 600,000 units/ 600,000 units.

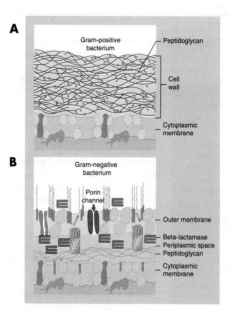

A Gram-positive bacterium — Peptidoglycan

Cell wall

Cytoplasmic membrane

B Gram-negative bacterium

Porin channel

Outer membrane

Beta-lactamase
Periplasmic space
Peptidoglycan

Cytoplasmic membrane

Mechanisms of Action: Penicillins

Generally, penicillins act by weakening the normally rigid cell walls of bacteria. A weakened wall causes the cell to absorb excess water, leading to cellular swelling and rupture. However, penicillins' effectiveness is determined by the bacterial cell wall, which differs in gram-positive and gram-negative bacteria.

Gram-positive bacteria (A) have a rigid cell wall composed of long strands of peptidoglycan. This peptidoglycan is held together by cross-bridges, which are formed by transpeptidase and give the cell wall its strength. In addition, autolysins (bacterial enzymes that adhere to cellular bonds in the wall) are present in the cell wall. Bacteria use these enzymes to break down portions of the cell wall to permit growth and cell division. Penicillins inhibit transpeptidases, thereby interfering with the creation of cross-bridges and weakening the cell wall. These drugs also activate autolysins, which then lead to cell wall breakdown—and cell destruction.

Gram-negative bacteria (B) have a different cell wall structure. Unlike gram-positive bacteria, which have two layers (a cell wall and a cytoplasmic membrane), gram-negative bacteria have three layers (an outer membrane, a thin cell wall, and a cytoplasmic membrane). Although penicillins can penetrate the cell wall, they must first penetrate the outer membrane. Only a few penicillins are small enough to pass through the tiny openings (porin channels) in the outer member to be effective against gram-negative bacteria.

In addition, gram-positive and gram-negative bacteria produce enzymes called beta-lactamases, which can render penicillins ineffective. Beta-lactamases that act specifically on penicillins are known as penicillinases. Gram-positive bacteria produce large amount of penicillinases, but release them into the environment around the cell. In contrast, gram-negative bacteria produce smaller amounts of these enzymes, but release them into the periplasmic space. So even if a penicillin can pass through the porin channel, it must also be resistant to penicillinase to achieve its therapeutic effect.

amoxicillin
ah-**mocks**-ih-sill-in
(Alphamox[AUS], Amohexal[AUS],
Amoxil, Apo-Amoxi[CAN],
Cilamox[AUS], Clamoxyl[AUS],
DisperMox, Fisamox[AUS],
Moxamox[AUS], Moxacin[AUS],
Novamoxin[CAN], Polymox,
Trimox, Wymox)
**Do not confuse with amoxapine
or Tylox.**

CATEGORY AND SCHEDULE
Pregnancy Risk Category: B

MECHANISM OF ACTION
A penicillin that acts as a bactericidal in susceptible microorganisms.
Therapeutic Effect: Inhibits bacterial
cell wall synthesis.

PHARMACOKINETICS
Well absorbed from gastrointestinal
(GI) tract. Protein binding: 20%.
Partially metabolized in liver. Primarily excreted in urine. Removed
by hemodialysis. **Half-life:** 1–1.3
hrs (half-life increased in reduced
renal function).

AVAILABILITY
Tablets (chewable): 125 mg,
200 mg, 250 mg, 400 mg.
Tablets: 500 mg, 875 mg.
Tablets for Oral Suspension: 200
mg, 400 mg.
Capsules: 250 mg, 500 mg.
Powder for PO Suspension: 50
mg/ml, 125 mg/5 ml, 200 mg/ml,
250 mg/5 ml, 400 mg/5 ml.

INDICATIONS AND DOSAGES
▸ **Ear, nose, throat, genitourinary
(GU), skin/skin-structure infections**
PO
*Adults, Elderly, Children weighing
more than 20 kg.* 250–500 mg q8h
(or 500–875 mg tablets 2 times/day).

Children weighing less than 20 kg.
20–40 mg/kg/day in divided doses
q8–12h.
▸ **Lower respiratory tract infections**
PO
*Adults, Elderly, Children weighing
more than 20 kg.* 500 mg q8h
(or 875 mg tablets 2 times/day).
Children weighing less than 20 kg.
40 mg/kg/day in divided doses
q8–12h.
▸ **Acute, uncomplicated gonorrhea**
PO
Adults. 3 g one time with 1 g pro-
benecid. Follow with tetracycline or
erythromycin therapy.
Children 2 yrs and older. 50 mg/kg
plus probenecid 25 mg/kg as a
single dose.
▸ **Acute otitis media**
PO
Children. 80–90 mg/kg/day in
divided doses q12h.
▸ **H. pylori**
PO
*Adults, Elderly (in combination with
other antibiotics).* 1 g 2 times/day
for 10 days.
▸ **Endocarditis**
PO
Adults, Elderly. 2 g 1 hr prior to
procedure.
Children. 50 mg/kg as above.
▸ **Usual pediatric dosage**
*Neonates, Children younger than
3 mos.* 20–30 mg/kg/day in divided
doses q12h.
▸ **Dosage in renal impairment**
Creatinine clearance 10–30 ml/min.
Administer q12h.
Creatinine clearance less than
10 ml/min. Administer q24h.

UNLABELED USES
Treatment of Lyme disease and
typhoid fever

CONTRAINDICATIONS
Hypersensitivity to any penicillin,
infectious mononucleosis

INTERACTIONS
Drug
Allopurinol: May increase incidence of rash.
Oral contraceptives: May decrease effects of oral contraceptives.
Probenecid: May increase amoxicillin blood concentration and risk for amoxicillin toxicity.
Herbal
None known.
Food
None known.

DIAGNOSTIC TEST EFFECTS
May increase BUN, LDH, serum bilirubin, serum creatinine, SGOT (AST), and SGPT (ALT) levels. May cause positive Coombs' test.

SIDE EFFECTS
Frequent
Gastrointestinal (GI) disturbances (mild diarrhea, nausea, or vomiting), headache, oral or vaginal candidiasis
Occasional
Generalized rash, urticaria

SERIOUS REACTIONS
• Altered bacterial balance may result in potentially fatal superinfections and antibiotic-associated colitis as evidenced by abdominal cramps, watery or severe diarrhea, and fever.
• Severe hypersensitivity reactions, including anaphylaxis and acute interstitial nephritis occur rarely.

NURSING CONSIDERATIONS
Baseline Assessment
• Determine the patient's history of allergies, especially to cephalosporins or penicillins, before giving the drug.

Lifespan Consideration
• Be aware that amoxicillin crosses the placenta, appears in cord blood and amniotic fluid, and is distributed in breast milk in low concentrations.
• Be aware that amoxicillin administration may lead to allergic sensitization, candidiasis, diarrhea, and skin rash in infants.
• Be aware that immature renal function in neonates and young infants may delay renal excretion of amoxicillin.
• In the elderly, age-related renal impairment may require dosage adjustment.
Precautions
• Use cautiously in patients with antibiotic-associated colitis or a history of allergies, especially to cephalosporins.
Administration and Handling
PO
• Store capsules or tablets at room temperature.
• After reconstitution, the oral solution is stable for 14 days whether at room temperature or refrigerated.
• Give without regard to meals.
• Instruct the patient to chew or crush chewable tablets thoroughly before swallowing.
Intervention and Evaluation
• Withhold amoxicillin and promptly notify the physician if the patient experiences a rash or diarrhea. Severe diarrhea with abdominal pain, blood or mucus in stool, and fever may indicate antibiotic-associated colitis.
• Monitor the patient for signs and symptoms of superinfection, including anal or genital pruritus, black hairy tongue, diarrhea, increased fever, sore throat, ulceration or changes of oral mucosa, and vomiting.

Patient Teaching
• Urge the patient to continue taking the antibiotic for the full length of treatment and to evenly space doses around the clock.
• Instruct the patient to take amoxicillin with meals if GI upset occurs.
• Stress to the patient that he or she must thoroughly chew or crush the chewable tablets before swallowing.
• Warn the patient to notify the physician if diarrhea, a rash, or other new symptoms occur.

amoxicillin/ clavulanate potassium
a-**mocks**-ih-sill-in/
klah-view-**lan**-ate
(Augmentin, Augmentin ES 600, Augmentin XR, Ausclav[AUS], Ausclav Duo Forte[AUS], Ausclav Duo 400[AUS], Clamoxyl[AUS], Clamoxyl Duo Forte[AUS], Clavulin[CAN], Clavulin Duo Forte[AUS])

CATEGORY AND SCHEDULE
Pregnancy Risk Category: B

MECHANISM OF ACTION
An antibiotic, amoxicillin is bactericidal in susceptible microorganisms while clavulanate inhibits bacterial beta-lactamase. *Therapeutic Effect:* Amoxicillin inhibits cell wall synthesis. Clavulanate protects amoxicillin from enzymatic degradation.

PHARMACOKINETICS
Well absorbed from the gastrointestinal (GI) tract. Protein binding: 20%. Partially metabolized in liver. Primarily excreted in urine. Removed by hemodialysis. **Half-life**: 1–1.3 hrs (half-life increased in reduced renal function).

AVAILABILITY
Tablets (chewable): 125 mg, 200 mg, 250 mg, 400 mg.
Tablets: 250 mg, 500 mg, 875 mg, 1000 mg.
Powder for PO Suspension: 125 mg/5 ml, 200 mg/5 ml, 250 mg/ 5 ml, 400 mg/5 ml, 600 mg/5 ml.

INDICATIONS AND DOSAGES
▸ **Mild to moderate infections**
PO
Adults, Elderly, Children weighing more than 40 kg. 250 mg q8h or 500 mg q12h.
Children weighing less than 40 kg. 20 mg/kg/day in divided doses q8h.
▸ **Respiratory tract infections, severe infections**
PO
Adults, Elderly, Children weighing more than 40 kg. 500 mg q8h or 875 mg q12h.
Children weighing less than 40 kg. 40 mg/kg/day in divided doses q8h.
▸ **Otitis media**
PO
Children. 90 mg/kg/day in divided doses q12h for 10 days.
▸ **Sinusitis, lower respiratory tract infections**
PO
Children. 40 mg/kg/day in divided doses q8h or 45 mg/kg/day in divided doses q12h.
▸ **Usual neonate dosage**
PO
Neonates, Children younger than 3 mos. 30 mg/kg/day in divided doses q12h.
▸ **Dosage in renal impairment**
Creatinine clearance 10–30 ml/min: 250–500 mg q12h.

Creatinine clearance less than 10 ml/min: 250–500 mg q24h.

UNLABELED USES
Treatment of bronchitis and chancroid

CONTRAINDICATIONS
Hypersensitivity to any penicillins, infectious mononucleosis

INTERACTIONS
Drug
Allopurinol: May increase incidence of rash.
Oral contraceptives: May decrease effects of oral contraceptives.
Probenecid: May increase amoxicillin and clavulanate blood concentration and risk of toxicity.
Herbal
None known.
Food
None known.

DIAGNOSTIC TEST EFFECTS
May increase SGOT (AST) and SGPT (ALT) levels. May cause positive Coombs' test.

SIDE EFFECTS
Frequent
GI disturbances (mild diarrhea, nausea, vomiting), headache, oral or vaginal candidiasis
Occasional
Generalized rash, urticaria

SERIOUS REACTIONS
• Altered bacterial balance may result in potentially fatal superinfections and antibiotic-associated colitis, as evidenced by abdominal cramps, watery or severe diarrhea, and fever.
• Severe hypersensitivity reactions, including anaphylaxis and acute interstitial nephritis occur rarely.

NURSING CONSIDERATIONS
Baseline Assessment
◀ALERT▶ Determine the patient's history of allergies, especially to cephalosporins and penicillins before you give the drug.
Lifespan Considerations
• Be aware that amoxicillin/clavulanate crosses the placenta, appears in cord blood and amniotic fluid, and is distributed in breast milk in low concentrations.
• Be aware that amoxicillin/clavulanate may lead to allergic sensitization, candidiasis, diarrhea, and skin rash in infants.
• Be aware that immature renal function in neonates and young infants may delay renal excretion of amoxicillin/clavulanate.
• In the elderly, age-related renal impairment may require dosage adjustment.
Precautions
• Use cautiously in patients with antibiotic-associated colitis or a history of allergies, especially to cephalosporins.
Administration and Handling
◀ALERT▶ Drug dosage is expressed in terms of amoxicillin. Be aware that an alternative dosing for adults is 500 to 875 mg 2 times/day and for children, 200 to 400 mg 2 times/day.
PO
• Store tablets at room temperature.
• After reconstitution, oral solution is stable for 14 days whether at room temperature or refrigerated.
• Give without regard to meals.
• Instruct the patient to chew or crush chewable tablets thoroughly before swallowing.
Intervention and Evaluation
• Withhold amoxicillin and promptly notify the physician if the patient experiences a rash or diar-

rhea. Immediately notify the physician if the patient develops severe diarrhea with abdominal pain, blood or mucus in stool, and fever. These symptoms may indicate antibiotic-associated colitis.
• Be alert for signs and symptoms of superinfection, including anal or genital pruritus, black hairy tongue, diarrhea, increased fever, sore throat, ulceration or changes of oral mucosa, and vomiting.

Patient Teaching
• Advise the patient to continue taking the antibiotic for the full length of treatment and to evenly space drug doses around the clock.
• Instruct the patient to take the drug with meals if gastrointestinal (GI) upset occurs.
• Stress that the patient should thoroughly chew or crush the chewable tablets before swallowing.
• Warn the patient to notify the physician if diarrhea, rash, or other new symptoms occur.

ampicillin sodium

amp-ih-**sill**-in
(Alphacin[AUS], Apo-Ampi[CAN], Novo-Ampicillin[CAN], Nu-Ampi[CAN], Polycillin)
Do not confuse with aminophylline, Imipenem, or Unipen.

CATEGORY AND SCHEDULE

Pregnancy Risk Category: B

MECHANISM OF ACTION

A penicillin that inhibits cell wall synthesis in susceptible microorganisms. *Therapeutic Effect:* Produces bactericidal effect.

PHARMACOKINETICS

Moderately absorbed from the gastrointestinal (GI) tract. Protein binding: 28%. Widely distributed. Partially metabolized in liver. Primarily excreted in urine. Removed by hemodialysis. **Half-life:** 1–1.5 hrs (half-life increased in impaired renal function).

AVAILABILITY

Capsules: 250 mg, 500 mg.
Powder for PO Suspension: 125 mg/5 ml, 250 mg/5 ml, 500 mg/5 ml.
Powder for Injection: 125 mg, 250 mg, 500 mg, 1 g, 2 g.

INDICATIONS AND DOSAGES

▸ **Respiratory tract, skin/skin-structure infections**
PO
Adults, Elderly, Children weighing more than 20 kg. 250–500 mg q6h.
Children weighing less than 20 kg. 50 mg/kg/day in divided doses q6h.
IM/IV
Adults, Elderly, Children weighing more than 40 kg. 250–500 mg q6h.
Children weighing less than 40 kg. 25–50 mg/kg/day in divided doses q6–8h.
▸ **Bacterial meningitis, septicemia**
IM/IV
Adults, Elderly. 2 g q4h or 3 g q6h.
Children. 100–200 mg/kg/day in divided doses q4h.
▸ **Gonococcal infections**
PO
Adults. 3.5 g one time with 1 g probenecid.
▸ **Perioperative prophylaxis**
IM/IV
Adults, Elderly. 2 g 30 min before procedure. May repeat in 8 hrs.
Children. 50 mg/kg using same dosage regimen.

▸ **Usual neonate dosage**
IM/IV
Neonates 7–28 days old. 75 mg/kg/day in divided doses q8h up to 200 mg/kg/day in divided doses q6h.
Neonates 0–7 days old. 50 mg/kg/day in divided doses q12h up to 150 mg/kg/day in divided doses q8h.

CONTRAINDICATIONS
Hypersensitivity to any penicillin, infectious mononucleosis

INTERACTIONS
Drug
Allopurinol: May increase incidence of rash.
Oral contraceptives: May decrease effectiveness of oral contraceptives.
Probenecid: May increase ampicillin blood concentration and risk of ampicillin toxicity.
Herbal
None known.
Food
None known.

DIAGNOSTIC TEST EFFECTS
May increase SGOT (AST) and SGPT (ALT) levels. May cause positive Coombs' test.

IV INCOMPATIBILITIES
Amikacin (Amikin), gentamicin, diltiazem (Cardizem), midazolam (Versed)

IV COMPATIBILITIES
Calcium gluconate, cefepime (Maxipime), dopamine (Inotropin), famotidine (Pepcid), furosemide (Lasix), heparin, hydromorphone (Dilaudid), insulin (regular), levofloxacin (Levaquin), magnesium sulfate, morphine, multivitamins, potassium chloride, propofol (Diprivan)

SIDE EFFECTS
Frequent
Pain at IM injection site, GI disturbances, including mild diarrhea, nausea, or vomiting, oral or vaginal candidiasis
Occasional
Generalized rash, urticaria, phlebitis, thrombophlebitis with IV administration, headache
Rare
Dizziness, seizures, especially with IV therapy

SERIOUS REACTIONS
• Altered bacterial balance may result in potentially fatal superinfections and antibiotic-associated colitis as evidenced by abdominal cramps, watery or severe diarrhea, and fever.
• Severe hypersensitivity reactions, including anaphylaxis and acute interstitial nephritis occur rarely.

NURSING CONSIDERATIONS
Baseline Assessment
◀ALERT▶ Determine the patient's history of allergies, especially to cephalosporins and penicillins, before you give the drug.
Lifespan Considerations
• Be aware that ampicillin readily crosses the placenta, appears in cord blood and amniotic fluid, and is distributed in breast milk in low concentrations.
• Ampicillin may lead to allergic sensitization, candidiasis, diarrhea, and skin rash in infants.
• Immature renal function in neonates and young infants may delay renal excretion of ampicillin.
◀ALERT▶ Keep in mind that higher dosages may be needed for neonatal meningitis.
• In the elderly, age-related renal

impairment may require dosage adjustment.

Precautions

• Use cautiously in patients with antibiotic-associated colitis or a history of allergies, particularly to cephalosporins.

Administration and Handling

PO

• Store capsules at room temperature.

• Oral suspension, after reconstituted, is stable for 7 days at room temperature, 14 days if refrigerated.

• Give orally 1 hour before or 2 hours after meals for maximum absorption.

IM

• Reconstitute each vial with Sterile Water for Injection or Bacteriostatic Water for Injection. Consult individual ampicillin vials for specific volumes of diluent. Reconstituted solution is stable for 1 hour.

• Give injection deeply in a large muscle mass.

IV

• An IV solution, diluted with 0.9% NaCl, is stable for 2 to 8 hours at room temperature or 3 days if refrigerated.

• An IV solution diluted with D_5W is stable for 2 hours at room temperature or 3 hours if refrigerated.

• Discard the IV solution if a precipitate forms.

• For IV injection, dilute each vial with 5 ml Sterile Water for Injection or 10 ml for 1- and 2-g vials.

• For intermittent IV infusion or piggyback, further dilute with 50 to 100 ml 0.9% NaCl or D_5W.

• For IV injection, give over 3 to 5 minutes or 10 to 15 minutes for a 1- to 2-g dose.

• For intermittent IV infusion or piggyback, infuse over 20 to 30 minutes.

• Because of the potential for hypersensitivity and anaphylaxis, start the initial dose at a few drops per minute, increase the dosage slowly to the prescribed rate; and stay with the patient for the first 10 to 15 minutes. Then assess the patient every 10 minutes for signs and symptoms of hypersensitivity or anaphylaxis.

• Expect to switch to the oral route as soon as possible.

Intervention and Evaluation

• Withhold ampicillin and promptly notify the physician if the patient experiences a rash or diarrhea. Although a rash is common with ampicillin, it also may indicate hypersensitivity. Severe diarrhea with abdominal pain, blood or mucus in stools, and fever may indicate antibiotic-associated colitis.

• Evaluate the IV site for phlebitis as evidenced by heat, pain, and red streaking over the vein.

• Check the IM injection site for pain and swelling.

• Monitor the patient's intake and output, renal function tests, and urinalysis results.

• Assess the patient for signs and symptoms of superinfection such as anal or genital pruritus, black hairy tongue, oral ulcerations or pain, diarrhea, increased fever, sore throat, and vomiting.

Patient Teaching

• Advise the patient to take the antibiotic for the full length of treatment and to evenly space doses around the clock.

• Explain that the antibiotic is more effective if taken 1 hour before or 2 hours after the patient consumes food or beverages.

• Instruct the patient that discomfort may occur with IM injection.

• Warn the patient to notify the physician if diarrhea, rash, or other new symptoms occur.

ampicillin/sulbactam sodium
amp-ih-**sill**-in/sull-**bak**-tam
(Unasyn)

CATEGORY AND SCHEDULE
Pregnancy Risk Category: B

MECHANISM OF ACTION
A penicillin that is bactericidal in susceptible microorganisms and inhibits bacterial beta-lactamase. *Therapeutic Effect:* Ampicillin inhibits cell wall synthesis. Sulbactam protects ampicillin from enzymatic degradation.

PHARMACOKINETICS
Protein binding: 28%–38%. Widely distributed. Partially metabolized in liver. Primarily excreted in urine. Removed by hemodialysis. **Half-life:** 1 hr (half-life increased in impaired renal function).

AVAILABILITY
Powder for Injection: 1.5 g, 3 g.

INDICATIONS AND DOSAGES
▸ **Skin/skin-structure, intra-abdominal, gynecologic infections**
IM/IV
Adults, Elderly. 1.5 g (1 g ampicillin/500 mg sulbactam) to 3 g (2 g ampicillin/1 g sulbactam) q6h.
▸ **Skin/skin-structure infections**
IV
Children 1–12 yrs. 150–300 mg/kg/day in divided doses q6h.
▸ **Dosage in renal impairment**
Modifications of dosage and frequency are based on creatinine clearance and the severity of infection.

Creatinine Clearance	Dosage
greater than 30 ml/min	0.5–3 g q6–8h
15–29 ml/min	1.5–3 g q12h
5–14 ml/min	1.5–3 g q24h
less than 5 ml/min	Not recommended

CONTRAINDICATIONS
Hypersensitivity to any penicillin, infectious mononucleosis

INTERACTIONS
Drug
Allopurinol: May increase incidence of rash.
Oral contraceptives: May decrease effectiveness of oral contraceptives.
Probenecid: May increase ampicillin blood concentration and risk of ampicillin toxicity.
Herbal
None known.
Food
None known.

DIAGNOSTIC TEST EFFECTS
May increase serum LDH, alkaline phosphatase, and creatinine and SGOT (AST) and SGPT (ALT) levels. May cause positive Coombs' test.

IV INCOMPATIBILITIES
Diltiazem (Cardizem), idarubicin (Idamycin), ondansetron (Zofran), sargramostim (Leukine)

IV COMPATIBILITIES
Famotidine (Pepcid), heparin, insulin (regular), morphine

SIDE EFFECTS
Frequent
Diarrhea and rash (most common),

urticaria, pain at IM injection site; thrombophlebitis with IV administration; oral or vaginal candidiasis
Occasional
Nausea, vomiting, headache, malaise, urinary retention

SERIOUS REACTIONS
• Severe hypersensitivity reactions, including anaphylaxis, acute interstitial nephritis, and blood dyscrasias may be noted.
• Altered bacterial balance may result in potentially fatal superinfections and antibiotic-associated colitis as evidenced by abdominal cramps, watery or severe diarrhea, and fever.
• Overdose may produce seizures.

NURSING CONSIDERATIONS
Baseline Assessment
• Determine the patient's history of allergies, especially to cephalosporins and penicillins before you give the drug.
Lifespan Considerations
• Be aware that ampicillin readily crosses the placenta, appears in cord blood and amniotic fluid, and is distributed in breast milk in low concentrations.
• Be aware that ampicillin may lead to allergic sensitization, candidiasis, diarrhea, and skin rash in infants.
• Be aware that the safety and efficacy of ampicillin have not been established in children younger than 1 year.
• In the elderly, age-related renal impairment may require dosage adjustment.
Precautions
• Use cautiously in patients with antibiotic-associated colitis or a history of allergies, particularly to cephalosporins.

Administration and Handling
IM
• Reconstitute each 1.5-g vial with 3.2 ml Sterile Water for Injection to provide concentration of 250 mg ampicillin/125 mg sulbactam/ml.
• Give injection deeply into a large muscle mass within 1 hour of preparation.
IV
• When reconstituted with 0.9% NaCl, IV solution is stable for 8 hours at room temperature or 48 hours if refrigerated. Stability may be different with other diluents.
• Discard IV solution if precipitate forms.
• For IV injection, dilute with 10 to 20 ml Sterile Water for Injection.
• For intermittent IV infusion or piggyback, further dilute with 50 to 100 ml D_5W or 0.9% NaCl.
• For IV injection, give slowly over minimum of 10 to 15 minutes.
• For intermittent IV infusion or piggyback, infuse over 15 to 30 minutes.
• Due to the potential for hypersensitivity and anaphylaxis, start the initial dose at a few drops per minute, the increase the dose slowly to the ordered rate. Stay with the patient for the first 10 to 15 minutes and assess for signs and symptoms of hypersensitivity or anaphylaxis, and then check the patient every 10 minutes during the infusion.
• Expect to switch to a PO antibiotic as soon as possible.
Intervention and Evaluation
• Withhold ampicillin and promptly notify the physician if the patient experiences a rash or diarrhea. Although a rash is common with ampicillin, it also may indicate hypersensitivity. Severe diarrhea with abdominal pain, blood or

mucus in stools, and fever may indicate antibiotic-associated colitis.
• Evaluate the IV site for phlebitis as evidenced by heat, pain, and red streaking over vein.
• Check the IM injection site for pain and swelling.
• Monitor the patient's intake and output, renal function test results, and urinalysis results.
• Assess the patient for signs and symptoms of superinfection such as anal or genital pruritus, black hairy tongue, changes in oral mucosa, diarrhea, increased fever, onset of sore throat, and vomiting.

Patient Teaching
• Advise the patient to take the antibiotic for the full length of therapy and to evenly space drug doses around the clock.
• Instruct the patient that discomfort may occur at the IM injection site.
• Warn the patient to notify the physician if diarrhea, rash, or other new symptoms occur.

oxacillin
ox-ah-**sill**-inn

CATEGORY AND SCHEDULE
Pregnancy Risk Category: B

MECHANISM OF ACTION
A penicillin that binds to bacterial membranes. *Therapeutic Effect:* Inhibits bacterial cell wall synthesis. Bactericidal.

AVAILABILITY
Powder for Injection: 1 g vials, 2 g vials.

INDICATIONS AND DOSAGES
▸ **Upper respiratory tract, skin/skin-structure infections**

IM/IV
Adults, Elderly, Children weighing more than 40 kg. 250–500 mg q4–6h.
Children weighing less than 40 kg. 50 mg/kg/day in divided doses q6h. Maximum: 12 g/day.
▸ **Lower respiratory tract, serious infections**

IM/IV
Adults, Elderly, Children weighing more than 40 kg. 1 g q4–6h. Maximum: 12 g/day.
Children weighing less than 40 kg. 100 mg/kg/day in divided doses q4–6h.

CONTRAINDICATIONS
Hypersensitivity to penicillin

INTERACTIONS
Drug
Probenecid: May increase oxacillin blood concentration and risk of toxicity.
Herbal
None known.
Food
None known.

DIAGNOSTIC TEST EFFECTS
May increase SGOT(AST) levels. May cause positive Coomb's test.

SIDE EFFECTS
Frequent
Mild hypersensitivity reaction including fever, rash, and pruritus, gastrointestinal (GI) effects including nausea, vomiting, and diarrhea
Occasional
Phlebitis, thrombophlebitis that's more common in elderly, liver toxicity with high IV oxacillin dosage

SERIOUS REACTIONS
• Superinfections and antibiotic-associated colitis may result from

altered bacteria balance and hypersensitivity reaction ranging from mild to severe may occur in those allergic to penicillin.

Baseline Assessment
• Determine if the patient has a history of allergies, especially to cephalosporins and penicillin.

Precautions
• Use cautiously in patients with a history of allergies, especially to cephalosporins, and with impaired renal function.

Administration and Handling
IV
• Store at room temperature.
• Once reconstituted, vials stable for 3 days at room temperature or 7 days refrigerated.
• Remember that the solution is stable for 24 hours when further diluted with D5W or NaCl.
• To each 1 g vial, add 10 ml sterile water for injection to provide concentration of 100 mg/ml.
• For piggyback administration, further dilute with 50 to 100 mg D5W or 0.9% NaCl.
• Administer IV push over 10 minutes; IV piggyback over 30 minutes.

Intervention and Evaluation
• Withhold the medication, as prescribed, and promptly report if the patient experiences diarrhea with abdominal pain, blood or mucus in stool, and fever or rash.
• Evaluate the patient's IV site frequently for phlebitis as evidenced by heat, pain, and red streaking over the vein.
• Monitor the patient's intake and output, renal function, and urinalysis.
• Be alert for patient development of anal or genital pruritus, black or hairy tongue, diarrhea, changes or ulcerations of the oral mucosa, signs and symptoms of superinfection, and vomiting.

Patient Teaching
• Tell the patient to immediately report burning or pain at the IV site
• Tell the patient to immediately report shortness of breath, chest tightness, or hives, signs of an allergic reaction.
• Encourage the patient to use good oral hygiene.

penicillin G benzathine
pen-ih-**sil**-lin G **benz**-ah-thene
(Bicillin LA, Permapen)

CATEGORY AND SCHEDULE
Pregnancy Risk Category: B

MECHANISM OF ACTION
A penicillin that binds to one or more of the penicillin-binding proteins of bacteria. *Therapeutic Effect:* Inhibits bacterial cell wall synthesis. Bactericidal.

AVAILABILITY
Injection (prefilled syringe): 600,000 units/ml.

INDICATIONS AND DOSAGES
▸ **Group A streptococcal infection**
IM
Adults, Elderly. 1.2 million units as a single dose.
Children. 25,000–50,000 units/kg as a single dose.
▸ **Prophylaxis for rheumatic fever**
IM
Adults, Elderly. 1.2 million units q3–4 wks or 600,000 units 2 times/mo.

Children. 25,000–50,000 units/kg
q3–4 wks.
▶ **Early syphilis**
IM
Adults, Elderly. 2.4 million
units as a single dose in 2 in-
jection sites.
▶ **Congenital syphilis**
IM
Children. 50,000 units/kg qwk
for 3 wks.
▶ **Syphilis greater than 1 yrs'
duration**
IM
Adults, Elderly. 2.4 million units as
a single dose in 2 injection sites
qwk for 3 doses.
Children. 50,000 units/kg qwk
for 3 doses.

CONTRAINDICATIONS
Hypersensitivity to any penicillin

INTERACTIONS
Drug
Erythromycin: May antagonize
effects of penicillin.
Probenecid: Increases serum con-
centration of penicillin.
Herbal
None known.
Food
None known.

DIAGNOSTIC TEST EFFECTS
May cause positive Coombs' test.

SIDE EFFECTS
Occasional
Lethargy, fever, dizziness, rash, pain
at injection site
Rare
Seizures, interstitial nephritis

SERIOUS REACTIONS
• Hypersensitivity reactions ranging
from chills, fever, and rash to anaphylaxis occur.

NURSING CONSIDERATIONS
Baseline Assessment
• Determine the patient's history of
allergies, particularly to aspirin,
cephalosporins, and penicillins
before beginning drug therapy.
Precautions
• Use cautiously in patients with a
hypersensitivity to cephalosporins,
impaired cardiac or renal function,
and seizure disorders.
Administration and Handling
IM
• Store in refrigerator. Do not freeze.
• Administer undiluted by deep IM
injection in the upper outer quadrant
of buttock for adolescents and
adults and the midlateral muscle of
the thigh for infants and children.
◀**ALERT**▶ Do not give IV, intra-
arterially, or subcutaneously as giving penicillin G via these routes may
cause death, heart attack, severe neu-
rovascular damage, and thrombosis.
Intervention and Evaluation
• Monitor the patient's complete
blood count (CBC) renal function
test, and urinalysis results.
Patient Teaching
• Warn the patient to immediately
report if he or she experiences,
chills, fever, rash, or any other
unusual sign or symptom.
• Explain to the patient that he or
she may experience temporary pain
at the injection site.

penicillin G potassium
pen-ih-**sil**-lin G
(Megacillin[CAN], Novepen-
G[CAN], Pfizerpen)

CATEGORY AND SCHEDULE
Pregnancy Risk Category: B

MECHANISM OF ACTION
A penicillin that binds to one or more of the penicillin-binding proteins of bacteria. *Therapeutic Effect:* Inhibits bacterial cell wall synthesis. Bactericidal.

AVAILABILITY
Injection: 5 million units.
Premixed dextrose solution: 1 million units, 2 million units, 3 million units.

INDICATIONS AND DOSAGES
▶ **Treatment of sepsis, meningitis, pericarditis, endocarditis, pneumonia due to susceptible gram-positive organisms (not *Staphylococcus aureus*), some gram-negative organisms**
IM/IV
Adults, Elderly. 2–24 million units/day in divided doses q4–6h.
Children. 100,000–400,000 units/kg/day in divided doses q4–6h.
▶ **Dosage in renal impairment**

Creatinine Clearance	Dosage Interval
10–30 ml/min	q8–12h
less than 10 ml/min	q12–18h

CONTRAINDICATIONS
Hypersensitivity to any penicillin

INTERACTIONS
Drug
Erythromycin: May antagonize effects of penicillin.
Probenecid: Increases serum concentration of penicillin.
Herbal
None known.
Food
Food or milk decreases absorption.

DIAGNOSTIC TEST EFFECTS
May cause positive Coombs' test.

IV INCOMPATIBILITIES
Amikacin (Amikin), aminophylline, amphotericin, dopamine (Intropin)

IV COMPATIBILITIES
Amiodarone (Cordarone), calcium gluconate, diltiazem (Cardizem), diphenhydramine (Benadryl), furosemide (Lasix), heparin, hydromorphone (Dilaudid), lidocaine, magnesium sulfate, methylprednisolone (Solu-Medrol), morphine, potassium chloride

SIDE EFFECTS
Occasional
Lethargy, fever, dizziness, rash, electrolyte imbalance, diarrhea, thrombophlebitis
Rare
Seizures, interstitial nephritis

SERIOUS REACTIONS
• Hypersensitivity reactions ranging from rash, fever, and chills to anaphylaxis occur.

NURSING CONSIDERATIONS
Baseline Assessment
◀ALERT▶ Determine the patient's history of allergies, particularly to aspirin, cephalosporins, and penicillins before beginning drug therapy.
Precautions
• Use cautiously in patients with a hypersensitivity to cephalosporins, impaired liver or renal function, and seizure disorders.
Administration and Handling
IV
• Reconstituted solution is stable for 7 days if refrigerated.
• Follow dilution guide per manufacturer.
• After reconstitution, further dilute with 50 to 100 ml D_5W or 0.9%

NaCl for a final concentration of 100 to 500,000 units/ml (50,000 units/ml for infants and neonates).
• Infuse over 15 to 60 minutes.
Intervention and Evaluation
• Monitor the patient's complete blood count (CBC), electrolytes, renal function test, and urinalysis results.
Patient Teaching
• Advise the patient to continue to take the drug for the full course of treatment.
• Explain to the patient that drug doses should be spaced evenly.
• Warn the patient to immediately notify the physician if he or she experiences diarrhea, a rash, fever or chills, or any other unusual sign or symptoms.

penicillin V potassium
pen-ih-**sil**-lin V
(Abbocillin VK[AUS], Apo-Pen-VK[CAN], Cilicaine VK[AUS], L.P.V.[AUS], Novo-Pen-VK[CAN], Pen-Vee K, V-Cillin-K)

CATEGORY AND SCHEDULE
Pregnancy Risk Category: B

MECHANISM OF ACTION
A penicillin that binds to bacterial cell membranes. *Therapeutic Effect:* Inhibits cell wall synthesis. Bactericidal.

PHARMACOKINETICS
Moderately absorbed from the gastrointestinal (GI) tract. Protein binding: 80%. Widely distributed. Metabolized in liver. Primarily

excreted in urine. **Half-life:** 1 hr (half-life is increased in those with impaired renal function).

AVAILABILITY
Tablets: 250 mg, 500 mg.
Powder for Oral Solution: 125 mg/5 ml, 250 mg/5 ml.

INDICATIONS AND DOSAGES
▶ **Mild to moderate respiratory tract or skin or skin-structure infections; otitis media; or necrotizing ulcerative gingivitis**
PO
Adults, elderly, children 12 yrs and older. 125–500 mg q6–8h.
Children younger than 12 yrs. 25–50 mg/kg/day in divided doses q6–8h. Maximum: 3 g/day.
▶ **Primary prevention of rheumatic fever**
PO
Adults, Elderly. 500 mg 2–3 times/day for 10 days.
Children. 250 mg 2–3 times/day for 10 days.
▶ **Prophylaxis for recurrent rheumatic fever**
PO
Adults, Elderly, Children. 250 mg 2 times/day.

CONTRAINDICATIONS
Hypersensitivity to any penicillin

INTERACTIONS
Drug
Probenecid: May increase penicillin V blood concentration and risk of toxicity.
Herbal
None known.
Food
None known.

DIAGNOSTIC TEST EFFECTS
May cause positive Coombs' test.

SIDE EFFECTS
Frequent
Mild hypersensitivity reaction (chills, fever, rash), nausea, vomiting, diarrhea
Rare
Bleeding, allergic reaction

SERIOUS REACTIONS
• Severe hypersensitivity reaction, including anaphylaxis, may occur.
• Nephrotoxicity, antibiotic-associated colitis (severe abdominal pain and tenderness, fever, and watery and severe diarrhea), and other superinfections may result from high dosages or prolonged therapy.

NURSING CONSIDERATIONS
Baseline Assessment
◀ALERT▶ Determine the patient's history of allergies, particularly to aspirin, cephalosporins and penicillins before beginning drug therapy.
Lifespan Considerations
• Be aware that penicillin V readily crosses the placenta, appears in amniotic fluid and cord blood, and is distributed in breast milk in low concentrations.
• Be aware that penicillin V use may lead to allergic sensitization, candidiasis, diarrhea, and skin rash in infants.
• Use caution when giving penicillin V to neonates and young infants as these patients may have a delayed renal elimination of the drug.
• In the elderly, age-related renal impairment may require dosage adjustment.
Precautions
• Use cautiously in patients with a history of allergies, particularly to aspirin or cephalosporins, a history of seizures, and renal impairment.
Administration and Handling
PO
• Store tablets at room temperature. Oral solution, after reconstitution, is stable for 14 days if refrigerated.
• Space drug doses evenly around the clock.
• Give without regard to meals.
Intervention and Evaluation
• Withhold penicillin V potassium and promptly notify the physician if the patient experiences any diarrhea (with abdominal pain, fever, mucus and blood in stool may indicate antibiotic-associated colitis) or rash (may indicate hypersensitivity).
• Monitor the patient's intake and output, renal function tests, and urinalysis for signs of nephrotoxicity.
• Be alert for signs and symptoms of superinfection including anal or genital pruritus, diarrhea, increased fever, nausea, sore throat, ulceration or changes of oral mucosa, vaginal discharge, and vomiting.
• Review the patient's blood Hgb levels.
• Check the patient for signs of bleeding including bruising, overt bleeding, and swelling of tissue.
Patient Teaching
• Advise the patient to continue penicillin V potassium for the full length of treatment and to evenly space drug doses around the clock.
• Warn the patient to immediately notify the physician if he or she experiences bleeding, bruising, diarrhea, rash, or any other new symptom.

piperacillin sodium/ tazobactam sodium
pip-ur-ah-**sill**-in/tay-zoe-**back**-tam
(Tazocin[CAN], Zosyn)
Do not confuse with Zofran or Zyvox.

CATEGORY AND SCHEDULE
Pregnancy Risk Category: B

MECHANISM OF ACTION
A penicillin antibiotic. Piperacillin: Binds to bacterial cell membranes. *Therapeutic Effect:* Inhibits cell wall synthesis. Bactericidal. Tazobactam: Inactivates bacterial beta-lactamase enzymes. *Therapeutic Effect:* Protects piperacillin from inactivation by beta-lactamase–producing organisms, extends spectrum of activity, prevents bacterial overgrowth.

PHARMACOKINETICS
Protein binding: 16%–30%. Widely distributed. Primarily excreted unchanged in urine. Removed by hemodialysis. **Half-life:** 0.7–1.2 hrs (half-life is increased in those with hepatic cirrhosis, impaired renal function).

AVAILABILITY
Powder for Injection: 2.25 g, 3.375 g, 4.5 g.
Premix ready to use: 2.25 g, 3.375 g, 4.5 g.

INDICATIONS AND DOSAGES
▸ **Severe infections**
IV
Adults, Elderly, Children older than 12 yrs. 4g/0.5g q8h or 3 g/ 0.375g q6h. Maximum: 18g/2.25g a day.

▸ **Moderate infections**
IV
Adults, Elderly, Children older than 12 yrs. 2 g/0.225g q6–8h.
▸ **Dosage in renal impairment**
Dosage and frequency are based on creatinine clearance.

Creatinine Clearance	Dosage
20–40 ml/min	8 g/1 g/day (2.25 g q6h)
less than 20 ml/min	6 g/0.75 g/day (2.25 g q8h)

▸ **Hemodialysis**
IV
Adults, Elderly. 2.25 g q8h with additional dose of 0.75 g after each dialysis.

CONTRAINDICATIONS
Hypersensitivity to any penicillin

INTERACTIONS
Drug
Hepatotoxic medications: May increase the risk of liver toxicity. *Probenecid:* May increase piperacillin blood concentration and risk of toxicity.
Herbal
None known.
Food
None known.

DIAGNOSTIC TEST EFFECTS
May increase serum alkaline phosphatase, serum bilirubin, serum LDH, SGOT (AST), SGPT (ALT), and serum sodium levels. May cause positive Coombs' test. May decrease serum potassium.

IV INCOMPATIBILITIES
Amphotericin (Fungizone), amphotericin B complex (Abelcet, AmBisome, Amphotec), chlorpromazine (Thorazine), dacarbazine (DTIC),

daunorubicin (Cerubidine), dobutamine (Dobutrex), doxorubicin (Adriamycin), doxorubicin liposome (Doxil), droperidol (Inapsine), famotidine (Pepcid), haloperidol (Haldol), hydroxyzine (Vistaril), idarubicin (Idamycin), minocycline (Minocin), nalbuphine (Nubain), prochlorperazine (Compazine), promethazine (Phenergan), vancomycin (Vancocin)

IV COMPATIBILITIES

Aminophylline, bumetanide (Bumex), calcium gluconate, diphenhydramine (Benadryl), dopamine (Intropin), enalapril (Vasotec), furosemide (Lasix), granisetron (Kytril), heparin, hydrocortisone (Solu-Cortef), hydromorphone (Dilaudid), lorazepam (Ativan), magnesium sulfate, methylprednisolone (Solu-Medrol), metoclopramide (Reglan), morphine, ondansetron (Zofran), potassium chloride

SIDE EFFECTS

Frequent
Diarrhea, headache, constipation, nausea, insomnia, rash
Occasional
Vomiting, dyspepsia, pruritus, fever, agitation, pain, moniliasis, dizziness, abdominal pain, edema, anxiety, dyspnea, rhinitis

SERIOUS REACTIONS

• Antibiotic-associated colitis as evidenced by severe abdominal pain and tenderness, fever, and watery and severe diarrhea may result from altered bacterial balance.
• Overdosage, more often with renal impairment, may produce seizures and neurologic reactions.
• Severe hypersensitivity reactions, including anaphylaxis, occur rarely.

NURSING CONSIDERATIONS

Baseline Assessment
◀ALERT▶ Determine the patient's history of allergies, especially to cephalosporins and penicillins before beginning drug therapy.
Lifespan Considerations
• Be aware that piperacillin readily crosses the placenta, appears in amniotic fluid and cord blood, and is distributed in breast milk in low concentrations.
• Piperacillin use in infants may lead to allergic sensitization, candidiasis, diarrhea, and skin rash.
• Be aware that piperacillin dosage has not been established for children younger than 12 years of age.
• In the elderly, age-related renal impairment may require dosage adjustment.
Precautions
• Use cautiously in patients with a history of allergies, especially to cephalosporins, preexisting seizure disorder, and renal impairment.
Administration and Handling
IV
• Reconstituted vial is stable for 24 hours at room temperature or 48 hours if refrigerated.
• After further dilution, the solution is stable for 24 hours at room temperature or 7 days if refrigerated.
• Reconstitute each 1 g with 5 ml D_5W or 0.9% NaCl. Shake vigorously to dissolve.
• Further dilute with at least 50 ml D_5W, 0.9% NaCl, D_5W 0.9% NaCl, or lactated Ringer's.
• Infuse over 30 minutes.
Intervention and Evaluation
• Assess the patient's pattern of daily bowel activity and stool consistency. Mild gastrointestinal (GI) effects may be tolerable, but in-

creasing severity may indicate onset of antibiotic-associated colitis.
- Be alert for signs and symptoms of superinfection including abdominal pain, moderate to severe diarrhea, severe anal or genital pruritus, and severe mouth soreness.
- Monitor the patient's electrolytes, especially potassium, intake and output, renal function test, and urinalysis results.

Patient Teaching
- Advise the patient to immediately notify the physician if he or she experiences severe diarrhea and to avoid taking antidiarrheals until directed to do so by the physician.
- Warn patient to notify the physician if he or she experiences pain, redness, or swelling at his or her infusion site.
- Explain to the patient that piperacillin contains 1.85 mEq of sodium and that they should discuss a reduction in salt intake with the physician.

ticarcillin disodium/ clavulanate potassium
tie-car-**sill**-in/klah-view-**lan**-ate (Timentin)

CATEGORY AND SCHEDULE
Pregnancy Risk Category: B

MECHANISM OF ACTION
A penicillin antibiotic. Ticarcillin: Binds to bacterial cell wall, inhibiting bacterial cell wall synthesis. *Therapeutic Effect:* Causes cell lysis, death. Bactericidal. Clavulanate: Inhibits action of bacterial beta-lactamase. *Therapeutic Effect:* Protects ticarcillin from enzymatic degradation.

PHARMACOKINETICS
Widely distributed. Protein binding: Ticarcillin: 45%–60%. Clavulanate: 9%–30%. Minimal metabolism in liver. Primarily excreted unchanged in urine. Removed by hemodialysis. **Half-life:** 1–1.2 hrs (half-life is increased in those with impaired renal function).

AVAILABILITY
Powder for Injection: 3.1 g.
Solution for Infusion: 3.1 g/100 ml.

INDICATIONS AND DOSAGES
▶ **Septicemia; skin and skin-structure, bone, joint, and lower respiratory tract infections; and endometriosis**
IV
Adults, Elderly. 3.1 g (3 g ticarcillin) q4–6h. Maximum: 18–24 g/day.
Children older than 3 mos. 200–300 mg (as ticarcillin) q4–6h.
▶ **Urinary tract infection (UTI)**
IV
Adults, Elderly. 3.1 g q6–8h.
▶ **Dosage in renal impairment**

Creatinine Clearance	Dosage Interval
10–30 ml/min	q8h
less than 10 ml/min	q12h

CONTRAINDICATIONS
Hypersensitivity to any penicillin

INTERACTIONS
Drug
Anticoagulants, heparin, NSAIDs, thrombolytics: May increase the risk of hemorrhage with high dosages of ticarcillin.
Probenecid: May increase ticarcillin blood concentration and risk of toxicity.
Herbal
None known.

Food
None known.

DIAGNOSTIC TEST EFFECTS
May cause positive Coombs' test. May increase bleeding time, serum alkaline phosphatase, serum bilirubin, serum creatinine, serum LDH, SGOT (AST), and SGPT (ALT) levels. May decrease serum potassium, sodium, and uric acid levels.

IV INCOMPATIBILITIES
Amphotericin B complex (Abelcet, AmBisome, Amphotec), vancomycin (Vancocin)

IV COMPATIBILITIES
Diltiazem (Cardizem), heparin, insulin, morphine, propofol (Diprivan)

SIDE EFFECTS
Frequent
Phlebitis, thrombophlebitis with IV dose, rash, urticaria, pruritus, smell or taste disturbances
Occasional
Nausea, diarrhea, vomiting
Rare
Headache, fatigue, hallucinations, bleeding or bruising

SERIOUS REACTIONS
• Overdosage may produce seizures and neurologic reactions.
• Superinfections, including potentially fatal antibiotic-associated colitis, may result from bacterial imbalance.
• Severe hypersensitivity reactions, including anaphylaxis, occur rarely.

NURSING CONSIDERATIONS

Baseline Assessment
◄ **ALERT** ► Determine the patient's history of allergies, especially to cephalosporins and penicillins before beginning drug therapy.

Lifespan Considerations
• Be aware that ticarcillin readily crosses the placenta, appears in amniotic fluid and cord blood, and is distributed in breast milk in low concentrations.
• Ticarcillin use in infants may lead to allergic sensitization, candidiasis, diarrhea, and skin rash.
• Be aware that the safety and efficacy of this drug have not been established in children younger than 3 months.
• In the elderly, age-related renal impairment may require dosage adjustment.

Precautions
• Use cautiously in patients with a history of allergies, especially to cephalosporins, and renal impairment.

Administration and Handling
IV
• Solution normally appears colorless to pale yellow (if solution darkens, this indicates loss of potency).
• Reconstituted IV infusion (piggyback) is stable for 24 hours at room temperature, 3 days if refrigerated.
• Discard if precipitate forms.
• Available in ready-to-use containers.
• For IV infusion (piggyback), reconstitute each 3.1-g vial with 13 ml Sterile Water for Injection or 0.9% NaCl to provide concentration of 200 mg ticarcillin and 6.7 mg clavulanic acid per ml.
• Shake vial to assist reconstitution.
• Further dilute with 50 to 100 ml D_5W or 0.9% NaCl.
• Infuse over 30 minutes.
• Because of the potential for hypersensitivity reactions such as anaphylaxis, start initial dose at a few drops per minute, increase

slowly to ordered rate; monitor the patient the first 10 to 15 minutes, then check the patient every 10 minutes.

Intervention and Evaluation
• Withhold the drug and promptly notify the physician of the patient experiences diarrhea (with fever, abdominal pain, mucus and blood in stool may indicate antibiotic-associated colitis) or rash (hypersensitivity).
• Assess the patient's food tolerance.
• Provide the patient with mouth care, sugarless gum or hard candy to offset the drug's taste and smell effects.
• Evaluate the patient's IV site for signs and symptoms of phlebitis as evidenced by heat, pain, and red streaking over the vein.
• Monitor the patient's intake and output, renal function tests, and urinalysis results.
• Assess the patient for signs and symptoms of bruising or tissue swelling and overt bleeding.
• Monitor the patient's hematology reports and serum electrolytes, particularly potassium.
• Be alert for signs and symptoms of superinfection including anal or genital pruritus, diarrhea, increased fever, sore throat, ulceration or other oral changes, and vomiting.

Patient Teaching
• Advise the patient to immediately notify the physician if he or she experiences pain, redness, or swelling at the infusion site.
• Warn the patient to immediately notify the physician if he or she experiences severe diarrhea, a rash or itching, or any other unusual sign or symptom.

10 Quinolones

ciprofloxacin
hydrochloride
gatifloxacin
gemifloxacin mesylate
levofloxacin
lomefloxacin
hydrochloride
moxifloxacin
hydrochloride
norfloxacin
ofloxacin

Uses: Quinolones are used primarily to treat lower respiratory infections, skin and skin structure infections, urinary tract infections (UTIs), and sexually transmitted diseases.

Action: Quinolones are bactericidal and act against a wide range of gram-negative and gram-positive organisms. In susceptible microorganisms, they inhibit deoxyribonucleic acid (DNA) gyrase, the enzyme responsible for unwinding and supercoiling DNA before it replicates. By inhibiting DNA gyrase, quinolones interfere with bacterial cell replication and repair and cause cell death. (See illustration, *Sites and Mechanisms of Action: Anti-infective Agents,* page 2.)

COMBINATION PRODUCTS
CIPRODEX OTIC: ciprofloxacin/
dexamethasone (a steroid)
0.3%/0.1%.
CIPRO HC OTIC: ciprofloxacin/
hydrocortisone (a steroid)
0.2%/1%.

ciprofloxacin
hydrochloride
sip-row-**flocks**-ah-sin
(C-Flox[AUS], Ciloquin[AUS],
Ciloxan, Cipro, Ciproxin[AUS])
**Do not confuse with cinoxacin
or Cytoxan.**

CATEGORY AND SCHEDULE
Pregnancy Risk Category: C

MECHANISM OF ACTION
A fluoroquinolone that inhibits DNA enzyme in susceptible bacteria. *Therapeutic Effect:* Interferes with bacterial DNA replication. Bactericidal.

PHARMACOKINETICS
Well absorbed from the gastrointestinal (GI) tract (absorption is delayed by food). Protein binding: 20%–40%. Widely distributed (including cerebrospinal fluid [CSF]). Metabolized in liver to active metabolite. Primarily excreted in urine. Minimal removal by hemodialysis. **Half-life:** 4–6 hrs (half-life is increased with impaired renal function, elderly).

AVAILABILITY
Tablets: 100 mg, 250 mg, 500 mg, 750 mg.
Tablets (extended-release): 500 mg.
Oral Suspension. 50 mg/ml, 100 mg/ml.
Injection: 200 mg, 400 mg.
Ophthalmic Solution: 0.03%.
Ophthalmic Ointment: 0.3%.

INDICATIONS AND DOSAGES
▶ **Mild to moderate urinary tract infections**
PO
Adults, Elderly. 250 mg q12h.

IV
Adults, Elderly. 200 mg q12h.
▸ **Complicated urinary tract infections, mild to moderate respiratory tract infections, bone and joint infections, skin and skin-structure infections; infectious diarrhea**
PO
Adults, Elderly. 500 mg q12h.
IV
Adults, Elderly. 400 mg q12h.
▸ **Severe, complicated infections**
PO
Adults, Elderly. 750 mg q12h.
IV
Adults, Elderly. 400 mg q12h.
▸ **Prostatitis**
PO
Adults, Elderly. 500 mg q12h for 28 days.
▸ **Uncomplicated bladder infection**
PO
Adults. 100 mg 2 times/day for 3 days.
▸ **Acute sinusitis**
PO
Adults. 500 mg q12h.
▸ **Uncomplicated gonorrhea**
PO
Adults. 250 mg as a single dose.
▸ **Usual pediatric dosage**
PO
Children. 20–30 mg/kg/day in 2 divided doses. Maximum: 1.5 g/day.
IV
Children. 20–30 mg/kg/day in 2 divided doses q12h. Maximum: 800 mg/day.
▸ **Corneal ulcer**
Ophthalmic
Adults, Elderly. 2 drops q15min for 6 hrs, then 2 drops q30min for the remainder of first day; 2 drops q1h for second day; then 2 drops q4h days 3–14.
▸ **Conjunctivitis**
Ophthalmic
Adults, Elderly. 1–2 drops q2h

for 2 days, then 2 drops q4h next 5 days.
▸ **Dosage in renal impairment**
The dosage and frequency are modified in patients based on the severity of infection and the degree of renal impairment.

Creatinine Clearance	Dosage Interval
less than 30 ml/min	q18–24h

Hemodialysis, peritoneal dialysis 250–500 mg q24h (after dialysis).

UNLABELED USES
Treatment of chancroid

CONTRAINDICATIONS
Hypersensitivity to ciprofloxacin, quinolones
Ophthalmic: Vaccinia, varicella, epithelial herpes simplex, keratitis, mycobacterial infection, fungal disease of ocular structure. Not for use after uncomplicated removal of foreign body.

INTERACTIONS
Drug
Antacids, iron preparations, sucralfate: May decrease ciprofloxacin absorption.
Oral anticoagulants: May increase the effects of oral anticoagulants.
Theophylline: Decreases clearance, and may increase blood concentration and risk of toxicity of this drug.
Herbal
None known.
Food
None known.

DIAGNOSTIC TEST EFFECTS
May increase BUN, serum alkaline phosphatase, serum bilirubin, serum creatinine, LDH, SGOT (AST), and SGPT (ALT) levels.

IV INCOMPATIBILITIES

Aminophylline, ampicillin/
sulbactam (Unasyn), cefepime
(Maxipime), dexamethasone
(Decadron), furosemide (Lasix),
heparin, hydrocortisone (Solu-
Cortef), methylprednisolone (Solu-
Medrol), phenytoin (Dilantin),
sodium bicarbonate

IV COMPATIBILITIES

Calcium gluconate, diltiazem
(Cardizem), dobutamine (Dobutrex),
dopamine (Intropin), lidocaine,
lorazepam (Ativan), magnesium,
midazolam (Versed), potassium
chloride

SIDE EFFECTS

Frequent (5%–2%)
Nausea, diarrhea, dyspepsia,
vomiting, constipation, flatulence,
confusion, crystalluria
Ophthalmic: Burning, crusting in
corner of eye
Occasional (less than 2%)
Abdominal pain or discomfort,
headache, rash
Ophthalmic: Bad taste, sense of
something in eye, redness of eyelids, eyelid itching
Rare (less than 1%)
Dizziness, confusion, tremors,
hallucinations, hypersensitivity
reaction, insomnia, dry mouth,
paresthesia

SERIOUS REACTIONS

• Superinfection (especially entero-
coccal, fungal), nephropathy, cardiopulmonary arrest, and cerebral
thrombosis may occur.
• Arthropathy may occur if the drug
is given to children younger than
18 yrs.
• Sensitization to the ophthalmic
form of the drug may contraindicate
later systemic use of ciprofloxacin.

NURSING CONSIDERATIONS

Baseline Assessment
◀ ALERT ▶ Determine the patient's
history of hypersensitivity to ciprofloxacin and quinolones before
beginning drug therapy.
Lifespan Considerations
• Be aware that it is unknown if
ciprofloxacin is distributed in breast
milk. If possible, do not use during
pregnancy or breast-feeding because
of the risk of arthropathy to the
fetus or infant.
• The safety and efficacy of ciprofloxacin have not been established
in children younger than 18 years
of age.
• In the elderly, age-related renal
impairment may require dosage
adjustment.
Precautions
• Use cautiously in patients with
central nervous system (CNS)
disorders, renal impairment, and
seizures, and those taking caffeine
or theophylline.
• Do not use the suspension in a
nasogastric (NG) tube.
Administration and Handling
PO
• May be given without regard
to meals (preferred dosing time:
2 hours after meals).
• Do not administer antacids (aluminum, magnesium) within 2 hours of
ciprofloxacin.
• Provide the patient with sufficient
amounts of citrus fruits and cranberry juice to acidify urine.
• Suspension may be stored for
14 days at room temperature.
IV
• Store at room temperature.
• Solution normally appears clear,
colorless to slightly yellow.
• Available prediluted in infusion
container ready for use.
• Infuse over 60 minutes.

Ophthalmic
• Tilt the patient's head back and place the solution in the conjunctival sac of the affected eye.
• Have the patient close his or her eye, then press gently on the lacrimal sac for 1 minute.
• Do not use ophthalmic solutions for injection.
• Unless the infection is very superficial, systemic administration generally accompanies ophthalmic use.

Intervention and Evaluation
• Evaluate the patient's food tolerance.
• Assess the patient's pattern of daily bowel activity and stool consistency.
• Evaluate the patient for dizziness, headache, tremors, and visual difficulties.
• Assess the patient for chest and joint pain.
• Observe patients receiving the ophthalmic form for therapeutic response.

Patient Teaching
• Advise the patient not to skip drug doses and to take ciprofloxacin for the full length of therapy.
• Instruct the patient to take ciprofloxacin during meals with 8 oz water and to drink several glasses of water between meals.
• Encourage the patient to eat and drink foods and liquids (citrus fruits, cranberry juice) that are high in ascorbic acid to prevent crystalluria.
• Warn the patient not to take antacids while taking this drug as antacids reduce or destroy ciprofloxacin's effectiveness.
• Teach the patient to shake the suspension well before using and not to chew the microcapsules in suspension.
• Explain to the patient that sugarless gum or hard candy may relieve ciprofloxacin's bad taste.
• In patients receiving the ophthalmic form of ciprofloxacin, explain to the patient that there is a possibility of crystal precipitate forming, usually resolving in 1 to 7 days.

gatifloxacin
gat-ih-**flocks**-ah-sin
(Tequin, Zymar)

CATEGORY AND SCHEDULE
Pregnancy Risk Category: C

MECHANISM OF ACTION
A fluoroquinolone that inhibits two enzymes, topoisomerase II and IV, in susceptible microorganisms. *Therapeutic Effect:* Interferes with bacterial DNA replication. Prevents or delays resistance emergence. Bactericidal.

PHARMACOKINETICS
Well absorbed from the gastrointestinal (GI) tract after PO administration. Protein binding: 20%. Widely distributed. Metabolized in liver. Primarily excreted in urine. **Half-life:** 7–14 hrs.

AVAILABILITY
Tablets: 200 mg, 400 mg.
Injection: 200-mg, 400-mg vials.
Ophthalmic Solution: 0.3%.

INDICATIONS AND DOSAGES
▶ **Chronic bronchitis, complicated urinary tract infections, pyelonephritis**
PO/IV
Adults, Elderly. 400 mg/day for 7–10 days (5 days for chronic bronchitis).

► **Sinusitis**
PO/IV
Adults, Elderly. 400 mg/day for 10 days.
► **Pneumonia**
PO/IV
Adults, Elderly. 400 mg/day for 7–14 days.
► **Cystitis**
PO/IV
Adults, Elderly. 400 mg as a single dose or 200 mg/day for 3 days.
► **Urethral gonorrhea in men and women, endocervical and rectal gonorrhea in women**
PO/IV
Adults, Elderly. 400 mg as a single dose.
► **Topical treatment of bacterial conjunctivitis due to susceptible strains of bacteria**
Ophthalmic
Adults, Elderly, Children older than 1 yr. 1 drop q2h while awake for 2 days, then 1 drop up to 4 times/day for days 3–7.
► **Dosage in renal impairment**

Creatinine Clearance	Dosage
40 ml/min	400 mg/day
less than 40 ml/min	Initially, 400 mg/day then 200 mg/day
Hemodialysis	Initially, 400 mg/day then 200 mg/day
Peritoneal dialysis	Initially, 400 mg/day then 200 mg/day

CONTRAINDICATIONS
Hypersensitivity to quinolones

INTERACTIONS
Drug
Antacids, digoxin, iron preparations: May decrease gatifloxacin plasma concentration and half-life.
Probenecid: May increase gatifloxacin plasma concentration and half-life.
Herbal
None known.
Food
None known.

DIAGNOSTIC TEST EFFECTS
None known.

IV INCOMPATIBILITIES
Amphotericin (Fungizone), potassium phosphate

IV COMPATIBILITIES
Aminophylline, calcium gluconate, hydromorphone (Dilaudid), lidocaine, lorazepam (Ativan), magnesium sulfate, methylprednisolone (Solu-Medrol), metoclopramide (Reglan), midazolam (Versed), morphine, nitroglycerin, potassium chloride, sodium phosphate

SIDE EFFECTS
Occasional (8%–3%)
Nausea, vaginitis, diarrhea, headache, dizziness
Ophthalmic: conjunctival irritation, increased tearing, corneal inflammation
Rare (3%–0.1%)
Abdominal pain, constipation, dyspepsia, stomatitis, edema, insomnia, abnormal dreams, diaphoresis, change in taste, rash
Ophthalmic: swelling around cornea, dry eye, eye pain, eyelid swelling, headache, red eye, reduced visual acuity, altered taste

SERIOUS REACTIONS
• Pseudomembranous colitis as evidenced by severe abdominal pain and cramps, severe watery diarrhea, and fever, may occur.
• Superinfection manifested as genital or anal pruritus, ulceration

or changes in oral mucosa, and moderate to severe diarrhea, may occur.

NURSING CONSIDERATIONS

Baseline Assessment
◀**ALERT**▶ Determine the patient's history of hypersensitivity to gatifloxacin and quinolones. before beginning drug therapy

Lifespan Considerations
* Be aware that it is unknown if gatifloxacin is distributed in breast milk.
* The safety and efficacy of gatifloxacin have not been established in children.
* In the elderly, age-related renal impairment may require dosage adjustment.

Precautions
* Use cautiously in patients with cerebral atherosclerosis, central nervous system (CNS) disorders, liver or renal impairment, seizures, and those with a prolonged QT interval.
* Use cautiously in patients taking other medications known to prolong the QT interval (e.g., erythromycin, tricyclic antidepressants).
* Use cautiously in patients with uncorrected hypokalemia and those receiving amiodarone, quinidine, procainamide, and sotalol.

Administration and Handling
PO
* Give without regard to meals.
* Administer oral gatifloxacin 4 hours before giving antacids, buffered tablets or solutions, ferrous sulfate, or multivitamins.

Ophthalmic
* Tilt the patient's head backward and have the patient look up.
* Gently pull the patient's lower eyelid down until a pocket is formed.

* Hold the dropper above the pocket, and without touching the eyelid or conjunctival sac, place drops into the center of the pocket.
* Close the patient's eye, then apply gentle digital pressure to the lacrimal sac at the inner canthus.
* Remove excess solution around the patient's eye with a tissue.

IV
* Know that the drug is available prediluted and ready for use and that it's also available in 20- and 40-ml vials, which must be diluted in 100–200 ml D_5W, 0.9% NaCl.
* Infuse over 60 minutes.
* Do not give by rapid or bolus IV.

Intervention and Evaluation
* Assess the patient's pattern of daily bowel activity and stool consistency.
* Assist the patient with ambulation if he or she experiences dizziness.
* Evaluate the patient for headache, nausea, signs of infection, and vaginitis.
* Monitor the patient's mental status and white blood cell (WBC) count.

Patient Teaching
* Advise the patient not to skip a drug dose and to take gatifloxacin for the full course of therapy.
* Instruct the patient to take gatifloxacin with 8 oz water and to drink several glasses of water between meals.
* Warn the patient not to take antacids within 4 hours of taking the medication as antacids would reduce or destroy gatifloxacin's effectiveness.
* Urge the patient to avoid exposure to direct sunlight during therapy and for several days after treatment.

gemifloxacin mesylate
gem-ih-**flocks**-ah-sin
(Factive)

CATEGORY AND SCHEDULE
Pregnancy Risk Category: C

MECHANISM OF ACTION
A fluoroquinolone that interferes with DNA-gyrase in susceptible microorganisms. *Therapeutic Effect:* Inhibits DNA replication and repair. Bactericidal.

PHARMACOKINETICS
Rapidly, well absorbed from the gastrointestinal (GI) tract. Widely distributed. Penetrates well into lung tissue and fluid. Protein binding: 70%. Undergoes limited liver metabolism. Primarily excreted in feces with a lesser amount eliminated in the urine. Partially removed by hemodialysis. **Half-life:** 4–12 hrs.

AVAILABILITY
Tablets: 320 mg.

INDICATIONS AND DOSAGES
▶ **Acute bacterial exacerbation of chronic bronchitis**
PO
Adults, Elderly. 320 mg once a day for 5 days.
▶ **Community-acquired pneumonia**
PO
Adults, Elderly. 320 mg once a day for 7 days.
▶ **Dosage in renal impairment**
The dosage and frequency are modified based on degree of renal impairment.

Creatinine Clearance	Dosage
greater than 40 ml/min	320 mg once a day
40 ml/min or less	160 mg once a day

CONTRAINDICATIONS
History of prolongation of the QTc interval, uncorrected electrolyte disorders, such as hypokalemia and hypomagnesemia, hypersensitivity to fluoroquinolone antibiotic agents, patients receiving amiodarone, quinidine, procainamide, sotalol

INTERACTIONS
Drug
Aluminum and magnesium-containing antacids, bismuth sub-salicylate, didanosine, iron salts, sucralfate, zinc salts, other metals: May decrease the absorption of gemifloxacin.
Class 1A and Class III antiarrhythmics, antipsychotics, tricyclic antidepressants, erythromycin: Concurrent use of these drugs may increase the risk of QTc prolongation and life-threatening arrhythmias.
Cyclosporine: Increases the risk of nephrotoxicity.
Probenecid: Increases gemifloxacin serum concentration.
Herbal
None known.
Food
None known.

DIAGNOSTIC TEST EFFECTS
May increase BUN, LDH concentrations, serum alkaline phosphatase, creatinine, SGOT (AST), and SGPT (ALT) levels.

SIDE EFFECTS
Occasional (4%–2%)
Diarrhea, rash, nausea

Rare (1% or less)
Headache, abdominal pain, dizziness

SERIOUS REACTIONS

• Antibiotic-associated colitis, marked by severe abdominal pain and tenderness, watery and severe diarrhea, and fungal overgrowth may result from altered bacterial balance.

NURSING CONSIDERATIONS

Baseline Assessment
• Determine if the patient's history of hypersensitivity to fluoroquinolone antibiotics.
• Measure the patient's baseline QT interval, and calculate the QTc.
• Plan to obtain baseline lab tests, especially serum electrolyte levels. Expect to administer supplements, as needed, for low electrolyte levels.

Lifespan Considerations
• Be aware that gemifloxacin has the potential for teratogenic effects. Substitute formula feedings for breast-feeding.
• Be aware that the safety and efficacy of gemifloxacin have not been established in children younger than 18 years of age.
• In the elderly, age-related renal impairment may require dosage adjustment.

Precautions
• Use cautiously in patients with acute myocardial ischemia, clinically significant bradycardia, and impaired liver or renal function.

Administration and Handling
PO
• Give gemifloxacin without regard to meals.
• Do not crush or break tablets.
• Do not administer antacids with or within 2 hours of gemifloxacin.

Intervention and Evaluation
• Monitor the patient's liver function test results and white blood cell (WBC) count.
• Monitor the patient for signs and symptoms of infection.
• Encourage the patient to maintain adequate fluid intake.
• Assess the patient's daily pattern of bowel activity and stool consistency.
• Examine the patient's skin for rash.
• Be alert to signs and symptoms of superinfection including genital pruritus and oral candidiasis.
• Measure and calculate the QT interval and QTc to check for prolongation.

Patient Teaching
• Instruct the patient to complete the full course of gemifloxacin therapy.
• Teach the patient to take each drug dose with 8 oz. of water. Explain to the patient that he or she may take gemifloxacin without regard to food.
• Encourage the patient to drink several glasses of water between meals.
• Warn the patient not to take antacids with or within 2 hours of a gemifloxacin dose as antacids destroy or reduce the drug's effectiveness.

levofloxacin
leave-oh-**flocks**-ah-sin
(Levaquin, Quixin)

CATEGORY AND SCHEDULE
Pregnancy Risk Category: C

MECHANISM OF ACTION
A fluoroquinolone that inhibits the DNA enzyme gyrase in susceptible

microorganisms, interfering with bacterial DNA replication and repair. *Therapeutic Effect:* Produces bactericidal activity.

PHARMACOKINETICS
Well absorbed after both PO and IV administration. Protein binding: 24%–38%. Penetrates rapidly and extensively into leukocytes, epithelial cells, and macrophages. Lung concentrations are 2–5 times higher than those of plasma. Eliminated unchanged in the urine. Partially removed by hemodialysis. **Half-life:** 8 hrs.

AVAILABILITY
Tablets: 250 mg, 500 mg, 750 mg.
Injection: 500 mg/20 ml vials.
Premix: 250 mg/50 ml, 500 mg/ 100 ml, 750 mg/150 ml.
Ophthalmic Solution: 0.5%.

INDICATIONS AND DOSAGES
▶ **Bronchitis**
PO/IV
Adults, Elderly. 500 mg q24h for 7 days.
▶ **Pneumonia**
PO/IV
Adults, Elderly. 500 mg q24h for 7–14 days.
▶ **Acute maxillary sinusitis**
PO/IV
Adults, Elderly. 500 mg q24h for 10–14 days.
▶ **Skin and skin-structure infections**
PO/IV
Adults, Elderly. 500 mg q24h for 7–10 days.
▶ **Urinary tract infection, acute pyelonephritis**
PO/IV
Adults, Elderly. 250 mg q24h for 10 days.
▶ **Bacterial conjunctivitis**
Ophthalmic
Adults, Elderly, Children 1 yr and

older. 1–2 drops q2h for 2 days (up to 8 times/day), then 1–2 drops q4h for 5 days.
▶ **Dosage in renal impairment**
Bronchitis, pneumonia, sinusitis, skin and skin-structure infections

Creatinine Clearance	Dosage
50–80 ml/min	No change
20–49 ml/min	500 mg initially, then 250 mg q24h
10–19 ml/min	500 mg initially, dialysis then 250 mg q48h

Urinary tract infection, pyelonephritis

Creatinine Clearance	Dosage
20 ml/min	No change
10–19 ml/min	250 mg initially, then 250 mg q48h

CONTRAINDICATIONS
History of hypersensitivity to cinoxacin, fluoroquinolones, nalidixic acid

INTERACTIONS
Drug
Antacids, iron preparations, sucralfate: Decrease levofloxacin absorption.
NSAIDs: May increase the risk of central nervous system (CNS) stimulation or seizures.
Herbal
None known.
Food
None known.

DIAGNOSTIC TEST EFFECTS
May alter blood glucose levels.

IV INCOMPATIBILITIES
Furosemide (Lasix), heparin, insulin, nitroglycerin, propofol (Diprivan)

IV COMPATIBILITIES

Aminophylline, dobutamine
(Dobutrex), dopamine (Intron),
fentanyl (Sublimaze), lidocaine,
lorazepam (Ativan), morphine

SIDE EFFECTS

Occasional (3%–1%)
Diarrhea, nausea, stomach pain,
dizziness, drowsiness, headache,
lightheadedness
Ophthalmic: Local burning or
discomfort, margin crusting, crystals
or scales, foreign body sensation,
itching, bad taste
Rare (less than 1%)
Flatulence, taste perversion, pain,
inflammation or swelling in calves,
hands, or shoulder
Ophthalmic: Corneal staining,
keratitis, allergic reaction, lid
edema, tearing, reduced vision

SERIOUS REACTIONS

• Pseudomembranous colitis as
evidenced by severe abdominal pain
and cramps, and severe watery
diarrhea, and fever, may occur.
• Superinfection manifested as genital or anal pruritus, ulceration or
changes in oral mucosa, and moderate to severe diarrhea, may occur.
• Hypersensitivity reactions, including photosensitivity as evidenced by
rash, pruritus, blistering, swelling,
and the sensation of the skin burning have occurred in patients receiving fluoroquinolone therapy.

NURSING CONSIDERATIONS

Baseline Assessment

◀ALERT▶ Determine the patient's
hypersensitivity to levofloxacin or
other fluoroquinolones before beginning drug therapy.

Lifespan Considerations

• Be aware that levofloxacin is
excreted in breast milk and that
levofloxacin use should be avoided
during pregnancy.
• The safety and efficacy of levofloxacin have not been established
in children younger than 18 years
of age.
• In the elderly, age-related renal
impairment may require dosage
adjustment.

Precautions

• Use cautiously in patients with
bradycardia, cardiomyopathy, hypokalemia, hypomagnesia, impaired
renal function, seizures disorder,
and suspected central nervous system (CNS) disorders.

Administration and Handling

PO
• Do not administer antacids (aluminum, magnesium), sucralfate, iron
and multivitamin preparations with
zinc within 2 hours of levofloxacin
administration as these drugs significantly reduces levofloxacin
absorption.
• Provide patient with citrus fruits
and cranberry juice to acidify urine.
• Give levofloxacin without regard
to food.
IV
• Know that the drug is available in
single-dose 20-ml (500-mg) vials
and premixed with D_5W and is
ready to infuse.
• For infusion using single-dose
vial, withdraw desired amount (10
ml for 250 mg, 20 ml for 500 mg).
Dilute each 10 ml (250 mg) with
minimum 40 ml 0.9% NaCl, D_5W.
• Administer slowly, over not less
than 60 minutes.
Ophthalmic
• Place a gloved finger on the
patient's lower eyelid and pull it out
until a pocket is formed between
the eye and lower lid.
• Hold the dropper above the pocket
and place the correct number of
drops into the pocket.

• Close the patient's eye gently. Apply digital pressure to the lacrimal sac for 1 to 2 minutes to minimize drainage of the medication into the patient's nose and throat, reducing the risk of systemic effects.

Intervention and Evaluation

• Monitor the patient's blood glucose levels and liver and renal function test results.

• Report any hypersensitivity reactions including photosensitivity, pruritus, skin rash, and urticaria promptly to the physician.

• Be alert for signs and symptoms of superinfection manifested as anal or genital pruritus, moderate to severe diarrhea, new or increased fever, and ulceration or changes in oral mucosa.

• Provide symptomatic relief for nausea.

• Evaluate the patient's food tolerance and change in taste sensation.

Patient Teaching

• Encourage the patient to drink 6 to 8 glasses of fluid a day. Citrus and cranberry juices acidify urine.

• Advise the patient to avoid tasks that require mental alertness or motor skills until his or her response to the drug is established.

• Warn the patient to notify the physician if he or she experiences chest pain, difficulty breathing, palpitations, persistent diarrhea, swelling, or tendon pain.

lomefloxacin hydrochloride

low-meh-**flocks**-ah-sin
(Maxaquin)

CATEGORY AND SCHEDULE

Pregnancy Risk Category: C

MECHANISM OF ACTION

A quinolone that inhibits the enzyme DNA-gyrase in susceptible microorganisms. *Therapeutic Effect:* Interferes with bacterial DNA replication and repair. Bactericidal.

PHARMACOKINETICS

Well absorbed from the gastrointestinal (GI) tract. Protein binding: 10%. Widely distributed. Metabolized in liver. Primarily excreted in urine. Not removed by hemodialysis. **Half-life:** 4–6 hrs (half-life is increased with impaired renal function, elderly).

AVAILABILITY

Tablets: 400 mg.

INDICATIONS AND DOSAGES

▸ **Urinary tract infection (UTI)**
PO
Adults, Elderly. 400 mg/day for 10–14 days.

▸ **Uncomplicated UTI**
PO
Adults (females). 400 mg/day for 3 days.

▸ **Lower respiratory tract infections**
PO
Adults, Elderly. 400 mg/day for 10 days.

▸ **Surgical prophylaxis**
PO
Adults, Elderly. 400 mg 2–6 hrs before surgery.

▸ **Dosage in renal impairment**
The dosage and frequency are modified in patients based on severity of renal impairment.

Creatinine Clearance	Dosage
greater than 40 ml/min	No change
10–40 ml/min	400 mg initially, then 200 mg/day for 10–14 days

CONTRAINDICATIONS
Hypersensitivity to quinolones

INTERACTIONS
Drug
Antacids, iron prep, sucralfate: May decrease lomefloxacin absorption.
Oral anticoagulants: May increase the effects of oral anticoagulants.
Theophylline: Decreases clearance, may increase blood concentration and risk of theophylline toxicity.
Herbal
None known.
Food
None known.

DIAGNOSTIC TEST EFFECTS
May increase BUN, serum alkaline phosphatase, serum bilirubin, serum creatinine, serum LDH, SGOT (AST), and SGPT (ALT) levels.

SIDE EFFECTS
Occasional (3%–2%)
Nausea, headache, photosensitivity, dizziness
Rare (1%)
Diarrhea

SERIOUS REACTIONS
• Antibiotic-associated colitis as evidenced by severe abdominal pain and tenderness, fever, and watery and severe diarrhea, and superinfection may result from altered bacterial balance.

NURSING CONSIDERATIONS

Baseline Assessment
◀ALERT▶ Determine the patient's history of hypersensitivity to lomefloxacin and quinolones before beginning drug therapy.
Lifespan Considerations
• Be aware that it is unknown if lomefloxacin is distributed in breast milk. If possible, do not use during pregnancy or breast-feeding because of the risk of arthropathy to the fetus or infant.
• Be aware that the safety and efficacy of lomefloxacin have not been established in children.
• In the elderly, age-related renal impairment may require dosage adjustment.
Precautions
• Use cautiously in patients with central nervous system (CNS) disorders, renal impairment, and seizures, and those taking caffeine or theophylline.
Administration and Handling
PO
• May be given without regard to meals, preferably 2 hours after meals.
• Do not administer antacids, such as aluminum, magnesium, within 2 hours of lomefloxacin.
• Provide the patient with citrus fruits and cranberry juice to acidify urine.
Intervention and Evaluation
• Monitor the patient for dizziness, headache, and signs and symptoms of infection.
• Monitor the patient's mental status and white blood cell (WBC) count.
• Be alert for signs and symptoms of superinfection manifested as anal or genital pruritus, fever, oral candidiasis, and vaginitis.
Patient Teaching
• Advise the patient not to skip drug doses and to take lomefloxacin for the full course of therapy.
• Warn the patient not to take antacids while on lomefloxacin because antacids reduce or destroy lomefloxacin's effectiveness.
• Urge the patient to avoid sunlight and ultraviolet light exposure and to wear sunscreen and protective clothing if photosensitivity develops.

moxifloxacin hydrochloride

mox-ih-**flocks**-ah-sin
(Avelox, Avelox IV, Vigamox)
Do not confuse with Avonex.

CATEGORY AND SCHEDULE
Pregnancy Risk Category: C

MECHANISM OF ACTION
A fluoroquinolone that inhibits two enzymes, topoisomerase II and IV, in susceptible microorganisms. *Therapeutic Effect:* Interferes with bacterial DNA replication. Prevents or delays emergence of resistant organisms. Bactericidal.

PHARMACOKINETICS
Well absorbed from the gastrointestinal (GI) tract after PO administration. Protein binding: 50%. Widely distributed throughout body with tissue concentration often exceeding plasma concentration. Metabolized in liver. Primarily excreted in urine with a lesser amount in feces.
Half-life: 10.7–13.3 hrs.

AVAILABILITY
Tablets: 400 mg.
Injection: 400 mg.
Ophthalmic Solution: 0.5%.

INDICATIONS AND DOSAGES
▶ **Acute bacterial sinusitis, community-acquired pneumonia**
IV/PO
Adults, Elderly. 400 mg q24h for 10 days.
▶ **Acute bacterial exacerbation of chronic bronchitis**
IV/PO
Adults, Elderly. 400 mg q24h for 5 days.
▶ **Skin and skin-structure infection**
IV/PO
Adults, Elderly. 400 mg once a day for 7 days.
▶ **Topical treatment of bacterial conjunctivitis due to susceptible strains of bacteria**
Ophthalmic
Adults, Elderly, Children older than 1 yr. 1 drop 3 times/day for 7 days.

CONTRAINDICATIONS
Hypersensitivity to quinolones

INTERACTIONS
Drug
Antacids, didanosine chewable, buffered tablets or pediatric powder for oral solution, iron preparations, sucralfate: May decrease moxifloxacin absorption.
Herbal
None known.
Food
None known.

DIAGNOSTIC TEST EFFECTS
None known.

IV INCOMPATIBILITIES
Do not add or infuse other drugs simultaneously through the same IV line. Flush line before and after use if same IV line is used with other medications.

SIDE EFFECTS
Frequent (8%–6%)
Nausea, diarrhea
Occasional (3%–2%)
Dizziness, headache, abdominal pain, vomiting
Ophthalmic (6%–1%): conjunctival irritation, reduced visual acuity, dry eye, keratitis, eye pain, ocular itching, swelling of tissue around cornea, eye discharge, fever, cough, pharyngitis, rash, rhinitis

Rare (1%)

Change in sense of taste, dyspepsia (heartburn, indigestion), photosensitivity

SERIOUS REACTIONS

• Pseudomembranous colitis as evidenced by fever, severe abdominal cramps or pain, and severe watery diarrhea may occur.

• Superinfection manifested as anal or genital pruritus, moderate to severe diarrhea, and ulceration or changes in oral mucosa may occur.

NURSING CONSIDERATIONS

Baseline Assessment

◀ALERT▶ Determine the patient's history of hypersensitivity to moxifloxacin and quinolones before beginning drug therapy.

Lifespan Considerations

• Be aware that moxifloxacin may be distributed in breast milk and may produce teratogenic effects.

• Be aware that the safety and efficacy of moxifloxacin have not been established in children.

• There are no age-related precautions noted in the elderly.

Precautions

• Use cautiously in patients with cerebral arthrosclerosis, central nervous system (CNS) disorders, liver or renal impairment; seizures, those with a prolonged QT interval, and uncorrected hypokalemia.

• Use cautiously in patients receiving amiodarone, procainamide, quinidine, and sotalol.

Administration and Handling

◀ALERT▶ Infuse IV over 60 minutes or more.

PO

• Give without regard to meals.

• Administer oral moxifloxacin 4 hours before or 8 hours after antacids, didanosine chewable, buffered tablets or pediatric powder for oral solution, iron preparations, multivitamins, or sucralfate.

Ophthalmic

• Tilt the patient's head back and instruct the patient to look up.

• With a gloved finger, gently pull the patient's lower eyelid down until a pocket is formed.

• Hold the dropper above the pocket and, without touching the eyelid or conjunctival sac, place drops into the center of the pocket.

• Close the patient's eye gently and apply gentle finger pressure to the lacrimal sac at the inner canthus.

• Remove excess solution around the patient's eye with a tissue.

IV

• Store at room temperature.

• Do not refrigerate.

• Available in ready-to-use containers.

• Give by IV infusion only.

• Avoid rapid or bolus IV infusion.

• Infuse over 60 minutes or more.

Intervention and Evaluation

• Assess the patient's pattern of daily bowel activity and stool consistency.

• Assist the patient with ambulation if he or she experiences dizziness.

• Evaluate the patient for abdominal pain, change in sense of taste, dyspepsia (heartburn, indigestion), headache, and vomiting.

• Monitor the patient for signs of infection.

• Monitor the patient's white blood cell (WBC) count.

Patient Teaching

• Explain to the patient that moxifloxacin may be taken without regard to food.

• Encourage the patient to drink plenty of fluids.

• Urge the patient to avoid exposure to direct sunlight as this may cause a photosensitivity reaction.

• Instruct the patient not take antacids 4 hours before or 8 hours after moxifloxacin dose.
• Advise the patient to take moxifloxacin for the full course of therapy.

norfloxacin
nor-**flocks**-ah-sin
(Insensye[AUS], Noroxin, Noroxin Ophthalmic)

CATEGORY AND SCHEDULE
Pregnancy Risk Category: C

MECHANISM OF ACTION
A quinolone that inhibits DNA replication and repair by interfering with DNA-gyrase in susceptible microorganisms. *Therapeutic Effect:* Produces bactericidal activity.

AVAILABILITY
Tablets: 400 mg.
Ophthalmic Solution 0.3%: 3 mg/ml.

INDICATIONS AND DOSAGES
▶ **Complicated or uncomplicated urinary tract infections**
PO
Adults, Elderly. 400 mg 2 times/day for 7–21 days.
▶ **Prostatitis**
PO
Adults. 400 mg 2 times/day for 28 days.
▶ **Uncomplicated gonococcal infections**
PO
Adults. 800 mg as a single dose.
▶ **Acute meibomianitis, blepharitis, blepharoconjunctivitis, conjunctival keratitis, corneal ulcers, dacryocystitis, keratoconjunctivitis**

Ophthalmic
Adults, Elderly. 1–2 drops 4 times/day up to 7 days. For severe infections, may give 1–2 drops q2h while awake the first day.
▶ **Dosage in renal impairment**
The dosage and frequency are modified based on the degree of renal impairment.

Creatinine Clearance	Dosage
30 ml/min or higher	400 mg twice a day
less than 30 ml/min	400 mg once a day

CONTRAINDICATIONS
Hypersensitivity to norfloxacin, quinolones, or any component of preparation. Do not use in children younger than 18 years of age as the drug may produce arthropathy in these patients. Ophthalmic: Epithelial herpes simplex, fungal disease of ocular structure, keratitis, mycobacterial infection, vaccinia, varicella. Do not use after uncomplicated removal of foreign body.

INTERACTIONS
Drug
Antacids, sucralfate: May decrease norfloxacin absorption.
Oral anticoagulants: May increase effects of oral anticoagulants.
Theophylline: Decreases clearance, may increase blood concentration and risk of theophylline toxicity.
Herbal
None known.
Food
None known.

DIAGNOSTIC TEST EFFECTS
May increase BUN, serum alkaline phosphatase, serum bilirubin, serum creatinine, serum LDH, SGOT (AST), and SGPT (ALT) levels.

SIDE EFFECTS
Frequent
Nausea, headache, dizziness
Ophthalmic: Bad taste in mouth
Occasional
Ophthalmic: Temporary blurring of vision, irritation, burning, stinging, itching
Rare
Vomiting, diarrhea, dry mouth, bitter taste, nervousness, drowsiness, insomnia, photosensitivity, tinnitus, crystalluria, rash, fever, seizures
Ophthalmic: Conjunctival hyperemia, photophobia, decreased vision, pain.

SERIOUS REACTIONS
• Superinfection, anaphylaxis, Stevens-Johnson syndrome, and arthropathy (joint disease) occur rarely.

NURSING CONSIDERATIONS
Baseline Assessment
◀ ALERT ▶ Determine the patient's history of hypersensitivity to norfloxacin and quinolones before beginning drug therapy.
Precautions
• Use cautiously in patients with impaired renal function and any predisposition to seizures.
Administration and Handling
PO
• Give 1 hour before or 2 hours after meals, with 8 oz of water.
• Encourage the patient to drink additional glasses of water between meals.
• Do not administer antacids with or within 2 hours of norfloxacin dose.

• Provide the patient with citrus fruits and cranberry juice acidify urine.
Ophthalmic
• Place a gloved finger on the patient's lower eyelid and pull it out until a pocket is formed between the eye and lower lid.
• Hold the dropper above the pocket and place the correct number of drops into the pocket.
• Close the patient's eye gently.
• Apply digital pressure to lacrimal sac for 1 to 2 minutes to minimize drainage into the patient's nose and throat, thereby reducing the risk of systemic effects.
Intervention and Evaluation
• Assess the patient for chest pain, dizziness, headache, joint pain, and nausea.
• Evaluate the patient's food tolerance.
• Evaluate patients taking norfloxacin's ophthalmic form for therapeutic response.
Patient Teaching
• Instruct the patient to take norfloxacin with 8 oz of water 1 hour before or 2 hours after meals.
• Advise the patient to complete the full course of norfloxacin therapy.
• Encourage the patient to drink several glasses of water between meals.
• Explain to the patient that norfloxacin may cause dizziness or drowsiness.
• Teach the patient not to take antacids with or within 2 hours of a norfloxacin dose as antacids reduce or destroy norfloxacin's effectiveness.

ofloxacin
oh-**flocks**-ah-sin
(Apo-Oflox[CAN], Floxin, Floxin
Otic, Ocuflox)
**Do not confuse with Flexeril,
Flexon, or Ocufen.**

CATEGORY AND SCHEDULE
Pregnancy Risk Category: C

MECHANISM OF ACTION
A fluoroquinolone that inhibits
DNA-gyrase in susceptible microorganisms. *Therapeutic Effect:* Interferes with bacterial DNA replication
and repair. Bactericidal.

PHARMACOKINETICS
Rapidly, well absorbed from the
gastrointestinal (GI) tract. Protein
binding: 20%–25%. Widely distributed (penetrates cerebrospinal fluid
[CSF]). Metabolized in liver. Primarily excreted in urine. Removed
by hemodialysis. **Half-life:** 4.7–7
hrs (half-life is increased with
impaired renal function, elderly,
cirrhosis).

AVAILABILITY
Tablets: 200 mg, 300 mg, 400 mg.
Premix Injection: 400 mg/100 D_5W.
Ophthalmic Solution: 3%.
Otic Solution: 0.3%.

INDICATIONS AND DOSAGES
▸ **Urinary tract infection (UTI)**
PO/IV infusion
Adults. 200 mg q12h.
▸ **Lower respiratory tract, skin and
skin-structure infections**
PO/IV infusion
Adults. 400 mg q12h for 10 days.
▸ **Prostatitis, sexually transmitted
diseases (cervicitis, urethritis)**
PO
Adults. 300 mg q12h.

▸ **Pelvic inflammatory disease (PID)**
PO
Adults. 400 mg q12h for 10–14 days.
▸ **Prostatitis**
IV infusion
Adults. 300 mg q12h.
▸ **Sexually transmitted diseases**
IV infusion
Adults. 400 mg as a single dose.
▸ **Acute, uncomplicated gonorrhea**
PO
Adults. 400 mg 1 time.
▸ **Usual elderly dosage**
PO
Elderly. 200–400 mg q12–24h for
7 days up to 6 wks.
▸ **Bacterial conjunctivitis**
Ophthalmic
Adults, Elderly. 1–2 drops q2–4h for
2 days, then 4 times/day for 5 days.
▸ **Corneal ulcers**
Ophthalmic
Adults. 1–2 drops q30min while
awake for 2 days, then q60min
while awake for 5–7 days, then
4 times/day.
▸ **Otitis externa, acute or chronic
otitis media.**
Adults, Elderly, Children. Twice a
day. Eardrops should be at body
temperature (wrap hand around
bottle).
▸ **Dosage in renal impairment**
After a normal initial dose, dosage
and interval are based on creatinine
clearance.

Creatinine Clearance	Adjusted Dose	Dosage Interval
greater than 50 ml/min	None	12 hrs
10–50 ml/min	None	24 hrs
less than 10 ml/min		24 hrs

CONTRAINDICATIONS
Children younger than 18 years
of age, hypersensitivity to any
quinolones

INTERACTIONS
Drug
Antacids, sucralfate: May decrease absorption and effects of ofloxacin.
Theophylline: May increase blood concentrations and risk of theophylline toxicity.
Herbal
None known.
Food
None known.

DIAGNOSTIC TEST EFFECTS
None known.

IV INCOMPATIBILITIES
Amphotericin B complex (Abelcet, AmBisome, Amphotec), cefepime (Maxipime), doxorubicin liposome (Doxil)

IV COMPATIBILITIES
Propofol (Diprivan)

SIDE EFFECTS
Frequent (10%–7%)
Nausea, headache, insomnia
Occasional (5%–3%)
Abdominal pain, diarrhea, vomiting, dry mouth, flatulence, dizziness, fatigue, drowsiness, rash, pruritus, fever
Rare (less than 1%)
Constipation, numbness of the feet and hands

SERIOUS REACTIONS
• Superinfection and severe hypersensitivity reaction occur rarely.
• Arthropathy manifested as swelling, pain, clubbing of fingers and toes, and degeneration of stress-bearing portion of a joint, may occur if the drug is given to children.

NURSING CONSIDERATIONS
Baseline Assessment
◀ALERT▶ Determine the patient's history of hypersensitivity to ofloxacin or any quinolones before beginning drug therapy.
Lifespan Considerations
• Be aware that ofloxacin is distributed in breast milk, has potentially serious adverse reactions in nursing infants, and presents a risk of arthropathy development to a fetus.
• Be aware that the safety and efficacy of ofloxacin have not been established in children. The safety and efficacy of the otic form of ofloxacin have not been established in children less than 1 year of age.
• There are no age-related precautions noted for the otic form of ofloxacin in the elderly.
• In the elderly, age-related renal impairment may require dosage adjustment for oral and parenteral administration.
Precautions
• Use cautiously in patients with central nervous system (CNS) disorders, renal impairment, and seizures, and those taking caffeine or theophylline.
• Use cautiously in patients with syphilis, ofloxacin may mask or delay symptoms of syphilis; serologic test for syphilis should be done at diagnosis and 3 months after treatment.
Administration and Handling
PO
• Do not give with food. The preferred dosing time is 1 hour before or 2 hours after meals.
• Do not administer antacids (aluminum, magnesium) or iron or zinc-containing products within 2 hours of ofloxacin.
• Provide the patient with citrus

fruits and cranberry juice to acidify urine.

• Give with 8 oz of water and encourage fluid intake.

Ophthalmic

• Tilt the patient's head back and place the solution in the conjunctival sac.

• Have the patient close his or her eye; then press gently on the lacrimal sac for 1 minute.

• Do not use ophthalmic solutions for injection.

• Unless the infection is very superficial, expect to also administer systemic drug therapy.

Otic

• Instruct the patient to lie down with his or her head turned so the affected ear is upright.

• Instill drops toward the canal wall, not directly on the eardrum.

• Pull the auricle down and posterior in children; up and posterior in adults.

IV

• Store at room temperature.

• After dilution, store IV solution for 72 hours at room temperature or refrigerate for 14 days.

• Discard unused portions.

• Know that ofloxacin is also available in premix ready-to-hang solutions.

• Be sure to dilute each 200 mg with 50 ml D_5W or 0.9% NaCl (400 mg with 100 ml) to provide concentration of 4 mg/ml.

• Give only by IV infusion over at least 60 minutes; avoid rapid or bolus IV administration.

• Do not add or infuse other medication through same IV line at same time.

Intervention and Evaluation

• Monitor the patient for signs and symptoms of infection.

• Monitor the patient's mental status and white blood cell (WBC) count.

• Assess the patient's skin for rash. Withhold the drug at the first sign of rash or other allergic reaction and promptly notify the physician.

• Assess the patient's pattern of daily bowel activity and stool consistency.

• Observe the patient during the night for insomnia.

• Evaluate the patient for dizziness, headache, tremors, and visual difficulties.

• Provide ambulation assistance as needed.

• Be alert for signs of superinfection manifested as anal or genital pruritus, discomfort in the mouth, fever, sores, and vaginitis.

Patient Teaching

• Instruct the patient not to take antacids within 6 hours before or 2 hours after taking ofloxacin. Teach the patient that ofloxacin is best taken 1 hour before or 2 hours after meals.

• Warn the patient that ofloxacin may cause dizziness, drowsiness, headache, and insomnia.

• Advise the patient to avoid tasks requiring mental alertness or motor skills until his or her response to ofloxacin is established.

11 Tetracyclines

demeclocycline
hydrochloride
doxycycline
minocycline
hydrochloride
tetracycline
hydrochloride

Uses: Tetracyclines are used to treat rickettsial diseases (such as typhus fever and Q fever), *Chlamydia trachomatis* infections, brucellosis, cholera, pneumonia caused by *Mycoplasma pneumoniae,* Lyme disease, *Helicobacter pylori* gastric infections (in combination therapy), and periodontal disease. Topical formulations are used to treat acne.

Action: Tetracyclines are bacteriostatic. They inhibit bacterial protein synthesis by binding to the 30S ribosomal subunit and preventing the binding of transfer ribonucleic acid (RNA) to messenger RNA. (See illustration, *Mechanism of Action: Tetracyclines,* page 211.)

demeclocycline hydrochloride
deh-meh-clo-sigh-clean
(Declomycin, Ledermycin[AUS])

CATEGORY AND SCHEDULE
Pregnancy Risk Category: D

MECHANISM OF ACTION
This tetracycline antibiotic produces bacteriostats by binding to ribosomal receptor sites; also inhibits ADH-induced water reabsorption. *Therapeutic Effect:* Inhibits bacterial protein synthesis. Produces water diuresis.

AVAILABILITY
Tablets: 150 mg, 300 mg.

INDICATIONS AND DOSAGES
▸ **Mild to moderate infections, including acne, pertussis, chronic bronchitis, and urinary tract infection (UTI)**
PO
Adults, Elderly. 600 mg/day in 2–4 divided doses.

Children older than 8 yrs.
6–12 mg/kg/day in 2–4 divided doses.
▸ **Uncomplicated gonorrhea**
PO
Adults. Initially, 600 mg, then 300 mg q12h for 4 days for total of 3 g.
▸ **Chronic form of syndrome of inappropriate ADH secretion (SIADH)**
PO
Adults, Elderly. 600 mg–1.2 g/day in 3–4 divided doses, or 3.25–3.75 mg/kg q6h.

CONTRAINDICATIONS
Last half of pregnancy, infants, children up to 8 yrs of age

INTERACTIONS
Drug
Antacids containing aluminum, calcium, or magnesium; laxatives containing magnesium; oral iron preparations: Impair the absorption of tetracyclines.
Cholestyramine, colestipol: May decrease demeclocycline absorption.
Oral contraceptives: May decrease the effects of these drugs.

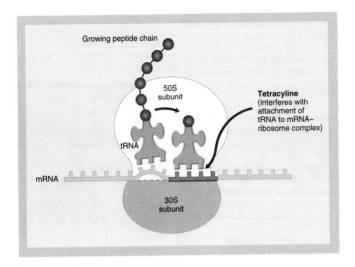

Mechanism of Action: Tetracyclines

Like certain other anti-infectives, tetracyclines work by interfering with bacterial protein synthesis. Protein synthesis normally occurs when the ribosomal subunits 50S and 30S bind to messenger ribonucleic acid (mRNA), which arranges amino acids into peptide chains that form proteins. Then transfer ribonucleic acid (tRNA) helps carry out genetic instructions from mRNA to arrange certain amino acids in a specific sequence to form a growing peptide chain. Once the peptide chain is complete, mRNA detaches from the ribosomal subunits, and the new protein is created.

Tetracyclines inhibit bacterial protein synthesis by attaching to the 30S ribosomal subunit. As a result, tRNA can't bind with the mRNA-ribosome complex, and no new amino acids can be synthesized or added to the growing peptide chain.

Herbal
None known.
Food
Milk, dairy products: May decrease demeclocycline absorption.

DIAGNOSTIC TEST EFFECTS

May increase BUN, serum alkaline phosphatase, serum amylase, serum bilirubin, SGOT (AST), and SGPT (ALT) levels.

SIDE EFFECTS
Frequent
Anorexia, nausea, vomiting, diarrhea, dysphagia. Exaggerated sunburn reaction may occur with moderate to high demeclocycline dosage.
Occasional
Urticaria, rash
Long-term therapy may result in diabetes insipidus syndrome: polydipsia, polyuria, and weakness.

SERIOUS REACTIONS
• Superinfection (especially fungal), anaphylaxis, and increased intracranial pressure occur rarely.
• Bulging fontanelles occur rarely in infants.

NURSING CONSIDERATIONS

Baseline Assessment
◀ALERT▶ Determine the patient's history of allergies, especially to tetracyclines, before beginning drug therapy.

Precautions
• Use cautiously in patients with renal impairment, and who cannot avoid sun or ultraviolet exposure, because this may produce a severe photosensitivity reaction.

Administration and Handling
• Give antacids containing aluminum, calcium, or magnesium; laxatives containing magnesium; or oral iron preparations, 1 to 2 hours before or after demeclocycline because they may impair the drug's absorption.

Intervention and Evaluation
• Assess the patient's pattern of daily bowel activity and stool consistency.
• Evaluate the patient's food intake and tolerance.
• Monitor the patient's intake and output and renal function test results.
• Assess the patient's skin for rash.
• Be alert to signs and symptoms of superinfection as evidenced by anal or genital pruritus, diarrhea, and ulceration or changes of oral mucosa or tongue.
• Monitor the patient's blood pressure (B/P) and level of consciousness (LOC) because of potential for increased intracranial pressure.

Patient Teaching
• Advise the patient to continue taking the antibiotic for the full length of treatment and to evenly space drug doses around the clock.
• Instruct the patient to take oral doses of demeclocycline on an empty stomach with a full glass of water.

• Encourage the patient to avoid overexposure to sun or ultraviolet light to prevent photosensitivity reactions.

doxycycline
dock-see-**sigh**-clean
(Adoxa, Apo-Doxy[CAN], Doryx, Doxsig[AUS], Doxycin[CAN], Doxylin[AUS], Periostat, Vibra-Tabs, Vibramycin)
Do not confuse with Dicyclomine or doxylamine.

CATEGORY AND SCHEDULE
Pregnancy Risk Category: D

MECHANISM OF ACTION
A tetracycline antibiotic that inhibits bacterial protein synthesis by binding to ribosomes. *Therapeutic Effect:* Prevents bacterial cell growth.

AVAILABILITY
Capsules: 50 mg, 100 mg.
Tablets: 20 mg, 100 mg.
Powder for Oral Suspension: 50 mg/5 ml.
Syrup: 50 mg/5 ml.
Powder for Injection: 100 mg, 200 mg.
Capsules (extended release): 75 mg, 100 mg.

INDICATIONS AND DOSAGES
▶ **Treatment of respiratory, skin and soft tissue, urinary tract infections; pelvic inflammatory disease(PID); rheumatic fever prophylaxis; brucellosis; trachoma; Rocky Mountain spotted fever; typhus; Q fever; rickettsia; severe acne (Adoxa); smallpox; psittacosis; ornithosis; granuloma inguinale; lymphogranuloma venereum; ad-**

junctive treatment of intestinal amebiasis
PO
Adults, Elderly. Initially, 200 mg in 2 divided doses of 100 mg q12h, then 100 mg/day as single dose or in 2 divided doses of 100 mg q12h for severe infections.
Children older than 8 yrs, weighing more than 45 kg. 2–4 mg/kg/day divided q12–24h. Maximum: 200 mg/day.
IV
Adults, Elderly. Initially, 200 mg as 1–2 infusions; then 100–200 mg/day (200 mg as 12 infusions).
Children 8 yrs and older. 2–4 mg/kg/day divided q12–24h. Maximum: 200 mg/day.
▸ **Acute gonococcal infections**
PO
Adults. Initially, 200 mg, then 100 mg at bedtime on first day; then 100 mg 2 times a day for 14 days.
▸ **Syphilis**
PO/IV
Adults. 200 mg/day in divided doses for 14–28 days.
▸ **Traveler's diarrhea**
PO
Adults, Elderly. 100 mg a day during a period of risk, up to 14 days, and for 2 days after returning home.
▸ **Periodontitis**
PO
Adults. 20 mg 2 times a day.

UNLABELED USES
Treatment of atypical mycobacterial infections, gonorrhea, malaria, prevention of Lyme disease, prophylaxis or treatment of traveler's diarrhea, rheumatoid arthritis

CONTRAINDICATIONS
Hypersensitivity to tetracyclines, sulfite, last half of pregnancy, children younger than 8 yrs, severe liver dysfunction

INTERACTIONS
Drug
Antacids containing aluminum, calcium, or magnesium; laxatives containing magnesium: Decrease doxycycline absorption.
Barbiturates, carbamazepine, phenytoin: May decrease doxycycline blood concentrations.
Cholestyramine, colestipol: May decrease doxycycline absorption.
Oral contraceptives: May decrease the effects of these drugs.
Oral iron preparations: Impair absorption of tetracyclines.
Herbal
None known.
Food
None known.

DIAGNOSTIC TEST EFFECTS
May increase serum alkaline phosphatase, serum amylase, serum bilirubin, SGOT (AST), and SGPT (ALT) levels. May alter complete blood count (CBC).

IV INCOMPATIBILITIES
Allopurinol (Aloprim), heparin, piperacillin/tazobactam (Zosyn)

IV COMPATIBILITIES
Amiodarone (Cordarone), diltiazem (Cardizem), hydromorphone (Dilaudid), magnesium sulfate, morphine, propofol (Diprivan)

SIDE EFFECTS
Frequent
Anorexia, nausea, vomiting, diarrhea, dysphagia, photosensitivity, which may be severe
Occasional
Rash, urticaria

SERIOUS REACTIONS

• Superinfection (especially fungal) and benign intracranial hypertension (headache, visual changes) may occur.

• Liver toxicity, fatty degeneration of liver, and pancreatitis occur rarely.

NURSING CONSIDERATIONS

Baseline Assessment

◀ALERT▶ Determine the patient's history of allergies, especially to sulfites and tetracyclines, before beginning drug therapy.

Precautions

• Use cautiously in patients who cannot avoid sun or ultraviolet light exposure because this may produce a severe photosensitivity reaction.

Administration and Handling

◀ALERT▶ Do not administer IM or subcutaneously. Space doses evenly around clock.

• Give doxycycline 1 to 2 hours before or after antacids that contain aluminum, calcium, or magnesium; laxatives that contain magnesium; or oral iron preparations because these drugs may impair doxycycline absorption.

PO

• Store capsules and tablets at room temperature.

• Store oral suspension for up to 2 weeks at room temperature.

• Give with full glass of fluid. Know that drug may be given with food or milk.

IV

• After reconstitution, store IV piggyback infusion for up to 12 hours at room temperature, or refrigerate for up to 72 hours.

• Protect from direct sunlight. Discard if precipitate forms.

• Reconstitute each 100-mg vial with 10 ml Sterile Water for Injection for concentration of 10 mg/ml.

• Further dilute each 100 mg with at least 100 ml D_5W, 0.9% NaCl, lactated Ringer's.

• Give by intermittent IV piggyback infusion.

• Infuse over more than 1 to 4 hours.

Intervention and Evaluation

• Assess the patient's pattern of daily bowel activity and stool consistency.

• Assess the patient's skin for rash.

• Monitor the patient's level of consciousness (LOC) because of the potential for increased intracranial pressure.

• Be alert for signs and symptoms of superinfection as evidenced by anal or genital pruritus, diarrhea, and ulceration or changes of the oral mucosa.

Patient Teaching

• Encourage the patient to avoid overexposure to sun or ultraviolet light to prevent photosensitivity reactions.

• Instruct the patient not to take doxycycline with antacids, dairy products, or iron products as these substances decrease the absorption of doxycycline.

• Advise the patient to continue taking doxycycline for the full course of therapy.

• Teach the patient that after application of the dental gel, he or she should avoid tooth brushing or flossing the treated areas for 7 days.

minocycline hydrochloride

min-know-**sigh**-clean
(Akamin[AUS], Dynacin, Minocin,
Novo Minocycline[CAN],
Minomycin[AUS])
**Do not confuse with Dynabac
or Mithracin.**

CATEGORY AND SCHEDULE
Pregnancy Risk Category: D

MECHANISM OF ACTION
A tetracycline antibiotic that binds
to ribosomes. *Therapeutic Effects:*
Inhibits bacterial protein synthesis.
Bacteriostatic.

AVAILABILITY
Capsules: 50 mg, 75 mg,
100 mg.
Tablets: 50 mg, 75 mg, 100 mg.
Powder for Injection: 100 mg.

INDICATIONS AND DOSAGES
▸ **Mild to moderate to severe prostate, urinary tract, and central
nervous system (CNS) infections
(excluding meningitis); uncomplicated gonorrhea; inflammatory
acne; brucellosis; skin granulomas;
cholera; trachoma; nocardiasis;
yaws; and syphilis when penicillins
are contraindicated**
PO
Adults, Elderly. Initially,
100–200 mg, then 100 mg q12h
or 50 mg q6h.
IV
Adults, Elderly. Initially,
200 mg, then 100 mg q12h up
to 400 mg/day.
PO/IV
Children older than 8 yrs. Initially, 4 mg/kg, then 2 mg/kg
q12h.

UNLABELED USES
Treatment of atypical mycobacterial
infections, rheumatoid arthritis,
scleroderma

CONTRAINDICATIONS
Hypersensitivity to tetracyclines,
last half of pregnancy, children
younger than 8 yrs

INTERACTIONS
Drug
Carbamazepine, phenytoin: May
decrease minocycline blood concen-
tration.
Cholestyramine, colestipol: May
decrease minocycline absorption.
Oral contraceptives: May decrease
the effects of these drugs.
Herbal
St. John's wort: May increase risk
of photosensitivity.
Food
None known.

DIAGNOSTIC TEST EFFECTS
May increase serum alkaline
phosphatase, serum amylase,
serum bilirubin, SGOT (AST),
and SGPT (ALT) levels.

IV INCOMPATIBILITIES
Piperacillin/tazobactam (Zosyn)

IV COMPATIBILITIES
Heparin, magnesium, potassium

SIDE EFFECTS
Frequent
Dizziness, lightheadedness, diarrhea, nausea, vomiting, stomach
cramps, photosensitivity (may be
severe)
Occasional
Pigmentation of skin, mucous
membranes; itching in rectal
and genital area; sore mouth or
tongue

SERIOUS REACTIONS
• Superinfection (especially fungal), anaphylaxis, and increased intracranial pressure may occur.
• Bulging fontanelles occur rarely in infants.

NURSING CONSIDERATIONS

Baseline Assessment
◄ALERT► Determine the patient's history of allergies, especially to sulfite and tetracyclines before beginning drug therapy.

Precautions
• Use cautiously in patients with renal impairment, and who cannot avoid sun or ultraviolet exposure because this may produce a severe photosensitivity reaction.

Administration and Handling
◄ALERT► Space drug doses evenly around the clock.

PO
• Store at room temperature.
• Give capsules and tablets with a full glass of water.

IV
• Store IV solution for up to 24 hours at room temperature.
• Use piggyback IV infusion immediately after reconstitution.
• Discard solution if precipitate forms.
• For intermittent piggyback IV infusion, reconstitute each 100-mg vial with 5 to 10 ml Sterile Water for Injection to provide concentration of 20 or 10 mg/ml, respectively.
• Further dilute with 500 to 1,000 ml D₅W or 0.9% NaCl.
• Infuse over 6 hours.

Intervention and Evaluation
• Assess the patient's ability to ambulate. Minocycline may cause dizziness, drowsiness, or vertigo.

• Assess the patient's pattern of daily bowel activity and stool consistency.
• Assess the patient's skin for rash.
• Check the patient's blood pressure (B/P) and level of consciousness (LOC) for increased intracranial pressure.
• Be alert for signs and symptoms of superinfection as evidenced by anal or genital pruritus, diarrhea, and ulceration or changes of the oral mucosa.

Patient Teaching
• Advise the patient to continue taking the antibiotic for the full length of treatment and to evenly space drug doses around the clock.
• Teach the patient to drink a full glass of water with minocycline capsules or tablets and to avoid bedtime doses.
• Warn the patient to avoid tasks that require mental alertness or motor skills until his or her response to the drug is established.
• Instruct the patient to notify the physician if diarrhea, rash, or other new symptoms occur.
• Encourage the patient to protect his or her skin from sun exposure.

tetracycline hydrochloride
tet-rah-**sigh**-klin
(Achromycin, Apo-Tetra[CAN], Latycin[AUS], Mysteclin[AUS], Novotetra[CAN], Sumycin, Tetrex[AUS])

CATEGORY AND SCHEDULE
Pregnancy Risk Category: D (B with topical)

MECHANISM OF ACTION
A tetracycline antibiotic that inhibits bacterial protein synthesis by binding to ribosomes. *Therapeutic Effect:* Prevents bacterial cell growth. Bacteriostatic.

PHARMACOKINETICS
Readily absorbed from the gastrointestinal (GI) tract. Protein binding: 30%–60%. Widely distributed. Excreted in urine; eliminated in feces via biliary system. Not removed by hemodialysis. **Half-life:** 6–11 hrs (half-life is increased with impaired renal function).

AVAILABILITY
Capsules: 250 mg, 500 mg.
Tablets: 250 mg, 500 mg.
Suspension: 125 mg/5 ml.
Topical Solution.
Topical Ointment: 3%.

INDICATIONS AND DOSAGES
▸ **Treatment of inflammatory acne vulgaris, Lyme disease, mycoplasma disease, *Legionella*, Rocky Mountain spotted fever, chlamydial infection in patients with gonorrhea**
PO
Adults, Elderly. 250–500 mg q6–12h.
Children older than 8 yrs. 25–50 mg/kg/day in 4 divided doses. Maximum: 3 g/day.
▸ *H. pylori*
PO
Adults, Elderly. 500 mg 2–4 times/ day (in combination).
▸ **Topical**
Adults, Elderly. Apply 2 times a day (once in the morning, once in the evening)

▸ **Dosage in renal impairment**

Creatinine Clearance	Dosage Interval
50–80 ml/min	q8–12h
10–50 ml/min	q12–24h
less than 10 ml/min	q24h

CONTRAINDICATIONS
Hypersensitivity to tetracyclines, sulfite, children 8 yrs and younger

INTERACTIONS
Drug
Carbamazepine, phenytoin: May decrease tetracycline blood concentration.
Cholestyramine, colestipol: May decrease tetracycline absorption.
Oral contraceptives: May decrease the effects of these drugs.
Herbal
St. John's wort: May increase risk of photosensitivity.
Food
Dairy products: Inhibit tetracycline absorption.

DIAGNOSTIC TEST EFFECTS
May increase BUN, serum alkaline phosphatase, serum amylase, serum bilirubin, SGOT (AST), and SGPT (ALT) levels.

SIDE EFFECTS
Frequent
Dizziness, lightheadedness, diarrhea, nausea, vomiting, stomach cramps, increased sensitivity of skin to sunlight
Topical: Dry scaly skin, stinging, burning sensation
Occasional
Pigmentation of skin, mucous membranes, itching in rectal or genital area, sore mouth or tongue
Topical: Pain, redness, swelling, other skin irritation.

SERIOUS REACTIONS
• Superinfection (especially fungal), anaphylaxis, and increased intracranial pressure may occur.
• Bulging fontanelles occur rarely in infants.

NURSING CONSIDERATIONS

Baseline Assessment
◄ALERT► Determine the patient's history of allergies, especially to sulfite and tetracyclines before beginning drug therapy.

Lifespan Considerations
• Be aware that tetracycline readily crosses the placenta and is distributed in breast milk.
• Avoid tetracycline use in women during the last half of pregnancy.
• Be aware that tetracycline use may produce permanent tooth discoloration or enamel hypoplasia and inhibit fetal skeletal growth in children 8 years of age or younger.
• Be aware that tetracycline use is not recommended in children 8 years of age and younger.
• There are no age-related precautions noted in the elderly.

Precautions
• Use cautiously in patients who cannot avoid sun or ultraviolet light exposure because this may produce a severe photosensitivity reaction.

Administration and Handling
◄ALERT► Space drug doses evenly around the clock.
PO
• Give capsules and tablets with a full glass of water 1 hour before or 2 hours after meals.
Topical
• Cleanse area gently before application.
• Wear gloves and apply only to the affected area. There is potential for skin staining.

Intervention and Evaluation
• Assess the patient's skin for rash.
• Assess the patient's pattern of daily bowel activity and stool consistency.
• Monitor the patient's food intake and tolerance.
• Be alert for signs and symptoms of superinfection as evidenced by anal or genital pruritus, diarrhea, and ulceration or changes of the oral mucosa.
• Monitor the patient's blood pressure (B/P) and level of consciousness (LOC) because of the potential for increased intracranial pressure.

Patient Teaching
• Advise the patient to continue taking the antibiotic for the full length of treatment and to evenly space drug doses around the clock.
• Instruct the patient to take oral tetracycline doses on an empty stomach 1 hour before or 2 hours after consuming beverages or food.
• Teach the patient to drink a full glass of water with tetracycline capsules and to avoid bedtime tetracycline doses.
• Warn the patient to notify the physician if diarrhea, rash, or any other new symptoms occur.
• Encourage the patient to protect his or her skin from sun exposure and to avoid overexposure to sun or ultraviolet light to prevent photosensitivity reactions.
• Explain to the patient that he or she should not take any medications, including over-the-counter (OTC) drugs, without consulting the physician.
• Explain to the patient that his or her skin may turn yellow with topical tetracycline application and that washing removes the solution. Also explain that fabrics may be stained by heavy topical application.
• Warn the patient not to apply topical tetracycline to deep or open wounds.

atovaquone
aztreonam
bacitracin
chloramphenicol
clindamycin
clofazimine
co-trimoxazole
  (sulfamethoxazole-
  trimethoprim)
dapsone
daptomycin
drotrecogin alfa
fosfomycin
  tromethamine
hydrochloroquine
  sulfate
linezolid
metronidazole
  hydrochloride
nitrofurantoin sodium
pentamidine
  isethionate
quinupristin-
  dalfopristin
sulfasalazine
trimethoprim
vancomycin
  hydrochloride

Uses: Miscellaneous anti-infective agents have a wide variety of uses because they belong to many different subclasses. Some agents, such as atovaquone, chloramphenicol, and linezolid, are used for serious infections when other, less toxic agents have failed or aren't appropriate. Others are prescribed to treat uncommon infections, such as malaria (with hydrochloroquine), leprosy (with dapsone), and trichomoniasis and amebiasis (with metronidazole). Several including aztreonam, clindamycin, and quinupristin combat a broad range of systemic infections; yet some are used for just one indication, such as fosfomycin and nitrofurantoin, which are given solely for urinary tract infections. In addition to treatment, some miscellaneous anti-infectives are used prophylactically, such as vancomycin (to prevent bacterial endocarditis) and co-trimoxazole and pentamidine (to prevent *Pneumocystis carinii* pneumonia).

Action: Miscellaneous anti-infective agents may be bacteriostatic or bactericidal and work in many different ways. (See illustration, *Sites and Mechanisms of Action: Anti-infective Agents*, page 2.) For details, see the specific drug entries.

COMBINATION PRODUCTS

BACTRIM: trimethoprim/ sulfamethoxazole (a sulfonamide) 16 mg/80 mg/ml (injection), 40 mg/200 mg/5 ml (suspension), 80 mg/400 mg or 160 mg/800 mg (tablets).

HELIDAC: metronidazole/bismuth (an antisecretory)/tetracycline (an anti-infective) 250 mg/262 mg/500 mg. MYCITRACIN: bacitracin/polymyxin B (an anti-infective)/neomycin (an aminoglycoside). 400 units/5,000 units/3.5 mg per/g, 500 units/5,000 units/3.5 mg/g.

NEOSPORIN OINTMENT, TRIPLE
ANTIBIOTIC: bacitracin (an anti-infective)/neomycin/polymyxin B (an anti-infective) 400 units/3.5 mg/5,000 units, 400 units/3.5 mg/10,000 units.

POLYSPORIN: bacitracin/polymyxin B (an anti-infective) 500 units/10,000 units/g.

SEPTRA: trimethoprim/sulfamethoxazole (a sulfonamide) 16 mg/80 mg/ml (injection), 40 mg/200 mg/5 ml (suspension), 80 mg/400 mg or 160 mg/800 mg (tablets).

ZOTRIM: trimethoprim/sulfamethoxazole (a sulfonamide)/phenazopyridine (a urinary analgesic) 160 mg/800 mg/200 mg.

atovaquone
ah-**tow**-vah-quon
(Mepron, Wellvone[AUS])

CATEGORY AND SCHEDULE
Pregnancy Risk Category: C

MECHANISM OF ACTION
A systemic anti-infective that inhibits the mitochondrial electron-transport system at the cytochrome bc_1 complex (Complex III). *Therapeutic Effect:* Interrupts nucleic acid and adenosine triphosphate (ATP) synthesis.

INDICATIONS AND DOSAGES
▶ **Pneumocystis carinii pneumonia (PCP)**
PO
Adults. 750 mg with food 2 times a day for 21 days.
▶ **Prevention of PCP**
PO
Adults. 1,500 mg once a day with food.

▶ **Usual pediatric dosage**
PO
Children. 40 mg/kg/day.

CONTRAINDICATIONS
Development or history of potentially life-threatening allergic reaction to the drug

INTERACTIONS
Drug
Rifampin: May decrease atovaquone blood concentration. Atovaquone may increase rifampin blood concentration.
Herbal
None known.
Food
None known.

DIAGNOSTIC TEST EFFECTS
May elevate serum alkaline phosphatase, serum amylase, SGOT (AST), and SGPT (ALT) levels. May decrease serum sodium levels.

SIDE EFFECTS
Frequent (greater than 10%)
Rash, nausea, diarrhea, headache, vomiting, fever, insomnia, cough
Occasional (less than 10%)
Abdominal discomfort, thrush, asthenia (loss of strength, energy), anemia, neutropenia

SERIOUS REACTIONS
• None known.

NURSING CONSIDERATIONS
Precautions
• Use cautiously in elderly patients and in patients with chronic diarrhea, malabsorption syndromes, or severe PCP.
Intervention and Evaluation
• Assess the patient for GI discomfort, nausea, and vomiting.
• Assess the patient's pattern of

daily bowel activity and stool consistency.
• Assess the patient's skin for rash.
• Monitor the patient's Hgb levels, intake and output, and renal function test results.
• Monitor elderly patients closely because of age-related decreased cardiac, liver, and renal function.

Patient Teaching
• Advise the patient to continue therapy for the full length of treatment.
• Warn the patient not to take any other medications without first notifying the physician.
• Urge the patient to notify his or her physician in the event of diarrhea, rash or other new symptom development.

aztreonam
az-**tree**-oh-nam
(Azactam)

CATEGORY AND SCHEDULE
Pregnancy Risk Category: B

MECHANISM OF ACTION
A monobactam bactericidal antibiotic that inhibits bacterial cell wall synthesis. *Therapeutic Effect:* Produces bacterial cell lysis and death.

PHARMACOKINETICS
Completely absorbed after IM administration. Protein binding: 56%–60%. Partially metabolized by hydrolysis. Primarily excreted unchanged in urine. Removed by hemodialysis. **Half-life:** 1.4–2.2 hrs (half-life increased in reduced renal, liver function).

AVAILABILITY
Injection: 500 mg, 1 g, 2 g.

INDICATIONS AND DOSAGES
▸ **Urinary tract infections**
IM/IV
Adults, Elderly. 500 mg–1 g q8–12h.
▸ **Moderate to severe systemic infections**
IM/IV
Adults, Elderly. 1–2 g q8–12h.
▸ **Severe or life-threatening infections**
IV
Adults, Elderly. 2 g q6–8h.
▸ **Mild to severe infections in children**
IV
Children. 30 mg/kg q6–8h.
Maximum: 120 mg/kg/day.
▸ **Dosage in renal impairment**
Dosage and frequency are modified based on creatinine clearance and the severity of infection:

Creatinine Clearance	Dosage
10–30 ml/min	1–2 g initially; then ½ the usual dose at usual intervals
less than 10 ml/min	1–2 g initially; then ¼ the usual dose at usual intervals

UNLABELED USES
Treatment of bone and joint infections

CONTRAINDICATIONS
None known.

INTERACTIONS
Drug
None known.
Herbal
None known.
Food
None known.

DIAGNOSTIC TEST EFFECTS

Positive Coombs' test. May increase serum alkaline phosphatase, serum creatinine, LDH, SGOT (AST), and SGPT (ALT) levels.

IV INCOMPATIBILITIES

Acyclovir (Zovirax), amphotericin (Fungizone), daunorubicin (Cerubidine), ganciclovir (Cytovene), lorazepam (Ativan), metronidazole (Flagyl), vancomycin (Vancocin)

IV COMPATIBILITIES

Aminophylline, bumetanide (Bumex), calcium gluconate, cimetidine (Tagamet), diltiazem (Cardizem), dobutamine (Dobutrex), dopamine (Intropin), famotidine (Pepcid), furosemide (Lasix), heparin, hydromorphone (Dilaudid), insulin (regular), magnesium sulfate, morphine, potassium chloride, propofol (Diprivan)

SIDE EFFECTS

Occasional (less than 3%)
Discomfort and swelling at IM injection site, nausea, vomiting, diarrhea, rash
Rare (less than 1%)
Phlebitis or thrombophlebitis at IV injection site, abdominal cramps, headache, hypotension

SERIOUS REACTIONS

• Superinfections and antibiotic-associated colitis, manifested as abdominal cramps, severe, watery diarrhea, and fever may result from altered bacterial balance.
• Severe hypersensitivity reactions, including anaphylaxis, occur rarely.

NURSING CONSIDERATIONS

Baseline Assessment

◀ALERT▶ Determine the patient's history of allergies, especially to antibiotics, before giving aztreonam.

Lifespan Considerations

• Be aware that aztreonam crosses the placenta, and is distributed in amniotic fluid as well as in low concentrations in breast milk.
• Be aware that the safety and efficacy of aztreonam have not been established in children less than 9 months old.
• In the elderly, age-related renal impairment may require dosage adjustment.

Precautions

• Use cautiously in patients with a history of allergy, especially to antibiotics, or liver or renal impairment.

Administration and Handling

IM
• Shake immediately and vigorously after adding diluent.
• Inject deeply into a large muscle mass.
• Following reconstitution for IM injection, solution is stable for 48 hours at room temperature, or 7 days if refrigerated.
IV
• Store vials at room temperature.
• Solution normally appears colorless to light yellow.
• Following reconstitution, the solution is stable for 48 hours at room temperature, or 7 days if refrigerated.
• Discard the solution if a precipitate forms. Discard unused portions of solution.
• For IV push, dilute each gram with 6–10 ml Sterile Water for Injection.
• For intermittent IV infusion, further dilute with 50 to 100 ml D_5W or 0.9% NaCl.
• For IV push, give over 3 to 5 minutes.

• For IV infusion, administer over 20 to 60 minutes.

Intervention and Evaluation

• Evaluate the patient for signs and symptoms of phlebitis, manifested as heat, pain, and red streaking over the vein and pain at the IM injection site.

• Observe the patient for GI discomfort, nausea, or vomiting.

• Assess the patient's pattern of daily bowel activity and stool consistency.

• Assess the patient's skin for rash.

• Be alert for signs and symptoms of superinfection, including anal or genital pruritus, black hairy tongue, diarrhea, increased temperature, sore throat, ulceration or changes of oral mucosa, and vomiting.

Patient Teaching

• Urge the patient to report any diarrhea, nausea, rash, or vomiting he or she experiences.

---

bacitracin
bah-cih-**tray**-sin
(Baciguent, Bacitracin, Baci-IM)
Do not confuse with Bactrim or Bactroban.

CATEGORY AND SCHEDULE
Pregnancy Risk Category: C
OTC

MECHANISM OF ACTION
An antibiotic that interferes with plasma membrane permeability in susceptible bacteria. *Therapeutic Effect:* Inhibits bacterial cell wall synthesis and is bacteriostatic.

AVAILABILITY
Powder for Irrigation: 50,000 units.
Ophthalmic Ointment.
Topical Ointment.

INDICATIONS AND DOSAGES
▶ **Superficial ocular infections**
Ophthalmic ointment
Adults. ½-inch ribbon in conjunctival sac q3–4h.
▶ **Skin abrasions, superficial skin infections**
Topical ointment
Adults, Children. Apply 1–5 times a day to the affected area.
▶ **Surgical treatment and prophylaxis**
Irrigation
Adults, Elderly. 50,000–150,000 units, as needed.

CONTRAINDICATIONS
None known

INTERACTIONS
Drug
None known.
Herbal
None known.
Food
None known.

DIAGNOSTIC TEST EFFECTS
None known.

SIDE EFFECTS
Rare
Topical: Hypersensitivity reaction as evidenced by allergic contact dermatitis, burning, inflammation, and itching
Ophthalmic: Burning, itching, redness, swelling, pain

SERIOUS EFFECTS
• Severe hypersensitivity reaction, including apnea and hypotension, occurs rarely.

NURSING CONSIDERATIONS
Precautions
◀ ALERT ▶ Familiarize yourself with the side effects of each of a drug's

components when bacitracin is used in a fixed-combination.

Administration and Handling
Ophthalmic
• Place a gloved finger on the patient's lower eyelid and pull it out until a pocket is formed between the eye and lower lid. Place ¼ to ½ inch ointment in the pocket.
• Have the patient close the eye gently for 1 to 2 minutes, rolling his or her eyeball to increase contact area of drug to eye.
• Remove excess ointment around the eye with a tissue.

Intervention and Evaluation
Topical
• Evaluate the patient for signs and symptoms of hypersensitivity as evidenced by burning, inflammation, and itching.
• With preparations containing corticosteroids, closely monitor the patient for any unusual signs or symptoms because corticosteroids may mask clinical signs.
Ophthalmic
• Assess the patient's eye for the therapeutic response or a hypersensitivity reaction manifested as increased burning, itching, redness, and swelling.

Patient Teaching
• Advise the patient to continue therapy for the full length of treatment and to evenly space drug doses around the clock.
• Urge the patient to report any burning, increased irritation, itching, and rash he or she experiences.

chloramphenicol
klor-am-**fen**-ih-call
(Chloromycetin, Chloroptic, Chlorsig [AUS])
Do not confuse with chlorambucil.

CATEGORY AND SCHEDULE
Pregnancy Risk Category: C

MECHANISM OF ACTION
A dichloroacetic acid derivative that acts as a bacteriostatic (may be bactericidal in high concentrations) by binding to bacterial ribosomal receptor sites. *Therapeutic Effect:* Inhibits bacterial protein synthesis.

AVAILABILITY
Capsules: 250 mg.
Oral Suspension: 150 mg/5 ml.
Powder for Injection: 100 mg/ml.
Ophthalmic Solution: 5 mg/ml.
Ophthalmic Ointment: 10 mg/g.

INDICATIONS AND DOSAGES
▶ **Mild to moderate infections from organisms resistant to other less toxic antibiotics**
PO/IV
Adults, Elderly, Children. 50 mg/kg/day in divided doses q6h.
Newborns. 25 mg/kg/day in 4 doses q6h.
Infants older than 2 wks. 50 mg/kg/day in 4 doses q6h.
Neonates weighing less than 2 kg. 25 mg/kg once a day.
Neonates younger than 7 days weighing more than 2 kg. 25 mg/kg once a day.
Neonates 7 days and older weighing more than 2 kg. 50 mg/kg/day in divided doses q12h.
Ophthalmic
Adults, Elderly, Children. Apply

thin strip of ointment to conjunctiva q3–4h.
Adults, Elderly, Children. 1–2 drops of solution 4–6 times/day.
Otic
Adults, Elderly, Children. 2–3 drops into ear 3 times/day.
▶ **Severe infections, infections due to moderately resistant organisms**
PO/IV
Adults, Elderly, Children. 50–100 mg/kg/day in divided doses q6h.
▶ **Dosage in liver or renal impairment**
Dosage is reduced on based on the degree of renal impairment and plasma concentration of the drug. Initially, 1 g, then 500 mg q6h.

CONTRAINDICATIONS
Hypersensitivity to chloramphenicol

INTERACTIONS
Drug
Anticonvulsants, bone marrow depressants: May increase bone marrow depression.
Clindamycin, erythromycin: May antagonize the effects of these drugs.
Oral hypoglycemics: May increase the effects of these drugs.
Phenobarbital, phenytoin, warfarin: May increase blood concentrations of these drugs.
Herbal
None known.
Food
None known.

DIAGNOSTIC TEST EFFECTS
None known. Therapeutic blood level: 10–20 mcg/ml; toxic level: greater than 25 mcg/ml.

SIDE EFFECTS
Occasional
Systemic: Nausea, vomiting, diarrhea

Ophthalmic: Blurred vision, burning, stinging, hypersensitivity reaction
Otic: Hypersensitivity reaction
Rare
"Gray baby" syndrome in neonates (abdominal distention, blue-gray skin color, cardiovascular collapse, unresponsiveness), rash, shortness of breath, confusion, headache, optic neuritis (blurred vision, eye pain), peripheral neuritis (numbness and weakness in feet and hands)

SERIOUS REACTIONS
• Superinfection due to bacterial or fungal overgrowth may occur.
• There is a narrow margin between effective therapy and toxic levels producing blood dyscrasias.
• Bone marrow depression with resulting aplastic anemia, hypoplastic anemia, and pancytopenia may occur weeks or months later.

NURSING CONSIDERATIONS
Baseline Assessment
• Be aware that chloramphenicol should not be given concurrently, if possible, with other drugs that cause bone marrow depression.
• Expect to obtain blood studies to establish the patient's baseline before beginning chloramphenicol therapy.
Precautions
• Use cautiously in patients with bone marrow depression, liver or renal impairment, previous cytotoxic drug therapy, and radiation therapy.
• Use cautiously in pediatric patients, infants and children younger than 2 years of age.
Intervention and Evaluation
• Assess the patient's nausea and monitor the patient for vomiting.

• Evaluate the patient's mental status.
• Test the patient to determine if he or she is experiencing visual disturbances.
• Assess the patient's skin for rash.
• Assess the patient's pattern of daily bowel activity and stool consistency.
• Be alert for signs and symptoms of superinfection manifested as anal or genital pruritus, a change in the oral mucosa, diarrhea, and increased fever.
• Monitor the patient's drug blood levels and know that the therapeutic blood level is 10 to 20 mcg/ml and the toxic level is greater than 25 mcg/ml.

Patient Teaching
• Advise the patient to continue taking chloramphenicol for the full length of treatment and to evenly space drug doses around the clock.
• Instruct the patient that ophthalmic treatment should continue at least 48 hours after the eye returns to normal appearance.
• Teach the patient to take oral doses on an empty stomach, 1 hour before or 2 hours after meals.
• Explain to the patient that gastrointestinal (GI) upset may occur while taking this drug. If GI upset occurs, tell the patient he or she may take the drug with food, but not with iron or vitamins.

clindamycin
klin-da-**my**-sin
(Cleocin, Dalacin[CAN])

CATEGORY AND SCHEDULE
Pregnancy Risk Category: B

MECHANISM OF ACTION
A lincosamide antibiotic that acts as a bacteriostatic by binding to bacterial ribosomal receptor sites. Topically, decreases fatty acid concentration on skin. *Therapeutic Effect:* Inhibits protein synthesis of the bacterial cell wall. Prevents outbreak of acne vulgaris.

PHARMACOKINETICS
Rapidly absorbed from the gastrointestinal (GI) tract. Protein binding: 92%–94%. Widely distributed. Metabolized in liver to some active metabolites. Primarily excreted in urine. Not removed by hemodialysis. **Half-life:** 2.4–3 hrs (half-life is increased with impaired renal function, premature infants).

AVAILABILITY
Capsules: 75 mg, 150 mg, 300 mg.
Oral Solution: 75 mg/5 ml.
Injection: 150 mg/ml.
Vaginal Cream: 2%.
Vaginal Suppository.
Lotion.
Topical Solution.

INDICATIONS AND DOSAGES
▶ **Treatment of chronic bone and joint, respiratory tract, and skin and soft tissue infections, intra-abdominal, female, genitourinary infections, endocarditis, septicemia**
IM/IV
Adults, Elderly. 1.2–1.8 g/day in 2–4 divided doses.
Children. 25–40 mg/kg/day in 3–4 divided doses. Maximum: 4.8 g/day.
PO
Adults, Elderly. 150–450 mg/dose q6–8h.
Children. 10–30 mg/kg/day in 3–4 divided doses. Maximum: 1.8 g/day.
▶ **Bacterial vaginosis**
Intravaginal
Adults. One applicatorful at bedtime

for 3–7 days or 1 suppository at bedtime for 3 days.
PO
Adults, Elderly. 300 mg 2 times/day for 7 days.
▶ **Acne vulgaris**
Topical
Adults. Apply thin layer 2 times/day to affected area.

UNLABELED USES
Treatment of malaria, otitis media, *Pneumocystis carinii* pneumonia (PCP), toxoplasmosis

CONTRAINDICATIONS
History of antibiotic-associated colitis, regional enteritis, or ulcerative colitis, hypersensitivity to clindamycin or lincomycin, known allergy to tartrazine dye

INTERACTIONS
Drug
Adsorbent antidiarrheals: May delay absorption of clindamycin.
Chloramphenicol, erythromycin: May antagonize the effects of clindamycin.
Neuromuscular blockers: May increase the effects of these drugs.
Herbal
None known.
Food
None known.

DIAGNOSTIC TEST EFFECTS
May increase serum alkaline phosphatase, SGOT (AST), and SGPT (ALT) levels.

IV INCOMPATIBILITIES
Allopurinol (Aloprim), filgrastim (Neupogen), fluconazole (Diflucan), idarubicin (Idamycin)

IV COMPATIBILITIES
Amiodarone (Cordarone), diltiazem (Cardizem), heparin, hydromor-

phone (Dilaudid), magnesium sulfate, midazolam (Versed), morphine, multivitamins, propofol (Diprivan)

SIDE EFFECTS
Frequent
Abdominal pain, nausea, vomiting, diarrhea
Vaginal: Vaginitis, itching
Topical: Dry scaly skin
Occasional
Phlebitis, thrombophlebitis with IV administration, pain, induration at IM injection site, allergic reaction, urticaria, pruritus
Vaginal: Headache, dizziness, nausea, vomiting, abdominal pain
Topical: Contact dermatitis, abdominal pain, mild diarrhea, burning or stinging
Rare
Vaginal: Hypersensitivity reaction

SERIOUS REACTIONS
• Antibiotic-associated colitis as evidenced by severe abdominal pain and tenderness, fever, and watery and severe diarrhea, may occur during and several weeks after clindamycin therapy, including the topical form.
• Blood dyscrasias (leukopenia, thrombocytopenia) and nephrotoxicity (proteinuria, azotemia, oliguria) occur rarely.

NURSING CONSIDERATIONS
Baseline Assessment
◀ ALERT ▶ Determine the patient's history of allergies, particularly to aspirin, clindamycin, and lincomycin before beginning drug therapy.
• Avoid, if possible, concurrent use of neuromuscular blocking agents.
Lifespan Considerations
• Be aware that clindamycin readily crosses the placenta and is distributed in breast milk.

• Be aware that it is unknown if the topical and vaginal forms of clindamycin are distributed in breast milk.

• Use cautiously in children less than 1 month old.

• There are no age-related precautions noted in the elderly.

Precautions

• Use cautiously in patients concomitantly using neuromuscular blocking agents.

• Use cautiously in patients with severe renal or liver dysfunction.

• Use cautiously in neonates.

• Use topical preparations cautiously; they should not be applied to abraded areas or near the eyes.

Administration and Handling

PO

• Store capsules at room temperature.

• After reconstitution, oral solution is stable for 2 weeks at room temperature.

• Do not refrigerate oral solution to avoid thickening the solution.

• Give with 8 oz water. May give without regard to food.

IM

• Do not exceed 600 mg/dose.

• Give by deep IM injection.

IV

• IV infusion (piggyback) is stable at room temperature for up to 16 days.

• Dilute 300 to 600 mg with 50 ml D_5W or 0.9% NaCl (900 to 1,200 mg with 100 ml). Never exceed concentration of 18 mg/ml.

• Infuse 50 ml (300–600 mg) piggyback over more than 10 to 20 minutes; Infuse 100 ml (900 mg to 1.2 g) piggyback over more than 30 to 40 minutes. Be aware that severe hypotension or cardiac arrest can occur with too rapid administration.

• Do not administer more than 1.2 g in a single infusion.

Intervention and Evaluation

• Assess the patient's pattern of daily bowel activity and stool consistency. Report diarrhea promptly to the physician because of the potential for developing serious colitis (even with topical or vaginal clindamycin).

• Assess the patient's skin for dryness, irritation, and rash with topical application.

• Be alert for signs and symptoms of superinfection manifested as anal or genital pruritus, a change in oral mucosa, increased fever, and severe diarrhea.

Patient Teaching

• Advise the patient to continue taking clindamycin for the full length of treatment and to evenly space drug doses around the clock.

• Teach the patient to take oral doses with 8 oz water.

• Warn the patient to use caution when applying topical clindamycin concurrently with abrasive, peeling acne agents, soaps, or alcohol-containing cosmetics to avoid cumulative effect.

• Instruct the patient not to apply topical preparations near the eyes or abraded areas.

• Teach the patient that in the event the vaginal form of clindamycin accidentally comes in contact with the eyes to rinse his or her eyes with copious amounts of cool tap water.

• Advise the patient not to engage in sexual intercourse during clindamycin treatment.

clofazimine
klo-**faze**-ih-mean
(Lamprene)

CATEGORY AND SCHEDULE
Pregnancy Risk Category: C

MECHANISM OF ACTION

An antibiotic that binds to mycobacterial DNA. Possesses anti-inflammatory action. *Therapeutic Effect:* Inhibits mycobacterial growth.

AVAILABILITY

Capsules: 50 mg.

INDICATIONS AND DOSAGES

▸ **Leprosy**
PO
Adults, Elderly. 100 mg/day in combination for 3 yrs, then 100 mg/day as single therapy.
Children. 1 mg/kg/day in combination with dapsone and rifampin.
▸ **Erythema nodosum**
PO
Adults, Elderly. 100–200 mg/day for up to 3 mos, then 100 mg/day.

CONTRAINDICATIONS

None significant.

INTERACTIONS

Drug
Dapsone: May decrease the effects of clofazimine.
Herbal
None significant.
Food
Food: May increase the absorption of clofazimine.

DIAGNOSTIC TEST EFFECTS

May increase blood glucose levels.

SIDE EFFECTS

Frequent (greater than 10%)
Dry skin, abdominal pain, nausea, vomiting, diarrhea, discoloration of the skin (pink to brownish-black)
Occasional (10%–1%)
Rash, itching, eye irritation, discoloration of sputum, sweat, urine

SERIOUS REACTIONS

• None significant.

NURSING CONSIDERATIONS

Baseline Assessment
• Assess the patient for sensitivity to clofazimine.
Precautions
• Use cautiously in patients with gastrointestinal problems, including abdominal pain and diarrhea.
Administration and Handling
PO
• May give clofazimine with food.
Intervention and Evaluation
• Monitor the patient's gastrointestinal signs and symptoms.
• Notify the physician if the patient complains of abdominal pain or colic.
Patient Teaching
• Advise the patient that clofazimine use may cause skin discoloration.
• Instruct the patient to take clofazimine with meals to decrease gastrointestinal discomfort.

co-trimoxazole (sulfamethoxazole-trimethoprim)

koe-try-**mox**-oh-zole
(Apo-Sulfatrim[CAN], Bactrim, Bactrim DS[AUS], Cosig Forte[AUS], Novotrimel[CAN], Resprim[AUS], Resprim Forte[AUS], Septra, Septrin[AUS], Septrin Forte[AUS])
Do not confuse with bacitracin, clotrimazole, Sectral, or Septa.

CATEGORY AND SCHEDULE

Pregnancy Risk Category: C

MECHANISM OF ACTION
A sulfonamide and folate antagonist that blocks bacterial synthesis of essential nucleic acids. *Therapeutic Effect:* Produces bactericidal action in susceptible microorganisms.

PHARMACOKINETICS
Rapidly, well absorbed from the gastrointestinal (GI) tract. Widely distributed. Protein binding: 45%–60%. Metabolized in liver. Excreted in urine. Minimally removed by hemodialysis. **Half-life:** 6–12 hrs (trimethoprim 8–10 hrs). Half-life is increased with impaired renal function.

AVAILABILITY
Tablets: 80 mg trimethoprim/ 400 mg sulfamethoxazole; 160 mg/ 800 mg.
Oral Suspension: 40 mg/200 mg per 5 ml.
Injection: 80 mg/400 mg per 5 ml.

INDICATIONS AND DOSAGES
▸ **Mild to moderate infections**
PO/IV
Adults, Elderly, Children older than 2 mos. 6–12 mg/kg/day in divided doses q12h.
▸ **Serious infections, *Pneumocystis Carinii* pneumonia**
PO/IV
Adults, Elderly, Children older than 2 mos. 15–20 mg/kg/day in divided doses q6–8 h.
▸ **Prevention of *Pneumocystis carinii* pneumonia**
PO
Adults. One double-strength tablet each day.
Children. 150 mg/m^2/day on 3 consecutive days/wk.
▸ **Traveler's diarrhea**
PO
Adults, Elderly. One double-strength tablet q12h for 5 days.

▸ **Acute exacerbation of chronic bronchitis**
PO
Adults, Elderly. One double-strength tablet q12h for 14 days.
▸ **Urinary tract infection prophylaxis**
PO
Adults, Elderly, children older than 2 mos. 2 mg/kg/dose once a day.
▸ **Dosage in renal impairment**
The dosage and frequency are modified based on the severity of infection, degree of renal impairment, and serum concentration of the drug. For those with creatinine clearance of 15–30 ml/min, a reduction in dose of 50% is recommended.

UNLABELED USES
Treatment of bacterial endocarditis, biliary tract, bone or joint, and chancroid infections, chlamydial infection, gonorrhea, intra-abdominal infection, meningitis, septicemia, sinusitis, skin and soft tissue infections

CONTRAINDICATIONS
Hypersensitivity to trimethoprim or any sulfonamides, megaloblastic anemia due to folate deficiency, infants younger than 2 mos

INTERACTIONS
Drug
Hemolytics: May increase the risk of toxicity with other hemolytics.
Hydantoin anticonvulsants, oral hypoglycemics, warfarin: May increase or prolong the effects of and increase the risk of toxicity with these drugs.
Liver toxic medications: May increase the risk of liver toxicity.
Methenamine: May form precipitate.
Methotrexate: May increase the effect of methotrexate.

Herbal
None known.
Food
None known.

DIAGNOSTIC TEST EFFECTS

May increase BUN, serum alkaline phosphatase, serum creatinine, serum potassium, SGOT (AST) and SGPT (ALT) levels.

IV INCOMPATIBILITIES

Fluconazole (Diflucan), foscarnet (Foscavir), midazolam (Versed), vinorelbine (Navelbine)

IV COMPATIBILITIES

Diltiazem (Cardizem), heparin, hydromorphone (Dilaudid), lorazepam (Ativan), magnesium sulfate, morphine

SIDE EFFECTS

Frequent
Anorexia, nausea, vomiting, rash (generally 7–14 days after therapy begins), urticaria
Occasional
Diarrhea, abdominal pain, local pain or irritation at IV site
Rare
Headache, vertigo, insomnia, seizures, hallucinations, depression

SERIOUS REACTIONS

• Rash, fever, sore throat, pallor, purpura, cough, and shortness of breath may be early signs of serious adverse reactions.
• Fatalities are rare but have occurred in sulfonamide therapy following Stevens-Johnson syndrome, toxic epidermal necrolysis, fulminant hepatic necrosis, agranulocytosis, aplastic anemia, and other blood dyscrasias.
• The elderly are at increased risk of developing adverse reactions: bone marrow suppression, decreased platelets, and severe dermatologic reactions.

NURSING CONSIDERATIONS

Baseline Assessment
◀ALERT▶ Determine the patient's history of bronchial asthma, hypersensitivity to trimethoprim or any sulfonamide, and sulfite sensitivity before beginning drug therapy.
• Expect to establish the patient's hematologic, liver, and renal baselines.
Lifespan Considerations
• Be aware that co-trimoxazole use is contraindicated during pregnancy at term and during lactation.
• Be aware that co-trimoxazole readily crosses the placenta and is distributed in breast milk.
• Be aware that co-trimoxazole use is contraindicated in children younger than 2 months and that co-trimoxazole use in newborns may produce kernicterus.
• In the elderly, there is an increased risk for bone marrow depression, decreased platelet count, and severe skin reaction.
Precautions
• Use cautiously in patients with G6PD deficiency and impaired renal or liver function.
Administration and Handling
◀ALERT▶ Be aware that drug potency is expressed in terms of trimethoprim content.
PO
• Store tablets and suspension at room temperature.
• Give to the patient on an empty stomach with 8 oz water and be sure to provide the patient with several extra glasses of water each day.
IV
• Be aware that the piggyback IV infusion solution is stable for 2 to 6 hours. Use the solution immediately.

• Discard the solution if it is cloudy or precipitate forms.
• For piggyback IV infusion, dilute each 5 ml with 75 to 125 ml D_5W.
• Do not mix co-trimoxazole with other drugs or solutions.
• Infuse over 60 to 90 minutes and avoid bolus or rapid infusion.
• Do not give IM.
• Ensure the patient is adequately hydrated.

Intervention and Evaluation
• Monitor the patient's intake and output.
• Assess the patient's pattern of daily bowel activity and stool consistency.
• Assess the patient's skin for pallor, purpura, and rash.
• Check the patient's IV site and flow rate.
• Monitor the patient's hematology, liver, and renal function test reports.
• Evaluate the patient for central nervous system (CNS) symptoms such as hallucinations, headache, insomnia, and vertigo.
• Monitor the patient's vital signs at least twice a day.
• Evaluate the patient for cough or shortness of breath.
• Assess the patient for signs and symptoms of bruising, overt bleeding, or swelling.

Patient Teaching
• Advise the patient to continue taking co-trimoxazole for the full length of treatment and to evenly space drug doses around the clock.
• Instruct the patient to take oral co-trimoxazole doses with 8 oz water and to drink several extra glasses of water each day.
• Warn the patient to notify the physician immediately if he or she experiences any new symptoms, especially bleeding, bruising, fever, rash or other skin changes, and sore throat.

dapsone
dap-sewn
(Dapsone)

CATEGORY AND SCHEDULE
Pregnancy Risk Category: C

MECHANISM OF ACTION
An antibiotic that is a competitive antagonist of para-aminobenzoic acid (PABA) and prevents normal bacterial utilization of PABA for synthesis of folic acid. *Therapeutic effect:* Inhibits bacterial growth.

AVAILABILITY
Tablets: 25 mg, 100 mg.

INDICATIONS AND DOSAGES
▶ **Leprosy**
PO
Adults, Elderly. 50–100 mg/day for 3–10 yrs.
Children. 1–2 mg/kg/24 hrs. Maximum: 100 mg/day.
▶ **Dermatitis herpetiformis**
PO
Adults, Elderly. Initially, 50 mg/day. May increase up to 300 mg/day.
▶ *Pneumocystis carinii* **pneumonia (PCP) treatment**
PO
Adults, Elderly. 100 mg/day in combination with trimethoprim for 21 days.
▶ **PCP prophylaxis**
PO
Adults, Elderly. 100 mg/day.
Children older than 1 mo. 2 mg/kg/day. Maximum: 100 mg/day.

UNLABELED USES
Treatment of inflammatory bowel disorder, malaria

CONTRAINDICATIONS
None significant.

INTERACTIONS
Drug
Methotrexate: May increase hematologic reactions.
Probenecid: May decrease the excretion of dapsone.
Protease inhibitors, including ritonavir: May increase dapsone blood concentration.
Rifampin: May decrease rifampin blood concentration.
Trimethoprim: May increase the risk of toxic effects.
Herbal
St. John's wort: May decrease dapsone blood concentration.
Food
None significant.

DIAGNOSTIC TEST EFFECTS
None significant.

SIDE EFFECTS
Frequent (greater than 10%)
Hemolytic anemia, methemoglobinemia, skin rash
Occasional (10%–1%)
Hemolysis, photosensitivity reaction

SERIOUS REACTIONS
• Agranulocytosis and blood dyscrasias may occur.

NURSING CONSIDERATIONS
Baseline Assessment
• As ordered, obtain the patient's baseline complete blood count (CBC).
• Determine if the patient has a hypersensitivity to sulfa.
Precautions
• Use cautiously in patients with agranulocytosis, aplastic anemia, G6PD deficiency, sensitivity to sulfa, and severe anemia.

Administration and Handling
PO
• May give dapsone with or without food.
Intervention and Evaluation
• Assess the patient's skin for a dermatologic reaction.
• Monitor the patient for signs and symptoms of hemolysis and jaundice.
• Monitor the patient's CBC.
Patient Teaching
• Explain to the patient that frequent blood tests are necessary, especially during early dapsone therapy.
• Instruct the patient to notify the physician and discontinue dapsone use if a rash develops.
• Warn the patient to report if he or she experiences persistent fatigue, fever, or sore throat.
• Encourage the patient to avoid overexposure to sun or ultraviolet light.

daptomycin
dap-toe-my-sin
(Cubicin)

CATEGORY AND SCHEDULE
Pregnancy Risk Category: B

MECHANISM OF ACTION
A lipopeptide antibacterial agent that binds to bacterial membranes and causes a rapid depolarization of membrane potential. *Therapeutic Effect:* Inhibits protein synthesis, resulting in bacterial cell death.

PHARMACOKINETICS
Widely distributed. Protein binding: 90%. Primarily excreted unchanged in urine. Moderately removed by hemodialysis. **Half-life:** 7–8 hrs,

half-life is increased in patients with impaired renal function.

AVAILABILITY
Powder for Injection: 250 mg/vial, 500 mg/vial.

INDICATIONS AND DOSAGES
▸ **Complicated skin and skin-structure infections**
IV infusion
Adults, Elderly. 4 mg/kg every 24 hrs for 7–14 days.

▸ **Severe renal function impairment, creatinine clearance less than 30 ml/min**
IV infusion
Adults, Elderly. 4 mg/kg every 48 hrs for 7–14 days.

CONTRAINDICATIONS
None known

INTERACTIONS
Drug
HMG-CoA reductase inhibitors: May cause myopathy.
Tobramycin: Increases the serum concentration of daptomycin.
Herbal
None known.
Food
None known.

DIAGNOSTIC TEST EFFECTS
May increase creatine phosphokinase (CPK) levels. May alter liver function test results.

IV INCOMPATIBILITIES
Incompatible with dextrose-containing diluents. If same IV line is used to administer different drugs, the line should be flushed with 0.9% NaCl.

SIDE EFFECTS
Frequent (6%–5%)
Constipation, nausea, peripheral injection site reactions, headache, diarrhea
Occasional (4%–3%)
Insomnia, rash, vomiting
Rare (less than 3%–2%)
Pruritus, dizziness, hypotension

SERIOUS REACTIONS
• Skeletal muscle myopathy, characterized by muscle pain and weakness, particularly of the distal extremities, occurs rarely.
• Antibiotic-associated colitis, marked by severe abdominal pain and tenderness, fever, watery and severe diarrhea, may result from altered bacterial balance.

NURSING CONSIDERATIONS
Baseline Assessment
• Obtain the patient's blood culture and sensitivity tests, as ordered, before giving the first dose of daptomycin. Therapy may begin before the test results are known.
Lifespan Considerations
• Be aware that it is unknown if daptomycin is distributed in breast milk.
• Be aware that the safety and efficacy of this drug have not been established in children younger than 18 years of age.
• There are no age-related precautions noted in the elderly.
Precautions
• Use cautiously in pregnant patients and patients with history of or current musculoskeletal disorders and renal impairment.
• Discontinue concurrent use with HMG-CoA reductase inhibitors because they may cause myopathy.
Administration and Handling
IV
• Store in refrigerator.
• Normally appears as a pale yellow to light brown lyophilized cake.

• Reconstituted solution is stable for 12 hours at room temperature or up to 48 hours if refrigerated.

• Inspect for particulate matter.

• Reconstitute 250 mg vial with 5 ml 0.9% NaCl; reconstitute 500 mg vial with 10 ml 0.9% NaCl. Further dilute in 50 ml 0.9% NaCl.

• For intermittent IV infusion (piggyback), infuse over 30 minutes.

Intervention and Evaluation

• Examine the patient's mouth for white patches on mucous membranes and tongue.

• Assess the patient's daily pattern of bowel activity and stool consistency. Mild gastrointestinal (GI) effects may be tolerable, but increasing severity may indicate the onset of antibiotic-associated colitis.

• Be alert for signs and symptoms of superinfection including abdominal pain, moderate to severe diarrhea, severe anal or genital pruritus, and severe mouth soreness.

• Monitor the patient for dizziness and institute appropriate safety measures.

Patient Teaching

• Warn the patient to notify the physician if he or she experiences headache, nausea, rash, or any new symptoms.

• Tell the patient to report any new development of muscle weakness, or severe diarrhea.

---

drotrecogin alfa
dro-trae-**coe**-gin alfa
(Xigris)

CATEGORY AND SCHEDULE
Pregnancy Risk Category: C

MECHANISM OF ACTION

An activated protein C that possesses anti-inflammatory, antithrombotic, and profibrinolytic effects. Recombinant-produced preparation of human-activated protein C. *Therapeutic Effect:* Interferes with some of the body's harmful responses to severe infection, including the formation of blood clots, that can lead to organ failure and death.

PHARMACOKINETICS

Inactivated by endogenous plasma protease inhibitors. Clearance occurs within 2 hrs of initiating infusion. **Half-life:** 1.6 hrs.

AVAILABILITY

Powder for Infusion: 5 mg, 20 mg.

INDICATIONS AND DOSAGES

▶ **Severe sepsis**
IV infusion
Adults, Elderly. 24 mcg/kg/hr given for 96 hrs.

CONTRAINDICATIONS

Active internal bleeding, evidence of cerebral herniation, presence of an epidural catheter, intracranial neoplasm or mass lesion, recent (within the past 3 mos) hemorrhage stroke, recent (within the last 2 mos) intracranial or intraspinal surgery or severe head trauma, trauma with an increased risk of life-threatening bleeding

INTERACTIONS

Drug
None known.
Use caution when used with other drugs that affect hemostasis.
Herbal
None known.
Food
None known.

DIAGNOSTIC TEST EFFECTS
May variably prolong activated partial thromboplastin time (APTT).

IV INCOMPATIBILITIES
Do not mix with other medications.

IV COMPATIBILITIES
0.9% NaCl, lactated Ringer's, dextrose are the only solutions that can be administered through the same line.

SIDE EFFECTS
None known.

SERIOUS REACTIONS
• Bleeding (intrathoracic, retroperitoneal, genitourinary[GU], gastrointestinal [GI], intra-abdominal, intracranial) rarely occurs (2%).

NURSING CONSIDERATIONS

Baseline Assessment
• Know the criteria that must be met before initiating drotrecogin alfa therapy, including 3 or greater systemic inflammatory response criteria (fever, heart rate greater than 90 beats/minute, respiratory rate greater than 20 breaths/minute, increased white blood cell [WBC] count); actual body weight less than 135 kg; older than 18 years of age; not pregnant or breast-feeding; and at least one sepsis-induced organ or system failure (cardiovascular, liver, renal, respiratory, or unexplained metabolic acidosis).

Lifespan Considerations
• Be aware that it is unknown if drotrecogin alfa causes fetal harm or is excreted in breast milk.
• Be aware that the safety and efficacy of drotrecogin alfa have not been established in children or the elderly.

Precautions
• Use cautiously in patients concurrently using heparin.
• Use cautiously in patients with chronic severe liver disease, intracranial aneurysm, a platelet count less than 30,000/mm^3, prolonged prothrombin time, and recent (within the past 6 weeks) gastrointestinal (GI) bleeding.
• Use cautiously in patients with recent (within the past 3 days) thrombolytic therapy and recent (within the past 7 days) anticoagulant or aspirin therapy.

Administration and Handling

IV
• Store unreconstituted vials at room temperature.
• Start infusion within 3 hours after reconstitution.
• Reconstitute 5-mg vials with 2.5 ml Sterile Water for Injection and 20-mg vials with 10 ml Sterile Water for Injection. Resulting concentration is 2 mg/ml.
• Slowly add the Sterile Water for Injection by swirling; do not shake or invert vial.
• Further dilute with 0.9% NaCl.
• Withdraw amount from vial and add to infusion bag containing 0.9% NaCl for a final concentration of between 100 and 200 mcg/ml.
• Direct the stream to the side of the bag to minimize agitation.
• Invert infusion bag to mix solution.
• Administer through a dedicated IV line or a dedicated lumen of a multilumen central venous catheter.
• Administer infusion rate of 24 mcg/kg/hr for 96 hours.
• If infusion is interrupted, restart drotrecogin alfa at 24 mcg/kg/hr as prescribed.

Intervention and Evaluation
• Monitor the patient closely for hemorrhagic complications.

Patient Teaching
• Warn the patient to immediately notify the physician if he or she experiences signs or symptoms of unusual bleeding
• Explain to the patient that bleeding may occur for up to 28 days after treatment.

fosfomycin tromethamine
foss-foe-**my**-sin
(Monurol)
Do not confuse with Monopril.

CATEGORY AND SCHEDULE
Pregnancy Risk Category: B

MECHANISM OF ACTION
An antibiotic and urinary tract infection agent that inhibits the synthesis of peptidoglycan. *Therapeutic Effect:* Prevents bacterial cell wall synthesis. Bactericidal.

AVAILABILITY
Powder: 3 g.

INDICATIONS AND DOSAGES
▶ **Urinary tract infection (UTI)**
PO
Females. 3 g mixed in 4 oz water as a single dose.
Males (complicated UTI). 3 g a day for 2–3 days.

CONTRAINDICATIONS
None known

INTERACTIONS
Drug
Metoclopramide: Lowers serum concentration and urinary excretion of fosfomycin.
Herbal
None known.

Food
None known.

DIAGNOSTIC TEST EFFECTS
May increase blood eosinophil count, serum alkaline phosphatase, serum bilirubin, SGOT (AST), and SGPT (ALT) levels. May alter platelet and white blood cell (WBC) counts. May decrease blood Hct and Hgb levels.

SIDE EFFECTS
Occasional (9%–3%)
Diarrhea, nausea, headache, back pain
Rare (less than 2%)
Dysmenorrhea, pharyngitis, abdominal pain, rash

SERIOUS REACTIONS
• None known.

NURSING CONSIDERATIONS
Administration and Handling
• Give without regard to food.
Patient Teaching
• Advise the patient that symptoms should improve 2 to 3 days after the initial dose of fosfomycin.
• Teach the patient to always mix fosfomycin with water before consuming.

hydroxychloroquine sulfate
hi-drocks-ee-**klor**-oh-kwin
(Plaquenil)
Do not confuse with hydrocortisone or hydroxyzine.

CATEGORY AND SCHEDULE
Pregnancy Risk Category: C

MECHANISM OF ACTION

An antimalarial and antirheumatic that concentrates in parasite acid vesicles, interfering with parasite protein synthesis, and increasing pH. Antirheumatic action unknown but may involve suppressing formation of antigens responsible for hypersensitivity reactions. *Therapeutic Effect:* Inhibits parasite growth.

AVAILABILITY

Tablets: 200 mg (155 mg base).

INDICATIONS AND DOSAGES

▶ **Suppression of malaria**
PO
• *Adults.* 310 mg base weekly on same day each week.
• *Children.* 5 mg base/kg/wk. Begin 2 wks before exposure; continue 6–8 wks after leaving endemic area or if therapy is not begun before exposure.

▶ **Treatment of malaria**
PO
Adults. 620 mg base.
Children. 10 mg base/kg given in 2 divided doses 6 hrs apart.

▶ **Treatment of malaria (acute attack; dose [mg base]):**

Dose	Times	Adults	Children
Initial	Day 1	620 mg	10 mg/kg
Second	6 hrs later	310 mg	5 mg/kg
Third	Day 2	310 mg	5 mg/kg
Fourth	Day 3	310 mg	5 mg/kg

▶ **Rheumatoid arthritis**
PO
Adults. Initially, 400–600 mg (310–465 mg base) a day for 5–10 days; gradually increase dosage to optimum response level. Maintenance (usually within 4–12 wks): Decrease dose by 50%, continue at level of 200–400 mg/day. Maximum effect may not be seen for several months.

▶ **Lupus erythematosus**
PO
Adults. Initially, 400 mg 1–2 times/day for several weeks or months. Maintenance: 200–400 mg/day.

UNLABELED USES

Treatment of juvenile arthritis, sarcoid-associated hypercalcemia

CONTRAINDICATIONS

Long-term therapy for children, porphyria, psoriasis, retinal or visual field changes

INTERACTIONS

Drug
Penicillamine: May increase blood concentration of this drug. May increase the risk of hematologic and renal or severe skin reaction when taken concurrently with this drug.
Herbal
None known.
Food
None known.

DIAGNOSTIC TEST EFFECTS

None known.

SIDE EFFECTS

Frequent
Mild transient headache, anorexia, nausea, vomiting
Occasional
Visual disturbances, nervousness, fatigue, pruritus (especially of palms, soles, scalp), irritability, personality changes, diarrhea
Rare
Stomatitis dermatitis, impaired hearing

SERIOUS REACTIONS

• Ocular toxicity, especially retinopathy, which may progress even after drug is discontinued, may occur.

• Prolonged therapy may result in peripheral neuritis, neuromyopathy, hypotension, electrocardiogram (EKG) changes, agranulocytosis, aplastic anemia, thrombocytopenia, seizures, and psychosis.
• Overdosage may result in headache, vomiting, visual disturbance, drowsiness, seizures, and hypokalemia followed by cardiovascular collapse and death.

NURSING CONSIDERATIONS

Baseline Assessment
• Evaluate the patient's complete blood count (CBC) and liver function test results.

Precautions
• Use cautiously in patients who abuse alcohol or have a history of alcohol abuse.
• Use cautiously in patients with G6PD deficiency and liver disease.
• Be aware that children are especially susceptible to hydroxychloroquine's fatal effects.

Administration and Handling
◀ALERT▶ 200 mg hydroxychloroquine = 155 mg base.

Intervention and Evaluation
• Monitor the patient and promptly report any visual disturbances experienced by the patient to the physician.
• Evaluate the patient for gastrointestinal (GI) distress.
• Give the drug dose with food for treatment of malaria.
• Monitor the patient's liver function test results.
• Assess the patient's buccal mucosa and skin. Evaluate the patient for pruritus.
• Report to the physician immediately if the patient experiences impaired hearing.

Patient Teaching
• Advise the patient to continue taking hydroxychloroquine sulfate for the full length of treatment.
• Explain to the patient that in long-term therapy, therapeutic response may not be evident for up to 6 months.
• Warn the patient to immediately notify the physician of any new symptom of decreased hearing, muscular weakness, tinnitus, and visual difficulties.

linezolid
lyn-eh-**zoe**-lid
(Zyvox)
Do not confuse with Vioxx.

CATEGORY AND SCHEDULE
Pregnancy Risk Category: C

MECHANISM OF ACTION
An oxalodinone that binds to a site on bacterial 23S ribosomal RNA This action prevents the formation of the complex that is an essential component of bacterial translation process. *Therapeutic Effect:* Bacteriostatic against enterococci and staphylococci, bactericidal against streptococci.

PHARMACOKINETICS
Rapidly, extensively absorbed after PO administration. Protein binding: 31%. Metabolized in liver by oxidation. Excreted in urine. **Half-life:** 4–5.4 hrs.

AVAILABILITY
Tablets: 400 mg, 600 mg.
Powder for Reconstitution (PO): 100 mg/5 ml.
Injection: 2 mg/ml in 100-ml, 300-ml bags.

INDICATIONS AND DOSAGES

▸ **Treatment of vancomycin-resistant** *Enterococcus faecium* **(VRE) infections**
PO/IV
Adults, Elderly, Children older than 12 yrs. 600 mg q12h for 14–28 days.

▸ **Nosocomial pneumonia, community-acquired pneumonia (CAP), complicated skin infections**
PO/IV
Adults, Elderly. 600 mg q12h for 10–14 days.

▸ **Uncomplicated skin infections**
PO/IV
Adults, Elderly. 400 mg q12h for 10–14 days.
Children older than 12 yrs. 600 mg q12h.
Children 5–11 yrs. 10 mg/kg/dose q12h.

CONTRAINDICATIONS
None known

INTERACTIONS
Drug
Adrenergic agents (sympathomimetics): Increase effects of linezolid.
MAOIs: Decreases the effects of these drugs.
Herbal
None known.
Food
None known.

DIAGNOSTIC TEST EFFECTS
May decrease blood Hgb, platelet count, white blood cell (WBC) count, and SGPT (ALT) levels.

IV INCOMPATIBILITIES
Amphotericin B complex (Abelcet, AmBisome, Amphotec), chlorpromazine (Thorazine), diazepam (Valium), erythromycin (Erythrocin), pentamidine (Pentam IV), phenytoin (Dilantin), sulfamethoxazole-trimethoprim (Bactrim)

SIDE EFFECTS
Occasional (5%–2%)
Diarrhea, nausea, headache
Rare (less than 2%)
Taste alteration, vaginal candidiasis (discharge, itching), fungal infection, dizziness, tongue discoloration

SERIOUS REACTIONS
• Thrombocytopenia occurs rarely.
• Myelosuppression occurs.
• Antibiotic-associated colitis manifested as severe abdominal pain and tenderness, fever, and watery and severe diarrhea may result from altered bacterial balance.

NURSING CONSIDERATIONS

Lifespan Considerations
• Be aware that it is unknown if linezolid is distributed in breast milk.
• Be aware that the safety and efficacy of linezolid have not been established in children.
• There are no age-related precautions noted in the elderly.
Precautions
• Use cautiously in patients with carcinoid syndrome, pheochromocytoma, severe renal or liver impairment, uncontrolled hypertension, and untreated hyperthyroidism.
Administration and Handling
PO
• Give without regard to meals.
• Use suspension within 21 days after reconstitution.
IV
◀**ALERT**▶ Do not mix with other medications. If same line is used, flush with compatible fluid (D_5W, 0.9% NaCl, lactated Ringer's).

• Store at room temperature and protect from light.
• Know that yellow color does not affect potency.
• Infuse over 30 to 120 minutes.

Intervention and Evaluation

• Assess the patient's pattern of daily bowel activity and stool consistency. Mild gastrointestinal (GI) effects may be tolerable, but increasing severity may indicate the onset of antibiotic-associated colitis.
• Be alert for signs and symptoms of superinfection manifested as abdominal pain, moderate to severe diarrhea, severe anal or genital pruritus, and severe mouth soreness.
• Monitor the patient's complete blood count (CBC) weekly.

Patient Teaching

• Advise the patient to continue linezolid therapy for the full length of treatment and to evenly space drug doses around the clock.
• Explain that linezolid may cause GI upset. Tell the patient that he or she may take linezolid with food or milk if GI upset occurs.
• Teach the patient to avoid excessive amounts of tyramine-containing foods (e.g., aged cheese, red wine). Give the patient a list of tyramine-containing foods.
• Warn the patient to notify the physician if symptoms of infection get persistently worse.

metronidazole hydrochloride

meh-trow-**nye**-dah-zoll
(Apo-Metronidazole[CAN], Flagyl, MetroCream, MetroGel, Metrogyl[AUS], MetroLotion, Metronide[AUS], NidaGel[CAN], Noritate, Novonidazol[CAN], Rozex[AUS], Satric 500)

CATEGORY AND SCHEDULE
Pregnancy Risk Category: B

MECHANISM OF ACTION
A nitroimidazole derivative that is an antibacterial and antiprotozoal. Disrupts bacterial and protozoal DNA and inhibits nucleic acid synthesis. *Therapeutic Effect:* Produces bactericidal, amebicidal, trichomonacidal effects. Produces anti-inflammatory, immunosuppressive effects when applied topically.

PHARMACOKINETICS
Well absorbed from the gastrointestinal (GI) tract, minimal absorption after topical application. Protein binding: less than 20%. Widely distributed, crosses blood-brain barrier. Metabolized in liver to active metabolite. Primarily excreted in urine; partially eliminated in feces. Removed by hemodialysis. **Half-life:** 8 hrs (half-life is increased in patients with alcoholic liver disease, neonates).

AVAILABILITY
Tablets: 250 mg, 500 mg.
Tablets (extended-release): 750 mg.
Capsules: 375 mg.
Powder for Injection: 500 mg.
Injection (Infusion): 500 mg/ 100 ml.
Lotion: 0.75%.
Vaginal Gel: 0.75%.

Topical Gel: 0.75%.
Topical Cream: 0.75%, 1%.

INDICATIONS AND ROUTES
▸ **Amebiasis**
PO
Adults, Elderly. 500–750 mg q8h.
Children. 35–50 mg/kg/day in divided doses q8h.
▸ **Parasitic infections**
PO
Adults, Elderly. 250 mg q8h or 2 g as a single dose.
Children. 15–30 mg/kg/day in divided doses q8h.
▸ **Anaerobic skin and skin-structure, central nervous system (CNS), lower respiratory tract, bone, joint, intra-abdominal, and gynecologic infections, endocarditis, and septicemia**
PO/IV
Adults, Elderly, Children. 30 mg/kg/day in divided doses q6h. Maximum: 4 g/day.
▸ **Antibiotic-associated pseudomembranous colitis (AAPC)**
PO
Adults, Elderly. 250–500 mg 3–4 times/day for 10–14 days.
Children. 30 mg/kg/day in divided doses q6h for 7–10 days.
▸ *Helicobacter pylori*
PO
Adults, Elderly. 250–500 mg 3 times/day (in combination).
Children. 15–20 mg/kg/day in 2 divided doses.
▸ **Bacterial vaginosis**
Intravaginal
Adults. One applicatorful 2 times/day or once a day at bedtime for 5 days.
PO
Adults. 750 mg at bedtime for 7 days.
▸ *Rosacea*
Topical
Adults. Thin application 2 times/day to affected area. Cream: Once a day. Lotion: Apply twice a day.

UNLABELED USES
Topical application in treatment of acne rosacea, treatment of bacterial vaginosis, treatment of grade III-IV decubitus ulcers with anaerobic infection, treatment of *H. pylori*–associated gastritis and duodenal ulcer, treatment of inflammatory bowel disease

CONTRAINDICATIONS
Hypersensitivity to metronidazole or other nitroimidazole derivatives (also parabens with topical application)

INTERACTIONS
Drug
Alcohol: May cause disulfiram-type reaction.
Disulfiram: May increase toxicity with disulfiram.
Oral anticoagulants: May increase the effects of these drugs.
Herbal
None known.
Food
None known.

DIAGNOSTIC TEST EFFECTS
May increase LDH concentrations, SGOT (AST), and SGPT (ALT) levels.

IV INCOMPATIBILITIES
Amphotericin B complex (Abelcet, AmBisome, Amphotec), filgrastim (Neupogen)

IV COMPATIBILITIES
Diltiazem (Cardizem), dopamine (Intropin), heparin, hydromorphone (Dilaudid), lorazepam (Ativan), magnesium sulfate, midazolam (Versed), morphine

SIDE EFFECTS

Frequent

Anorexia, nausea, dry mouth, metallic taste

Vaginal: Symptomatic cervicitis and vaginitis, abdominal cramps, uterine pain

Occasional

Diarrhea or constipation, vomiting, dizziness, erythematous rash, urticaria, reddish brown or dark urine

Topical: Transient redness, mild dryness, burning, irritation, stinging, tearing when applied too close to eyes

Vaginal: Vaginal, perineal, vulvar itching; vulvar swelling

Rare

Mild, transient leukopenia, thrombophlebitis with IV therapy

SERIOUS REACTIONS

• Oral therapy may result in furry tongue, glossitis, cystitis, dysuria, pancreatitis, and flattening of T waves with electrocardiogram (EKG) readings.

• Peripheral neuropathy, manifested as numbness, tingling, and paresthesia, which is usually reversible if treatment is stopped immediately after neurologic symptoms appear, occurs.

• Seizures occur occasionally.

NURSING CONSIDERATIONS

Baseline Assessment

• Determine the patient's history of hypersensitivity to metronidazole or other nitroimidazole derivatives (and parabens with topical).

• Obtain patient specimens for diagnostic tests before giving the first dose of metronidazole. Therapy may begin before the test results are known.

Lifespan Considerations

• Be aware that metronidazole readily crosses the placenta and is distributed in breast milk.

• Be aware that metronidazole use is contraindicated during the first trimester of pregnancy in women with trichomoniasis. Topical use during pregnancy or during breast-feeding is discouraged.

• There are no age-related precautions noted in children.

• In the elderly, age-related liver impairment may require dosage adjustment.

Precautions

• Use cautiously in patients with blood dyscrasias, central nervous system (CNS) disease, predisposition to edema, and severe liver dysfunction.

• Use cautiously in those patients concurrently on corticosteroid therapy.

• Be aware that the safety and efficacy of topical administration in those younger than 21 years of age have not been established.

Administration and Handling

PO

• Give metronidazole without regard to meals. Give with food to decrease gastrointestinal (GI) irritation.

IV

• Store ready-to-use infusion bags at room temperature.

• Infuse over more than 30 to 60 minutes. Do not give as a bolus.

Intervention and Evaluation

• Avoid prolonged use of indwelling catheters.

• Assess the patient's pattern of daily bowel activity and stool consistency.

• Monitor the patient's intake and output and assess the patient for urinary problems.

• Be alert for neurologic symptoms,

such as dizziness or numbness, tingling, or paresthesia of the extremities.

• Assess the patient for rash and urticaria.

• Be alert for signs and symptoms of superinfection manifested as anal or genital pruritus, furry tongue, ulceration or change of oral mucosa, and vaginal discharge.

Patient Teaching

• Explain to the patient that his or her urine may be red-brown or dark during drug therapy.

• Urge the patient to avoid alcohol and alcohol-containing preparations (e.g., cough syrups, elixirs) while taking metronidazole.

• Warn the patient to avoid tasks requiring mental alertness or motor skills until his or her response to the drug is established. Metronidazole may cause dizziness.

• Stress to patients taking metronidazole for trichomoniasis that they should refrain from sexual intercourse until the physician advises otherwise.

• In amebiasis patients, check stool specimens frequently.

• Warn patients taking the topical version of metronidazole to avoid drug contact with eyes.

• Tell the patient that he or she may apply cosmetics after topical drug application.

• Explain to the patient that metronidazole acts on papules, pustules, and redness, but has no effect on ocular problems (conjunctivitis, keratitis, blepharitis), rhinophyma (hypertrophy of nose), or telangiectasia.

• Urge rosacea patients to avoid alcohol, excessive sunlight, exposure to extremes of hot and cold temperatures, and hot and spicy foods.

nitrofurantoin sodium

ny-tro-feur-**an**-twon
(Apo-Nitrofurantoin[CAN],
Furadantin, Macrobid,
Macrodantin, Novo-Furan[CAN],
Ralodantin[AUS])

CATEGORY AND SCHEDULE
Pregnancy Risk Category: B

MECHANISM OF ACTION
An antibacterial, urinary tract infection agent. Inhibits bacterial enzyme systems that may alter ribosomal proteins. *Therapeutic Effect:* Inhibits protein, DNA, RNA, cell wall synthesis. Bacteriostatic (bactericidal at high concentration).

PHARMACOKINETICS
Microcrystalline: rapidly, completely absorbed; macrocrystalline: more slowly absorbed. Food increases absorption. Protein binding: 40%. Primarily concentrated in urine, kidneys. Metabolized in most body tissues. Primarily excreted in urine. Removed by hemodialysis.
Half-life: 20–60 min.

AVAILABILITY
Capsules (Macrodantin): 25 mg, 50 mg, 100 mg
Capsules (Macrobid): 100 mg.
PO Suspension (Furadantin): 25 mg/5 ml.

INDICATIONS AND DOSAGES
▶ **Initial or recurrent urinary tract infection (UTI)**
PO
Adults, Elderly. 50–100 mg 4 times/day. Maximum: 400 mg/day.
Children younger than 1 mo. 5–7 mg/kg in 4 divided doses. Maximum: 400 mg/day.

▶ **Long-term prophylactic therapy of urinary tract infection (UTI)**
PO
Adults, Elderly. 50–100 mg as a single evening dose.
Children. 1–2 mg/kg in 1–2 divided doses.

UNLABELED USES
Prophylaxis of bacterial UTIs

CONTRAINDICATIONS
Infants younger than 1 mo because of hemolytic anemia, anuria, oliguria, substantial renal impairment (creatinine clearance less than 40 ml/min)

INTERACTIONS
Drug
Hemolytics: May increase the risk of nitrofurantoin toxicity.
Neurotoxic medications: May increase the risk of neurotoxicity.
Probenecid: May increase blood concentration and toxicity of nitrofurantoin.
Herbal
None known.
Food
None known.

DIAGNOSTIC TEST EFFECTS
None known.

SIDE EFFECTS
Frequent
Anorexia, nausea, vomiting, dark yellow or brown urine
Occasional
Abdominal pain, diarrhea, rash, pruritus, urticaria, hypertension, headache, dizziness, drowsiness
Rare
Photosensitivity, transient alopecia, asthmatic attack in those with history of asthma

SERIOUS REACTIONS
• Superinfection, liver toxicity, peripheral neuropathy (may be irreversible), Stevens-Johnson syndrome, permanent pulmonary function impairment, and anaphylaxis occur rarely.

NURSING CONSIDERATIONS
Baseline Assessment
• Determine the patient's history of asthma.
• Evaluate the patient's laboratory test results for renal and liver baselines.
Lifespan Considerations
• Be aware that nitrofurantoin readily crosses the placenta and is distributed in breast milk.
• Be aware that nitrofurantoin use is contraindicated at term and during breast-feeding when an infant is suspected of having G6PD deficiency.
• There are no age-related precautions noted in children older than 1 month of age.
• The elderly are more likely to develop acute pneumonitis and peripheral neuropathy.
• In the elderly, age-related renal impairment may require dosage adjustment.
Precautions
• Use cautiously in patients with anemia, debilitated (greater risk of peripheral neuropathy), diabetes mellitus, electrolyte imbalance, G6PD deficiency (greater risk of hemolytic anemia), renal impairment, and vitamin B deficiency.
Administration and Handling
PO
• Give nitrofurantoin with food or milk to enhance absorption and reduce gastrointestinal (GI) upset.
Intervention and Evaluation
• Monitor the patient's intake and

output and renal function test results.

• Assess the patient's pattern of daily bowel activity and stool consistency.

• Assess the patient's skin for rash and urticaria.

• Be alert for signs and symptoms of peripheral neuropathy, such as numbness or tingling, especially of the lower extremities.

• Observe the patient for signs and symptoms of liver toxicity manifested as arthralgia, fever, hepatomegaly, and rash.

• Perform a respiratory assessment of the patient. Auscultate the patient's lungs, check for chest pain, cough, and difficulty breathing.

Patient Teaching

• Explain to the patient that his or her urine may become dark yellow or brown with nitrofurantoin use.

• Teach the patient to take nitrofurantoin with food or milk for best results and to reduce GI upset.

• Advise the patient to continue taking nitrofurantoin for the full length of therapy.

• Urge the patient to avoid sun and ultraviolet light, to use sunscreens, and wear protective clothing.

• Warn the patient to notify the physician if chest pain, cough, difficult breathing, fever, or numbness and tingling of fingers or toes occurs.

• Explain to the patient that alopecia is a rare occurrence and is only temporary.

pentamidine isethionate
pen-**tam**-ih-deen
(NebuPent, Pentacarinat[CAN], Pentam-300)

CATEGORY AND SCHEDULE
Pregnancy Risk Category: C

MECHANISM OF ACTION
An anti-infective, antiprotozoal that interferes with nuclear metabolism and incorporation of nucleotides. *Therapeutic Effect:* Inhibits DNA, RNA, phospholipid, protein synthesis.

PHARMACOKINETICS
Minimal absorption after inhalation, well absorbed after IM administration. Widely distributed. Primarily excreted in urine. Minimally removed by hemodialysis. **Half-life:** 6.5 hrs (half-life is increased with impaired renal function).

AVAILABILITY
Injection (Pentam-300): 300 mg.
Powder for Nebulization (Nebupent): 300 mg.

INDICATIONS AND DOSAGES
▸ *Pneumocystis carinii* **pneumonia (PCP) treatment**
IV/IM
Adults, Elderly. 4 mg/kg/day once a day for 14–21 days.
Children. 4 mg/kg/day once daily for 10–14 days.
▸ **PCP prevention**
Inhalation
Adults, Elderly. 300 mg once q4wks.
Children 5 yrs and older. 300 mg q3–4wks.
Children younger than 5 yrs. 8 mg/kg/dose q3–4wks.

UNLABELED USES
Treatment of African trypanosomiasis, cutaneous or visceral leishmaniasis

CONTRAINDICATIONS
Do not use concurrently with didanosine.

INTERACTIONS
Drug
Blood dyscrasia–producing medication, bone marrow depressants: May increase abnormal hematologic effects of pentamidine.
Didanosine: May increase the risk of pancreatitis.
Foscarnet: May increase the risk of hypocalcemia, hypomagnesemia, and nephrotoxicity of pentamidine.
Nephrotoxic medications: May increase the risk of nephrotoxicity.
Herbal
None known.
Food
None known.

DIAGNOSTIC TEST EFFECTS
May increase BUN, serum alkaline phosphatase, serum bilirubin, serum creatinine, SGOT (AST), and SGPT (ALT) levels. May decrease serum calcium and magnesium levels. May alter blood glucose levels.

IV INCOMPATIBILITIES
Interleukin (Proleukin), cefazolin (Ancef), cefotaxime (Claforan), ceftazidime (Fortaz), ceftriaxone (Rocephin), fluconazole (Diflucan), foscarnet (Foscavir)

IV COMPATIBILITIES
Diltiazem (Cardizem), zidovudine (AZT, Retrovir)

SIDE EFFECTS
Frequent

Injection (greater than 10%): Abscess, pain at injection site
Inhalation (greater than 5%): Fatigue, metallic taste, shortness of breath, decreased appetite, dizziness, rash, cough, nausea, vomiting, chills
Occasional
Injection (10%–1%): Nausea, decreased appetite, hypotension, fever, rash, bad taste, confusion
Inhalation (5%–1%): Diarrhea, headache, anemia, muscle pain
Rare
Injection (less than 1%): Neuralgia, thrombocytopenia, phlebitis, dizziness

SERIOUS REACTIONS
• Life-threatening or fatal hypotension, arrhythmias, hypoglycemia, or leukopenia, nephrotoxicity and renal failure, anaphylactic shock, Stevens-Johnson syndrome, and toxic epidural necrolysis occur rarely.
• Hyperglycemia and insulin-dependent diabetes mellitus (often permanent) may occur even months after therapy.

NURSING CONSIDERATIONS
Baseline Assessment
• Avoid concurrent use of nephrotoxic drugs.
• Establish the patient's baseline blood glucose and blood pressure (B/P).
• Obtain patient specimens for diagnostic tests before giving the first dose of pentamidine.
Lifespan Considerations
• Be aware that it is unknown if pentamidine crosses the placenta or is distributed in breast milk.
• There are no age-related precautions noted in children.
• There is no information regarding pentamidine use in the elderly.

Precautions
• Use cautiously in patients with diabetes mellitus, hypertension, hypotension, and liver or renal impairment.

Administration and Handling
◄ALERT▶ Patient must be in the supine position during administration, with frequent B/P checks until the patient is stable because of the potential for developing a life-threatening hypotensive reaction. Have resuscitative equipment immediately available.

IM
• Reconstitute 300-mg vial with 3 ml Sterile Water for Injection to provide concentration of 100 mg/ml.

IV
• Store vials at room temperature.
• After reconstitution, IV solution is stable at room temperature for 48 hours.
• Discard unused portion.
• For intermittent IV infusion (piggyback), reconstitute each vial with 3 to 5 ml D_5W or Sterile Water for Injection.
• Withdraw desired dose and further dilute with 50 to 250 ml D_5W.
• Infuse over 60 minutes.
• Do not give by IV injection or rapid IV infusion as this increases the potential for severe hypotension development.

Aerosol (Nebulizer)
• Store aerosol at room temperature for 48 hours.
• Reconstitute 300-mg vial with 6 ml Sterile Water for Injection. Avoid NaCl as this may cause precipitate to form.
• Do not mix with other medications in nebulizer reservoir.

Intervention and Evaluation
• Monitor the patient's B/P during pentamidine administration until stable for both IM and IV adminis-

tration. The patient should remain supine until stable.
◄ALERT▶ Check the patient's blood glucose levels. Also assess the patient for signs and symptoms of hypoglycemia as evidenced by diaphoresis, double vision, headache, incoordination, lightheadedness, nervousness, numbness of lips, palpitation, tachycardia, and tremor, and hyperglycemia manifested as abdominal pain, headache, malaise, nausea, polydipsia, polyphagia, polyuria, visual changes, and vomiting.
• Evaluate the patient's IM sites for induration, pain, and redness.
• Evaluate the patient's IV sites for phlebitis as evidenced by heat, pain, and red streaking over the vein.
• Monitor the patient's hematology, liver, and renal function test results.
• Assess the patient's skin for rash.
• Evaluate the patient's equilibrium during ambulation.
• Be alert for respiratory difficulty when administering pentamidine by inhalation route.

Patient Teaching
• Teach the patient to remain flat in bed during administration of this medication and to get up slowly and with assistance only when his or her B/P becomes stable.
• Warn the patient to notify the nurse immediately if he or she experiences lightheadedness, palpitations, shakiness, or sweating.
• Advise the patient that even several months after therapy stops, anorexia, drowsiness, and increased thirst and urination may develop.
• Instruct the patient to drink plenty of water to maintain adequate fluid intake.
• Warn the patient to notify the physician if cough, fever, or shortness of breath occurs.

• Urge the patient to avoid consuming alcohol.

quinupristin-dalfopristin
quin-you-pris-tin/**dal**-foh-pris-tin
(Synercid)

CATEGORY AND SCHEDULE
Pregnancy Risk Category: B

MECHANISM OF ACTION
A streptogramin that acts as a bactericidal (in combination). Two chemically distinct compounds that, when given together, bind to different sites on bacterial ribosomes forming a drug-ribosome complex. Protein synthesis is interrupted. *Therapeutic Effect:* Results in bacterial cell death.

PHARMACOKINETICS
After IV administration, both are extensively metabolized in the liver, with dalfopristin to active metabolite. Protein binding:(quinupristin) 23%–32%, (dalfopristin) 50%–56%. Primarily eliminated in feces. **Half-life:** Quinupristin: 0.85 hr. Dalfopristin: 0.7 hr.

AVAILABILITY
Injection: 500-mg vial (350 mg dalfopristin/150 mg quinupristin).

INDICATIONS AND DOSAGES
▸ **Vancomycin-resistant enterococcus**
IV infusion
Adults, Elderly. 7.5 mg/kg/dose q8h.
▸ **Skin/skin-structure infections**
IV infusion
Adults, Elderly. 7.5 mg/kg/dose q12h.

CONTRAINDICATIONS
None known

INTERACTIONS
Drug
None known.
Herbal
None known.
Food
None known.

DIAGNOSTIC TEST EFFECTS
May increase serum bilirubin, creatinine, LDH, SGOT (AST), and SGPT (ALT) levels.

IV INCOMPATIBILITIES
Heparin, sodium chloride

IV COMPATIBILITIES
Aztreonam (Azactam), ciprofloxacin (Cipro), fluconazole (Diflucan), haloperidol (Haldol), metoclopramide (Reglan), morphine, potassium chloride

SIDE EFFECTS
Generally well tolerated.
Frequent
Mild erythema, itching, pain, or burning at infusion site for doses 7 mg/kg or higher
Occasional
Headache, diarrhea
Rare
Vomiting, arthralgia, myalgia

SERIOUS REACTIONS
• Superinfection, including antibiotic-associated colitis, may result from bacterial imbalance.
• Liver function abnormalities and peripheral venous intolerability may occur.

NURSING CONSIDERATIONS

Baseline Assessment
• Assess the patient's blood pressure

(B/P), body temperature, pulse, and respiratory rate.
• Expect to obtain the patient's baseline BUN, complete blood count (CBC), liver function tests, and urinalysis.

Lifespan Considerations
• Be aware that it is unknown if quinupristin-dalfopristin crosses the placenta or is distributed in breast milk.
• Be aware that the safety and efficacy of quinupristin-dalfopristin have not been established in children.
• There are no age-related precautions noted in the elderly.

Precautions
• Use cautiously in patients with liver or renal dysfunction.

Administration and Handling
IV
• Refrigerate unopened vials.
• Reconstituted vials are stable for 1 hour at room temperature. Diluted infusion bag is stable for 6 hours at room temperature or refrigerate for 54 hours.
• Reconstitute vial by slowly adding 5 ml D$_5$W or Sterile Water for Injection to make a 100 mg/ml solution.
• Gently swirl vial contents to minimize foaming.
• Further dilute with D$_5$W to final concentration of 2 mg/ml (5 mg/ml if using a central line).
• Infuse over 60 minutes.
• After infusion, flush line with D$_5$W to minimize vein irritation. Do not flush with 0.9% NaCl as this is incompatible.

Intervention and Evaluation
• Monitor the patient's CBC and liver function tests.
• Observe the infusion site for redness and vein irritation.
• Withhold the medication and promptly inform the physician if diarrhea occurs. Know that diar-

rhea with abdominal pain, fever, and mucus or blood in stool may indicate antibiotic-associated colitis.
• Evaluate the patient's IV site for burning, itching, mild erythema, and pain.
• Be alert for signs and symptoms of superinfection manifested as anal or genital pruritus, diarrhea, increased fever, nausea, onset of sore throat, ulceration or changes of oral mucosa, and vomiting.

Patient Teaching
• Advise patient to immediately notify the physician if he or she experiences pain, redness, or swelling at infusion site.
• Warn patient to immediately notify the physician if he or she experiences severe diarrhea and to avoid taking antidiarrheals until instructed to do so by the physician.

sulfasalazine
sul-fah-**sal**-ah-zeen
(Azulfidine, Azulfidine EN-tabs, Pyralin EN[AUS], Salazopyrin[CAN], SAS-500[CAN])
Do not confuse with azathioprine, sulfadiazine, or sulfisoxazole.

CATEGORY AND SCHEDULE
Pregnancy Risk Category: B (D if given near term)

MECHANISM OF ACTION
A sulfonamide that inhibits prostaglandin synthesis. Acts locally in the colon. *Therapeutic Effect:* Decreases inflammatory response, interferes with gastrointestinal (GI) secretion. Effect may be result of antibacterial action with change in intestinal flora.

PHARMACOKINETICS

Poorly absorbed from the GI tract. Cleaved in colon by intestinal bacterial forming sulfapyridine and mesalamine (5-ASA). Absorbed in colon. Widely distributed. Metabolized in liver. Primarily excreted in urine. **Half-life:** sulfapyridine: 6–14 hrs; 5-ASA: 0.6–1.4 hrs.

AVAILABILITY

Tablets (Azulfidine): 500 mg.
Tablets (delayed-release) (Azulfidine EN-Tabs): 500 mg.

INDICATIONS AND DOSAGES
▸ **Ulcerative colitis**
PO
Adults, Elderly. 1 g 3–4 times/day in divided doses q4–6h. Maximum: 6 g/day. Maintenance: 2 g/day in divided doses q6–12h.
Children. 40–75 mg/kg/day in divided doses q4–6h. Maximum: 6 g/day. Maintenance: 30–50 mg/kg/day in divided doses q4–8h. Maximum: 2 g/day.
▸ **Rheumatoid arthritis**
PO
Adults, Elderly. Initially, 0.5–1 g/day for 1 wk. Increase by 0.5 g/wk, up to 3 g/day.
▸ **Juvenile rheumatoid arthritis**
PO
Children. Initially, 10 mg/kg/day. May increase by 10 mg/kg/day at weekly intervals. Range: 30–50 mg/kg/day. Maximum: 2 g/day.

UNLABELED USES

Treatment of ankylosing spondylitis

CONTRAINDICATIONS

Children younger than 2 years of age; hypersensitivity to carbonic anhydrase inhibitors, local anesthetics, salicylates, sulfonamides, sulfonylureas, sunscreens containing PABA, thiazide or loop diuretics; intestinal or urinary tract obstruction; porphyria; pregnancy at term; severe liver or renal dysfunction

INTERACTIONS
Drug
Anticonvulsants, oral anticoagulants, oral hypoglycemics, methotrexate: May increase the effects of these drugs.
Hemolytics: May increase toxicity of sulfasalazine.
Liver toxic medications: May increase the risk of liver toxicity of sulfasalazine.
Herbal
None known.
Food
None known.

DIAGNOSTIC TEST EFFECTS

None known.

SIDE EFFECTS

Frequent (33%)
Anorexia, nausea, vomiting, headache, oligospermia (generally reversed by withdrawal of drug)
Occasional (3%)
Hypersensitivity reaction: rash, urticaria, pruritus, fever, anemia
Rare (less than 1%)
Tinnitus, hypoglycemia, diuresis, photosensitivity

SERIOUS REACTIONS

• Anaphylaxis, Stevens-Johnson syndrome, hematologic toxicity (leukopenia, agranulocytosis), liver toxicity, and nephrotoxicity occur rarely.

▮ NURSING CONSIDERATIONS

Baseline Assessment
◂ALERT▸ Determine the patient's hypersensitivity to medications (see Contraindications) before beginning drug therapy.

• Check the patient's initial complete blood count (CBC), liver and renal function, and urinalysis test results.

Lifespan Considerations

• Be aware that sulfasalazine may produce infertility and oligospermia in men while taking the medication.

• Be aware that sulfasalazine readily crosses the placenta and is excreted in breast milk. Do not breast-feed premature infants or those with hyperbilirubinemia or G6PD deficiency.

• Be aware that if sulfasalazine is given near term, it may produce hemolytic anemia, jaundice, and kernicterus in the newborn.

• There are no age-related precautions noted in children older than 2 years of age or the elderly.

Precautions

• Use cautiously in patients with bronchial asthma, G6PD deficiency, impaired liver or renal function, and severe allergies.

Administration and Handling

PO

• Space drug doses evenly at intervals not to exceed 8 hours.

• Administer the drug after meals, if possible, to prolong intestinal passage.

• Have the patient swallow enteric-coated tablets whole; do not chew or crush.

• Give with 8 oz of water; encourage several glasses of water between meals.

Intervention and Evaluation

• Monitor the patient's intake and output and renal function and urinalysis test results.

• Ensure that the patient drinks plenty of water to maintain adequate hydration (minimum output 1,500 ml/24 hour) to prevent nephrotoxicity.

• Assess the patient's skin for rash.

Withhold the drug and notify the physician at first sign of rash.

• Assess the patient's pattern of daily bowel activity and stool consistency. Drug dosage may need to be increased if diarrhea continues or recurs.

• Monitor the patient's complete blood count (CBC) closely.

• Assess the patient for hematologic effects: bleeding, bruising, fever, jaundice, pallor, purpura, sore throat, and weakness. If hematologic effects occur, notify the physician immediately.

Patient Teaching

• Explain to the patient that sulfasalazine may cause orange-yellow discoloration of the skin and urine.

• Advise the patient to continue sulfasalazine therapy for the full length of treatment and to evenly space drug doses around the clock. Explain to the patient that it may be necessary to continue taking the drug even after symptoms are relieved.

• Instruct the patient to take sulfasalazine after food with 8 oz of water and to drink several glasses of water between meals.

• Stress to the patient the importance of follow-up and lab tests.

• Tell the patient that if he or she is to have dental or other surgery, that he or she must inform the dentist or surgeon of sulfasalazine therapy.

• Urge the patient to avoid exposure to sun and ultraviolet light until his or her photosensitivity is determined. Explain to the patient that photosensitivity may last for months after the last dose of sulfasalazine.

trimethoprim
try-**meth**-oh-prim
(Primsol, Proloprim, Trimpex)

CATEGORY AND SCHEDULE
Pregnancy Risk Category: C

MECHANISM OF ACTION
A folate antagonist that blocks bacterial biosynthesis of nucleic acids and proteins by interfering with metabolism of folinic acid. *Therapeutic Effect:* Produces antibacterial activity.

PHARMACOKINETICS
Rapidly, completely absorbed from the gastrointestinal (GI) tract. Protein binding: 42%–46%. Widely distributed, including cerebrospinal fluid (CSF). Metabolized in liver. Primarily excreted in urine. Moderately removed by hemodialysis.
Half-life: 8–10 hrs (half-life is increased with impaired renal function, newborns; decreased in children).

AVAILABILITY
Tablets: 100 mg, 200 mg.
Oral Solution: 50 mg/5 ml.

INDICATIONS AND DOSAGES
▶ **Acute, uncomplicated urinary tract infections (UTIs)**
PO
Adults, Elderly, Children 12 yrs and older. 100 mg q12h or 200 mg once a day for 10 days.
Children younger than 12 yrs. 4–6 mg/kg/day in 2 divided doses for 10 days.
▶ **Dosage in renal impairment**

Creatinine Clearance	Dosage Interval
greater than 30 ml/min	No change
15–30 ml/min	50 mg q12h

UNLABELED USES
Prophylaxis of bacterial UTIs, treatment of pneumonia caused by *Pneumocystis carinii*

CONTRAINDICATIONS
Infants younger than 2 mos, megaloblastic anemia due to folic acid deficiency

INTERACTIONS
Drug
Folate antagonists, including methotrexate: May increase the risk of myeloblastic anemia.
Herbal
None known.
Food
None known.

DIAGNOSTIC TEST EFFECTS
May increase BUN, serum bilirubin, serum creatinine, SGOT (AST), and SGPT (ALT) levels.

SIDE EFFECTS
Occasional
Nausea, vomiting, diarrhea, decreased appetite, stomach cramps, headache
Rare
Hypersensitivity reaction (pruritus, rash), methemoglobinemia (blue color on fingernails, lips, or skin, fever, pale skin, sore throat, unusual tiredness)

SERIOUS REACTIONS
• Stevens-Johnson syndrome, erythema multiforme, exfoliative dermatitis, and anaphylaxis occur rarely.
• Hematologic toxicity (thrombocytopenia, neutropenia, leukopenia, megaloblastic anemia) is more likely to occur in the elderly, debilitated, alcoholics, and patients with impaired renal function or receiving prolonged high dosage.

NURSING CONSIDERATIONS

Baseline Assessment
• Assess the patient's baseline hematology and renal function test reports.

Lifespan Considerations
• Be aware that trimethoprim readily crosses the placenta and is distributed in breast milk.
• Be aware that the safety and efficacy of trimethoprim have not been established in children.
• There are no age-related precautions noted in the elderly.
• The elderly may have an increased incidence of thrombocytopenia.

Precautions
• Use cautiously in those with impaired liver or renal function, in children who have X chromosome with mental retardation, and patients who have folic acid deficiency.

Administration and Handling
PO
• Space doses evenly around the clock to maintain constant drug level in urine.
• Give without regard to meals (if stomach upset occurs, give with food).

Intervention and Evaluation
• Assess the patient's skin for rash.
• Evaluate the patient's food tolerance.
• Monitor the patient's hematology reports and liver or renal function test results, if ordered.
• Observe the patient for signs and symptoms of hematologic toxicity manifested as bleeding, bruising, fever, malaise, pallor, and sore throat.

Patient Teaching
• Advise patients to complete the full course of trimethoprim therapy, usually 10–14 days, and to evenly space drug doses around the clock.

• Instruct the patient that trimethoprim may be taken on an empty stomach or with food if stomach upset occurs.
• Urge the patient to avoid sun and ultraviolet light, to use sunscreen, and wear protective clothing.
• Warn the patient to immediately report any bleeding, bruising, discoloration of the skin, fever, pallor, rash, sore throat, and tiredness he or she experiences to the physician.

vancomycin hydrochloride
van-koe-**my**-sin
(Vancocin, Vancoled)

CATEGORY AND SCHEDULE
Pregnancy Risk Category: B

MECHANISM OF ACTION
A tricyclic glycopeptide antibiotic that binds to bacterial cell wall, altering cell membrane permeability, inhibiting RNA synthesis. *Therapeutic Effect:* Inhibits cell wall synthesis, produces bacterial cell death. Bactericidal.

PHARMACOKINETICS
PO: Poorly absorbed from the gastrointestinal (GI) tract. Primarily eliminated in feces. Parenteral: Widely distributed. Protein binding: 55%. Primarily excreted unchanged in urine. Not removed by hemodialysis. **Half-life:** 4–11 hrs (half-life is increased with impaired renal function).

AVAILABILITY
Capsules: 125 mg, 250 mg.
Powder for Injection: 500 mg, 1 g.
Infusion (Premix): 500 mg/100 ml, 1 g/200 ml.

INDICATIONS AND DOSAGES
▶ **Treatment of bone, respiratory tract, skin and soft tissue infections, endocarditis, peritonitis, septicemia. Given prophylactically to those at risk for bacterial endocarditis (if penicillin contraindicated) when undergoing biliary, dental, GI, genitourinary (GU), respiratory surgery or invasive procedures.**
IV
Adults, Elderly. 500 mg q6h or 1 g q12h.
Children older than 1 mo. 40 mg/kg/day in divided doses q6–8h. Maximum: 3–4 g/day.
Neonates. 15 mg/kg initially, then 10 mg/kg q8–12h.
▶ **Dosage in renal impairment**
After a loading dose, subsequent dosages and frequency are modified based on the degree of renal impairment, severity of infection, and serum concentration of drug.
Staphylococcal enterocolitis, antibiotic-associated pseudomembranous colitis caused by *Clostridium Difficile*
PO
Adults, Elderly. 0.5–2 g/day in 3–4 divided doses for 7–10 days.
Children. 40 mg/kg/day in 3–4 divided doses for 7–10 days. Maximum: 2 g/day.

UNLABELED USES
Treatment of brain abscess, perioperative infections, staphylococcal or streptococcal meningitis

CONTRAINDICATIONS
None known

INTERACTIONS
Drug
Aminoglycosides, amphotericin, aspirin, bumetanide, carmustine, cisplatin, cyclosporine, ethacrynic acid, furosemide, streptozocin: May increase ototoxicity and nephrotoxicity of parenteral vancomycin.
Cholestyramine, colestipol: May decrease the effects of oral vancomycin.
Herbal
None known.
Food
None known.

DIAGNOSTIC TEST EFFECTS
May increase BUN. Therapeutic peak blood level is 20–40 mcg/ml; trough level is 5–15 mcg/ml. Toxic peak blood level is greater than 40 mcg/ml; trough level is greater than 15 mcg/ml.

IV INCOMPATIBILITIES
Albumin, amphotericin B complex (Abelcet, AmBisome, Amphotec), aztreonam (Azactam), cefazolin (Ancef), cefepime (Maxipime), cefotaxime (Claforan), cefotetan (Cefotan), cefoxitin (Mefoxin), ceftazidime (Fortaz), ceftriaxone (Rocephin), cefuroxime (Zinacef), foscarnet (Foscavir), heparin, idarubicin (Idamycin), nafcillin (Nafcil), piperacillin/tazobactam (Zosyn), ticarcillin/clavulanate (Timentin)

IV COMPATIBILITIES
Amiodarone (Cordarone), calcium gluconate, diltiazem (Cardizem), hydromorphone (Dilaudid), insulin, lorazepam (Ativan), magnesium sulfate, midazolam (Versed), morphine, potassium chloride, propofol (Diprivan)

SIDE EFFECTS
Frequent
PO: Bitter or unpleasant taste, nausea, vomiting, mouth irritation (oral solution)
Rare
Systemic: Phlebitis, thrombophlebi-

tis, pain at peripheral IV site; necrosis may occur with extravasation, dizziness, vertigo, tinnitus, chills, fever, rash
PO: Rash.

SERIOUS REACTIONS

• Nephrotoxicity (a change in the amount or frequency of urination, nausea, vomiting, increased thirst, anorexia), ototoxicity (deafness due to damage to auditory branch of eighth cranial nerve), and red-neck syndrome (from too rapid injection–redness on face, neck, arms, back) may occur.
• Chills, fever, tachycardia, nausea, vomiting, itching, rash, and unpleasant taste may occur.

NURSING CONSIDERATIONS

Baseline Assessment

• Know that vancomycin should not be given while administering other ototoxic and nephrotoxic medications, if possible.
• Obtain patient culture and sensitivity tests before giving the first dose of vancomycin. Therapy may begin before test results are known.

Lifespan Considerations

• Be aware that vancomycin crosses the placenta and that it is unknown if vancomycin is distributed in breast milk.
• Be aware that close monitoring of drug serum levels is recommended in premature neonates and young infants.
• In the elderly, age-related renal impairment may increase the risk of ototoxicity and nephrotoxicity. Dosage adjustment is recommended.

Precautions

• Use cautiously in patients with preexisting hearing impairment and renal dysfunction.
• Use cautiously in patients concurrently taking other ototoxic or nephrotoxic medications.

Administration and Handling

PO
• Be aware that vancomycin is usually not given for systemic infections because of poor absorption from GI tract; however, some patients with colitis may effectively absorb the drug.
• Reconstitute powder for oral solution as appropriate and give it PO or nasogastric (NG) tube. Do not use powder for oral solution for IV administration.
• Refrigerated oral solution is stable for 2 weeks.

IV
◀ALERT▶ Give by intermittent IV infusion (piggyback) or continuous IV infusion. Do not give IV push as this may result in exaggerated hypotension.
• After reconstitution, IV solution may be refrigerated; use within 14 days.
• Discard if precipitate forms.
• For intermittent IV infusion (piggyback), reconstitute each 500-mg vial with 10 ml Sterile Water for Injection (20 ml for 1-g vial) to provide concentration of 50 mg/ml.
• Further dilute to a final concentration not to exceed 5 mg/ml.
• Administer over 60 minutes or more.
• Monitor the patient's blood pressure (B/P) closely during IV infusion.
• ADD-Vantage vials should not be used in neonates, infants, children requiring less than 500-mg dose.

Intervention and Evaluation

• Monitor the patient's intake and output and renal function test results.
• Assess the patient's skin for rash.
• Evaluate the patient's balance and hearing acuity.

• Monitor the patient's B/P carefully during infusion.

• Evaluate the patient's IV site for phlebitis as evidenced by heat, pain, and red streaking over the vein.

• Know that the vancomycin therapeutic peak blood level is 20 to 40 mcg/ml; trough level is 5 to15 mcg/ml. Toxic peak blood level is greater than 40 mcg/ml; trough level is greater than 15 mcg/ml.

Patient Teaching

• Advise the patient to continue vancomycin therapy for the full length of treatment and to evenly space drug doses around the clock.

• Warn the patient to notify the physician if he or she experiences rash, signs and symptoms of nephrotoxicity, or tinnitus.

• Stress to the patient that lab tests are an important part of total therapy.

13 Alkylating Agents

busulfan
carboplatin
carmustine
chlorambucil
cisplatin
cyclophosphamide
estramustine
  phosphate sodium
ifosfamide
lomustine
melphalan
oxaliplatin
thiotepa

Uses: Alkylating agents are used to treat many types of cancer, including acute and chronic leukemias, lymphomas, multiple myeloma, and solid tumors in the breasts, ovaries, uterus, lungs, bladder, and stomach.

Action: Alkylating agents form cross-links on deoxyribonucleic acid (DNA) strands, which disturb DNA synthesis and cell division. In this way, these agents interfere with DNA integrity and function in rapidly proliferating tissues. They affect all phases of the cell cycle.

busulfan
bew-**sull**-fan
(Busulfex, Myleran)
Do not confuse with Alkeran or Leukeran.

CATEGORY AND SCHEDULE
Pregnancy Risk Category: D

MECHANISM OF ACTION
An alkylating agent that interferes with DNA replication, RNA synthesis, and is cell cycle–phase nonspecific. *Therapeutic Effect:* Disrupts nucleic acid function. Myelosuppressant.

PHARMACOKINETICS
Completely absorbed from the gastrointestinal (GI) tract. Protein binding: 33%. Metabolized in liver. Primarily excreted in urine. Minimal removal by hemodialysis.
Half-life: 2.5 hrs.

AVAILABILITY
Tablets: 2 mg.
Injection: 60 mg ampoule.

INDICATIONS AND DOSAGES
▶ **Treatment of chronic myelogenous leukemia (CML); remission induction**
PO
Adults. 4–8 mg/day. Drug withdrawn when white blood cell (WBC) count falls below 15,000/mm^3.
Children. 0.06–0.12 mg/kg once a day.
▶ **Treatment of CML; maintenance therapy**
PO
Adults. Induction dose (4–8 mg/day) when total leukocyte count reaches 50,000/mm^3. If remission occurs in less than 3 mos, 1–3 mg/day may produce satisfactory response.
Elderly. Initially, lowest dosage for adults.
▶ **Conditioning regimen before allogeneic hematopoietic cell transplantation in patients with CML**
IV
Adults. 0.8 mg/kg q6h (as 2-hr infusion) for total of 16 doses.

Children. 60–120 mcg/kg/day or 1.8–4.6 mg/m²/day.

UNLABELED USES
Treatment of acute myelocytic leukemia (AML)

CONTRAINDICATIONS
Disease resistance to previous therapy with this drug

INTERACTIONS
Drug
Antigout medications: May decrease the effects of these drugs.
Bone marrow depressants: May increase the risk of bone marrow depression.
Live virus vaccines: May potentiate virus replication, increase vaccine side effects, and decrease the patient's antibody response to the vaccine.
Herbal
None known.
Food
None known.

DIAGNOSTIC TEST EFFECTS
May decrease serum magnesium, potassium, phosphates, and sodium. May increase blood glucose, BUN, serum calcium, serum alkaline phosphatase, serum bilirubin, serum creatinine, and SGPT (ALT) levels.

IV INCOMPATIBILITIES
Do not mix with any other medications.

SIDE EFFECTS
Expected (98%–72%)
Nausea, stomatitis, vomiting, anorexia, insomnia, diarrhea, fever, abdominal pain, anxiety
Frequent (69%–44%)
Headache, rash, asthenia (loss of energy, strength), infection, chills, tachycardia, dyspepsia

Occasional (38%–16%)
Constipation, dizziness, edema, pruritus, cough, dry mouth, depression, abdominal enlargement, pharyngitis, hiccups, back pain, alopecia, myalgia
Rare (13%–5%)
Injection site pain, arthralgia, confusion, hypotension, lethargy

SERIOUS REACTIONS
• Busulfan's major adverse reaction is bone marrow depression resulting in hematologic toxicity as evidenced by severe leukopenia, anemia, and severe thrombocytopenia.
• Very high busulfan dosages may produce blurred vision, muscle twitching, and tonic-clonic seizures.
• Long-term therapy (more than 4 yrs) may produce pulmonary syndrome or "busulfan lung" which is characterized by persistent cough, congestion, rales, and dyspnea.
• Hyperuricemia may produce uric acid nephropathy, renal stones, and acute renal failure.

NURSING CONSIDERATIONS

Baseline Assessment
• Expect to perform hematologic studies, including blood Hct and Hgb, white blood cell (WBC) count, differential, platelet count, and liver and renal function tests weekly. Know that busulfan's dosage is based on hematologic values.
• Teach the patient and family about the expected effects of busulfan treatment.
Lifespan Considerations
• If possible, busulfan use should be avoided during pregnancy, especially in the first trimester.
• Be aware that busulfan use may cause fetal harm and it is unknown if the drug is distributed in breast

milk. Breast-feeding is not recommended in this patient population.

• There are no age-related precautions noted in children or the elderly.

Precautions

• Use extremely cautiously in patients with compromised bone marrow reserve.

• Use cautiously in patients with chickenpox, herpes zoster, history of gout, or infection.

Administration and Handling

◀ALERT▶ Busulfan dosage is individualized based on the patient's clinical response and tolerance of the drug's adverse effects. When used in combination therapy, consult specific protocols for optimum dosage and sequence of drug administration.

◀ALERT▶ Busulfan may be carcinogenic, mutagenic, or teratogenic. Handle with extreme care during administration. Use of gloves recommended. If contact occurs with skin or mucosa, wash thoroughly with water.

PO

• Give at same time each day.

• Give to the patient on an empty stomach if nausea or vomiting occur.

IV Infusion

◀ALERT▶ Premedicate the patient with phenytoin to decrease the risk of seizures.

• Refrigerate ampoules.

• Following dilution, the solution is stable for 8 hours at room temperature, 12 hours if refrigerated when diluted with 0.9% NaCl.

• Dilute with 0.9% NaCl or D_5W only. The diluent quantity must be 10 times the volume of busulfan (e.g., 9.3 ml busulfan must be diluted with 93 ml diluent).

• Use filter to withdraw busulfan from ampoule.

• Add busulfan to calculated diluent.

• Lock infusion pump when administering busulfan.

• Infuse over 2 hours.

• Prior to and after infusion, flush catheter line with 5 ml 0.9% NaCl or D_5W.

Intervention and Evaluation

• Monitor the patient's lab values diligently for evidence of bone marrow depression.

• Assess the patient's mouth for onset of stomatitis as evidenced by difficulty swallowing, gum inflammation, and redness or ulceration of the oral mucous membranes.

• Give the patient antiemetic medications to prevent nausea or vomiting.

• Assess the patient's pattern of daily bowel activity and stool consistency.

Patient Teaching

• Instruct the patient to maintain adequate daily fluid intake to protect against renal impairment.

• Warn the patient to report congestion, consistent cough, difficulty breathing, easy bruising, fever, signs of local infection, sore throat, or unusual bleeding from any site.

• Stress to the patient that he or she should not receive vaccinations without the physician's approval as busulfan lowers the body's resistance and that he or she should avoid contact with anyone who recently received a live virus vaccine.

• Teach the patient to take busulfan at the same time each day.

• Caution women of childbearing age to avoid pregnancy. Educate the patient regarding contraception options.

carboplatin
car-bow-**play**-tin
(Paraplatin)
**Do not confuse with Cisplatin
or Platinol.**

CATEGORY AND SCHEDULE
Pregnancy Risk Category: D

MECHANISM OF ACTION
A platinum coordination complex
that inhibits DNA synthesis by
cross-linking with DNA strands.
Cell cycle–phase nonspecific. *Therapeutic Effect:* Prevents cellular
division, interferes with DNA function.

PHARMACOKINETICS
Protein binding: Low. Hydrolyzed
in solution to active form. Primarily
excreted in urine. **Half-life:** 2.6–5.9
hrs.

AVAILABILITY
Powder for Injection: 50 mg, 150
mg, 450 mg.

INDICATIONS AND DOSAGES
▶ **Ovarian carcinoma (single agent)**
IV
Adults. 360 mg/m^2 on day 1,
q4wks. Do not repeat dose until
neutrophil and platelet counts are
within acceptable levels. Adjust
drug dosage in patients previously
treated based on lowest post-
treatment platelet or neutrophil
value. Make only one escalation,
not greater than 125% of starting
dose.
▶ **Ovarian carcinoma (combination
therapy)**
IV
Adults. 300 mg/m^2 (with cyclophosphamide) on day 1, q4wks. Do not
repeat dose until neutrophil and

platelet counts are within acceptable
levels.
Children. Solid tumor: 300–600
mg/m^2 q4wks. Brain tumor: 175
mg/m^2 q4wks.
▶ **Dosage in renal impairment**
Initial dosage is based on creatinine
clearance; subsequent dosages are
based on the patient's tolerance and
degree of myelosuppression.

Creatinine Clearance	Dosage Day 1
greater than 60 ml/min	360 mg/m^2
41–59 ml/min	250 mg/m^2
16–40 ml/min	200 mg/m^2

UNLABELED USES
Treatment of bony and soft tissue
sarcomas; germ cell tumors;
neuroblastoma; pediatric brain
tumor; small cell lung cancer; solid
tumors of the bladder, cervix, and
testes; squamous cell carcinoma of
the esophagus

CONTRAINDICATIONS
History of severe allergic reaction
to cisplatin, platinum compounds,
mannitol; severe bleeding, severe
myelosuppression

INTERACTIONS
Drug
Bone marrow depressants: May
increase bone marrow depression.
Live virus vaccines: May potentiate
virus replication, increase vaccine
side effects, and decrease the pa-
tient's antibody response to the
vaccine.
*Nephrotoxic-, ototoxic-producing
agents:* May increase the risk of
toxicity.
Herbal
None known.
Food
None known.

DIAGNOSTIC TEST EFFECTS

May decrease serum electrolytes, including calcium, magnesium, potassium, and sodium. High dosages (greater than 4 times the recommended dosage) may elevate BUN, serum alkaline phosphatase, serum bilirubin, serum creatinine, and SGOT (AST) levels.

IV INCOMPATIBILITIES

Amphotericin B complex (AmBisome, Amphotec, Abelcet)

IV COMPATIBILITIES

Etoposide (VePesid), granisetron (Kytril), ondansetron (Zofran), paclitaxel (Taxol)

SIDE EFFECTS

Frequent
Nausea (75%–80%), vomiting (65%)
Occasional
Generalized pain (17%), diarrhea or constipation (6%), peripheral neuropathy (4%)
Rare (3%-2%)
Alopecia, asthenia (loss of energy, strength), hypersensitivity reaction (erythema, pruritus, rash, urticaria)

SERIOUS REACTIONS

• Bone marrow suppression may be severe, resulting in anemia, infection, and bleeding (gastrointestinal bleeding, sepsis, pneumonia).
• Prolonged treatment may result in peripheral neurotoxicity.

NURSING CONSIDERATIONS

Baseline Assessment
• Offer the patient emotional support.
• Be aware that treatment should not be repeated until the patient's white blood cell (WBC) count recovers from previous therapy.

• Expect to administer transfusions in those patients receiving prolonged therapy.

Lifespan Considerations
• If possible, carboplatin use should be avoided during pregnancy, especially in the first trimester.
• Be aware that carboplatin use may cause fetal harm and that it is unknown if the drug is distributed in breast milk. Breast-feeding is not recommended in this patient population.
• Be aware that the safety and efficacy of carboplatin have not been established in children.
• In the elderly, the peripheral neurotoxicity risk is increased and myelotoxicity may be more severe.
• In the elderly, age-related decreased renal function may require decreased dosage and more careful monitoring of blood counts.

Precautions
• Use cautiously in patients with chickenpox, herpes zoster, infection, and renal function impairment.

Administration and Handling
◀ALERT▶ Be aware that carboplatin dosage is individualized based on the patient's clinical response and tolerance of the drug's adverse effects. Also, know that platelets must be greater than 100,000 mm^3 and neutrophils greater than 2,000 mm^3 before giving any dosage.
◀ALERT▶ Know that carboplatin may be carcinogenic, mutagenic, or teratogenic. Handle with extreme care during preparation and administration.

IV
• Store vials at room temperature.
• After reconstitution, solution is stable for 8 hours. Discard unused portion after 8 hours.
• Reconstitute immediately before use.

• Do not use aluminum needles or administration sets that come in contact with drug because this may produce black precipitate and a loss of potency.
• Reconstitute each 50 mg with 5 ml Sterile Water for Injection, D_5W, or 0.9% NaCl to provide concentration of 10 mg/ml.
• Further dilute solution with D_5W or 0.9% NaCl to provide concentration as low as 0.5 mg/ml, if needed.
• Infuse over 15 to 60 minutes.
• Be aware that rarely, an anaphylactic reaction may occur minutes after administration. Use epinephrine and corticosteroid, as prescribed, to alleviate symptoms.

Intervention and Evaluation
• Monitor the patient's hematologic status, pulmonary function studies, and liver and renal function tests. Be aware that myelosuppression is increased in those who have received previous carboplatin therapy or have impaired renal function.
• Assess the patient for easy bruising, fever, signs of local infection, sore throat, symptoms of anemia (excessive fatigue, weakness) and unusual bleeding from any site.

Patient Teaching
• Advise the patient that nausea or vomiting is a side effect of carboplatin that generally abates in less than 24 hours.
• Stress to the patient that he or she should not receive vaccinations without the physician's approval as carboplatin lowers the body's resistance. Also advise patient to avoid contact with anyone who recently received a live virus vaccine.

carmustine
car-**muss**-teen
(BiCNU, Gliadel)

CATEGORY AND SCHEDULE
Pregnancy Risk Category: D

MECHANISM OF ACTION
An alkylating agent and nitrosourea that inhibits DNA, RNA synthesis by cross-linking with DNA, RNA strands, preventing cellular division. Cell cycle–phase nonspecific. *Therapeutic Effect:* Interferes with DNA and RNA function.

AVAILABILITY
Powder for Injection: 100 mg.
Wafer: 7.7 mg.

INDICATIONS AND DOSAGES
▸ **As a single agent in previously untreated patients with disseminated Hodgkin's disease, multiple myeloma, non-Hodgkin's lymphoma, primary and metastatic brain tumors**
IV infusion
Adults, Elderly. 150–200 mg/m² as single dose or 75–100 mg/m² on 2 successive days. *Children.* 200–250 mg/m² q4–6wks as a single dose.

UNLABELED USES
Treatment of hepatic, gastrointestinal (GI) carcinoma; malignant melanoma; mycosis fungoides

CONTRAINDICATIONS
None known

INTERACTIONS
Drug
Bone marrow depressants, cimetidine: May enhance carmustine's myelosuppressive effect.
Live virus vaccines: May potentiate

virus replication, increase vaccine side effects, and decrease the patient's antibody response to the vaccine.

Hepatotoxic, nephrotoxic drugs:
May increase the risk of hepatotoxicity or nephrotoxicity.

Herbal
None known.

Food
None known.

DIAGNOSTIC TEST EFFECTS

May increase BUN, serum alkaline phosphatase, serum bilirubin, SGOT (AST), and SGPT (ALT) levels.

IV INCOMPATIBILITIES

Allopurinol (Aloprim)

SIDE EFFECTS

Frequent
Nausea and vomiting within minutes to 2 hrs after administration (may last up to 6 hrs)
Occasional
Diarrhea, esophagitis, anorexia, dysphagia
Rare
Thrombophlebitis

SERIOUS REACTIONS

• Hematologic toxicity, because of bone marrow depression, occurs frequently.
• Thrombocytopenia occurs at about 4 weeks and lasts 1 to 2 weeks.
• Leukopenia is evident at about 5 to 6 weeks after carmustine treatment begins and lasts 1 to 2 weeks.
• Anemia occurs less frequently and is less severe.
• Mild, reversible liver toxicity also occurs frequently.
• Prolonged carmustine therapy with high dosage may produce impaired renal function and pulmonary toxicity (pulmonary infiltrate or fibrosis).

NURSING CONSIDERATIONS

Baseline Assessment
• Expect to perform liver function studies periodically during therapy.
• Monitor the patient's blood counts weekly during and for at least 6 weeks after carmustine therapy ends.

Precautions
• Use cautiously in patients with decreased erythrocyte, leukocyte, and platelet counts.

Administration and Handling
◀ALERT▶ Be aware that carmustine dosage is individualized based on the patient's clinical response and tolerance of the drug's adverse effects. When using this drug in combination therapy, consult specific protocols for optimum dosage and sequence of drug administration.

◀ALERT▶ Know that carmustine may be carcinogenic, mutagenic, or teratogenic. Wear protective gloves during preparation of the drug; may cause transient burning and brown staining of the skin.

IV
• Refrigerate unopened vials of dry powder.
• Reconstituted vials are stable at room temperature for up to 8 hours or up to 24 hrs if refrigerated.
• Know that solutions further diluted to 0.2 mg/ml with D_5W or 0.9% NaCl are stable for 48 hours if refrigerated or an additional 8 hours at room temperature.
• Solutions normally appear clear, colorless to yellow.
• Discard if precipitate forms, color change occurs, or oily film develops on bottom of vial.
• Reconstitute 100-mg vial with 3 ml sterile dehydrated (absolute) alcohol, followed by 27 ml Sterile Water for Injection to provide concentration of 3.3 mg/ml.

• Further dilute with 50 to 250 ml
D_5W or 0.9% NaCl.
• Infuse over 1 to 2 hours (shorter
duration may produce intense burning pain at injection site, intense
flushing of skin, conjunctiva).
• Flush IV line with 5 to 10 ml
0.9% NaCl or D_5W before and after
administration to prevent irritation
at injection site.

Intervention and Evaluation
• Monitor the patient's BUN, complete blood count (CBC), serum
alkaline phosphatase, bilirubin,
transaminase, and pulmonary and
renal function tests.
• Monitor the patient for signs and
symptoms of hematologic toxicity
as evidenced by easy bruising,
fever, signs of local infection, sore
throat, symptoms of anemia, such as
excessive fatigue, weakness, and
unusual bleeding from any site.
• Evaluate the patient for signs and
symptoms, including dyspnea and
fine lung rales.

Patient Teaching
• Instruct the patient to maintain
adequate daily fluid intake to protect against renal impairment.
• Stress to the patient that he or she
should not receive vaccinations
without the physician's approval as
carmustine lowers the body's resistance and that he or she should
avoid contact with anyone who
recently received a live virus vaccine.
• Warn the patient to contact the
physician if nausea or vomiting
continues at home.

chlorambucil
klor-**am**-bew-sill
(Leukeran)
**Do not confuse with Alkeran,
Chloromycetin, or Myleran.**

CATEGORY AND SCHEDULE
Pregnancy Risk Category: D

MECHANISM OF ACTION
An alkylating agent and nitrogen
mustard that inhibits DNA, RNA
synthesis by cross-linking with DNA
and RNA strands. Cell cycle–phase
nonspecific. *Therapeutic Effect:* Interferes with nucleic acid function.

PHARMACOKINETICS
Rapidly, completely absorbed from
the gastrointestinal (GI) tract. Protein binding: 99%. Rapidly metabolized in liver to active metabolite.
Not removed by hemodialysis.
Half-life: 1.5 hrs; metabolite:
2.5 hrs.

AVAILABILITY
Tablets: 2 mg.

INDICATIONS AND DOSAGES
▶ **Palliative treatment of advanced
Hodgkin's disease, advanced malignant (non-Hodgkin's) lymphomas,
chronic lymphocytic leukemia,
giant follicular lymphomas, and
lymphosarcoma**
PO
Adults, Elderly, Children. Initial or
short-course therapy: 0.1–0.2 mg/
kg/day as single or divided dose for
3–6 wks. Average dose is 4–10
mg/day. Single daily dose q2wks is
0.4 mg/kg initially. Increase by 0.1
mg/kg q2wks until response and
myelosuppression occurs. Maintenance dose: 0.03–0.1 mg/kg/day.
Average dose is 2–4 mg/day.

UNLABELED USES

Treatment of hairy cell leukemia; nephrotic syndrome; ovarian, testicular carcinoma; polycythemia vera

CONTRAINDICATIONS

Previous allergic reaction, disease resistance to previous therapy with drug

INTERACTIONS
Drug

Antigout medications: May decrease the effect of these drugs.
Bone marrow depressants: May increase bone marrow depression.
Live virus vaccines: May potentiate virus replication, increase vaccine side effects, or decrease the patient's antibody response to the vaccine.
Other immunosuppressants, including steroids: May increase the risk of infection or development of neoplasms.
Herbal
None known.
Food
None known.

DIAGNOSTIC TEST EFFECTS

May increase serum alkaline phosphatase, serum uric acid, and SGOT (AST) levels.

SIDE EFFECTS
Expected
Gastrointestinal (GI) effects such as nausea, vomiting, anorexia, diarrhea, and abdominal distress are generally mild, last less than 24 hours, and occur only if single dose exceeds 20 mg.
Occasional
Rash or dermatitis, pruritus, cold sores
Rare
Alopecia, urticaria (hives), erythema, hyperuricemia

SERIOUS REACTIONS

• Bone marrow depression manifested as hematologic toxicity, including neutropenia, leukopenia, progressive lymphopenia, anemia, thrombocytopenia, may occur.
• After discontinuation of therapy, thrombocytopenia, and leukopenia usually occur at 1 to 3 weeks and last 1 to 4 weeks.
• Neutrophil count decreases up to 10 days after last dose.
• Toxicity appears to be less severe with intermittent rather than continuous drug administration.
• Overdosage may produce seizures in children.
• Excessive serum uric acid level and liver toxicity occurs rarely.

NURSING CONSIDERATIONS
Baseline Assessment
• Expect to obtain a complete blood count (CBC) each week during chlorambucil therapy.
• Expect to obtain a white blood cell (WBC) count 3 to 4 days after each weekly CBC during the first 3 to 6 weeks of chlorambucil therapy or 4 to 6 weeks if the patient is on an intermittent dosing schedule.
Lifespan Considerations
• If possible, chlorambucil use should be avoided during pregnancy, especially in the first trimester.
• Be aware that breast-feeding is not recommended in this patient population.
• There are no age-related precautions noted in children and the elderly.
• Be aware that when chlorambucil is taken for nephritic syndrome, seizures may increase.
Precautions
• Use extremely cautiously in patients within 4 weeks after full-

course radiation therapy or myelo-suppressive drug regimen.

Administration and Handling
◀ ALERT ▶ Be aware that chlorambucil may be carcinogenic, mutagenic, or teratogenic. Handle with extreme care during administration. Know that dosage is individualized on the basis of the patient's clinical response and tolerance of the drug's adverse effects. When using this drug in combination therapy, consult specific protocols for optimum dosage and sequence of drug administration.

PO
• Give chlorambucil without regard to food.

Intervention and Evaluation
• Monitor the patient for signs and symptoms of hematologic toxicity as evidenced by easy bruising, fever, signs of local infection, sore throat, symptoms of anemia (excessive fatigue, weakness) or unusual bleeding from any site.
• Assess the patient's skin for rash, pruritus, and urticaria.

Patient Teaching
• Instruct the patient to maintain adequate daily fluid intake to protect against hyperuricemia.
• Stress to the patient that he or she should not receive vaccinations without the physician's approval because chlorambucil lowers the body's resistance. Also advise patient to avoid contact with anyone who recently received a live virus vaccine.
• Warn the patient to report congestion, consistent cough, difficulty breathing, easy bruising, fever, signs of local infection, sore throat, or unusual bleeding from any site.

cisplatin
sis-**plah**-tin
(Platinol-AQ)
Do not confuse with carboplatin, Paraplatin, or Patanol.

CATEGORY AND SCHEDULE
Pregnancy Risk Category: D

MECHANISM OF ACTION
A platinum coordination complex that inhibits DNA, and to lesser extent, RNA, protein synthesis by cross-linking with DNA strands. Cell cycle–phase nonspecific. *Therapeutic Effect:* Prevents cellular division.

PHARMACOKINETICS
Widely distributed. Protein binding: greater than 90%. Undergoes rapid nonenzymatic conversion to inactive metabolite. Excreted in urine. Removed by hemodialysis. **Half-life:** 58–73 hrs (half-life is increased with impaired renal function).

AVAILABILITY
Injection: 50-mg, 100-mg vials.

INDICATIONS AND DOSAGES
▸ **Treatment of advanced bladder carcinoma, metastatic ovarian tumors, metastatic testicular tumors**
IV
Adults, Elderly, Children. Intermittent dosage schedule: $37–75 \text{ mg/m}^2$ once every 2–3 wks or $50–100 \text{ mg/m}^2$ over 4–8 hrs once every 21–28 days.
IV
Adults, Elderly, Children. Daily dosage schedule: $15–20 \text{ mg/m}^2$/day for 5 days every 3–4 wks.

▶ **Dosage in renal impairment**

Creatinine Clearance	% of Dose
10–50 ml/min	75%
less than 10 ml/min	50%

UNLABELED USES

Treatment of carcinoma of breast, cervical, endometrial, gastric, head and neck, lung, prostate; germ cell tumors, neuroblastoma, osteosarcoma

CONTRAINDICATIONS

Hearing impairment, myelosuppression, pregnancy

INTERACTIONS
Drug

Antigout medications: May decrease the effects of these drugs.
Bone marrow depressants: May increase bone marrow depression.
Live virus vaccines: May potentiate virus replication, increase vaccine side effects, and decrease the patient's antibody response to the vaccine.
Nephrotoxic, ototoxic agents: May increase the risk of respective toxicities.
Herbal
None known.
Food
None known.

DIAGNOSTIC TEST EFFECTS

May cause positive Coombs' test. May increase BUN, serum creatinine, serum uric acid, and SGOT (AST) levels. May decrease creatinine clearance and serum calcium, magnesium, phosphate, potassium, and sodium levels.

IV INCOMPATIBILITIES

Amifostine (Ethyol), amphotericin B complex (AmBisome, Amphotec, Abelcet), cefepime (Maxipime), piperacillin/tazobactam (Zosyn), thiotepa

IV COMPATIBILITIES

Etoposide (VePesid), granisetron (Kytril), heparin, hydromorphone (Dilaudid), lorazepam (Ativan), magnesium sulfate, mannitol, morphine, ondansetron (Zofran)

SIDE EFFECTS
Frequent
Nausea, vomiting (begins 1–4 hrs after administration, generally last up to 24 hrs). Myelosuppression occurs in 25%–30% of patients. Recovery can generally be expected in 18–23 days.
Occasional
Peripheral neuropathy (numbness, tingling of face, fingers, toes) may occur with prolonged therapy (4–7 mos).
Pain or redness at injection site, loss of taste or appetite
Rare
Hemolytic anemia, blurred vision, stomatitis

SERIOUS REACTIONS

• Anaphylactic reaction manifested as facial edema, wheezing, tachycardia, and hypotension may occur in the first few minutes of IV administration in patients previously exposed to cisplatin.
• Nephrotoxicity occurs in 28%–36% of patients treated with single dose of cisplatin, usually during second week of therapy.
• Ototoxicity, including tinnitus and hearing loss, occurs in 31% of patients treated with a single dose of cisplatin (more severe in children). Ototoxicity may become more frequent or severe with repeated doses.

NURSING CONSIDERATIONS

Baseline Assessment
• Keep patients well hydrated before and 24 hours after receiving this drug to ensure good urinary output and decrease the risk of nephrotoxicity.

Lifespan Considerations
• If possible, cisplatin use should be avoided during pregnancy, especially in the first trimester.
• Be aware that breast-feeding is not recommended in this patient population.
• Be aware that the ototoxic effects of this drug may be more severe in children.
• In the elderly, age-related renal impairment may require dosage adjustment.

Precautions
• Use cautiously in patients with previous therapy with other antineoplastic agents or radiation.

Administration and Handling
◀ALERT▶ Verify any cisplatin dose exceeding 120 mg/m² per course. Know that the dosage is individualized based on the patient's clinical response and tolerance of the drug's adverse effects. When used in combination therapy, consult specific protocols for optimum dosage and sequence of drug administration. Be aware that repeat courses should not be given more frequently than every 3 to 4 weeks. Also, know that the course should not be repeated unless the patient's auditory acuity is within normal limits, serum creatinine less than 1.5 mg/dl, BUN less than 25 mg/dl, and platelet count and white blood cell (WBC) count are within acceptable levels.
◀ALERT▶ Wear protective gloves during handling of cisplatin. Cisplatin may be carcinogenic, mutagenic, or teratogenic. Handle with extreme care during preparation and administration.

IV
• Following reconstitution, solution normally appears clear, colorless.
• Protect from direct sunlight; do not refrigerate because the solution may form a precipitate. Discard if precipitate forms.
• Reconstituted solution is stable for up to 20 hours at room temperature.
• Reconstitute 10-mg vial with 10 ml Sterile Water for Injection (50 ml for 50-mg vial) to provide concentration of 1 mg/ml.
• For IV infusion, dilute desired dose in up to 1,000 ml D_5W, 0.33% or 0.45% NaCl containing 12.5 to 50 g mannitol/L.
• Infuse over 2 to 24 hours.
• Avoid rapid infusion as this increases the risk of nephrotoxicity and ototoxicity.
• Monitor for anaphylactic reaction during first few minutes of IV infusion.

Intervention and Evaluation
• Measure all of the patient's vomitus. If the patient vomits 750 ml or more over 8 hours, notify the physician immediately.
• Monitor the patient's intake and output every 1 to 2 hours, beginning with pretreatment hydration, and continuing for 48 hours after cisplatin therapy. If the patient has a urinary output less than 100 ml each hour, notify the physician immediately.
• Assess the patient's vital signs every 1 to 2 hours during cisplatin infusion.
• Monitor the patient's urinalysis and renal function test results for evidence of nephrotoxicity.

Patient Teaching
• Warn the patient to report signs and symptoms of ototoxicity, including hearing loss or ringing or roaring in the ears.
• Stress to the patient that he or she should not receive vaccinations without the physician's approval as cisplatin lowers the body's resistance and that he or she should avoid contact with anyone who recently received an oral polio vaccine.
• Warn the patient to contact the physician if nausea or vomiting continues at home.
• Teach the patient to recognize signs and symptoms of peripheral neuropathy.

cyclophosphamide
sigh-klo-**phos**-fah-mide
(Cycloblastin[AUS], Cytoxan, Endoxan Asta[AUS], Endoxon Asta[AUS], Neosar, Procytox[CAN])
Do not confuse with cefoxitin, Ciloxan, or Cytotec.

CATEGORY AND SCHEDULE
Pregnancy Risk Category: D

MECHANISM OF ACTION
An alkylating agent that inhibits DNA, RNA protein synthesis by cross-linking with DNA, RNA strands. *Therapeutic Effect:* Inhibits protein synthesis, prevents cell growth. Potent immunosuppressant.

PHARMACOKINETICS
Well absorbed from the gastrointestinal (GI) tract. Crosses blood-brain barrier. Protein binding: Low. Metabolized in liver to active metabolites. Primarily excreted in urine.

Removed by hemodialysis. **Half-life:** 3–12 hrs.

AVAILABILITY
Tablets: 25 mg, 50 mg.
Powder for Injection: 100 mg, 200 mg, 500 mg, 1 g, 2 g.

INDICATIONS AND DOSAGES
▸ **Treatment of adenocarcinoma of ovary, carcinoma of breast, disseminated neuroblastoma, Hodgkin's disease, multiple myeloma, leukemia (acute lymphoblastic, acute myelogenous, acute monocytic, chronic granulocytic, chronic lymphocytic), mycosis fungoides, non-Hodgkin's lymphomas, retinoblastoma**
PO
Adults. 1–5 mg/kg/day.
Children. Initially, 2–8 mg/kg/day. Maintenance: 2–5 mg/kg 2 times/wk.
IV
Adults. 40–50 mg/kg in divided doses over 2–5 days; or 10–15 mg/kg q7–10 days or 3–5 mg/kg 2 times/wk.
Children. Initially, 40–50 mg/kg in divided doses over 2–5 days. Maintenance: 10–15 mg/kg q7–10 days or 3–5 mg/kg 2 times/wk.
▸ **Biopsy-proven minimal-change nephrotic syndrome**
PO
Adults, Children. 2.5–3 mg/kg/day for 60–90 days.

UNLABELED USES
Treatment of carcinoma of bladder, cervix, endometrium, lung, prostate, testicles; germ cell ovarian tumors; osteosarcoma; rheumatoid arthritis; systemic lupus erythematosus

CONTRAINDICATIONS
None known

INTERACTIONS
Drug
Allopurinol, bone marrow depressants: May increase bone marrow depression.

Antigout medications: May decrease the effects of these drugs.

Cytarabine: May increase risk of cardiomyopathy.

Immunosuppressants: May increase the risk of infection and development of neoplasms.

Live virus vaccines: May potentiate virus replication, increase vaccine side effects, and decrease the patient's antibody response to the vaccine.

Herbal
None known.

Food
None known.

DIAGNOSTIC TEST EFFECTS
May increase serum uric acid levels.

IV INCOMPATIBILITIES
Amphotericin B complex (Abelcet, AmBisome, Amphotec)

IV COMPATIBILITIES
Granisetron (Kytril), heparin, hydromorphone (Dilaudid), lorazepam (Ativan), morphine, ondansetron (Zofran), propofol (Diprivan)

SIDE EFFECTS
Expected
Marked leukopenia 8–15 days after initial therapy

Frequent
Nausea, vomiting begins about 6 hrs after administration and lasts about 4 hrs; alopecia (33%)

Occasional
Diarrhea, darkening of skin and fingernails, stomatitis (may include oral ulceration), headache, diaphoresis

Rare
Pain or redness at injection site

SERIOUS REACTIONS
• Cyclophosphamide's major toxic effect is bone marrow depression resulting in blood dyscrasias manifested as leukopenia, anemia, thrombocytopenia, and hypoprothrombinemia.

• Thrombocytopenia may occur 10–15 days after drug initiation.

• Anemia generally occurs after large doses of the drug or prolonged therapy.

• Hemorrhagic cystitis occurs commonly in long-term therapy, especially in pediatric patients.

• Pulmonary fibrosis and cardiotoxicity have been noted with high doses.

• Amenorrhea, azoospermia, and hyperkalemia may also occur.

NURSING CONSIDERATIONS
Baseline Assessment
• Expect to obtain the patient's white blood cell (WBC) count weekly during cyclophosphamide therapy or until the drug's maintenance dose is established, then at 2- to 3-week intervals.

Precautions
• Use cautiously in patients with severe leukopenia, thrombocytopenia, tumor infiltration of bone marrow, or previous therapy with other antineoplastic agents or radiation.

Lifespan Considerations
• Know that cyclophosphamide use should be avoided during pregnancy because of the risk of malformations such as cardiac anomalies, hernias, and limb abnormalities.

• Be aware that cyclophosphamide is distributed in breast milk and that breast-feeding is not recommended in this patient population.

• There are no age-related precautions noted in children.
• In the elderly, age-related renal impairment may require caution.

Administration and Handling

◀ALERT▶ Be aware that cyclophosphamide dosage is individualized based on the patient's clinical response and tolerance of the drug's adverse effects. When used in combination therapy, consult specific protocols for optimum dosage and sequence of drug administration.

◀ALERT▶ Because cyclophosphamide may be carcinogenic, mutagenic, or teratogenic, handle the drug with extreme care during drug preparation and administration.

PO
• Give on an empty stomach. If gastrointestinal (GI) upset occurs, give with food.

IV
• Reconstituted solution is stable for up to 24 hours at room temperature or up to 6 days if refrigerated.
• For IV push, reconstitute each 100 mg with 5 ml Sterile Water for Injection or Bacteriostatic Water for Injection to provide concentration of 20 mg/ml.
• Shake to dissolve. Allow solution to stand until clear.
• Give by IV push or further dilute with 250 ml D_5W, 0.9% NaCl, 0.45% NaCl, lactated Ringer's (LR) solution or D_5W/LR.
• Infuse each 100 mg or fraction thereof over 15 minutes or more.
• Be aware that IV route may produce diaphoresis, facial flushing, faintness, and oropharyngeal sensation.

Intervention and Evaluation
• Monitor the patient's blood chemistries, complete blood count (CBC), and serum uric acid concentration.

• Monitor the patient's WBC closely during initial therapy.
• Monitor the patient for signs and symptoms of anemia, such as excessive fatigue and weakness, and hematologic toxicity, such as, easy bruising, fever, signs of local infection, sore throat, and unusual bleeding from any site.
• Expect recovery from marked leukopenia because of bone marrow depression in 17 to 28 days.

Patient Teaching
• To help prevent cystitis, encourage the patient to drink fluids 24 hours before, during, and after therapy and to void frequently.
• Stress to the patient that he or she should not receive vaccinations without the physician's approval because cyclophosphamide lowers the body's resistance. Also warn the patient to avoid contact with anyone who recently received a live virus vaccine.
• Warn the patient to report easy bruising, fever, signs of local infection, sore throat, or unusual bleeding from any site.
• Explain to the patient that hair loss (alopecia) is reversible, but new hair growth may have a different color or texture.

estramustine phosphate sodium
es-trah-mew-steen
(Emcyt)
Do not confuse with Eryc.

CATEGORY AND SCHEDULE
Pregnancy Risk Category: C

MECHANISM OF ACTION
An alkylating agent, estrogen and nitrogen mustard, that binds to

microtubule-associated proteins, causing their disassembly. *Therapeutic Effect:* Reduces serum testosterone concentration.

PHARMACOKINETICS

Well absorbed from the gastrointestinal (GI) tract. Highly localized in prostatic tissue. Rapidly dephosphorylated during absorption into peripheral circulation. Metabolized in liver. Primarily eliminated in feces via biliary system. **Half-life:** 20 hrs.

AVAILABILITY

Capsules: 140 mg.

INDICATIONS AND DOSAGES
▸ **Prostatic carcinoma**
PO
Adults, Elderly. 10–16 mg/kg/day (140 mg for each 10 kg weight) in 3–4 doses/day.

CONTRAINDICATIONS

Active thrombophlebitis or thrombolic disorders unless the tumor is the cause of the thrombolic disorders and the benefits outweigh the risk; hypersensitivity to estradiol or nitrogen mustard

INTERACTIONS
Drug
Liver toxic drugs: May increase the risk of liver toxicity.
Herbal
None known.
Food
None known.

DIAGNOSTIC TEST EFFECTS

May increase serum bilirubin, blood glucose, serum cortisol, serum LDH, serum phospholipids, serum prolactin, SGOT (AST), serum sodium, and serum triglyceride levels. May decrease serum levels of antithrombin III, folate, and phosphate and urine levels of pregnanediol. May alter thyroid function tests.

SIDE EFFECTS
Frequent
Peripheral edema of lower extremities, breast tenderness or enlargement, diarrhea, flatulence, nausea
Occasional
Increase in blood pressure (B/P), thirst, dry skin, easy bruising, flushing, thinning hair, night sweats
Rare
Headache, rash, fatigue, insomnia, vomiting

SERIOUS REACTIONS

• Estramustine use may exacerbate congestive heart failure (CHF), and increase the risk of pulmonary emboli, thrombophlebitis, and cerebrovascular accident.

NURSING CONSIDERATIONS

Lifespan Considerations
• Be aware that estramustine is not used in pregnant women or in children.
• In the elderly, age-related renal impairment and peripheral vascular disease may require cautious use of this drug.
Precautions
• Use cautiously in patients with cerebrovascular or coronary artery disease; a history of thrombophlebitis, thrombosis, or thromboembolic disorders; impaired liver function; and metabolic bone disease in those with hypercalcemia or renal insufficiency.
Administration and Handling
PO
• Refrigerate capsules. The drug may be maintained at room temperature for 24 to 48 hours without loss of potency.

• Give with water 1 hour before or 2 hours after meals.

Intervention and Evaluation
• Monitor the patient's B/P periodically.

Patient Teaching
• Instruct the patient not to take estramustine with calcium-containing antacids, calcium-rich food, milk, or milk products.
• Encourage the patient to use contraceptive measures during estramustine therapy.
• Warn the patient to notify the physician if he or she experiences calf pain, disturbed speech or vision, dizziness, headache (migraine or severe), heaviness in chest, numbness, shortness of breath, unexplained cough, or vomiting.

ifosfamide
eye-**fos**-fah-mid
(Holoxan[AUS], Ifex)

CATEGORY AND SCHEDULE
Pregnancy Risk Category: D

MECHANISM OF ACTION
An alkylating agent that is converted to active metabolite and binds with intracellular structures. Action primarily due to cross-linking strands of DNA, RNA. *Therapeutic Effect:* Inhibits protein synthesis.

PHARMACOKINETICS
Metabolized in liver to active metabolite. Crosses blood-brain barrier (limited). Primarily excreted in urine. Removed by hemodialysis.
Half-life: 15 hrs.

AVAILABILITY
Powder for Injection: 1 g, 3 g.

INDICATIONS AND DOSAGES
▸ **Germ cell testicular carcinoma**
IV
Adults. 700–2,000 mg/m²/day for 5 consecutive days. Repeat q3wks or after recovery from hematologic toxicity. Administer with mesna.
Children. 1,200–1,800 mg/m²/day for 5 days q21–28 days.

UNLABELED USES
Treatment of Ewing's sarcoma; non-Hodgkin's lymphomas; lung, pancreatic, and soft tissue carcinoma

CONTRAINDICATIONS
Pregnancy, severely depressed bone marrow function

INTERACTIONS
Drug
Bone marrow depressants: May increase bone marrow depression.
Live virus vaccines: May potentiate virus replication, increase vaccine side effects, and decrease the patient's antibody response to vaccine.
Herbal
None known.
Food
None known.

DIAGNOSTIC TEST EFFECTS
May increase BUN, serum bilirubin, serum creatinine, serum uric acid, SGOT (AST), and SGPT (ALT) levels.

IV INCOMPATIBILITIES
Cefepime (Maxipime), methotrexate

IV COMPATIBILITIES
Granisetron (Kytril), ondansetron (Zofran)

SIDE EFFECTS
Frequent
Alopecia (83%); nausea, vomiting (58%)

Occasional (15%–5%)
Confusion, somnolence, hallucinations, infection
Rare (less than 5%)
Dizziness, seizures, disorientation, fever, malaise, stomatitis (mucosal irritation, glossitis, gingivitis)

SERIOUS REACTIONS

• Hemorrhagic cystitis with hematuria, dysuria occurs frequently if a protective agent (mesna) is not used.
• Myelosuppression characterized as leukopenia, and, to a lesser extent, thrombocytopenia, occurs frequently.
• Pulmonary toxicity, liver toxicity, nephrotoxicity, cardiotoxicity, central nervous system (CNS) toxicity manifested as confusion, hallucinations, somnolence, and coma may require discontinuation of therapy.

NURSING CONSIDERATIONS

Baseline Assessment
• Obtain the patient's urinalysis test results, as appropriate, before each dose. If hematuria occurs, evidenced by greater than 10 red blood cells per field, notify physician because therapy should be withheld until resolution occurs.
• Expect to obtain the patient's white blood cell (WBC) count, platelet count, and blood Hgb levels before each dose.
Precautions
• Use cautiously in patients with compromised bone marrow function and impaired liver or renal function.
Lifespan Considerations
• If possible, ifosfamide use should be avoided during pregnancy, especially in the first trimester.
• Be aware that ifosfamide may cause fetal harm.
• Be aware that ifosfamide is dis-

tributed in breast milk. Breast-feeding is not recommended in this patient population.
• Be aware that ifosfamide is not intended for use in children.
• In the elderly, age-related renal impairment may require dosage adjustment.

Administration and Handling
◀ALERT▶ Be aware that ifosfamide dosage is individualized based on the patient's clinical response and tolerance of the drug's adverse effects. When used in combination therapy, consult specific protocols for optimum dosage and sequence of drug administration.
◀ALERT▶ Because ifosfamide may be carcinogenic, mutagenic, or teratogenic, handle the drug with extreme care during preparation and administration.
◀ALERT▶ Hemorrhagic cystitis may occur if mesna is not given concurrently with ifosfamide. Mesna should always be given with ifosfamide.
IV
• Store vial at room temperature.
• After reconstitution with Bacteriostatic Water for Injection, store solution for up to 1 week at room temperature, or refrigerate for up to 3 weeks. Refrigerate further diluted solution for up to 6 weeks.
• Use solution prepared with other diluents within 6 hours.
• Reconstitute 1-g vial with 20 ml Sterile Water for Injection or Bacteriostatic Water for Injection to provide a concentration of 50 mg/ml. Shake to dissolve.
• Further dilute with D_5W or 0.9% NaCl to provide concentration of 0.6 to 20 mg/ml.
• Infuse over a minimum of 30 minutes.
• Give with at least 2,000 ml PO or IV fluid to prevent bladder toxicity.

• Give with a prescribed protectant against hemorrhagic cystitis, such as mesna. Be aware that mesna should always be given with ifosfamide to prevent other adverse reactions, including chills, fever, jaundice, joint pain, sore throat, stomatitis, or unusual bleeding or bruising.

Intervention and Evaluation

• Monitor the patient's hematologic studies and urinalysis results diligently.

• Assess the patient for easy bruising, fever, signs of local infection, sore throat, symptoms of anemia, such as excessive fatigue, weakness, and unusual bleeding from any site.

Patient Teaching

• Encourage the patient to drink fluids to protect against cystitis.

• Stress to the patient that he or she should not receive vaccinations without the physician's approval because ifosfamide lowers the body's resistance. Also warn the patient to avoid contact with anyone who recently received a live virus vaccine. Explain to the patient that he or she should avoid crowds and those with known infection.

• Warn the patient to notify the physician if he or she experiences chills, fever, joint pain, sores in the mouth or on the lips, sore throat, yellowing of the skin or eyes, unusual bleeding or bruising.

lomustine
low-**meuw**-steen
(CeeNU)

CATEGORY AND SCHEDULE
Pregnancy Risk Category: D

MECHANISM OF ACTION
An alkylating agent and nitrosourea that inhibits DNA, RNA synthesis by cross-linking with DNA, RNA strands, preventing cellular division. Cell cycle–phase nonspecific. *Therapeutic Effect:* Interferes with DNA and RNA function.

AVAILABILITY
Capsules: 10 mg, 40 mg, 100 mg, 300 mg.

INDICATIONS AND DOSAGES
▸ **Treatment of disseminated Hodgkin's disease; primary and metastatic brain tumors**
PO
Adults, Elderly. 100–130 mg/m^2 as single dose. Repeat dose at intervals of at least 6 wks but not until circulating blood elements have returned to acceptable levels. Adjust dose based on hematologic response to previous dose.
Children. 75–150 mg/m^2 as single dose q6wks.

UNLABELED USES
Treatment of breast, gastrointestinal (GI), lung, renal carcinoma; malignant melanoma; multiple myeloma

CONTRAINDICATIONS
Pregnancy

INTERACTIONS
Drug
Bone marrow depressants: May increase bone marrow depression.
Live virus vaccines: May potentiate virus replication, increase vaccine side effects, and decrease a patient's antibody response to the vaccine.
Herbal
None known.
Food
None known.

DIAGNOSTIC TEST EFFECTS

May cause elevated liver function test results.

SIDE EFFECTS

Frequent

Nausea, vomiting occur 45 min–6 hrs after dosing, lasts 12–24 hrs. Anorexia often follows for 2–3 days.

Occasional

Neurotoxicity (confusion, slurred speech), stomatitis, darkening of skin, diarrhea, skin rash, itching, hair loss

SERIOUS REACTIONS

• Bone marrow depression manifested as hematologic toxicity (principally leukopenia, mild anemia, thrombocytopenia) may occur.

• Leukopenia occurs at about 6 weeks, thrombocytopenia at about 4 weeks, and persists for 1–2 weeks.

• Refractory anemia and thrombocytopenia occur commonly if lomustine therapy is continued for more than 1 year.

• Liver toxicity occurs infrequently.

• Large cumulative doses of lomustine may result in renal damage.

NURSING CONSIDERATIONS

Baseline Assessment

• As ordered, obtain weekly blood counts and know that this is recommended by the manufacturer. Be aware that experts recommend that the first blood count be obtained 2 to 3 weeks after initial therapy and that subsequent blood counts should be obtained based on prior hematologic toxicity.

• Give antiemetics, as prescribed, to reduce the duration and frequency of nausea or vomiting.

Precautions

• Use cautiously in patients with depressed erythrocyte, leukocyte, or platelet counts.

Administration and Handling

◄ALERT► Be aware that lomustine dosage is individualized based on the patient's clinical response and tolerance of the drug's adverse effects. When used in combination therapy, consult specific protocols for optimum dosage and sequence of drug administration.

Intervention and Evaluation

• Monitor the patient's complete blood count (CBC) with differential; platelet count; and liver, renal, and pulmonary function tests.

• Assess the patient for stomatitis as evidenced by burning or erythema of the oral mucosa at the inner margin of lips, difficulty swallowing, and sore throat.

• Monitor for the patient for signs and symptoms of anemia, including excessive fatigue and weakness, and hematologic toxicity, including easy bruising, fever, signs of local infection, sore throat, and unusual bleeding from any site.

Patient Teaching

• Explain that nausea or vomiting usually abates in less than 1 day. Further explain that fasting before therapy can reduce the frequency and duration of GI effects.

• Teach the patient to maintain fastidious oral hygiene to prevent stomatitis.

• Stress to the patient that he or she should not receive vaccinations without the physician's approval as lomustine lowers the body's resistance. Warn patient to avoid contact with anyone who recently received a live virus vaccine. Explain to the patient that he or she should avoid crowds and those with known illness.

• Warn the patient to notify the physician if he or she experiences easy bruising, fever, jaundice, signs of local infection, sore throat, swelling of the legs and feet, and unusual bleeding from any site.

melphalan
mel-fah-lan
(Alkeran)
Do not confuse with Leukeran, Mephyton, or Myleran.

CATEGORY AND SCHEDULE
Pregnancy Risk Category: D

MECHANISM OF ACTION
An alkylating agent that primarily cross-links strands of DNA and RNA. Cell cycle–phase nonspecific. *Therapeutic Effect:* Inhibits protein synthesis, producing cell death.

AVAILABILITY
Tablets: 2 mg.
Powder for Injection: 50 mg.

INDICATIONS AND DOSAGES
▸ **Ovarian carcinoma**
PO
Adults, Elderly. 0.2 mg/kg/day for 5 successive days. Repeat at 4- to 6-wk intervals.
▸ **Multiple myeloma**
PO
Adults. 6 mg once a day, initially adjusted as indicated or 0.15 mg/kg/day for 7 days or 0.25 mg/kg/day for 4 days. Repeat at 4- to 6-wk intervals.
IV
Adults. 16 mg/m²/dose q2wks for 4 doses; then repeat monthly as per protocol.

UNLABELED USES
Treatment of breast carcinoma, neuroblastoma, rhabdomyosarcoma, testicular carcinoma

CONTRAINDICATIONS
Pregnancy, severe bone marrow suppression

INTERACTIONS
Drug
Antigout medications: May decrease the effects of these drugs.
Bone marrow depressants: May increase bone marrow depression.
Live virus vaccines: May potentiate virus replication, increase vaccine side effects, and decrease the patient's antibody response to vaccine.
Herbal
None known.
Food
None known.

DIAGNOSTIC TEST EFFECTS
May increase serum uric acid and cause a positive direct Coombs test.

IV INCOMPATIBILITIES
Do not mix with any other medications.

SIDE EFFECTS
Frequent
Nausea, vomiting (may be severe with large dose)
Occasional
Diarrhea, stomatitis (burning or erythema of oral mucosa, sore throat, difficulty swallowing, oral ulceration), rash, pruritus, alopecia

SERIOUS REACTIONS
• Bone marrow depression manifested as hematologic toxicity (principally leukopenia, thrombocytopenia, and to lesser extent, anemia, pancytopenia, and agranulocytosis) may occur.

• Leukopenia may occur as early as 5 days following drug initiation.
• White blood cell (WBC) and platelet counts return to normal levels during fifth week, but leukopenia or thrombocytopenia may last more than 6 weeks after discontinuing this drug.
• Hyperuricemia noted by hematuria, crystalluria, and flank pain may occur.

NURSING CONSIDERATIONS

Baseline Assessment
• Expect to obtain blood counts weekly. Expect dosage to be decreased or discontinued if WBC falls below 3,000/mm³ or platelet count falls below 100,000/mm³.
• Expect to give antiemetics, if ordered, to prevent and treat nausea and vomiting.

Precautions
• Use cautiously in patients with bone marrow suppression, impaired renal function, and a leukocyte count less than 3,000/mm³ or platelet count less than 100,000/mm³.

Administration and Handling
◀ ALERT ▶ Because melphalan may be carcinogenic, mutagenic, or teratogenic, handle the drug with extreme care during preparation and administration. Know that melphalan dosage is individualized on the basis of the patient's clinical response and tolerance of the drug's adverse effects. When used in combination therapy, consult specific protocols for optimum dosage and sequence of drug administration. Be aware that leukocyte count is usually maintained between 3,000 to 4,000/mm³.
◀ ALERT ▶ Expect to decrease melphalan dosage by 50% in patients with BUN greater than 30 mg/dl or

serum creatinine greater than 1.5 mg/dl.
IV
• Store melphalan at room temperature and protect from light.
• Once reconstituted, the solution is stable for up to 90 minutes at room temperature. Do not refrigerate.
• Reconstitute 50-mg vial with diluent supplied by manufacturer to yield a 5 mg/ml solution.
• Further dilute with 0.9% NaCl to a final concentration, not to exceed 2 mg/ml for a central line or 0.45 mg/ml for a peripheral line.
• Infuse over 15 to 30 minutes at a rate not to exceed 10 mg/min.

Intervention and Evaluation
• Monitor the patient's blood Hgb, complete blood count (CBC) with differential, serum electrolytes, and platelet count.
• Evaluate the patient for signs and symptoms of stomatitis.
• Monitor the patient for signs and symptoms of anemia, including excessive fatigue and weakness, hematologic toxicity, including easy bruising, fever, signs of local infection, sore throat, and unusual bleeding from any site, and hyperuricemia, including hematuria and flank pain).

Patient Teaching
• Teach the patient to avoid IM injections, rectal temperatures, or other traumatic procedures that may induce bleeding.
• Encourage the patient to increase his or her fluid intake to protect against hyperuricemia development.
• Teach the patient to maintain fastidious oral hygiene.
• Advise the patient that alopecia is reversible, but new hair growth may have a different color or texture.
• Stress to the patient that he or she

avoid crowds and those with known infections.

• Warn the patient to notify the physician if bleeding, bruising, cough, fever, shortness of breath, or sore throat occurs.

oxaliplatin
ox-**ale**-ee-plah-tin
(Eloxatin)

CATEGORY AND SCHEDULE
Pregnancy Risk Category: D

MECHANISM OF ACTION
A platinum-containing complex that inhibits DNA replication by cross-linking with DNA strands. Cell cycle–phase nonspecific. *Therapeutic Effect:* Prevents cellular division.

PHARMACOKINETICS
Rapidly distributed. Undergoes rapid, extensive nonenzymatic biotransformation. Protein binding: greater than 90%. Excreted in urine. **Half-life:** 70 hrs.

AVAILABILITY
Powder for Injection: 50-mg, 100-mg vials.

INDICATIONS AND DOSAGES
▸ **Metastatic colon or rectal cancer in patients whose disease has recurred or progressed during or within 6 months of completion of first-line therapy with bolus 5-fluorouracil (5-FU)/leucovorin and irinotecan.**
IV
Adults. Day 1: Oxaliplatin 85 mg/m² in 250–500 ml D_5W and leucovorin 200 mg/m², both given more than 120 min at the same time in separate bags using a Y-line,

followed by 5-FU 400 mg/m² IV bolus given over 2–4 min, followed by 5-FU 600 mg/m² IV infusion in 500 ml D_5W as a 22-hr continuous infusion. Day 2: Leucovorin 200 mg/m² IV infusion given over more than 120 min, followed by 5-FU 400 mg/m² IV bolus given over 2–4 min, followed by 5-FU 600 mg/m² IV infusion in 500 ml D_5W as a 22-hr continuous infusion.
▸ **Ovarian cancer**
IV
Adults. Cisplatin 100 mg/m² and oxaliplatin 130 mg/m² q3wks.

UNLABELED USES
Treatment of ovarian cancer

CONTRAINDICATIONS
History of allergy to platinum compounds

INTERACTIONS
Drug
Live virus vaccines: May potentiate virus replication, increase vaccine side effects, and decrease the patient's antibody response to vaccine. *Nephrotic agents:* May decrease the clearance of oxaliplatin.
Herbal
None known.
Food
None known.

DIAGNOSTIC TEST EFFECTS
May alter serum bilirubin, SGOT (AST), and SGPT (ALT) levels. May decrease blood Hgb and Hct levels and platelet count.

IV INCOMPATIBILITIES
Do not infuse with alkaline medications.

SIDE EFFECTS
Frequent (76%–20%)
Peripheral or sensory neuropathy

usually occurs in hands, feet, peri-oral area, throat but may present as jaw spasm, abnormal tongue sensation, eye pain, chest pressure, difficulty walking, swallowing, writing; nausea (occurs in 64%), fatigue, diarrhea, vomiting, constipation, abdominal pain, fever, anorexia
Occasional (14%–10%)
Stomatitis, earache, insomnia, cough, difficulty breathing, back-ache, edema
Rare (7%–3%)
Dyspepsia (indigestion, heartburn), dizziness, rhinitis, flushing, alopecia

SERIOUS REACTIONS
• Peripheral or sensory neuropathy can occur without any prior event, but ice or drinking, or holding a glass of cold liquid during IV infusion phase can precipitate or exacerbate this neurotoxicity.
• Pulmonary fibrosis characterized as nonproductive cough, dyspnea, crackles, and radiologic pulmonary infiltrates may warrant discontinuation of drug therapy.
• Hypersensitivity reaction (rash, hives, itching) occurs rarely.

NURSING CONSIDERATIONS
Baseline Assessment
• Ensure that the patient doesn't suck on ice, drink or touch a glass of cold liquid during IV infusion because this can precipitate or exacerbate neurotoxicity, which occurs within hours or 1 to 2 days of dosing and lasts up to 14 days.
• Assess the patient's baseline BUN, serum creatinine, blood platelet count, and white blood cell (WBC) count.
Lifespan Considerations
• Know that oxaliplatin use should be avoided, if possible, during pregnancy, especially in the first trimester because it may cause fetal harm. Breast-feeding is not recommended in this patient population.
• Be aware that the safety and efficacy of oxaliplatin have not been established in children.
• In the elderly, there is an increased incidence of dehydration, diarrhea, fatigue, and hypokalemia.
Precautions
• Use cautiously in patients that have had previous therapy with other antineoplastic agents or radiation.
• Use cautiously in patients with impaired renal function, infection, or who are pregnant or immunosuppressed.
• Use cautiously in patients with peripheral neuropathy or a history of peripheral neuropathy.
Administration and Handling
◀ALERT▶ Pretreat the patient with antiemetics (5-HT$_3$ antagonists), if ordered. Know that repeat courses should not be given more frequently than every 2 weeks.
◀ALERT▶ Wear protective gloves during handling of oxaliplatin. If solution comes in contact with skin, wash skin immediately with soap and water. Do not use aluminum needles or administration sets that may come in contact with drug because they may cause degradation of platinum compounds.
◀ALERT▶ Have the patient avoid ice or drinking or touching cold objects during infusion because this can exacerbate acute neuropathy.
◀ALERT▶ Never reconstitute oxaliplatin with sodium chloride solution or chloride-containing solutions.
IV
• Following reconstitution, solution is stable up to 24 hours in the refrigerator and for up to 6 hours at room temperature.

• Reconstitute 50-mg vial with 10 ml sterile Water for Injection or D_5W (20 ml for 100-mg vial). Further dilute with 150 to 500 ml D_5W.

• Administer differing infusion rates as a 2-hour or 22-hour rate, according to protocol orders.

Intervention and Evaluation

• Although myelosuppression is minimal, monitor the patient for a decrease in platelet or white blood cell (WBC) counts.

• Evaluate the patient for diarrhea and gastrointestinal (GI) bleeding as evidenced by bright red or tarry stool.

• Monitor the patient's intake and output.

• Assess the patient for signs and symptoms of stomatitis, including mucosal erythema of the oral mucosa, sore throat, and ulceration of the inner margin of lips and mouth.

Patient Teaching

• Encourage the patient not to consume cold drinks or ice and to avoid holding cold objects during the IV infusion phase because this can produce neuropathy.

• Warn the patient to promptly report if he or she experiences easy bruising, fever, signs of local infection, sore throat, or unusual bleeding from any site.

• Stress to the patient that he or she should not receive vaccinations and should avoid contact with anyone who recently received oral polio vaccine.

thiotepa
thigh-oh-**teh**-pah
(Thiotepa)

CATEGORY AND SCHEDULE
Pregnancy Risk Category: D

MECHANISM OF ACTION
An alkylating agent that binds with many intracellular structures. Crosslinks strands of DNA and RNA. Cell cycle–phase nonspecific. *Therapeutic Effect:* Disrupts protein synthesis, producing cell death.

AVAILABILITY
Powder for Injection: 15 mg, 30 mg.

INDICATIONS AND DOSAGES
▸ **Treatment of adenocarcinoma of breast and ovary, Hodgkin's disease, lymphosarcoma, superficial papillary carcinoma of urinary bladder**
IV
Adults, Elderly. Initially, 0.3–0.4 mg/kg q1–4wks. Maintenance dose adjusted weekly on basis of blood counts.
Children. 25–65 mg/m² as a single dose q3–4wks.
▸ **Control pericardial, peritoneal, or pleural effusions due to metastatic tumors**
Intracavitary injection
Adults, Elderly. 0.6–0.8 mg/kg q1–4wks.

UNLABELED USES
Treatment of lung carcinoma

CONTRAINDICATIONS
Pregnancy, severe myelosuppression (leukocyte count less than 3,000/mm³ or platelet count less than 150,000 mm³)

INTERACTIONS
Drug
Antigout medications: May decrease the effects of these drugs.
Bone marrow depressants: May increase bone marrow depression.
Live virus vaccines: May potentiate virus replication, increase vaccine side effects, and decrease the patient's antibody response to vaccine.
Herbal
None known.
Food
None known.

DIAGNOSTIC TEST EFFECTS
May increase serum uric acid levels.

IV INCOMPATIBILITIES
Cisplatin (Platinol AQ), filgrastim (Neupogen)

IV COMPATIBILITIES
Allopurinol (Aloprim), bumetanide (Bumex), calcium gluconate, carboplatin (Paraplatin), cyclophosphamide (Cytoxan), dexamethasone (Decadron), diphenhydramine (Benadryl), doxorubicin (Adriamycin), etoposide (VePesid), fluorouracil, gemcitabine (Gemzar), granisetron (Kytril), heparin, hydromorphone (Dilaudid), leucovorin, lorazepam (Ativan), magnesium sulfate, morphine, ondansetron (Zofran), paclitaxel (Taxol), potassium chloride, vincristine (Oncovin), vinorelbine (Navelbine)

SIDE EFFECTS
Occasional
Pain at injection site, headache, dizziness, hives, rash, nausea, vomiting, anorexia, stomatitis
Rare
Alopecia, cystitis, hematuria following intravesical dosing

SERIOUS REACTIONS
• Hematologic toxicity manifested as leukopenia, anemia, thrombocytopenia, and pancytopenia due to bone marrow depression may occur.
• Although white blood cell (WBC) count falls to lowest point at 10–14 days after initial therapy, bone marrow effects are not evident for 30 days.
• Stomatitis and ulceration of intestinal mucosa may be noted.

NURSING CONSIDERATIONS
Baseline Assessment
• Expect the patient to undergo hematologic testing at least weekly during therapy and for 3 weeks after therapy is discontinued.
Precautions
• Use cautiously in patients with bone marrow dysfunction and liver or renal impairment.
Administration and Handling
◀ALERT▶ Know that thiotepa dosage is individualized based on the patient's clinical response and tolerance of the drug's adverse effects. When used in combination therapy, consult specific protocols for optimum thiotepa dosage and sequence of drug administration.
◀ALERT▶ Because thiotepa may be carcinogenic, mutagenic, or teratogenic, handle the drug with extreme care during preparation and administration.
◀ALERT▶ Know that the drug may be given by intrapericardial, intraperitoneal, intrapleural, intratumoral, or IV injection and by intravesical instillation.
IV
• Refrigerate unopened vials.
• Reconstituted solution normally appears clear to slightly opaque. Store refrigerated solution for up to 5 days. Discard if solution ap-

pears grossly opaque or precipitate forms.

• Reconstitute 15-mg vial with 1.5 ml Sterile Water for Injection to provide concentration of 10 mg/ml. Shake solution gently; let stand to clear.

• Withdraw reconstituted drug through a 0.22-micron filter before administering. For IV push, give over 5 minutes at concentration of 10 mg/ml. Give IV infusion at concentration of 1 mg/ml.

Intervention and Evaluation

• Interrupt thiotepa therapy if the patient's platelet count falls below 150,000/mm^3 and WBC falls below 3,000/mm^3 or if the patient's platelet or WBC count declines rapidly.

• Monitor the patient's hematology tests and serum uric acid levels.

• Assess the patient for signs and symptoms of stomatitis, such as burning or erythema of the oral mucosa at the inner margin of lips, difficulty swallowing, oral ulceration, and sore throat.

• Monitor the patient for signs and symptoms of symptoms of anemia, including excessive fatigue and weakness, and hematologic toxicity, including easy bruising, fever, signs of local infection, sore throat, or unusual bleeding from any site).

• Assess the patient's skin for hives and rash.

Patient Teaching

• Teach the patient to maintain fastidious oral hygiene to guard against developing stomatitis.

• Stress to the patient that he or she should not receive vaccinations and should avoid contact with crowds and anyone with known infection or who recently received a live virus vaccine.

• Warn the patient to promptly notify the physician if he or she experiences easy bruising, fever, signs of local infection, sore throat, or unusual bleeding from any site.

bleomycin sulfate
daunorubicin
doxorubicin
epirubicin
idarubicin
  hydrochloride
mitomycin
plicamycin
valrubicin

Uses: Antineoplastic antibiotics are cytotoxic and are therefore only used to treat cancer and not infections. *Bleomycin* is prescribed for germ cell tumors of the testes and ovaries. *Daunorubicin* is effective in acute lymphocytic and acute myelogenous leukemias. *Doxorubicin* is used in acute leukemias, malignant lymphomas, and breast cancer. *Epirubicin* is used only in breast cancer. *Idarubicin* is active against acute myelogenous leukemia. *Mitomycin* may be prescribed for carcinoma of cervix, stomach, breasts, bladder, head, or neck. *Plicamycin* provides treatment for testicular carcinoma. *Valrubicin* is a useful treatment for urinary bladder cancer.

Action: Originally isolated from cultures of *Streptomyces,* antineoplastic antibiotics act by inhibiting ribonucleic acid synthesis and binding with deoxyribonucleic acid (DNA). These actions cause fragmentation of DNA molecules.

bleomycin sulfate
blee-oh-**my**-sin
(Blenoxane)

CATEGORY AND SCHEDULE
Pregnancy Risk Category: D

MECHANISM OF ACTION
A glycopeptide antibiotic whose mechanism of action is unknown. Most effective in G_2 phase of cell division. *Therapeutic Effect:* Appears to inhibit DNA synthesis and, to a lesser extent, RNA and protein synthesis.

AVAILABILITY
Powder for Injection: 15 units, 30 units.

INDICATIONS AND DOSAGES
▶ **As single agent therapy to treat lymphomas, including Hodgkin's disease, choriocarcinoma, reticulum cell sarcoma, lymphosarcoma and squamous cell carcinomas of the head and neck, including mouth, tongue, tonsil, nasopharynx, oropharynx, sinus, palate, lip, buccal mucosa, gingiva, epiglottis, and larynx, and testicular carcinoma.**
IV/IM/Subcutaneous
Adults, Elderly. 10–20 units/m^2 (0.25–0.5 units/kg) 1–2 times/wk.
IV
Adults, Elderly. 15 units/m^2 over 24 hrs for 4 days.
▶ **In combination therapy to treat lymphomas, including Hodgkin's disease, choriocarcinoma, reticulum cell sarcoma, lymphosarcoma and squamous cell carcinomas of**

the head and neck, including mouth, tongue, tonsil, nasopharynx, oropharynx, sinus, palate, lip, buccal mucosa, gingiva, epiglottis, and larynx, and testicular carcinoma.
IV/IM
Adults, Elderly. 3–4 units/m²
▸ **Pleural sclerosing**
IV infusion
Adults, Elderly. 60–240 units as a single infusion.

UNLABELED USES
Treatment of mycosis fungoides, osteosarcoma, ovarian tumors, renal carcinoma, soft tissue sarcoma

CONTRAINDICATIONS
Previous allergic reaction

INTERACTIONS
Drug
Antineoplastics: May increase risk of bleomycin toxicity.
Cisplatin: Cisplatin-induced renal impairment may decrease bleomycin clearance and increase the risk of bleomycin toxicity.
Herbal
None known.
Food
None known.

DIAGNOSTIC TEST EFFECTS
None known.

IV INCOMPATIBILITIES
None known via Y-site administration.

IV COMPATIBILITIES
Cefepime (Maxipime), dacarbazine (DTIC), dexamethasone (Decadron), diphenhydramine (Benadryl), fludarabine (Fludara), gemcitabine (Gemzar), ondansetron (Zofran), paclitaxel (Taxol), piperacillin/

tazobactam (Zosyn), vinblastine (Velban), vinorelbine (Navelbine)

SIDE EFFECTS
Frequent
Anorexia, weight loss, erythematous skin swelling, urticaria, rash, striae (streaking), vesiculation (small blisters), hyperpigmentation (particularly at areas of pressure, skin folds, nail cuticles, IM injection sites, scars), mucosal lesions of lips, tongue (stomatitis, which is usually evident 1 to 3 wks after initial therapy). May also be accompanied by decreased skin sensitivity followed by hypersensitivity of skin, nausea, vomiting, alopecia, fever or chills with parenteral form (particularly noted a few hours after large single dose, lasts 4–12 hrs).

SERIOUS REACTIONS
• Interstitial pneumonitis occurs in 10% of patients, occasionally progressing to pulmonary fibrosis. This condition appears to be dose or age-related, particularly in patients older than 70 years of age or those receiving a total dose greater than 400 units.
• Renal and liver toxicity occur infrequently.

NURSING CONSIDERATIONS
Baseline Assessment
• Expect the patient to have chest x-rays performed every 1 to 2 weeks during bleomycin therapy.
Precautions
• Use cautiously in patients with severe pulmonary or renal impairment.
Administration and Handling
◀ALERT▶ Know that bleomycin dosage is individualized based on the patient's clinical response and tolerance of the drug's adverse

effects. When used in combination therapy, consult specific protocols for optimum dosage and sequence of drug administration. Be aware that cumulative doses greater than 400 units increase the risk of developing pulmonary toxicity. For lymphoma patients, administer test doses of 2 units or less for the first 2 doses, as ordered, because of the increased possibility of an anaphylactoid reaction.

◀ALERT▶ Because bleomycin may be carcinogenic, mutagenic, or teratogenic, handle the drug with extreme care during drug preparation and administration.

Subcutaneous/IM
• Refrigerate powder.
• After reconstitution with 0.9% NaCl, the solution is stable for up to 24 hours at room temperature.
• Reconstitute 15-unit vial with 1 to 5 ml (30-unit vial with 2 to 10 ml) Sterile Water for Injection, 0.9% NaCl injection, or Bacteriostatic Water for Injection to provide concentration of 3 to 15 units/ml. Do not use D_5W.

IV
• Refrigerate powder.
• After reconstitution with 0.9% NaCl, store solution for up to 24 hours at room temperature.
• Reconstitute 15-unit vial with at least 5 ml (30-unit vial with at least 10 ml) 0.9% NaCl to provide a concentration not greater than 3 unit/ml.
• Administer over at least 10 minutes for IV injection.

Intervention and Evaluation
• Monitor the patient's lung sounds for pulmonary toxicity as evidenced by dyspnea, fine lung rales, and rhonchi.
• Monitor the patient's hematologic and oxygen saturation tests and liver and renal function test results, including BUN, serum bilirubin, creatinine, SGOT (AST), and SGPT (ALT) levels.
• Assess the patient's skin each day for cutaneous toxicity.
• Monitor the patient for signs and symptoms of anemia, including excessive fatigue and weakness, hematologic toxicity, including easy bruising, fever, signs of local infection, sore throat, unusual bleeding, and stomatitis, including burning or erythema of oral mucosa at inner margin of lips, palate, and tongue.

Patient Teaching
• Advise the patient that the fever and chills reaction occurs less frequently with continued bleomycin therapy.
• Explain to the patient that improvement of Hodgkin's disease and testicular tumors is usually noted within 2 weeks of bleomycin treatment and improvement of squamous cell carcinoma is usually noted within 3 weeks of bleomycin treatment.
• Stress to the patient that he or she should not receive vaccinations and should avoid contact with anyone who recently received a live virus vaccine.

daunorubicin
dawn-oh-**rue**-bih-sin
(Cerubidine, DaunoXome)
Do not confuse with dactinomycin or doxorubicin

CATEGORY AND SCHEDULE
Pregnancy Risk Category: D

MECHANISM OF ACTION
An anthracycline antibiotic that is cell cycle–phase nonspecific. Most active in S phase of cell division. Appears to bind to DNA. *Therapeutic Effect:* Inhibits DNA, DNA-dependent RNA synthesis.

PHARMACOKINETICS

Widely distributed. Does not cross blood-brain barrier. Protein binding: High. Metabolized in liver to active metabolite. Excreted in urine, eliminated by biliary excretion. **Half-life:** 18.5 hrs; metabolite: 26.7 hrs.

AVAILABILITY

Cerubidine
Powder for Injection: 20 mg.
Solution for Injection: 5 mg/ml.
DaunoXome
Injection: 2 mg/ml.

INDICATIONS AND DOSAGES

▸ **Acute lymphocytic leukemia (ALL)**
IV
Adults. 45 mg/m^2 on days 1–3 of induction course.
Children. 25–45 mg/m^2 on days 1 and 8 of cycle.
▸ **Acute myeloid leukemia (AML)**
IV
Adults. 45 mg/m^2/day for 3 days first cycle then for 2 days thereafter.
Children. 30–60 mg/m^2 on days 1–3 of cycle.
▸ **Kaposi's sarcoma (DaunoXome)**
IV
Adults. 20–40 mg/m^2 over 1 hr. Repeat q2wks or 100 mg/m^2 q3wks.

UNLABELED USES

Treatment of chronic myelocytic leukemia, Ewing's sarcoma, neuroblastoma, non-Hodgkin's lymphoma, Wilms' tumor

CONTRAINDICATIONS

Arrhythmias, congestive heart failure (CHF), left ventricular ejection fraction less than 40%, preexisting bone marrow suppression

INTERACTIONS

Drug
Antigout medications: May decrease the effects of these drugs.
Bone marrow depressants: May enhance myelosuppression.
Live virus vaccines: May potentiate virus replication, increase vaccine side effects, and decrease the patient's antibody response to vaccine.
Herbal
None known.
Food
None known.

DIAGNOSTIC TEST EFFECTS

May increase serum alkaline phosphatase, serum bilirubin, serum uric acid, and SGOT (AST) levels.

IV INCOMPATIBILITIES

Allopurinol (Aloprim), aztreonam (Azactam), cefepime (Maxipime), fludarabine (Fludara), piperacillin/tazobactam (Zosyn)
DaunoXome: Do not mix with any other solution, especially NaCl or bacteriostatic agents (e.g., benzyl alcohol).

IV COMPATIBILITIES

Cytarabine (Cytosar), etoposide (VePesid), filgrastim (Neupogen), granisetron (Kytril), ondansetron (Zofran)

SIDE EFFECTS

Frequent
Complete alopecia (scalp, axillary, pubic hair), nausea, vomiting begins a few hrs after administration, lasts 24–48 hrs
DaunoXome: Mild to moderate nausea, fatigue, fever
Occasional
Diarrhea, abdominal pain, esophagitis, stomatitis (redness or burning of oral mucous membranes, inflammation of gums or tongue), transverse

pigmentation of fingernails and toenails
Rare
Transient fever, chills

SERIOUS REACTIONS

• Bone marrow depression manifested as hematologic toxicity (severe leukopenia, anemia, and thrombocytopenia) may occur.
• A decrease in platelet count and white blood cell (WBC) count occurs in 10 to 14 days and returns to normal levels by the third week of daunorubicin treatment.
• Cardiotoxicity noted as either acute with transient abnormal EKG findings or as chronic with cardiomyopathy manifested as congestive heart failure (CHF). The risk of cardiotoxicity increases when the cumulative dose exceeds 550 mg/m^2 in adults and 300 mg/m^2 in children older than 2 yrs, or the total dosage is greater than 10 mg/kg in children younger than 2 yrs.

NURSING CONSIDERATIONS

Baseline Assessment
• Expect to obtain the patient's erythrocyte, platelet, and white blood cell (WBC) counts before beginning and at frequent intervals during daunorubicin therapy.
• Obtain the patient's baseline EKG before beginning daunorubicin therapy.
• Give antiemetics, if ordered, to the patient to prevent and treat nausea.
Precautions
• Use cautiously in patients with biliary, liver, or renal impairment.
Lifespan Considerations
• Be aware that daunorubicin use should be avoided during pregnancy, especially in the first trimes-

ter because it may cause fetal harm. Know that breast-feeding is not recommended in this patient population.
• Be aware that the safety and efficacy of daunorubicin have not been established in children.
• In the elderly, cardiotoxicity may be more frequent and reduced bone marrow reserves requires caution.
• In the elderly, age-related renal impairment may require dosage adjustment.
Administration and Handling
◀ALERT▶ Be aware that daunorubicin dosage is individualized based on the patient's clinical response and tolerance of the drug's adverse effects. When used in combination therapy, consult specific protocols for optimum dosage and sequence of drug administration. Do not exceed total dosage of 500 to 600 mg/m^2 in adults, 400 to 450 mg/m^2 in those who received irradiation of the cardiac region, 300 mg/m^2 in children older than 2 years, or 10 mg/kg in children younger than 2 years (increases risk of cardiotoxicity). Expect to reduce dosage in those with liver or renal impairment. Use body weight to calculate dose in children younger than 2 years or with a body surface area less than 0.5 m^2.
◀ALERT▶ Give daunorubicin by IV push or IV infusion. IV infusion is not recommended due to the risk of thrombophlebitis and vein irritation. Avoid areas overlying joints and tendons, small veins, and swollen or edematous extremities. Because daunorubicin may be carcinogenic, mutagenic, or teratogenic, handle the drug with extreme care during preparation and administration.
IV
Cerubidine
• Store reconstituted solution for up

to 24 hours at room temperature or up to 48 hours if refrigerated.

• Discard the solution if the color changes from red to blue-purple because this indicates decomposition.

• Reconstitute each 20-mg vial with 4 ml Sterile Water for Injection to provide concentration of 5 mg/ml.

• Gently agitate vial until completely dissolved.

• For IV push, withdraw desired dose into syringe containing 10 to 15 ml 0.9% NaCl. Inject over 2 to 3 minutes into tubing of running IV solution of D_5W or 0.9% NaCl.

• For IV infusion, further dilute with 100 ml D_5W or 0.9% NaCl. Infuse over 30 to 45 minutes.

• Know that extravasation produces immediate pain and severe local tissue damage. Aspirate as much infiltrated drug as possible, then infiltrate the area with hydrocortisone sodium succinate injection (50 to 100 mg hydrocortisone) or isotonic sodium thiosulfate injection or 1 ml of 5% ascorbic acid injection, as ordered. Apply cold compresses. DaunoXome

• Refrigerate unopened vials.

• Be aware that reconstituted solution is stable for 6 hours refrigerated.

• Do not use solution if it is opaque.

• Must dilute with equal part D_5W to provide concentration of 1 mg/ml.

• Do not use any other diluent.

• Infuse over 60 minutes.

Intervention and Evaluation

• Monitor the patient for signs and symptoms of stomatitis, including (burning and erythema of oral mucosa. Know that stomatitis may lead to ulceration within 2 to 3 days.

• Assess the patient's skin and nailbeds for hyperpigmentation.

• Monitor the patient's hematologic status, liver and renal function studies, and serum uric acid level.

• Assess the patient's pattern of daily bowel activity and stool consistency.

• Monitor the patient for signs and symptoms of anemia, including excessive fatigue and weakness, and hematologic toxicity, including easy bruising, fever, signs of local infection, sore throat, or unusual bleeding from any site.

Patient Teaching

• Advise the patient that his or her urine may turn a reddish color for 1 to 2 days after beginning daunorubicin therapy.

• Explain to the patient that alopecia is reversible, but new hair growth may have different color or texture. Tell the patient that new hair growth resumes about 5 weeks after last daunorubicin therapy dose.

• Teach the patient to maintain fastidious oral hygiene.

• Stress to the patient that he or she should not receive vaccinations and should avoid contact with anyone who recently received a live virus vaccine.

• Warn the patient to notify the physician if he or she experiences easy bruising, fever, signs of local infection, sore throat, or unusual bleeding from any site.

• Urge the patient to increase his or her fluid intake to help protect against hyperuricemia development.

• Caution the patient to notify the physician if nausea and vomiting persist at home.

doxorubicin
dox-o-**roo**-bi-sin
(Adriamycin, Caelyx, Doxil)
**Do not confuse with
Daunorubicin, Idamycin, or
Idarubicin.**

CATEGORY AND SCHEDULE
Pregnancy Risk Category: D

MECHANISM OF ACTION
An anthracycline antibiotic that
inhibits DNA and DNA-dependent
RNA synthesis by binding with
DNA strands. Liposomal encapsula-
tion increases uptake by tumors,
prolongs action, and may decrease
toxicity. *Therapeutic Effect:* Prevents cellular division.

PHARMACOKINETICS
Widely distributed. Does not cross
blood-brain barrier. Protein binding:
74%–76%. Metabolized rapidly in
liver to active metabolite. Primarily
eliminated via biliary system. Not
removed by hemodialysis. **Half-life:**
16 hrs; metabolite: 32 hrs.

AVAILABILITY
Powder for Injection: 10 mg,
20 mg, 50 mg, 200 mg.
Lipid Complex (Doxil): 2 mg/ml.

INDICATIONS AND DOSAGES
Treatment of breast, bronchogenic,
gastric, ovarian, thyroid, and transitional cell bladder carcinoma; lymphomas of Hodgkin's and non-
Hodgkin's type; neuroblastoma;
primary liver cancer; soft tissue and
bone sarcomas; Wilms' tumor;
regression in acute lymphoblastic
and myeloblastic leukemia
IV
Adults. 60–75 mg/m^2 single dose
q21 days, 20 mg/m^2 once weekly,

or 25–30 mg/m^2 a day on 2–3
successive days q4wks. Due to risk
of cardiotoxicity, do not exceed
cumulative dose of 550 mg/m^2 or
400–450 mg/m^2 for those whose
previous therapy included related
compounds or irradiation of cardiac
region.
Children. 35–75 mg/m^2 as single
dose q3wks or 20–30 mg/m^2
weekly or 60–90 mg/m^2 as continuous infusion over 96 hrs q3–4wks.
Kaposi's Sarcoma (Doxil)
IV infusion
Adults. 20 mg/m^2 q3wks; infuse
over 30 min.
Ovarian Cancer (Doxil)
IV infusion
Adults. 50 mg/m^2 q4wks.
Dosage in liver impairment

Serum Bilirubin Concentration	Dosage
1.2–3 mg/dl	50% usual dose
greater than 3 mg/dl	25% usual dose

UNLABELED USES
Treatment of cervical, head or neck,
endometrial, liver, pancreatic, prostatic, and testicular carcinoma;
treatment of germ cell tumors,
multiple myeloma

CONTRAINDICATIONS
Cardiomyopathy; preexisting
myelosuppression; previous or
concomitant treatment with cyclophosphamide, idarubicin, mitoxantrone, or irradiation of the cardiac region, severe congestive heart
failure (CHF)

INTERACTIONS
Drug
Antigout medications: May decrease
the effects of these drugs.
Bone marrow depressants: May
increase bone marrow depression.

Daunorubicin: May increase the risk of cardiotoxicity.
Live virus vaccines: May potentiate virus replication, increase vaccine side effects, and decrease the patient's antibody response to vaccine.
Herbal
None known.
Food
None known.

DIAGNOSTIC TEST EFFECTS
May cause EKG changes. May increase serum uric acid.
Doxil: May reduce neutrophil and red blood cell (RBC) count.

IV INCOMPATIBILITIES
Doxil: Do not mix with any other medications.
Doxorubicin: Allopurinol (Aloprim), amphotericin B complex (Abelcet, AmBisome, Amphotec), cefepime (Maxipime), furosemide (Lasix), ganciclovir (Cytovene), heparin, piperacillin/tazobactam (Zosyn), propofol (Diprivan)

IV COMPATIBILITIES
Dexamethasone (Decadron), diphenhydramine (Benadryl), etoposide (Vepesid), granisetron (Kytril), hydromorphone (Dilaudid), lorazepam (Ativan), morphine, ondansetron (Zofran), paclitaxel (Taxol), propofol (Diprivan)

SIDE EFFECTS
Frequent
Complete alopecia (scalp, axillary, pubic hair), nausea, vomiting, stomatitis, esophagitis (especially if drug is given each day on several successive days), reddish urine
Doxil: Nausea
Occasional
Anorexia, diarrhea, hyperpigmentation of nailbeds, phalangeal and dermal creases

Rare
Fever, chills, conjunctivitis, lacrimation

SERIOUS REACTIONS
• Bone marrow depression manifested as hematologic toxicity (principally leukopenia and, to lesser extent, anemia, thrombocytopenia) may occur. Generally occurs within 10–15 days and returns to normal levels by third week.
• Cardiotoxicity noted as either acute, transient abnormal EKG findings and cardiomyopathy manifested as CHF may occur.

NURSING CONSIDERATIONS
Baseline Assessment
• As ordered, obtain the patient's blood Hct and Hgb, platelet, and white blood cell (WBC) counts before beginning and at frequent intervals during doxorubicin therapy.
• Obtain a baseline EKG of the patient before doxorubicin therapy.
• As ordered, obtain liver function studies of the patient before administering each doxorubicin dose.
• Give antiemetics, if ordered, to the patient to prevent or treat nausea.
Lifespan Considerations
• Know that doxorubicin use should be avoided, if possible, during pregnancy, especially in the first trimester and that breast-feeding is not recommended in this patient population.
• Be aware that cardiotoxicity may be more frequent in children younger than 2 years or in elderly over 70 years of age.
Precautions
• Use cautiously in patients with impaired liver function.
Administration and Handling
◀ALERT▶ Know that doxorubicin

dosage is individualized based on the patient's clinical response and tolerance of the drug's adverse effects. When used in combination therapy, consult specific protocols for optimum dosage and sequence of drug administration.

◀ALERT▶ Wear gloves. If doxorubicin powder or solution comes in contact with skin, wash thoroughly. When accessing a vein for infusion, avoid areas overlying joints and tendons, small veins, and swollen or edematous extremities. For Doxil, don't use with in-line filter or mix with any diluent except D_5W. Because Doxil may be carcinogenic, mutagenic, or teratogenic, handle the drug with extreme care during preparation and administration.

IV
• Store at room temperature.
• Reconstituted solution is stable for up to 24 hours at room temperature or up to 48 hours if refrigerated.
• Protect from prolonged exposure to sunlight; discard unused solution.
• Reconstitute each 10-mg vial with 5 ml preservative-free 0.9% NaCl (10 ml for 20 mg; 25 ml for 50 mg) to provide concentration of 2 mg/ml.
• Shake vial; allow contents to dissolve.
• Withdraw appropriate volume of air from vial during reconstitution to avoid excessive pressure build-up.
• Further dilute with 50 ml D_5W or 0.9% NaCl, if necessary, and give as a continuous infusion through a central venous line.
• For IV push, administer into the tubing of a freely running IV infusion of D_5W or 0.9% NaCl, preferably through a butterfly needle. To avoid local erythematous streaking along the vein and facial flushing, administer at a rate no faster than 3 to 5 minutes.

• Test for flashback every 30 seconds to be certain the needle remains in the vein during injection.
• Be aware that extravasation produces immediate pain, severe local tissue damage. If extravasation occurs, terminate drug administration immediately; withdraw as much medication as possible, obtain extravasation kit, and follow protocol.

Doxil
• Refrigerate unopened vials.
• After solution is diluted, use within 24 hours.
• Dilute each dose in 250 ml D_5W.
• Give as infusion over more than 30 minutes.
• Do not use in-line filters.

Intervention/Evaluation
• Monitor the patient for signs and symptoms of stomatitis, including burning or erythema of oral mucosa at inner margin of lips and difficulty swallowing. Be aware that stomatitis may lead to ulceration of mucous membranes within 2 to 3 days.
• Assess the patient's nailbeds and skin for hyperpigmentation.
• Monitor the patient's hematologic status, liver and renal function studies, and serum uric acid levels.
• Assess the patient's pattern of daily bowel activity and stool consistency.
• Monitor the patient for signs and symptoms of anemia, including excessive fatigue and weakness, and hematologic toxicity, including easy bruising, fever, signs of local infection, sore throat, and unusual bleeding from any site.

Patient Teaching
• Explain to the patient that alopecia is reversible, but new hair growth may have a different color or texture. Tell the patient that new hair growth resumes 2 to 3 months

after the last doxorubicin therapy dose.
• Teach the patient to maintain fastidious oral hygiene.
• Stress to the patient that he or she should not receive vaccinations and should avoid contact with anyone who recently received a live virus vaccine.
• Warn the patient to notify the physician if he or she experiences easy bruising, fever, signs of local infection, sore throat, or unusual bleeding from any site.
• Caution the patient to notify the physician if nausea and vomiting persist after discharge.
• Urge the patient to avoid consuming alcohol during doxorubicin therapy.

epirubicin
eh-pea-**rew**-bih-sin
(Ellence)

CATEGORY AND SCHEDULE
Pregnancy Risk Category: D

MECHANISM OF ACTION
An anthracycline antibiotic whose exact mechanism is unknown but may include formation of a complex with DNA by intercalation of its planar rings with consequent inhibition of DNA, RNA, protein synthesis. Inhibits DNA helicase activity, preventing enzymatic separation of double-stranded DNA and interfering with replication and transcription. *Therapeutic Effect:* Produces antiproliferative and cytotoxic activity.

PHARMACOKINETICS
Widely distributed into tissues. Protein binding: 77%. Metabolized in liver, red blood cells (RBCs). Primarily eliminated through biliary excretion. Not removed by hemodialysis. **Half-life:** 33 hrs.

AVAILABILITY
Injection: 2 mg/ml single-use vial.

INDICATIONS AND DOSAGES
▸ **Breast cancer**
IV infusion
Adults. Initially, 100– 120 mg/m^2 in repeated cycles of 3–4 wks, in combination with 5-FU and Cytoxan. Total dose may be given day 1 of each cycle or divided equally on days 1 and 8 of each cycle.

UNLABELED USES
Lung, ovarian carcinoma; non-Hodgkin's lymphoma; sarcomas

CONTRAINDICATIONS
Baseline neutrophil count less than 1,500 cells/mm^3, hypersensitivity to epirubicin, previous treatment with anthracyclines up to maximum cumulative dose, recent myocardial infarction (MI), severe liver impairment, severe myocardial insufficiency

INTERACTIONS
Drug
Cimetidine: May increase epirubicin serum concentrations.
Herbal
None known.
Food
None known.

DIAGNOSTIC TEST EFFECTS
None known.

IV INCOMPATIBILITIES
Heparin, 5-fluorouracil (5-FU)
Do not mix with other medications in same syringe.

SIDE EFFECTS
Frequent (83%–70%)
Nausea, vomiting alopecia, amenorrhea
Occasional (9%–5%)
Stomatitis (burning or erythema of oral mucosa, oral ulceration of mucous membranes, difficulty swallowing), diarrhea, hot flashes
Rare (2%–1%)
Rash, pruritus, fever, lethargy, conjunctivitis

SERIOUS REACTIONS
• Cardiotoxicity noted as either acute, transient abnormal EKG findings and cardiomyopathy manifested as congestive heart failure (CHF) may occur. Risk increased with total cumulative dose in excess of 900 mg/m^2.
• Severe local tissue necrosis will occur if extravasation occurs during administration.
• Bone marrow depression manifested as hematologic toxicity (principally leukopenia and, to lesser extent, anemia, thrombocytopenia) may occur.

NURSING CONSIDERATIONS
Baseline Assessment
• As ordered, obtain the patient's blood Hct and Hgb, platelet, and white blood cell (WBC) counts before and at frequent intervals during epirubicin therapy.
• Obtain a baseline EKG of the patient, if ordered, before starting epirubicin therapy.
• As ordered, obtain liver function studies before each epirubicin dose.
• Give antiemetics, if ordered, to the patient to prevent or treat nausea.
Lifespan Considerations
• Be aware that epirubicin may cause fetal harm and it is unknown if epirubicin is distributed in breast milk.

• Be aware that the safety and efficacy of epirubicin have not been established in children.
• In the elderly, no age-related precautions are noted, but monitor for toxicity.
Precautions
• Use cautiously in patients with liver or renal function impairment.
Administration and Handling
◀ALERT▶ Be aware that there is a dosage adjustment necessary for patients with bone marrow dysfunction, hematologic toxicities, liver dysfunction, and severe renal impairment.
◀ALERT▶ Exclude pregnant staff from working with epirubicin; wear protective clothing. If accidental contact with skin or eyes occurs, flush area immediately with copious amounts of water.
◀ALERT▶ Know that venous sclerosis may result if epirubicin is infused into a small vein.
IV
• Refrigerate vial and protect from light.
• Use within 24 hours of first penetration of rubber stopper.
• Discard unused portion.
• Ready-to-use vials require no reconstitution.
• Infuse medication into tubing of free-flowing IV of 0.9% NaCl or D$_5$W over 3 to 5 minutes.
Intervention and Evaluation
• Monitor the patient for signs and symptoms of stomatitis because this condition may lead to ulceration of mucous membranes within 2 to 3 days.
• Monitor the patient's blood Hct and Hgb, platelet, and white blood cell (WBC) counts for signs of myelosuppression. Also monitor the patient's cardiac function and results of liver and renal function studies.

• Assess the patient's pattern of daily bowel activity and stool consistency.
• Monitor the patient for signs and symptoms of anemia, including excessive fatigue and weakness, and hematologic toxicity, including easy bruising, fever, signs of local infection, sore throat, and unusual bleeding from any site.

Patient Teaching

• Explain to the patient that alopecia is reversible, but new hair growth may have a different color or texture. Tell the patient that new hair growth resumes 2 to 3 months after last epirubicin therapy dose.
• Teach the patient to maintain fastidious oral hygiene.
• Stress to the patient that he or she should not receive vaccinations and should avoid contact with anyone who recently received a live virus vaccine.
• Warn the patient to notify the physician if he or she experiences easy bruising, fever, signs of local infection, sore throat, or unusual bleeding from any site.

idarubicin hydrochloride
eye-dah-**roo**-bi-sin
(Idamycin PFS, Zavedos)
Do not confuse with Adriamycin or doxorubicin.

CATEGORY AND SCHEDULE
Pregnancy Risk Category: D

MECHANISM OF ACTION
An anthracycline antibiotic that inhibits nucleic acid synthesis by interacting with the enzyme topoisomerase II, which promotes DNA strand supercoiling. *Therapeutic*

Effect: Produces death of rapidly dividing cells.

PHARMACOKINETICS
Widely distributed. Protein binding: 97%. Rapidly metabolized in liver to active metabolite. Primarily eliminated via biliary excretion. Not removed by hemodialysis. **Half-life:** 4–46 hrs; metabolite: 8–92 hrs.

AVAILABILITY
Injection: 5 mg, 10 mg, 20 mg.

INDICATIONS AND DOSAGES
▸ **Treatment of acute myeloid leukemia (AML)**
IV
Adults. 8–12 mg/m^2/day for 3 days in combination with Ara-C).
Children (solid tumor). 5 mg/m^2 once a day for 3 days.
Children (leukemia). 10–12 mg/m^2 once a day for 3 days.
▸ **Dosage in liver or renal impairment**

Serum Level	Dose Reduction
Serum creatinine 2 mg/dl or more	25%
Serum bilirubin greater than 2.5 mg/dl	50%
Serum bilirubin greater than 5 mg/dl	Do not give

CONTRAINDICATIONS
Preexisting arrhythmias, bone marrow suppression, cardiomyopathy, pregnancy, severe congestive heart failure (CHF)

INTERACTIONS
Drug
Antigout medications: May decrease the effects of these drugs.
Bone marrow depressants: May increase bone marrow depression.

Live virus vaccines: May potentiate virus replication, increase vaccine side effects, and decrease the patient's antibody response to vaccine.
Herbal
None known.
Food
None known.

DIAGNOSTIC TEST EFFECTS

May increase serum alkaline phosphatase, serum bilirubin, SGOT (AST), SGPT (ALT), and serum uric acid levels. May cause EKG changes.

IV INCOMPATIBILITIES

Acyclovir (Zovirax), allopurinol (Aloprim), ampicillin-sulbactam (Unasyn), cefazolin (Ancef, Kefzol), cefepime (Maxipime), ceftazidime (Fortaz), clindamycin (Cleocin), dexamethasone (Decadron), furosemide (Lasix), hydrocortisone (Solu-Cortef), lorazepam (Ativan), meperidine (Demerol), methotrexate, piperacillin/tazobactam (Zosyn), sodium bicarbonate, teniposide (Vumon), vancomycin (Vancocin), vincristine (Oncovin)

IV COMPATIBILITIES

Diphenhydramine (Benadryl), granisetron (Kytril), magnesium, potassium

SIDE EFFECTS

Frequent
Nausea, vomiting (82%); complete alopecia (scalp, axillary, pubic hair) (77%); abdominal cramping, diarrhea (73%); mucositis (50%)
Occasional
Hyperpigmentation of nailbeds, phalangeal and dermal creases (46%); fever (36%); headache (20%)
Rare
Conjunctivitis, neuropathy

SERIOUS REACTIONS

• Bone marrow depression manifested as hematologic toxicity (principally leukopenia and, to lesser extent, anemia, thrombocytopenia) generally occurs within 10 to 15 days, returns to normal levels by third week.
• Cardiotoxicity noted as either acute, transient abnormal EKG findings and cardiomyopathy manifested as CHF may occur.

NURSING CONSIDERATIONS

Baseline Assessment

• Evaluate the patient's baseline complete blood count (CBC) results and liver and renal function test results.
• Obtain an EKG of the patient, as ordered, before starting idarubicin therapy.
• Give an antiemetic, if ordered, to the patient before and during idarubicin therapy to prevent or treat nausea and vomiting.
• Inform the patient of the high potential for alopecia development.

Lifespan Considerations

• Know that idarubicin use should be avoided during pregnancy because the drug may be embryotoxic.
• Be aware that it is unknown if idarubicin is distributed in breast milk and the patient should discontinue breast-feeding before starting idarubicin therapy.
• Be aware that the safety and efficacy of idarubicin have not been established in children.
• In the elderly, cardiotoxicity may be more frequent with idarubicin use.
• Use idarubicin with caution in elderly with inadequate bone marrow reserves.
• In the elderly, age-related renal

impairment may require dosage adjustment.

Precautions

• Use cautiously in patients receiving concurrent radiation therapy or with impaired liver or renal function.

Administration and Handling

◀ALERT▶ Know that idarubicin dosage is individualized based on the patient's clinical response and tolerance of the drug's adverse effects. When used in combination therapy, consult specific protocols for optimum dosage and sequence of drug administration.

◀ALERT▶ Give idarubicin by free-flowing IV infusion and never by the subcutaneous or IM route. Use gloves, gowns, and eye goggles during the preparation and administration of this medication. If powder or solution comes in contact with skin, wash thoroughly. Avoid areas overlying joints and tendons, small veins, and swollen or edematous extremities.

◀ALERT▶ Be aware that Idamycin pre-filled syringe does not require reconstitution and is stored refrigerated.

IV

• Reconstituted solution is stable for up to 72 hours, or 3 days, at room temperature or up to 168 hours, or 7 days, if refrigerated.

• Discard unused solution.

• Reconstitute each 10-mg vial with 10 ml or each 5 mg-vial with 5 ml of 0.9% NaCl to provide a concentration of 1 mg/ml.

• Administer into the tubing of a freely running IV infusion of D_5W or 0.9% NaCl, preferably through a butterfly needle, slowly over more than 10 to 15 minutes.

• Monitor for signs and symptoms of extravasation, such as immediate pain and severe local tissue damage.

Terminate the infusion immediately. Apply cold compresses for a half hour immediately, then half an hour 4 times a day for 3 days. Keep affected extremity elevated.

Intervention and Evaluation

• Monitor the patient's complete blood count (CBC) with differential, EKG, platelet count, and liver and renal function tests.

• Monitor the patient for signs and symptoms of anemia, including excessive fatigue and weakness, and hematologic toxicity, including easy bruising, fever, signs of local infection, sore throat, or unusual bleeding from any site.

• Avoid giving the patient IM injections, rectal medications, and causing other trauma that may precipitate bleeding.

• Check the patient's infusion site frequently for evidence extravasation, which causes severe local necrosis.

• Assess the patient for potentially fatal congestive heart failure (CHF) (dyspnea, edema, and rales) and life-threatening arrhythmias.

Patient Teaching

• Explain to the patient that total body alopecia may occur and that it is reversible. Take measures to help the patient cope with hair loss. Tell the patient that new hair growth resumes 2 to 3 months after last idarubicin dose and that new hair may have a different color or texture than the original.

• Teach the patient to maintain fastidious oral hygiene.

• Stress to the patient that he or she should avoid crowds and those with known infections.

• Teach the patient and family how to recognize the early signs and symptoms of bleeding and infection.

• Warn the patient to notify the physician if he or she experiences

easy bruising, bleeding, fever, or
sore throat.
• Advise the patient that idarubicin
use may turn his or her urine pink
or red.
• Explain to the patient that he or
she should use contraceptive measures during idarubicin therapy.

mitomycin
my-toe-**my**-sin
(Mutamycin, Mytomycin
C-Kyowa)

CATEGORY AND SCHEDULE
Pregnancy Risk Category: Safety
in pregnancy has not been
established.

MECHANISM OF ACTION
An antibiotic that acts as an alkylating agent and cross-links the strands
of DNA. *Therapeutic Effect:* Inhibits DNA and RNA synthesis.

PHARMACOKINETICS
Widely distributed. Does not cross
blood-brain barrier. Primarily metabolized in liver and excreted in
urine. **Half-life:** 50 min.

AVAILABILITY
Powder for Injection: 5 mg, 20 mg,
40 mg.

INDICATIONS AND DOSAGES
▸ **Treatment of disseminated
adenocarcinoma of pancreas and
stomach**
IV
Adults, Elderly, Children. Initial
dosage: 10–20 mg/m^2 as single
dose. Repeat q6–8wks. Give additional courses only after platelet and
white blood cell (WBC) counts are
within acceptable levels.

▸ **Dosage in renal impairment**

Creatinine Clearance	% Normal Dose
less than 10 ml/min	75%

Leukocytes/ mm^3	Platelets/ mm^3	% of Prior Dose to Give
4,000	more than 100,000	100
3,000–3,999	75,000–99,000	100
2,000–2,999 1,999 or less	25,000–74,999 less than 25,000	70 50

UNLABELED USES
Treatment of biliary, bladder, breast,
cervical, colorectal, head and neck,
lung carcinoma and chronic myelocytic leukemia

CONTRAINDICATIONS
Coagulation disorders and bleeding
tendencies, platelet count less than
75,000/mm^3, serious infection,
serum creatinine greater than 1.7
mg/dl, white blood cell (WBC)
count less than 3,000/mm^3

INTERACTIONS
Drug
Bone marrow depressants: May
increase bone marrow depression.
Live virus vaccines: May potentiate
virus replication, increase vaccine
side effects, decrease the patient's
antibody response to vaccine.
Herbal
None known.
Food
None known.

DIAGNOSTIC TEST EFFECTS
May increase BUN and serum
creatinine levels.

IV INCOMPATIBILITIES
Do not mix with any other medications.

IV COMPATIBILITIES
Cisplatin (Platinol AQ), cyclophosphamide (Cytoxan), doxorubicin (Adriamycin), fluorouracil, granisetron (Kytril), leucovorin, methotrexate, ondansetron (Zofran), vinblastine (Velban), vincristine (Oncovin)

SIDE EFFECTS
Frequent (greater than 10%)
Fever, anorexia, nausea, vomiting
Occasional (10%–2%)
Stomatitis, numbness of fingers and toes, purple color bands on nails, skin rash, alopecia, unusual tiredness
Rare (less than 1%)
Thrombophlebitis, cellulitis, extravasation

SERIOUS REACTIONS
• Marked bone marrow depression results in hematologic toxicity manifested as leukopenia, thrombocytopenia, and to a lesser extent, anemia, which generally occurs within 2–4 wks after initial therapy.
• Renal toxicity, evidenced by a rise in BUN and serum creatinine, may occur.
• Pulmonary toxicity, manifested as dyspnea, cough, hemoptysis, pneumonia, may occur.
• Long-term therapy may produce hemolytic uremic syndrome (HUS), characterized by hemolytic anemia, thrombocytopenia, renal failure, and hypertension.

NURSING CONSIDERATIONS

Baseline Assessment
• If ordered, obtain the patient's bleeding time, CBC and prothrombin time before and periodically during mitomycin therapy.
• Give antiemetics, if ordered, to the patient before and during mitomycin therapy to prevent or treat nausea and vomiting.

Lifespan Considerations
• Be aware that mitomycin use should be avoided during pregnancy, especially in the first trimester and that breast-feeding is not recommended in this patient population.
• There are no age-related precautions noted in children.
• In the elderly, age-related renal impairment may require cautious use.

Precautions
• Use cautiously in patients with impaired liver or renal function and myelosuppression.

Administration and Handling
◀ALERT▶ Be aware that mitomycin dosage is individualized based on the patient's clinical response and tolerance of the drug's adverse effects. When used in combination therapy, consult specific protocols for optimum dosage and sequence of drug administration.
◀ALERT▶ Because mitomycin may be carcinogenic, mutagenic, or teratogenic, handle the drug with extreme care during preparation and administration. Be aware that this drug is extremely irritating to veins and may produce pain during infusion with induration, paresthesia, and thrombophlebitis.
IV
• Use only clear, blue-gray solutions.
• Concentration of 0.5 mg/ml is stable for up to 7 days at room temperature or up to 2 weeks if refrigerated.
• If solution is further diluted with

D_5W, solution is stable for up to 3 hours, or if diluted with 0.9% NaCl, is stable for up to 24 hours at room temperature.
• Reconstitute 5-mg vial with 10 ml and a 20-mg vial with 40 ml of Sterile Water for Injection to provide solution containing 0.5 mg/ml.
• Do not shake vial to dissolve. Allow vial to stand at room temperature until complete dissolution occurs.
• For IV infusion, further dilute with 50 to 100 ml D_5W or 0.9% NaCl.
• Give IV push over 5 to 10 minutes.
• Give IV through tubing running IV infusion.
• Monitor for signs and symptoms of extravasation, which may produce cellulitis, tissue sloughing, and ulceration. If extravasation occurs, terminate the infusion immediately and inject the ordered antidote, as appropriate. Apply ice intermittently for up to 72 hours and keep the affected area elevated.
Intervention and Evaluation
• Monitor the patient's BUN, hematologic status, and serum creatinine.
• Assess the patient's IV site for evidence of extravasation and phlebitis.
• Monitor the patient for signs and symptoms of anemia, including excessive fatigue and weakness, hematologic toxicity, including easy bruising, fever, signs of local infection, sore throat, and unusual bleeding from any site, and renal toxicity, including rise in BUN and serum creatinine.
Patient Teaching
• Teach the patient to maintain fastidious oral hygiene.
• Warn the patient to immediately

report any burning or pain felt at the injection site.
• Stress to the patient that he or she should not receive vaccinations and should avoid contact with anyone who recently received a live virus vaccine.
• Warn the patient to notify the physician if he or she experiences bleeding, easy bruising, burning or painful urination, increased urinary frequency, fever, nausea, signs of local infection, shortness of breath, sore throat, unusual bleeding from any site, and vomiting.
• Explain to the patient that alopecia is reversible, but new hair growth may have a different color or texture.

plicamycin
ply-kah-**my**-sin
(Mithracin)
Do not confuse with Minocin.

CATEGORY AND SCHEDULE
Pregnancy Risk Category: X

MECHANISM OF ACTION
An antibiotic that forms complexes with DNA, inhibiting DNA-directed RNA synthesis. May inhibit parathyroid hormone effect on osteoclasts and inhibit bone resorption. *Therapeutic Effect:* Lowers serum calcium concentration. Blocks hypercalcemic action of vitamin D and blocks action of parathyroid hormone. Decreases serum calcium and phosphate levels.

PHARMACOKINETICS

Route	Onset	Peak	Duration
IV	1–2 days	2–3 days	3–15 days

Protein binding: None. Localized in liver, kidney, formed bone surfaces. Crosses blood-brain barrier, enters cerebrospinal fluid (CSF). Primarily excreted in urine.

AVAILABILITY
Powder for Injection: 2,500 mcg.

INDICATIONS AND DOSAGES
▸ **Testicular tumors**
IV
Adults, Elderly. 25–30 mcg/kg/day for 8–10 days. Repeat at monthly intervals.
▸ **Hypercalcemia, hyperuricemia**
IV
Adults, Elderly. 25 mcg/kg as a single dose. May repeat in 48 hrs if no response occurs or 25 mcg/kg/day for 3–4 days or 25–50 mcg/kg/dose every other day for 3–8 doses.
▸ **Paget's disease**
IV
Adults, Elderly. 15 mcg/kg/day for 10 days.

UNLABELED USES
Treatment of Paget's disease refractory to other therapy

CONTRAINDICATIONS
Coagulation disorders, existing thrombocytopathy, thrombocytopenia, impaired bone marrow function, tendency to hemorrhage

INTERACTIONS
Drug
Aspirin, dipyridamole, NSAIDs, sulfinpyrazone, valproic acid: May increase risk of hemorrhage.
Bone marrow depressants, hepatotoxic and nephrotoxic medications: May increase risk of toxicity.
Calcium-containing medications, vitamin D: May decrease plicamycin's effects.

Heparin, oral anticoagulants, thrombolytics: May increase the effects of these drugs.
Live virus vaccines: May potentiate virus replication, increase vaccine side effects, and decrease the patient's antibody response to vaccine.
Herbal
None known.
Food
None known.

DIAGNOSTIC TEST EFFECTS
None known.

IV INCOMPATIBILITIES
Cefepime (Maxipime)

IV COMPATIBILITIES
Allopurinol (Aloprim), etoposide (VePesid), filgrastim (Neupogen), gemcitabine (Gemzar), granisetron (Kytril), teniposide (Vumon), vinorelbine (Navelbine)

SIDE EFFECTS
Frequent
Nausea, vomiting, anorexia, diarrhea, stomatitis
Occasional
Fever, drowsiness, weakness, lethargy, malaise, headache, mental depression, nervousness, dizziness, rash, acne

SERIOUS REACTIONS
• Hematologic toxicity noted by marked facial flushing, persistent nosebleeds, hemoptysis, purpura, ecchymoses, leukopenia, and thrombocytopenia may occur.
• Risk of bleeding tendencies increases with higher dosages and when more than 10 doses are given.
• Plicamycin therapy may produce electrolyte imbalance.

NURSING CONSIDERATIONS

Baseline Assessment
• Determine whether the patient is pregnant before initiating plicamycin therapy as this drug is pregnancy risk category X.
• Give antiemetics, if ordered, to prevent and treat nausea.
• Expect to discontinue plicamycin therapy if the patient's platelet count falls below 150,000/mm^3, if the patient's white blood cell (WBC) count falls below 4,000/mm^3, or if the patient's prothrombin time is 4 seconds higher than the control.
• Expect patients with liver or renal impairment to undergo liver and renal function studies daily.

Lifespan Considerations
• Be aware that plicamycin use is contraindicated during pregnancy and that breast-feeding is not recommended in this patient population.
• Information is unavailable on plicamycin use in children or the elderly.

Precautions
• Use extremely cautiously in patients with liver or renal impairment.
• Use cautiously in patients with electrolyte imbalance.

Administration and Handling
◀ALERT▶ Be aware that plicamycin dosage is individualized based on the patient's clinical response and tolerance of the drug's adverse effects and that dosage is based on actual body weight. Use ideal body weight for edematous or obese patients. Do not exceed 30 mcg/kg/day or more than 10 daily doses as this increases the potential for hemorrhage.
◀ALERT▶ Because plicamycin may be carcinogenic, mutagenic, or teratogenic handle the drug with extreme care during preparation and administration.

IV
• Refrigerate vials.
• Freshly prepare solution before use and discard unused portions.
• Reconstitute 2,500-mcg (2.5-mg) vial with 4.9 ml Sterile Water for Injection to provide concentration of 500 mcg/ml (0.5 mg/ml).
• Dilute with 500 to 1,000 ml D$_5$W or 0.9% NaCl.
• Infuse over 4 to 6 hours.
• Monitor for signs and symptoms of extravasation, which produces painful inflammation, induration, and possible sloughing. If extravasation occurs, aspirate as much drug as possible and apply warm compresses.

Intervention and Evaluation
• Monitor the patient's hematologic, liver, and renal function studies; platelet count; prothrombin and bleeding times; and serum calcium, phosphorus, and potassium levels.
• Assess the patient's pattern of daily bowel activity and stool consistency.
• Monitor the patient for signs and symptoms of stomatitis, including burning or erythema of the oral mucosa at the inner margin of the lips, difficulty swallowing, oral ulceration, or sore throat, and evidence of thrombocytopenia, including bleeding from gums, petechiae, small subcutaneous hemorrhages, and tarry stool.
• Avoid giving the patient IM injections, rectal medications, or performing any traumatic procedures that may induce bleeding.

Patient Teaching
• Teach the patient to maintain fastidious oral hygiene.
• Stress to the patient that he or she should not receive vaccinations and

should avoid contact with anyone who recently received a live virus vaccine.
• Warn the patient to notify the physician if he or she experiences bleeding, bruising, fever, nausea and vomiting that continue at home, pain upon urination, shortness of breath, signs of local infection, and sore throat.
• Urge the patient to use nonhormonal contraception.

valrubicin
val-**rue**-bih-sin
(Valstar)
Do not confuse with valsartan.

CATEGORY AND SCHEDULE
Pregnancy Risk Category: C

MECHANISM OF ACTION
An anthracycline antibiotic that following intracellular penetration, inhibits incorporation of nucleosides into nucleic acids. *Therapeutic Effect:* Causes chromosomal damage, arresting cell cycle in G_2 phase, interfering with DNA synthesis.

AVAILABILITY
Solution for Intravesical Instillation: 40 mg/ml.

INDICATIONS AND DOSAGES
▸ **Bladder cancer**
Intravesical
Adults, Elderly. 800 mg once weekly for 6 wks.

CONTRAINDICATIONS
Perforated bladder, sensitivity to valrubicin, severe irritated bladder, small bladder capacity, urinary tract infection

SIDE EFFECTS
Frequent
Local intravesical reaction (10%): Local bladder symptoms, urinary frequency, dysuria, urinary urgency, hematuria, bladder pain, cystitis, bladder spasms
Systemic (15%–5%): Abdominal pain, nausea, urinary tract infection
Occasional
Local intravesical reaction (less than 10%): Nocturia, local burning, urethral pain, pelvic pain, gross hematuria
Systemic (5%–2%): Diarrhea, vomiting, urinary retention, microscopic hematuria, asthenia, headache, malaise, back pain, chest pain, dizziness, rash, anemia, fever, vasodilation
Rare
Systemic (1%): Flatus, peripheral edema, increased glucose, pneumonia, myalgia

NURSING CONSIDERATIONS
Baseline Assessment
• Determine if the patient is breastfeeding, pregnant, and sensitive to valrubicin before beginning therapy.
• Establish the patient's other conditions and medications.
Lifespan Considerations
• Breast-feeding is not recommended in this patient population.
Administration and Handling
◀ALERT▶ Valrubicin is not for IM/IV use.
Patient Teaching
• Warn patient to use reliable contraceptive measures during drug therapy.
• Explain that red-tinged urine may occur during the first 24 hours after drug administration.
• Advise patient to report consistent red-colored urine to the physician.

15 Antimetabolites

capecitabine
cytarabine
fludarabine phosphate
fluorouracil
gemcitabine
  hydrochloride
hydroxyurea
mercaptopurine
methotrexate sodium

Uses: Antimetabolites produce the best response in patients with lymphomas, acute leukemias, cancer of the gastrointestinal tract, or breast cancer.

Action: Structurally similar to natural metabolites, antimetabolites act by disrupting critical metabolic processes. Some agents inhibit enzymes that synthesize essential cellular components; others are incorporated into deoxyribonucleic acid (DNA), interfering with DNA replication and function. By altering DNA synthesis and metabolism, antimetabolites affect the S phase of the cell cycle.

capecitabine
cap-eh-**site**-ah-bean
(Xeloda)
Do not confuse with Xenical.

CATEGORY AND SCHEDULE
Pregnancy Risk Category: D

MECHANISM OF ACTION
An antimetabolite that is enzymatically converted to 5-fluorouracil. Inhibits enzymes necessary for synthesis of essential cellular components. *Therapeutic Effect:* Interferes with DNA synthesis, RNA processing, and protein synthesis.

PHARMACOKINETICS
Readily absorbed from the gastrointestinal (GI) tract. Protein binding: less than 60%. Metabolized in the liver. Primarily excreted in urine. **Half-life:** 45 min.

AVAILABILITY
Tablets: 150 mg, 500 mg.

INDICATIONS AND DOSAGES
▶ **Metastatic breast cancer, colon cancer**
PO
Adults, Elderly. Initially, 2,500 mg/m^2/day in 2 equally divided doses approximately 12 hrs apart for 2 wks. Follow with a 1-wk rest period; given in 3-wk cycles.

CONTRAINDICATIONS
Severe renal function impairment

INTERACTIONS
Drug
Warfarin: May alter the effects of warfarin.
Herbal
None known.
Food
None known.

DIAGNOSTIC TEST EFFECTS
May increase serum alkaline phosphatase, serum bilirubin, SGOT (AST), and SGPT (ALT) levels. May decrease blood Hct, Hgb, and white blood cell (WBC) count.

SIDE EFFECTS

Frequent (greater than 5%)
Diarrhea (sometimes severe), nausea, vomiting, stomatitis (painful erythema, ulcers of mouth or tongue), hand and foot syndrome (painful palmar-plantar erythema and swelling with paresthesia, tingling, blistering), fatigue, anorexia, dermatitis
Occasional (less than 5%)
Constipation, dyspepsia, nail disorder, headache, dizziness, insomnia, edema, myalgia

SERIOUS REACTIONS

• Bone marrow depression evidenced by neutropenia, thrombocytopenia, and anemia, cardiovascular toxicity noted as angina, cardiomyopathy, and deep vein thrombosis (DVT), and lymphedema may occur.
• Respiratory toxicity is noted as dyspnea, epistaxis, pneumonia.

NURSING CONSIDERATIONS

Baseline Assessment

• Assess the patient's history of sensitivity to capecitabine or 5-fluorouracil.
• As ordered, obtain the patient's baseline Hct and Hgb blood levels.

Lifespan Considerations

• Be aware that capecitabine may be harmful to a fetus and that it is unknown if capecitabine is distributed in breast milk.
• Be aware that the safety and efficacy of capecitabine in children younger than 18 years of age have not been established.
• Be aware that the elderly may be more sensitive to capecitabine's GI side effects.

Precautions

• Use cautiously in patients with chickenpox, existing bone marrow depression, herpes zoster, liver function impairment, moderate renal function impairment, and previous cytotoxic or radiation therapy.

Administration and Handling

• Give 30 minutes before a meal.

Intervention and Evaluation

• Evaluate the patient for severe diarrhea. If dehydration occurs, fluid and electrolyte replacement therapy should be ordered.
• Assess the patient's hands and feet for chemotherapy induced erythema.
• Monitor the patient's complete blood count (CBC) for evidence of bone marrow depression.
• Monitor the patient for signs and symptoms of anemia, including excessive fatigue, weakness, and blood dyscrasias, including easy bruising, fever, signs of local infection, sore throat, or unusual bleeding from any site.

Patient Teaching

• Teach the patient that he or she has the potential to develop hand-and-foot syndrome, nausea, severe diarrhea, stomatitis, and vomiting. Warn the patient to notify the physician if he or she experiences any of these conditions.
• Stress to the patient that he or she should not receive vaccinations and should avoid contact with anyone who recently received a live virus vaccine.
• Warn the patient to notify the physician if he or she develops easy bruising, a fever higher than 100.5°F, signs of local infection, sore throat, or unusual bleeding from any site.

cytarabine

sigh-**tar**-ah-bean
(Ara-C, Cytosar[CAN], Cytosar-U)
**Do not confuse with Cytadren,
Cytovene, or vidarabine.**

CATEGORY AND SCHEDULE
Pregnancy Risk Category: D

MECHANISM OF ACTION
An antimetabolite that is converted
intracellularly to a nucleotide. Cell
cycle–specific for S phase of cell
division. Potent immunosuppressive
activity. *Therapeutic Effect:* May
inhibit DNA synthesis.

PHARMACOKINETICS
Widely distributed; moderate
amount crosses blood-brain barrier.
Protein binding: 15%. Primarily
excreted in urine. **Half-life:** 1–3 hrs.

AVAILABILITY
Powder for Injection: 100 mg, 1 g,
2 g.

INDICATIONS AND DOSAGES
▸ **Treatment of acute lymphocytic
leukemia, acute and chronic myelocytic leukemia, meningeal leukemia, non-Hodgkin's lymphoma in
children; Induction remission**
IV
Adults, Elderly, Children. 200 mg/
m²/day for 5 days at 2-wk intervals
as a single agent. 100–200 mg/m²/
day for 5-to 10-day therapy course
every 2–4 wks in combination
therapy.
Intrathecal
Adults, Elderly, Children. 5–7.5
mg/m² q2–7 days.
▸ **Treatment of acute lymphocytic
leukemia, acute and chronic myelocytic leukemia, meningeal leukemia, non-Hodgkin's lymphoma in
children; Maintenance remission**
IV
Adults, Elderly, Children. 70–200
mg/m²/day for 2–5 days every
month.
IM, Subcutaneous
Adults, Elderly, Children. 1–1.5
mg/m² as single dose at 1- to 4-wk
intervals.
Intrathecal
Adults, Elderly, Children. 5–7.5
mg/m² q2–7 days.

UNLABELED USES
Treatment of Hodgkin's lymphoma,
myelodysplastic syndrome

CONTRAINDICATIONS
None known.

INTERACTIONS
Drug
Antigout medications: May decrease
the effects of these drugs.
Bone marrow depressants: May
increase bone marrow depression.
Cyclophosphamide: May increase
risk of developing cardiomyopathy.
Live virus vaccines: May potentiate
virus replication, increase vaccine
side effects, and decrease the pa-
tient's antibody response to vaccine.
Herbal
None known.
Food
None known.

DIAGNOSTIC TEST EFFECTS
May increase serum alkaline phos-
phatase, serum bilirubin, SGOT
(AST), and serum uric acid levels.

IV INCOMPATIBILITIES
Amphotericin B complex (AmBisome, Amphotec, Abelcet), ganciclovir (Cytovene), heparin, insulin
(regular)

IV COMPATIBILITIES

Dexamethasone (Decadron), diphenhydramine (Benadryl), filgrastim (Neupogen), granisetron (Kytril), heparin, hydromorphone (Dilaudid), lorazepam (Ativan), morphine, ondansetron (Zofran), potassium chloride, propofol (Diprivan)

SIDE EFFECTS

Frequent

Subcutaneous, IV (33%–16%): Asthenia, fever, pain, change in taste and smell, nausea, vomiting (risk of nausea and vomiting greater with IV push than with continuous IV infusion)

Intrathecal (28%–11%): Headache, asthenia, change in taste and smell, confusion, somnolence, nausea, vomiting

Occasional

Subcutaneous, IV (11%–7%): Abnormal gait, somnolence, constipation, back pain, urinary incontinence, peripheral edema, headache, confusion

Intrathecal (7%–3%): Peripheral edema, back pain, constipation, abnormal gait, urinary incontinence

SERIOUS REACTIONS

• The major toxic effect of cytarabine use is bone marrow depression resulting in blood dyscrasias, including leukopenia, anemia, thrombocytopenia, megaloblastosis, reticulocytopenia, occurring minimally after single IV dose.

• Leukopenia, anemia, and thrombocytopenia should be expected with daily or continuous IV therapy.

• Cytarabine syndrome, evidenced by fever, myalgia, rash, conjunctivitis, malaise, or chest pain, and hyperuricemia may be noted.

• High-dose cytarabine therapy may produce severe central nervous system (CNS), gastrointestinal (GI), and pulmonary toxicity.

NURSING CONSIDERATIONS

Baseline Assessment

• Expect the patient's leukocyte count to decrease within 24 hours after the initial cytarabine dose; continue to decrease for 7 to 9 days; show a brief rise at 12 days; decrease again at 15 to 24 days; and finally rise rapidly for the next 10 days.

• Expect the patient's platelet count to decrease 5 days after cytarabine initiation to a low count at 12 to 15 days, then rise rapidly for the next 10 days.

Lifespan Considerations

• Know that cytarabine use should be avoided during pregnancy as the drug may cause fetal malformations.

• Be aware that it is unknown if cytarabine is distributed in breast milk. Breast-feeding is not recommended in this patient population.

• There are no age-related precautions noted in children.

• In the elderly, age-related renal impairment may require dosage adjustment.

Precautions

• Use cautiously in patients with impaired liver function.

Administration and Handling

◄ALERT► Know that cytarabine dosage is individualized based on the patient's clinical response and tolerance of the drug's adverse effects. When used in combination therapy, consult specific protocols for optimum dosage and sequence of drug administration. Expect to modify the dosage when serious hematologic depression occurs.

◄ALERT► May give cytarabine by subcutaneous injection, IV infusion, IV push, or intrathecally. Because cytarabine may be carcinogenic, mutagenic, or teratogenic, causing embryonic deformity, handle the drug with extreme care during preparation and administration.

Subcutaneous, IV, Intrathecal

• Reconstituted solution is stable for up to 48 hours at room temperature.

• IV infusion solutions at concentration up to 0.5 mg/ml are stable for up to 7 days at room temperature.

• Discard if slight haze develops.

• Reconstitute 100-mg vial with 5 ml Bacteriostatic Water for Injection with benzyl alcohol (10 ml for 500 mg vial) to provide concentration of 20 mg/ml and 50 mg/ml, respectively.

• Further dilute the dose, if necessary, with up to 1,000 ml D_5W or 0.9% NaCl for IV infusion.

• For intrathecal use, reconstitute vial with preservative-free 0.9% NaCl or patient's spinal fluid. Be aware that the dose is usually administered in 5 to 15 ml of solution, after equivalent volume of cerebrospinal fluid (CSF) removed.

• For IV push, give over 1 to 3 minutes. For IV infusion, give over 30 minutes to 24 hours.

Intervention and Evaluation

• Monitor the patient's complete blood count (CBC) for signs of bone marrow depression.

• Monitor the patient for signs and symptoms of anemia, including excessive tiredness and weakness, and blood dyscrasias, including easy bruising, fever, signs of local infection, sore throat, or unusual bleeding from any site.

• Evaluate the patient for neuropathy as evidenced by gait disturbances, handwriting difficulties, and numbness.

Patient Teaching

• Instruct the patient to increase his or her fluid intake to help protect against hyperuricemia development.

• Stress to the patient that he or she should not receive vaccinations and should avoid contact with anyone who recently received a live virus vaccine.

• Warn the patient to promptly report if he or she experiences easy bruising, fever, signs of local infection, sore throat, or unusual bleeding from any site.

fludarabine phosphate
flew-**dare**-ah-been
(Fludara)
Do not confuse with FUDR.

CATEGORY AND SCHEDULE
Pregnancy Risk Category: D

MECHANISM OF ACTION
An antimetabolite that interferes with DNA polymerase alpha, ribonucleotide reductase, and DNA primase. *Therapeutic Effect:* Inhibits DNA synthesis, induces cell death.

PHARMACOKINETICS
Rapidly dephosphorylated in serum, then phosphorylated intracellularly to active triphosphate. Primarily excreted in urine. **Half-life:** 7–20 hrs.

AVAILABILITY
Injection: 50 mg.

INDICATIONS AND DOSAGES
▶ **Chronic lymphocytic leukemia**
IV
Adults. 25 mg/m^2 daily for 5 consecutive days. Continue up to 3 additional cycles. Begin each course of treatment q28 days.

▸ **Acute leukemia**
IV
Children. 10 mg/m^2 bolus (over 15 min), then IV infusion of 30.5 mg/m^2/day.
▸ **Solid tumors**
IV
Children. 9 mg/m^2 bolus, then 27 mg/m^2/day for 5 days as continuous infusion.
▸ **Non-Hodgkin's lymphoma**
IV
Adults, Elderly. Initially, 20 mg/m^2, then 30 mg/m^2/day for 48 hrs.
▸ **Dosage in renal impairment**

Creatinine Clearance	Dosage
30–70 ml/min	decrease dose by 20%
less than 30 ml/min	not recommended

CONTRAINDICATIONS

Concomitant administration with pentostatin

INTERACTIONS

Drug
Antigout medications: May decrease the effects of these drugs.
Bone marrow depressants: May increase risk of bone marrow depression.
Live virus vaccines: May potentiate virus replication, increase vaccine side effects, and decrease the patient's antibody response to the vaccine.
Herbal
None known.
Food
None known.

DIAGNOSTIC TEST EFFECTS

May increase serum alkaline phosphatase, SGOT (AST), and uric acid levels.

IV INCOMPATIBILITIES

Acyclovir (Zovirax), amphotericin (Fungizone), hydroxyzine (Vistaril), prochlorperazine (Compazine)

IV COMPATIBILITIES

Heparin, hydromorphone (Dilaudid), lorazepam (Ativan), magnesium sulfate, morphine, multivitamins, potassium chloride

SIDE EFFECTS

Frequent
Fever (60%), nausea and vomiting (36%), chills (11%)
Occasional (20%–10%)
Fatigue, generalized pain, rash, diarrhea, cough, weakness, stomatitis (burning or erythema of oral mucosa, sore throat, difficulty swallowing), dyspnea, weakness, peripheral edema
Rare (7%–3%)
Anorexia, sinusitis, dysuria, myalgia, paresthesia, headaches, visual disturbances

SERIOUS REACTIONS

• Pneumonia occurs frequently.
• Severe bone marrow toxicity as evidenced by anemia, thrombocytopenia, and neutropenia may occur.
• Tumor lysis syndrome may occur with onset of flank pain and hematuria. This syndrome may include hypercalcemia, hyperphosphatemia, hyperuricemia and result in renal failure.
• Gastrointestinal (GI) bleeding may occur.
• High fludarabine dosage may produce acute leukemia, blindness, and coma.

▮ NURSING CONSIDERATIONS

Baseline Assessment
• Assess the patient's baseline complete blood count (CBC) and serum creatinine level.

• Expect to discontinue fludarabine if intractable diarrhea, GI bleeding, stomatitis, or vomiting occur.

Lifespan Considerations
• Know that fludarabine use should be avoided during pregnancy, if possible, especially in the first trimester.
• Be aware that fludarabine may cause fetal harm and it is unknown if it is distributed in breast milk. Breast-feeding is not recommended in this patient population.
• The safety and efficacy of fludarabine have not been established in children.
• In the elderly, age-related renal impairment may require dosage adjustment.

Precautions
• Use cautiously in patients with preexisting bone marrow suppression, neurologic problems, and renal insufficiency.

Administration and Handling
◀ALERT▶ Be aware that fludarabine dosage is individualized on the basis of the patient's clinical response and tolerance of the drug's adverse effects. When used in combination therapy, consult specific protocols for optimum dosage and sequence of drug administration. Drug dosage is based on the patient's actual weight. Use ideal body weight in edematous or obese patients.
◀ALERT▶ Give fludarabine by IV infusion. Do not add to other IV infusions. Avoid areas overlying joints and tendons, small veins, and swollen or edematous extremities.
IV
• Store in refrigerator.
• Handle with extreme care during preparation and administration.

If contact with skin or mucous membranes occurs, wash thoroughly with soap and water; rinse eyes profusely with plain water.
• After reconstitution, use within 8 hours; discard unused portion.
• Reconstitute 50-mg vial with 2 ml Sterile Water for Injection to provide a concentration of 25 mg/ml.
• Further dilute with 100 to 125 ml 0.9% NaCl or D_5W.
• Infuse over 30 minutes.

Intervention and Evaluation
• Assess the patient for onset of peripheral edema, pneumonia, visual disturbances, and weakness.
• Monitor the patient for cough, dyspnea, GI bleeding, including bright red or tarry stools, intractable diarrhea, and rapidly falling white blood cell (WBC) count.
• Examine the patient for difficulty swallowing, mucosal erythema, sore throat, and ulceration at inner margin of lips, which indicate the presence of stomatitis.
• Assess the patient's skin for rash.
• Be alert to signs and symptoms of possible tumor lysis syndrome manifested as hematuria and onset of flank pain.

Patient Teaching
• Stress to the patient to avoid crowds and exposure to those with known infection.
• Teach the patient to maintain fastidious oral hygiene.
• Warn the patient to notify the physician if he or she experiences easy bruising, fever, signs of local infection, sore throat, or unusual bleeding from any site.
• Caution the patient to contact the physician if nausea and vomiting continue at home.

fluorouracil

phlur-oh-**your**-ah-sill
(Adrucil, Efudex, Efudix[AUS],
Fluoroplex)
Do not confuse with Efidac.

CATEGORY AND SCHEDULE

Pregnancy Risk Category: D

MECHANISM OF ACTION

An antimetabolite that blocks formation of thymidylic acid. *Therapeutic Effect:* Inhibits DNA, RNA synthesis. Topical: Destroys rapidly proliferating cells. Cell cycle–specific for S phase of cell division.

PHARMACOKINETICS

Crosses blood-brain barrier. Widely distributed. Rapidly metabolized in tissues to active metabolite, which is localized intracellularly. Primarily excreted via lungs as CO_2. Removed by hemodialysis. **Half-life:** 20 hrs.

AVAILABILITY

Injection: 50 mg/ml.
Cream: 1%, 5%.
Topical Solution: 1%, 2%, 5%.

INDICATIONS AND DOSAGES

▶ **Treatment of carcinoma of breast, colon, pancreas, rectum, and stomach; in combination with levamisole after surgical resection in patients with Duke's stage C colon cancer**
IV
Adults, Elderly, Children. Initially, 12 mg/kg/day for 4–5 days. Maximum: 800 mg/day.
Maintenance: 6 mg/kg every other day for 4 doses. Repeat in 4 wks or 15 mg/kg as a single bolus dose. Or, 5–15 mg/kg/wk as a single dose, not to exceed 1 g.

▶ **Treatment of multiple actinic or solar keratoses and superficial basal cell carcinomas**
Topical
Adults. Apply 2 times/day to cover lesions.

UNLABELED USES

Parenteral: Treatment of bladder, cervical, endometrial, head and neck, liver, lung, ovarian, prostate carcinomas; treatment of pericardial, peritoneal, pleural effusions
Topical: Treatment of actinic cheilitis, radiodermatitis

CONTRAINDICATIONS

Depressed bone marrow function, major surgery within previous month, poor nutritional status, potentially serious infections

INTERACTIONS

Drug
Bone marrow depressants: May increase risk of bone marrow depression.
Live virus vaccines: May potentiate virus replication, increase vaccine side effects, and decrease the patient's antibody response to vaccine.
Herbal
None known.
Food
None known.

DIAGNOSTIC TEST EFFECTS

May decrease serum albumin. May increase excretion of 5-HIAA in urine. Topical: May cause eosinophilia, leukocytosis, thrombocytopenia, and toxic granulation.

IV INCOMPATIBILITIES

Amphotericin B complex (Abelcet, Amphotec, AmBisome), droperidol (Inapsine), filgrastim (Neupogen), ondansetron (Zofran), vinorelbine (Navelbine)

IV COMPATIBILITIES

Granisetron (Kytril), heparin, hydromorphone (Dilaudid), leucovorin, morphine, ondansetron (Zofran), potassium chloride, propofol (Diprivan)

SIDE EFFECTS

Occasional

Anorexia, diarrhea, minimal alopecia, fever, dry skin, fissuring, scaling, erythema
Topical: Pain, pruritus, hyperpigmentation, irritation, inflammation, burning at application site

Rare

Nausea, vomiting, anemia, esophagitis, proctitis, gastrointestinal (GI) ulcer, confusion, headache, lacrimation, visual disturbances, angina, allergic reactions

SERIOUS REACTIONS

• The earliest sign of toxicity, which may occur 4–8 days after beginning of therapy, is stomatitis as evidenced by dry mouth, burning sensation, mucosal erythema, and ulceration at inner margin of lips.
• Most common dermatologic toxicity is pruritic rash that generally appears on extremities, less frequently on trunk.
• Leukopenia generally occurs within 9–14 days after drug administration and may occur as late as the 25th day.
• Thrombocytopenia occasionally occurs within 7–17 days after administration.
• Hematologic toxicity may also manifest itself as pancytopenia or agranulocytosis.

NURSING CONSIDERATIONS

Baseline Assessment

• Monitor the patient's complete blood count (CBC) with differential, liver and renal function tests, and platelet count.

Lifespan Considerations

• Be aware that fluorouracil use should be avoided during pregnancy, if possible, especially in the first trimester.
• Be aware that fluorouracil may cause fetal harm and it is unknown whether fluorouracil is distributed in breast milk. Breast-feeding is not recommended in this patient population.
• There are no age-related precautions noted in children.
• In the elderly, age-related renal impairment may require dosage adjustment.

Precautions

• Use cautiously in patients with a history of high-dose pelvic irradiation, impaired liver or renal function, and metastatic cell infiltration of bone marrow.

Administration and Handling

◀ALERT▶ Know that fluorouracil dosage is individualized on the basis of the patient's clinical response and tolerance of the drug's adverse effects. When used in combination therapy, consult specific protocols for optimum dosage and sequence of drug administration. Be aware that dosage is based on the patient's actual weight. Use ideal body weight in edematous or obese patients.

◀ALERT▶ Give fluorouracil by IV injection or IV infusion. Do not add to other IV infusions. Avoid areas overlying joints and tendons, small veins, and swollen or edematous extremities. Because fluorouracil may be carcinogenic, mutagenic, or teratogenic, handle the drug with extreme care during preparation and administration.

IV

• Solution normally appears color-

less to faint yellow. Slight discoloration does not adversely affect potency or safety.
• If precipitate forms, redissolve by heating, shaking vigorously; allow to cool to body temperature.
• Administer IV push as undiluted or unreconstituted, as appropriate. Inject through Y-tube or 3-way stopcock of free-flowing solution.
• For IV infusion, further dilute with D$_5$W or 0.9% NaCl.
• Give IV push slowly over 1 to 2 minutes.
• Administer IV infusion over 30 minutes to 24 hours.
• Monitor patient for signs and symptoms of extravasation, including immediate pain and severe local tissue damage. If this occurs, follow your facility's protocol.

Intervention and Evaluation
• Monitor the patient for signs of GI bleeding, including bright red or tarry stool, intractable diarrhea, and rapidly falling white blood cell (WBC) count.
• Assess the patient for signs and symptoms of stomatitis, including difficulty swallowing, mucosal erythema, sore throat, and ulceration of inner margin of lips.
• Discontinue fluorouracil if intractable diarrhea, GI bleeding, or stomatitis occurs.
• Assess the patient's skin for rash.

Patient Teaching
• Teach the patient to maintain fastidious oral hygiene.
• Warn the patient to notify the physician if he or she experiences bleeding, bruising, chest pain, diarrhea, nausea, palpitations, signs and symptoms of infection, or visual changes.

• Encourage the patient to avoid overexposure to sun or ultraviolet light and to wear protective clothing, sunglasses, and sunscreen.
• Instruct patients using topical fluorouracil to apply the drug only to the affected area and not to use occlusive coverings. Explain to the patient that he or she needs to be careful when applying topical drug near the eyes, mouth, and nose. Teach the patient to wash hands thoroughly after topical drug application. Explain to the patient that treated areas may be unsightly for several weeks after therapy.

gemcitabine hydrochloride
gem-**cih**-tah-bean
(Gemzar)

CATEGORY AND SCHEDULE
Pregnancy Risk Category: D

MECHANISM OF ACTION
An antimetabolite that inhibits ribonucleotide reductase, the enzyme necessary for catalyzing DNA synthesis. *Therapeutic Effect:* Produces cell death in those cells undergoing DNA synthesis.

PHARMACOKINETICS
After IV infusion, not extensively distributed (increased with length of infusion). Protein binding: less than 10%. Excreted primarily in urine as metabolite. **Half-life:** 42–94 min (influenced by gender of patient and duration of infusion).

AVAILABILITY
Powder for Reconstitution: 200 mg, 1-g vial.

INDICATIONS AND DOSAGES
▶ **Non small cell lung cancer (in combination with cisplatin)**
IV
Adults, Elderly, Children. 1000 mg/m² days 1, 8, 15. Repeat q28 days or 1250 mg/m² day 1 and 8. Repeat q21 days.
▶ **Pancreatic cancer**
IV infusion
Adults. 1,000 mg/m² once weekly for up to 7 wks, or until toxicity necessitates decreasing or holding the dose, followed by 1 wk of rest. Subsequent cycles should consist of once weekly for 3 consecutive wks out of every 4 wks. For patients completing cycles at 1,000 mg/m², increase dose to 1,250 mg/m² as tolerated. Dose for next cycle may be increased to 1,500 mg/m².
▶ **Dose reduction guidelines**

AGC (10⁶/L)		Platelets (10⁶/L)	% Full Dose
1,000	and	100,000	100
500–999	or	50,000–99,000	75
less than 500	or	less than 50,000	Hold

CONTRAINDICATIONS
None known.

INTERACTIONS
Drug
Bone marrow depressants: May increase risk of bone marrow depression.
Live virus vaccines: May potentiate virus replication, increase vaccine side effects, and decrease the patient's antibody response to vaccine.
Herbal
None known.
Food
None known.

DIAGNOSTIC TEST EFFECTS
May increase serum alkaline phosphatase, serum bilirubin, BUN, serum creatinine, SGOT (AST), and SGPT (ALT) levels.

IV INCOMPATIBILITIES
Acyclovir (Zovirax), amphotericin (Fungizone), cefoperazone (Cefobid), furosemide (Lasix), ganciclovir (Cytovene), imipenem-cilastatin (Primaxin), irinotecan (Camptosar), methotrexate, methylprednisolone (Solu-Medrol), mitomycin (Mutamycin), piperacillin/tazobactam (Zosyn), prochlorperazine (Compazine)

IV COMPATIBILITIES
Bumetanide (Bumex), calcium gluconate, dexamethasone (Decadron), diphenhydramine (Benadryl), dobutamine (Dobutrex), dopamine (Intropin), granisetron (Kytril), heparin, hydrocortisone (Solu-Cortef), lorazepam (Ativan), ondansetron (Zofran), potassium

SIDE EFFECTS
Frequent
Nausea and vomiting (69%); generalized pain (48%); fever (41%); mild to moderate pruritic rash (30%); mild to moderate dyspnea, constipation (23%); peripheral edema (20%)
Occasional (19%–10%)
Diarrhea, petechiae, alopecia, stomatitis (burning or erythema of oral mucosa, sore throat, difficulty swallowing), infection, somnolence, paresthesia
Rare
Diaphoresis, rhinitis, insomnia, malaise

SERIOUS REACTIONS
• Severe bone marrow suppression evidenced by anemia, thrombocyto-

penia, and leukopenia commonly occurs.

Baseline Assessment

• Expect to perform complete blood count (CBC) and liver and renal function tests before initiating gemcitabine therapy and periodically thereafter.

• Expect to stop or modify the gemcitabine dosage if bone marrow suppression is detected.

Lifespan Considerations

• Know that gemcitabine use should be avoided during pregnancy, if possible, especially in the first trimester.

• Be aware that gemcitabine may cause fetal harm and it is unknown if gemcitabine is distributed in breast milk. Breast-feeding is not recommended in this patient population.

• The safety and efficacy of gemcitabine have not been established in children.

• In the elderly, there is an increased risk of hematologic toxicity.

Precautions

• Use cautiously in patients with impaired renal function and liver insufficiency.

Administration and Handling

◀ALERT▶ Be aware that gemcitabine dosage is individualized on the basis of the patient's clinical response and tolerance of the drug's adverse effects. When used in combination therapy, consult specific protocols for optimum dosage and sequence of drug administration.

◀ALERT▶ Increase gemcitabine dose, as prescribed, provided the absolute granulocyte count (AGC) and platelet nadirs exceed $1,500 \times 10^6$/L and $100,000 \times 10^6$/L, respectively.

IV

• Store unreconstituted form at room temperature because refrigeration may cause crystallization.

• Reconstituted solution is stable for up to 24 hours at room temperature.

• Use gloves when handling and preparing gemcitabine.

• Reconstitute 200-mg or 1-g vial with 0.9% NaCl injection without preservative, 5 ml or 25 ml, respectively, to provide a concentration of 40 mg/ml.

• Shake to dissolve and give without further dilution, as appropriate.

• Further dilute with 0.9% NaCl to a concentration as low as 0.1 mg/ml if desired.

• Infuse over 30 minutes. Do not infuse over longer than 1 hour because this increases the risk of toxicity.

Intervention and Evaluation

• Evaluate all of the patient's lab results before each gemcitabine dose is given.

• Monitor the patient for dehydration from vomiting, dyspnea, fever, and pruritic rash.

• Assess the patient for signs and symptoms of stomatitis, including difficulty swallowing, erythema, sore throat, and ulceration at inner margin of lips.

• Assess the patient's skin for rash.

• Monitor the patient for diarrhea and report if diarrhea develops.

• Provide antiemetics as needed, if ordered.

Patient Teaching

• Stress to the patient to avoid crowds and exposure to those with known infection.

• Teach the patient to maintain fastidious oral hygiene.

• Warn the patient to notify the physician if he or she experiences easy bruising, fever, signs of local infection, rash, or sore throat.

• Caution the patient to notify the physician if nausea or vomiting continues at home.

hydroxyurea
high-**drocks**-ee-your-e-ah
(Droxia, Hydrea, Mylocel)

CATEGORY AND SCHEDULE
Pregnancy Risk Category: D

MECHANISM OF ACTION
A synthetic urea analogue that is cell cycle–specific for S phase. Inhibits DNA synthesis without interfering with RNA synthesis or protein. *Therapeutic Effect:* Interferes with the normal repair process of cells damaged by irradiation.

AVAILABILITY
Capsules: 200 mg, 300 mg, 400 mg, 500 mg.
Tablets: 1,000 mg.

INDICATIONS AND DOSAGES
▶ **Treatment of melanoma; recurrent, metastatic, or inoperable ovarian carcinoma. Also used in combination with radiation therapy for local control of primary squamous cell carcinoma of head and neck, excluding lip**
PO
Adults, Elderly. 80 mg/kg q3 days or 20–30 mg/kg/day as a single dose each day.
▶ **Control of primary squamous cell carcinoma of the head and neck, excluding lip, in combination with radiation therapy**
PO
Adults, Elderly. 80 mg/kg q3 days beginning at least 7 days before starting radiation therapy.

▶ **Resistant chronic myelocytic leukemia (CML)**
PO
Adults, Elderly. 20–30 mg/kg once a day.
Children. Initially, 10–20 mg/kg once a day.
▶ **HIV Infection**
PO
Adults, Elderly. 500 mg 2 times/day with didanosine.
▶ **Sickle cell anemia**
PO
Adults, Elderly, Children. Initially, 15 mg/kg once a day. May increase by 5 mg/kg/day. Maximum: 35 mg/kg/wk.

UNLABELED USES
Treatment of cervical carcinoma, polycythemia vera. Long-term suppression of HIV.

CONTRAINDICATIONS
White blood cell (WBC) count less than $2,500/mm^3$ or platelet count less than $100,000/mm^3$

INTERACTIONS
Drug
Antigout medications: May decrease the effects of these drugs.
Bone marrow depressants: May increase bone marrow depression.
Live virus vaccines: May potentiate virus replication, increase vaccine side effects, and decrease the patient's antibody response to vaccine.
Herbal
None known.
Food
None known.

DIAGNOSTIC TEST EFFECTS
May increase BUN, serum creatinine, and serum uric acid.

SIDE EFFECTS
Frequent
Nausea, vomiting, anorexia, constipation or diarrhea
Occasional
Mild reversible rash, facial flushing, pruritus, fever, chills, malaise
Rare
Alopecia, headache, drowsiness, dizziness, disorientation

SERIOUS REACTIONS
• Bone marrow depression manifested as hematologic toxicity (leukopenia, and to lesser extent, thrombocytopenia, anemia) may occur.

NURSING CONSIDERATIONS
Baseline Assessment
• Expect the patient to undergo bone marrow studies and liver and kidney function tests before hydroxyurea therapy begins and periodically thereafter.
• Obtain baseline blood Hgb and serum uric acid levels and platelet and white blood cell counts weekly during hydroxyurea therapy.
• Know that those patients with marked renal impairment may develop auditory or visual hallucinations and marked hematologic toxicity.
Precautions
• Use cautiously in patients with impaired liver or renal function, who have had previous radiation therapy, or who are using other cytotoxic drugs.
Administration and Handling
◀ALERT▶ Be aware that hydroxyurea dosage is individualized based on the patient's clinical response and tolerance of the drug's adverse effects. When used in combination therapy, consult specific protocols for optimum dosage and sequence

of drug administration. Know that dosage is based on actual or ideal body weight, whichever is less. Expect therapy to be interrupted when platelets fall below 100,000/mm^3 or leukocytes fall below 2,500/mm^3 and to resume when counts rise toward normal.
Intervention and Evaluation
• Assess the patient's pattern of daily bowel activity and stool consistency.
• Monitor the patient for signs and symptoms of anemia, including excessive tiredness and weakness, and hematologic toxicity, including easy bruising, fever, signs of local infection, sore throat, or unusual bleeding from any site.
• Assess the patient's skin for erythema or rash.
• Monitor the patient's blood Hgb, complete blood count (CBC) with differential, liver function test results, platelet count, renal function studies, and serum uric acid levels.
Patient Teaching
• Warn the patient to notify the physician if he or she experiences easy bruising, fever, signs of local infection, sore throat, or unusual bleeding from any site.

mercaptopurine
mur-cap-**tow**-pure-een
(Purinethol)

CATEGORY AND SCHEDULE
Pregnancy risk category: D

MECHANISM OF ACTION
An antimetabolite that is incorporated into RNA and DNA. Blocks purine synthesis. *Therapeutic effect:* Inhibits DNA and RNA synthesis.

AVAILABILITY
Tablets: 50 mg.

INDICATIONS AND DOSAGES
▶ **Acute lymphoblastic leukemia (ALL)**
PO (induction)
Adults, Elderly, Children. 2.5–5 mg/kg/day once a day.
PO (maintenance)
Adults, Elderly, Children. 1.5–2.5 mg/kg/day.
▶ **Dosage in renal impairment: Creatinine clearance less than 50 ml/min.** Administer q48 hrs.

CONTRAINDICATIONS
Pregnancy, severe bone marrow suppression, severe liver disease

INTERACTIONS
Drug
Allopurinol, doxorubicin, liver toxic drugs: May increase the effects and risk of toxicity of mercaptopurine.
Warfarin: May decrease the effects of this drug.
Herbal
None known.
Food
Decreases bioavailability of mercaptopurine.

DIAGNOSTIC TEST EFFECTS
None known.

SIDE EFFECTS
Frequent (greater than 10%)
Myelosuppression, leukopenia, thrombocytopenia, anemia, intrahepatic cholestasis, focal centrilobular necrosis
Occasional (10%–1%)
Drug fever, hyperpigmentation, rash, hyperuricemia, nausea, vomiting, diarrhea, stomatitis, anorexia, stomach pain, mucositis

SERIOUS REACTIONS
• Nausea, vomiting, bone marrow suppression, liver necrosis, and gastroenteritis may occur.

NURSING CONSIDERATIONS
Baseline Assessment
• Determine if the patient is pregnant or breast-feeding (not recommended) and taking other medication, especially allopurinol, other bone marrow suppressants, and other liver toxic medications, before beginning mercaptopurine therapy.
Precautions
• Use cautiously in patients with history of gout, infection, liver impairment, prior bone marrow suppression, and renal impairment.
Administration and Handling
PO
• Do not administer with meals.
Intervention and Evaluation
• Monitor the patient's liver function tests, platelet count, renal function, and serum uric acid.
Patient Teaching
• Urge the patient to avoid consuming alcohol during mercaptopurine therapy. Explain to the patient that alcohol may increase the risk of toxicity with this drug.
• Stress to the patient that he or she should not receive vaccinations and should avoid contact with anyone with known infection.
• Warn the patient to notify the physician if he or she experiences unusual bleeding or bruising.

methotrexate sodium

meth-oh-**trex**-ate
(Ledertrexate[AUS],
Methoblastin[AUS], Rheumatrex)

CATEGORY AND SCHEDULE

Pregnancy Risk Category: D
(X for psoriasis or rheumatoid
arthritis patients)

MECHANISM OF ACTION

An antimetabolite that competes
with enzymes necessary to reduce
folic acid to tetrahydrofolic acid, a
component essential to DNA, RNA,
and protein synthesis. *Therapeutic
Effect:* Inhibits DNA, RNA, and
protein synthesis.

PHARMACOKINETICS

Variably absorbed from the gastrointestinal (GI) tract. Completely
absorbed after IM administration.
Protein binding: 50%–60%. Widely
distributed. Metabolized in liver,
intracellularly. Primarily excreted in
urine. Removed by hemodialysis;
not removed by peritoneal dialysis.
Half-life: 8–12 hrs (large doses:
8–15 hrs).

AVAILABILITY

Tablets: 2.5 mg, 5 mg, 7.5 mg, 10
mg, 15 mg.
Powder for Injection: 20 mg, 1 g.
Injection: 25 mg/ml.
Injection (preservative-free): 25
mg/ml.

INDICATIONS AND DOSAGES

▸ **Trophoblastic neoplasms**
PO/IM
Adults, Elderly. 15–30 mg/day for 5
days; repeat in 7 days for 3–5
courses.

▸ **Head and neck cancer**
PO/IM/IV
Adults, Elderly. 25–50 mg/m^2 once
weekly.

▸ **Rheumatoid arthritis**
PO
Adults, Elderly. 7.5 mg once weekly
or 2.5 mg q12h for 3 doses/wk.
Maximum: 20 mg/wk.

▸ **Psoriasis**
PO
Adults, Elderly. 2.5–5 mg/dose q12h
for 3 doses/wk given once weekly.
PO/IM
Adults, Elderly. 10–25 mg once
weekly.

▸ **Choriocarcinoma, chorioadenoma
destruens, hydatidiform mole**
IM/PO
Adults, Elderly. 15–30 mg/day for 5
days; repeat 3–5 times with 1–2
wks between courses.

▸ **Acute lymphocytic leukemia (ALL)**
IM/IV/PO
Adults, Elderly. Induction: 3.3
mg/m^2/day in combination with
other chemotherapeutic agents.
IM/PO
Adults, Elderly. Maintenance: 30
mg/m^2/wk in divided doses.
IV
Adults, Elderly. 2.5 mg/kg q14
days.

▸ **Burkitt's lymphoma**
PO
Adults. 10–25 mg/day for 4–8 days;
repeat with 7-to 10-day rest between courses.

▸ **Lymphosarcoma**
PO
Adults, Elderly. 0.625–2.5 mg/kg/
day.

▸ **Mycosis fungoides**
PO
• *Adults, Elderly.* 2.5–10 mg/day.
IM
Adults, Elderly. 50 mg/wk or 25 mg
2 times/wk.

▸ **Juvenile rheumatoid arthritis**
PO/IM/Subcutaneous
Children. 5–15 mg/m^2/wk as a
single dose or in 3 divided doses
given 12 hrs apart.
▸ **Antineoplastic dosage for children**
PO/IM
Children. 7.5–30 mg/m^2/wk or
q2wks.
IV
Children. 10–33,000 mg/m^2 bolus
or continuous infusion over 6–42
hrs.

UNLABELED USES
Treatment of acute myelocytic
leukemia, bladder, cervical, ovarian,
prostatic, renal, and testicular carcinoma, psoriatic arthritis, systemic
dermatomyositis

CONTRAINDICATIONS
Preexisting bone marrow suppression, severe liver or renal impairment

INTERACTIONS
Drug
Asparaginase: May decrease the
effects of methotrexate.
Bone marrow depressants: May
increase bone marrow depression.
Live virus vaccines: May potentiate
virus replication, increase vaccine
side effects, and decrease the patient's antibody response to vaccine.
Liver toxic medications: May increase liver toxicity.
NSAIDs: May increase risk of
methotrexate toxicity.
Parenteral acyclovir: May increase
risk of neurotoxicity.
Probenecid, salicylates: May increase blood methotrexate concentration and risk of toxicity.
Herbal
None known.

Food
Alcohol: May increase risk of liver
toxicity.

DIAGNOSTIC TEST EFFECTS
May increase serum uric acid and
SGOT (AST) levels.

IV INCOMPATIBILITIES
Chlorpromazine (Thorazine), dro-
peridol (Inapsine), gemcitabine
(Gemzar), idarubicin (Idamycin),
midazolam (Versed), nalbuphine
(Nubain)

IV COMPATIBILITIES
Cisplatin (Platinol AQ), cyclophosphamide (Cytoxan), daunorubicin
(DaunoXome), doxorubicin (Adriamycin), etoposide (VePesid), fluorouracil, granisetron (Kytril), leucovorin, mitomycin (Mutamycin),
ondansetron (Zofran), paclitaxel
(Taxol), vinblastine (Velban), vincristine (Oncovin), vinorelbine
(Navelbine)

SIDE EFFECTS
Frequent (10%–3%)
Nausea, vomiting, stomatitis
In patients with psoriasis, burning,
erythema at psoriatic site.
Occasional (3%–1%)
Diarrhea, rash, dermatitis, pruritus,
alopecia, dizziness, anorexia, mal-
aise, headache, drowsiness, blurred
vision

SERIOUS REACTIONS
• There is a high potential for
various, severe toxicity development.
• Gastrointestinal (GI) toxicity may
produce oral ulcers of mouth, gingivitis, glossitis, pharyngitis, stomatitis, enteritis, and hematemesis.
• Liver toxicity occurs more frequently with frequent, small doses
than with large, intermittent doses.

• Pulmonary toxicity is characterized as interstitial pneumonitis.
• Hematologic toxicity, which may develop rapidly, resulting from marked bone marrow depression may be manifested as leukopenia, thrombocytopenia, anemia, and hemorrhage.
• Skin toxicity produces rash, pruritus, urticaria, pigmentation, photosensitivity, petechiae, ecchymosis, and pustules.
• Severe nephropathy produces azotemia, hematuria, and renal failure.

Baseline Assessment
• Determine if the patient with psoriasis or rheumatoid arthritis is pregnant before initiating methotrexate therapy because the drug has a Pregnancy Category rating of X.
• Evaluate diagnostic test results, including renal and liver function tests, Hgb and Hct levels and platelet count, before methotrexate therapy and throughout therapy.
• Give antiemetics, if ordered, to prevent and treat nausea and vomiting.

Lifespan Considerations
• Know that pregnancy should be avoided during methotrexate therapy and for a minimum of 3 months after therapy is completed in males or at least one ovulatory cycle after therapy is completed in females.
• Be aware that methotrexate may cause congenital anomalies and fetal death.
• Be aware that methotrexate is distributed in breast milk and that breast-feeding is not recommended in this patient population.
• In children and the elderly, decreased liver and renal function

requires caution and may require dosage adjustment.

Precautions
• Use cautiously in patients with ascites, bone marrow suppression, peptic ulcer disease, pleural effusion, and ulcerative colitis.

Administration and Handling
◀ALERT▶ Because methotrexate may be carcinogenic, mutagenic, or teratogenic, handle the drug with extreme care during preparation and administration. Wear gloves when preparing solution. If powder or solution comes in contact with skin, wash immediately, thoroughly with soap, water.
• Be aware that the drug may be given IM, IV, intra-arterially, intrathecally.
IV
• Store vials at room temperature.
• Reconstitute each 5 mg with 2 ml Sterile Water for Injection or 0.9% NaCl to provide a concentration of 2.5 mg/ml up to a maximum concentration of 25 mg/ml.
• May further dilute with D_5W or 0.9% NaCl.
• For intrathecal use, dilute with preservative-free 0.9% NaCl to provide a 1 mg/ml concentration.
• Give IV push at rate of 10 mg/min.
• Give IV infusion over 30 minutes to 4 hours.

Intervention and Evaluation
• Monitor the patient's blood Hgb and Hct levels, chest x-ray results, liver and renal function tests, platelet count, serum uric acid level, urinalysis, and white blood cell (WBC) count with differential.
• Monitor the patient for signs and symptoms of anemia, including excessive fatigue and weakness, and hematologic toxicity, including easy bruising, fever, signs of local

infection, sore throat, and unusual bleeding from any site.

• Assess the patient's skin for evidence of dermatologic toxicity.

• As prescribed, administer IV fluids to keep the patient well hydrated and medication, such as bicarbonate, to alkalinize the urine.

• Avoid giving IM injections, taking rectal temperatures, and performing traumatic procedures that induce bleeding.

• Apply 5 full minutes of pressure to the patient's IV sites after discontinuation.

Patient Teaching

• Teach the patient to maintain fastidious oral hygiene.

• Stress to the patient that he or she should not receive vaccinations and should avoid contact with crowds and those with known infection.

• Urge the patient to avoid alcohol and salicylates during methotrexate therapy.

• Encourage the patient to avoid overexposure to sun or ultraviolet light.

• Instruct the male patient in the use of contraceptive measures during therapy and for 3 months or, for the female patient, one ovulatory cycle after therapy.

• Warn the patient to report if he or she experiences easy bruising, fever, signs of local infection, sore throat, and unusual bleeding from any site.

• Explain to the patient that alopecia is reversible, but new hair growth may have a different color or texture.

• Caution the patient to notify the physician if nausea and vomiting continues at home.

16 Antimitotic Agents

docetaxel
paclitaxel
vinblastine sulfate
vincristine sulfate
vinorelbine

Uses: Antimitotic agents are used to treat lymphoma, lymphosarcomas, neuroblastomas, multiple myeloma, and cancer of testes, breasts, kidneys, lungs, or ovaries.

Action: Antimitotic agents include two groups that act in different ways—vinca alkaloids and taxoids. *Vinca alkaloids*, which include vinblastine and vincristine, block mitosis during metaphase (M phase) by disrupting the assembly of microtubules (filaments that move chromosomes during cell division). This action prevents cell division. *Taxoids,* such as docetaxel and paclitaxel, act during the late G_2 phase to enhance the formation of stable microtubules, which prevents cell division.

docetaxel
dox-eh-**tax**-el
(Taxotere)
Do not confuse with Taxol.

CATEGORY AND SCHEDULE
Pregnancy Risk Category: D

MECHANISM OF ACTION
This antimitotic agent belongs to the taxoid family and disrupts the microtubular cell network, which is essential for cellular function. *Therapeutic Effect:* Inhibits cell mitosis.

PHARMACOKINETICS
Distributed into peripheral compartments. Protein binding: 94%. Extensively metabolized. Excreted primarily in feces with lesser amount in urine. **Half-life:** 11.1 hrs.

AVAILABILITY
Injection: 20 mg in 0.5 ml with diluent, 80 mg in 2 ml with diluent.

INDICATIONS AND DOSAGES
▸ **Breast carcinoma**
IV infusion
Adults. 60–100 mg/m^2 given over 1 hr q3wks. Those dosed initially at 100 mg/m^2 who experience febrile neutropenia, neutrophils less than 500 cells/mm^3 for more than 1 wk, severe or cumulative cutaneous reactions, or severe peripheral neuropathy during therapy should have dose adjusted from 100 to 75 mg/m^2. If reaction continues, lower dose from 75 to 55 mg/m^2 or stop therapy. Those patients dosed at 60 mg/m^2 who do not experience the above symptoms may tolerate an increased docetaxel dose.
▸ **Non–small cell lung carcinoma**
IV infusion
Adults. 75 mg/m^2 q3wks. Adjust dosage if toxicity occurs.

UNLABELED USES
Treatment of small cell bladder, head and neck, lung, ovarian, prostate cancer

CONTRAINDICATIONS

History of severe hypersensitivity to docetaxel or other drugs formulated with polysorbate 80, neutrophil count less than 1,500 cells/mm^3

INTERACTIONS
Drug
Cyclosporine, erythromycin, ketoconazole: May significantly modify docetaxel metabolism.
Live virus vaccines: May potentiate replication, increase side effects, and decrease the patient's antibody responses to the vaccine virus.
Herbal
None known.
Food
None known.

DIAGNOSTIC TEST EFFECTS

May significantly increase BUN, serum alkaline phosphatase, serum bilirubin, serum creatinine, and serum transaminase. Reduces blood neutrophil, thrombocyte, and white blood cell (WBC) counts.

IV INCOMPATIBILITIES

Amphotericin (Fungizone), doxorubicin liposome (DaunoXome), methylprednisolone (Solu-Medrol), nalbuphine (Nubain)

IV COMPATIBILITIES

Bumetanide (Bumex), calcium gluconate, dexamethasone (Decadron), diphenhydramine (Benadryl), dobutamine (Dobutrex), dopamine (Inotropin), furosemide (Lasix), granisetron (Kytril), heparin, hydromorphone (Dilaudid), lorazepam (Ativan), magnesium sulfate, mannitol, morphine, ondansetron (Zofran), potassium chloride

SIDE EFFECTS
Frequent
Alopecia (80%), asthenia (loss of strength) (62%), hypersensitivity reaction (i.e., dermatitis) (59%) [Hypersensitivity reaction decreases to 16% in those treated with premedicated oral corticosteroids], fluid retention (49%), stomatitis (redness or burning of oral mucous membranes, gum or tongue inflammation) (43%), nausea, diarrhea (40%), fever (30%), nail changes (28%), vomiting (24%), myalgia (19%)
Occasional
Hypotension, edema, anorexia, headache, weight gain, infection (urinary tract, injection site, catheter tip), dizziness
Rare
Dry skin, sensory disorders (vision, speech, taste), arthralgia, myalgia, weight loss, conjunctivitis, hematuria, proteinuria

SERIOUS REACTIONS
• In those with normal liver function tests, neutropenia, less than 2,000 cells/mm^3, and leukopenia, less than 4,000 cells/mm^3, occurs in 96% of patients.
• Anemia, less than 11 g/dl, occurs in 90% of patients.
• Thrombocytopenia, less than 100,000 cells/mm^3, occurs in 8% of patients.
• Infection occurs in 28% of patients.
• Neurosensory and neuromotor effects such as distal paresthesias, occur in 54% and 13% of patients, respectively.

NURSING CONSIDERATIONS
Baseline Assessment
• Offer emotional support to the patient and family.
• Give antiemetics, if ordered, to prevent or treat nausea and vomiting.

• Pretreat the patient with corticosteroids, as ordered, before initiating docetaxel therapy to reduce the risks of fluid retention and hypersensitivity reaction.

Lifespan Considerations
• Be aware that docetaxel may cause fetal harm and it is unknown if docetaxel is distributed in breast milk. Patients receiving docetaxel should not breast-feed.
• Be aware that the safety and efficacy of docetaxel have not been established in children younger than 16 years of age.
• There are no age-related precautions noted in the elderly.

Precautions
• Use cautiously in patients with bone marrow depression, chemotherapy or radiation, chickenpox, herpes zoster, infection, impaired liver function, and preexisting pleural effusion.

Administration and Handling
◀ALERT▶ Dilute the drug before administration. If prescribed, premedicate the patient with oral corticosteroids, such as dexamethasone 16 mg/day for 5 days beginning day 1 before docetaxel therapy, to reduce the severity of fluid retention and hypersensitivity reaction.
IV
• Refrigerate vial and know that freezing does not adversely affect drug.
• Protect the drug from bright light.
• Stand vial at room temperature for 5 minutes before administering. Do not store the drug in PVC bags.
• Reconstituted solution is stable for up to 8 hours either at room temperature or refrigerated.
• Withdraw contents of diluent provided by manufacturer and add to vial of docetaxel.
• Gently rotate to ensure thorough mixing with a resulting solution of 10 mg/ml.
• Withdraw dose and add to 250 ml 0.9% NaCl or D_5W glass or polyolefin container to provide a final concentration of 0.3 to 0.9 mg/ml.
• Administer as a 1-hour infusion.
• Monitor the patient closely for signs and symptoms of a hypersensitivity reaction, including bronchospasm, flushing, and localized skin reaction that may occur within a few minutes after beginning the infusion.

Intervention and Evaluation
• Frequently monitor the patient's blood counts, particularly liver and renal function studies, neutrophil count, and serum uric acid levels. A neutrophil count of less than 1,500 cells/mm^3 requires discontinuation of docetaxel therapy.
• Observe the patient for cutaneous reactions characterized by rash with eruptions, mainly on the feet or hands.
• Assess the patient for extravascular fluid accumulation manifested as dependent edema, dyspnea at rest, pronounced abdominal distention from ascites, and rales in lungs.

Patient Teaching
• Explain to the patient that alopecia is reversible, but new hair growth may have a different color or texture. Tell the patient that new hair growth resumes 2 to 3 months after last docetaxel therapy dose.
• Teach the patient to maintain fastidious oral hygiene.
• Stress to the patient that he or she should not receive vaccinations and should avoid contact with anyone who recently received a live virus vaccine.

paclitaxel
pass-leh-**tax**-ell
(Anzatax[AUS], Onxol, Taxol)
Do not confuse with Paxil or Taxotere.

CATEGORY AND SCHEDULE
Pregnancy Risk Category: D

MECHANISM OF ACTION
An antimitotic agent in the taxoid family that promotes the assembly of microtubules and stabilizes them by preventing depolymerization. *Therapeutic Effect:* Inhibits mitotic cellular functions and cell replication. Blocks cells in late G_2 phase/M phase of cell cycle.

PHARMACOKINETICS
Does not readily cross blood-brain barrier. Protein binding: 89%–98%. Metabolized in liver (active metabolites); eliminated via bile. Not removed by hemodialysis. **Half-life:** 1.3–8.6 hrs.

AVAILABILITY
Injection: 30 mg/5 ml, 100 mg/17 ml, 150 mg/25 ml, 300 mg/50 ml.

INDICATIONS AND DOSAGES
▶ **Ovarian cancer**
IV infusion
Adults. 135–175 mg/m^2/dose over 1–24 hrs q3wks.
▶ **Breast carcinoma**
IV infusion
Adults, Elderly. 175 mg/m^2 over 3 hrs q3wks.
▶ **Non–small cell lung carcinoma**
IV infusion
Adults, Elderly. 135 mg/m^2 over 24 hrs, then cisplatin 75 mg/m^2 q3wks.
▶ **Kaposi's sarcoma**
IV infusion
Adults, Elderly. 135 mg/m^2/dose

over 3 hrs q3wks or 100 mg/m^2/dose over 3 hrs q2wks.
▶ **Dosage in liver impairment**

Total Bilirubin	Total Dose
1.5 mg/dl or less	less than 135 mg/m^2
1.6–3 mg/dl	less than 75 mg/m^2
more than 3 mg/dl	less than 50 mg/m^2

UNLABELED USES
Treatment of adenocarcinoma of upper gastrointestinal (GI) tract, head and neck cancer, hormone-refractory prostate cancer, non-Hodgkin's lymphoma, small cell lung cancer, transitional cell cancer of urothelium

CONTRAINDICATIONS
Baseline neutropenia less than 1,500 cells/mm^3, hypersensitivity to drugs developed with Cremophor EL (polyoxyethylated castor oil)

INTERACTIONS
Drug
Bone marrow depressants: May increase bone marrow depression. *Live virus vaccines:* May potentiate virus replication, increase vaccine side effects, and decrease the patient's antibody response to vaccine virus.
Herbal
None known.
Food
None known.

DIAGNOSTIC TEST EFFECTS
May elevate serum alkaline phosphatase, serum bilirubin, SGOT (AST), and SGPT (ALT) levels. Decreases blood Hgb and Hct levels, and platelet, red blood cell (RBC), and white blood cell (WBC) counts.

IV INCOMPATIBILITIES

Amphotericin B complex (Abelcet, AmBisome, Amphotec), chlorpromazine (Thorazine), doxorubicin liposome (Doxil), hydroxyzine (Vistaril), methylprednisolone (Solu-Medrol), mitoxantrone (Novantrone)

IV COMPATIBILITIES

Carboplatin (Paraplatin), cisplatin (Platinol AQ), cyclophosphamide (Cytoxan), cytarabine (Cytosar), dacarbazine (DTIC-Dome), dexamethasone (Decadron), diphenhydramine (Benadryl), doxorubicin (Adriamycin), etoposide (VePesid), gemcitabine (Gemzar), granisetron (Kytril), hydromorphone (Dilaudid), magnesium sulfate, mannitol, methotrexate, morphine, ondansetron (Zofran), potassium chloride, vinblastine (Velban), vincristine (Oncovin)

SIDE EFFECTS

Expected (90%–70%)
Diarrhea, alopecia, nausea, vomiting
Frequent (48%–46%)
Myalgia or arthralgia, peripheral neuropathy
Occasional (20%–13%)
Mucositis, hypotension during infusion, pain or redness at injection site
Rare (3%)
Bradycardia

SERIOUS REACTIONS

• Neutropenic nadir occurs at the median of 11 days.
• Anemia and leukopenia occur commonly.
• Thrombocytopenia occurs occasionally.
• Severe hypersensitivity reaction, including dyspnea, severe hypotension, angioedema, an generalized urticaria occurs rarely.

Baseline Assessment
• Offer emotional support to the patient and family.
• Use strict asepsis and protect the patient from infection.
• Assess the patient's blood counts, particularly neutrophil and platelet counts, before each course of paclitaxel therapy or as clinically indicated.

Lifespan Considerations
• Be aware that paclitaxel may produce fetal harm and it is unknown if paclitaxel is distributed in breast milk. Paclitaxel use should be avoided during pregnancy.
• Be aware that the safety and efficacy of paclitaxel have not been established in children.
• There are no age-related precautions noted in the elderly.

Precautions
• Use cautiously in patients with liver impairment, peripheral neuropathy, and severe neutropenia.

Administration and Handling
◀ALERT▶ Pretreat the patient with corticosteroids, diphenhydramine, and H_2 antagonists, as prescribed.
◀ALERT▶ Wear gloves during handling of the drug; if contact with skin occurs, wash hands thoroughly with soap and water. If drug comes in contact with mucous membranes, flush with water.

IV
• Refrigerate unopened vials.
• Reconstituted solution is stable at room temperature for up to 24 hours.
• Store diluted solutions in bottles or plastic bags and administer through polyethylene-lined administration sets. Avoid storing diluted solutions in plasticized PVC equipment or devices.
• Dilute with 0.9% NaCl, D_5W to

final concentration of 0.3 to 1.2 mg/ml.
• Administer at rate as ordered by physician through in-line filter not greater than 0.22 microns.
• Monitor the patient's vital signs during infusion, especially during the first hour.
• Discontinue paclitaxel administration and notify the physician if the patient experiences severe hypersensitivity reaction.

Intervention and Evaluation
• Monitor the patient's complete blood count (CBC), liver enzymes, platelets, and vital signs.
• Monitor the patient for signs and symptoms of anemia, including excessive fatigue and weakness, and hematologic toxicity, including easy bruising, fever, signs of local infection, sore throat, and unusual bleeding.
• Assess the patient's response to medication. Monitor the patient for and report diarrhea.
• Avoid giving the patient IM injections, rectal medications, and other traumas that may induce bleeding.
• Put pressure to the patient's injection sites for a full 5 minutes.

Patient Teaching
• Explain to the patient that alopecia is reversible, but new hair may have a different color or texture.
• Stress to the patient that he or she should not receive vaccinations and should avoid contact with crowds and those with known infection.
• Warn the patient to immediately notify the physician if he or she experiences signs of infection, including fever and flu-like symptoms.
• Caution the patient to notify the physician if nausea and vomiting continue at home.
• Teach the patient to recognize the

signs and symptoms of peripheral neuropathy.
• Warn the patient to avoid pregnancy during paclitaxel therapy. Teach the patient about various contraception methods.

vinblastine sulfate
vin-**blass**-teen
(Velbe[CAN])
Do not confuse with vincristine or vinorelbine.

CATEGORY AND SCHEDULE
Pregnancy Risk Category: D

MECHANISM OF ACTION
A vinca alkaloid and antineoplastic agent that binds to microtubular protein of mitotic spindle. *Therapeutic Effect:* Causes metaphase arrest. Inhibits cellular division.

PHARMACOKINETICS
Does not cross blood-brain barrier. Protein binding: 75%. Metabolized in liver to active metabolite. Primarily eliminated in feces via biliary system. **Half-life:** 24.8 hrs.

AVAILABILITY
Powder for Injection: 10 mg.
Injection: 1 mg/ml.

INDICATIONS AND DOSAGES
▸ **Induction of remission of advanced carcinoma of testis, advanced stage of mycosis fungoides, breast carcinoma, choriocarcinoma, disseminated Hodgkin's disease, Kaposi's sarcoma, Letterer-Siwe disease, non-Hodgkin's lymphoma**
IV
Adults, Elderly. Initially, 3.7 mg/m^2 as single dose. Increase dose at weekly intervals of about 1.8

mg/m^2 until desired therapeutic response is attained, white blood cell (WBC) count falls below 3,000/mm^3, or the maximum weekly dose of 18.5 mg/m^2 is reached.
Children. Initially, 2.5 mg/m^2 as single dose. Increase dose at weekly intervals of about 1.25 mg/m^2 until desired therapeutic response is attained, WBC count falls below 3,000/mm^3, or maximum weekly dose of 7.5–12.5 mg/m^2 is reached.

▶ **Maintenance dose for treatment of advanced carcinoma of testis, advanced stage of mycosis fungoides, breast carcinoma, choriocarcinoma, disseminated Hodgkin's disease, Kaposi's sarcoma, Letterer-Siwe disease, non-Hodgkin's lymphoma**
IV
Adults, Elderly, Children. Use one increment less than dose required to produce leukocyte count of 3,000/mm^3. Each subsequent dose given when leukocyte count returns to 4,000/mm^3 and at least 7 days has elapsed since previous dose.

UNLABELED USES
Treatment of carcinoma of bladder, head and neck, kidneys, lungs, chronic myelocytic leukemia, germ cell ovarian tumors, neuroblastoma

CONTRAINDICATIONS
Bacterial infection, severe leukopenia, significant granulocytopenia unless a result of disease being treated

INTERACTIONS
Drug
Antigout medications: May decrease the effects of these drugs.
Bone marrow depressants: May increase bone marrow depression.
Live virus vaccines: May potentiate virus replication, increase vaccine side effects, and decrease the patient's antibody response to vaccine.
Herbal
None known.
Food
None known.

DIAGNOSTIC TEST EFFECTS
May increase serum uric acid levels.

IV INCOMPATIBILITIES
Cefepime (Maxipime), furosemide (Lasix)

IV COMPATIBILITIES
Allopurinol (Aloprim), cisplatin (Platinol AQ), cyclophosphamide (Cytoxan), doxorubicin (Adriamycin), etoposide (VePesid), fluorouracil, gemcitabine (Gemzar), granisetron (Kytril), heparin, leucovorin, methotrexate, ondansetron (Zofran), paclitaxel (Taxol), vinorelbine (Navelbine)

SIDE EFFECTS
Frequent
Nausea, vomiting, alopecia
Occasional
Constipation or diarrhea, rectal bleeding, paresthesia, headache, malaise, weakness, dizziness, pain at tumor site, jaw or face pain, mental depression, dry mouth. Gastrointestinal (GI) distress, headache, paresthesia (occurs 4–6 hrs after administration, persists for 2–10 hrs)
Rare
Dermatitis, stomatitis, phototoxicity, hyperuricemia

SERIOUS REACTIONS
• Hematologic toxicity manifested most commonly as leukopenia, less frequently as anemia, may occur. The white blood cell (WBC) count falls to its lowest point 4 to 10 days

after initial therapy with recovery within another 7 to 14 days. High vinblastine dosages may require a 21-day recovery period.

• Thrombocytopenia is usually slight and transient, with rapid recovery within few days.

• Liver insufficiency may increase the risk of toxicity.

• Acute shortness of breath or bronchospasm may occur, particularly when vinblastine is administered concurrently with mitomycin.

NURSING CONSIDERATIONS

Baseline Assessment

• Give antiemetics, if ordered, to control nausea and vomiting. Be aware that usually these side effects are easily controlled by antiemetics.

• Expect to discontinue therapy if WBC and thrombocyte counts fall abruptly. However, be aware that the physician may continue the drug if it is clearly destroying tumor cells in bone marrow.

• Expect to obtain a complete blood count (CBC) weekly or before each vinblastine dosing.

Lifespan Considerations

• Know that vinblastine use should be avoided during pregnancy, if possible, and especially in the first trimester. Breast-feeding is not recommended in this patient population.

• There are no age-related precautions noted in children or the elderly.

Precautions

• Use cautiously in patients with liver function impairment, neurotoxicity, and recent exposure to radiation therapy or chemotherapy.

Administration and Handling

◀ALERT▶ Know that vinblastine dosage is individualized based on the patient's clinical response and tolerance of the drug's adverse effects. When used in combination

therapy, consult specific protocols for optimum dosage and sequence of drug administration. Reduce dosage if serum bilirubin is greater than 3 mg/dl. Repeat dosage at intervals of no less than 7 days and if the WBC count is at least 4,000/mm^3.

◀ALERT▶ Because vinblastine may be carcinogenic, mutagenic, or teratogenic, handle the drug with extreme care during preparation and administration. Give by IV injection. Leakage from IV site into surrounding tissue may produce extreme irritation. Avoid eye contact with solution as severe eye irritation and possible corneal ulceration may result. If eye contact occurs, immediately irrigate eye with water.

IV

• Refrigerate unopened vials.

• Solutions normally appears clear, colorless.

• Following reconstitution, solution is stable for up to 30 days if refrigerated.

• Discard if precipitate forms, discoloration occurs.

• Reconstitute 10-mg vial with 10 ml 0.9% NaCl preserved with phenol or benzyl alcohol to provide concentration of 1 mg/ml.

• Inject into tubing of running IV infusion or directly into vein over 1 minute.

• Do not inject into extremity with impaired or potentially impaired circulation caused by compression or invading neoplasm, phlebitis, or varicosity.

• After completing administration directly into a vein, withdraw a minute amount of venous blood before withdrawing the needle to minimize the possibility of extravasation.

• Be aware that extravasation may result in cellulitis and phlebitis and that a large amount of extravasation may result in tissue sloughing. If extravasation occurs, give local injection of hyaluronidase, if ordered, and apply warm compresses to the affected area.

Intervention and Evaluation

• Assess the patient diligently for signs and symptoms of infection if his or her WBC falls below 2,000/mm³.

• Assess the patient for signs and symptoms of stomatitis, including burning or erythema of oral mucosa at inner margin of lips, difficulty swallowing, oral ulceration, and sore throat.

• Monitor the patient for signs and symptoms of anemia, including excessive fatigue and weakness, and hematologic toxicity, including easy bruising, fever, signs of local infection, sore throat, and unusual bleeding from any site.

• Assess the patient's pattern of daily bowel activity and stool consistency. Practice measures to prevent the patient from becoming constipated.

Patient Teaching

• Warn the patient to immediately notify the physician if he or she experiences any pain or burning at injection site during administration.

• Advise the patient that pain at the tumor site may occur during or shortly after vinblastine injection.

• Stress to the patient that he or she should not receive vaccinations and should avoid contact with crowds and those with known infection.

• Caution the patient to promptly notify the physician if he or she experiences easy bruising, fever, signs of local infection, sore throat, or unusual bleeding from any site.

• Explain to the patient that alopecia is reversible, but new hair growth may have a different color or texture.

• Instruct the patient to notify the physician if nausea and vomiting continue at home.

• Urge the patient increase his or her fluid intake and bulk in diet, as well as exercise as tolerated, to avoid constipation.

vincristine sulfate
vin-**cris**-teen
(Vincasar PFS)
Do not confuse with Ancobon or vinblastine.

CATEGORY AND SCHEDULE
Pregnancy Risk Category: D

MECHANISM OF ACTION
A vinca alkaloid and antineoplastic agent that binds to microtubular protein of mitotic spindle. *Therapeutic Effect:* Causes metaphase arrest. Inhibits cellular division.

PHARMACOKINETICS
Does not cross blood-brain barrier. Protein binding: 75%. Metabolized in liver. Primarily eliminated in feces via biliary system. **Half-life:** 10–37 hrs.

AVAILABILITY
Injection: 1 mg/ml.

INDICATIONS AND DOSAGES
▶ **Treatment of acute leukemia, advanced non-Hodgkin's lymphomas, disseminated Hodgkin's disease, neuroblastoma, rhabdomyosarcoma, Wilms' tumor (administer at weekly intervals)**
IV
Adults, Elderly. 0.4–1.4 mg/m². Maximum: 2 mg.

Children. 1–2 mg/m^2.
Children weighing less than 10 kg or with a body surface area less than 1 m^2. 0.05 mg/kg.
▶ **Liver function impairment**
Reduce dosage by 50% in those patients with a direct serum bilirubin concentration less than 3 mg/dl.

UNLABELED USES
Treatment of breast, cervical, colorectal, lung, and ovarian carcinoma, chronic lymphocytic, germ cell ovarian tumors, idiopathic thrombocytopenia purpura, malignant melanoma, multiple myeloma, mycosis fungoides, myelocytic leukemia

CONTRAINDICATIONS
Patients receiving radiation therapy through ports that include the liver

INTERACTIONS
Drug
Asparaginase, neurotoxic medications: May increase the risk of neurotoxicity.
Antigout medications: May decrease the effects of these drugs.
Doxorubicin: May increase myelosuppression.
Live virus vaccines: May potentiate virus replication, increase vaccine side effects, and decrease the patient's antibody response to vaccine.
Herbal
None known.
Food
None known.

DIAGNOSTIC TEST EFFECTS
May increase serum uric acid levels.

IV INCOMPATIBILITIES
Cefepime (Maxipime), furosemide (Lasix), idarubicin (Idamycin)

IV COMPATIBILITIES
Allopurinol (Aloprim), cisplatin (Platinol AQ), cyclophosphamide (Cytoxan), cytarabine (Ara-C, Cytosar), doxorubicin (Adriamycin), etoposide (VePesid), fluorouracil, gemcitabine (Gemzar), granisetron (Kytril), leucovorin, methotrexate, ondansetron (Zofran), paclitaxel (Taxol), vinorelbine (Navelbine)

SIDE EFFECTS
Expected
Peripheral neuropathy occurs in nearly every patient. Its first clinical sign is depression of Achilles tendon reflex.
Frequent
Peripheral paresthesia, alopecia, constipation or obstipation (upper colon impaction with empty rectum), abdominal cramps, headache, jaw pain, hoarseness, double vision, ptosis or drooping of eyelid, urinary tract disturbances
Occasional
Nausea, vomiting, diarrhea, abdominal distention, stomatitis, fever
Rare
Mild leukopenia, mild anemia, thrombocytopenia

SERIOUS REACTIONS
• Acute shortness of breath and bronchospasm may occur, especially when vincristine is used in combination with mitomycin.
• Prolonged or high-dose therapy may produce foot or wrist drop, difficulty walking, slapping gait, ataxia, and muscle wasting.
• Acute uric acid nephropathy may be noted.

NURSING CONSIDERATIONS

Baseline Assessment
• Monitor the patient's hematologic

status, liver and renal function tests, and serum uric acid levels.
• Assess the patient's Achilles tendon reflex for evidence of peripheral neuropathy.
• Assess the patient's pattern of daily bowel activity and stool consistency.
• Monitor the patient for development of blurred vision or ptosis.
• Evaluate the patient's urine output for changes.

Lifespan Considerations
• Be aware that vincristine use should be avoided during pregnancy, especially in the first trimester because it may cause fetal harm. Breast-feeding is not recommended in this patient population.
• There are no age-related precautions noted in children.
• The elderly are more susceptible to the drug's neurotoxic effects.

Precautions
• Use cautiously in patients with liver function impairment, neurotoxicity, and preexisting neuromuscular disease.

Administration and Handling
◄ALERT► Know that vincristine dosage is individualized based on the patient's clinical response and tolerance of the drug's adverse effects. When used in combination therapy, consult specific protocols for optimum dosage and sequence of drug administration.
◄ALERT► Because vincristine may be carcinogenic, mutagenic, or teratogenic, handle the drug with extreme care during preparation and administration. Give by IV injection. Use extreme caution in calculating and administering vincristine and know that overdose may result in serious or fatal outcomes.
IV
• Refrigerate unopened vials.

• Solutions normally appears clear, colorless.
• Discard if precipitate forms or discoloration occurs.
• May give undiluted.
• Inject dose into tubing of running IV infusion or directly into vein over more than 1 minute.
• Do not inject vincristine into an extremity with impaired or potentially impaired circulation caused by compression or invading neoplasm, phlebitis, varicosity.
• Be aware that extravasation produces burning, edema, and stinging at the injection site. If this occurs, terminate injection immediately, notify the physician, locally inject hyaluronidase, if ordered, and apply heat to the affected area to disperse vincristine and minimizes cellulitis and discomfort.

Patient Teaching
• Warn the patient to immediately notify the physician of any pain or burning at the injection site during administration.
• Explain to the patient that alopecia is reversible, but new hair growth may have a different color and texture.
• Caution the patient to notify the physician if nausea and vomiting continue at home.
• Teach the patient to recognize the signs of peripheral neuropathy.
• Warn the patient to notify the physician if he or she experiences easy bruising, fever, signs of infection, sore throat, shortness of breath, or unusual bleeding for any site.

vinorelbine

vin-oh-**rell**-bean
(Navelbine)
**Do not confuse with
vinblastine.**

CATEGORY AND SCHEDULE
Pregnancy Risk Category: D

MECHANISM OF ACTION
An antineoplastic that interferes
with mitotic microtubule assembly.
Therapeutic Effect: Prevents cellular
division.

PHARMACOKINETICS
After IV administration, widely
distributed. Protein binding:
80%–90%. Metabolized in liver.
Primarily eliminated via biliary or
fecal route. **Half-life:** 28–43 hrs.

AVAILABILITY
Injection: 10 mg/ml (1-ml, 5-ml
vials).

INDICATIONS AND DOSAGES
▸ **Single agent or in combination
with cisplatin for treatment of
unresectable, advanced, non–small
cell lung cancer (NSCLC)**
IV injection
Adults, Elderly. 30 mg/m^2, given
over 6–10 min, administered
weekly.
Dosage adjustments should be based
on granulocyte count obtained on
day of treatment, as follows:

Granulocytes (cells/mm^3) on Day of Treatment	Dose (mg/m^2)
1,500 or higher	30
1,000–1,499	15
less than 1,000	Do not administer

UNLABELED USES
Treatment of breast cancer,
cisplatin-resistant ovarian carcinoma, Hodgkin's disease

CONTRAINDICATIONS
Pretreatment granulocyte count less
than 1,000 cells/mm^3

INTERACTIONS
Drug
Bone marrow depressants: May
increase the risk of bone marrow
depression.
Cisplatin: Significantly increases the
risk of granulocytopenia.
Live virus vaccines: May potentiate
virus replication, increase vaccine
side effects, and decrease the patient's antibody response to vaccine.
Mitomycin: May produce acute
pulmonary reaction.
Herbal
None known.
Food
None known.

DIAGNOSTIC TEST EFFECTS
May increase total serum bilirubin
and SGOT (AST) levels, and liver
function test results. Decreases
granulocyte, leukocyte, thrombocyte
counts, and red blood cells (RBCs)
levels.

IV INCOMPATIBILITIES
Acyclovir (Zovirax), allopurinol
(Aloprim), amphotericin B (Fungizone), amphotericin B complex
(Abelcet, AmBisome, Amphotec),
ampicillin (Omnipen), cefazolin
(Ancef), cefoperazone (Cefobid),
cefotetan (Cefotan), ceftriaxone
(Rocephin), cefuroxime (Zinacef),
fluorouracil, furosemide (Lasix),
ganciclovir (Cytovene), methylprednisolone (Solu-Medrol), sodium
bicarbonate

IV COMPATIBILITIES

Calcium gluconate, carboplatin (Paraplatin), cisplatin (Platinol AQ), cyclophosphamide (Cytoxan), cytarabine (ARA-C, Cytosar), dacarbazine (DTIC-Dome), daunorubicin (Cerubidine), dexamethasone (Decadron), diphenhydramine (Benadryl), doxorubicin (Adriamycin), etoposide (VePesid), gemcitabine (Gemzar), granisetron (Kytril), hydromorphone (Dilaudid), idarubicin (Idamycin), methotrexate, morphine, ondansetron (Zofran), teniposide (Vumon), vinblastine (Velban), vincristine (Oncovin)

SIDE EFFECTS

Frequent
Asthenia (35%), mild or moderate nausea (34%), constipation (29%), injection site reaction manifested as erythema, pain, vein discoloration (28%), fatigue (27%), peripheral neuropathy manifested as paresthesia and hyperesthesia (25%), diarrhea (17%), alopecia (12%)
Occasional
Phlebitis (10%), dyspnea (7%), loss of deep tendon reflexes (5%)
Rare
Chest pain, jaw pain, myalgia, arthralgia, rash

SERIOUS REACTIONS

• Bone marrow depression is manifested mainly as granulocytopenia which may be severe. Other hematologic toxicity, including neutropenia, thrombocytopenia, leukopenia, and anemia increases the risk of infection and bleeding.
• Acute shortness of breath and severe bronchospasm occur infrequently, particularly manifesting in patients with preexisting pulmonary dysfunction.

NURSING CONSIDERATIONS

Baseline Assessment

• Review the patient's medication history.
• Assess the patient's hematology values, including blood Hgb and platelet count before giving each vinorelbine dose.
• Know that granulocyte count should be 1,000 cells/mm^3 or more before vinorelbine administration and that granulocyte nadirs occur 7–10 days after dosing.
• Be aware that hematologic growth factors should not be given within 24 hours before administration of chemotherapy or no earlier than 24 hours after cytotoxic chemotherapy.
• Advise females with childbearing potential to avoid pregnancy during drug therapy.

Lifespan Considerations

• Know that vinorelbine use should be avoided during pregnancy, if possible, and especially during the first trimester because vinorelbine may cause fetal harm. Breast-feeding is not recommended in this patient population.
• Be aware that it is unknown if vinorelbine is excreted in breast milk.
• The safety and efficacy of vinorelbine have not been established in children.
• There are no age-related precautions noted in the elderly.

Precautions

• Use extremely cautiously in patients who are immunocompromised.
• Use cautiously in patients with existing or recent chickenpox, herpes zoster, impaired pulmonary function, infection, leukopenia, and severe liver injury or impairment.

Administration and Handling

◀ALERT▶ Know that the patient's granulocyte count should be 1,000 cells/mm³ or more before vinorelbine administration.

◀ALERT▶ It is extremely important to correctly position the IV needle or catheter before vinorelbine administration because leakage into surrounding tissue produces extreme irritation, local tissue necrosis, or thrombophlebitis. Wear gloves when preparing the solution. If solution comes in contact with skin or mucosa, wash immediately and thoroughly with soap, water.

• Refrigerate unopened vials.

• Protect from light.

• Unopened vials are stable at room temperature for up to 72 hours.

• Do not administer if particulate matter is noted.

• Diluted vinorelbine may be used for up to 24 hours under normal room light when stored in polypropylene syringes or polyvinyl chloride bags at room temperature.

• Know that vinorelbine must be diluted and administered via a syringe or IV bag.

• Dilute calculated vinorelbine dose with D_5W or 0.9% NaCl to a concentration of 1.5 to 3 mg/ml for syringe administration.

• Dilute calculated vinorelbine dose with D_5W, 0.45% or 0.9% NaCl, Ringer's or lactated Ringer's to a concentration of 0.5 to 2 mg/ml for IV bag administration.

• Administer diluted vinorelbine over 6 to 10 minutes into the side port of free-flowing IV closest to IV bag followed by flushing with 75 to 125 ml of one of the solutions.

• If extravasation occurs, stop injection immediately; give remaining portion of the dose into another vein.

Intervention and Evaluation

• Diligently monitor the patient's injection site for pain, redness, and swelling.

• Frequently monitor the patient for signs and symptoms of myelosuppression both during and after vinorelbine therapy.

• Assess the patient for signs and symptoms of anemia, including excessive fatigue and weakness, and hematologic toxicity, including easy bruising, fever, signs of local infection, sore throat, and unusual bleeding from any site.

• Monitor patients developing severe granulocytopenia for evidence of infection or fever.

• Give the patient crackers, dry toast, and sips of cola to help relieve nausea.

• Assess the patient's pattern of daily bowel activity and stool consistency.

• Check the patient's injection site for reaction.

• Determine if the patient experiences burning, numbness, or tingling of the feet and hands, which are symptoms of peripheral neuropathy, or complains of feeling like "walking on glass" which is a symptom of hyperesthesia.

Patient Teaching

• Warn the patient immediately report pain, redness, or swelling occur at the injection site.

• Stress to the patient that he or she should not receive vaccinations and should avoid contact with crowds and those with known infection.

• Warn the patient to notify the physician if he or she experiences difficulty breathing, easy bruising, fever, signs of local infection, sore throat, or unusual bleeding from any site.

• Caution the patient to avoid pregnancy during vinorelbine therapy.
• Explain to the patient that alopecia is reversible, but new hair growth may have a different color or texture.

17 Cytoprotective Agents

**amifostine
dexrazoxane
mesna**

Uses: During antineoplastic therapy, specific cytoprotective agents are used to help prevent or reduce the severity of specific adverse reactions. For example, *amifostine* may be used to reduce nephrotoxicity caused by cisplatin and other alkylating agents and to minimize xerostomia caused by radiation therapy. *Dexrazoxane* reduces the risk of cardiomyopathy related to doxorubicin therapy. *Mesna* protects against hemorrhagic cystitis, which may result from cyclophosphamide or ifosfamide.

Action: Each cytoprotective agent works by a different action. *Amifostine* is converted to an active metabolite that binds with and detoxifies the reactive metabolites of cisplatin and other alkylating agents. In myocardial cell membranes, *dexrazoxane* binds with intracellular iron, preventing the generation of free radicals by the anthracycline doxorubicin. *Mesna* binds with and detoxifies the urotoxic metabolites of cyclophosphamide and ifosfamide.

amifostine
am-ih-**fos**-teen
(Ethyol)
Do not confuse with ethanol.

CATEGORY AND SCHEDULE
Pregnancy Risk Category: C

MECHANISM OF ACTION
An antineoplastic adjunct and cytoprotective agent that is converted to an active metabolite by alkaline phosphatase in tissues. The active metabolite binds to and detoxifies metabolites of cisplatin. These actions occur more readily in normal tissues than in tumor tissue. *Therapeutic Effect:* Reduces the toxic effect of the chemotherapeutic agent cisplatin.

AVAILABILITY
Powder for Injection: 500 mg in a 10-ml single-use vial.

INDICATIONS AND DOSAGES
▸ **Cytoprotective (chemotherapy)**
IV infusion
Adults. 910 mg/m^2 once a day as 15-min infusion, beginning 30 min before chemotherapy. A 15-min infusion is better tolerated than extended infusions. If the full dose can't be administered, dose for subsequent cycles should be 740 mg/m^2.
▸ **Treatment of dry mouth**
IV infusion
Adults. 200 mg/m^2 once a day as 3-min infusion, starting 15–30 min before radiation therapy.

UNLABELED USES
Protects lung fibroblasts from damaging effects of chemotherapeutic agent paclitaxel

CONTRAINDICATIONS
Sensitivity to aminothiol compounds or mannitol

INTERACTIONS
Drug
Antihypertensive medications or drugs that may potentiate hypotension: May increase risk of hypotension.
Herbal
None known.
Food
None known.

DIAGNOSTIC TEST EFFECTS
May reduce serum calcium levels, especially in those patients with nephrotic syndrome.

IV INCOMPATIBILITIES
Do not mix in solution other than 0.9% NaCl

IV COMPATIBILITIES
Mannitol, potassium chloride

SIDE EFFECTS
Frequent (62%)
Transient reduction in blood pressure (B/P) with onset 14 min into infusion and lasts about 6 min. B/P generally returns to normal in 5–15 min; severe nausea, vomiting
Occasional (20%–10%)
Flushing or feeling of warmth or chills or feeling of coldness; dizziness, hiccups, sneezing, somnolence
Rare (less than 1%)
Clinically relevant hypocalcemia, mild skin rash

SERIOUS REACTIONS
• A pronounced drop in B/P may require temporary cessation of amifostine.

NURSING CONSIDERATIONS
Baseline Assessment
• Be sure the patient is adequately hydrated before beginning infusion.
• Keep the patient in the supine position during the infusion.
• Expect to monitor B/P every 5 minutes during IV infusion.
• Stop the IV infusion if systolic B/P decreases significantly from baseline. Significant decreases are for a baseline of less than 100, B/P drop by 20 mm Hg; for a baseline of 100 to 119, a drop by 25 mm Hg; for a baseline of 120 to 139, a drop by 30 mm Hg; for a baseline of 140 to 179, a drop by 40 mm Hg; for a baseline of greater than 180, a drop by 50 mm Hg. If systolic B/P returns to normal within 5 minutes and the patient appears asymptomatic, begin infusion again so that full dose can be administered.
Precautions
• Use cautiously in patients with preexisting cardiovascular or cerebrovascular conditions such as arrhythmias, congestive heart failure (CHF), history of cerebrovascular accident (CVA) or transischemic attack (TIA), and ischemic heart disease.
• Use cautiously in patients with uncorrected dehydration or hypotension.
• Use cautiously in patients receiving antihypertensive therapy that cannot be discontinued 24 hours before amifostine treatment begins.
• Use cautiously in patients receiving chemotherapy for malignancies that are potentially curable.

Administration and Handling
IV
• Do not use the solution if it is discolored or contains particulate matter.
• Reconstitute with 9.7 ml 0.9% NaCl. Reconstituted solution stays stable for 5 hours at room temperature, 24 hours under refrigeration.
• Further dilute with 0.9% NaCl for a concentration of 5 to 40 mg/ml.
• Administer over 15 minutes about 30 minutes before chemotherapy.
◀ALERT▶ If hypotension requires interruption of therapy, place the patient in the Trendelenburg position and give an infusion of normal saline using a separate IV line.
• An antiemetic, dexamethasone 20 mg IV and serotonin 5-HT$_3$, a receptor antagonist, should be given before and concurrently with amifostine.

Intervention and Evaluation
• Expect to carefully monitor the patient's fluid balance to ensure adequate hydration.
• Monitor serum calcium levels in those patients at risk of hypocalcemia or nephrotic syndrome.
• Monitor B/P every 5 minutes during infusion.

Patient Teaching
• Advise patient to immediately report chills, nausea, skin rash, vomiting, or other side effects.
• Explain that he or she must remain in a lying position during the infusion and that the B/P will be monitored frequently.

dexrazoxane
dex-rah-**zox**-ann
(Zinecard)

CATEGORY AND SCHEDULE
Pregnancy Risk Category: C

MECHANISM OF ACTION
A cytoprotective agent antineoplastic adjunct that rapidly penetrates myocardial cell membrane. Binds intracellular iron and prevents generation of oxygen free radicals by anthracyclines, which may be responsible for anthracycline-induced cardiomyopathy. *Therapeutic Effect:* Protects against anthracycline-induced cardiomyopathy.

PHARMACOKINETICS
Rapidly distributed after IV administration. Not bound to plasma proteins. Primarily excreted in urine. Removed by peritoneal dialysis. Elimination **half-life:** 2.1–2.5 hrs.

AVAILABILITY
Powder for Injection: 250 mg (10 mg/ml reconstituted in 25 ml single-use vial), 500 mg (10 mg/ml reconstituted in 50-ml single-use vial).

INDICATIONS AND DOSAGES
▶ **Reduction of incidence and severity of cardiomyopathy associated with doxorubicin therapy in women with metastatic breast cancer; cardioprotective**
IV
Adults, Children. Recommended dosage ratio of dexrazoxane to doxorubicin is 10:1 (e.g., 500 mg/m^2 dexrazoxane, 50 mg/m^2 doxorubicin).

CONTRAINDICATIONS
Chemotherapy regimens that do not contain an anthracycline

INTERACTIONS
Drug
Concurrent FAC therapy (cyclophosphamide, adriamycin,

fluorouracil): May produce severe blood dyscrasias.

Herbal

None known.

Food

None known.

DIAGNOSTIC TEST EFFECTS

Concurrent FAC (cyclophosphamide, adriamycin, fluorouracil) therapy may produce abnormal liver or renal function test results.

IV INCOMPATIBILITIES

Do not mix with other medications.

SIDE EFFECTS

Frequent

Alopecia, nausea, vomiting, fatigue, malaise, anorexia, stomatitis, fever, infection, diarrhea

Occasional

Pain with injection, neurotoxicity, phlebitis, dysphagia, streaking or erythema

Rare

Urticaria, skin reaction

SERIOUS REACTIONS

• FAC therapy with dexrazoxane may produce more severe leukopenia, granulocytopenia, and thrombocytopenia than those receiving FAC without dexrazoxane.

• Dexrazoxane overdosage can be removed with peritoneal or hemodialysis.

NURSING CONSIDERATIONS

Baseline Assessment

• Give antiemetics, if ordered, to prevent and treat nausea.

Lifespan Considerations

• Be aware that dexrazoxane may be embryotoxic or teratogenic and it is unknown if dexrazoxane is distributed in breast milk. Breast-

feeding is not recommended in this patient population.

• The safety and efficacy of dexrazoxane have not been established in children.

• There is no information available on dexrazoxane use in the elderly.

Precautions

• Use cautiously in patients taking chemotherapeutic agents that increase the risk of myelosuppression or those also receiving FAC therapy (cyclophosphamide, adriamycin, fluorouracil).

Administration and Handling

◀**ALERT**▶ Be aware that dexrazoxane should be used only in those patients who have received a cumulative doxorubicin dose of 300 mg/m^2 and are continuing with doxorubicin therapy.

◀**ALERT**▶ Do not mix dexrazoxane with other drugs. Use caution and wear gloves during the handling and preparation of reconstituted solution. If powder or solution comes in contact with skin, wash immediately with soap and water.

IV

• Store vials at room temperature.

• Reconstituted solution is stable for up to 6 hours at room temperature or if refrigerated. Discard unused solution.

• Reconstitute with 0.167 molar (M/6) sodium lactate injection to give concentration of 10 mg dexrazoxane for each ml of sodium lactate.

• May further dilute with 0.9% NaCl or D$_5$W. Concentration should range from 1.3 to 5 mg/ml.

• Give reconstituted solution by slow IV push or IV infusion over 15 to 30 minutes.

• After infusion is completed, and before a total elapsed time of 30 minutes from beginning of dexrazoxane infusion, give IV injection of doxorubicin.

Intervention and Evaluation
• Frequently monitor the patient's blood counts for evidence of blood dyscrasias.
• Monitor the patient for signs and symptoms of stomatitis, including burning or erythema of oral mucosa at inner margin of lips, difficulty swallowing, and sore throat.
• Monitor the patient's cardiac function, hematologic status, and liver and renal function studies.
• Assess the patient's pattern of daily bowel activity and stool consistency.
• Monitor the patient for signs and symptoms of hematologic toxicity, including easy bruising, fever, signs of local infection, sore throat, and unusual bleeding from any site.

Patient Teaching
• Explain to the patient that alopecia is reversible, but new hair growth may have a different color or texture. Tell the patient that new hair growth resumes 2 to 3 months after last dexrazoxane therapy dose.
• Teach the patient to maintain fastidious oral hygiene.
• Warn the patient to notify the physician if he or she experiences fever, signs of local infection, or sore throat.
• Caution the patient to notify the physician if nausea and vomiting persist at home.

mesna
mess-nah
(Mesnex, Uromitexan[CAN])

CATEGORY AND SCHEDULE
Pregnancy Risk Category: B

MECHANISM OF ACTION
A cytoprotective agent and antineoplastic adjunct that binds with and detoxifies urotoxic metabolites of ifosfamide and cyclophosphamide. *Therapeutic Effect:* Inhibits ifosfamide-and cyclophosphamide-induced hemorrhagic cystitis.

PHARMACOKINETICS
Rapidly metabolized after IV administration to mesna disulfide, which is reduced to mesna in kidney. Excreted in urine. **Half-life:** 24 min.

AVAILABILITY
Injection: 100 mg/ml.
Tablets: 400 mg.

INDICATIONS AND DOSAGES
▶ **To prevent hemorrhagic cystitis in patients receiving ifosfamide**
IV
Adults, Elderly. 20% of ifosfamide dose at time of ifosfamide administration and 4 and 8 hrs after each dose of ifosfamide. Total dose: 60% of ifosfamide dosage.
▶ **To prevent hemorrhagic cystitis in patients receiving cyclophosphamide**
IV
Adults, Elderly. 20% of cyclophosphamide dose at time of cyclophosphamide administration and q3h for 3–4 doses.
PO
Adults, Elderly. 40% of antineoplastic agent dose in 3 doses at 4-hr intervals.

CONTRAINDICATIONS
None known.

INTERACTIONS
Drug
None known.

Herbal
None known.
Food
None known.

DIAGNOSTIC TEST EFFECTS

May produce false-positive test for urinary ketones.

IV INCOMPATIBILITIES

Amphotericin B complex (Abelcet, AmBisome, Amphotec)

IV COMPATIBILITIES

Allopurinol (Aloprim), docetaxel (Taxotere), doxorubicin (Adriamycin), etoposide (VP-16, VePesid), gemcitabine (Gemzar), granisetron (Kytril), methotrexate, ondansetron (Zofran), paclitaxel (Taxol), vinorelbine (Navelbine)

SIDE EFFECTS

Frequent (more than 17%)
Bad taste in mouth, soft stools
Large doses: Diarrhea, limb pain, headache, fatigue, nausea, hypotension, allergic reaction

SERIOUS REACTIONS

• Hematuria occurs rarely.

NURSING CONSIDERATIONS

Baseline Assessment
• Administer each mesna dose with ifosfamide, as prescribed.
Lifespan Considerations
• Be aware that it is unknown if mesna crosses placenta or is distributed in breast milk.
• Be aware that the safety and efficacy of mesna have not been established in children.

• There is no information available on mesna use in the elderly.
Administration and Handling
PO
• Dilute mesna solution before oral administration to decrease sulfur odor. If desired, dilute in carbonated cola drinks, fruit juices, or milk.
IV
• Store parenteral form at room temperature.
• After reconstitution, the solution is stable up to 24 hours at room temperature. Recommended use is within 6 hours. Discard unused medication.
• Dilute with D_5W or 0.9% NaCl to concentration of 1 to 20 mg/ml, as appropriate.
• Add to solutions containing ifosfamide or cyclophosphamide, as appropriate.
• Administer by IV infusion (piggyback) over 15 to 30 minutes or by continuous infusion.
Intervention and Evaluation
• Test the patient's morning urine specimen for hematuria. If hematuria occurs, mesna dosage reduction or discontinuation may be necessary.
• Assess the patient's pattern of daily bowel activity and stool consistency. Record time of evacuation.
• Monitor the patient's blood pressure (B/P) for hypotension.
Patient Teaching
• Warn the patient to notify the physician or nurse if he or she experiences headache, limb pain, or nausea.

18 Hormones

ANTINEOPLASTIC AGENTS

anastrozole
bicalutamide
exemestane
flutamide
fulvestrant
goserelin acetate
letrozole
leuprolide acetate
megestrol acetate
nilutamide
tamoxifen citrate
toremifene citrate
triptorelin pamoate

Uses: In antineoplastic therapy, hormones are used to treat cancers that are hormone dependent, including cancer of the breasts, endometrium, and prostate. Antineoplastic hormones are less toxic than other antineoplastic agents.

Action: Antineoplastic hormones may act as agonists that inhibit tumor cell growth or as antagonists that compete with endogenous hormones. These agents include *antiandrogens,* such as bicalutamide and flutamide; *antiestrogens,* such as fulvestrant and tamoxifen; *aromatase inhibitors,* such as anastrozole and letrozole; *progestins,* such as megestrol; and *gonadotropin-releasing hormone analogues,* such as goserelin and leuprolide.

Specifically, antiandrogens act primarily by inhibiting androgen uptake or binding to androgen receptors in target tissue. Antiestrogens compete with endogenous estrogen and estrogen-receptor binding sites. Aromatase inhibitors interfere with aromatase, the enzyme that catalyzes the final step in estrogen production; this, in turn, decreases circulating estrogen. Progestins suppress the release of luteinizing hormone (LH) from the anterior pituitary gland. Gonadotropin-releasing hormone analogues stimulate the release of LH and follicle-stimulating hormone from the anterior pituitary gland.

---

anastrozole
ah-**nas**-trow-zole
(Arimidex)
Do not confuse with Imitrex.

CATEGORY AND SCHEDULE
Pregnancy Risk Category: D

MECHANISM OF ACTION
Decreases circulating estrogen by inhibiting aromatase, an enzyme that catalyzes the final step in estrogen production. *Therapeutic Effect:* Because growth of many breast cancers are stimulated by estrogens, drug significantly lowers serum estradiol (estrogen) concentration.

PHARMACOKINETICS
Well absorbed into systemic circulation. Protein binding: 40%. Food does not affect extent of absorption. Extensively metabolized. Eliminated

by liver metabolism and, to a lesser extent, renal excretion. **Mean half-life:** 50 hrs in postmenopausal women. Plasma concentrations reach steady-state levels at about 7 days.

AVAILABILITY
Tablets: 1 mg.

INDICATIONS AND DOSAGES
▸ **Breast cancer**
PO
Adults, Elderly. 1 mg once a day.

CONTRAINDICATIONS
None known

INTERACTIONS
Drug
None known.
Herbal
None known.
Food
None known.

DIAGNOSTIC TEST EFFECTS
May elevate serum GGT level in those with liver metastases. May increase LDL cholesterol, serum alkaline phosphate, SGOT (AST), SGPT (ALT), and total cholesterol levels.

SIDE EFFECTS
Frequent (16%–8%)
Asthenia (loss of strength and energy), nausea, headache, hot flashes, back pain, vomiting, cough, diarrhea
Occasional (6%–4%)
Constipation, abdominal pain, anorexia, bone pain, pharyngitis, dizziness, rash, dry mouth, peripheral edema, pelvic pain, depression, chest pain, paresthesia
Rare (2%–1%)
Weight gain, increased sweating

SERIOUS REACTIONS
• Thrombophlebitis, anemia, and leukopenia occur rarely.
• Vaginal hemorrhage occurs rarely (2%).

NURSING CONSIDERATIONS
Lifespan Considerations
• Be aware that anastrozole crosses the placenta and may cause fetal harm.
• Be aware that it is unknown if anastrozole is excreted in breast milk.
• The safety and efficacy of anastrozole have not been established in children.
• There are no age-related precautions noted in the elderly.
Administration and Handling
PO
• May give without regard to food.
Intervention and Evaluation
• Monitor the patient for asthenia or dizziness. If present, do not let the patient ambulate without assistance.
• Determine if the patient is experiencing diarrhea, headache, nausea, or vomiting. If the patient has diarrhea, give an antidiarrheal medication, as prescribed. If the patient is nauseous or vomiting, give the patient an antiemetic medication, as prescribed.
Patient Teaching
• Warn the patient to notify the physician if asthenia, hot flashes, and nausea become unmanageable.

bicalutamide
by-kale-**yew**-tah-myd
(Casodex, Cosudex[AUS])

CATEGORY AND SCHEDULE
Pregnancy Risk Category: X

MECHANISM OF ACTION
An antiandrogen hormone and antineoplastic agent that competitively inhibits androgen action by binding to androgen receptors in target tissue. *Therapeutic Effect:* Decreases growth of prostatic carcinoma.

PHARMACOKINETICS
Well absorbed from the gastrointestinal (GI) tract. Protein binding: 96%. Metabolized in liver to inactive metabolite. Excreted in urine, feces. Not removed by hemodialysis. **Half-life:** 5.8 days.

AVAILABILITY
Tablets: 50 mg.

INDICATIONS AND DOSAGES
▸ **Prostatic carcinoma**
PO
Adults, Elderly. 50 mg once a day, morning or evening. Use concurrently with a luteinizing hormone-releasing hormone (LHRH) analogue or after surgical castration.

CONTRAINDICATIONS
None known.

INTERACTIONS
Drug
Warfarin: May displace this drug from protein-binding sites and increase its effects.
Herbal
None known.
Food
None known.

DIAGNOSTIC TEST EFFECTS
May increase BUN, serum alkaline phosphatase, serum bilirubin, SGOT (AST), and SGPT (ALT) levels. May increase blood Hgb levels and white blood cell (WBC) count.

SIDE EFFECTS
Frequent
Hot flashes (49%), breast pain (38%), muscle pain (27%), constipation (17%), diarrhea (10%), asthenia (15%), nausea (11%)
Occasional (9%–8%)
Nocturia, abdominal pain, peripheral edema
Rare (7%–3%)
Vomiting, weight loss, dizziness, insomnia, rash, impotence, gynecomastia

SERIOUS REACTIONS
• Sepsis, congestive heart failure (CHF), hypertension, and iron deficiency anemia may be noted.

NURSING CONSIDERATIONS
Lifespan Considerations
• Be aware that bicalutamide may inhibit spermatogenesis and is not used in women.
• Be aware that the safety and efficacy of bicalutamide have not been established in children.
• There are no age-related precautions noted in the elderly.
Precautions
• Use cautiously in patients with moderate to severe liver impairment.
Administration and Handling
PO
• May be given without regard to food.
• Take at same time each day.
Intervention and Evaluation
• Assess the patient for diarrhea, nausea, and vomiting.
Patient Teaching
• Caution the patient against abruptly discontinuing the drug. Explain that both bicalutamide and the LHRH analogue must be continued to achieve desired therapeutic effect.

• Instruct the patient to take the bicalutamide at the same time each day.
• Advise the patient of the possible and frequent side effects.
• Warn the patient to notify the physician if he or she experiences persistent nausea and vomiting.

exemestane
x-eh-**mess**-tane
(Aromasin)

CATEGORY AND SCHEDULE
Pregnancy Risk Category: D

MECHANISM OF ACTION
A hormone and antineoplastic agent that acts as an irreversible, steroidal aromatase inactivator. Aromatase is the principal enzyme that converts androgens to estrogens in both pre-menopausal and postmenopausal women. Acts as false substrate for aromatase enzyme; binds irrevers-ibly to active site of enzyme, causing its inactivation. *Therapeutic Effect:* Lowers circulating estrogens in those with breast cancers in which tumor growth is estrogen dependent.

PHARMACOKINETICS
Rapidly absorbed after PO administration. Distributed extensively into tissues. Protein binding: 90%. Metabolized in liver; eliminated in urine and feces. **Half-life:** 24 hrs.

AVAILABILITY
Tablets: 25 mg.

INDICATIONS AND DOSAGES
▸ **Breast cancer**
PO
Adults, Elderly. 25 mg once a day after a meal.

UNLABELED USES
Prevention of prostate cancer

CONTRAINDICATIONS
Hypersensitivity to exemestane

INTERACTIONS
Drug
None known.
Herbal
None known.
Food
None known.

DIAGNOSTIC TEST EFFECTS
May increase serum alkaline phosphatase, SGOT (AST), and SGPT (ALT) levels.

SIDE EFFECTS
Frequent (22%–10%)
Fatigue, nausea, depression, hot flashes, pain, insomnia, anxiety, dyspnea
Occasional (8%–5%)
Headache, dizziness, vomiting, edema (peripheral, leg), abdominal pain, anorexia, flu-like symptoms, diaphoresis, constipation, hypertension
Rare (4%)
Diarrhea

SERIOUS REACTIONS
• None known.

NURSING CONSIDERATIONS
Lifespan Considerations
• Be aware that exemestane is indicated for postmenopausal women.
• Be aware that this drug is not used in children.
• There are no age-related precautions noted in the elderly.
Precautions
• Do not give exemestane to pre-menopausal women.

Administration and Handling
PO
• Give drug after a meal.
Intervention and Evaluation
• Monitor the patient for the onset of depression.
• Assess the patient's sleep pattern.
• Monitor the patient for dizziness and assist the patient with ambulation if dizziness occurs.
• Evaluate the patient for headache.
• Give antiemetics, if ordered, to the patient to prevent and treat nausea and vomiting.
Patient Teaching
• Caution the patient to notify the physician if nausea or hot flashes become unmanageable.
• Warn the patient to avoid tasks that require mental alertness or motor skills until his or her response to the drug is established.
• Instruct the patient that exemestane is best taken after meals and at the same time each day.

---

flutamide
flew-tah-myd
(Euflex[CAN], Eulexin, Flugerel[AUS], Novo-Flutamide[CAN])
Do not confuse with Flumadine.

CATEGORY AND SCHEDULE
Pregnancy Risk Category: D

MECHANISM OF ACTION
An antiandrogen hormone that inhibits androgen uptake and binding of androgen in tissues. Interferes with testosterone at cellular level, complements leuprolide. *Therapeutic Effect:* Suppresses testicular androgen production.

PHARMACOKINETICS
Completely absorbed from the gastrointestinal (GI) tract. Protein binding: 94%–96%. Metabolized in liver to active metabolite. Primarily excreted in urine. Not removed by hemodialysis. **Half-life:** 6 hrs (half-life is increased in elderly).

AVAILABILITY
Capsules: 125 mg.

INDICATIONS AND DOSAGES
▶ **Prostatic carcinoma**
PO
Adults, Elderly. 250 mg q8h.

CONTRAINDICATIONS
Severe liver impairment

INTERACTIONS
Drug
None known.
Herbal
None known.
Food
None known.

DIAGNOSTIC TEST EFFECTS
May increase blood glucose, serum estradiol, serum testosterone, serum bilirubin, serum creatinine, SGOT (AST), and SGPT (ALT) levels.

SIDE EFFECTS
Frequent
Hot flashes (50%); loss of libido, impotence, diarrhea (24%); generalized pain (23%); asthenia (loss of strength, energy) (17%); constipation (12%); nausea, nocturia (11%)
Occasional (8%–6%)
Dizziness, paresthesia, insomnia, impotence, peripheral edema, gynecomastia
Rare (5%–4%)
Rash, sweating, hypertension, hematuria, vomiting, urinary inconti-

nence, headache, flu syndrome, photosensitivity

SERIOUS REACTIONS
• Liver toxicity, including liver encephalopathy, and hemolytic anemia may be noted.

NURSING CONSIDERATIONS
Lifespan Considerations
• Be aware that flutamide is not used in pregnant women or in children.
• There are no age-related precautions noted in the elderly.
Administration and Handling
PO
• Give flutamide without regard to food.
Intervention and Evaluation
• Periodically monitor liver function test results in patients on long-term flutamide therapy.
Patient Teaching
• Caution the patient against abruptly discontinuing the drug.
• Advise the patient that his or her urine color may change to an amber or yellow-green during flutamide therapy.
• Encourage the patient to avoid overexposure to sun or ultraviolet light and to wear protective clothing until his or her tolerance to ultraviolet exposure is determined.

fulvestrant
full-**ves**-trant
(Faslodex)

CATEGORY AND SCHEDULE
Pregnancy Risk Category: D

MECHANISM OF ACTION
An estrogen antagonist that competes with endogenous estrogen at estrogen receptor binding sites.

Therapeutic Effect: Inhibits tumor growth.

PHARMACOKINETICS
Extensively and rapidly distributed after IM administration. Protein binding: 99%. Metabolized in the liver. Eliminated by hepatobiliary route; excreted in the feces. **Half-life:** 40 days in postmenopausal women. Peak serum levels occur in 7–9 days.

AVAILABILITY
Prefilled Syringe: 50 mg/ml in 5- and 2.5-ml syringes.

INDICATIONS AND DOSAGES
▶ **Breast cancer**
IM
Adults, Elderly. 250 mg given once monthly.

CONTRAINDICATIONS
Known or suspected pregnancy

INTERACTIONS
Drug
None known.
Herbal
None known.
Food
None known.

DIAGNOSTIC TEST EFFECTS
None known.

SIDE EFFECTS
Frequent (26%–13%)
Nausea, hot flashes, pharyngitis, asthenia (loss of strength, energy), vomiting, vasodilatation, headache
Occasional (12%–5%)
Injection site pain, constipation, diarrhea, abdominal pain, anorexia, dizziness, insomnia, paresthesia, bone or back pain, depression, anxiety, peripheral edema, rash, sweating, fever

Rare (2%–1%)
Vertigo, weight gain

SERIOUS REACTIONS

• Urinary tract infection occurs occasionally.
• Vaginitis, anemia, thromboembolic phenomena, and leukopenia occur rarely.

NURSING CONSIDERATIONS

Baseline Assessment

• Expect the patient to have an estrogen receptor assay test performed before initiating fulvestrant therapy.
• Also expect the patient to undergo a baseline computed tomography (CT) scan initially and periodically thereafter to evaluate tumor regression.

Lifespan Considerations

• Do not administer fulvestrant to pregnant women.
• Be aware that it is unknown if fulvestrant is excreted in breast milk.
• Be aware that fulvestrant is not for use in children.
• There are no age-related precautions noted in the elderly.

Precautions

• Use cautiously in patients on anticoagulant therapy and those with bleeding diathesis, estrogen receptor-negative breast cancer, liver disease or reduced hepatic flow, and thrombocytopenia.

Administration and Handling

IM
• Administer slowly into the buttock as a single 5-ml injection or 2 concurrent 2.5-ml injections.

Intervention and Evaluation

• Monitor the patient's blood chemistry and plasma lipid levels.
• Evaluate the patient's level of bone pain and ensure adequate pain relief if pain levels increase.

• Assess the patient for edema, especially in dependent areas.
• Monitor the patient for asthenia and dizziness and provide assistance with ambulation if these symptoms occur.
• Assess the patient for headache.
• Offer the patient an antiemetic, if ordered, to prevent and treat nausea and vomiting.

Patient Teaching

• Warn the patient to notify the physician if asthenia, hot flashes, or nausea become unmanageable.

goserelin acetate

gos-**er**-ah-lin
(Zoladex, Zoladex LA)

CATEGORY AND SCHEDULE

Pregnancy Risk Category: D (advanced breast cancer), X (endometriosis, endometrial thinning)

MECHANISM OF ACTION

A gonadotropin-releasing hormone analogue and antineoplastic agent that stimulates the release of luteinizing hormone (LH) and follicle-stimulating hormone (FSH) from anterior pituitary. *Therapeutic Effect:* Increases testosterone concentrations. After initial increase, decreases release of LH, FSH, testosterone.

AVAILABILITY

Implant: 3.6 mg, 10.8 mg.

INDICATIONS AND DOSAGES

▶ **Prostatic carcinoma**
Subcutaneous/Implant
Adults older than 18 yrs, Elderly.
3.6 mg q28 days or 10.8 mg q12wks into upper abdominal wall.

▸ **Breast carcinoma, endometriosis**
Subcutaneous/Implant
Adults. 3.6 mg q28 days into upper abdominal wall.
▸ **Endometrial thinning**
Subcutaneous
Adults. 3.6 mg once or 4 wks apart in 2 doses.

CONTRAINDICATIONS
Pregnancy

INTERACTIONS
Drug
None known.
Herbal
None known.
Food
None known.

DIAGNOSTIC TEST EFFECTS
May increase serum acid phosphatase and testosterone levels.

SIDE EFFECTS
Frequent
Headache (60%), hot flashes (55%), depression (54%), sweating (45%), sexual dysfunction (21%), decreased erection (18%), lower urinary tract symptoms (13%)
Occasional (10%-5%)
Nausea, pain, lethargy, dizziness, insomnia, anorexia, nausea, rash, upper respiratory infection, hair growth, abdominal pain
Rare
Pruritus

SERIOUS REACTIONS
• Arrhythmias, congestive heart failure (CHF), and hypertension occur rarely.
• Ureteral obstruction and spinal cord compression have been observed. Immediate orchiectomy may be necessary if these conditions occur.

NURSING CONSIDERATION
Intervention and Evaluation
• Monitor the patient for worsening signs and symptoms of prostatic cancer, especially during the first month of goserelin therapy.
Patient Teaching
• Encourage the patient to use nonhormonal contraceptive measures during goserelin therapy. Teach the patient about forms of nonhormonal contraception.
• Warn the patient to notify the physician if regular menstruation persists or she becomes pregnant.
• Advise the patient that breakthrough menstrual bleeding may occur if a goserelin dose is missed.

letrozole
leh-troe-zoll
(Femara)

CATEGORY AND SCHEDULE
Pregnancy Risk Category: D

MECHANISM OF ACTION
This hormone and antineoplastic agent decreases circulating estrogen by inhibiting aromatase, an enzyme that catalyzes the final step in estrogen production. *Therapeutic Effect:* Suppresses estrogen biosynthesis in hormonally responsive breast cancers.

PHARMACOKINETICS
Rapidly and completely absorbed. Metabolized in liver. Primarily eliminated via the kidneys. Unknown if removed by hemodialysis.
Half-life: Approximately 2 days.

AVAILABILITY
Tablets: 2.5 mg.

INDICATIONS AND DOSAGES
▶ **Breast cancer**
PO
Adults, Elderly. 2.5 mg a day. Continue until tumor progression is evident.

CONTRAINDICATIONS
None known

INTERACTIONS
Drug
None known.
Herbal
None known.
Food
None known.

DIAGNOSTIC TEST EFFECTS
May increase serum calcium, serum cholesterol, serum GGT, SGOT (AST), and SGPT (ALT) levels.

SIDE EFFECTS
Frequent (21%–9%)
Musculoskeletal pain (back, arm, leg), nausea, headache
Occasional (8%–5%)
Constipation, arthralgia, fatigue, vomiting, hot flashes, diarrhea, abdominal pain, cough, rash, anorexia, hypertension, peripheral edema
Rare (4%–1%)
Asthenia (loss of strength, energy), somnolence, dyspepsia (heartburn, indigestion, epigastric pain), weight increase, pruritus

SERIOUS REACTIONS
• None known.

NURSING CONSIDERATIONS
Lifespan Considerations
• Be aware that it is unknown if letrozole is distributed in breast milk.
• Be aware that the safety and

efficacy of letrozole have not been established in children.
• There are no age-related precautions noted in the elderly.
Precautions
• Use cautiously in patients with liver or renal impairment.
Administration and Handling
PO
• Give letrozole without regard to food.
Intervention and Evaluation
• Monitor the patient for asthenia and dizziness and assist the patient with ambulation if either condition occurs.
• Assess the patient for headache.
• Offer the patient an antiemetic, if ordered, to prevent or treat nausea and vomiting.
• Monitor the patient's complete blood count (CBC), serum electrolytes, liver and renal function test results, and thyroid function.
• Evaluate the patient for evidence of musculoskeletal pain. Offer the patient analgesics, if ordered, to provide pain relief.
Patient Teaching
• Advise the patient to notify the physician if asthenia, hot flashes, or nausea become unmanageable.

leuprolide acetate
leu-pro-lied
(Eligard, Lucrin[AUS], Lupron, Lupron Depot Ped, Viadur)
Do not confuse with Lopurin or Nuprin.

CATEGORY AND SCHEDULE
Pregnancy Risk Category: X

MECHANISM OF ACTION
A gonadotropin-releasing hormone analogue and antineoplastic agent

whose initial or intermittent administration stimulates release of luteinizing hormone (LH) and follicle-stimulating hormone (FSH) from anterior pituitary, increasing testosterone level in males and estradiol in premenopausal women within 1 wk. Continuous daily administration suppresses secretion of gonadotropin-releasing hormone. *Therapeutic Effect:* Produces fall within 2 to 4 wks in testosterone levels to castrate level in males, estrogen level in premenopausal women to postmenopausal levels. In central precocious puberty, gonadotropins reduced to prepubertal levels.

PHARMACOKINETICS
Rapidly, well absorbed after subcutaneous administration. Slow absorption after IM administration. Protein binding: 43%–49%. **Half-life:** 3–4 hrs.

AVAILABILITY
Implant: 65 mg (Viadur).
Injection solution: 5 mg/ml (Lupron).
Injection depot formulation: 3.75 mg (Lupron Depot), 7.5 mg (Eligard), 7.5 mg (Lupron Depot), 7.5 mg, 22.5 mg, 30 mg, (Lupron Depot-Ped), 11.25 mg (Lupron Depot monthly), 11.25 mg (Lupron Depot-Ped), 15 mg (Lupron Depot-Ped), 22.5 mg (Lupron Depot monthly), 30 mg (Lupron Depot monthly).

INDICATIONS AND DOSAGES
▸ **Prostatic carcinoma**
Subcutaneous
Adults, Elderly. 1 mg a day.
IM
Adults, Elderly. Depot: 7.5 mg q28–33 days or 22.5 mg q3mos or 30 mg q4mos.

▸ **Endometriosis, uterine leiomyomata**
IM
Adults. Depot: 3.75 mg monthly or 11.25 mg as single injection.
▸ **Central precocious puberty**
Subcutaneous
Children. Initially, 35–50 mcg/kg/day; if down regulation not achieved, titrate upward by 10 mcg/kg/day.
IM
Children. Initially, 0.15–0.3 mg/kg/4 wks (minimum: 7.5 mg); if down regulation not achieved, titrate upward in 3.75-mg increments q4wks.

CONTRAINDICATIONS
Pernicious anemia, pregnancy

INTERACTIONS
Drug
None known.
Herbal
None known.
Food
None known.

DIAGNOSTIC TEST EFFECTS
May increase serum acid phosphatase levels. Initially increases testosterone, then decreases testosterone concentration.

SIDE EFFECTS
Frequent
Hot flashes (ranging from mild flushing to diaphoresis)
Females: Amenorrhea, spotting
Occasional
Arrhythmias, palpitations, blurred vision, dizziness, edema, headache, burning or itching, swelling at injection site, nausea, insomnia, increased weight
Females: Deepening voice, increased hair growth, decreased

libido, increased breast tenderness, vaginitis, altered mood
Males: Constipation, decreased testicle size, gynecomastia, impotence, decreased appetite, angina
Rare
Males: Thrombophlebitis

SERIOUS REACTIONS

• Occasionally, a worsening of signs and symptoms of prostatic carcinoma occurs 1 to 2 wks after initial dosing but subsides during continued therapy.
• Increased bone pain and less frequently dysuria or hematuria, weakness or paresthesia of lower extremities, may be noted.
• Myocardial infarction and pulmonary embolism occur rarely.

NURSING CONSIDERATIONS

Baseline Assessment
• Determine if the patient is pregnant before initiating leuprolide therapy.
• Expect to obtain serum testosterone and prostatic acid phosphatase (PAP) levels periodically during leuprolide therapy. Be aware that serum testosterone and PAP levels should increase during first week of therapy. Testosterone level then should decrease to baseline level or less within 2 weeks, PAP level within 4 weeks.
Lifespan Considerations
• Be aware that Depot use is contraindicated in pregnancy. Depot may cause spontaneous abortion.
• Be aware that the long-term safety of leuprolide has not been established in children.
• There are no age-related precautions noted in the elderly.
Precautions
• Use cautiously in children for long-term use.

Administration and Handling
◄ALERT► Because leuprolide may be carcinogenic, mutagenic, or teratogenic, handle with extreme care during preparation and administration.
Subcutaneous
• Solution normally appears clear, colorless.
• Refrigerate.
• Store opened vial at room temperature.
• Discard if precipitate forms or solution appears discolored.
• Store Depot vials at room temperature. Reconstitute only with diluent provided; use immediately. Do not use needles less than 22 gauge.
• Use syringes provided by manufacturer or use a 0.5-ml low-dose insulin syringe as an alternative.
Intervention and Evaluation
• Monitor the patient for arrhythmias and palpitations.
• Assess the patient for peripheral edema behind the medial malleolus or in sacral area in bedridden patients.
• Evaluate the patient's sleep pattern.
• Monitor the patient for visual difficulties.
• Assist the patient with ambulation if dizziness occurs.
• Offer the patient antiemetics, if ordered, to treat any nausea and vomiting he or she experiences.
Patient Teaching
• Advise the patient that hot flashes tend to decrease in frequency during continued leuprolide therapy.
• Explain to the patient that a temporary exacerbation of signs and symptoms of the disease may occur during the first few weeks of leuprolide therapy.
• Encourage the patient to use contraceptive measures during leuprolide therapy.

• Warn the patient to notify the physician if regular menstruation persists or she becomes pregnant.

megestrol acetate
meh-**geh**-stroll
(Apo-Megestrol[CAN], Megace, Megase OS, Megostat[AUS])

CATEGORY AND SCHEDULE
Pregnancy Risk Category: X

MECHANISM OF ACTION
A hormone and antineoplastic agent that suppresses release of luteinizing hormone from anterior pituitary by inhibiting pituitary function. *Therapeutic Effect:* Regresses tumor size. Increases appetite, mechanism unknown.

PHARMACOKINETICS
Well absorbed from the gastrointestinal (GI) tract. Metabolized in liver; excreted in urine.

AVAILABILITY
Tablets: 20 mg, 40 mg.
Suspension: 40 mg/ml.

INDICATIONS AND DOSAGES
▶ **Palliative treatment of advanced breast cancer**
PO
Adults, Elderly. 160 mg/day in 4 equally divided doses.
▶ **Palliative treatment of advanced endometrial carcinoma**
PO
Adults, Elderly. 40–320 mg/day in divided doses. Maximum: 800 mg/day in 1-4 divided doses.
▶ **Anorexia, cachexia, weight loss**
PO
Adults, Elderly. 800 mg (20 ml)/day.

UNLABELED USES
Appetite stimulant, treatment of hormonally-dependent or advanced prostate carcinoma

CONTRAINDICATIONS
None known

INTERACTIONS
Drug
None known.
Herbal
None known.
Food
None known.

DIAGNOSTIC TEST EFFECTS
May increase blood glucose levels.

SIDE EFFECTS
Frequent
Weight gain secondary to increased appetite
Occasional
Nausea, breakthrough bleeding, backache, headache, breast tenderness, carpal tunnel syndrome
Rare
Feeling of coldness

SERIOUS REACTIONS
• Thrombophlebitis and pulmonary embolism occur rarely.

NURSING CONSIDERATIONS
Baseline Assessment
• Determine if the patient is pregnant before initiating megestrol therapy. Advise the patient that megestrol is Pregnancy Risk Category X in suspension form, Pregnancy Risk Category D in tablet form.
• Provide support to the patient and family, recognizing this drug is palliative, not curative.
Lifespan Considerations
• Know that megestrol use should be avoided during pregnancy, if

possible, especially in the first 4 months.
• Be aware that breast-feeding is not recommended in this patient population.
• Be aware that the safety and efficacy of megestrol have not been established in children.
• There are no age-related precautions noted in the elderly.
Precautions
• Use cautiously in patients with a history of thrombophlebitis.
Intervention and Evaluation
• Monitor the patient for signs and symptoms of a therapeutic response to the drug.
Patient Teaching
• Caution the patient that contraception is imperative. Megestrol is a Pregnancy Risk Category X drug in suspension form, a Pregnancy Risk Category D drug in tablet form.
• Instruct the patient to notify the physician if he or she experiences any calf pain, difficulty breathing, or vaginal bleeding.
• Advise the patient that megestrol may cause backache, breast tenderness, headache, nausea, and vomiting.

nilutamide
nih-**lute**-ah-myd
(Anandron[CAN], Nilandron)

CATEGORY AND SCHEDULE
Pregnancy Risk Category: C

MECHANISM OF ACTION
A hormone and antineoplastic agent that competitively inhibits androgen action by binding to androgen receptors in target tissue. *Therapeutic Effect:* Decreases growth of prostatic carcinoma.

AVAILABILITY
Tablets: 150 mg.

INDICATIONS AND DOSAGES
▸ **Prostatic carcinoma**
PO
Adults, Elderly. 300 mg once a day for 30 days, then 150 mg once a day. Begin on same day or day after surgical castration.

CONTRAINDICATIONS
Severe liver impairment, severe respiratory insufficiency

INTERACTIONS
Drug
None known.
Herbal
None known.
Food
None known.

DIAGNOSTIC TEST EFFECTS
May increase serum bilirubin, serum creatinine, SGOT (AST), and SGPT (ALT) levels.

SIDE EFFECTS
Frequent (greater than 10%)
Hot flashes, delay in recovering vision after bright illumination (sun, television, bright lights), loss of libido or sexual potency, mild nausea, gynecomastia, alcohol intolerance
Occasional (less than 10%)
Constipation, hypertension, dizziness, dyspnea, urinary tract infections

SERIOUS REACTIONS
• Interstitial pneumonitis occurs rarely.

NURSING CONSIDERATIONS

Baseline Assessment
• Expect to obtain a baseline chest x-ray and liver enzyme levels before beginning nilutamide therapy.

Precautions
• Use cautiously in patients with hepatitis and a marked increase in liver enzymes.

Intervention and Evaluation
• Monitor the patient's blood pressure (B/P) and liver function test results periodically during long-term nilutamide therapy.

Patient Teaching
• Warn the patient to notify the physician if he or she experiences any side effects at home, especially signs of liver toxicity, including abdominal pain, dark urine, fatigue, and jaundice.
• Caution the patient about driving at night. Recommend tinted glasses to help decrease the visual effect of bright headlights and streetlights.

tamoxifen citrate
tam-**ox**-ih-fen
(Apo-Tamox[CAN], Genox[AUS], Istubol, Nolvadex, Nolvadex-D[CAN], Novo-Tamoxifen[CAN], Tamofen[CAN], Tamone[CAN], Tamosin[AUS])

CATEGORY AND SCHEDULE
Pregnancy Risk Category: D

MECHANISM OF ACTION
This nonsteroidal antiestrogen competes with estradiol for binding to estrogen in tissues that contain a high concentration of receptors, including the breasts, uterus, and vagina. *Therapeutic Effect:* Reduces DNA synthesis, inhibits estrogen response.

PHARMACOKINETICS
Well absorbed from the gastro-intestinal (GI) tract. Metabolized in liver. Primarily eliminated in feces via biliary system. **Half-life:** 7 days.

AVAILABILITY
Tablets: 10 mg, 20 mg.

INDICATIONS AND DOSAGES
▸ **Treatment of metastatic breast cancer, delaying recurrence of metastatic breast cancer after total mastectomy and axillary dissection or segmental mastectomy, axillary dissection, and breast irradiation in women with axillary node-negative breast carcinoma.**
PO
Adults, Elderly. 20–40 mg/day. Give doses greater than 20 mg/day in divided doses.
▸ **Prevention of breast cancer in high-risk women**
PO
Adults, Elderly. 20 mg/day.

UNLABELED USES
Induction of ovulation

CONTRAINDICATIONS
None known

INTERACTIONS
Drug
Estrogens: May decrease the effects of tamoxifen.
Herbal
None known.
Food
None known.

DIAGNOSTIC TEST EFFECTS
May increase serum cholesterol, calcium, and triglyceride levels.

SIDE EFFECTS
Frequent
Women (greater than10%): Hot flashes, nausea, vomiting

Occasional

Women (9%–1%): Changes in menstruation, genital itching, vaginal discharge, endometrial hyperplasia or polyps

Males: Impotence, decreased sexual libido

Men and women: Headache, nausea, vomiting, rash, bone pain, confusion, weakness, sleepiness

SERIOUS REACTIONS

• Retinopathy, corneal opacity, and decreased visual acuity have been noted in those receiving extremely high dosages (240–320 mg/day) for longer than 17 mos.

NURSING CONSIDERATIONS

Baseline Assessment

• Check the results of the patient's estrogen receptor assay test, if ordered, before beginning tamoxifen therapy.

• Monitor the patient's complete blood count (CBC) and serum calcium levels before beginning and periodically during tamoxifen therapy.

Lifespan Considerations

• Know that tamoxifen use should be avoided during pregnancy, if possible, especially during the first trimester. Also know that tamoxifen may cause fetal harm and that it's unknown if tamoxifen is distributed in breast milk. Be aware that breast-feeding is not recommended in this patient population.

• Be aware that tamoxifen use is safe and effective in girls aged 2 to 10 years with McCune Albright syndrome and precocious puberty.

• There are no age-related precautions noted in the elderly.

Precautions

• Use cautiously in patients with leukopenia and thrombocytopenia.

Administration and Handling

PO

• Give tamoxifen without regard to food.

Intervention and Evaluation

• Be alert to reports from the patient of increased bone pain and provide adequate pain relief.

• Monitor the patient's intake and output and weight.

• Examine the patient for dependent edema.

• Assess the patient for signs and symptoms of hypercalcemia, including constipation, deep bone or flank pain, excessive thirst, hypotonicity of muscles, increased urine volume, nausea, renal stones, and vomiting.

Patient Teaching

• Warn the patient to notify the physician if he or she experiences leg cramps, weakness, weight gain, or vaginal bleeding, itching, or discharge.

• Advise the patient that he or she may initially experience an increase in bone and tumor pain and that this appears to indicate good tumor response to tamoxifen.

• Caution the patient to notify the physician if nausea and vomiting continue at home.

• Teach the patient about the use of nonhormonal contraception during tamoxifen treatment.

toremifene citrate

tore-mih-feen

(Fareston)

CATEGORY AND SCHEDULE

Pregnancy Risk Category: D

MECHANISM OF ACTION

A nonsteroidal antiestrogen and antineoplastic agent that binds to estrogen receptors on tumors, producing a complex that decreases DNA synthesis and inhibits estrogen effects. *Therapeutic Effect:* Blocks growth-stimulating effects of estrogen in breast cancer.

PHARMACOKINETICS
Well absorbed after PO administration. Metabolized in the liver. Eliminated in feces. **Half-life:** Approximately 5 days.

AVAILABILITY
Tablets: 60 mg.

INDICATIONS AND DOSAGES
▶ **Breast cancer**
PO
Adults. 60 mg a day until disease progression is observed.

CONTRAINDICATIONS
History of thromboembolic disease

INTERACTIONS
Drug
Carbamazepine, phenobarbital, phenytoin: May decrease toremifene blood concentration.
Warfarin: May increase prothrombin time.
Herbal
None known.
Food
None known.

DIAGNOSTIC TEST EFFECTS
May increase serum alkaline phosphatase, serum bilirubin, serum calcium, and SGOT (AST) levels.

SIDE EFFECTS
Frequent
Hot flashes (35%); sweating (20%); nausea (14%); vaginal discharge (13%); dizziness, dry eyes (9%)
Occasional (5%–2%)
Edema, vomiting, vaginal bleeding

Rare
Nausea, vomiting, fatigue, depression, lethargy, anorexia

SERIOUS REACTIONS
• Cataracts, glaucoma, and decreased visual acuity may occur.
• May produce hypercalcemia.

NURSING CONSIDERATIONS
Baseline Assessment
• Expect to perform an estrogen receptor assay of the patient before initiating toremifene therapy.
• Monitor the patient's complete blood count (CBC) and serum calcium levels before and periodically during toremifene therapy.
Lifespan Considerations
• Be aware that it is unknown if toremifene is distributed in breast milk.
• Be aware that the safety and efficacy of toremifene have not been established in children and that this drug is not prescribed in this patient population.
• There are no age-related precautions noted in the elderly.
Precautions
• Use cautiously in patients with preexisting endometrial hyperplasia, leukopenia, and thrombocytopenia.
Administration and Handling
PO
• Give toremifene without regard to food.
Intervention and Evaluation
• Assess the patient for signs and symptoms of hypercalcemia, including constipation, deep bone or flank pain, excessive thirst, hypotonicity of muscles, increased urine volume, nausea, renal stones, and vomiting.
• Monitor the patient's complete blood count (CBC), leukocyte, liver

function test results, and serum calcium levels.

Patient Teaching
• Advise the patient that he or she may experience an initial flare-up of disease, including bone pain and hot flashes, that will subside with continued therapy.
• Warn the patient to notify the physician if he or she experiences leg cramps, shortness of breath, vaginal bleeding, discharge, or itching, weakness, and weight gain.
• Caution the patient to notify the physician if nausea and vomiting continue at home.
• Encourage the patient to use nonhormonal methods of contraception during toremifene therapy.

triptorelin pamoate
trip-toe-**ree**-linn
(Trelstar Depot, Trelstar LA)

CATEGORY AND SCHEDULE
Pregnancy Risk Category: X

MECHANISM OF ACTION
A gonadotropin-releasing hormone (GnRH) analogue and antineoplastic agent that through a negative feedback mechanism inhibits gonadotropin hormone secretion. Initially, a transient surge in circulating levels of luteinizing hormone (LH), follicle-stimulating hormone (FSH), testosterone, and estradiol occurs. Chronic administration results in decreased LH and FSH, marked reduction in testosterone and estradiol levels. *Therapeutic Effect:* Suppresses abnormal growth of prostate tissue.

AVAILABILITY
Powder for Injection: 3.75 mg once q28 days (Trelstar Depot), 11.25 mg every 3 mos (Trelstar LA).

INDICATIONS AND DOSAGES
▸ **Prostate cancer**
IM
Adults, Elderly. 3.75 mg once monthly.

CONTRAINDICATIONS
Hypersensitivity to luteinizing hormone-releasing hormone (LHRH) agonists or LHRH

INTERACTIONS
Drug
Hyperprolactinemic drugs: Reduce number of pituitary GnRH receptors.
Herbal
None known.
Food
None known.

DIAGNOSTIC TEST EFFECTS
May alter pituitary-gonadal function test results. Increases transient testosterone levels, usually during first week of treatment, and levels decline thereafter.

SIDE EFFECTS
Frequent (greater than 5%)
Hot flashes, skeletal pain, headache, impotence
Occasional (5%–2%)
Insomnia, vomiting, leg pain, fatigue
Rare (less than 2%)
Dizziness, emotional lability, diarrhea, urinary retention, urinary tract infection (UTI), anemia, pruritus

SERIOUS REACTIONS
• Bladder outlet obstruction, bone pain, hematuria, and spinal cord compression with weakness or

paralysis of lower extremities may occur.

NURSING CONSIDERATIONS

Intervention and Evaluation

• Expect to obtain prostatic acid phosphatase (PAP), prostate-specific antigen (PSA), and serum testosterone levels periodically during therapy. Know that serum testosterone and PAP levels should increase during first week of therapy. Also, be aware that the testosterone level then should decrease to baseline level or less within 2 weeks and PAP level within 4 weeks.

• Monitor the patient closely for worsening signs and symptoms of prostatic cancer, especially during the first week of therapy due to a transient increase in testosterone.

Patient Teaching

• Caution the patient against missing monthly injections.

• Advise the patient that he or she may experience blood in urine, increased bone pain, and urinary retention initially, which usually subsides within 1 week.

• Explain to the patient that he or she may have hot flashes during triptorelin therapy.

• Warn the patient to notify the physician if he or she experiences difficulty breathing, infection at the injection site, numbness of arms or legs, pain or swelling of breasts, persistent nausea or vomiting, and rapid heartbeat.

19 Monoclonal Antibodies

Uses: Each monoclonal antibody is used to treat different types of cancer, including breast cancer, low-grade B-cell non-Hodgkin's lymphoma, and B-cell chronic lymphocytic leukemia. For details, see the specific drug entries.

Action: Although their exact mechanism of action is unknown, monoclonal antibodies may act by binding to specific cell-surface antigens. The agents' cytotoxic effects may be related to T-cell mediated recognition of the bound antibody and interference with cell proliferation.

ANTINEOPLASTIC AGENTS

alemtuzumab
al-lem-**two**-zoo-mab
(Campath)

CATEGORY AND SCHEDULE
Pregnancy Risk Category: C

MECHANISM OF ACTION
A monoclonal antibody that binds to CD52, a cell surface glycoprotein, found on the surface of all B and T lymphocytes, most monocytes, macrophages, NK cells, and granulocytes. *Therapeutic Effect:* Produces cytotoxicity, reduces tumor size.

PHARMACOKINETICS
Half-life: About 12 days. Peak and trough levels rise during first few weeks of therapy, approach steady state by about week 6.

AVAILABILITY
Solution for Injection: 30 mg/3 ml.

INDICATIONS AND DOSAGES
▸ Chronic lymphocytic leukemia (B-CLL)
IV infusion
Adults, Elderly. Initially, 3 mg/day given as a 2-hr infusion. When the 3-mg daily dose is tolerated (low grade or no infusion-related toxicities), increase daily dose to 10 mg. When the 10 mg/day dose is tolerated, maintenance dose of 30 mg/day may be initiated. Maintenance Dose: 30 mg/day 3 times/ wk on alternate days (Mon., Wed., Fri. or Tues., Thurs., Sat.) for up to 12 wks. The increase to 30 mg/day is usually achieved in 3–7 days.

CONTRAINDICATIONS
Active systemic infections, anaphylactic reaction, immunosuppression, or known hypersensitivity

INTERACTIONS
Drug
None known.
Herbal
None known.
Food
None known.

DIAGNOSTIC TEST EFFECTS
May decrease Hgb level, platelet count, and white blood cell count.

IV INCOMPATIBILITIES
Do not mix with any other medications.

SIDE EFFECTS
Frequent
Rigors (86%); fever (85%); nausea (54%); vomiting (41%); rash (40%); fatigue (34%); hypotension (32%); urticaria (30%); pruritus, skeletal pain, headache (24%); diarrhea (22%); anorexia (20%)
Occasional (less than 10%)
Myalgia, dizziness, abdominal pain, throat irritation, vomiting, neutropenia, rhinitis, bronchospasm, urticaria

SERIOUS REACTIONS
• Neutropenia occurs in 85% of patients.
• Anemia occurs in 80% of patients.
• Thrombocytopenia occurs in 72% of patients.
• A rash occurs in 40% of patients.
• Respiratory toxicity (16%–26%) occurs and is manifested as dyspnea, cough, bronchitis, pneumonitis, and pneumonia.

NURSING CONSIDERATIONS

Baseline Assessment
◀ALERT▶ Expect to pretreat the patient with 650 mg acetaminophen and 50 mg diphenhydramine before each infusion to prevent infusion-related side effects.
• Expect to obtain complete blood count (CBC) frequently during and after therapy to assess for anemia, neutropenia, and thrombocytopenia.
Lifespan Considerations
• Alemtuzumab has the potential to cause fetal B- and T-lymphocyte depletion. Advise the patient to discontinue breast-feeding during treatment and for at least 3 months after the last dose.

• Be aware that the safety and efficacy have not been established in children.
• There are no age-related precautions noted in the elderly.
Administration and Handling
IV
• Do not give by IV push or bolus.
• Prior to dilution, refrigerate ampoules. Do not freeze.
• Use within 8 hours after dilution. Diluted solution may be stored at room temperature or refrigerated.
• Discard if particulate matter is present or if solution is discolored.
• Withdraw needed amount from ampoule into a syringe.
• Inject into 100-ml 0.9% NaCl or D_5W using a low-protein binding, nonfiber-releasing 5-micron filter.
• Invert bag to mix; do not shake.
• Give the 100 ml solution as a 2-hour IV infusion.
Intervention and Evaluation
• Monitor for any infusion-related symptoms complex consisting mainly of chills, fever, hypotension, and rigors generally occurring 30 minutes to 2 hours from the beginning of the first infusion. The symptoms may resolve by slowing the drip rate of the infusion.
• Monitor for signs and symptoms of hematologic toxicity, including easy bruising, fever, signs of local infection, sore throat or unusual bleeding from any site.
• Monitor for signs and symptoms of anemia, such as excessive fatigue or weakness.
Patient Teaching
• Instruct the patient to avoid crowds and those with known infection.
• Stress to the patient that he or she should not receive vaccinations and should avoid contact with anyone who recently received a live virus vaccine.

bexarotene
becks-**aye**-row-teen
(Targretin)

CATEGORY AND SCHEDULE
Pregnancy Risk Category: X

MECHANISM OF ACTION
This retinoid antineoplastic agent binds to and activates retinoid X receptor subtypes, which regulate the genes that control cellular differentiation and proliferation. *Therapeutic Effect:* Inhibits growth of tumor cell lines of hematopoietic and squamous cell and induces tumor regression.

PHARMACOKINETICS
Metabolized in liver. Moderately absorbed from the gastrointestinal (GI) tract. Protein binding: greater than 99%. Primarily eliminated through hepatobiliary system.
Half-life: 7 hrs.

AVAILABILITY
Capsules, soft gelatin: 75 mg.

INDICATIONS AND DOSAGES
▸ **Cutaneous T-cell lymphoma (CTCL) refractory to at least one prior systemic therapy**
PO
Adults. 300 mg/m²/day. If no response and initial dose well tolerated, may be increased to 400 mg/m²/day. If not tolerated, may decrease to 200 mg/m²/day then to 100 mg/m²/day.

UNLABELED USES
Treatment of diabetes mellitus, head, neck, lung, and renal cell carcinomas, Kaposi's sarcoma

CONTRAINDICATIONS
None known.

INTERACTIONS
Drug
Antidiabetic agents: Bexarotene may enhance the effects of these drugs.
Erythromycin, itraconazole, ketoconazole: May increase bexarotene blood concentrations.
Phenytoln, rifampin: May decrease bexarotene blood concentrations.
Herbal
None known.
Food
Grapefruit juice: May increase bexarotene blood concentration and risk of toxicity.

DIAGNOSTIC TEST EFFECTS
CA-125 in ovarian cancer may be increased. May produce abnormal liver function test results, increase serum cholesterol, triglycerides, and total and LDL cholesterol levels. May decrease serum HDL cholesterol levels.

SIDE EFFECTS
Frequent
Hyperlipemia (79%), headache (30%), hypothyroidism (29%), asthenia (loss of strength and energy) (20%)
Occasional
Rash (17%), nausea (15%), peripheral edema (13%), dry skin, abdominal pain (11%), chills, exfoliative dermatitis (10%), diarrhea (7%)

SERIOUS REACTIONS
• Pancreatitis, liver failure, and pneumonia occur rarely.

NURSING CONSIDERATIONS
Baseline Assessment
• Assess the patient's baseline lipid profile, liver function, thyroid function, and white blood cell (WBC) count.
• Determine if the patient is pregnant.

Lifespan Considerations
• Be aware that bexarotene may cause fetal harm and it is unknown if bexarotene is distributed in breast milk.
• Be aware that the safety and efficacy of bexarotene have not been established in children.
• There are no age-related precautions noted in the elderly.

Precautions
• Use cautiously in patients with diabetes mellitus, lipid abnormalities, and liver impairment.

Administration and Handling
PO
• Give bexarotene with food.

Intervention and Evaluation
• Monitor the patient's serum cholesterol level, complete blood count (CBC), liver and thyroid function test results, and serum triglyceride levels.

Patient Teaching
• Advise the patient not to use abrasive, drying, or medicated soaps. Instruct the patient to wash with bland soap.
• Warn female patients of childbearing age about the potential fetal risk if pregnancy occurs and to notify the physician if she plans to become or becomes pregnant.
• Instruct female patients, even infertile, premenopausal women, to use reliable forms of contraceptives concurrently during bexarotene therapy and for 1 month after discontinuation of therapy.

---

bortezomib
bor-**teh**-zoe-mib
(Velcade)

CATEGORY AND SCHEDULE
Pregnancy Risk Category: D

MECHANISM OF ACTION
A proteasome inhibitor, antineoplastic agent that degrades conjugated proteins required for cell-cycle progression and mitosis; disrupts cell proliferation. *Therapeutic Effect:* Produces antitumor and chemosensitizing activity and cell death.

PHARMACOKINETICS
Distributed to tissues and organs, with highest level in the gastrointestinal (GI) tract and liver. Protein binding: 83%. Primarily metabolized by enzymatic action. Rapidly cleared from the circulation. Significant biliary excretion, with lesser amount excreted in the urine. **Half-life:** 9–15 hrs.

AVAILABILITY
Powder for Injection: 3.5 mg.

INDICATIONS AND DOSAGES
▸ **Multiple myeloma**
IV injection
Adults, Elderly. Treatment cycle consists of 1.3 mg/m^2/dose twice weekly on days 1, 4, 8, and 11 for 2 weeks followed by a 10-day rest period on days 12 to 21. Consecutive doses separated by at least 72 hrs. Dose modification: Therapy withheld at onset of grade 3 nonhematological or grade 4 hematological toxicities, excluding neuropathy. When symptoms resolve, therapy restarted at a 25% reduced dosage.
▸ **Neuropathic pain, peripheral sensory neuropathy**
IV injection
Adults, Elderly. For grade 1 with pain or grade 2 (interfering with function but not activities of daily living), reduce dose to 1 mg/m^2. For grade 2 with pain or grade 3 (interfering with activities of daily living), withhold until toxicity

resolved then reinitiate with 0.7 mg/m^2. For grade 4 (permanent sensory loss that interferes with function), discontinue bortezomib.

CONTRAINDICATIONS

Hypersensitivity to boron or mannitol

INTERACTIONS

Drug
Oral hypoglycemics: May alter the response of these drugs.
Food
None known.
Herbal
None known.

DIAGNOSTIC TEST EFFECTS

May significantly decrease blood Hgb and Hct levels, and neutrophil, platelet, and white blood cell (WBC) counts.

SIDE EFFECTS

Expected (65%–36%)
Fatigue, malaise, weakness, nausea, diarrhea, anorexia, constipation, fever, vomiting
Frequent (28%–21%)
Headache, insomnia, arthralgia, limb pain, edema, paresthesia, dizziness, rash
Occasional (18%–11%)
Dehydration, cough, anxiety, bone pain, muscle cramps, myalgia, back pain, abdominal pain, taste alteration, dyspepsia (heartburn, epigastric distress), pruritus, hypotension, rigors, blurred vision

SERIOUS REACTIONS

• Thrombocytopenia occurs in 40% of patients, peaks at day 11, and returns to baseline by day 21. GI and intracerebral hemorrhage are associated with drug-induced thrombocytopenia.
• Anemia occurs in 32% of patients.

• New onset or worsening of existing neuropathy occurs in 37% of patients. Symptoms may improve or return to baseline in some patients when bortezomib is discontinued.
• Pneumonia occurs occasionally.

NURSING CONSIDERATIONS

Baseline Assessment
• Keep in mind that bortezomib is used to treat patients with refractory or relapsed multiple myeloma, who have received at least 2 prior therapies, and who have demonstrated disease progression with the last therapy.
• As ordered, obtain and monitor the patient's baseline complete blood count (CBC), especially the platelet count, throughout bortezomib treatment.
• Give the patient antiemetics, if ordered, to prevent and treat nausea and vomiting.
• Administer antidiarrheals, if ordered, to prevent and treat diarrhea.

Lifespan Considerations
• Be aware that bortezomib may induce degenerative effects in the ovaries and testes and may affect male and female fertility. Know that breast-feeding is not recommended for patients receiving this drug.
• Be aware that the safety and efficacy of bortezomib have not been established in children.
• Note that an increased incidence of grade 3 and 4 thrombocytopenia occurs in the elderly.

Precautions
• Use cautiously in patients with a history of syncope.
• Use cautiously in patients receiving any medication that increases the risk of dehydration, hypotension, and liver or renal function impairment.

Administration and Handling
IV
• Store unopened vials at room temperature.
• Reconstituted solution is stable at room temperature for up to 8 hours.
• Reconstitute vial with 3.5 ml 0.9% NaCl.
• Give bortezomib as a bolus IV injection.

Intervention and Evaluation
• Routinely assess the patient's blood pressure (B/P). Monitor the patient for signs and symptoms of orthostatic hypotension.
• Maintain strict intake and output procedures.
• Monitor the patient's temperature and be alert to the high potential for fever.
• Assess the patient for signs and symptoms of peripheral neuropathy, including a burning sensation, hyperesthesia, neuropathic pain, and paresthesia of the extremities.
• Avoid giving the patient IM injections, rectal medications, patient positioning, and performing other procedures that may induce trauma and bleeding.

Patient Teaching
• Caution women of childbearing age to avoid pregnancy while taking bortezomib. Discuss the importance of pregnancy testing. Teach the patient about effective forms of contraception.
• Instruct the patient to increase his or her fluid intake to prevent dehydration.
• Warn the patient to avoid tasks that require mental alertness or motor skills until his or her response to the drug is established.

gefitinib
geh-**fih**-tih-nib
(Iressa)

CATEGORY AND SCHEDULE
Pregnancy Risk Category: D

MECHANISM OF ACTION
This antineoplastic agent blocks the signaling pathway that binds to a receptor (epidermal growth factor receptor [EGFR]) on the surface of cells. The purpose of EGFR is to activate an enzyme, tyrosine kinase, to send signals inside the cell, instructing the cell to grow. *Therapeutic Effect:* Inhibits the activation of tyrosine kinase, effectively inhibiting signaling at the receptor, preventing the growth signal within the cancer cell.

PHARMACOKINETICS
Slowly absorbed, extensively distributed throughout the body. Protein binding: 90%. Undergoes extensive liver metabolism. Excreted in the feces. **Half-life:** 48 hrs.

AVAILABILITY
Tablets: 250 mg.

INDICATIONS AND DOSAGES
▸ **Non–small cell lung cancer**
PO
Adults, Elderly. Give one 250 mg tablet a day. In those receiving rifampin or phenytoin, may increase gefitinib dose to 500 mg a day.

CONTRAINDICATIONS
None known.

INTERACTIONS
Drug
Cimetidine, phenytoin, rifampin, ranitidine, sodium bicarbonate: May decrease gefitinib blood concentration and effectiveness.
Itraconazole, ketoconazole: Increases gefitinib blood concentration.
Metoprolol: Increases the effect of metoprolol.
Warfarin: Increases risk of bleeding.
Herbal
None known.
Food
None known.

DIAGNOSTIC TEST EFFECTS
May increase serum alkaline phosphatase, serum bilirubin, SGOT (AST), and SGPT (ALT) levels.

SIDE EFFECTS
Frequent (48%–25%)
Diarrhea, rash, acne
Occasional (13%–8%)
Dry skin, nausea, vomiting, pruritus
Rare (7%–2%)
Anorexia, asthenia (loss of strength, energy), weight loss, peripheral edema, eye pain

SERIOUS REACTIONS
• Pancreatitis and ocular hemorrhage occur rarely.
• Hypersensitivity reaction produces angioedema and urticaria.

NURSING CONSIDERATIONS
Baseline Assessment
• Give the patient antidiarrheals and antiemetics, if ordered, to help prevent and treat diarrhea, nausea, and vomiting. For patients who are unable to tolerate diarrhea, expect to briefly interrupt gefitinib therapy for up to 14 days and then resume gefitinib therapy, as ordered.

Lifespan Considerations
• Be aware that gefitinib has the potential to cause fetal harm and may result in termination of pregnancy. Know that breast-feeding is not recommended for patients receiving this drug. Substitute formula feedings for breast feedings.
• Be aware that the safety and efficacy of gefitinib have not been established in children.
• There are no age-related precautions noted in the elderly.
Precautions
• Use cautiously in patients with impaired liver function and severe renal impairment.
Administration and Handling
• Give gefitinib without regard to food. Do not crush or break filmcoated tablets.
Intervention and Evaluation
• Encourage the patient to drink adequate fluids.
• Assess the patient's bowel sounds for hyperactivity.
• Assess the patient's pattern of daily bowel activity and stool consistency.
• Examine the patient's skin for evidence of rash.
Patient Teaching
• Stress to the patient that he or she should not receive vaccinations without the physician's approval and should avoid crowds and those with known infection.
• Warn the patient to immediately notify the physician if he or she experiences signs and symptoms of infection, including fever and flulike symptoms.
• Advise the patient to notify the physician if he or she experiences anorexia, nausea, vomiting, or persistent or severe diarrhea.
• Caution female patients to avoid becoming pregnant during gefitinib therapy, and to use contraceptive

methods during treatment and for up to 12 months after therapy.

gemtuzumab ozogamicin
gem-**too**-zoo-mab
(Mylotarg)

CATEGORY AND SCHEDULE
Pregnancy Risk Category: D

MECHANISM OF ACTION
A monoclonal antibody, antineoplastic agent that's composed of an antibody conjoined with a cytotoxic antitumor antibody. The antibody portion binds to an antigen on surface of leukemic blast cells in over 80% of patients with acute myeloid leukemia (AML), resulting in the formation of a complex. This releases the antibiotic inside the lysosomes of the myeloid cells. *Therapeutic Effect:* Binds to DNA, resulting in DNA double-strand breaks and cell death. Produces inhibition of colony formation in cultures of adult leukemic bone marrow cells.

PHARMACOKINETICS
After first infusion, elimination **half-life:** 45 hrs; after second dose, elimination **half-life:** increased to 60 hrs.

AVAILABILITY
Powder for Injection: 5 mg.

INDICATIONS AND DOSAGES
▸ **CD33 positive acute myeloid leukemia (AML)**
IV infusion
Adults 60 yrs and older. 9 mg/m^2; repeat in 14 days for total of 2 doses.

CONTRAINDICATIONS
None known.

INTERACTIONS
Drug
None known.
Herbal
None known.
Food
None known.

DIAGNOSTIC TEST EFFECTS
May increase serum bilirubin, SGOT (AST), SGPT (ALT), and serum transaminase levels. May decrease blood Hgb and Hct levels, platelet count, serum magnesium, serum potassium, and white blood cell (WBC) count.

IV INCOMPATIBILITIES
Do not mix with any other medications.

SIDE EFFECTS
◂**ALERT**▸ Most patients experience a postinfusion symptom complex of fever (85%), chills (73%), nausea (70%), vomiting (63%) that resolves within 2–4 hrs with supportive therapy.
Frequent (44%–31%)
Asthenia (loss of strength, energy), diarrhea, abdominal pain, headache, stomatitis (burning or erythema of oral mucosa, ulceration, sore throat, difficulty swallowing), dyspnea, epistaxis
Occasional (25%–15%)
Constipation, neutropenic fever, nonspecific rash, herpes simplex infection, hypertension, hypotension, petechiae, peripheral edema, dizziness, insomnia, back pain
Rare (14%–10%)
Pharyngitis, ecchymosis, dyspepsia, tachycardia, hematuria, rhinitis

SERIOUS REACTIONS

• Severe myelosuppression occurs in 98% of all patients, and is characterized as neutropenia, anemia, and thrombocytopenia.
• Sepsis occurs in 25% of patients.
• Hepatotoxicity may occur.

NURSING CONSIDERATIONS

Baseline Assessment

• Monitor the patient's baseline serum chemistry levels, complete blood count (CBC), and liver function studies for the expected myelosuppression and to evaluate for severe myelosuppression.
• Use strict aseptic technique to protect the patient from infection.

Lifespan Considerations

• Be aware that gemtuzumab may cause fetal harm and it is unknown if gemtuzumab is excreted in breast milk.
• The safety and efficacy of gemtuzumab have not been established in children.
• There are no age-related precautions noted in the elderly.

Precautions

• Use cautiously in patients with liver impairment.

Administration and Handling

◀ALERT▶ Give diphenhydramine 50 mg and acetaminophen 650 to 1,000 mg 1 hour before administering gemtuzumab, as prescribed. Follow with acetaminophen 650 to 1,000 mg every 4 hours for 2 doses, then every 4 hours as prescribed and as needed. Know that full recovery from hematologic toxicities is not a requirement for giving second gemtuzumab dose.

IV

• Protect the drug from direct and indirect sunlight and unshielded fluorescent light during preparation and administration.
• Refrigerate, do not freeze.
• Following reconstitution in vial, protect solution from light. Solution is stable for up to 8 hours if refrigerated.
• Once diluted with 100 ml 0.9% NaCl, use immediately.
• Prepare in a biologic safety hood with fluorescent light off.
• Allow vials to come to room temperature.
• Reconstitute each vial with 5 ml Sterile Water for Injection using sterile syringes to provide concentration of 1 mg/ml.
• Gently swirl, then inspect for particulate matter or discoloration.
• Withdraw desired volume from each vial and inject into 100 ml 0.9% NaCl and place into a UV protectant bag.
• Do not give by IV push or bolus.
• Infuse over 2 hours.
• Use separate line equipped with a low protein binding 1.2-micron filter.
• Administer through peripheral or central line.

Intervention and Evaluation

• Monitor the patient's blood chemistries, complete blood count (CBC), and liver function studies.
• Assess the patient for signs and symptoms of anemia, including excessive fatigue and weakness, and myelosuppression, including easy bruising, fever, signs of local infection, sore throat, or unusual bleeding from any site.
• Evaluate the patient for signs and symptoms of stomatitis.
• Monitor the patient's blood pressure (B/P) for evidence of hypertension or hypotension.

Patient Teaching

• Stress to the patient that he or she should not receive vaccinations and should avoid contact with anyone who recently received a live virus vaccine.

• Warn the patient to notify the physician if he or she experiences easy bruising, fever, signs of local infection, sore throat, or unusual bleeding from any site.

imatinib mesylate
ih-**mah**-tin-ib
(Gleevec, Glivec[AUS])

CATEGORY AND SCHEDULE
Pregnancy Risk Category: D

MECHANISM OF ACTION
An antineoplastic that inhibits the Bcr-Abl tyrosine kinase, a translocation-created enzyme, created by the Philadelphia chromosome abnormality noted in chronic myeloid leukemia (CML). *Therapeutic Effect:* Inhibits proliferation and inhibiting tumor growth during the three stages of CML, including CML in myeloid blast crisis, CML in accelerated phase, and CML in chronic phase.

PHARMACOKINETICS
Well absorbed after PO administration. Binds to plasma proteins, particularly albumin. Metabolized in the liver. Eliminated mainly in the feces as metabolites. **Half-life:** 18 hrs.

AVAILABILITY
Tablets: 100 mg, 400 mg.

INDICATIONS AND DOSAGES
▸ **Chronic myeloid leukemia (CML)**
PO
Adults, Elderly. 400 mg/day for patients in chronic-phase CML; 600 mg/day for patients in accelerated

phase or blast crisis. May increase dose 400–600 mg/day in patients in chronic phase or 600–800 mg (given as 400 mg twice/day) in patients in accelerated phase/blast crisis in absence of severe drug reaction or severe neutropenia or thrombocytopenia in the following circumstances: progression of the disease, failure to achieve satisfactory hematologic response after 3 months or more of treatment, or loss of previously achieved hematologic response.
Children. 260 mg/m^2 a day as a single daily dose or 2 divided doses.

CONTRAINDICATIONS
Known hypersensitivity to imatinib

INTERACTIONS
Drug
Calcium channel blockers, dihydropyridine, simvastatin, triazolobenzodiazepines: Increase the blood concentration of these drugs.
Carbamazepine, dexamethasone, phenobarbital, phenytoin, rifampicin: Decrease imatinib plasma concentration.
Clarithromycin, erythromycin, itraconazole, ketoconazole: Increase imatinib plasma concentration.
Cyclosporine, pimozide: May alter the therapeutic effects of these drugs.
Warfarin: Reduces the effect of warfarin.
Herbal
St. John's wort: Decreases imatinib concentration.
Food
None known.

DIAGNOSTIC TEST EFFECTS
May increase serum bilirubin and transaminase levels. May decrease

platelet count, serum potassium level, and white blood cell (WBC) count.

SIDE EFFECTS
Frequent (68%–24%)
Nausea, diarrhea, vomiting, headache, fluid retention (periorbital, lower extremities), rash, musculoskeletal pain, muscle cramps, arthralgia
Occasional (23%–10%)
Abdominal pain, cough, myalgia, fatigue, pyrexia, anorexia, dyspepsia (heartburn, gastric upset), constipation, night sweats, pruritus
Rare (less than 10%)
Nasopharyngitis, petechiae, weakness, epistaxis

SERIOUS REACTIONS
• Severe fluid retention manifested as pleural effusion, pericardial effusion, pulmonary edema, and ascites, and hepatotoxicity occur rarely.
• Neutropenia and thrombocytopenia are expected responses to the drug.
• Respiratory toxicity, manifested as dyspnea and pneumonia, may occur.

NURSING CONSIDERATIONS
Baseline Assessment
• Expect to obtain the patient's complete blood count (CBC) weekly for first month, biweekly for second month, and periodically thereafter.
• Monitor the patient's liver function tests, including serum alkaline phosphatase, bilirubin, and transaminase, before imatinib treatment begins and monthly thereafter.
Lifespan Considerations
• Be aware that imatinib has the potential for severe teratogenic effects. Female patients should

avoid breast-feeding while taking this drug.
• Be aware that the safety and efficacy of imatinib have not been established in children.
• In the elderly, there is an increased frequency of fluid retention noted.
Precautions
• Use cautiously in patients with liver or renal impairment.
Administration and Handling
PO
• Give imatinib with a meal and a large glass of water.
Intervention and Evaluation
• Assess the patient's eye area and lower extremities for early evidence of fluid retention.
• Weigh and monitor the patient for unexpected rapid weight gain.
• Administer antiemetics, if ordered, to the patient to control nausea and vomiting.
• Assess the patient's pattern of daily bowel activity and stool consistency.
• Monitor the patient's complete blood count (CBC) for evidence of neutropenia and thrombocytopenia and liver function tests for hepatotoxicity. Duration of neutropenia and thrombocytopenia ranges from 2 to 4 weeks.
Patient Teaching
• Stress to the patient that he or she should not receive vaccinations and should avoid contact with anyone who recently received a live virus vaccine, crowds, and those with known infection.
• Instruct the patient to take imatinib with food and a full glass of water.

rituximab
rye-**tucks**-ih-mab
(Mabthera[AUS], Rituxan)

CATEGORY AND SCHEDULE
Pregnancy Risk Category: C

MECHANISM OF ACTION
A monoclonal antibody and antineoplastic agent that binds to CD20, the antigen found on surface of B lymphocytes and B-cell non-Hodgkin's lymphomas. *Therapeutic Effect:* Produces cytotoxicity, reducing tumor size.

PHARMACOKINETICS
Rapidly depletes B cells. **Half-life:** 59.8 hrs after first infusion and 174 hrs after fourth infusion.

AVAILABILITY
Injection: 10 mg/ml.

INDICATIONS AND DOSAGES
▸ **Non-Hodgkin's lymphoma**
IV infusion
Adults. 375 mg/m^2 given once weekly for 4–8 wks. May be retreated with second 4-wk course.

CONTRAINDICATIONS
Hypersensitivity to murine proteins

INTERACTIONS
Drug
None known.
Herbal
None known.
Food
None known.

DIAGNOSTIC TEST EFFECTS
None known.

IV INCOMPATIBILITIES
Do not mix with any other medications.

SIDE EFFECTS
Frequent
Fever (49%), chills (32%), asthenia (16%), headache (14%), angioedema (13%), hypotension (10%), nausea (18%), rash or pruritus (10%)
Occasional (less than 10%)
Myalgia, dizziness, abdominal pain, throat irritation, vomiting, neutropenia, rhinitis, bronchospasm, urticaria

SERIOUS REACTIONS
• Hypersensitivity reaction, producing hypotension, bronchospasm, and angioedema, may occur.
• Arrhythmias may occur, particularly in those with history of preexisting cardiac conditions.

NURSING CONSIDERATIONS
Baseline Assessment
• Pretreat the patient with acetaminophen and diphenhydramine, as prescribed, before each infusion to help prevent infusion-related effects.
• Expect to obtain the patient's complete blood count (CBC) at regular intervals during therapy.
Lifespan Considerations
• Be aware that rituximab has the potential to cause fetal B-cell depletion.
• Be aware that it is unknown if rituximab is distributed in breast milk.
• Know that female patients with childbearing potential should use contraceptive methods during treatment and up to 12 months following therapy.
• Be aware that the safety and efficacy of rituximab have not been established in children.

• There are no age-related precautions noted in the elderly.

Precautions

• Use cautiously in patients with a history of cardiac disease.

Administration and Handling

◄ALERT► Know that pretreatment with acetaminophen and diphenhydramine before each infusion may prevent infusion-related effects.

◄ALERT► Do not give by IV push or bolus.

IV

• Refrigerate vials.

• Store diluted solution for up to 24 hours refrigerated and at room temperature for an additional 12 hours.

• Dilute with 0.9% NaCl or D_5W to provide a final concentration of 1 to 4 mg/ml into infusion bag.

• Infuse at rate of 50 mg/hr. Increase infusion rate, as necessary, in 50 mg/hr increments every 30 minutes to maximum 400 mg/hr.

• Subsequent infusion can be given at 100 mg/hr and increased by 100 mg/hr increments every 30 minutes to maximum 400 mg/hr.

Intervention and Evaluation

• Monitor the patient for an infusion-related symptoms complex consisting mainly of chills, fever, and rigors that generally occurs 30 minutes to 2 hours after beginning the first rituximab infusion. Slowing the infusion resolves these symptoms.

Patient Teaching

• Instruct female patients of childbearing age to use contraceptive methods during rituximab treatment and up to 12 months following therapy.

• Advise the patient to immediately report chills, fever, or rigors.

tositumomab and iodine 131 I-tositumomab

toe-sit-**two**-mo-mab
(Bexxar)

CATEGORY AND SCHEDULE

Pregnancy Risk Category: X

MECHANISM OF ACTION

A monoclonal antibody composed of an antibody conjoined with a radiolabeled antitumor antibody. The antibody portion binds specifically to the CD20 antigen, found on the pre-B and B lymphocytes. It is also found on more than 90% of B-cell Non-Hodgkin lymphoma, resulting in formation of a complex. *Therapeutic Effect:* Induces cytotoxicity and cell death associated with ionizing radiation from the radioisotope.

PHARMACOKINETICS

Depletes circulating CD20 positive cells. Elimination of iodine 131 occurs by decay and excretion in the urine. **Half-life:** 8 days. Patients with high tumor burden, splenomegaly, or bone marrow involvement have a faster clearance, shorter half-life, larger volume of distribution.

AVAILABILITY

Tositumomab
Injection: 14 mg/ml.
Iodine ^{131}I-Tositumomab
Injection: 0.1 mg/ml, 1.1 mg/ml.

INDICATIONS AND DOSAGES

▶ **Non-Hodgkin's lymphoma**
IV infusion
Adults 60 yrs and older. 9 mg/m^2 repeat in 14 days for total of 2 doses.

◀**ALERT**▶ Diphenhydramine 50 mg and acetaminophen 650-1000 mg given 1 hr prior to administering; follow by acetaminophen 650-1000 mg q4h for 2 doses, then q4h as needed. Full recovery from hematological toxicities is not a requirement for giving second dose.

CONTRAINDICATIONS

Hypersensitivity to murine proteins

INTERACTIONS
Drug

Anticoagulants, medications that interfere with platelet function: Due to occurrence of severe and prolonged thrombocytopenia, the benefits of these drugs should be weighed against the increased risk of bleeding and hemorrhage.
Herbal
None known.
Food
None known.

DIAGNOSTIC TEST EFFECTS

May decrease blood Hct and Hgb, platelet count, thyroid stimulating hormone, and white blood cell (WBC) count.

SIDE EFFECTS

Frequent (46%–18%)
Asthenia (loss of strength, energy), fever, nausea, cough, chills
Occasional (17%–10%)
Rash, headache, abdominal pain, vomiting, anorexia, myalgia, diarrhea, pharyngitis, arthralgia, rhinitis, pruritus
Rare (9%–5%)
Peripheral edema, diaphoresis, constipation, dyspepsia, such as heartburn and epigastric distress, back pain, hypotension, vasodilation, dizziness, somnolence

SERIOUS REACTIONS

• Infusion toxicity characterized by fever, rigors, diaphoresis, hypotension, dyspnea, and nausea occurs during or within 48 hrs of infusions.
• Severe, prolonged myelosuppression occurs in 71% of all patients and is characterized by neutropenia, anemia, and thrombocytopenia.
• Sepsis occurs in 45% of patients.
• Hemorrhage occurs in 12% of patients.
• Myelodysplastic syndrome occurs in 8% of patients.

NURSING CONSIDERATIONS
Baseline Assessment
• Pre-treat the patient, as prescribed, with acetaminophen and diphenhydramine before administering the infusion to help prevent infusion-related side effects.
• Plan to obtain the patient's baseline complete blood count (CBC) before beginning therapy and at least weekly following administration for a minimum of 10 weeks.
• Use strict aseptic technique to protect the patient from infection.
• Follow radiation safety protocols.
• Know that time to nadir is 4 to 7 weeks and the duration of cytopenias is approximately 30 days.
Lifespan Considerations
• Be aware that use of the iodine[131]I-tositumomab component is contraindicated during pregnancy and causes severe, possibly irreversible hypothyroidism in neonates.
• Be aware that radioiodine is excreted in breast milk. Breast-feeding should be avoided in this patient population.
• Be aware that the safety and efficacy of this drug have not been established in children.
• Be aware that the response rate and duration of severe hematologic

toxicity is lower in elderly patients older than 65 years of age.

Precautions

• Use cautiously in patients with active systemic infection, immuno-suppression, and impaired renal function.

Administration and Handling

◀ **ALERT** ▶ Be aware that the regimen consists of 4 components given in 2 separate steps: the dosimetric step, followed 7 to 14 days later by a therapeutic step. When infusing, use IV tubing with an in-line 0.22 micron filter and use the same tubing throughout the entire dosimetric or therapeutic step because changing the filter results in drug loss. Plan to reduce infusion rate by 50% for mild to moderate infusion toxicity; interrupt infusion for severe infusion toxicity. Expect to resume therapy at 50% reduction rate of infusion when resolution of toxicity occurs.

◀ **ALERT** ▶ Initiate thyroid protective agents, such as potassium iodide, 24 hours before administration of iodine ^{131}I-tositumomab dosimetric step and continue until 2 weeks following administration of the iodine ^{131}I-tositumomab therapeutic step, as prescribed. Plan to pre-treat the patient against infusion reactions with 650 mg acetaminophen and 50 mg diphenhydramine 30 min before beginning therapy.

◀ **ALERT** ▶ Remember that reconstitution amounts and rates of administration are the same for both dosimetric and therapeutic step.

IV

• Refrigerate tositumomab vials before dilution. Protect from strong light.

• Following dilution, tositumomab solution is stable for 24 hours if refrigerated, up to 8 hours at room temperature. Discard any unused portion left in the vial. Do not shake.

• Reconstitute 450 mg tositumomab in 50 ml 0.9% NaCl.

• Infuse tositumomab over 60 minutes.

• Store iodine ^{131}I-tositumomab frozen until it is removed for thawing before drug administration.

• Thawed iodine ^{131}I-tositumomab doses are stable for 8 hours if refrigerated. Discard any unused portion.

• Reconstitute iodine ^{131}I-tositumomab in 30 ml 0.9% NaCl.

• Infuse iodine ^{131}I-tositumomab over 20 minutes.

Intervention and Evaluation

• Monitor the patient's lab values for possibly severe and prolonged anemia, neutropenia, and thrombocytopenia.

• Monitor the patient for signs and symptoms of anemia, including excessive tiredness, and weakness, hematologic toxicity, marked by chills, easy bruising, fever, and unusual bleeding from any site, and hypothyroidism.

Patient Teaching

• Caution the female patient against becoming pregnant while receiving this drug. Explain to the patient that this drug is pregnancy risk category X.

• Stress to the patient that he or she should not receive immunizations without the physician's prior approval as this drug lowers the body's resistance. Tell the patient to avoid contact with those who recently received a live virus vaccine.

• Warn the patient to notify the physician if he or she experiences easy bruising, fever, signs of local infection, sore throat, or unusual bleeding from any site.

trastuzumab
traz-**two**-zoo-mab
(Herceptin)

CATEGORY AND SCHEDULE
Pregnancy Risk Category: B

MECHANISM OF ACTION
A monoclonal antibody and antineoplastic agent that mediates antibody-dependent cellular cytotoxicity. *Therapeutic Effect:* Inhibits proliferation of human tumor cells that overexpress HER-2 (HER-2 protein overexpression is seen in 25%–30% of primary breast cancer patients).

PHARMACOKINETICS
Half-life: 5.8 days (Range: 1–32 days).

AVAILABILITY
Lyophilized Powder: 440 mg.

INDICATIONS AND DOSAGES
▸ **Breast cancer**
IV infusion
Adults, Elderly. Initially, 4 mg/kg as 30–90-min infusion, then weekly infusion of 2 mg/kg as 30-min infusion.

CONTRAINDICATIONS
Preexisting cardiac disease

INTERACTIONS
Drug
Cyclophosphamide, doxorubicin, epirubicin: May increase the risk of developing cardiac dysfunction.
Herbal
None known.
Food
None known.

DIAGNOSTIC TEST EFFECTS
None known.

IV INCOMPATIBILITIES
Avoid use with D_5W. Do not mix with any other medications.

SIDE EFFECTS
Frequent (greater than 20%)
Pain, asthenia, fever, chills, headache, abdominal pain, back pain, infection, nausea, diarrhea, vomiting, cough, dyspnea
Occasional (15%–5%)
Tachycardia, congestive heart failure (CHF), flu-like symptoms, anorexia, edema, bone pain, arthralgia, insomnia, dizziness, paresthesia, depression, rhinitis, pharyngitis, sinusitis
Rare (less than 5%)
Allergic reaction, anemia, leukopenia, neuropathy, herpes simplex

SERIOUS REACTIONS
• Cardiomyopathy, development of ventricular dysfunction, and CHF occur rarely.
• Pancytopenia may occur.

NURSING CONSIDERATIONS
Baseline Assessment
• Evaluate the patient's left ventricular function.
• Expect the patient to have a baseline echocardiogram, EKG, and multigated acquisition (MUGA) scan performed.
• Expect to obtain the patient's baseline and periodic complete blood count (CBC) at regular intervals during therapy.
Lifespan Considerations
• Be aware that it is unknown if trastuzumab is distributed in breast milk.
• Be aware that the safety and

efficacy of trastuzumab have not been established in children.

• In the elderly, age-related cardiac dysfunction may require cautious use.

Precautions

• Use cautiously in patients with previous cardiotoxic drug or radiation therapy to chest wall and those with known hypersensitivity to trastuzumab.

Administration and Handling

◀ALERT▶ Do not give as IV bolus or IV push. Do not use dextrose solutions.

IV

• Refrigerate vial.

• Reconstituted solution normally appears colorless to pale yellow.

• Solution is stable for up to 28 days if refrigerated after reconstitution with Bacteriostatic Water for Injection. If using Sterile Water for Injection without preservative, use immediately; discard unused portions.

• Reconstituted solution with 0.9% NaCl is stable for up to 24 hours if refrigerated.

• Reconstitute with 20 ml Bacteriostatic Water for Injection to yield concentration of 21 mg/ml.

• Add calculated dose to 250 ml 0.9% NaCl (do not use D_5W).

• Gently mix contents in bag.

• Give loading dose (4 mg/kg) over 90 minutes. Give maintenance infusion (2 mg/kg) over 30 minutes.

Intervention and Evaluation

• Frequently monitor the patient for signs and symptoms of deteriorating cardiac function.

• Assess the patient for asthenia, which is a loss of strength or energy. Assist the patient with ambulation if asthenia occurs.

• Monitor the patient for abdominal pain, back pain, chills, and fever.

• Offer antiemetics, if ordered, to the patient to treat any nausea or vomiting experienced.

• Assess the patient's pattern of daily bowel activity and stool consistency.

Patient Teaching

• Stress to the patient that he or she should not receive vaccinations and should avoid contact with anyone who recently received oral polio vaccine, crowds, and those with known infection.

20 Miscellaneous Antineoplastic Agents

abarelix
arsenic trioxide
asparaginase
BCG, intravesical
dacarbazine
etoposide, VP-16
interleukin-2
irinotecan
mitotane
mitoxantrone
pegaspargase
procarbazine
  hydrochloride
temozolomide
teniposide
topotecan

Uses: Miscellaneous antineoplastic agents have a wide range of specific uses. *Aldesleukin* is prescribed to treat metastatic renal cell carcinoma and metastatic melanoma. *Arsenic trioxide* is used in patients with acute promyelocytic leukemia who don't respond to other treatments. The enzyme *asparaginase* and its derivative *pegaspargase* are used to treat acute lymphocytic leukemia; asparaginase is also given with other drugs for lymphoma. *BCG, intravesical* is used to treat and prevent carcinoma in situ of the urinary bladder. *Dacarbazine* is used for metastatic malignant melanoma and, with other drugs, for Hodgkin's disease. The podophyllotoxins *etoposide* and *teniposide* are used in acute lymphocytic leukemia; etoposide is also used to treat testicular tumors, small-cell lung carcinoma, and other cancers. Of the deoxyribonucleic acid topoisomerase inhibitors, *irinotecan* is used for metastatic colon or rectal cancer, whereas *topotecan* is used for metastatic ovarian cancer and small-cell lung cancer. Because of its antiadrenal activity, *mitotane* is used to treat adrenocortical carcinoma as well as Cushing's syndrome. *Mitoxantrone* is not only helpful in leukemias and prostate cancer, but also in multiple sclerosis. *Procarbazine* is used primarily to treat advanced Hodgkin's disease. *Temozolomide* is prescribed for gliomas, metastatic melanoma, and some types of anaplastic astrocytoma.

Action: Because miscellaneous antineoplastic agents belong to many different subcategories, their mechanisms of action are diverse. For details, see the specific drug entries.

---

abarelix
ah-**bar**-eh-lex
(Plenaxis)

CATEGORY AND SCHEDULE
Pregnancy Risk Category: X

MECHANISM OF ACTION
A luteinizing hormone-releasing hormone (LHRH) antagonist that inhibits gonadotropin and androgen production by blocking gonadotropin releasing-hormone receptors in the pituitary. *Therapeutic Effect:* Suppresses luteinizing hormone, follicle stimulating hormone secre-

tion, reducing the secretion of testosterone by the testes.

AVAILABILITY

Powder for Injection: 113 mg kit containing 10 ml 0.9% NaCl, 18-gauge needle, 22-gauge needle.

INDICATIONS AND DOSAGES
▶ **Prostate cancer**
IM
Adults, Elderly. 100 mg on days 1, 15, 29 and every 4 weeks thereafter. Treatment failure can be detected by obtaining serum testosterone concentration prior to abarelix administration, day 19 and every 8 weeks thereafter.

CONTRAINDICATIONS
None known

INTERACTIONS
Drug
None known.
Herbal
None known.
Food
None known.

DIAGNOSTIC TEST EFFECTS
May increase SGOT (AST), SGPT (ALT), and serum triglyceride levels. May slightly decrease blood hemoglobin concentrations. Extended treatment may decrease bone mineral density.

SIDE EFFECTS
Frequent (79%–20%)
Hot flashes, sleep disturbances, breast enlargement, nipple tenderness
Occasional (17%–12%)
Back pain, constipation, peripheral edema, dizziness, headache, upper respiratory tract infection
Rare (11%–10%)
Diarrhea, nausea, urinary retention/

frequency, dysuria, urinary tract infection, fatigue

SERIOUS REACTIONS
• Serious or life-threatening allergic reaction characterized by periorbital edema, tightening of throat, tongue swelling, wheezing, shortness of breath, and low blood pressure occur rarely.

NURSING CONSIDERATIONS

Baseline Assessment
• Plan to perform a baseline EKG, to measure the QT interval, and calculate the QTc.
Lifespan Considerations
• Be aware that this drug is not for use in women or children.
Precautions
• Use cautiously in patients with asthma, eczema, hayfever, impaired liver or renal function, prolonged QT interval, and urticaria.
Administration and Handling
IM
• Shake abarelix vial gently before reconstituting.
• Withdraw 2.2 ml of 0.9% NaCl using 18-gauge needle and a 3-ml syringe.
• Insert the needle into the abarelix vial and inject the diluent.
• Before withdrawing the needle, remove 2.2 ml of air.
• Shake immediately for 15 seconds.
• Allow vial to stand for 2 minutes.
• Shake the vial again for 15 seconds and allow to stand again for 2 minutes.
• Tap the vial to reduce foaming and swirl the vial.
• Insert 18-gauge needle, invert the vial, and draw up some of the suspension into the syringe. Without removing the needle from the vial, re-inject it at any remaining solids

in the vial. Repeat this process until all solids are dispersed.
• Swirl the vial before withdrawal, then withdraw the entire contents, about 2.2 ml.
• Reconstitution will provide a concentration of 50 mg/ml and should be used within 1 hour of reconstitution.
• Exchange the 18-gauge needle with the 22-gauge needle and give entire suspension IM into the upper, outer quadrant of the buttock.
Patient Teaching
• Make sure the patient and care-giver know about preparing and injecting the drug, if the patient is to take it at home.
• Tell the patient about potential side effects, including hot flashes, sleep disturbances, breast enlarge-ment, and nipple tenderness.

interleukin-2 (aldesleukin)
in-tur-lew-kin
(IL-2, Proleukin)
Do not confuse with inter-feron 2.

CATEGORY AND SCHEDULE
Pregnancy Risk Category: C

MECHANISM OF ACTION
A biologic response modifier that acts as an antineoplastic and modi-fies human recombinant inter-leukin-2. *Therapeutic Effect:* Pro-motes proliferation, differentiation, recruitment of T and B cells, natural killer cells, thymocytes. Causes cytolytic activity in lymphocytes.

PHARMACOKINETICS
Primarily distributed into plasma, lymphocytes, lungs, liver, kidney, and spleen. Metabolized to amino acids in the cells lining the kidney. **Half-life:** 85 min.

AVAILABILITY
Powder for Injection: 22 million units (1.3 mg).

INDICATIONS AND DOSAGES
▶ **Metastatic melanoma, metastatic renal cell carcinoma**
IV
Adults older than 18 yrs. 600,000 units/kg q8h for 14 doses; rest 9 days, repeat 14 doses. Total: 28 doses. May repeat treatment no sooner than 7 wks from date of hospital discharge.

UNLABELED USES
Treatment of colorectal cancer, Kaposi's sarcoma, non-Hodgkin's lymphoma.

CONTRAINDICATIONS
Abnormal pulmonary function tests or thallium stress test, bowel is-chemia or perforation, coma or toxic psychosis longer than 48 hrs, gastrointestinal bleeding requiring surgery, intubation more than 72 hrs, organ allografts, pericardial tamponade, renal dysfunction re-quiring dialysis longer than 72 hrs, repetitive or difficult-to-control seizures, retreatment in those who experience the following toxicities: angina, myocardial infarction, recurrent chest pain with EKG changes, sustained ventricular tachycardia, uncontrolled or unre-sponsive cardiac rhythm distur-bances

INTERACTIONS
Drug
Antihypertensives: May increase hypotensive effect.
Cardiotoxic-, liver toxic-, nephro-toxic-, myelotoxic-producing

medications: May increase the risk of toxicity.

Glucocorticoids: May decrease the effects of interleukin.

Herbal

None known.

Food

None known.

DIAGNOSTIC TEST EFFECTS

May increase BUN, serum alkaline phosphatase, bilirubin, creatinine, and transaminase. May decrease serum calcium, magnesium, phosphorus, potassium, and sodium.

IV INCOMPATIBILITIES

Ganciclovir (Cytovene), pentamidine (Pentam), prochlorperazine (Compazine), promethazine (Phenergan)

IV COMPATIBILITIES

Calcium gluconate, dopamine (Intropin), heparin, lorazepam (Ativan), magnesium, potassium

SIDE EFFECTS

Side effects generally self-limiting and reversible within 2–3 days after discontinuation of therapy.

Frequent (89%–48%)

Fever, chills, nausea, vomiting, hypotension, diarrhea, oliguria or anuria, mental status changes, irritability, confusion, depression, sinus tachycardia, pain (abdomen, chest, back), fatigue, dyspnea, pruritus

Occasional (47%–17%)

Edema, erythema, rash, stomatitis, anorexia, weight gain, infection (urinary tract, injection site, catheter tip), dizziness

Rare (15%–4%)

Dry skin, sensory disorders (vision, speech, taste), dermatitis, headache, arthralgia, myalgia, weight loss, hematuria, conjunctivitis, proteinuria

SERIOUS REACTIONS

• Anemia, thrombocytopenia, and leukopenia occur commonly.

• GI bleeding and pulmonary edema occur occasionally.

• Capillary leak syndrome results in hypotension (less than 90 mm Hg or a 20 mm Hg drop from baseline systolic pressure) and extravasation of plasma proteins and fluid into extravascular space and loss of vascular tone. May result in cardiac arrhythmias, angina, MI, and respiratory insufficiency.

• Fatal malignant hyperthermia, cardiac arrest or stroke, pulmonary emboli as well as bowel perforation or gangrene, and severe depression leading to suicide have occurred in less than 1% of patients.

NURSING CONSIDERATIONS

Baseline Assessment

• Treat patients with bacterial infection and those with indwelling central lines with antibiotic therapy before beginning interleukin therapy.

• Confirm that the patient is neurologically stable with a negative CT scan before beginning interleukin therapy.

• Obtain results of blood chemistries (including electrolytes), chest x-ray, complete blood count (CBC), and liver and renal function tests before beginning interleukin therapy and every day thereafter.

Lifespan Considerations

• Be aware that interleukin use should be avoided in patients of either sex not practicing effective contraception.

• Be aware that the safety and efficacy of interleukin have not been established in children.

• In the elderly, age-related decreased renal function may require caution.

• Be aware that the elderly will not tolerate toxicity.

Precautions

• Use extremely cautiously in patients with normal thallium stress tests and pulmonary function tests who have history of prior cardiac or pulmonary disease.

• Use cautiously in patients with fixed requirements for large volumes of fluid (e.g., those with hypercalcemia) or a history of seizures.

Administration and Handling

◀ALERT▶ Withhold the drug in patients who develop moderate to severe lethargy or somnolence (continued administration may result in coma).

◀ALERT▶ Restrict interleukin therapy to patients with normal cardiac and pulmonary functions as defined by thallium stress testing, pulmonary function testing. Dosage is individualized based on the patient's clinical response and tolerance of the drug's adverse effects.

IV

• Refrigerate vials, do not freeze.

• Reconstituted solution is stable for 48 hours refrigerated or at room temperature (refrigerated preferred).

• Reconstitute 22-million-unit vial with 1.2 ml Sterile Water for Injection to provide concentration of 18 million units/ml. Do not use Bacteriostatic Water for Injection or 0.9% NaCl.

• During reconstitution, direct the Sterile Water for Injection at the side of vial. Swirl contents gently to avoid foaming. Do not shake. Bacteriostatic Water for Injection or NaCl should not be used to reconstitute because of increased aggregation.

• Further dilute dose in 50 ml D$_5$W and infuse over 15 minutes. Do not use an in-line filter.

• Solution should be warmed to room temperature before infusion.

• Monitor diligently for drop in mean arterial blood pressure (B/P), a sign of capillary leak syndrome (CLS). Continued treatment may result in edema, pleural effusion, mental status changes, and significant hypotension (less than 90 mm Hg or a 20 mm Hg drop from baseline systolic pressure).

Intervention and Evaluation

• Monitor the patient's CBC, electrolytes, liver function, platelets, pulse oximetry, renal function, and weight.

• Determine the patient's serum amylase concentration frequently during therapy.

• Discontinue interleukin at the first sign of hypotension and withhold the drug for moderate to severe lethargy (physician must decide whether therapy should continue).

• Assess the patient's mental status changes (irritability, confusion, depression) and weight gain or loss.

• Maintain strict intake and output protocols.

• Assess the patient for extravascular fluid accumulation evidenced by dependent edema and rales in lungs.

Patient Teaching

• Advise the patient that nausea may decrease during continued therapy.

• Instruct the patient to increase his or her fluid intake to protect against renal impairment.

• Warn the patient against receiving immunizations without the physician's approval as interleukin lowers the body's resistance.

• Urge the patient to avoid contact with those who have recently taken live virus vaccine.

arsenic trioxide
are-sih-nic try-**ox**-ide
(Trisenox)

CATEGORY AND SCHEDULE
Pregnancy Risk Category: D

MECHANISM OF ACTION
An antineoplastic that produces morphologic changes and DNA fragmentation in promyelocytic leukemia cells. *Therapeutic Effect:* Produces cell death.

AVAILABILITY
Injection: 1 mg/ml.

INDICATIONS AND DOSAGES
▸ **Acute promyelocytic leukemia (APL), induction treatment**
IV
Adults, Elderly. 0.15 mg/kg/day until bone marrow suppression occurs. Total induction dose should not exceed 60 doses.
▸ **Acute promyelocytic leukemia, consolidation treatment**
IV
Adults, Elderly. Consolidation treatment should begin 3–6 wks after completion of induction therapy. Give dose of 0.15 mg/kg/day for 25 doses up to 5 wks.

CONTRAINDICATIONS
None known

INTERACTIONS
Drug
Amphotericin B, diuretics: May produce electrolyte abnormalities.
Antiarrhythmics, thioridazine: May prolong QT interval in those taking these drugs.
Herbal
None known.

Food
None known.

DIAGNOSTIC TEST EFFECTS
May decrease Hgb levels, serum calcium levels, serum magnesium levels, platelet count, and white blood cell (WBC) count. May increase SGOT (AST) and SGPT (ALT) levels.

IV INCOMPATIBILITIES
Do not mix with any other medications.

SIDE EFFECTS
Expected (75%–50%)
Nausea, cough, fatigue, fever, headache, vomiting, abdominal pain, tachycardia, diarrhea, dyspnea
Frequent (43%–30%)
Dermatitis, insomnia, edema, rigors, prolonged QT interval, sore throat, pruritus, arthralgia, paresthesia, anxiety
Occasional (28%–20%)
Constipation, myalgia, hypotension, epistaxis, anorexia, dizziness, sinusitis
Occasional (15%–8%)
Ecchymosis, nonspecific pain, weight gain, herpes simplex, wheezing, flushing, increased sweating, tremor, hypertension, palpitations, dyspepsia, eye irritation, blurred vision, weakness, decreased breath sounds, rales
Rare
Confusion, petechiae, dry mouth oral candidiasis, incontinence, rhonchi

SERIOUS REACTIONS
• Seizures, gastrointestinal (GI) hemorrhage, renal impairment or failure, pleural or pericardial effusion, hemoptysis, and sepsis occur rarely.
• Prolonged QT interval, complete

atrioventricular (AV) block, unexplained fever, dyspnea, weight gain, and effusion are evidence of arsenic toxicity. If arsenic toxicity is apparent, arsenic trioxide treatment should be halted and steroid treatment instituted.

NURSING CONSIDERATIONS

Baseline Assessment
• Establish and monitor the patient's blood Hct and Hgb levels, platelet count, and WBC before and frequently during treatment.
• Determine if the patient is breastfeeding, pregnant, or planning to become pregnant, because arsenic trioxide may cause fetal harm.
Precautions
• Use cautiously in patients with cardiac abnormalities or renal impairment.
Administration and Handling
IV
◀ALERT▶ A central venous line is not required for drug administration; the drug may be infused through a peripheral line
• Store the drug at room temperature.
• Diluted solution is stable for 24 hours at room temperature, 48 hours if refrigerated.
• After withdrawing the drug from ampoule, dilute it with 100 to 250 ml D₅W or 0.9% NaCl.
• Infuse the solution over 1 to 2 hours. The duration of infusion may be extended up to 4 hrs.
Intervention and Evaluation
• Monitor the patient's complete blood count (CBC), liver function test results, and blood chemistry values. Check serum potassium levels because the patient is more likely to develop hypokalemia than hyperkalemia. Also check blood glucose levels. The patient is more

likely to develop hyperglycemia than hypoglycemia.
• Monitor the patient for any signs and symptoms of arsenic toxicity syndrome, including confusion, dyspnea, fever, muscle weakness, seizures, and weight gain.
Patient Teaching
• Advise the patient to avoid crowds and those with known infection.
• Warn the patient not to receive live virus vaccinations and to avoid contact with anyone who recently received a live virus vaccine.

asparaginase
ah-spa-**raj**-in-ace
(Elspar, Kidrolase[CAN], Leunase[AUS])

CATEGORY AND SCHEDULE
Pregnancy Risk Category: C

MECHANISM OF ACTION
Asparaginase is an enzyme that inhibits protein synthesis by deaminating asparagines, thus depriving tumor cells of this essential amino acid. *Therapeutic Effect:* Interferes with DNA, RNA, and protein synthesis in leukemic cells. Cell cycle-specific for G_1 phase of cell division.

PHARMACOKINETICS
Metabolized via slow sequestration by reticuloendothelial system. **Half-life:** 39–49 hrs IM; 8–30 hrs IV.

AVAILABILITY
Powder for Injection: 10,000 units.

INDICATIONS AND DOSAGES
▶ **Acute lymphocytic leukemia (ALL)**
IV
Adults, Elderly, Children (combina-

tion therapy). 1,000 units/kg/day for 10 days.
Adults, Elderly, Children (single drug therapy). 200 units/kg/day for 28 days.
IM
Adults, Elderly, Children (combination therapy). 6,000–10,000 units/m²/dose 3 times/wk for 3 wks.

UNLABELED USES
Treatment of acute myelocytic leukemia, acute myelomonocytic leukemia, chronic lymphocytic leukemia, Hodgkin's disease, lymphosarcoma, melanosarcoma, and reticulum cell sarcoma

CONTRAINDICATIONS
Hypersensitivity to *Eserichia coli*, pancreatitis

INTERACTIONS
Drug
Antigout medications: May decrease effect of antigout medications.
Live virus vaccines: May decrease patient's antibody response to vaccine, increase vaccine side effects, and potentiate virus replication.
Methotrexate: May block effects of methotrexate.
Steroids, vincristine: May increase disturbances of erythropoiesis, hyperglycemia, and risk of neuropathy.
Herbal
None known.
Food
None known.

DIAGNOSTIC TEST EFFECTS
May increase serum alkaline phosphatase, blood ammonia, serum bilirubin, BUN, blood glucose, activated partial thromboplastin time (APTT), platelet count, prothrombin time (PT), thrombin time (TT), serum uric acid, SGOT (AST), and SGPT (ALT) levels. May decrease blood-clotting factors, including antithrombin, plasma fibrinogen, and plasminogen, as well as blood levels of albumin, calcium, and cholesterol.

IV INCOMPATIBILITIES
None known. Consult pharmacy.

SIDE EFFECTS
Frequent
Allergic reaction, manifested as rash, urticaria, arthralgia, facial edema, hypotension, and respiratory distress; pancreatitis as evidenced by severe stomach pain with nausea and vomiting
Occasional
CNS effects, including confusion, drowsiness, depression, nervousness, and tiredness; stomatitis, as evidenced by sores in the mouth and on lips; hypoalbuminemia or uric acid nephropathy, manifested as swelling of the feet or lower legs; hyperglycemia
Rare
Hyperthermia, including fever or chills; thrombosis, seizures

SERIOUS REACTIONS
• Hepatotoxicity usually occurs within 2 weeks of initial treatment.
• There is an increased risk of allergic reaction, including anaphylaxis, after repeated therapy, and severe bone marrow depression.

NURSING CONSIDERATIONS

Baseline Assessment
◄ALERT► Be sure to keep antihistamines, epinephrine, and an IV corticosteroid readily available as well as oxygen equipment, before administering asparaginase.
• Assess baseline central nervous system function and expect to

obtain blood chemistry, complete blood count (CBC), and liver, pancreatic, and renal function tests and results before therapy begins and when longer than 1 week has elapsed between doses.

Lifespan Considerations

• Be aware that asparaginase use should be avoided during pregnancy, especially during the first trimester, and in patients who are breast-feeding.

• There are no age-related precautions noted in children and the elderly.

Precautions

• Use cautiously in patients with diabetes mellitus, existing or recent chickenpox, gout, herpes zoster, infection, liver or renal function impairment, or recent cytotoxic and radiation therapy.

Administration and Handling

◀ALERT▶ This drug's dosage is individualized based on clinical response and the patient's tolerance to adverse effects. When used in combination therapy, consult specific protocols for optimum drug dosage and sequence of drug administration.

◀ALERT▶ Asparaginase may be carcinogenic, mutagenic, or teratogenic. Handle with extreme care during preparation and administration. Urine should be treated as infectious waste. Asparaginase powder or solution may irritate the skin on contact. Wash the affected area for 15 minutes if contact occurs.

IM

• Add 2 ml 0.9% NaCl to 10,000 international units vial to provide a concentration of 5,000 international units/ml.

• Administer no more than 2 ml at any one site.

IV

• Refrigerate the powder for the injected form.

• Reconstituted solutions are stable for 8 hours if refrigerated.

• Gelatinous fiber-like particles may develop in the solution. If this occurs, remove the particles using a 5-micron filter during administration.

◀ALERT▶ Administer intradermal test dose (2 units) before beginning therapy or when longer than 1 week has elapsed between doses. Observe the patient for any appearance of erythema or of a wheal for 1 hour after drug administration.

• For a test solution reconstitute 10,000-units vial with 5 ml Sterile Water for Injection or 0.9% NaCl. Shake to dissolve. Withdraw 0.1 ml, inject into vial containing 9.9 ml of the same diluent for concentration of 20 units/ml.

• Reconstitute 10,000-units vial with 5 ml Sterile Water for Injection or 0.9% NaCl to provide a concentration of 2,000 units/ml.

• Shake gently to ensure complete dissolution. Vigorous shaking will produce foam and cause some loss of potency.

• For IV injection, administer asparaginase solution into the tubing of freely running IV solution of D_5W or 0.9% NaCl over at least 30 minutes.

• For IV infusion, further dilute with up to 1,000 ml D_5W or 0.9% NaCl.

Intervention and Evaluation

• As appropriate, monitor serum amylase levels frequently during therapy.

◀ALERT▶ Expect to discontinue asparaginase at the first sign or symptom of renal failure (oliguria, anuria) or pancreatitis, as evidenced by abdominal pain, nausea, and vomiting, or elevated serum amylase and lipase levels.

• Monitor the patient for signs and

symptoms of hematologic toxicity, manifested as easy bruising, fever, signs of local infection, sore throat, and unusual bleeding, as well as for signs and symptoms of anemia, including excessive fatigue and weakness.

Patient Teaching

• Advise the patient to increase his or her fluid intake to protect against any kidney problems.

• Explain to the patient that any nausea he or she experiences may decrease during therapy.

• Caution the patient to avoid contact with those who have recently received a live virus vaccine and to avoid receiving any immunizations without his or her physician's approval.

BCG, intravesical
(TheraCys, Tice BCG)

CATEGORY AND SCHEDULE
Pregnancy Risk Category: D

MECHANISM OF ACTION
An antineoplastic that promotes local inflammation reaction with histiocytic and leukocytic infiltration in urinary bladder. *Therapeutic Effect:* Promotes inflammatory effects associated with apparent elimination and reduction of superficial cancerous lesions of urinary bladder.

AVAILABILITY
Parenteral Vials: 50 mg, 81 mg

INDICATIONS AND DOSAGES
▶ **Intravesical treatment and prophylaxis for carcinoma in situ of urinary bladder**
Parenteral (TheraCys)
Adults, Elderly. One dose in 50 ml

0.9% sodium chloride once weekly for 6 wks, then one treatment at 3, 6, 12, 18 and 24 months after initial treatment. Begin 7–14 days after biopsy or transurethral resection.
Parenteral (Tice BCG)
Adults, Elderly. One dose in 50 ml 0.9% sodium chloride once weekly for 6 wks. May repeat once. Thereafter, continue monthly for 6–12 months.

CONTRAINDICATIONS
Compromised immune system, concurrent corticosteroid or immunosuppressive therapy, positive HIV virus, positive Mantoux test, undetermined fever or fever due to infection, urinary tract infection

INTERACTIONS
Drug
Bone marrow depressants, immunosuppressants: May decrease immune response, increase the risk of osteomyelitis and disseminated BCG infection.
Live virus vaccines: May decrease the patient's antibody response to the vaccine, increase the vaccine side effects, and potentiate virus replication.
Herbal
None known.
Food
None known.

DIAGNOSTIC TEST EFFECTS
None known.

SIDE EFFECTS
Frequent
Dysuria, urinary frequency, hematuria, hypersensitivity reaction, manifested as malaise, fever, chills
Occasional
Cystitis, urinary urgency, nausea, vomiting, anorexia, diarrhea, myalgia, arthralgia

SERIOUS REACTIONS
• Systemic BCG infection manifested as fever higher than 103°F or persistent fever higher than 101°F for more than 2 days, or severe malaise may occur.

NURSING CONSIDERATIONS

Baseline Assessment
• Establish the patient's baseline renal status.
• Plan to obtain a urine specimen for culture and sensitivity tests to rule out a urinary tract infection.
• Assess any medications that patient is taking concurrently, especially corticosteroids and immunosuppressants.
• Determine if the patient has a compromised immune system, fever, or is HIV positive.
• Instruct the patient to avoid drinking fluids within 4 hours of administration. Have the patient void immediately before the drug is given.

Administration and Handling
◀ALERT▶ Be aware that the drug contains live, attenuated mycobacteria. Treat the drug as infectious material, and use protective gear when reconstituting. Avoid contact with the drug if you are immunocompromised.
• Reconstitute powder immediately before administration. Discard within 2 hours of reconstitution.
• After adding diluent to powder, gently swirl the solution, or repeatedly inject and withdraw the solution from the vial until the solution is mixed. Avoid vigorous shaking that could cause foaming.
• Do not give intravenously or subcutaneously; plan to deliver drug by urethral catheter.

Intervention and Evaluation
• During the first hour of drug administration, ask the patient to roll from side to side, and from supine to prone at 15 minute intervals to allow the drug to come in contact with all areas of the bladder. Ask the patient to try to retain the solution for 2 hours.
• Instruct patients to sit while voiding after medication instillation, to avoid spraying or splashing the infected urine.
• Disinfect the patient's expelled urine for 6 hours postinstillation, with an equal volume 5% hypochlorite solution, undiluted household bleach, before flushing.
• Diligently monitor the patient's renal status.
• Assess the patient for dysuria, hematuria, urinary frequency, and urinalysis for bacterial urinary tract infection.
• Monitor the patient for BCG infection.

Patient Teaching
• Warn the patient to notify the physician if his or her symptoms persist or increase or if he or she experiences blood in urine, chills, fever, frequent urge to urinate, joint pain, nausea, painful urination, or vomiting.
• Advise the patient to get the physician's approval before receiving any immunizations during BCG treatment. Explain to the patient that the drug lowers the body's resistance.
• Caution the patient to avoid contact with those who have recently taken live virus vaccine.

dacarbazine

day-**car**-bah-zeen
(DTIC[CAN], DTIC-Dome)
**Do not confuse with Dicarbosil
or procarbazine.**

MECHANISM OF ACTION

An alkylating, antineoplastic
agent that forms methyldiazonium
ions, which attack nucleophilic
groups in DNA. Cross-links
DNA strands. *Therapeutic Effect:*
Inhibits DNA, RNA, and protein
synthesis.

PHARMACOKINETICS

Minimally crosses blood-brain
barrier. Protein binding: 5%.
Metabolized in liver. Excreted in
urine. **Half-life:** 5 hrs (half-life is
increased in those with impaired
renal function).

AVAILABILITY

Powder for Injection: 100-mg,
200-mg vials.

INDICATIONS AND DOSAGES

▸ **Malignant melanoma**
IV
Adults, Elderly. 2–4.5 mg/kg/
day for 10 days, repeated at
4-wk intervals, or 250 mg/m²
a day for 5 days, repeated
q3wks.
▸ **Hodgkin's disease**
IV
Adults, Elderly. Combination
therapy: 150 mg/m² a day for
5 days, repeated q4wks, or 375
mg/m² once, repeated q15 days.
Children. 375 mg/m² on days
1 and 15; repeat q28 days.

▸ **Solid tumors**
IV
Children. 200–470 mg/m²/day over
5 days q21–28 days.
▸ **Neuroblastoma**
IV
Children. 800–900 mg/m² as single
dose on day 1 of therapy q3–4wks
in combination therapy.

UNLABELED USES

Treatment of islet cell carcinoma,
neuroblastoma, soft tissue sarcoma

CONTRAINDICATIONS

Demonstrated hypersensitivity to
dacarbazine

INTERACTIONS

Drug
Bone marrow depressants: May
enhance myelosuppression.
Live virus vaccines: May potentiate
virus replication, increase vaccine
side effects, and decrease the pa-
tient's antibody response to vaccine.
Herbal
None known.
Food
None known.

DIAGNOSTIC TEST EFFECTS

May increase BUN, serum alkaline
phosphatase, SGOT (AST), and
SGPT (ALT) levels.

IV INCOMPATIBILITIES

Allopurinol (Aloprim), cefepime
(Maxipime), heparin, piperacillin/
tazobactam (Zosyn)

IV COMPATIBILITIES

Etoposide (VePesid), granisetron
(Kytril), ondansetron (Zofran),
paclitaxel (Taxol)

SIDE EFFECTS

Frequent (90%)
Nausea, vomiting, anorexia (occurs

within 1 hr of initial dose, may last up to 12 hrs)

Occasional

Facial flushing, paresthesia, alopecia, flu-like syndrome (fever, myalgia, malaise), dermatologic reactions, central nervous system (CNS) symptoms (confusion, blurred vision, headache, lethargy)

Rare

Diarrhea, stomatitis (redness or burning of oral mucous membranes, gum or tongue inflammation), photosensitivity

SERIOUS REACTIONS

• Bone marrow depression resulting in blood dyscrasias, such as leukopenia and thrombocytopenia, generally appears 2–4 wks after last dacarbazine dose.
• Liver toxicity occurs rarely.

NURSING CONSIDERATIONS

Baseline Assessment

• Hydrate the patient prior to treatment to avoid dehydration from vomiting.

Lifespan Considerations

• Be aware that dacarbazine use should be avoided during pregnancy, if possible, especially during the first trimester and that breastfeeding is not recommended in this patient population.
• The safety and efficacy of dacarbazine have not been established in children.
• In the elderly, age-related renal impairment may require dosage adjustment.

Precautions

• Use cautiously in patients with impaired liver function.

Administration and Handling

◀ALERT▶ Know that dacarbazine dosage is individualized based on the patient's clinical response and tolerance of the drug's adverse effects. When used in combination therapy, consult specific protocols for optimum dosage and sequence of drug administration.

◀ALERT▶ Give dacarbazine by IV push or IV infusion, as prescribed. Because dacarbazine may be carcinogenic, mutagenic, or teratogenic, handle the drug with extreme care during preparation and administration.

IV

• Protect from light; refrigerate vials.
• Discard if the color changes from ivory to pink because this indicates decomposition.
• Reconstituted solution containing 10 mg/ml is stable for up to 8 hours at room temperature or up to 72 hours if refrigerated.
• Store solution diluted with up to 500 ml D_5W or 0.9% NaCl for up to 8 hours at room temperature or up to 24 hours if refrigerated.
• Reconstitute 100-mg vial with 9.9 ml Sterile Water for Injection (19.7 ml for 200-mg vial) to provide concentration of 10 mg/ml.
• Give IV push over 2 to 3 minutes.
• For IV infusion, further dilute with up to 250 ml D_5W or 0.9% NaCl. Infuse over 15 to 30 minutes.
• Apply hot packs if a burning sensation, irritation, or local pain at the injection site occurs.
• Monitor for signs and symptoms of extravasation, including coolness, slight or no blood return at the injection site, and stinging, and swelling at the injection site.

Intervention and Evaluation

• Monitor the patient's erythrocyte, leukocyte, and platelet counts for evidence of bone marrow depression.
• Monitor the patient for signs and symptoms of hematologic toxicity including easy bruising, fever, signs

of local infection, sore throat, and unusual bleeding from any site.
Patient Teaching
• Advise the patient that the gastro-intestinal side effects are usually better tolerated after 1 to 2 days of treatment.
• Stress to the patient that he or she should not receive vaccinations and should avoid contact with anyone who recently received a live virus vaccine.
• Advise the patient to notify the physician if he or she experiences easy bruising, fever, signs of local infection, sore throat, and unusual bleeding from any site.
• Explain that the patient should notify the physician if nausea and vomiting persist at home.

etoposide, VP-16
eh-**toe**-poe-side
(Etopophos, VePesid)
Do not confuse with Pepcid or Versed.

CATEGORY AND SCHEDULE
Pregnancy Risk Category: D

MECHANISM OF ACTION
An epipodophyllotoxin that induces single- and double-stranded breaks in DNA. Cell cycle–dependent and phase specific with maximum effect on S, G_2 phase of cell division. *Therapeutic Effect:* Inhibits or alters DNA synthesis.

PHARMACOKINETICS
Variably absorbed from the gastro-intestinal (GI) tract. Rapidly distributed. Low concentrations in cerebrospinal fluid (CSF). Protein binding: 97%. Metabolized in liver. Primarily excreted in urine. Not removed by hemodialysis. **Half-life:** 3–12 hrs.

AVAILABILITY
Capsules: 50 mg.
Injection: 20 mg/ml.
Injection (water soluble): 100 mg/ml (Etopophos).

INDICATIONS AND DOSAGES
▸ **Refractory testicular tumors**
IV
Adults. Combination therapy: 50–100 mg/m^2/day on days 1 to 5 or 100 mg/m^2/day on days 1, 3, 5.
▸ **Small cell lung carcinoma**
PO
Adults. 2 times IV dose rounded to nearest 50 mg.
IV
Adults. Combination therapy: 35 mg/m^2 a day for 4 consecutive days up to 50 mg/m^2 a day for 5 consecutive days.
▸ **Usual pediatric dosage**
Children. 60–150 mg/m^2/day for 2–5 days q3–6wks.

UNLABELED USES
Treatment of acute myelocytic leukemia, AIDS-associated Kaposi's sarcoma, bladder carcinoma, Ewing's sarcoma, Hodgkin's and non-Hodgkin's lymphoma

CONTRAINDICATIONS
Pregnancy

INTERACTIONS
Drug
Bone marrow depressants: May increase bone marrow depression.
Live virus vaccines: May potentiate virus replication, increase vaccine side effects, and decrease the patient's antibody response to vaccine.
Herbal
None known.
Food
None known.

DIAGNOSTIC TEST EFFECTS
None known.

IV INCOMPATIBILITIES
Cefepime (Maxipime), filgrastim (Neupogen), idarubicin (Idamycin). Etopophos: amphotericin (Fungizone), cefepime (Maxipime), chlorpromazine (Thorazine), methylprednisolone (Solu-Medrol), prochlorperazine (Compazine)

IV COMPATIBILITIES
Carboplatin (Paraplatin), cisplatin (Platinol), cytarabine (Cytosar), daunorubicin (Cerubidine), doxorubicin (Adriamycin), granisetron (Kytril), mitoxantrone (Novantrone), ondansetron (Zofran)

Etopophos

Carboplatin (Paraplatin), cisplatin (Platinol), cytarabine (Cytosar), dacarbazine (DTIC-Dome), daunorubicin (Cerubidine), dexamethasone (Decadron), diphenhydramine (Benadryl), doxorubicin (Adriamycin), granisetron (Kytril), magnesium sulfate, mannitol, mitoxantrone (Novantrone), ondansetron (Zofran), potassium chloride

SIDE EFFECTS
Frequent (66%–43%)
Mild to moderate nausea and vomiting, alopecia
Occasional (13%–6%)
Diarrhea, anorexia, stomatitis (redness or burning of oral mucous membranes, gum or tongue inflammation)
Rare (2% or less)
Hypotension, peripheral neuropathy

SERIOUS REACTIONS
• Bone marrow depression manifested as hematologic toxicity, principally anemia, leukopenia, and thrombocytopenia, and, to lesser extent, pancytopenia, may occur. Leukopenia occurs within 7–14 days after drug administration. Thrombocytopenia occurs within 9–16 days after administration. Bone marrow recovery occurs by day 20.
• Liver toxicity occurs occasionally.

NURSING CONSIDERATIONS
Baseline Assessment
• Monitor the patient's hematology test results before and at frequent intervals during etoposide therapy.
• Administer antiemetics, if ordered, to readily control nausea and vomiting.
Lifespan Considerations
• Be aware that etoposide use should be avoided during pregnancy, especially during the first trimester because of the risk of fetal harm and that breast-feeding is not recommended.
• Be aware that the safety and efficacy of etoposide have not been established in children.
• In the elderly, age-related renal impairment may require dosage adjustment.
Precautions
• Use cautiously in patients with bone marrow suppression and liver or renal impairment.
Administration and Handling
◄ALERT► Be aware that etoposide dosage is individualized based on the patient's clinical response and tolerance of the drug's adverse effects and that treatment is repeated at 3- to 4-week intervals.
◄ALERT► Administer etoposide by slow IV infusion. Wear gloves when preparing solution. If powder or solution comes in contact with skin, wash immediately and thoroughly with soap, water. Because etoposide may be carcinogenic, mutagenic, or teratogenic, handle the drug with

extreme care during preparation and administration.

PO

• Refrigerate gelatin capsules.

IV

• Store VePesid injection at room temperature before dilution.

• Know that VePesid concentrate for injection normally is clear, yellow.

• Reconstituted VePesid solution is stable at room temperature for up to 96 hours at 0.2 mg/ml and 48 hours at 0.4 mg/ml.

• Discard VePesid solution if crystallization occurs.

• Dilute each 100 mg (5 ml) of VePesid with at least 250 ml D_5W or 0.9% NaCl to provide a concentration of 0.4 mg/ml (500 ml for a concentration of 0.2 mg/ml).

• Infuse VePesid slowly, over 30 to 60 minutes. Rapid IV infusion may produce marked hypotension.

• Monitor the patient receiving VePesid for an anaphylactic reaction manifested as back, chest, or throat pain, chills, diaphoresis, dyspnea, fever, lacrimation, and sneezing.

• Refrigerate Etopophos vials.

• Etopophos is stable for up to 24 hours after reconstitution.

• Reconstitute each 100 mg of Etopophos with 5 to 10 ml Sterile Water for Injection, D_5W, or 0.9% NaCl to provide concentration of 20 mg/ml or 10 mg/ml, respectively.

• As desired, give Etopophos without further dilution or further dilute to concentration as low as 0.1 mg/ml with 0.9% NaCl or D_5W.

• Administer Etopophos over at least 5 minutes or up to 210 minutes, as appropriate.

Intervention and Evaluation

• Monitor the patient's blood Hgb and Hct levels and platelet and white blood cell (WBC) counts.

• Assess the patient's pattern of daily bowel activity and stool consistency.

• Monitor the patient for signs and symptoms of anemia, including excessive fatigue and weakness, and hematologic toxicity, including easy bruising, fever, signs of local infection, sore throat, or unusual bleeding from any site.

• Assess the patient for signs and symptoms of paresthesias and peripheral neuropathy.

• Monitor the patient for signs and symptoms of stomatitis manifested as burning or redness of the oral mucous membranes and gum or tongue inflammation.

Patient Teaching

• Explain to the patient that alopecia is reversible, but new hair growth may have a different color or texture.

• Stress to the patient that he or she should not receive vaccinations and should avoid contact with anyone who recently received a live virus vaccine.

• Warn the patient to notify the physician if he or she experiences easy bruising, fever, signs of local infection, sore throat, or unusual bleeding from any site.

irinotecan
eye-rin-**oh**-teh-can
(Camptosar)

CATEGORY AND SCHEDULE
Pregnancy Risk Category: C (first trimester), D (second and third trimester)

MECHANISM OF ACTION
This DNA topoisomerase inhibitor interacts with topoisomerase I, an enzyme, and relieves torsional strain

in DNA by inducing reversible single-strand breaks. Binds to topoisomerase-DNA complex preventing relegation of these single-strand breaks. *Therapeutic Effect:* Produces cytotoxic effect due to double-strand DNA damage produced during DNA synthesis.

PHARMACOKINETICS

After IV administration, metabolized to active metabolite in liver. Protein binding (metabolite): 95%. Excreted in urine and eliminated via biliary route. **Half-life:** 6 hrs (metabolite: 10 hrs).

AVAILABILITY

Injection: 20 mg/ml vial.

INDICATIONS AND DOSAGES
▶ **Carcinoma of colon and rectum with recurrent or progressive disease after 5-fluorouracil-based therapy**
IV infusion
Adults, Elderly. Initially, 125 mg/m² once weekly for 4 wks. Rest 2 wks. Additional courses may be repeated q6wks. Subsequent doses adjusted in 25–50 mg/m² increments as high as 150 mg/m², as low as 50 mg/m².

CONTRAINDICATIONS

None known

INTERACTIONS
Drug
Diuretics: May increase risk of dehydration from vomiting and diarrhea.
Laxatives: May increase severity of diarrhea.
Live virus vaccines: May potentiate virus replication, increase vaccine side effects, and decrease the patient's antibody response to vaccine.
Other myelosuppressants: May increase risk of myelosuppression.

Prochlorperazine: May increase akathisia.
Herbal
None known.
Food
None known.

DIAGNOSTIC TEST EFFECTS

May increase serum alkaline phosphatase and SGOT (AST) levels.

IV INCOMPATIBILITIES

Gemcitabine (Gemzar)

SIDE EFFECTS
Expected
Nausea (64%), alopecia (49%), vomiting (45%), diarrhea (32%)
Frequent
Constipation, fatigue (29%), fever (28%), asthenia (loss of strength, energy) (25%), skeletal pain (23%), abdominal pain, dyspnea (22%)
Occasional
Anorexia (19%), headache, stomatitis (18%), rash (16%)

SERIOUS REACTIONS

• Expect myelosuppression characterized as neutropenia in 97% of patients.
• Expect a neutrophil count less than 500/mm³ in 78% of patients.
• Thrombocytopenia, anemia, and sepsis occur frequently.

NURSING CONSIDERATIONS

Baseline Assessment
• Assess the patient's complete blood count (CBC), serum electrolytes, and hydration status before giving each irinotecan dose.
• Premedicate the patient with antiemetics on the day of irinotecan treatment, as prescribed, prior to at least 30 minutes before irinotecan administration.

Lifespan Considerations
• Be aware that irinotecan may cause fetal harm and it is unknown if irinotecan is distributed in breast milk. Also know that breast-feeding is not recommended in patients taking this drug.
• Be aware that the safety and efficacy of irinotecan have not been established in children.
• The risk of diarrhea is significantly increased in the elderly.

Precautions
• Use cautiously in patients previously receiving abdominal or pelvic irradiation as this increases the risk of myelosuppression.
• Use cautiously in elderly patients older than 65 years of age.

Administration and Handling
◀ALERT▶ As prescribed, begin a new irinotecan course when the patient's granulocyte count recovers to more than 1,500/mm^3, platelet count recovers to more than 100,000/mm^3, and treatment-related diarrhea fully resolves.

IV
• Store vials at room temperature, protect from light.
• Dilute in D$_5$W, which is the preferred method, or 0.9% NaCl to a concentration of 0.12 to 1.1 mg/ml for up to 48 hours if refrigerated.
• Reconstituted solution in D$_5$W is stable.
• Recommended for use within 24 hours if refrigerated or 6 hours if kept at room temperature.
• Do not refrigerate solution if diluted with 0.9% NaCl.
• Administer all doses as IV infusion over 90 minutes.
• Assess the patient for signs or symptoms of extravasation. If extravasation occurs, flush site with sterile water and apply ice.

Intervention and Evaluation
• Assess the patient for early signs and symptoms of diarrhea, usually preceded by abdominal cramping and complaints of diaphoresis.
• Monitor the patient's blood Hgb levels, CBC, and electrolytes. Also assess the patient's hydration status, including intake and output.
• Monitor the patient's infusion site for signs and symptoms of inflammation.
• Examine the patient's skin for evidence of rash.
• Offer the patient and family emotional support.

Patient Teaching
• Teach the patient how to recognize signs and symptoms of electrolyte depletion and dehydration.
• Advise the patient to use an antiemetic or antidiarrheal regimen if prescribed.
• Stress to the patient that he or she should not receive vaccinations and should avoid contact with anyone who recently received a live virus vaccine, crowds, and those with known infection.
• Explain to the patient that hair loss may occur.

mitotane
my-tow-tain
(Lysodren)

CATEGORY AND SCHEDULE
Pregnancy Risk Category: C

MECHANISM OF ACTION
A hormonal agent that inhibits activity of the adrenal cortex. *Therapeutic Effect:* Suppresses functional and nonfunctional adrenocortical neoplasms by direct cytoxic effect.

AVAILABILITY
Tablets: 500 mg.

INDICATIONS AND DOSAGES
▶ **Adrenocortical carcinomas**
PO
Adults, Elderly. Initially, 2–6 g/day in 3–4 divided doses. Increase by 2–4 g/day every 3–7 days up to 9–10 g/day. Range: 2–16 g/day.

UNLABELED USES
Treatment of Cushing's syndrome

CONTRAINDICATIONS
Known hypersensitivity to mitotane

INTERACTIONS
Drug
Central nervous system (CNS) depressants: May increase CNS depression.
Herbal
None known.
Food
None known.

DIAGNOSTIC TEST EFFECTS
May decrease plasma cortisol, urinary 17-OH, protein-bound iodine (PBI), and serum uric acid.

SIDE EFFECTS
Frequent (greater than 15%)
Anorexia, nausea, vomiting, diarrhea, lethargy, somnolence, adrenocortical insufficiency, dizziness, vertigo, maculopapular rash, hypouricemia
Occasional (less than 15%)
Blurred or double vision, retinopathy, decreased hearing, excessive salivation, urine abnormalities (hematuria, cystitis, albuminuria) hypertension, orthostatic hypotension, flushing, wheezing, shortness of breath, generalized aching, fever

SERIOUS REACTIONS
• Brain damage and functional impairment may occur with long-term, high dosage therapy.

NURSING CONSIDERATIONS
Baseline Assessment
• Discontinue mitotane therapy immediately following shock or trauma as the drug produces adrenal suppression.
• Expect to initiate steroid replacement therapy during therapy.
Precautions
• Use cautiously in patients with impaired liver function.
Administration and Handling
◀ **ALERT** ▶ Mitotane may be carcinogenic, mutagenic, or teratogenic. Handle with extreme care during administration.
Intervention and Evaluation
• Monitor the patient's liver function, serum uric acid levels, and urine tests.
• Perform neurologic and behavioral assessments periodically in patients receiving prolonged therapy (over 2 years).
• Assess the patient's pattern of daily bowel activity and stool consistency.
• Assess the patient's skin for maculopapular rash.
Patient Teaching
• Warn the patient to immediately notify the physician if he or she experiences infection, injury, or other illnesses.
• Stress to the patient that he or she should not receive vaccinations as mitotane lowers the body's resistance.
• Urge the patient to increase his or her fluid intake to help protect against urine abnormalities.
• Advise the patient to notify the physician if nausea and vomiting continue at home.

• Warn the patient to avoid tasks that require mental alertness or motor skills as dizziness and drowsiness may occur.

• Advise the patient that contraception is recommended during therapy. Teach the patient about various forms of contraception.

• Caution the patient to notify the physician if he or she experiences darkening of the skin, diarrhea, depression, loss of appetite, or rash.

mitoxantrone
my-toe-**zan**-trone
(Novantrone, Onkotrone[AUS])

CATEGORY AND SCHEDULE
Pregnancy Risk Category: D

MECHANISM OF ACTION
An anthracenedione that inhibits DNA and RNA synthesis. Active throughout entire cell cycle. *Therapeutic Effect:* Inhibits B-cell, T-cell, and macrophage proliferation. Causes cell death.

PHARMACOKINETICS
Protein binding: 78%. Widely distributed. Metabolized in liver. Primarily eliminated in feces via biliary system. Not removed by hemodialysis. **Half-life:** 2.3–13 days.

AVAILABILITY
Injection: 2 mg/ml.

INDICATIONS AND DOSAGES
▸ **Leukemias**
IV
Adults, Elderly, Children older than 2 yrs. 12 mg/m^2/day once a day for 2–3 days.

Children younger than 2 yrs. 0.4 mg/kg/day once a day for 3–5 days.
▸ **Acute leukemia in relapse**
Adults, Elderly, Children older than 2 yrs. 8–12 mg/m^2/day once a day for 4–5 days. Acute, nonlymphocytic leukemia (ANLL)
Adults, Elderly, Children older than 2 yrs. 10 mg/m^2/day once a day for 3–5 days.
▸ **Solid tumors**
IV
Adults, Elderly. 12–14 mg/m^2 once q3–4wks.
Children. 18–20 mg/m^2 once q3–4wks.
▸ **Multiple sclerosis**
IV
Adults, Elderly. 12 mg/m^2/dose q3mos.

UNLABELED USES
Treatment of breast carcinoma, liver carcinoma, non-Hodgkin's lymphoma

CONTRAINDICATIONS
Baseline left ventricular ejection fraction less than 50%, cumulative lifetime mitoxantrone dose 140 mg/m^2 or more, multiple sclerosis with liver impairment

INTERACTIONS
Drug
Antigout medications: May decrease the effects of these drugs.
Bone marrow depressants: May increase bone marrow depression.
Live virus vaccines: May potentiate virus replication, increase vaccine side effects, and decrease the patient's antibody response to vaccine.
Herbal
None known.
Food
None known.

DIAGNOSTIC TEST EFFECTS

May increase serum bilirubin and uric acid, SGOT (AST), and SGPT (ALT) levels.

IV INCOMPATIBILITIES

Heparin, paclitaxel (Taxol), piperacillin/tazobactam (Zosyn)

IV COMPATIBILITIES

Allopurinol (Aloprim), etoposide (VePesid), gemcitabine (Gemzar), granisetron (Kytril), ondansetron (Zofran), potassium chloride

SIDE EFFECTS

Frequent (greater than 10%)
Nausea, vomiting, diarrhea, cough, headache, stomatitis, abdominal discomfort, fever, alopecia
Occasional (9%–4%)
Easy bruising, fungal infection, conjunctivitis, urinary tract infection
Rare (3%)
Arrhythmias

SERIOUS REACTIONS

• Bone marrow suppression may be severe, resulting in gastrointestinal (GI) bleeding, sepsis, and pneumonia.
• Renal failure, seizures, jaundice, and congestive heart failure (CHF) may occur.

NURSING CONSIDERATIONS

Baseline Assessment

• Offer the patient and family emotional support.
• Assess the patient's baseline body temperature, complete blood count (CBC), as ordered, respiratory status including lung sounds, and pulse quality and rate.

Lifespan Considerations

• Know that mitoxantrone use should be avoided during pregnancy, if possible, especially during the first trimester because it can cause fetal harm. Also know that breast-feeding is not recommended in this patient population.
• Be aware that the safety and efficacy of mitoxantrone have not been established in children.
• There are no age-related precautions noted in the elderly.

Precautions

• Use cautiously in patients with impaired hepatobiliary function, preexisting bone marrow suppression, and previous treatment with cardiotoxic medications.

Administration and Handling

◀ALERT▶ Because mitoxantrone may be carcinogenic, mutagenic, or teratogenic, handle the drug with extreme care during preparation and administration. Give by IV injection, IV infusion following dilution before administration.

IV

• Store vials at room temperature.
• Dilute with at least 50 ml D_5W or 0.9% NaCl.
• Do not administer by subcutaneous, IM, intrathecal, or intra-arterial injection. Do not give IV push over less than 3 minutes. Give IV bolus over more than 3 minutes or intermittent IV infusion over 15 to 60 minutes. Administer continuous IV infusion of 0.02 to 0.5 mg/ml in D_5W or 0.9% NaCl.

Intervention and Evaluation

• Monitor the patient's hematologic status, liver and renal function test results, and pulmonary function studies.
• Monitor the patient for signs and symptoms of hematologic toxicity, including easy bruising, fever, signs of local infection, and unusual bleeding from any site, and stomatitis, including burning or erythema of oral mucosa, difficulty swallow-

ing, oral ulcerations, and sore throat.
• Evaluate the patient for signs and symptoms of extravasation including blue discoloration of skin, burning, pain, and swelling.
Patient Teaching
• Advise the patient that his or her urine will appear blue or green 24 hours after mitoxantrone administration. Explain to the patient that a blue tint to the sclera may also appear.
• Urge the patient to drink plenty of fluids to maintain adequate hydration and protect against renal impairment.
• Stress to the patient that he or she should not receive vaccinations and should avoid contact with crowds and those with known infection.
• Instruct the patient to use contraceptive measures during mitoxantrone therapy.

pegasparagase
peg-ah-spa-**raj**-ace
(Oncaspar)

CATEGORY AND SCHEDULE
Pregnancy Risk Category: C

MECHANISM OF ACTION
An enzyme that breaks down extracellular supplies of the amino acid asparagines that are necessary for survival of leukemic cells. Normal cells produce own asparagines. Binding to polyethylene glycol causes asparaginase to be less antigenic, less likely to cause hypersensitive reaction. *Therapeutic Effect:* Interferes with DNA, RNA, protein synthesis in leukemic cells. Cell cycle specific for G_1 phase of cell division.

AVAILABILITY
Injection: 7,500 international units/ml vial.

INDICATIONS AND DOSAGES
▶ **Acute lymphocytic leukemia**
IM/IV
Adults, Elderly, Children with a body surface area 0.6 m^2 or greater. 2,500 international units/m^2 every 14 days.
Children with a body surface area less than 0.6 m^2. 82.5 international units/kg every 14 days.

CONTRAINDICATIONS
Previous anaphylactic reaction or significant hemorrhagic event associated with prior L-asparaginase therapy, pancreatitis, history of pancreatitis

INTERACTIONS
Drug
Antigout medications: May decrease the effects of antigout medications.
Methotrexate: May block the effects of methotrexate.
Live virus vaccine: May potentiate virus replication, increase vaccine side effects, and decrease the patient's antibody response to vaccine.
Steroids, vincristine: May increase hyperglycemia, risk of neuropathy, disturbances of erythropoiesis.
Herbal
None known.
Food
None known.

DIAGNOSTIC TEST EFFECTS
May increase blood ammonia levels, blood glucose levels, BUN, uric acid levels, activated partial thromboplastin time (APTT), serum alkaline phosphatase, bilirubin, uric acid, thrombin time (TT), SGOT (AST), and SGPT (ALT) levels. May decrease blood clotting factors,

including plasma fibrinogen, anti-thrombin, and plasminogen, serum albumin, calcium, and cholesterol levels.

SIDE EFFECTS

Frequent

Allergic reaction, including rash, urticaria, arthralgia, facial edema, hypotension, and respiratory distress

Occasional

Central nervous system (CNS) effects, including confusion, drowsiness, depression, nervousness, and tiredness, stomatitis or sores to mouth or lips, hypoalbuminemia, uric acid nephropathy or pedal or lower extremity edema, hyperglycemia

Rare

Hyperthermia (fever or chills)

SERIOUS REACTIONS

• There is a risk of hypersensitivity reaction including anaphylaxis.
• An increased risk of blood coagulopathies occurs occasionally.
• Seizures occur rarely.
• Pancreatitis, evidenced by severe abdominal pain with nausea and vomiting, occurs frequently.

NURSING CONSIDERATIONS

Baseline Assessment

• Keep agents for adequate airway and allergic reaction readily available before giving and during administration.
• Closely monitor the patient following drug administration.
• Assess the patient's complete blood count (CBC), bone marrow tests, fibrinogen, liver, pancreatic, and renal function tests, prothrombin time (PT), partial thromboplastin time (pTT) before beginning the drug and when a week or more has elapsed between drug doses.

Precautions

• Use cautiously in patients concurrently taking aspirin or NSAIDs and those on concurrent anticoagulant therapy, and NSAIDs.

Administration and Handling

◀**ALERT**▶ Avoid inhalation of vapors. Wear gloves when handling pegasparagase and avoid contact with skin or mucous membranes (drug is a contact irritant). In case of contact, wash with copious amount of water for at least 15 minutes. Avoid excessive agitation of vial, do not shake. IM route preferred because of decreased risk of coagulopathy, gastrointestinal disorders, liver toxicity, and renal disorders.

• Refrigerate, do not freeze.
• Discard if cloudy, if precipitate is present, if stored at room temperature for longer than 48 hours, or if vial has been previously frozen because freezing destroys activity.
• Use one dose per vial, do not re-enter vial. Discard unused portion.

IM

• Administer no more than 2 ml at any one IM site.
• Use multiple injection sites if more than 2 ml is administered.

IV

• Add 100 ml 0.9% NaCl or D_5W and administer through an infusion that is already running.
• Infuse over 1 to 2 hours.

Intervention and Evaluation

• Monitor the patient's response and toxicity.
• Obtain the patient's serum amylase and lipase concentrations frequently during and following therapy for evidence of pancreatitis.
• Monitor the patient's BUN and serum creatinine for signs of renal failure.
• Discontinue the drug at the first sign of pancreatitis or renal failure.

• Monitor the patient for signs and symptoms of anemia, such as excessive fatigue and weakness, infection, and hematologic toxicity, including easy bruising, fever, signs of local infection, sore throat, and unusual bleeding.

Patient Teaching

• Urge the patient to increase his or her fluid intake to protect against renal impairment.

• Explain to the patient that nausea may decrease during therapy.

• Stress to the patient that he or she should not receive vaccinations and should avoid contact with anyone who recently received a live virus vaccine.

• Warn the patient to notify the physician if nausea and vomiting continue at home.

---

procarbazine hydrochloride

pro-**car**-bah-zeen
(Matulane, Natulan[CAN])
Do not confuse with dacarbazine.

CATEGORY AND SCHEDULE

Pregnancy Risk Category: D

MECHANISM OF ACTION

A methylhydrazine derivative that inhibits DNA, RNA, and protein synthesis. May also directly damage DNA. Cell cycle–specific for S phase of cell division. *Therapeutic Effect:* Cell death.

AVAILABILITY

Capsules: 50 mg.

INDICATIONS AND DOSAGES

▸ **Advanced Hodgkin's disease**
PO
Adults, Elderly. Initially, 2–4 mg/ kg/day as single or divided dose for 1 wk, then 4–6 mg/kg/day.

Maintenance: 1–2 mg/kg/day.
Children. 50–100 mg/m²/day for 10–14 days of a 28 day cycle. Continue until maximum response, leukocyte count falls below 4,000/ mm³, or platelets fall below 100,000/mm³. Maintenance: 50 mg/m²/day.

UNLABELED USES

Treatment of lung carcinoma, malignant melanoma, multiple myeloma, non-Hodgkin's lymphoma, polycythemia vera, primary brain tumors

CONTRAINDICATIONS

Inadequate bone marrow reserve

INTERACTIONS

Drug

Alcohol: May cause disulfiram reaction.

Anticholinergics, antihistamines: May increase anticholinergic effects of these drugs.

Bone marrow depressants: May increase bone marrow depression.

Buspirone, caffeine-containing medications: May increase blood pressure (B/P) with these drugs.

Carbamazepine, cyclobenzaprine, MAOIs, maprotiline,: May cause hyperpyretic crisis, seizures, or death with these drugs.

Central nervous system (CNS) depressants: May increase CNS depression.

Insulin, oral hypoglycemics: May increase the effects of these drugs.

Meperidine: May produce coma, convulsions, immediate excitation, rigidity, severe hypertension or hypotension, severe respiratory distress, sweating, and vascular collapse.

Sympathomimetics: May increase cardiac stimulant and vasopressor effects.

Tricyclic antidepressants: May increase anticholinergic effects, cause convulsions, and hyperpyretic crisis.

Herbal
None known.

Food
None known.

DIAGNOSTIC TEST EFFECTS
None known.

SIDE EFFECTS
Frequent
Severe nausea, vomiting, respiratory disorders (cough, effusion), myalgia, arthralgia, drowsiness, nervousness, insomnia, nightmares, sweating, hallucinations, seizures
Occasional
Hoarseness, tachycardia, nystagmus, retinal hemorrhage, photophobia, photosensitivity, urinary frequency, nocturia, hypotension, diarrhea, stomatitis, paresthesia, unsteadiness, confusion, decreased reflexes, foot drop
Rare
Hypersensitivity reaction (dermatitis, pruritus, rash, urticaria), hyperpigmentation, alopecia

SERIOUS REACTIONS
• Procarbazine's major toxic effects are bone marrow depression manifested as hematologic toxicity (mainly leukopenia, thrombocytopenia, anemia) and liver toxicity manifested as jaundice and ascites.
• Urinary tract infection (UTI) secondary to leukopenia may occur.
• Therapy should be discontinued if stomatitis, diarrhea, paresthesia, neuropathies, confusion, or hypersensitivity reaction occurs.

NURSING CONSIDERATIONS
Baseline Assessment
• Expect the patient to undergo bone marrow tests. Monitor the patient's leukocyte count, differential, platelet count, and reticulocyte count Also, check the results of the patient's urinalysis, blood Hgb and Hct levels, BUN, serum alkaline phosphatase and transaminase levels before beginning procarbazine therapy and periodically thereafter.
• Be aware that therapy should be interrupted if the patient's white blood cell (WBC) count falls below 4,000/mm^3 or platelet count falls below 100,000/mm^3.

Precautions
• Use cautiously in patients with impaired liver or renal function.

Intervention and Evaluation
• Monitor the results of the patient's hematologic tests and liver and renal function studies.
• Assess the patient for signs and symptoms of stomatitis, including burning or erythema of the oral mucosa at inner margin of lips, difficulty swallowing, oral ulceration, and sore throat.
• Monitor for the patient for signs and symptoms of anemia, including excessive fatigue and weakness, and hematologic toxicity, including easy bruising, fever, signs of local infection, sore throat, and unusual bleeding from any site.

Patient Teaching
• Warn the patient to notify the physician if he or she experiences bleeding, easy bruising, fever, or sore throat.
• Caution the patient to avoid consuming alcohol as it may cause a disulfiram reaction characterized by nausea, sedation, severe headache, visual disturbances, and vomiting.

temozolomide

teh-moe-**zoll**-oh-mide
(Temodal[AUS], Temodar)

CATEGORY AND SCHEDULE
Pregnancy Risk Category: D

MECHANISM OF ACTION
An imidazotetrazine derivative that acts as a prodrug, and is converted to highly active cytotoxic metabolite. Cytotoxic effect associated with methylation of DNA. *Therapeutic Effect:* Inhibits DNA replication, causing cell death.

PHARMACOKINETICS
Rapidly, completely absorbed after PO administration. Protein binding: 15%. Peak plasma concentration occurs in 1 hr. Weakly bound to plasma proteins. Penetrates across blood-brain barrier. Primarily eliminated in urine and, to a much lesser extent, in feces. **Half-life:** 1.6–1.8 hrs.

AVAILABILITY
Capsules: 5 mg, 20 mg, 100 mg, 250 mg.

INDICATIONS AND DOSAGES
▸ **Anaplastic astrocytoma**
PO
Adults. Initially, 150 mg/m² a day for 5 consecutive days of a 28-day treatment cycle. If myelosuppression is not severe on day 22, dose may increase to 200 mg/m² and be repeated at 4-wk intervals.

CONTRAINDICATIONS
Hypersensitivity to dacarbazine, pregnancy

INTERACTIONS
Drug
Live virus vaccines: May potentiate virus replication, increase vaccine side effects, and decrease the patient's antibody response to vaccine. *Valproic acid:* Decreases the clearance of temozolomide.
Herbal
None known.
Food
Food: Decreases the rate of absorption.

DIAGNOSTIC TEST EFFECTS
May decrease blood Hgb levels and neutrophil, platelet, and white blood cell (WBC) counts.

SIDE EFFECTS
Frequent (53%–33%)
Nausea, vomiting, headache, fatigue, constipation
Occasional (16%–10%)
Diarrhea, asthenia (loss of strength, energy), fever, dizziness, peripheral edema, incoordination, insomnia
Rare (9%–5%)
Paresthesia, drowsiness, anorexia, urinary incontinence, anxiety, pharyngitis, cough

SERIOUS REACTIONS
• Myelosuppression is characterized by neutropenia and thrombocytopenia with the elderly and women showing a higher incidence of developing severe myelosuppression. Usually occurs within the first few cycles; is not cumulative. Nadir occurs approximately 26–28 days, with recovery 14 days of nadir.

NURSING CONSIDERATIONS
Baseline Assessment
• Know that before dosing, the patient's absolute neutrophil count (ANC) must be 1,500/mm³ or higher and platelet count 100,000/ mm³ or higher.
• Administer antiemetics, as or-

dered, to control the patient's nausea and vomiting.

Lifespan Considerations
• Be aware that temozolomide use should be avoided during pregnancy. Although it's unknown if temozolomide is excreted in breast milk, the drug may cause fetal harm and produce malformation of external organs, soft tissue, and skeleton.
• Be aware that the safety and efficacy of temozolomide have not been established in children.
• Elderly patients older than 70 years of age may experience a higher risk of developing grade 4 neutropenia and grade 4 thrombocytopenia.

Precautions
• Use cautiously in patients with severe liver or renal impairment.

Administration and Handling
◀**ALERT**▶ Because temozolomide is cytotoxic, avoid touching the ingredients of an open capsule during preparation and administration.
• Administer temozolomide on an empty stomach because food reduces the drug's rate and extent of absorption as well as increases the risk of nausea and vomiting.
• For best results, give temozolomide at the patient's bedtime.
• Have the patient swallow the capsule whole with a glass of water. If the patient is unable to swallow, open temozolomide capsule and mix with applesauce or apple juice. Do not touch the ingredients of an open capsule as the drug is cytotoxic.

Intervention and Evaluation
• If ordered, obtain and monitor the results of the patient's complete blood count (CBC) on day 22, which is 21 days after the first dose, or within 48 hours of that day and then weekly until the ANC is 1,500/mm³ or higher and the platelet count is 100,000/mm³ or higher.

• Monitor the patient for signs and symptoms of anemia, including excessive fatigue and weakness, and hematologic toxicity, including easy bruising, fever, signs of local infection, sore throat, and unusual bleeding from any site.

Patient Teaching
• Advise the patient to take temozolomide on an empty stomach to reduce nausea and vomiting.
• Warn the patient not to touch the ingredients of open capsules and explain that the drug is cytotoxic.
• Warn the patient to notify the physician if he or she experiences easy bruising, fever, signs of local infection, sore throat, or unusual bleeding from any site.
• Caution women of childbearing age to avoid pregnancy while taking temozolomide. Teach the patient about effective contraception methods.
• Stress to the patient that he or she should not receive vaccinations and should avoid contact with crowds and those with known infection.

teniposide
ten-**ih**-poe-side
(Vumon)

CATEGORY AND SCHEDULE
Pregnancy Risk Category: D

MECHANISM OF ACTION
An epipodophyllotoxin that induces single and double stranded breaks in DNA, inhibiting or altering DNA synthesis. *Therapeutic Effect:* Prevents cells from entering mitosis. Phase specific acting in late S and early G_2 phases of cell cycle.

AVAILABILITY
Injection: 50 mg.

INDICATIONS AND DOSAGES
▸ **In combination with other anti-neoplastic agents, induction therapy in patients with refractory childhood acute lymphoblastic leukemia (ALL)**

Dosage is individualized based on the patient's clinical response and tolerance of the drug's adverse effects. When used in combination therapy, consult specific protocols for optimum dosage or sequence of drug administration.

CONTRAINDICATIONS
Absolute neutrophil count less than 500/mm^3, hypersensitivity to Cremophor EL (polyoxyethylated castor oil), etoposide, teniposide, platelet count less than 50,000/mm^3

INTERACTIONS
Drug
Bone marrow depressants: May increase bone marrow depression.
Live virus vaccines: May potentiate virus replication, increase vaccine side effects, and decrease the patient's antibody response to vaccine.
Methotrexate: May increase intracellular accumulation of this drug.
Vincristine: May increase severity of peripheral neuropathy with this drug.
Herbal
None known.
Food
None known.

DIAGNOSTIC TEST EFFECTS
None significant.

SIDE EFFECTS
Frequent (greater than 30%)
Mucositis, nausea, vomiting, diarrhea, anemia

Occasional (5%–3%)
Alopecia, rash
Rare (less than 3%)
Liver dysfunction, fever, renal dysfunction, peripheral neurotoxicity

SERIOUS REACTIONS
• Bone marrow depression manifested as hematologic toxicity (principally leukopenia, neutropenia, thrombocytopenia) with increased risk of infection or bleeding may occur.
• Hypersensitivity reaction including anaphylaxis (chills, fever, tachycardia, bronchospasm, dyspnea, facial flushing) may occur.

NURSING CONSIDERATIONS
Baseline Assessment
• Assess the patient's hematology, liver function tests, and renal function tests before beginning and frequently during teniposide therapy.
Precautions
• Use cautiously in patients with brain tumors, decreased liver function, Down's syndrome, and neuroblastoma (increases risk of anaphylaxis).
Administration and Handling
IV
• Refrigerate unopened ampoules.
• Protect from light.
• Reconstituted solutions are stable for 24 hours at room temperature.
• Discard if precipitation occurs.
• Use 1 mg/ml solutions within 4 hrs of preparation to reduce the potential for precipitation.
• Do not refrigerate reconstituted solutions.
• Wear gloves when preparing solution. If solution comes in contact with skin, wash immediately and thoroughly with soap, water.

• Dilute with 0.9% NaCl or D_5W to provide a concentration of 0.1 to 1 mg/ml.

• Prepare and administer in containers such as glass or polyolefin plastic bags or containers. Avoid use of PVC containers.

• Give over at least 30 to 60 minutes. Avoid rapid IV injection.

Intervention and Evaluation

• Have medication and supportive measures readily available for first dose as life threatening anaphylaxis characterized by bronchospasm, chills, dyspnea, facial flushing, fever, and tachycardia may occur.

• Monitor the patient for signs and symptoms of myelosuppression, including anemia, infection, and unusual bleeding or bruising.

Patient Teaching

• Stress to the patient that he or she should not receive vaccinations without physician approval and should avoid contact with crowds and anyone with known infection.

• Warn the patient to notify the physician if he or she experiences easy bruising, difficulty breathing, fever, signs of infection, or unusual bleeding from any site.

• Caution the patient to avoid becoming pregnant during teniposide therapy. Teach the patient about various methods of contraception.

• Explain to the patient that hair loss is reversible but new growth may have a different color or texture.

---

topotecan
toe-**poh**-teh-can
(Hycamtin)

CATEGORY AND SCHEDULE
Pregnancy Risk Category: D

MECHANISM OF ACTION
A DNA topoisomerase inhibitor that interacts with topoisomerase I, an enzyme, which relieves torsional strain in DNA by inducing reversible single-strand breaks. Binds to topoisomerase-DNA complex preventing relegation of these single-strand breaks. *Therapeutic Effect:* Double-strand DNA damage occurring during DNA synthesis produces cytotoxic effect.

PHARMACOKINETICS
Protein binding: 35%. After IV administration, hydrolyzed to active form. Excreted in urine. **Half-life:** 2–3 hrs (half-life is increased in those with impaired renal function).

AVAILABILITY
Powder for Injection: 4 mg (single-dose vial).

INDICATIONS AND DOSAGES
▸ **Carcinoma of ovary; small cell lung cancer**
IV infusion
Adults, Elderly. 1.5 mg/m² over 30 min a day for 5 consecutive days, beginning on day 1 of a 21-day course. Minimum of four courses recommended. If severe neutropenia occurs during treatment, reduce dose by 0.25 mg/m² for subsequent courses or as an alternative, give the medication following the subsequent course beginning day 6 of the course (24 hrs after completion of topotecan administration).
▸ **Dosage in renal impairment**
No dosage adjustment is necessary in patients with mild renal impairment with a creatinine clearance 40–60 ml/min. For moderate renal impairment with a creatinine clearance 20–39 ml/min, give 0.75 mg/m².

CONTRAINDICATIONS

Baseline neutrophil count less than 1,500 cells/mm³, breast-feeding, pregnancy, severe bone marrow depression

INTERACTIONS
Drug

Cisplatin: May increase severity of myelosuppression.

Live virus vaccines: May potentiate virus replication, increase vaccine side effects, and decrease the patient's antibody response to vaccine.

Other myelosuppressants: May increase risk of myelosuppression.

Herbal

None known.

Food

None known.

DIAGNOSTIC TEST EFFECTS

May increase serum bilirubin, SGOT (AST), and SGPT (ALT), levels. May decrease leukocyte count, neutrophil count, red blood cell (RBC) level, and thrombocyte (platelet) count.

IV INCOMPATIBILITIES

Dexamethasone (Decadron), fluorouracil, mitomycin (Mutamycin)

IV COMPATIBILITIES

Carboplatin (Paraplatin), cisplatin (Platinol AQ), cyclophosphamide (Cytoxan), doxorubicin (Adriamycin), etoposide (VePesid), gemcitabine (Gemzar), granisetron (Kytril), ondansetron (Zofran), paclitaxel (Taxol), vincristine (Oncovin)

SIDE EFFECTS

Frequent
Nausea (77%); vomiting (58%); diarrhea, total alopecia (42%); headache (21%); dyspnea (21%)

Occasional
Paresthesia (9%); constipation, abdominal pain (3%)
Rare
Anorexia, malaise, arthralgia, asthenia, myalgia

SERIOUS REACTIONS

• Severe neutropenia (less than 500 cells/mm³) occurs in 60% of patients and usually develops at median of 11 days after day 1 of initial therapy.
• Thrombocytopenia (less than 25,000/mm³) occurs in 26% of patients and severe anemia (less than 8 g/dl) occurs in 40% of patients, usually developing at median of 15 days after day 1 of initial therapy.

NURSING CONSIDERATIONS

Baseline Assessment

• Offer emotional support to the patient and family.
• Assess the patient's complete blood count (CBC), especially blood Hgb levels, and platelet count before each topotecan dose.
• Know that myelosuppression may precipitate life-threatening anemia, hemorrhage, and infection.
• If the patient's platelet count drops, minimize trauma to the patient (IM injections, rectal medications, patient positioning, etc.).
• Premedicate the patient with antiemetics, if ordered, on day of treatment, starting at least 30 minutes before topotecan administration.

Lifespan Considerations

• Be aware that topotecan may cause fetal harm and that patients taking topotecan should avoid pregnancy and breast-feeding.
• Be aware that the safety and efficacy of topotecan have not been established in children.

• In the elderly, age-related renal impairment may require dosage adjustment.

Precautions

• Use cautiously in patients with liver or renal impairment and mild bone marrow depression.

Administration and Handling

◀ **ALERT** ▶ As prescribed, do not give topotecan if the patient's baseline neutrophil count is less than 1,500 cells/mm^3 and platelet count is less than 100,000/mm^3.

IV

• Store vials at room temperature in original cartons.

• Reconstituted vials diluted for infusion are stable at room temperature in ambient lighting for up to 24 hours.

• Reconstitute each 4-mg vial with 4 ml Sterile Water for Injection.

• Further dilute with 50 to 100 ml 0.9% NaCl or D$_5$W.

• Administer all doses as IV infusion over 30 minutes.

• Be aware that extravasation is associated with only mild local reactions, such as bruising and erythema.

Intervention and Evaluation

• Monitor the patient's CBC, particularly blood Hgb and white blood cell (WBC) count with differential, and platelet count frequently during topotecan treatment for evidence of myelosuppression.

• Assess the patient for anemia, bleeding, and signs of infection.

• Monitor the patient's serum electrolyte levels, hydration status, and intake and output because diarrhea and vomiting are common side effects of topotecan administration.

• Assess the patient's therapeutic response to medication.

• Provide interventions to help the patient manage the drug's side effects, such as small, frequent meals and antiemetics to help prevent or treat nausea and vomiting.

• Assess the patient for the onset of headaches.

• Assess the patient's breathing pattern for evidence of dyspnea.

Patient Teaching

• Explain to the patient that alopecia is reversible but that new hair may have a different color or texture.

• Explain that diarrhea may develop late in therapy. Teach the patient to watch for signs and symptoms of dehydration and electrolyte depletion.

• If ordered, instruct the patient in the use of an antiemetic and antidiarrheal.

• Warn the patient to notify the physician if diarrhea and vomiting continue at home.

• Stress to the patient that he or she should not receive vaccinations and should avoid contact with anyone who recently received a live virus vaccine.

21 Angiotensin-Converting Enzyme (ACE) Inhibitors

benazepril
captopril
enalapril maleate
fosinopril
lisinoprll
moexipril
  hydrochloride
perindopril erbumine
quinapril
  hydrochloride
ramipril
trandolapril

Uses: Angiotensin-converting enzyme (ACE) inhibitors are used to treat hypertension and, as adjuncts, to treat congestive heart failure.

Action: ACE inhibitors act primarily by suppressing the renin-angiotensin-aldosterone system. (See illustration, *Site of Action: ACE Inhibitors,* page 412.) They reduce peripheral arterial resistance and increase cardiac output, but produce little or no change in the heart rate.

COMBINATION PRODUCTS

ACCURETIC: quinapril/hydrochlorothiazide (a diuretic) 10 mg/12.5 mg; 20 mg/12.5 mg; 20 mg/25 mg.

CAPOZIDE: captopril/hydrochlorothiazide (a diuretic) 25 mg/15 mg; 25 mg/25 mg; 50 mg/15 mg; 50 mg/25 mg.

LEXXEL: enalapril/felodipine (a calcium channel blocker) 5 mg/2.5 mg; 5 mg/5 mg.

LOTENSIN HCT: benazepril/hydrochlorothiazide (a diuretic) 5 mg/6.25 mg; 10 mg/12.5 mg; 20 mg/12.5 mg; 20 mg/25 mg.

LOTREL: benazepril/amlodipine (a calcium channel blocker) 2.5 mg/10 mg; 5 mg/10 mg; 5 mg/20 mg; 10 mg/20 mg.

PRINZIDE: lisinopril/hydrochlorothiazide (a diuretic) 10 mg/12.5 mg; 20 mg/12.5 mg; 20 mg/25 mg.

TARKA: trandolapril/verapamil (a calcium channel blocker) 1 mg/240 mg; 2 mg/180 mg; 2 mg/240 mg; 4 mg/240 mg.

TECZEM: enalapril/diltiazem (a calcium channel blocker) 5 mg/180 mg.

UNIRETIC: moexipril/hydrochlorothiazide (a diuretic) 7.5 mg/12.5 mg; 15 mg/12.5 mg; 15 mg/25 mg.

VASERETIC: enalapril/hydrochlorothiazide (a diuretic) 5 mg/12.5 mg; 10 mg/25 mg.

ZESTORETIC: lisinopril/hydrochlorothiazide (a diuretic) 10 mg/12.5 mg; 20 mg/12.5 mg; 20 mg/25 mg.

benazepril
ben-**ayz**-ah-prill
(Lotensin)
Do not confuse with Benadryl, Loniten, or lovastatin.

CATEGORY AND SCHEDULE
Pregnancy Risk Category: C (D if used in second or third trimester)

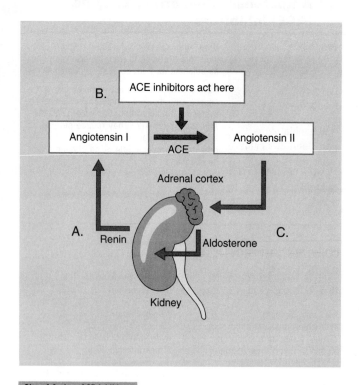

Site of Action: ACE Inhibitors

The renin-angiotensin-aldosterone system plays a major role in regulating blood pressure. Any condition that decreases renal blood flow, reduces blood pressure, or stimulates beta$_1$-adrenergic receptors prompts the kidneys to release renin (A). Renin acts on angiotensinogen, which is converted to angiotensin I, a weak vasoconstrictor. Angiotensin-converting enzyme (ACE) converts angiotensin I to angiotensin II, which causes systemic and renal blood vessels to constrict (B). Systemic vasoconstriction increases peripheral vascular resistance, raising the blood pressure. Renal vasoconstriction decreases glomerular filtration, resulting in sodium and water retention and increasing blood volume and blood pressure. In addition, angiotensin II also acts on the adrenal cortex causing it to release aldosterone (C). This makes the kidneys retain additional sodium and water, which further increases the blood pressure.

ACE inhibitors, such as captopril, enalapril, and lisinopril, block the action of ACE. As a result, angiotensin II can't form, which prevents systemic and renal vasoconstriction and the release of aldosterone.

MECHANISM OF ACTION

An angiotensin-converting enzyme (ACE) inhibitor that decreases the rate of conversion of angiotensin I to angiotensin II, a potent vasoconstrictor. Reduces peripheral arterial resistance. *Therapeutic Effect:* Lowers blood pressure (B/P).

PHARMACOKINETICS

Route	Onset	Peak	Duration
PO	1 hr	2–4 hrs	24 hrs

Partially absorbed from the gastrointestinal (GI) tract. Protein binding: 97%. Metabolized in liver to active metabolite. Primarily excreted in urine. Minimal removal by hemodialysis. **Half-life:** 35 min; metabolite: 10–11 hrs.

AVAILABILITY

Tablets: 5 mg, 10 mg, 20 mg, 40 mg.

INDICATIONS AND DOSAGES

▶ **Hypertension (used alone)**
PO
Adults. Initially, 10 mg/day. Maintenance: 20–40 mg/day as single dose. Maximum: 80 mg/day.
Elderly. Initially, 5–10 mg/day. Range: 20–40 mg/day.
▶ **Hypertension (combination therapy)**
PO
Adults. Initially, 5 mg/day titrated to patient's needs.
▶ **Dosage in renal impairment (Creatinine clearance less than 30 ml/min)**
Adults. Initially, 5 mg/day titrated up to maximum of 40 mg/day.

UNLABELED USES

Treatment of congestive heart failure (CHF)

CONTRAINDICATIONS

History of angioedema with previous treatment with ACE inhibitors

INTERACTIONS

Drug

Alcohol, diuretics, hypotensive agents: May increase the effects of benazepril.
Lithium: May increase the concentration and risk of toxicity with this drug.
NSAIDs: May decrease the effects of benazepril.
Potassium-sparing diuretics, potassium supplements: May cause hyperkalemia.

Herbal

None known.

Food

None known.

DIAGNOSTIC TEST EFFECTS

May increase BUN, serum alkaline phosphatase, serum bilirubin, serum potassium, SGOT (AST), and SGPT (ALT) levels. May decrease serum sodium levels. May cause positive ANA titer.

SIDE EFFECTS

Frequent (6%–3%)
Cough, headache, dizziness
Occasional (2%)
Fatigue, somnolence or drowsiness, nausea
Rare (less than 1%)
Skin rash, fever, joint pain, diarrhea, loss of taste

SERIOUS REACTIONS

• Excessive hypotension ("first-dose syncope") may occur in patients with CHF and who are severely salt or volume depleted.
• Angioedema (swelling of face and lips) and hyperkalemia occur rarely.
• Agranulocytosis and neutropenia may be noted in those with collagen

vascular disease, including scleroderma and systemic lupus erythematosus, and impaired renal
function.
• Nephrotic syndrome may be noted
in patients with history of renal
disease.

NURSING CONSIDERATIONS

Baseline Assessment
• Assess the patient's B/P immediately before giving each benazepril
dose, in addition to regular monitoring. Be alert to fluctuations in B/P.
If an excessive reduction in B/P
occurs, place the patient in the
supine position with legs elevated.
• As ordered, obtain a complete
blood count (CBC) and blood
chemistry before beginning
benazepril therapy, then every
2 weeks for the next 3 months, and
periodically thereafter in patients
with autoimmune disease, renal
impairment, or who are taking
drugs that affect immune response
or leukocyte count.

Lifespan Considerations
• Be aware that benazepril crosses
the placenta and it is unknown if
benazepril is distributed in breast
milk. Know that benazepril may
cause fetal or neonatal morbidity or
mortality.
• Be aware that the safety and
efficacy of benazepril have not been
established in children.
• The elderly may be more sensitive
to the hypotensive effects.

Precautions
• Use cautiously in patients with
cerebrovascular or coronary insufficiency, diabetes mellitus, hypovolemia, renal impairment, and sodium
depletion.
• Use cautiously in patients on
dialysis and diuretic therapy.

Administration and Handling
◀ALERT▶ Expect the physician to
discontinue diuretics 2 to 3 days
before beginning benazepril therapy.
• May give without regard to food.

Intervention and Evaluation
• Assist the patient with ambulation
if he or she experiences dizziness.
• Monitor the patient's B/P, BUN,
CBC, serum creatinine, and urinary
protein.

Patient Teaching
• Advise the patient to rise slowly
from lying to sitting position and to
permit legs to dangle from the bed
momentarily before standing to
reduce the hypotensive effect of
benazepril.
• Explain to the patient that the full
therapeutic effect of benazepril may
take 2 to 4 weeks to appear.
• Caution the patient against noncompliance with drug therapy or
skipping drug doses as this may
produce severe, rebound hypertension.

captopril
cap-toe-prill
(Acenorm[AUS], Capoten,
Captohexal[AUS], Novo-
Captoril[CAN], Topace[AUS])
Do not confuse with Capitrol.

CATEGORY AND SCHEDULE
Pregnancy Risk Category: C
(D if used in second or third
trimester)

MECHANISM OF ACTION
This angiotensin-converting enzyme
(ACE) inhibitor suppresses the
renin-angiotensin-aldosterone system and prevents conversion of
angiotensin I to angiotensin II, a

potent vasoconstrictor; may also inhibit angiotensin II at local vascular and renal sites. Decreases plasma angiotensin II, increases plasma renin activity, decreases aldosterone secretion. *Therapeutic Effect:* Reduces peripheral arterial resistance, pulmonary capillary wedge pressure; improves cardiac output, exercise tolerance.

PHARMACOKINETICS

Route	Onset	Peak	Duration
PO	0.25 hrs	0.5–1.5 hrs	Dose related

Rapidly, well absorbed from the gastrointestinal (GI) tract (absorption is decreased in the presence of food). Protein binding: 25%–30%. Metabolized in liver. Primarily excreted in urine. Removed by hemodialysis. **Half-life:** less than 3 hrs (half-life is increased in those with impaired renal function).

AVAILABILITY

Tablets: 12.5 mg, 25 mg, 50 mg, 100 mg.

INDICATIONS AND DOSAGES
▸ **Hypertension**
PO
Adults, Elderly. Initially, 12.5–25 mg 2–3 times/day. After 1–2 wks, may increase to 50 mg 2–3 times/day. Diuretic may be added if no response in additional 1–2 wks. If taken in combination with diuretic, may increase to 100–150 mg 2–3 times/day after 1–2 wks. Maintenance: 25–150 mg 2–3 times/day. Maximum: 450 mg/day.
▸ **Congestive heart failure (CHF)**
PO
Adults, Elderly. Initially, 6.25–25 mg 3 times/day. Increase to 50 mg

3 times/day. After at least 2 wks, may increase to 50–100 mg 3 times/day. Maximum: 450 mg/day.
▸ **Post-myocardial infarction (MI), impaired liver function**
PO
Adults, Elderly. 6.25 mg a day, then 12.5 mg 3 times/day. Increase to 25 mg 3 times/day over several days up to 50 mg 3 times/day over several weeks.
▸ **Diabetic nephropathy and prevention of kidney failure**
PO
Adults, Elderly. 25 mg 3 times/day. *Children.* Initially 0.3–0.5 mg/kg/dose titrated up to a maximum of 6 mg/kg/day in 2–4 divided doses. *Neonates.* Initially, 0.05–0.1 mg/kg/dose q8-24h titrated up to 0.5 mg/kg/dose given q6-24h.

UNLABELED USES
Diagnosis of anatomic renal artery stenosis, hypertensive crisis, rheumatoid arthritis

CONTRAINDICATIONS
History of angioedema and previous treatment with ACE inhibitors

INTERACTIONS
Drug
Alcohol, diuretics, hypotensive agents: May increase the effects of captopril.
Lithium: May increase lithium blood concentration and risk of toxicity.
NSAIDs: May decrease the effects of captopril.
Potassium-sparing diuretics, potassium supplements: May cause hyperkalemia.
Herbal
None known.
Food
None known.

DIAGNOSTIC TEST EFFECTS

May increase BUN, serum alkaline phosphatase, serum bilirubin, serum creatinine, serum potassium, SGOT (AST), and SGPT (ALT) levels. May decrease serum sodium levels. May cause positive ANA titer.

SIDE EFFECTS

Frequent (7%–4%)
Rash
Occasional (4%–2%)
Pruritus, dysgeusia (change in sense of taste)
Rare (less than 2%–0.5%)
Headache, cough, insomnia, dizziness, fatigue, paresthesia, malaise, nausea, diarrhea or constipation, dry mouth, tachycardia

SERIOUS REACTIONS

• Excessive hypotension ("first-dose syncope") may occur in those with CHF and who are severely salt and volume depleted.
• Angioedema (swelling of face and lips) and hyperkalemia occur rarely.
• Agranulocytosis and neutropenia may be noted in those with collagen vascular disease, including scleroderma and systemic lupus erythematosus, and impaired renal function.
• Nephrotic syndrome may be noted in those with history of renal disease.

NURSING CONSIDERATIONS

Baseline Assessment
• Expect to obtain the patient's blood pressure (B/P) immediately before each captopril dose, in addition to regular monitoring. Be alert to fluctuations in B/P. If an excessive reduction in B/P occurs, place the patient in the supine position with legs elevated and notify the physician.
• Test the patient's first urine of the day for protein by dipstick method before beginning captopril therapy and periodically thereafter in patients with prior renal disease or receiving captopril dosages greater than 150 mg/day.
• As ordered, obtain a complete blood count (CBC) and blood chemistry before beginning captopril therapy, then every 2 weeks for the next 3 months, and periodically thereafter in patients with autoimmune disease, renal impairment, or who are taking drugs that affect immune response or leukocyte count.

Lifespan Considerations
• Be aware that captopril crosses the placenta, is distributed in breast milk, and may cause fetal or neonatal morbidity or mortality.
• Be aware that the safety and efficacy of captopril have not been established in children.
• The elderly may be more sensitive to the hypotensive effects of captopril. Use captopril cautiously in the elderly.

Precautions
• Use cautiously in patients with cerebrovascular or coronary insufficiency, hypovolemia, renal impairment, and sodium depletion.
• Use cautiously in patients on dialysis or diuretic therapy.

Administration and Handling
PO
• Give captopril 1 hour before meals for maximum absorption because food significantly decreases drug absorption.
• Crush tablets if necessary.

Intervention and Evaluation
• Examine the patient's skin for pruritus and rash.
• Assist the patient with ambulation if he or she experiences dizziness.
• Check the patient's urinalysis test results for proteinuria.

• Assess the patient for anorexia due to decreased taste perception.
• Monitor the BUN, CBC, serum creatinine, and serum potassium levels in patient's also receiving a diuretic.

Patient Teaching
• Explain that the full therapeutic effect of captopril may not occur for several weeks.
• Warn the patient that noncompliance with drug therapy or skipping captopril doses may cause severe, rebound hypertension.
• Urge the patient not to consume alcohol while taking captopril.

enalapril maleate
en-**al**-ah-prill
(Alphapril[AUS], Amprace[AUS], Apo-Enalapril[CAN], Auspril[AUS], Renitec[AUS], Vasotec)
Do not confuse with Anafranil, Eldepryl, or ramipril.

CATEGORY AND SCHEDULE
Pregnancy Risk Category: D
(C if used in first trimester)

MECHANISM OF ACTION
This angiotensin-converting enzyme (ACE) inhibitor suppresses the renin-angiotensin-aldosterone system, and prevents conversion of angiotensin I to angiotensin II, a potent vasoconstrictor; may inhibit angiotensin II at local vascular, renal sites. Decreases plasma angiotensin II, increases plasma renin activity, decreases aldosterone secretion. *Therapeutic Effect:* In hypertension, reduces peripheral arterial resistance. In congestive heart failure (CHF), increases cardiac output; decreases peripheral

vascular resistance, blood pressure (B/P), pulmonary capillary wedge pressure, heart size.

PHARMACOKINETICS

Route	Onset	Peak	Duration
PO	1 hr	4–6 hrs	24 hrs
IV	15 min	1–4 hrs	6 hrs

Readily absorbed from the gastrointestinal (GI) tract (not affected by food). Protein binding: 50%–60%. Converted to active metabolite. Primarily excreted in urine. Removed by hemodialysis. **Half-life:** 11 hrs (half-life is increased in those with impaired renal function).

AVAILABILITY
Tablets: 2.5 mg, 5 mg, 10 mg, 20 mg.
Injection: 1.25 mg/ml.

INDICATIONS AND DOSAGES
▶ **Hypertension alone or in combination with other antihypertensives**
PO
Adults, Elderly. Initially, 2.5–5 mg/day. Range: 10–40 mg/day in 1–2 divided doses.
Children. 0.1 mg/kg/day in 1–2 divided doses. Maximum: 0.5 mg/kg/day.
Neonates. 0.1 mg/kg/day q24h.
IV
Adults, Elderly. 0.625–1.25 mg q6h up to 5 mg q6h.
Children, Neonates. 5–10 mcg/kg/dose q8–24h.
▶ **Adjunctive therapy for CHF**
PO
Adults, Elderly. Initially, 2.5–5 mg/day. Range: 5–20 mg/day in 2 divided doses.

▸ **Dosage in renal impairment**

Creatinine Clearance	% Usual Dose
10–50 ml/min	75–100
less than 10 ml/min	50

UNLABELED USES
Treatment of diabetic nephropathy or renal crisis in scleroderma

CONTRAINDICATIONS
History of angioedema and previous treatment with ACE inhibitors

INTERACTIONS
Drug
Alcohol, diuretics, hypotensive agents: May increase the effects of enalapril.
Herbal
None known.
Food
None known.

DIAGNOSTIC TEST EFFECTS
May increase BUN and serum alkaline phosphatase, serum bilirubin, serum creatinine, serum potassium, SGOT (AST), and SGPT (ALT) levels. May decrease serum sodium levels. May cause positive ANA titer.

IV INCOMPATIBILITIES
Amphotericin (Fungizone), amphotericin B complex (Abelcet, AmBisome, Amphotec), cefepime (Maxipime), phenytoin (Dilantin)

IV COMPATIBILITIES
Calcium gluconate, dobutamine (Dobutrex), dopamine (Inotropin), fentanyl (Sublimaze), heparin, lidocaine, magnesium sulfate, morphine, nitroglycerin, potassium chloride, potassium phosphate, propofol (Diprivan)

SIDE EFFECTS
Frequent (7%–5%)
Postural hypotension, headache, dizziness
Occasional (3%–2%)
Orthostatic hypotension, fatigue, diarrhea, cough, syncope
Rare (less than 2%)
Angina, abdominal pain, vomiting, nausea, rash, asthenia (loss of strength, energy), syncope

SERIOUS REACTIONS
• Excessive hypotension (first-dose syncope) may occur in those with CHF and those who are severely salt or volume depleted.
• Angioedema (swelling of face, lips) and hyperkalemia occur rarely.
• Agranulocytosis and neutropenia may be noted in patients with collagen vascular diseases, including scleroderma and systemic lupus erythematosus, and impaired renal function.
• Nephrotic syndrome may be noted in those with history of renal disease.

NURSING CONSIDERATIONS
Baseline Assessment
• Assess the patient's blood pressure (B/P) immediately before each enalapril dose. Be alert to fluctuations in B/P.
• As ordered, obtain a complete blood count (CBC) and blood chemistry before beginning enalapril therapy, then every 2 weeks for 3 months, and periodically thereafter in patients with autoimmune disease, renal impairment, or who are taking drugs that affect immune or leukocyte responses.
Lifespan Considerations
• Be aware that enalapril crosses the placenta and is distributed in breast milk. Enalapril may cause fetal or neonatal morbidity or mortality.

• Be aware that the safety and efficacy of enalapril have not been established in children.
• The elderly may be more susceptible to the hypotensive effects of enalapril.

Precautions

• Use cautiously in patients with cerebrovascular or coronary insufficiency, hypovolemia, renal impairment, and sodium depletion.
• Use cautiously in patients who are receiving dialysis and diuretic therapy.

Administration and Handling

PO
• Give enalapril without regard to food.
• Crush tablets if necessary.

IV
• Store parenteral form at room temperature.
• Use only clear, colorless solution.
• Diluted IV solution is stable for up to 24 hours at room temperature.
• Give undiluted or dilute with D_5W or 0.9% NaCl.
• For IV push, give undiluted over 5 minutes.
• For IV piggyback, infuse over 10 to 15 minutes.

Intervention and Evaluation

• Assist the patient with ambulation if he or she experiences dizziness.
• Monitor the patient's B/P, BUN, and serum creatinine and potassium levels.
• Assess the patient's pattern of daily bowel activity and stool consistency.

Patient Teaching

• Advise the patient to rise slowly from lying to sitting position and to permit legs to dangle from the bed momentarily before standing to reduce the hypotensive effect of enalapril.

• Explain to the patient that the full therapeutic effect of blood pressure reduction may take several weeks to appear.
• Caution the patient against noncompliance with drug therapy or skipping drug doses because this may produce severe, rebound hypertension.
• Urge the patient to limit consumption of alcohol while taking enalapril.
• Warn the patient to notify the physician if diarrhea, difficulty breathing, excessive perspiration, swelling of the face, lips, or tongue, and vomiting occur.

fosinopril
foh-**sin**-oh-prill
(Monopril)
Do not confuse with Monurol.

CATEGORY AND SCHEDULE
Pregnancy Risk Category: C
(D if used in second or third trimester)

MECHANISM OF ACTION
This angiotensin-converting enzyme (ACE) inhibitor suppresses renin-angiotensin-aldosterone system and prevents conversion of angiotensin I to angiotensin II, a potent vasoconstrictor; may also inhibit angiotensin II at local vascular and renal sites. Decreases plasma angiotensin II, increases plasma renin activity, decreases aldosterone secretion. *Therapeutic Effect:* Reduces peripheral arterial resistance, pulmonary capillary wedge pressure; improves cardiac output, exercise tolerance.

PHARMACOKINETICS

Route	Onset	Peak	Duration
PO	1 hr	2–6 hrs	24 hrs

Slowly absorbed from the gastrointestinal (GI) tract. Protein binding: 97%–98%. Metabolized in liver, GI mucosa to active metabolite. Primarily excreted in urine. Minimal removal by hemodialysis. **Half-life:** 11.5 hrs.

AVAILABILITY

Tablets: 10 mg, 20 mg, 40 mg.

INDICATIONS AND DOSAGES
▸ **Hypertension (used alone)**
PO
Adults, Elderly. Initially, 10 mg/day. Maintenance: 20–40 mg/day. Maximum: 80 mg/day.
▸ **Hypertension (with diuretic)**
PO
Adults, Elderly. Initially, 10 mg/day titrated to patient's needs.
▸ **Heart failure**
PO
Adults, Elderly. Initially, 5–10 mg. Maintenance: 20–40 mg/day.

UNLABELED USES

Treatment of diabetic and nondiabetic nephropathy, post-myocardial infarction (MI) left ventricular dysfunction, renal crisis in scleroderma

CONTRAINDICATIONS

History of angioedema with previous treatment of ACE inhibitors

INTERACTIONS
Drug
Alcohol, diuretics, hypotensive agents: May increase the effects of fosinopril.
Lithium: May increase lithium blood concentration and risk of toxicity.
NSAIDs: May decrease the effects of fosinopril.
Potassium-sparing diuretics, potassium supplements: May cause hyperkalemia.
Herbal
None known.
Food
None known.

DIAGNOSTIC TEST EFFECTS

May increase BUN, serum alkaline phosphatase, serum bilirubin, serum creatinine, serum potassium, SGOT (AST), and SGPT (ALT) levels. May decrease serum sodium levels. May cause positive ANA titer.

SIDE EFFECTS

Frequent (12%–9%)
Dizziness, cough
Occasional (4%–2%)
Hypotension, nausea, vomiting, upper respiratory infection

SERIOUS REACTIONS

• Excessive hypotension ("first-dose syncope") may occur in patients with congestive heart failure (CHF) and who are severely salt and volume depleted.
• Angioedema (swelling of face and lips) and hyperkalemia occur rarely.
• Agranulocytosis and neutropenia may be noted in those with collagen vascular disease, including scleroderma and systemic lupus erythematosus, and impaired renal function.
• Nephrotic syndrome may be noted in those with history of renal disease.

NURSING CONSIDERATIONS
Baseline Assessment
• Obtain the patient's blood pressure (B/P) immediately before each

fosinopril dose regularly monitoring. Be alert to fluctuations in B/P.
• Expect the patient to undergo renal function tests before beginning fosinopril therapy.
• As ordered, obtain a complete blood count (CBC) and blood chemistry before beginning fosinopril therapy, then every 2 weeks for 3 months, and periodically thereafter in patients with autoimmune disease, renal impairment, or who are taking drugs that affect immune response or leukocyte count.

Lifespan Considerations
• Be aware that fosinopril crosses the placenta and is distributed in breast milk and may cause fetal or neonatal morbidity or mortality.
• Be aware that the safety and efficacy of fosinopril have not been established in children.
• Be aware that neonates and infants may be at increased risk for neurologic abnormalities and oliguria.
• The elderly may be more sensitive to the hypotensive effects of fosinopril.

Precautions
• Use cautiously in patients with coronary or cerebrovascular insufficiency, hypovolemia, renal impairment, and sodium depletion.
• Use cautiously in patients receiving dialysis or diuretic therapy.

Administration and Handling
◀ALERT▶ Expect to discontinue diuretics 2 to 3 days before beginning fosinopril therapy.
PO
• Give fosinopril without regard to food.
• Crush tablets if necessary.

Intervention and Evaluation
• Place the patient in the supine position with legs elevated and notify physician if an excessive reduction in B/P occurs.

• Assist the patient with ambulation if he or she experiences dizziness.
• Assess the patient's intake and output, as appropriate.
• Auscultate lung sounds for rales and wheezes in patients with CHF.
• Monitor the patient's urinalysis results for proteinuria.
• Monitor the BUN, serum creatinine, and serum potassium levels in patients on concurrent diuretic therapy.

Patient Teaching
• Warn the patient to report any sign or symptom of infection, such as fever or sore throat.
• Explain that the full therapeutic effect of fosinopril may take several weeks to appear.
• Warn the patient that noncompliance with drug therapy or skipping fosinopril doses may cause severe, rebound hypertension.
• Advise the patient to rise slowly from lying to sitting position and to permit legs to dangle from the bed momentarily before standing to reduce the hypotensive effect of fosinopril.
• Caution the patient to notify the physician if he or she experiences excessive perspiration, persistent cough, or vomiting.

lisinopril
lih-**sin**-oh-prill
(Fibsol[AUS], Lisodur[AUS], Prinivil, Zestril)
Do not confuse with Desyrel, fosinopril, Lioresal, Plendil, Prilosec, Proventil, Restoril, or Zostrix.

CATEGORY AND SCHEDULE
Pregnancy Risk Category: C
(D if used in second or third trimester)

MECHANISM OF ACTION

This angiotensin-converting enzyme (ACE) inhibitor suppresses the renin-angiotensin-aldosterone system and prevents conversion of angiotensin I to angiotensin II, a potent vasoconstrictor; may also inhibit angiotensin II at local vascular and renal sites. Decreases plasma angiotensin II, increases plasma renin activity, and decreases aldosterone secretion. *Therapeutic Effect:* Reduces peripheral arterial resistance, blood pressure (B/P), afterload, pulmonary capillary wedge pressure (preload), pulmonary vascular resistance. In those with heart failure, also decreases heart size, increases cardiac output, and exercise tolerance time.

PHARMACOKINETICS

Route	Onset	Peak	Duration
PO	1 hr	6 hrs	24 hrs

Incompletely absorbed from the gastrointestinal (GI) tract. Protein binding: 25%. Primarily excreted unchanged in urine. Removed by hemodialysis. **Half-life:** 12 hrs (half-life is prolonged in those with impaired renal function).

AVAILABILITY

Tablets: 2.5 mg, 5 mg, 10 mg, 20 mg, 30 mg, 40 mg.

INDICATIONS AND DOSAGES
▶ **Hypertension (used alone)**
PO
Adults. Initially, 10 mg/day. May increase by 5–10 mcg/day at 1–2 wk intervals. Maximum: 40 mg/day.
Elderly. Initially, 2.5–5 mg/day. May increase by 2.5–5 mg/day at

1- to 2-wk intervals. Maximum: 40 mg/day.
▶ **Hypertension (used in combination with other antihypertensives)**
PO
• *Adults.* Initially, 2.5–5 mg/day titrated to patient's needs.
▶ **Adjunctive therapy for management of heart failure**
PO
Adults, Elderly. Initially, 2.5–5 mg/day. May increase by no more than 10 mg/day at intervals of at least 2 wks. Maintenance: 5–40 mg/day.
▶ **Improve survival in patients after a myocardial infarction (MI)**
PO
Adults, Elderly. Initially, 5 mg, then 5 mg after 24 hrs, 10 mg after 48 hrs, then 10 mg/day for 6 wks. For patients with low systolic B/P, give 2.5 mg/day for 3 days, then 2.5–5 mg/day.
▶ **Dosage in renal impairment**
Titrate to patient's needs after giving the following initial dose:

Creatinine Clearance	% Normal Dose
10–50 ml/min	50–75
less than 10 ml/min	25–50

UNLABELED USES

Treatment of hypertension or renal crises with scleroderma

CONTRAINDICATIONS

History of angioedema from previous treatment with ACE inhibitors

INTERACTIONS
Drug
Alcohol, diuretics, hypotensive agents: May increase the effects of lisinopril.
Lithium: May increase lithium blood concentration and risk of toxicity.

NSAIDs: May decrease the effects of lisinopril.
Potassium-sparing diuretics, potassium supplements: May cause hyperkalemia.
Herbal
None known.
Food
None known.

DIAGNOSTIC TEST EFFECTS

May increase BUN, serum alkaline phosphatase, serum bilirubin, serum creatinine, serum potassium, SGOT (AST), and SGPT (ALT) levels. May decrease serum sodium levels. May cause positive ANA titer.

SIDE EFFECTS

Frequent (12%–5%)
Headache, dizziness, postural hypotension
Occasional (4%–2%)
Chest discomfort, fatigue, rash, abdominal pain, nausea, diarrhea, upper respiratory infection
Rare (1% or less)
Palpitations, tachycardia, peripheral edema, insomnia, paresthesia, confusion, constipation, dry mouth, muscle cramps

SERIOUS REACTIONS

• Excessive hypotension ("first-dose syncope") may occur in patients with congestive heart failure (CHF) and severe salt and volume depletion.
• Angioedema (swelling of face and lips) and hyperkalemia occurs rarely.
• Agranulocytosis and neutropenia may be noted in patients with collagen vascular disease, including scleroderma and systemic lupus erythematosus, and impaired renal function.
• Nephrotic syndrome may be noted

in patients with history of renal disease.

NURSING CONSIDERATIONS

Baseline Assessment
• Assess the patient's apical pulse and B/P immediately before each lisinopril dose, and regularly throughout therapy. Be alert to fluctuations in apical pulse and B/P. If an excessive reduction in B/P occurs, place the patient in the supine position with legs elevated and notify the physician.
• Check the results of a complete blood count (CBC) and blood chemistry before beginning lisinopril therapy, then every 2 weeks for the next 3 months, and periodically thereafter in patients with autoimmune disease, renal impairment, or who are taking drugs that affect immune response or leukocyte count.
Lifespan Considerations
• Be aware that lisinopril crosses the placenta and that it is unknown if lisinopril is distributed in breast milk. Lisinopril has caused fetal or neonatal morbidity or mortality.
• Be aware that the safety and efficacy of lisinopril have not been established in children.
• The elderly may be more sensitive to the hypotensive effects of lisinopril.
Precautions
• Use cautiously in patients with cerebrovascular or coronary insufficiency, hypovolemia, renal impairment, severe congestive heart failure, and sodium depletion.
• Use cautiously in patients on dialysis or diuretic therapy.
Administration and Handling
◀ALERT▶ Expect to discontinue diuretics, as prescribed, 2 to 3 days before beginning lisinopril therapy.

PO
• Give lisinopril without regard to food.
• Crush tablets if necessary.
Intervention and Evaluation
• Examine the patient for edema.
• Auscultate the patient's lungs for rales.
• Monitor the patient's intake and output and daily weights.
• Assess the patient's pattern of daily bowel activity and stool consistency.
• Assist the patient with ambulation if he or she experiences dizziness.
• Monitor the patient's B/P, BUN, serum creatinine, and potassium levels, renal function tests, and white blood cell (WBC) count.
Patient Teaching
• Advise the patient to rise slowly from lying to sitting position and to permit legs to dangle from the bed momentarily before standing to reduce the hypotensive effect of lisinopril.
• Urge the patient to limit consumption of alcohol while taking lisinopril.
• Warn the patient to notify the physician if he or she experiences diarrhea, difficulty breathing, excessive perspiration, swelling of the face, lips, or tongue, or vomiting.

---

moexipril hydrochloride
mow-**ex**-ih-prill
(Univasc)

CATEGORY AND SCHEDULE
Pregnancy Risk Category: C
(D if used during second and third trimesters)

MECHANISM OF ACTION
This angiotensin-converting enzyme (ACE) inhibitor suppresses the renin-angiotensin-aldosterone system and prevents conversion of angiotensin I to angiotensin II, a potent vasoconstrictor; may also inhibit angiotensin II at local vascular and renal sites. *Therapeutic Effect:* Reduces peripheral arterial resistance, blood pressure (B/P).

PHARMACOKINETICS

Route	Onset	Peak	Duration
PO	1 hr	3–6 hrs	24 hrs

Incompletely absorbed from the gastrointestinal (GI) tract. Food decreases drug absorption. Rapidly converted to active metabolite. Protein binding: 50%. Primarily recovered in feces, partially excreted in urine. Unknown if removed by dialysis. **Half-life:** 1 hr (metabolite 2–9 hrs).

AVAILABILITY
Tablets: 7.5 mg, 15 mg.

INDICATIONS AND DOSAGES
◀**ALERT**▶ To reduce the risk of hypotension in patients receiving concurrent diuretic therapy, expect to discontinue the diuretic 2 to 3 days before beginning moexipril therapy. However, if the B/P is not controlled, resume diuretic therapy. If diuretics can't be discontinued, administer an initial moexipril dose of 3.75 mg.
▶ **Hypertension**
PO
Adults, Elderly. For patients not receiving diuretics, initial dose is 7.5 mg once a day 1 hr before meals. Adjust according to B/P effect. Maintenance: 7.5–30 mg a

day in 1–2 divided doses 1 hr before meals.

▶ **Hypertension in patients with impaired renal function**

PO

Adults, Elderly. 3.75 mg once a day in patients with creatinine clearance of 40 ml/min/1.73 m^2. Maximum: May titrate up to 15 mg/day.

CONTRAINDICATIONS

History of angioedema from previous treatment with ACE inhibitors

INTERACTIONS

Drug

Alcohol, diuretics, hypotensive agents: May increase the effects of moexipril.

Lithium: May increase lithium blood concentration and risk for toxicity.

NSAIDs: May decrease the effects of moexipril.

Potassium-sparing diuretics, potassium supplements: May cause hyperkalemia.

Herbal

None known.

Food

None known.

DIAGNOSTIC TEST EFFECTS

May increase BUN, serum alkaline phosphatase, serum bilirubin, serum creatinine, serum potassium, SGOT (AST), and SGPT (ALT) levels. May decrease serum sodium levels. May cause positive ANA titer.

SIDE EFFECTS

Occasional

Cough, headache (6%); dizziness (4%); nausea, fatigue (3%)

Rare

Flushing, rash, myalgia, nausea, vomiting

SERIOUS REACTIONS

• Excessive hypotension (first-dose syncope) may occur in those with congestive heart failure (CHF) and who are severely salt or volume depleted.

• Angioedema (swelling of face and lips) and hyperkalemia occur rarely.

• Agranulocytosis and neutropenia may be noted in those with collagen vascular disease, including scleroderma and systemic lupus erythematosus, and impaired renal function.

• Nephrotic syndrome may be noted in those with a history of renal disease.

NURSING CONSIDERATIONS

Baseline Assessment

• Assess the patient's apical pulse and B/P immediately before each moexipril dose, and regularly monitoring throughout therapy. Be alert for fluctuations in apical pulse and B/P. If an excessive reduction in B/P occurs, place the patient in the supine position with legs elevated and notify the physician.

• Expect the patient to have renal function tests done before beginning moexipril therapy.

• Assess the patient's complete blood count (CBC) and blood chemistry, if ordered, before beginning moexipril therapy, then every 2 weeks for the next 3 months, and periodically thereafter in patients with autoimmune disease, renal impairment, or who are taking drugs that affect immune response or leukocyte count.

Lifespan Considerations

• Be aware that moexipril crosses the placenta and it is unknown if moexipril is distributed in breast milk. Also know that moexipril has caused fetal or neonatal morbidity or mortality.

* Be aware that the safety and efficacy of moexipril have not been established in children.
* In the elderly, age-related renal impairment may require cautious use of moexipril.

Precautions
* Use cautiously in patients with angina, aortic stenosis, cerebrovascular disease, cerebrovascular or coronary insufficiency, hypovolemia, ischemic heart disease, renal impairment, severe CHF, and sodium depletion.
* Use cautiously in patients receiving dialysis or diuretic therapy.

Administration and Handling
◄ALERT► To reduce the risk of hypotension, expect to discontinue diuretics 2 to 3 days before initiating moexipril therapy. If B/P is not controlled, resume diuretic as ordered. If diuretic cannot be discontinued, prepare to give an initial dose of 3.75 mg moexipril.
PO
* Give moexipril 1 hour before meals.
* Crush tablets if necessary.

Intervention and Evaluation
* Monitor the patient's B/P, BUN, serum creatinine, serum potassium levels, and white blood cell (WBC) count.
* Assess the patient for hypotension for 1 to 3 hours after the first moexipril dose or after an increase in dose.
* Assess the patient for an irregular heart rate.
* Assist the patient with ambulation if he or she experiences dizziness.

Patient Teaching
* Caution the patient against abruptly discontinuing the drug.
* Warn the patient to notify the physician if he or she experiences chest pain, cough, difficulty breathing, fever, or sore throat.

* Warn the patient to notify the physician if he or she experiences symptoms of angioedema (swelling of eyes, face, feet, hands, lips, or tongue).
* Advise the patient that he or she should stand up slowly from a sitting or lying position to avoid the hypotensive effect of moexipril.
* Explain to the patient that moexipril may alter his or her sense of taste.

perindopril
per-**inn**-doe-prill
(Aceon)

CATEGORY AND SCHEDULE
Pregnancy risk category: C
(D if used in second or third trimesters)

MECHANISM OF ACTION
An antihypertensive that suppresses renin-angiotensin-aldosterone system, prevents conversion of angiotensin I to angiotensin II, a potent vasoconstrictor. May also inhibit angiotensin II at local vascular and renal sites. *Therapeutic Effect:* Reduces peripheral arterial resistance, blood pressure (B/P).

AVAILABILITY
Tablets: 2 mg, 4 mg, 8 mg.

INDICATIONS AND DOSAGES
▶ **Hypertension**
PO
Adults, Elderly. 2–8 mg/day as single dose or in 2 divided doses. Maximum: 16 mg/day.

UNLABELED USES
Management of heart failure

CONTRAINDICATIONS
History of angioedema with previous treatment with ACE inhibitors

INTERACTIONS
Drug
Alcohol, diuretics, hypotensive agents: May increase the effects of perindopril.
Herbal
None known.
Food
None known.

DIAGNOSTIC TEST EFFECTS
May increase BUN, serum alkaline phosphatase, bilirubin, creatinine, potassium, SGOT (AST), and SGPT (ALT) levels. May decrease serum sodium levels. May cause positive ANA titer.

SIDE EFFECTS
Occasional (5%–1%)
Cough, back pain, sinusitis, upper extremity pain, dyspepsia, fever, palpitations, hypotension, dizziness, fatigue, syncope

SERIOUS REACTIONS
• Excessive hypotension or first-dose syncope may occur in patients with congestive heart failure (CHF) or severe salt or volume depleted.
• Angioedema, marked by swelling of face and lips, and hyperkalemia occur rarely.
• Agranulocytosis and neutropenia may be noted in those with collagen vascular disease, scleroderma and systemic lupus erythematosus, and impaired renal function.
• Nephrotic syndrome may be noted in those with history of renal disease.

NURSING CONSIDERATIONS
Baseline Assessment
• Obtain the patient's B/P immediately before giving each drug dose. Be alert to B/P fluctuations.
• Expect to obtain baseline liver and renal function studies.
Precautions
• Use cautiously in those on dialysis or diuretic therapy.
• Use cautiously in patients with cerebrovascular insufficiency, coronary insufficiency, hypovolemia, renal impairment and sodium depletion.
Intervention and Evaluation
• Assist the patient with ambulation if he or she experiences dizziness.
• Monitor the patient's BUN, serum creatinine, serum potassium levels, SGOT (AST) and SGPT (ALT).
• Assess the patient's pattern of daily bowel activity and stool consistency.
Patient Teaching
• Instruct the patient to rise slowly from lying to sitting position and permit legs to dangle from bed momentarily before standing to avoid the hypotensive effect of the drug.
• Caution the patient that skipping doses or voluntarily discontinuing the drug may produce severe, rebound hypertension.

quinapril hydrochloride
quin-ah-prill
(Accupril, Asig[AUS])
Do not confuse with Accolate or Accutane.

CATEGORY AND SCHEDULE
Pregnancy Risk Category: C (D if used in second or third trimester)

MECHANISM OF ACTION

This angiotensin-converting enzyme (ACE) inhibitor suppresses the renin-angiotensin-aldosterone system and prevents the conversion of angiotensin I to angiotensin II, a potent vasoconstrictor; may also inhibit angiotensin II at local vascular and renal sites. *Therapeutic Effect:* Reduces peripheral arterial resistance, blood pressure (B/P), pulmonary capillary wedge pressure; improves cardiac output.

PHARMACOKINETICS

Route	Onset	Peak	Duration
PO	1 hr	N/A	24 hrs

Readily absorbed from the gastrointestinal (GI) tract. Protein binding: 97%. Metabolized in liver, GI tract, extravascular tissue to active metabolite. Primarily excreted in urine. Minimal removal by hemodialysis. **Half-life:** 1–2 hrs; metabolite half-life is 3 hrs (half-life is increased in those with impaired renal function).

AVAILABILITY

Tablets: 5 mg, 10 mg, 20 mg, 40 mg.

INDICATIONS AND DOSAGES

▸ **Hypertension (used alone)**
PO
Adults. Initially, 10–20 mg/day. May adjust dosage after at least 2-wk intervals. Maintenance: 20–80 mg/day as single dose or 2 divided doses. Maximum: 80 mg/day.
Elderly. Initially, 2.5–5 mg/day. May increase by 2.5–5 mg q1–2wks.
▸ **Hypertension (combination therapy)**
PO
Adults. Initially, 5 mg/day titrated to patient's needs.

Elderly. Initially, 2.5–5 mg/day. May increase by 2.5–5 mg q1–2wks.
▸ **Adjunct to manage heart failure**
PO
Adults, Elderly. Initially, 5 mg 2 times/day. Range: 20–40 mg/day.
▸ **Dosage in renal impairment**
Titrate to patient need after initial doses:

Creatinine Clearance	Initial Dose
more than 60 ml/min	10 mg
30–60 ml/min	5 mg
10–29 ml/min	2.5 mg

UNLABELED USES

Treatment of hypertension and renal crisis in scleroderma

CONTRAINDICATIONS

Bilateral renal artery stenosis

INTERACTIONS
Drug

Alcohol, diuretics, hypotensive agents: May increase the effects of quinapril.
Lithium: May increase lithium blood concentration and risk of toxicity.
NSAIDs: May decrease the effects of quinapril.
Potassium-sparing diuretics, potassium supplements: May cause hyperkalemia.
Herbal
Ginseng, yohimbe: May worsen hypertension.
Garlic: May increase antihypertensive effect.
Food
None known.

DIAGNOSTIC TEST EFFECTS

May increase BUN, serum alkaline phosphatase, serum bilirubin, serum creatinine, serum potassium, SGOT

(AST), and SGPT (ALT) levels.
May decrease serum sodium levels.
May cause positive ANA titer.

SIDE EFFECTS
Frequent (7%–5%)
Headache, dizziness
Occasional (4%–2%)
Fatigue, vomiting, nausea, hypotension, chest pain, cough, syncope
Rare (less than 2%)
Diarrhea, cough, dyspnea, rash, palpitations, impotence, insomnia, drowsiness, malaise

SERIOUS REACTIONS
• Excessive hypotension (first-dose syncope) may occur in those with congestive heart failure (CHF) and who are severely salt or volume depleted.
• Angioedema (swelling of face and lips) and hyperkalemia occur rarely.
• Agranulocytosis and neutropenia may be noted in those with collagen vascular disease, including scleroderma and systemic lupus erythematosus, and impaired renal function.
• Nephrotic syndrome may be noted in those with history of renal disease.

NURSING CONSIDERATIONS

Baseline Assessment
• Assess the patient's B/P immediately before each quinapril dose and regularly during therapy. Be alert to fluctuations in B/P. If an excessive reduction in B/P occurs, place the patient in the supine position with legs slightly elevated and notify the physician.
• Monitor the results of the patient's renal function tests before beginning quinapril therapy.
• For patient's with a history of renal disease, test the first urine of the day for protein by dipstick

method before beginning quinapril therapy and periodically thereafter.
• If ordered, monitor the patient's complete blood count (CBC) and blood chemistry before beginning quinapril therapy, then every 2 weeks for 3 months, and periodically thereafter in patients with autoimmune disease, renal impairment, or who are taking drugs that affect immune response or leukocyte count.

Lifespan Considerations
• Be aware that quinapril crosses the placenta and it is unknown if quinapril is distributed in breast milk. Also know that quinapril may cause fetal or neonatal morbidity or mortality.
• Be aware that the safety and efficacy of quinapril have not been established in children.
• The elderly may be more sensitive to the hypotensive effects of quinapril.

Precautions
• Use cautiously in patients with CHF, collagen vascular disease, hyperkalemia, hypovolemia, renal impairment, and renal stenosis.

Administration and Handling
◀ALERT▶ Expect to discontinue diuretics 2–3 days before beginning quinapril therapy.
PO
• Give quinapril without regard to food.
• Crush tablets as desired.

Intervention and Evaluation
• Monitor the patient's BUN, serum creatinine, serum potassium, and white blood cell (WBC) count.
• Assist the patient with ambulation if he or she experiences dizziness.
• Evaluate the patient for headache.
• Give the patient dry toast, non-cola carbonated beverages, or un-

salted crackers to help relieve nausea.

Patient Teaching
• To reduce the risk of orthostatic hypotension, advise the patient to rise slowly from the lying to the sitting position and to permit legs to dangle from the bed momentarily before standing.
• Explain to the patient that the full therapeutic effect of quinapril may take 1 to 2 weeks to appear.
• Warn the patient to notify the physician if he or she experiences signs or symptoms of infection, including fever and sore throat.
• Caution the patient that discontinuing the drug or skipping doses of quinapril may produce severe, rebound hypertension.
• Urge the patient to avoid tasks that require mental alertness or motor skills until his or her response to the drug is established.

ramipril
ram-ih-prill
(Altace, Ramace[AUS], Tritace[AUS])
Do not confuse with Alteplase or Artane.

CATEGORY AND SCHEDULE
Pregnancy Risk Category: C (D if used in second or third trimester)

MECHANISM OF ACTION
A renin-angiotensin system antagonist that suppresses the renin-angiotensin-aldosterone system. Decreases plasma angiotensin II, increases plasma renin activity, and decreases aldosterone secretion. *Therapeutic Effect:* Reduces peripheral arterial resistance, decreasing blood pressure (B/P).

PHARMACOKINETICS

Route	Onset	Peak	Duration
PO	1–2 hrs	3–6 hrs	24 hrs

Well absorbed from the gastrointestinal (GI) tract. Protein binding: 73%. Metabolized in liver to active metabolite. Primarily excreted in urine. Not removed by hemodialysis. **Half-life:** 5.1 hrs.

AVAILABILITY
Capsules: 1.25 mg, 2.5 mg, 5 mg, 10 mg.

INDICATIONS AND DOSAGES
▶ **Hypertension (used alone)**
PO
Adults, Elderly. Initially, 2.5 mg/day. Maintenance: 2.5–20 mg/day as single dose or in 2 divided doses.
▶ **Hypertension (in combination with other antihypertensives)**
PO
Adults, Elderly. Initially, 1.25 mg/day titrated to patient's needs.
▶ **Congestive heart failure (CHF)**
PO
Adults, Elderly. Initially, 1.25–2.5 mg 2 times/day. Maximum: 5 mg 2 times/day.
▶ **Risk reduction for myocardial infarction (MI), stroke**
PO
Adults, Elderly. Initially, 2.5 mg/day for 7 days, then 5 mg/day for 21 days, then 10 mg/day as a single dose or in divided doses.
▶ **Dosage in renal impairment**
Creatinine clearance less than 40 ml/min. 25% of normal dose.
Hypertension. Initially, 1.25 mg/day titrated upward.

CHF. Initially, 1.25 mg/day, titrate up to 2.5 mg twice a day.

UNLABELED USES
Prevention of heart attacks, stroke; treatment of hypertension and renal crisis in scleroderma

CONTRAINDICATIONS
Bilateral renal artery stenosis

INTERACTIONS
Drug
Alcohol, diuretics, hypotensive agents: May increase the effects of ramipril.
Lithium: May increase lithium blood concentration and risk of toxicity.
NSAIDs: May decrease the effects of ramipril.
Potassium-sparing diuretics, potassium supplements: May cause hyperkalemia.
Herbal
Ginseng, yohimbe: May worsen hypertension.
Garlic: May increase antihypertensive effect.
Food
None known.

DIAGNOSTIC TEST EFFECTS
May increase BUN, serum alkaline phosphatase, serum bilirubin, serum creatinine, serum potassium, SGOT (AST), and SGPT (ALT) levels. May decrease serum sodium levels. May cause positive ANA titer.

SIDE EFFECTS
Frequent (12%–5%)
Cough, headache
Occasional (4%–2%)
Dizziness, fatigue, nausea, asthenia (loss of strength)
Rare (less than 2%)
Palpitations, insomnia, nervousness, malaise, abdominal pain, myalgia

SERIOUS REACTIONS
• Excessive hypotension (first-dose syncope) may occur in those with CHF and who are severely salt or volume depleted.
• Angioedema (swelling of face and lips) and hyperkalemia occur rarely.
• Agranulocytosis and neutropenia may be noted in those with collagen vascular disease, including scleroderma and systemic lupus erythematosus, and impaired renal function.
• Nephrotic syndrome may be noted in those with a history of renal disease.

NURSING CONSIDERATIONS
Baseline Assessment
• Assess the patient's B/P immediately before each ramipril dose and regularly throughout therapy. Be alert to fluctuations in B/P. If an excessive reduction in B/P occurs, place the patient in the supine position with legs elevated and notify the physician.
• Check the patient's BUN, renal function test results, serum creatinine levels if ordered, before beginning ramipril therapy.
• For patients with a history of renal disease, test the patient's urine for protein by dipstick method before beginning ramipril therapy and periodically thereafter.
• Check the results of the patients complete blood count (CBC) and blood chemistry before beginning ramipril therapy, then every 2 weeks for 3 months, and periodically thereafter in patients with autoimmune disease, renal impairment, or who are taking drugs that affect immune response or leukocyte count.
Lifespan Considerations
• Be aware that ramipril crosses the placenta and is distributed in breast

milk. Also know that the drug may cause fetal or neonatal morbidity or mortality.
• Be aware that the safety and efficacy of ramipril have not been established in children.
• The elderly may be more sensitive to the hypotensive effects of ramipril.

Precautions
• Use cautiously in patients with CHF, collagen vascular disease, hyperkalemia, hypovolemia, renal impairment, and renal stenosis.

Administration and Handling
◀ALERT▶ Expect to discontinue diuretics 2 to 3 days before beginning ramipril therapy.
PO
• Give ramipril without regard to food.
• Have the patient swallow the capsules whole and not chew or break them.
• Mix with apple juice, applesauce, or water as needed.

Intervention and Evaluation
• Monitor the patient's BUN, serum creatinine and potassium levels, and white blood cell (WBC) count.
• Assess the patient for cough, which frequently occurs.
• Assist the patient with ambulation if he or she experiences dizziness.
• Assess the CHF patient's lung sounds for rales and wheezing.
• Monitor the patient's urinalysis for proteinuria.
• Monitor serum potassium levels in those patients also receiving diuretic therapy.

Patient Teaching
• Caution the patient against discontinuing the drug without physician approval.
• Warn the patient to notify the physician if he or she experiences chest pain, cough, and palpitations.

• Advise the patient that dizziness or lightheadedness may occur in the first few days after ramipril administration.
• Warn the patient to avoid tasks that require mental alertness or motor skills until his or her response to the drug is established.

trandolapril
tran-**doal**-ah-prill
(Gopten[AUS], Mavik, Odrik[AUS])

CATEGORY AND SCHEDULE
Pregnancy Risk Category: C
(D if used in second or third trimester)

MECHANISM OF ACTION
This angiotensin-converting enzyme (ACE) inhibitor suppresses the renin-angiotensin-aldosterone system and prevents the conversion of angiotensin I to angiotensin II, a potent vasoconstrictor; may also inhibit angiotensin II at local vascular and renal sites. Decreases plasma angiotensin II, increases plasma renin activity, decreases aldosterone secretion. *Therapeutic Effect:* Reduces peripheral arterial resistance, pulmonary capillary wedge pressure; improves cardiac output, exercise tolerance.

PHARMACOKINETICS
Slowly absorbed from the gastrointestinal (GI) tract. Protein binding: 80%. Metabolized in liver, GI mucosa to active metabolite. Primarily excreted in urine. Removed by hemodialysis. **Half-life:** 24 hrs.

AVAILABILITY
Tablets: 1 mg, 2 mg, 4 mg.

INDICATIONS AND DOSAGES
▶ **Hypertension (without diuretic)**
PO
Adults, Elderly. Initially, 1 mg once a day in nonblack patients, 2 mg once a day in black patients. Adjust dose at least at 7-day intervals.
Maintenance: 2–4 mg/day.
Maximum: 8 mg/day.
▶ **Congestive heart failure (CHF)**
PO
Adults, Elderly. Initially, 0.5–1 mg, titrated to target dose of 4 mg/day.

CONTRAINDICATIONS
History of angioedema from previous treatment with ACE inhibitors

INTERACTIONS
Drug
Alcohol, diuretics, hypotensive agents: May increase the effects of trandolapril.
Lithium: May increase lithium blood concentration and risk for toxicity.
NSAIDs: May decrease the effects of trandolapril.
Potassium-sparing diuretics, potassium supplements: May cause hyperkalemia.
Herbal
None known.
Food
None known.

DIAGNOSTIC TEST EFFECTS
May increase BUN, serum alkaline phosphatase, serum bilirubin, serum creatinine, serum potassium, SGOT (AST), and SGPT (ALT) levels.
May decrease serum sodium levels.
May cause positive ANA titer.

SIDE EFFECTS
Frequent (35%–23%)
Dizziness, cough
Occasional (11%–3%)
Hypotension, dyspepsia (heartburn, epigastric pain, indigestion), syncope, asthenia (loss of strength), tinnitus
Rare (less than 1%)
Palpitations, insomnia, drowsiness, nausea, vomiting, constipation, flushed skin

SERIOUS REACTIONS
• Excessive hypotension (first-dose syncope) may occur in those with CHF and who are severely salt or volume depleted.
• Angioedema (swelling of face and lips) and hyperkalemia occur rarely.
• Agranulocytosis and neutropenia may be noted in those with collagen vascular disease, including scleroderma and systemic lupus erythematosus, and impaired renal function.
• Nephrotic syndrome may be noted in those with a history of renal disease.

NURSING CONSIDERATIONS
Baseline Assessment
• Assess the patient's blood pressure (B/P) immediately before each trandolapril dose and regularly monitor throughout therapy. Be alert to fluctuations in B/P.
• Check the BUN renal function, and serum creatinine levels of the patient, if ordered, before beginning trandolapril therapy.
• Monitor the results of a complete blood count (CBC) and blood chemistries before beginning trandolapril therapy, then every 2 weeks for the next 3 months, and periodically thereafter in patients with autoimmune disease, renal impairment, or who are taking drugs that affect immune response or leukocyte count.
Lifespan Considerations
• Be aware that trandolapril crosses the placenta and is distributed in

breast milk. Also, know that trandolapril may cause fetal or neonatal morbidity or mortality.
• Be aware that the safety and efficacy of trandolapril have not been established in children.
• There are no age-related precautions noted in the elderly.

Precautions
• Use cautiously in patients with CHF, hyperkalemia, renal impairment, and valvular stenosis.

Administration and Handling
PO
• Give trandolapril without regard to meals.
• Crush tablets as necessary.

Intervention and Evaluation
• If an excessive reduction in B/P occurs, place the patient in the supine position with legs elevated and notify the physician.
• Assist the patient with ambulation if he or she experiences dizziness.
• Evaluate the patient's intake and output and urinary frequency.
• Auscultate lung sounds for rales and wheezing in patients with CHF.
• Monitor the patient's urinalysis for proteinuria.

• Monitor serum potassium levels in patients also receiving diuretic therapy.
• Assess the patient's pattern of daily bowel activity and stool consistency.

Patient Teaching
• Caution the patient against abruptly discontinuing the drug.
• Warn the patient to notify the physician if he or she experiences chest pain, cough, diarrhea, difficulty swallowing, fever, palpitations, sore throat, swelling of the face, or vomiting.
• Explain to the patient that trandolapril may cause altered taste perception.
• Advise the patient to rise slowly from lying to sitting position and to permit legs to dangle from the bed momentarily before standing to reduce the hypotensive effect of trandolapril.
• Stress to the patient that he or she should avoid potassium supplements and salt substitutes during trandolapril therapy.

22 Angiotensin II Receptor Antagonists

candesartan cilexetil
eprosartan
irbesartan
losartan
olmesartan
  medoxomil
telmisartan
valsartan

Uses: Angiotensin II receptor antagonists (AIIRAs) are used to treat hypertension alone or in combination with other antihypertensives.

Action: AIIRAs block the vasoconstricting and aldosterone-secreting effects of angiotensin II, a potent vasoconstrictor. By selectively blocking the binding of angiotensin II to AT_1 receptors in vascular smooth muscle and the adrenal gland, AIIRAs cause vasodilation, decrease aldosterone effects, and reduce blood pressure.

COMBINATION PRODUCTS

ATACAND HCT: candesartan/
hydrochlorothiazide (a diuretic)
16 mg/12.5 mg; 32 mg/
12.5 mg.
AVALIDE: irbesartan/
hydrochlorothiazide (a diuretic)
150 mg/12.5 mg; 300 mg/
12.5 mg.
BENICAR HCT: olmesartan/
hydrochlorothiazide (a diuretic)
20 mg/12.5 mg; 40 mg/
12.5 mg; 40 mg/25 mg.
DIOVAN HCT: valsartan/
hydrochlorothiazide (a diuretic)
80 mg/12.5 mg; 160 mg/
12.5 mg; 160 mg/25 mg.
HYZAAR: losartan/
hydrochlorothiazide (a diuretic)
50 mg/12.5 mg; 100 mg/
25 mg.
MICARDIS HCT: telmisartan/
hydrochlorothiazide (a diuretic)
40 mg/12.5 mg; 80 mg/
12.5 mg.
TEVETEN HCT: eprosartan/
hydrochlorothiazide (a diuretic)
600 mg/12.5 mg; 600 mg/
25 mg.

candesartan cilexetil
can-deh-**sar-tan sill-ex**-eh-til
(Atacand)

CATEGORY AND SCHEDULE
Pregnancy Risk Category: C
(D if used in second or third trimester)

MECHANISM OF ACTION
This angiotensin II receptor, type AT_1, antagonist blocks the vasoconstrictor and aldosterone-secreting effects of angiotensin II, inhibiting the binding of angiotensin II to the AT_1 receptors. *Therapeutic Effect:* Produces vasodilation, decreases peripheral resistance, decreases blood pressure (B/P).

PHARMACOKINETICS

Route	Onset	Peak	Duration
PO	2–3 hrs	6–8 hrs	Greater than 24 hrs

Rapidly, completely absorbed. Protein binding: greater than 99%. Undergoes minor hepatic metabolism to inactive metabolite. Excreted unchanged in urine and feces via biliary system. Not removed by hemodialysis. **Half-life:** 9 hrs.

AVAILABILITY
Tablets: 4 mg, 8 mg, 16 mg, 32 mg.

INDICATIONS AND DOSAGES
▸ **Hypertension alone or in combination with other antihypertensives**
PO
Adults, Elderly, Patient with mildly impaired liver or renal function.
Initially, 16 mg once a day in those who are not volume depleted. Can be given once or twice a day with total daily doses 8–32 mg. Give lower dosage in those treated with diuretics or with severely impaired renal function.

UNLABELED USES
Treatment of heart failure

CONTRAINDICATIONS
Hypersensitivity to candesartan

INTERACTIONS
Drug
None known.
Herbal
None known.
Food
None known.

DIAGNOSTIC TEST EFFECTS
May increase BUN, serum alkaline phosphatase, serum bilirubin, serum creatinine, SGOT (AST), and SGPT (ALT) levels. May decrease blood Hgb and Hct levels.

SIDE EFFECTS
Occasional (6%–3%)
Upper respiratory tract infection, dizziness, back and leg pain
Rare (2%–1%)
Pharyngitis, rhinitis, headache, fatigue, diarrhea, nausea, dry cough, peripheral edema

SERIOUS REACTIONS
• Overdosage may manifest as hypotension and tachycardia. Bradycardia occurs less often. Institute supportive measures.

NURSING CONSIDERATIONS
Baseline Assessment
• Assess the patient's apical pulse and B/P immediately before each candesartan dose, in addition to regular monitoring. Be alert to fluctuations in apical pulse and B/P. If an excessive reduction in B/P occurs, place the patient in the supine position with feet slightly elevated and notify physician.
• Assess the patient for pregnancy.
• Determine if the patient has a history of liver or renal impairment or renal artery stenosis.
• Assess the patient's medication history, especially for diuretics.
• Expect to obtain the patient's blood Hgb and Hct, BUN, and serum alkaline phosphatase, serum bilirubin, serum creatinine, SGOT (AST), and SGPT (ALT) levels.
Lifespan Considerations
• Be aware that it is unknown if candesartan is distributed in breast milk. Know that candesartan may cause fetal or neonatal morbidity or mortality.
• Be aware that the safety and efficacy of candesartan have not been established in children.
• There are no age-related precautions noted in the elderly.
Precautions
• Use cautiously in dehydrated patients because they are at risk for developing hypotension.
• Use cautiously in patients with liver or renal impairment, renal artery stenosis, and severe congestive heart failure (CHF).

Administration and Handling
PO
• Give candesartan without regard to food.
Intervention and Evaluation
• Offer the patient fluids frequently to maintain hydration.
• Assess the patient for evidence of an upper respiratory infection.
• Assist the patient with ambulation if he or she experiences dizziness.
• Monitor all of the patient's blood serum levels.
• Assess the patient's B/P for hypertension and hypotension.
Patient Teaching
• Advise female patients of the consequences of second- and third-trimester exposure to candesartan. Urge female patients to immediately notify the physician of pregnancy.
• Stress to the patient that he or she should avoid tasks that require mental alertness or motor skills until his or her response to the drug is established.
• Warn the patient to notify the physician if he or she experiences any sign of infection, including fever and sore throat.
• Caution the patient against discontinuing the drug because candesartan is necessary for lifelong control of hypertension.
• Encourage the patient not to exercise outside during hot weather to avoid the risks of dehydration and hypotension development.

eprosartan
eh-pro-**sar**-tan
(Teveten)

CATEGORY AND SCHEDULE
Pregnancy Risk Category: C
(D if used in second or third trimester)

MECHANISM OF ACTION
An angiotensin II receptor antagonist that blocks the vasoconstrictor and aldosterone-secreting effects of angiotensin II, inhibiting the binding of angiotensin II to the AT_1 receptors. *Therapeutic Effect:* Causes vasodilation, decreased peripheral resistance, decrease in blood pressure (B/P).

PHARMACOKINETICS
Rapidly absorbed after PO administration. Protein binding: 98%. Undergoes first-pass metabolism in liver to active metabolites. Excreted in urine and biliary system. Minimally removed by hemodialysis. **Half-life:** 5–9 hrs.

AVAILABILITY
Tablets: 400 mg, 600 mg.

INDICATIONS AND DOSAGES
▶ **Hypertension**
PO
Adults, Elderly. Initially, 600 mg/ day. Range: 400–800 mg/day.

CONTRAINDICATIONS
Bilateral renal artery stenosis, hyperaldosteronism

INTERACTIONS
Drug
None known.
Herbal
None known.

Food
None known.

DIAGNOSTIC TEST EFFECTS
May increase BUN, serum alkaline phosphatase, serum bilirubin, serum creatinine, SGOT (AST), and SGPT (ALT) levels. May decrease blood Hgb and Hgb levels.

SIDE EFFECTS
Occasional (5%–2%)
Headache, cough, dizziness
Rare (less than 2%)
Muscle pain, fatigue, diarrhea, upper respiratory infection, dyspepsia

SERIOUS REACTIONS
• Overdosage may manifest as hypotension and tachycardia. Bradycardia occurs less often.

NURSING CONSIDERATIONS

Baseline Assessment
• Assess the patient's apical pulse and B/P immediately before each eprosartan dose, in addition to regular monitoring. Be alert to fluctuations in apical pulse and B/P.
• Determine if the patient is pregnant or has a history of liver or renal impairment or renal artery stenosis.
• Assess the patient's medication history, especially for diuretics.
Lifespan Considerations
• Be aware that eprosartan has caused fetal or neonatal morbidity or mortality. Also, know that because of the potential for adverse effects on the infant, patients taking eprosartan should not breast-feed.
• Be aware that the safety and efficacy of eprosartan have not been established in children.
• There are no age-related precautions noted in the elderly.

Precautions
• Use cautiously in patients with preexisting renal insufficiency, significant aortic or mitral stenosis, and unilateral renal artery stenosis.
Administration and Handling
PO
• Give eprosartan without regard to food.
• Do not crush or break tablets.
Intervention and Evaluation
• Monitor the patient's BUN, serum electrolytes, and serum creatinine levels. Also, assess the patient's supine B/P, heart rate for tachycardia, and urinalysis results.
Patient Teaching
• Advise female patients of the consequences of second- and third-trimester exposure to eprosartan.
• Warn the patient to avoid tasks that require mental alertness or motor skills until his or her response to the drug is established.
• Urge the patient to restrict his or her alcohol and sodium consumption while taking eprosartan. Stress to the patient the he or she should adhere to the provided diet and control weight.
• Caution the patient against discontinuing the drug because eprosartan is necessary for lifelong control of hypertension.
• Encourage the patient not to exercise outside during hot weather to avoid the risks of dehydration and hypotension.
• Instruct the patient to check his or her B/P regularly.

irbesartan
ir-beh-**sar**-tan
(Avapro, Karvea[AUS])

CATEGORY AND SCHEDULE
Pregnancy Risk Category: C
(D if used in second or third
trimester)

MECHANISM OF ACTION
This angiotensin II receptor, type
AT_1, antagonist blocks the vasoconstrictor and aldosterone-secreting
effects of angiotensin II, inhibiting
the binding of angiotensin II to the
AT_1 receptors. *Therapeutic Effect:*
Produces vasodilation, decreases
peripheral resistance, decreases
blood pressure (B/P).

PHARMACOKINETICS
Rapidly and completely absorbed
after PO administration. Protein
binding: 90%. Undergoes hepatic
metabolism to inactive metabolite.
Recovered primarily in feces and, to
a lesser extent, in urine. Not removed by hemodialysis. **Half-life:**
11–15 hrs.

AVAILABILITY
Tablets: 75 mg, 150 mg, 300 mg.

INDICATIONS AND DOSAGES
▶ **Hypertension alone or in combi-
nation with other antihypertensives**
PO
*Adults, Elderly, Children 13 yrs and
older.* Initially, 75–150 mg/day.
May increase to 300 mg/day.
Children 6–12 yrs. Initially, 75
mg/day. May increase to 150 mg/
day.

UNLABELED USES
Treatment of heart failure

CONTRAINDICATIONS
Bilateral renal artery stenosis, biliary cirrhosis or obstruction, primary
hyperaldosteronism, severe liver
insufficiency

INTERACTIONS
Drug
Hydrochlorothiazide: Produces
further reduction in B/P.
Herbal
None known.
Food
None known.

DIAGNOSTIC TEST EFFECTS
Minor increase in BUN and serum
creatinine levels. May decrease
blood Hgb levels.

SIDE EFFECTS
Occasional (9%–3%)
Upper respiratory infection, fatigue,
diarrhea, cough
Rare (2%–1%)
Heartburn, dizziness, headache,
nausea, rash

SERIOUS REACTIONS
• Overdosage may manifest as
hypotension and tachycardia. Bradycardia occurs less often.

NURSING CONSIDERATIONS
Baseline Assessment
• Obtain the patient's apical pulse
and B/P immediately before each
irbesartan dose and monitor regularly throughout therapy. Be alert to
fluctuations in apical pulse and B/P.
If an excessive reduction in B/P
occurs, place the patient in the
supine position with feet slightly
elevated.
• Determine if the patient is pregnant before beginning therapy.
• Assess the patient's medication
history, especially for diuretics.

Lifespan Considerations
• Be aware that it is unknown if irbesartan is distributed in breast milk. Irbesartan may cause fetal or neonatal morbidity or mortality.
• Be aware that the safety and efficacy of irbesartan have not been established in children.
• There are no age-related precautions noted in the elderly.

Precautions
• Use cautiously in patients with congestive heart failure (CHF), coronary artery disease, mild to moderate liver dysfunction, sodium or water depletion, and unilateral renal artery stenosis.

Administration and Handling
◀ALERT▶ Know that irbesartan may be given concurrently with other antihypertensives and if the B/P is not controlled by irbesartan alone, a diuretic may also be prescribed.
PO
• Give irbesartan without regard to meals.

Intervention and Evaluation
• Offer the patient fluids frequently to maintain hydration.
• Assess the patient for signs and symptoms of an upper respiratory infection.
• Assist the patient with ambulation if he or she experiences dizziness.
• Monitor the patient's B/P and pulse rate. Also check the results of serum electrolyte tests, liver and renal function tests, and urinalysis.
• Assess the patient for signs and symptoms of hypotension.

Patient Teaching
• Advise female patients of the consequences of second- and third-trimester exposure to irbesartan.
• Stress to the patient that he or she should avoid tasks that require mental alertness or motor skills until his or her response to the drug is established.

• Warn the patient to report signs or symptoms of infection, including fever and sore throat.
• Encourage the patient to avoid outdoor exercise during hot weather to avoid the risks of dehydration and hypotension.

losartan
loh-**sar**-tan
(Cozaar)
Do not confuse with Zocor.

CATEGORY AND SCHEDULE
Pregnancy Risk Category: C
(D if used in second or third trimesters)

MECHANISM OF ACTION
An angiotensin II receptor, type AT_1, antagonist that blocks vasoconstrictor and aldosterone-secreting effects of angiotensin II, inhibiting the binding of angiotensin II to the AT_1 receptors. *Therapeutic Effect:* Causes vasodilation, decreased peripheral resistance, decrease in blood pressure (B/P).

PHARMACOKINETICS

Route	Onset	Peak	Duration
PO	N/A	6 hrs	24 hrs

Well absorbed after PO administration. Protein binding: greater than 98%. Undergoes first-pass metabolism in liver to active metabolites. Excreted in urine and via biliary system. Not removed by hemodialysis. **Half-life:** 2 hrs (metabolite: 6–9 hrs).

AVAILABILITY
Tablets: 25 mg, 50 mg, 100 mg.

INDICATIONS AND DOSAGES
▶ **Hypertension**
PO
Adults, Elderly. Initially, 50 mg once a day. Maximum: May be given once or twice a day with total daily doses ranging from 25–100 mg.
▶ **Nephropathy**
PO
Adults, Elderly. Initially, 50 mg/day. May increase to 100 mg/day based on B/P response.
▶ **Hypertension in patients with impaired liver function**
PO
Adults, Elderly. Initially, 25 mg a day.

CONTRAINDICATIONS
None known

INTERACTIONS
Drug
Cimetidine: May increase the effects of losartan.
Ketoconazole, troleandomycin: May inhibit the effects of these drugs.
Lithium: May increase lithium blood concentration and risk of toxicity.
Phenobarbital, rifampin: May decrease the effects of losartan.
Herbal
None known.
Food
Grapefruit juice: May alter the absorption of losartan.

DIAGNOSTIC TEST EFFECTS
May increase BUN, serum alkaline phosphatase, serum bilirubin, serum creatinine, SGOT (AST), and SGPT (ALT) levels. May decrease blood Hgb and Hct levels.

SIDE EFFECTS
Frequent (8%)
Upper respiratory infection

Occasional (4%–2%)
Dizziness, diarrhea, cough
Rare (1% or less)
Insomnia, dyspepsia, heartburn, back and leg pain, muscle cramps or aches, nasal congestion, sinusitis

SERIOUS REACTIONS
• Overdosage may manifest as hypotension and tachycardia. Bradycardia occurs less often.

NURSING CONSIDERATIONS
Baseline Assessment
• Assess the patient's apical pulse and B/P immediately before each dose and regularly throughout therapy. Be alert to fluctuations in apical pulse and B/P. If an excessive reduction in B/P occurs, place the patient in the supine position with feet slightly elevated and notify the physician.
• Determine if the patient is pregnant.
• Assess the patient's medication history, especially for diuretics.
Lifespan Considerations
• Be aware that losartan has caused fetal or neonatal morbidity or mortality and has the potential for adverse effects on the breast-fed infant. Patients should not breast-feed while taking losartan.
• Be aware that the safety and efficacy of losartan have not been established in children.
• There are no age-related precautions noted in the elderly.
Precautions
• Use cautiously in patients with liver or renal function impairment and renal arterial stenosis.
Administration and Handling
PO
• Give losartan without regard to food.
• Do not crush or break tablets.

Intervention and Evaluation
• Offer the patient fluids frequently to maintain hydration.
• Assess the patient for evidence of cough and upper respiratory infection.
• Assist the patient with ambulation if he or she experiences dizziness.
• Assess the patient's pattern of daily bowel activity and stool consistency.
• Monitor the patient's B/P and pulse.

Patient Teaching
• Advise female patients of the consequences of second- and third-trimester exposure to losartan.
• Stress to the female patient that she should immediately notify the physician if she becomes pregnant.
• Warn the patient to avoid tasks that require mental alertness or motor skills until his or her response to the drug is established.
• Caution the patient to notify the physician if he or she experiences any chest pain, or signs and symptoms of infection (fever, sore throat).
• Explain to the patient that he or she should not take cold preparations or nasal decongestants while on losartan therapy.
• Caution the patient against abruptly discontinuing the drug.

olmesartan medoxomil
ol-**mess**-er-tan
(Benicar)

CATEGORY AND SCHEDULE
Pregnancy Risk Category: C
(D if used in second or third trimester)

MECHANISM OF ACTION
An angiotensin II receptor, type AT_1, antagonist that blocks the vasoconstrictor and aldosterone-secreting effects of angiotensin II, inhibiting the binding of angiotensin II to the AT_1 receptors. *Therapeutic Effect:* Produces vasodilation; decreases peripheral resistance, blood pressure (B/P).

PHARMACOKINETICS
Rapidly and completely absorbed after PO administration. Metabolized in the liver. Recovered primarily in feces and, to a lesser extent, in urine. Not removed by hemodialysis. **Half-life:** 13 hrs.

AVAILABILITY
Tablets: 5 mg, 20 mg, 40 mg.

INDICATIONS AND DOSAGES
▸ **Hypertension**
PO
Adults, Elderly, Mildly impaired liver or renal function. 20 mg once a day in patients who are not volume depleted. After 2 weeks of therapy, if further reduction in B/P is needed, may increase dosage to 40 mg/day.

CONTRAINDICATIONS
Bilateral renal artery stenosis

INTERACTIONS
Drug
Diuretics: Produce further reduction in B/P.
Herbal
None known.
Food
None known.

DIAGNOSTIC TEST EFFECTS
May increase blood Hgb and Hct levels.

SIDE EFFECTS

Occasional (3%)
Dizziness
Rare (less than 2%)
Headache, diarrhea, upper respiratory tract infection

SERIOUS REACTIONS

• Overdosage may manifest as hypotension and tachycardia. Bradycardia occurs less often.

NURSING CONSIDERATIONS

Baseline Assessment
• Assess the patient's apical pulse and B/P immediately before each olmesartan dose, and regularly monitor throughout therapy. Be alert to fluctuations in apical pulse and B/P. If an excessive reduction in B/P occurs, place the patient in the supine position with feet slightly elevated and notify the physician.
• Determine if the patient is pregnant.
• Assess the patient's medication history, especially for diuretics.

Lifespan Considerations
• Be aware that is unknown if olmesartan is distributed in breast milk. Know that olmesartan may cause fetal or neonatal morbidity or mortality.
• Be aware that the safety and efficacy of olmesartan have not been established in children.
• There are no age-related precautions noted in the elderly.

Precautions
• Use cautiously in patients with liver or renal function impairment and renal arterial stenosis.

Administration and Handling
PO
• Give olmesartan without regard to meals.

Intervention and Evaluation
• Offer the patient fluids frequently to maintain hydration.
• Assess the patient for signs and symptoms of an upper respiratory infection.
• Assist the patient with ambulation if he or she experiences dizziness.
• Monitor the results of the patient's diagnostic tests.
• Assess the patient's B/P for hypertension or hypotension.

Patient Teaching
• Advise female patients of the consequences of second- and third-trimester exposure to olmesartan.
• Urge the patient to avoid tasks that require mental alertness or motor skills until his or her response to the drug is established.
• Warn the patient to notify the physician if he or she experiences any signs or symptoms of infection, including fever and sore throat.
• Explain to the patient that olmesartan will be needed for lifelong control of hypertension.
• Caution the patient against exercising outside during hot weather because of the risks of dehydration and hypotension.

telmisartan

tell-mih-**sar**-tan
(Micardis, Pritor[AUS])

CATEGORY AND SCHEDULE

Pregnancy Risk Category: C
(D if used in second or third trimester)

MECHANISM OF ACTION

An angiotensin II receptor, type AT_1, antagonist; blocks vasoconstrictor and aldosterone-secreting effects of angiotensin II, inhibiting the binding of angiotensin II to the AT_1 receptors. *Therapeutic Effect:* Causes vasodilation, decreased peripheral resistance, decrease in blood pressure (B/P).

PHARMACOKINETICS
Rapidly and completely absorbed after PO administration. Protein binding: greater than 99%. Undergoes liver metabolism to inactive metabolite. Excreted in feces. Unknown if removed by hemodialysis. **Half-life:** 24 hrs.

AVAILABILITY
Tablets: 20 mg, 40 mg, 80 mg.

INDICATIONS AND DOSAGES
▶ **Hypertension**
PO
Adults, Elderly. 40 mg once a day. Range: 20–80 mg.

UNLABELED USES
Treatment of congestive heart failure (CHF)

CONTRAINDICATIONS
None known

INTERACTIONS
Drug
Digoxin: Increases digoxin plasma concentrations.
Warfarin: Slightly decreases warfarin plasma concentrations.
Herbal
None known.
Food
None known.

DIAGNOSTIC TEST EFFECTS
May increase serum creatinine levels. May decrease blood Hgb and Hct levels.

SIDE EFFECTS
Occasional (7%–3%)
Upper respiratory tract infection, sinusitis, back or leg pain, diarrhea
Rare (1%)
Dizziness, headache, fatigue, nausea, heartburn, myalgia, cough, peripheral edema

SERIOUS REACTIONS
• Overdosage may manifest as hypotension and tachycardia. Bradycardia occurs less often.

NURSING CONSIDERATIONS
Baseline Assessment
• Assess the patient's apical pulse and B/P immediately before each telmisartan dose and regularly throughout therapy. Be alert to fluctuations in apical pulse and B/P. If an excessive reduction in B/P occurs, place the patient in the supine position with feet slightly elevated and notify physician.
• Assess the patient's medication history, especially for diuretics.
• Determine if the patient has a history of liver or renal impairment or renal artery stenosis.
• Monitor the results of the patient's blood Hgb, BUN, and serum creatinine tests. Also monitor the patient's BP, pulse rate, and other vital signs.
Lifespan Considerations
• Be aware that telmisartan may cause fetal harm and it is unknown if telmisartan is excreted in breast milk.
• Be aware that the safety and efficacy of telmisartan have not been established in children.
• There are no age-related precautions noted in the elderly.
Precautions
• Use cautiously in patients with liver and renal impairment, renal

artery stenosis (bilateral or unilateral), and volume depletion.

Administration and Handling

◀ALERT▶ May be given concurrently with other antihypertensives. If B/P is not controlled by telmisartan alone, a diuretic may be added.

PO

• Give telmisartan without regard to meals.

Intervention and Evaluation

• Monitor the patient's B/P, BUN, pulse, serum creatinine, and serum electrolyte levels.

• Monitor the patient for signs and symptoms of hypotension during the initial telmisartan doses.

Patient Teaching

• Encourage the patient to drink fluids frequently to maintain proper hydration.

• Advise female patients of the consequences of second- and third-trimester exposure to telmisartan. Emphasize that she should immediately notify the physician if she becomes pregnant.

• Urge the patient to avoid tasks that require mental alertness or motor skills until his or her response to the drug is established.

• Caution the patient to notify the physician if he or she experiences any signs or symptoms of infection, including fever and sore throat.

• Explain to the patient that telmisartan is needed for lifelong control of hypertension.

• Caution the patient against excessive exertion during hot weather because of the risks of dehydration and hypotension.

valsartan
val-**sar**-tan
(Diovan)

CATEGORY AND SCHEDULE
Pregnancy Risk Category: C (D if used in second or third trimester)

MECHANISM OF ACTION
An angiotensin II receptor, type AT_1, antagonist; blocks vasoconstrictor and aldosterone-secreting effects of angiotensin II, inhibiting the binding of angiotensin II to the AT_1 receptors. *Therapeutic Effect:* Produces vasodilation, decreased peripheral resistance, decrease in blood pressure (B/P).

PHARMACOKINETICS
Poorly absorbed after PO administration. Food decreases peak plasma concentration. Protein binding: 95%. Metabolized in the liver. Recovered primarily in feces and, to a lesser extent, in urine. Unknown if removed by hemodialysis. **Half-life:** 6 hrs.

AVAILABILITY
Tablets: 40 mg, 80 mg, 160 mg, 320 mg.

INDICATIONS AND DOSAGES
▶ **Hypertension**
PO
Adults, Elderly. Initially, 80–160 mg/day in patients who are not volume depleted. May increase up to a maximum 320 mg/day.
▶ **Congestive heart failure (CHF)**
PO
Adults, Elderly. Initially, 40 mg 2 times/day. May increase up to 160 mg 2 times/day. Maximum: 320 mg/day.

CONTRAINDICATIONS
Biliary cirrhosis or obstruction, bilateral renal artery stenosis, hypoaldosteronism, severe liver impairment

INTERACTIONS
Drug
Diuretics: Produces additive hypotensive effects.
Herbal
None known.
Food
Food: Decreases peak plasma concentration of valsartan.

DIAGNOSTIC TEST EFFECTS
May increase SGOT (AST), SGPT (ACT), and serum bilirubin, creatinine, and potassium. May decrease blood Hgb and Hct.

SIDE EFFECTS
Rare (2%–1%)
Insomnia, fatigue, heartburn, abdominal pain, dizziness, headache, diarrhea, nausea, vomiting, arthralgia, edema

SERIOUS REACTIONS
• Overdosage may manifest as hypotension and tachycardia. Bradycardia occurs less often.
• Viral infection and upper respiratory infection (cough, pharyngitis, sinusitis, rhinitis) occur rarely.

NURSING CONSIDERATIONS
Baseline Assessment
• Assess the patient's apical pulse and B/P immediately before each valsartan dose and regularly monitor throughout therapy. Be alert to fluctuations in apical pulse and B/P. If an excessive reduction in B/P occurs, place the patient in the supine position with feet slightly elevated and notify the physician.

• Determine if the patient is pregnant.
• Assess the patient's medication history, especially for diuretics.
• Determine if the patient has a history of liver and renal impairment, renal artery stenosis, or severe CHF.
• Monitor the results of the patient's blood Hgb and Hct, BUN, serum alkaline phosphatase, serum bilirubin, serum creatinine, SGOT (AST) and SGPT (ALT) levels, and vital signs, particularly B/P and pulse rate.
Lifespan Considerations
• Be aware that valsartan may cause fetal harm and it is unknown if valsartan is distributed in breast milk.
• Be aware that the safety and efficacy of valsartan have not been established in children.
• There are no age-related precautions noted in the elderly.
Precautions
• Use cautiously in patients also receiving potassium-sparing diuretics or potassium supplements.
• Use cautiously in patients with CHF, coronary artery disease, mild to moderate liver impairment, and unilateral renal artery stenosis.
Administration and Handling
◀ALERT▶ Know that valsartan may be given concurrently with other antihypertensives. If B/P is not controlled by valsartan alone, expect to administer a diuretic, as prescribed.
PO
• Give valsartan without regard to meals.
Intervention and Evaluation
• Offer the patient fluids frequently to maintain hydration.
• Assess the patient for signs and symptoms of an upper respiratory infection.

• Monitor the patient's B/P, serum electrolyte levels, liver and renal function tests, and urinalysis.
• Regularly assess the patient's B/P and pulse rate.
• Observe the patient for signs and symptoms of hypotension.

Patient Teaching

• Advise female patients of the consequences of second- and third-trimester exposure to valsartan.
• Stress to the female patient that she should immediately notify the physician if she becomes pregnant.

• Caution the patient to notify the physician if he or she experiences signs or symptoms of infection, including fever and sore throat.
• Explain to the patient that he or she should not stop taking valsartan because this drug will be needed for lifelong control of hypertension.
• Caution the patient against exercising outside during hot weather because of the risks of dehydration and hypotension.

23 Antiarrhythmic Agents

adenosine
amiodarone
  hydrochloride
atropine sulfate
disopyramide
  phosphate
dofetilide
flecainide
ibutilide fumarate
lidocaine
  hydrochloride
mexiletine
  hydrochloride
moricizine
  hydrochloride
procainamide
  hydrochloride
propafenone
  hydrochloride
quinidine
tocainide
  hydrochloride

Uses: Antiarrhythmics are used to prevent and treat cardiac arrhythmias, such as premature ventricular contractions, ventricular tachycardia, premature atrial contractions, paroxysmal atrial tachycardia, atrial fibrillation, and atrial flutter.

Action: Antiarrhythmic agents affect certain ion channels and receptors on the myocardial cell membrane. They're divided into four classes: Class I drugs are further divided into three subclasses (IA, IB, IC) based on the drugs' electrophysiologic effects.
  Class I: Blocks cardiac sodium channels and slows conduction velocity, prolonging refractoriness and decreasing automaticity of sodium-dependent tissue.
  Class IA: Blocks sodium and potassium channels.
  Class IB: Shortens the repolarization phase.
  Class IC: Doesn't affect the repolarization phase, but slows conduction velocity.
  Class II: Slows sinoatrial (SA) and atrioventricular (AV) nodal conduction.
  Class III: Blocks cardiac potassium channels, prolonging the repolarization phase of electrical cells.
  Class IV: Inhibits the influx of calcium through its channels, causing slower conduction through the SA and AV nodes.

COMBINATION PRODUCTS

EMLA: lidocaine/prilocaine (an anesthetic) 2.5%/2.5%.
LIDOCAINE WITH EPINEPHRINE: lidocaine/epinephrine (a vasopressor) 2%/1:50,000; 1%/1:100,000; 1%/1:200,000; 0.5%/1:200,000.
LOMOTIL: atropine/diphenoxylate (an antidiarrheal) 0.025 mg/2.5 mg.

adenosine
ah-**den**-oh-seen
(Adenocard, Adenocor[AUS])

CATEGORY AND SCHEDULE
Pregnancy Risk Category: C

MECHANISM OF ACTION
A cardiac agent that slows impulse formation in the sinoatrial (SA) node and conduction time through the atrioventricular (AV) node. Adenosine also acts as a diagnostic aid in myocardial perfusion imaging

or stress echocardiography. *Therapeutic Effect:* Depresses left ventricular function and restores normal sinus rhythm.

AVAILABILITY
Injection. 3 mg/ml in 6 mg and 12 mg syringes.

INDICATIONS AND DOSAGES
▸ **Paroxysmal supraventricular tachycardia (PSVT)**
Rapid IV bolus
Adults, Elderly. Initially, 6 mg given over 1–2 sec. If first dose does not convert within 1–2 min, give 12 mg; may repeat 12-mg dose in 1–2 min if no response has occurred. *Children.* Initially 0.1 mg/kg (maximum 6 mg). If ineffective, may give 0.2 mg/kg (maximum 12 mg).
▸ **Diagnostic testing**
IV infusion
Adults. 140 mcg/kg/min for 6 min.

CONTRAINDICATIONS
Atrial fibrillation or flutter, second-or third-degree AV block or sick sinus syndrome (with functioning pacemaker), ventricular tachycardia

INTERACTIONS
Drug
Carbamazepine: May increase degree of heart block caused by adenosine.
Dipyridamole: May increase effect of adenosine.
Methylxanthines (e.g., caffeine, theophylline): May decrease effect of adenosine.
Herbal
None known.
Food
None known.

DIAGNOSTIC TEST EFFECTS
None known.

IV INCOMPATIBILITIES
Any other drug or solution other than 0.9% NaCl or D_5W.

SIDE EFFECTS
Frequent (18%–12%)
Facial flushing, shortness of breath or dyspnea
Occasional (7%–2%)
Headache, nausea, lightheadedness, chest pressure
Rare (less than or equal to 1%)
Numbness or tingling in arms, dizziness, sweating, hypotension, palpitations, chest, jaw, or neck pain

SERIOUS REACTIONS
• May produce short-lasting heart block.

NURSING CONSIDERATIONS
Baseline Assessment
• Identify the arrhythmia on a 12-lead electrocardiogram (EKG). Also assess the patient's heart rate and rhythm on a continuous cardiac monitor and evaluate the apical pulse rate, rhythm, and quality.
Precautions
• Use cautiously in patients with arrhythmias at time of conversion, asthma, heart block, or liver or renal failure.
Administration and Handling
IV
• Store at room temperature. Solution normally appears clear.
• Crystallization occurs if refrigerated; if crystallization occurs, dissolve crystals by warming to room temperature. Discard unused portion.
• Administer very rapidly, over 1 to 2 seconds, undiluted directly into vein, or if using an IV line, use the closest port to the insertion site. If the IV line is infusing any fluid other than 0.9% NaCl, flush the line

first before administering adenosine.
• Follow the rapid bolus injection with a rapid 0.9% NaCl flush.

Intervention and Evaluation
• Continue to assess the patient's heart rate and rhythm with continuous cardiac monitoring.
• Monitor the patient's apical pulse rate, rhythm, and strength, blood pressure (B/P), and the quality of the respirations.
• Monitor the patient's intake and output.
• Assess the patient for fluid retention.
• Check serum electrolytes.

Patient Teaching
• Advise the patient to report unusual signs or symptoms, including chest pain, chest pounding or palpitations, or difficulty breathing or shortness of breath.
• Explain that facial flushing, headache, and nausea may occur and that these symptoms will resolve.

amiodarone hydrochloride

ah-me-**oh**-dah-roan
(Aratac[AUS], Cordarone, Cordarone X[AUS], Pacerone)
Do not confuse with amiloride or Cardura.

CATEGORY AND SCHEDULE
Pregnancy Risk Category: D

MECHANISM OF ACTION
A cardiac agent that prolongs myocardial cell action potential duration and refractory period by acting directly on all cardiac tissue. *Therapeutic Effect:* Decreases atrioventricular (AV) conduction and sinus node function.

PHARMACOKINETICS

Route	Onset	Peak	Duration
PO	3 days– 3 wks	1 wk– 5 mos	7–50 days after discontinuation

Slowly, variably absorbed from gastrointestinal (GI) tract. Protein binding: 96%. Extensively metabolized in liver to active metabolite. Excreted via bile; not removed by hemodialysis. **Half-life:** 26–107 days; metabolite half-life is 61 days.

AVAILABILITY
Tablets: 200 mg, 400 mg.
Injection: 50 mg/ml.

INDICATIONS AND DOSAGES
▶ **Life-threatening recurrent ventricular fibrillation or hemodynamically unstable ventricular tachycardia**
PO
Adults, Elderly. Initially, 800–1,600 mg/day in 2–4 divided doses for 1–3 wks. After arrhythmias controlled or side effects occur, reduce to 600–800 mg/day for about 4 wks.
Maintenance: 200–600 mg/day.
Children. Initially, 10–15 mg/kg/day for 4–14 days, then 5 mg/kg/day for several wks. Maintenance: 2.5 mg/kg minimal dose for 5 of 7 days/wk.
IV infusion
Adults. Initially, 1,050 mg over 24 hrs: 150 mg over 10 min, follow by 360 mg over 6 hrs, follow by 540 mg over 18 hrs. May continue at 0.5 mg/min up to 2–3 wks regardless of age or renal or left ventricular function.

UNLABELED USES
Treatment and prophylaxis of supraventricular arrhythmias refractory to

conventional treatment and symptomatic atrial flutter

CONTRAINDICATIONS
Bradycardia-induced syncope (except in the presence of a pacemaker), second- and third-degree AV block, severe liver disease, severe sinus-node dysfunction

INTERACTIONS
Drug
Antiarrhythmics: May increase cardiac effects.
Beta blockers, oral anticoagulants: May increase effect of beta-blockers and oral anticoagulants.
Digoxin, phenytoin: May increase drug concentration and risk of toxicity of digoxin and phenytoin.
Herbal
None known.
Food
None known.

DIAGNOSTIC TEST EFFECTS
May increase ANA titer, serum alkaline phosphatase levels, SGOT (AST), and SGPT (ALT). May cause changes in electrocardiogram (EKG) and thyroid function tests. Therapeutic blood serum level is 0.5–2.5 mcg/ml; toxic serum level has not been established.

IV INCOMPATIBILITIES
Aminophylline (Theophylline), cefazolin (Ancef), heparin, sodium bicarbonate

IV COMPATIBILITIES
Dobutamine (Dobutrex), dopamine (Intropin), furosemide (Lasix), insulin (regular), labetalol (Normodyne), lidocaine, midazolam (Versed), morphine, nitroglycerin, norepinephrine (Levophed), phenylephrine (Neo-Synephrine), potassium chloride, vancomycin

SIDE EFFECTS
Expected
Corneal microdeposits are noted in almost all patients treated for more than 6 mos (can lead to blurry vision).
Frequent (greater than 3%)
Parenteral: Hypotension, nausea, fever, bradycardia.
Oral: Constipation, headache, decreased appetite, nausea, vomiting, numbness of fingers and toes, photosensitivity, muscular incoordination.
Occasional (less than 3%)
Oral: Bitter or metallic taste; decreased sexual ability and interest; dizziness; facial flushing; blue-gray coloring of skin of face, arms, neck; blurred vision; slow heartbeat; asymptomatic corneal deposits.
Rare (less than 1%)
Oral: Skin rash, vision loss, blindness.

SERIOUS REACTIONS
• Serious, potentially fatal pulmonary toxicity (alveolitis, pulmonary fibrosis, pneumonitis, acute respiratory distress syndrome) may begin with progressive dyspnea and cough with rales, decreased breath sounds, pleurisy, congestive heart failure (CHF) or liver toxicity.
• Amiodarone may worsen existing arrhythmias or produce new arrhythmias called proarrhythmias.

NURSING CONSIDERATIONS
Baseline Assessment
• Expect to patient to undergo baseline chest x-ray, EKG, and pulmonary function tests. Also, if ordered, check the results of baseline liver enzyme tests, serum alkaline phosphatase, SGOT (AST), and SGPT (ALT).
• Assess the apical pulse and blood

pressure (B/P) immediately before giving the drug. Withhold the medication and notify the physician if the pulse is 60 beats per minute or lower or the systolic B/P is less than 90 mm Hg.

Lifespan Considerations

• Be aware that amiodarone crosses the placenta and is distributed in breast milk. Know that fetal development is adversely affected by amiodarone.

• Be aware that the safety and efficacy of amiodarone have not been established in children.

• The elderly may be more sensitive to amiodarone's effects on thyroid function and may experience increased incidence of ataxia or other neurotoxic effects.

Precautions

• Use cautiously in patients with thyroid disease.

Administration and Handling

PO

• Give with meals to reduce gastrointestinal (GI) distress.

• Crush tablets may if necessary.

IV

◀**ALERT**▶ Be aware that solution concentrations greater than 3 mg/ml can cause peripheral vein phlebitis.

• Store at room temperature.

• Use glass or polyolefin containers for dilution. Dilute the loading dose of 150 mg in 100 ml D$_5$W to yield a solution of 1.5 mg/ml. Dilute the maintenance dose of 900 mg in 500 ml D$_5$W to yield a solution of 1.8 mg/ml.

• Use solutions held in PVC containers within 2 hours of dilution. Use solutions in glass or polyolefin containers within 24 hours of dilution.

• Give the drug through a central venous catheter (CVC) if possible, using an in-line filter. The solution does not need protection from light during administration.

• Give a bolus over 10 minutes (15 mg/min) not to exceed 30 mg/min; then 1 mg/min over 6 hours; then 0.5 mg/min over 18 hours. For infusions lasting longer than 1 hour, drug concentration should not exceed 2 mg/ml, unless a CVC is used.

Intervention and Evaluation

◀**ALERT**▶ Assess the patient for signs and symptoms of pulmonary toxicity, including progressively worsening cough and dyspnea. Expect to discontinue or reduce the drug dosage if toxicity occurs.

• Monitor the patient's serum alkaline phosphatase, SGOT (AST), and SGPT (ALT) levels as well as liver and thyroid function tests for evidence of toxicity. Expect to reduce or discontinue the drug dose if toxicity is evident or liver enzyme levels are elevated.

• Monitor the patient's amiodarone blood level. Know that the drug's therapeutic blood level is 0.5 to 2.5 mcg/ml and that the drug's toxic level has not been established.

• Assess the patient's pulse for bradycardia and an irregular rhythm as well as its quality. Monitor the patient's EKG for changes, particularly widening of the QRS complex and prolonged PR and QT intervals. Notify the physician of any significant interval changes.

• Assess the patient for signs and symptoms of hyperthyroidism, such as breathlessness, bulging eyes (exophthalmos), eyelid edema, frequent urination, hot and dry skin, and weight loss. Also assess the patient for signs and symptoms of hypothyroidism, such as cool and pale skin, lethargy, night cramps, periorbital edema, and pudgy hands and feet.

• Assess the patient for nausea and vomiting.
• Check for bluish discoloration of the skin and cornea in patients receiving therapy for longer than 2 months.

Patient Teaching
• Urge the patient not to abruptly discontinue the medication. Explain that compliance with the prescribed therapy is essential to control arrhythmias.
• Teach outpatients to monitor their pulse before taking the drug.
• Instruct the patient to report shortness of breath, cough, or vision changes.
• Warn the patient to limit his or her exposure to sunlight to protect against photosensitivity.
• Inform the patient that the bluish skin and cornea discoloration gradually disappear after the drug is discontinued.
• Encourage the patient to restrict his or her salt and alcohol intake.
• Recommend the patient seek ophthalmic exams every 6 months. Advise the patient to report any vision changes to the physician.

atropine sulfate
ah-trow-peen
(Atropine Sulfate, Atropisol[CAN], Atropt[AUS])

CATEGORY AND SCHEDULE
Pregnancy Risk Category: C

MECHANISM OF ACTION
An acetylcholine antagonist that competes with acetylcholine for common binding sites on muscarinic receptors, which are located on exocrine glands, cardiac and smooth muscle ganglia, and intramural neurons. This action blocks all muscarinic effects. *Therapeutic Effect:* Inhibits the action of acetylcholine, decreases gastrointestinal (GI) motility and secretory activity, genitourinary (GU) muscle tone (ureter, bladder); produces ophthalmic cycloplegia, mydriasis.

AVAILABILITY
Injection: 0.05 mg/ml, 0.1 mg/ml, 0.4 mg/0.5 ml, 0.4 mg/ml, 0.5 mg/ml, 1 mg/ml.

INDICATIONS AND DOSAGES
▸ **Asystole, slow pulseless electrical activity**
IV
Adults, Elderly. 1 mg, may repeat q3-5min up to total dose of 0.04 mg/kg.
▸ **Pre-anesthetic**
IV/IM/Subcutaneous
Adults, Elderly. 0.4-0.6 mg 30-60 min pre-op.
Children weighing 5 kg and more. 0.01-0.02 mg/kg/dose to maximum of 0.4 mg/dose.
Children weighing less than 5 kg. 0.02 mg/kg/dose 30-60 min pre-op.
▸ **Bradycardia**
IV
Adults, Elderly. 0.5-1 mg q5min not to exceed 2 mg or 0.04 mg/kg.
Children. 0.02 mg/kg with a minimum of 0.1 mg to a maximum of 0.5 mg in children and 1 mg in adolescents. May repeat in 5 min. Maximum total dose: 1 mg in children, 2 mg in adolescents.

CONTRAINDICATIONS
Bladder neck obstruction due to prostatic hypertrophy, cardiospasm, intestinal atony, myasthenia gravis in those not treated with neostigmine, narrow-angle glaucoma, obstructive disease of GI tract, paralytic ileus, severe ulcerative

colitis, tachycardia secondary to cardiac insufficiency or thyrotoxicosis, toxic megacolon, unstable cardiovascular status in acute hemorrhage

INTERACTIONS
Drug
Antacids, antidiarrheals: May decrease absorption of atropine.
Anticholinergics: May increase effects of atropine.
Ketoconazole: May decrease absorption of ketoconazole.
Potassium chloride: May increase severity of GI lesions with KCl (wax matrix).
Herbal
None known.
Food
None known.

DIAGNOSTIC TEST EFFECTS
None known.

IV INCOMPATIBILITIES
Pentothal (Thiopental)

IV COMPATIBILITIES
Diphenhydramine (Benadryl), droperidol (Inapsine), fentanyl (Sublimaze), glycopyrrolate (Robinul), heparin, hydromorphone (Dilaudid), midazolam (Versed), morphine, potassium chloride, propofol (Diprivan)

SIDE EFFECTS
Frequent
Dry mouth, nose, and throat that may be severe, decreased sweating, constipation, irritation at subcutaneous or IM injection site
Occasional
Swallowing difficulty, blurred vision, bloated feeling, impotence, urinary hesitancy
Rare
Allergic reaction, including rash and urticaria, mental confusion or excitement, particularly in children, fatigue

SERIOUS REACTIONS
• Overdosage may produce tachycardia, palpitations, hot, dry or flushed skin, absence of bowel sounds, increased respiratory rate, nausea, vomiting, confusion, drowsiness, slurred speech, and central nervous system (CNS) stimulation.
• Overdosage may produce psychosis as evidenced by agitation, restlessness, rambling speech, visual hallucinations, paranoid behavior, and delusions, followed by depression.

NURSING CONSIDERATIONS
Baseline Assessment
• Instruct the patient to urinate before giving this drug to reduce the risk of urinary retention.
Precautions
◀ALERT▶ Use extremely cautiously in patients with autonomic neuropathy, diarrhea, known or suspected GI infections, and mild to moderate ulcerative colitis.
• Use cautiously in patients with chronic obstructive pulmonary disease (COPD), congestive heart failure (CHF), coronary artery disease, esophageal reflux or hiatal hernia associated with reflux esophagitis, gastric ulcer, liver or renal disease, hypertension, hyperthyroidism, and tachyarrhythmias.
• Use atropine cautiously in the elderly and in infants.
Administration and Handling
◀ALERT▶ Notify physician and expect to discontinue this medication immediately if blurred vision, dizziness, or increased pulse occurs.

IM
• May be given by subcutaneous or IM injection.
IV
• To prevent paradoxical slowing of the heart rate, give the drug rapidly.
Intervention and Evaluation
• Monitor for changes in the patient's blood pressure (B/P), pulse, and temperature.
• Monitor the patient with heart disease for signs of tachycardia.
• Assess the patient's skin turgor and mucous membranes to evaluate his or her hydration status. Encourage the patient to drink fluids unless the patient is to have nothing by mouth for surgery.
• Assess the patient's bowel sounds for the presence of peristalsis and be alert for diminished bowel sounds.
• Monitor the patient for fever because patients receiving atropine are at an increased risk of hyperthermia.
• Monitor the patient's intake and output and palpate his or her bladder to assess for urinary retention.
• Assess the patient's stool frequency and consistency.
Patient Teaching
• If atropine is being given preoperatively, explain to the patient that a warm, dry, flushing feeling may occur upon administration.
• Remind the patient to remain in bed and not to eat or drink anything before surgery.

disopyramide phosphate
dye-so-**peer**-ah-myd
(Norpace, Norpace CR, Rythmodan[CAN])
Do not confuse with desipramine, dipyridamole, or Rythmol.

CATEGORY AND SCHEDULE
Pregnancy Risk Category: C

MECHANISM OF ACTION
An antiarrhythmic that prolongs the refractory period of the cardiac cell by direct effect, decreasing myocardial excitability and conduction velocity. *Therapeutic Effect:* Depresses myocardial contractility. Has anticholinergic and negative inotropic effects.

AVAILABILITY
Capsules: 100 mg, 150 mg.
Capsules (extended-release): 100 mg, 150 mg.

INDICATIONS AND DOSAGES
▶ **Suppression and prevention of ventricular ectopy, unifocal or multifocal premature ventricular contractions, paired ventricular contractions (couplets), and episodes of ventricular tachycardia**
PO
Adults, Elderly weighing more than 50 kg. 150 mg q6h (300 mg q12h with extended-release).
Adults, Elderly weighing less than 50 kg. 100 mg q6h (200 mg q12h with extended-release).
Children 12–18 yrs. 6–15 mg/kg/day in divided doses q6h.
Children 5–11 yrs. 10–15 mg/kg/day in divided doses q6h.
Children 1–4 yrs. 10–20 mg/kg/day in divided doses q6h.

Children younger than 1 yr. 10–30 mg/kg/day in divided doses q6h.
▸ **Rapid control of arrhythmias**
PO
◀**ALERT**▸ Do not use extended-release capsules.
Adults, elderly weighing 50 kg and more. Initially, 300 mg, then 150 mg q6h.
Adults, elderly weighing less than 50 kg. Initially, 200 mg, then 100 mg q6h.
▸ **Severe refractory arrhythmias**
PO
Adults, Elderly. Up to 400 mg q6h.
Children 12–18 yrs. 6–15 mg/kg/day.
Children 4–12 yrs. 10–15 mg/kg/day.
Children 1–4 yrs. 10–20 mg/kg/day.
Children younger than 1 yr. 10–30 mg/kg/day.
▸ **Dosage in renal impairment**
With or without loading dose of 150 mg:

Creatinine Clearance	Dosage
greater than 40 ml/min	100 mg q6h (extended-release 200 mg q12h)
30–40 ml/min	100 mg q8h
15–30 ml/min	100 mg q12h
less than 15 ml/min	100 mg q24h

▸ **Dosage in liver impairment**
Adults, Elderly weighing 50 kg and more. 100 mg q6h (200 mg q12h with extended-release).
▸ **Dosage in cardiomyopathy, cardiac decompensation**
Adults, Elderly weighing 50 kg and more. No loading dose; 100 mg q6–8h with gradual dosage adjustments.

UNLABELED USES
Prophylaxis and treatment of supraventricular tachycardia

CONTRAINDICATIONS
Cardiogenic shock, narrow-angle glaucoma (unless patient is undergoing cholinergic therapy), preexisting second- or third-degree atrioventricular (AV) block, preexisting urinary retention

INTERACTIONS
Drug
Other antiarrhythmics, including diltiazem, propranolol, verapamil: May prolong cardiac conduction, decrease cardiac output.
Pimozide: May increase cardiac arrhythmias.
Herbal
None known.
Food
None known.

DIAGNOSTIC TEST EFFECTS
May decrease blood glucose levels. May cause EKG changes. May increase serum cholesterol and triglyceride levels. Therapeutic blood level is 2 to 8 mcg/ml and the toxic blood level is greater than 8 mcg/ml.

SIDE EFFECTS
Frequent (greater than 9%)
Dry mouth (32%), urinary hesitancy, constipation
Occasional (9%–3%)
Blurred vision, dry eyes, nose, or throat, urinary retention, headache, dizziness, fatigue, nausea
Rare (less than 1%)
Impotence, hypotension, edema, weight gain, shortness of breath, syncope, chest pain, nervousness, diarrhea, vomiting, decreased appetite, rash, itching

SERIOUS REACTIONS
• May produce or aggravate congestive heart failure (CHF).
• May produce severe hypotension,

shortness of breath, chest pain, syncope (especially in patients with primary cardiomyopathy or CHF).
• Hepatotoxicity occurs rarely.

NURSING CONSIDERATIONS

Baseline Assessment
• Have the patient empty his or her bladder before administering disopyramide to reduce the risk of urine retention.

Precautions
• Use cautiously in patients with bundle-branch block, CHF, impaired liver or renal function, myasthenia gravis, prostatic hypertrophy, sick sinus syndrome (sinus bradycardia alternating with tachycardia), and Wolff-Parkinson-White syndrome.

Intervention and Evaluation
• Monitor the patient's EKG for cardiac changes, particularly widening of the QRS complex and prolongation of the PR and QT intervals.
• Monitor the patient's blood glucose, liver enzyme, and serum alkaline phosphatase, bilirubin, and potassium, SGOT (AST), and SGPT (ALT) levels. Also monitor the patient's blood pressure (B/P). Be aware that disopyramide's therapeutic blood level is 2–8 mcg/ml and toxic blood level is greater than 8 mcg/ml.
• Monitor the patient's intake and output for signs of urine retention.
• Assess the patient for signs and symptoms of CHF including cough, dyspnea (particularly on exertion), fatigue, and rales at the base of the lungs.
• Assist the patient with ambulation if he or she experiences dizziness.

Patient Teaching
• Warn the patient to notify the physician if he or she has a productive cough or shortness of breath.
• Explain to the patient that he or she should not take nasal decongestants or over-the-counter (OTC) cold preparations, especially those containing stimulants, without consulting the physician for approval.
• Encourage the patient to restrict his or her alcohol and salt consumption while taking disopyramide.

dofetilide
doe-**fet**-ill-ide
(Tikosyn)

CATEGORY AND SCHEDULE
Pregnancy Risk Category: C

MECHANISM OF ACTION
This selective potassium channel blocker prolongs repolarization without affecting conduction velocity by blocking one or more time-dependent potassium currents. Dofetilide has no effect on sodium channels or adrenergic alpha or beta receptors. *Therapeutic Effect:* Terminates reentrant tachyarrhythmias, preventing reinduction.

AVAILABILITY
Capsules: 125 mcg, 250 mcg, 500 mcg.

INDICATIONS AND DOSAGES
▸ **Maintain normal sinus rhythm after conversion from atrial fibrillation or flutter**
PO
Adults, Elderly. Individualized using a seven-step dosing algorithm dependent upon calculated creatinine clearance and QT measurements.

CONTRAINDICATIONS
Concurrent use of drugs that prolong the QT interval, concurrent use

of amiodarone, megestrol, prochlorperazine, verapamil, congenital or
acquired long QT syndrome, paroxysmal atrial fibrillation, severe renal
impairment

INTERACTIONS
Drug
*Amiloride, megestrol, metformin,
prochlorperazine, triamterene:* May
increase serum levels of dofetilide.
*Bepridil, phenothiazines, tricyclic
antidepressants:* May cause a prolonged QT interval.
Cimetidine, verapamil: Increases
plasma levels of dofetilide.
Ketoconazole, trimethoprim: Increases maximum plasma concentration of dofetilide.
Herbal
None known.
Food
Grapefruit juice: Can increase
dofetilide levels.

DIAGNOSTIC TEST EFFECTS
None known.

SIDE EFFECTS
Occasional (less than 5%)
Headache, chest pain, dizziness,
dyspnea, nausea, insomnia, back
and abdominal pain, diarrhea,
rash

SERIOUS REACTIONS
• Angioedema, bradycardia, cerebral
ischemia, facial paralysis, and
serious ventricular arrhythmias or
various forms of heart block may be
noted.

NURSING CONSIDERATIONS
Baseline Assessment
• Be prepared to institute continu-
ous cardiac and blood pressure
(B/P) monitoring.

Intervention and Evaluation
• Monitor the patient's EKG
for ventricular arrhythmias and
for prolongation of the QT
interval.
• Monitor the patient's serum
creatinine for changes.
Patient Teaching
• Explain to the patient that he or
she may take dofetilide without
regard to food.
• Advise the patient that dofetilide
therapy compliance is essential and
that the dosing instructions must be
followed diligently.
• Warn the patient to notify the
physician if he or she experiences
diaphoresis, dizziness, increased
thirst, loss of appetite, severe diarrhea, tachycardia, or vomiting.

flecainide
fleh-kun-eyed
(Tambocor)

CATEGORY AND SCHEDULE
Pregnancy Risk Category: C

MECHANISM OF ACTION
An antiarrhythmic that slows atrial,
atrioventricular (AV), His-Purkinje,
intraventricular conduction. *Therapeutic Effect:* Decreases excitability, conduction velocity, automaticity.

AVAILABILITY
Tablets: 50 mg, 100 mg.

INDICATIONS AND DOSAGES
▶ **Life threatening ventricular arrhythmias, sustained ventricular
tachycardia**
PO
Adults, Elderly. Initially, 100 mg
q12h, increased by 100 mg (50 mg

2 times/day) every 4 days until effective dose or maximum of 400 mg/day is attained.

▸ **Paroxysmal supraventricular tachycardias (PSVT), paroxysmal atrial fibrillation (PAF)**
PO
Adults, Elderly. Initially, 50 mg q12h, increased by 100 mg (50 mg 2 times/day) every 4 days until effective dose or maximum of 300 mg/day is attained.

CONTRAINDICATIONS
Cardiogenic shock, pre-existing second- or third-degree AV block, right bundle branch block—without presence of a pacemaker

INTERACTIONS
Drug
Beta blockers: May increase negative inotropic effects.
Digoxin: May increase blood concentrations of digoxin.
Other anti-arrhythmics: May have additive effects.
Urinary acidifiers: May increase the excretion of flecainide.
Urinary alkalinizers: May decrease the excretion of flecainide.
Herbal
None known.
Food
None known.

DIAGNOSTIC TEST EFFECTS
None significant.

SIDE EFFECTS
Frequent (19%–10%)
Dizziness, dyspnea, headache
Occasional (9%–4%)
Nausea, fatigue, palpitations, chest pain, asthenia (loss of strength, energy), tremor, constipation

SERIOUS REACTIONS
• This drug has the ability to worsen existing arrhythmias or produce new ones.
• May also produce or worsen congestive heart failure (CHF).
• Overdose may increase QRS duration, QT interval and conduction disturbances, reduce myocardial contractility, conduction disturbances, and hypotension.

NURSING CONSIDERATIONS
Baseline Assessment
• Establish the patient's cardiovascular history and medication history, especially the use of other antiarrhythmics.
• Make sure that the patient receives continuous cardiac monitoring when instituting this drug.
• Perform baseline measurements of the EKG tracing, including QRS duration and QT interval.
Precautions
• Use cautiously in patients with CHF, impaired myocardial function, second or third degree AV block—with pacemaker, and sick sinus syndrome.
Administration and Handling
PO
• Crush scored tablets as needed.
Intervention and Evaluation
• Assess pulse the patient's pulse for irregular rate and quality.
• Monitor the patient's electrocardiogram (EKG) for cardiac changes, particularly widening of QRS or prolongation of the QT interval.
• Assess the patient for evidence of CHF, including weight gain, pulmonary crackles, and dyspnea.
• Monitor the patient's intake and output. Any decrease in urine output may indicate CHF.
• Monitor the patient for therapeutic serum level, 0.2–1 mcg/ml.

Patient Teaching
• Tell the patient that side effects generally disappear with continued use or decreased dosage.
• Caution the patient against abruptly discontinuing the medication.
• Warn the patient not to use nasal decongestants or over-the-counter cold preparations without physician approval.
• Urge the patient to restrict his or her alcohol and salt intake.
• Instruct the patient to use caution when performing tasks that require mental alertness or motor skills.
• Warn the patient to notify the physician if he or she experiences chest pain, faintness, or palpitations.

ibutilide fumarate
eye-**byewt**-ih-lied
(Corvert)

CATEGORY AND SCHEDULE
Pregnancy Risk Category: C

MECHANISM OF ACTION
An antiarrhythmic that prolongs both atrial and ventricular action potential duration and increases the atrial and ventricular refractory period. *Therapeutic Effect:* Activates slow, inward current (mostly of sodium), produces mild slowing of sinus node rate and atrioventricular (AV) conduction, dose-related prolongation of QT interval. Converts arrhythmias to sinus rhythm.

PHARMACOKINETICS
After IV administration, highly distributed, rapidly cleared. Protein binding: 40%. Primarily excreted in urine as metabolite. **Half-life:** 2–12 hrs (average: 6 hrs).

AVAILABILITY
Injection: 0.1 mg/ml solution.

INDICATIONS AND DOSAGES
▸ **Rapid conversion of atrial fibrillation or flutter of recent onset to normal sinus rhythm**
IV infusion
Adults, Elderly weighing 60 kg or more. One vial (1 mg) given over 10 min. If arrhythmia does not stop within 10 min after end of initial infusion, a second 1mg/10 min infusion may be given.
Adults, Elderly weighing less than 60 kg. 0.01 mg/kg given over 10 min. If arrhythmia does not stop within 10 min after end of initial infusion, a second 0.01 mg/kg, 10-min infusion may be given.

CONTRAINDICATIONS
None known

INTERACTIONS
Drug
Class IA antiarrhythmics (disopyramide, moricizine, procainamide, quinidine), Class III antiarrhythmics (amiodarone, bretylium, sotalol): Do not give concurrently with these drugs or give these drugs within 4 hrs after infusing ibutilide.
H_1 *receptor antagonists, phenothiazines, tricyclic and tetracyclic antidepressants:* May prolong QT interval.
Herbal
None known.
Food
None known.

DIAGNOSTIC TEST EFFECTS
None known.

IV INCOMPATIBILITIES
No information is available for Y-site administration.

SIDE EFFECTS

Generally well tolerated.
Occasional
Ventricular extrasystoles (5.1%),
ventricular tachycardia (4.9%),
headache (3.6%), hypotension,
postural hypotension (2%)
Rare
Bundle-branch block, AV block,
bradycardia, hypertension

SERIOUS REACTIONS

• Sustained polymorphic ventricular
tachycardia, occasionally with QT
prolongation (torsades de pointes)
occurs rarely.
• Overdosage results in central
nervous system (CNS) toxicity
including CNS depression,
rapid gasping breathing, and
seizures.
• May exaggerate expected prolongation of repolarization.
• May worsen existing arrhythmias
or produce new arrhythmias.

NURSING CONSIDERATIONS

Baseline Assessment
• For patients with atrial fibrillation
lasting more than 2 to 3 days,
expect to administer an anticoagulant for at least 2 weeks before
ibutilide therapy.
• Be prepared with advanced cardiac life support equipment, medications, and trained personnel
during and after ibutilide administration.
• Know that proarrhythmias may
develop.
Lifespan Considerations
• Be aware that ibutilide is embryo-
cidal and teratogenic in animals and
that breast-feeding is not recommended during drug therapy.
• Be aware that the safety and
efficacy of ibutilide have not been
established in children.

• There are no age-related precau-
tions noted in the elderly.
Precautions
• Use cautiously in patients with
abnormal liver function and heart
block.
Administration and Handling
IV
• Compatible with D_5W, 0.9%
NaCl. Compatible with polyvinyl
chloride plastic and polyolefin bag
admixtures.
• Admixtures with diluent are stable
at room temperature for up to 24
hours or up to 48 hours if refrigerated.
• Give undiluted or may dilute in
50 ml diluent.
• Give over 10 minutes.
Intervention and Evaluation
• Institute continuous EKG monitoring, as ordered, for at least 4 hours
following the ibutilide infusion or
until the QT interval has returned to
baseline. Continue EKG monitoring
if the patient develops arrhythmias.
• Monitor the patient for signs and
symptoms of serum electrolytes for
abnormalities, especially magnesium
and potassium, and for arrhythmias
requiring overdrive cardiac pacing,
electrical cardioversion, or defibrillation.
Patient Teaching
• Explain to the patient that his or
her blood pressure and EKG will be
continuously monitored during
therapy.
• Warn the patient to immediately
report palpitations or other adverse
reactions.

lidocaine hydrochloride
lie-**doe**-cane
(Lidoderm, Lignocaine[AUS], Xylocaine, Xylocard[CAN], Zilactin-L[CAN])

CATEGORY AND SCHEDULE
Pregnancy Risk Category: B

MECHANISM OF ACTION
An amide anesthetic that inhibits conduction of nerve impulses. *Therapeutic Effect:* Causes temporary loss of feeling and sensation. Also an antiarrhythmic that decreases depolarization, automaticity, excitability of the ventricle during diastole by direct action. *Therapeutic Effect:* Reverses ventricular arrhythmias.

PHARMACOKINETICS

Route	Onset	Peak	Duration
IV	30–90 sec	N/A	10–20 min
Local anesthetic	2.5 min	N/A	30–60 min

Completely absorbed after IM administration. Protein binding: 60%–80%. Widely distributed. Metabolized in liver. Primarily excreted in urine. Minimally removed by hemodialysis. **Half-life:** 1–2 hrs.

AVAILABILITY
IM Injection: 300 mg/3 ml.
Direct IV Injection: 10 mg/ml, 20 mg/ml.
IV Admixture Injection: 40 mg/ml, 100 mg/ml, 200 mg/ml.
IV Infusion: 2 mg/ml, 4 mg/ml, 8 mg/ml.

Injection (anesthesia): 0.5%, 1%, 1.5%, 2%, 4%.
Liquid: 2.5%, 5%.
Ointment: 2.5%, 5%.
Cream: 0.5%.
Gel: 0.5%, 2.5%.
Topical Spray: 0.5%.
Topical Solution: 2%, 4%.
Topical Jelly: 2%.
Dermal Patch: 5%.

INDICATIONS AND DOSAGES
▸ **Rapid control of acute ventricular arrhythmias after an MI, cardiac catheterization, cardiac surgery, or digitalis-induced ventricular arrhythmias**
IM
Adults, Elderly. 300 mg (or 4.3 mg/kg). May repeat in 60–90 min.
IV
Adults, Elderly. Initially, 50–100 mg (1 mg/kg) IV bolus at rate of 25–50 mg/min. May repeat in 5 min. Give no more than 200–300 mg in 1 hr. Maintenance: 20–50 mcg/kg/min (1–4 mg/min) as IV infusion.
Children, Infants. Initially, 0.5–1 mg/kg IV bolus; may repeat but total dose not to exceed 3–5 mg/kg. Maintenance: 10–50 mcg/kg/min as IV infusion.
▸ **Dental or surgical procedures, childbirth**
Infiltration or nerve block
Adults. Local anesthetic dosage varies with procedure, degree of anesthesia, vascularity, duration. Maximum dose: 4.5 mg/kg. Do not repeat within 2 hrs.
▸ **Local skin disorders (minor burns, insect bites, prickly heat, skin manifestations of chickenpox, abrasions), and mucous membrane disorders (local anesthesia of oral, nasal, and laryngeal mucous membranes; local anesthesia of respiratory, urinary tract; relief of**

discomfort of pruritus ani, hemorrhoids, pruritus vulvae)
Topical
Adults, Elderly. Apply to affected
areas as needed.

▶ **Treatment of shingles-related skin
pain**
Topical (Dermal patch)
Adults, Elderly. Apply to intact skin
over most painful area (up to 3
applications once for up to 12 hrs in
a 24-hr period).

CONTRAINDICATIONS
Adams-Stokes syndrome, hypersensitivity to amide-type local anesthetics, septicemia (spinal anesthesia),
supraventricular arrhythmias, Wolff-
Parkinson-White syndrome

INTERACTIONS
Drug
Anticonvulsants: May increase
cardiac depressant effects.
Beta-adrenergic blockers: May
increase risk of toxicity.
Other antiarrhythmics: May in-
crease cardiac effects.
Herbal
None known.
Food
None known.

DIAGNOSTIC TEST EFFECTS
IM lidocaine may increase
CPK level (used in diagnostic
test for presence of acute MI).
Therapeutic blood level is 1.5–6
mcg/ml; toxic blood level is
greater than 6 mcg/ml.

IV INCOMPATIBILITIES
Amphotericin B complex (Abelcet,
AmBisome, Amphotec), thiopental

IV COMPATIBILITIES
Aminophylline, amiodarone (Cor-
darone), calcium gluconate, digoxin
(Lanoxin), diltiazem (Cardizem),

dobutamine (Dobutrex), dopamine
(Intropin), enalapril (Vasotec),
furosemide (Lasix), heparin, insulin,
nitroglycerin, potassium chloride

SIDE EFFECTS
CNS effects are generally dose
related and of short duration.
Occasional
IM: Pain at injection site
Topical: Burning, stinging, tenderness
Rare
Generally with high dose: Drowsiness, dizziness, disorientation,
lightheadedness, tremors, apprehension, euphoria, sensation of heat or
cold or numbness, blurred or double
vision, ringing or roaring in ears
(tinnitus), nausea

SERIOUS REACTIONS
• Although serious adverse reactions
to lidocaine are uncommon, high
dosage by any route may produce
cardiovascular depression, bradycardia, somnolence, hypotension,
arrhythmias, heart block, cardiovascular collapse, and cardiac arrest.
• Potential for malignant hyperthermia.
• CNS toxicity may occur, especially
with regional anesthesia use, progressing rapidly from mild side effects to tremors, convulsions, vomiting, and respiratory depression.
• Methemoglobinemia (evidenced
by cyanosis) has occurred following
topical application of lidocaine for
teething discomfort and laryngeal
anesthetic spray.
• Overuse of oral lidocaine has
caused seizures in children.
• Allergic reactions are rare.

NURSING CONSIDERATIONS
Baseline Assessment
• Determine if the patient has a
hypersensitivity to amide anesthetics

and lidocaine before beginning drug therapy.

• Obtain the patient's baseline blood pressure (B/P), pulse, respirations, EKG, and serum electrolytes.

Lifespan Considerations

• Be aware that lidocaine crosses the placenta and is distributed in breast milk.

• There are no age-related precautions noted in children.

• The elderly are more sensitive to the adverse effects of lidocaine. Lidocaine dose and rate of infusion should be reduced in the elderly.

• In the elderly, age-related renal impairment may require dosage adjustment.

Precautions

• Use cautiously in patients with atrial fibrillation, bradycardia, heart block, hypovolemia, liver disease, marked hypoxia, and severe respiratory depression.

Administration and Handling

◀ALERT▶ Keep resuscitative equipment and drugs, including O_2, readily available when administering lidocaine by any route.

◀ALERT▶ Know that lidocaine's therapeutic blood level is 1.5–6 mcg/ml and the toxic blood level is greater than 6 mcg/ml.

IM

• Use 10% (100 mg/ml) and clearly identify that the lidocaine preparation is for IM use.

• Give injection in deltoid muscle because the blood level will be significantly higher than if the injection is given in gluteus muscle or lateral thigh.

IV

◀ALERT▶ Use only lidocaine without preservative, clearly marked for IV use.

• Store at room temperature.

• For IV infusion, prepare solution by adding 1 g to 1 L D_5W to pro-

vide concentration of 1 mg/ml (0.1%).

• Know that commercially available preparations of 0.2%, 0.4%, and 0.8% may be used for IV infusion. Be aware that the maximum concentration is 4 g/250 ml.

• For IV push, use 1% (10 mg/ml) or 2% (20 mg/ml).

• Administer IV push at rate of 25 to 50 mg/min.

• Administer for IV infusion at rate of 1 to 4 mg/min (1 to 4 ml) and use a volume control IV set.

Topical

• Be aware that the topical form is not for ophthalmic use.

• For skin disorders, apply directly to affected area or put on a gauze or bandage, which is then applied to the skin.

• For mucous membrane use, apply to desired area using manufacturer's insert.

• Administer the lowest dosage possible that still provides anesthesia.

Intervention and Evaluation

• Monitor the patient's EKG and vital signs closely for cardiac performance during and following lidocaine administration.

• Inform the physician immediately if the patient's EKG shows arrhythmias or prolongation of the PR interval or QRS complex.

• Assess the patient's pulse for its quality and for bradycardia and irregularity.

• Assess the patient's B/P for signs of hypotension.

• Monitor the patient for therapeutic blood levels, which is 1.5 to 6 mcg/ml.

• For lidocaine given by all routes, monitor the patient's level of consciousness and vital signs. Be aware that drowsiness may signal high lidocaine blood levels.

Patient Teaching

• Ensure that the patient receiving lidocaine as a local anesthetic understands that he or she will experience a loss of feeling or sensation and will need protection until anesthetic wears off.
• Warn the patient not to chew gum, drink, or eat for 1 hour after oral mucous membrane lidocaine application. The swallowing reflex may be impaired, increasing risk of aspiration; and numbness of tongue or buccal mucosa may lead to biting trauma.

mexiletine hydrochloride

mex-ill-eh-teen
(Mexitil)

CATEGORY AND SCHEDULE
Pregnancy Risk Category: C

MECHANISM OF ACTION

An antiarrhythmic that shortens duration of action potential, decreases effective refractory period in His-Purkinje system of myocardium by blocking sodium transport across myocardial cell membranes. *Therapeutic Effect:* Suppresses ventricular arrhythmias.

AVAILABILITY
Capsules: 150 mg, 200 mg, 250 mg.

INDICATIONS AND DOSAGES
▶ **Arrhythmias:**
PO
Adults, Elderly. Initially, 200 mg q8h. Adjust dose by 50–100 mg at 2–3 day intervals. Maximum: 1,200 mg/day.

UNLABELED USES
Treatment of diabetic neuropathy

CONTRAINDICATIONS

Cardiogenic shock, pre-existing second- or third-degree atrioventricular (AV) block, right bundle branch block without presence of pacemaker

SIDE EFFECTS
Frequent (greater than 10%)
Gastrointestinal (GI) distress, including nausea, vomiting, and heartburn, dizziness, lightheadedness, tremor
Occasional (10%–1%)
Nervousness, change in sleep habits, headache, visual disturbances, paresthesia, diarrhea or constipation, palpitations, chest pain, rash, respiratory difficulty, edema

SERIOUS REACTIONS
• Mexiletine has the ability to worsen existing arrhythmias or produce new ones.
• May produce or worsen congestive heart failure (CHF).

NURSING CONSIDERATIONS

Baseline Assessment
• Establish the patient's cardiovascular history and medication history, especially the use of other antiarrhythmics.
• Expect to obtain a baseline EKG.
Precautions
• Use cautiously in patients with CHF, impaired myocardial function, second- or third-degree AV block, with pacemaker, and sick sinus syndrome.
Administration and Handling
◀ALERT▶ If 300 mg every 8 hours or less controls arrhythmias, may give dose every 12 hours.
PO
• Do not crush, open, or break capsules.

Intervention and Evaluation
• Monitor the patient's electrocardiogram (EKG) and vital signs closely for cardiac side effects.
• Assess the patient's pulse for irregular rate and quality.
• Evaluate the patient for GI disturbances.
• Assess the patient's daily pattern of bowel activity and stool consistency.
• Assess the patient for dizziness and syncope.
• Evaluate the patient's hand movement for evidence of tremor.
• Evaluate the patient for signs and symptoms of CHF.
• Check the patient for therapeutic serum level (0.5 to 2 mcg/ml).

Patient Teaching
• Warn the patient to notify the physician if he or she experiences dark urine, cough, generalized fatigue, nausea, pale stools, severe or persistent abdominal pain, shortness of breath, unexplained sore throat or fever, vomiting, or yellowing of the eyes or skin.
• Caution the patient against using nasal decongestants and over-the-counter cold preparations without physician approval.
• Urge the patient to restrict his or her alcohol and salt intake.

moricizine hydrochloride
mor-ih-**see**-zeen
(Ethmozine)

CATEGORY AND SCHEDULE
Pregnancy Risk Category: B

MECHANISM OF ACTION
An antiarrhythmic that prevents sodium current across myocardial cell membranes. Has potent local anesthetic activity and membrane stabilizing effects. Slows atrioventricular (AV), Purkinje conduction, decreases action potential duration, effective refractory period. *Therapeutic Effect:* Suppresses ventricular arrhythmias.

AVAILABILITY
Tablets: 200 mg, 250 mg, 300 mg.

INDICATIONS AND DOSAGES
‣ **Arrhythmias**
PO
Adults, Elderly. 200–300 mg q8h. May increase by 150 mg/day at no less than 3-day intervals.

UNLABELED USES
Atrial arrhythmias, complete and non-sustained ventricular arrhythmias, premature ventricular contractions (PVCs)

CONTRAINDICATIONS
Cardiogenic shock, pre-existing second or third degree AV block or right bundle branch block without pacemaker

INTERACTIONS
Drug
Cimetidine: May increase moricizine blood concentrations.
Theophylline: May decrease blood concentrations of theophylline.
Herbal
None known.
Food
None known.

DIAGNOSTIC TEST EFFECTS
May cause electrocardiogram (EKG) changes, such as prolonged PR and QT intervals.

SIDE EFFECTS
Frequent (15%–5%)
Dizziness, nausea, headache, fatigue, dyspnea

Occasional (5%–2%)
Nervousness, paresthesia, sleep disturbances, dyspepsia, vomiting, diarrhea

SERIOUS REACTIONS
• May worsen existing arrhythmias or produce new ones.
• Jaundice with hepatitis occurs rarely.
• Overdose produces vomiting, lethargy, syncope, hypotension, conduction disturbances, exacerbation of congestive heart failure (CHF), myocardial infarction (MI), and sinus arrest.

NURSING CONSIDERATIONS

Baseline Assessment
• Correct electrolyte imbalances, as prescribed, before administering medication.
• Expect to obtain a baseline EKG. Measure the PR and QT intervals.
Precautions
• Use cautiously in patients with CHF, electrolyte imbalance, impaired liver or renal function, and sick sinus syndrome.
Administration and Handling
PO
• May be given without regard to food but give with food if gastrointestinal (GI) upset occurs.
• Taking 30 minutes after a meal decreases absorption, serum levels.
Intervention and Evaluation
• Monitor the patient's EKG for cardiac changes especially increase in PR and QRS intervals.
• Assess the patient's pulse for irregular rate and quality.
• Evaluate the patient for dizziness, GI upset, headache, and nausea.
• Monitor the patient's electrolytes, intake and output, and liver and renal function tests.

Patient Teaching
• Caution the patient against abruptly discontinuing the drug.
• Warn the patient to notify the physician if he or she experiences any chest pain or irregular heartbeats.

procainamide hydrochloride
pro-**cane**-ah-myd
(Apo-Procainamide[CAN], Procanbid, Procan-SR, Pronestyl)
Do not confuse with Ponstel or probenecid.

CATEGORY AND SCHEDULE
Pregnancy Risk Category: C

MECHANISM OF ACTION
An antiarrhythmic that increases the electrical stimulation threshold of the ventricles and His-Purkinje system. Possesses direct cardiac effects. *Therapeutic Effect:* Decreases myocardial excitability and conduction velocity and depresses myocardial contractility. Produces antiarrhythmic effect.

PHARMACOKINETICS
Rapidly, completely absorbed from the gastrointestinal (GI) tract. Protein binding: 15%–20%. Widely distributed. Metabolized in liver to active metabolite. Primarily excreted in urine. Removed by hemodialysis. **Half-life:** 2.5–4.5 hrs; metabolite: 6 hrs.

AVAILABILITY
Capsules: 250 mg, 375 mg, 500 mg.
Tablets: 250 mg, 375 mg, 500 mg.
Tablets (extended-release): 500 mg, 750 mg, 1,000 mg.
Injection: 100 mg/ml, 500 mg/ml.

INDICATIONS AND DOSAGES

▸ **Maintain normal sinus rhythm after conversion of atrial fibrillation or flutter; treat premature ventricular contractions, paroxysmal atrial tachycardia, atrial fibrillation, and ventricular tachycardia**

IV

Adults, Elderly. Loading Dose: 50–100 mg/dose. May repeat q5–10min or 15–18 mg/kg (Maximum: 1–1.5 g) then maintenance infusion of 3–4 mg/min. Range: 1–6 mg/min.

Children. Loading Dose: 3–6 mg/kg/dose over 5 min (Maximum: 100 mg). May repeat q5–10min to maximum total dose of 15 mg/kg then maintenance dose of 20–80 mcg/kg/min. Maximum: 2 g/day.

PO

Adults, Elderly. 250–500 mg of immediate-release tablets q3–6h. 0.5–1 g of sustained-release tablets q6h. 1–2 g of Procanbid q12h.

Children. 15–50 mg/kg/day of immediate-release tablets in divided doses q3–6h. Maximum: 4 g/day.

▸ **Dosage in renal impairment**

Creatinine Clearance	Dosage Interval
10–50 ml/min	q6–12h
less than 10 ml/min	q8–24h

UNLABELED USES

Conversion and management of atrial fibrillation

CONTRAINDICATIONS

Complete heart block, myasthenia gravis, preexisting QT prolongation, second- or third-degree heart block, systemic lupus erythematosus, torsades de pointes

INTERACTIONS

Drug

Antihypertensives (IV procainamide), neuromuscular blockers: May increase the effects of these drugs. May decrease antimyasthenic effect on skeletal muscle.

Other antiarrhythmics, pimozide: May increase cardiac effects.

Herbal

None known.

Food

None known.

DIAGNOSTIC TEST EFFECTS

May cause EKG changes and positive ANA titers and Coombs' test. May increase SGOT (AST), SGPT (ALT), serum alkaline phosphatase, serum bilirubin, and serum LDH levels. Therapeutic serum level is 4–8 mcg/ml and toxic serum level is greater than 10 mcg/ml.

IV INCOMPATIBILITIES

Milrinone (Primacor)

IV COMPATIBILITIES

Amiodarone (Cordarone), dobutamine (Dobutrex), heparin, lidocaine, potassium chloride

SIDE EFFECTS

Frequent

PO: Abdominal pain or cramping, nausea, diarrhea, vomiting

Occasional

Dizziness, giddiness, weakness, hypersensitivity reaction (rash, urticaria, pruritus, flushing)

IV: Transient, but at times, marked hypotension

Rare

Confusion, mental depression, psychosis

SERIOUS REACTIONS

• Paradoxical, extremely rapid ventricular rate may occur during

treatment of atrial fibrillation or flutter.
• Systemic lupus erythematosus–like syndrome (fever, joint pain, pleuritic chest pain) with prolonged therapy.
• Cardiotoxic effects occur most commonly with IV administration, observed as conduction changes (50% widening of QRS complex, frequent ventricular premature contractions, ventricular tachycardia, complete atrioventricular [AV] block).
• Prolonged PR and QT intervals, flattened T waves occur less frequently.

NURSING CONSIDERATIONS

Baseline Assessment
• Check the patient's blood pressure (B/P) and pulse for 1 full minute before giving procainamide unless the patient is on a continuous EKG monitor.

Lifespan Considerations
• Be aware that procainamide crosses the placenta and it is unknown if procainamide is distributed in breast milk.
• There are no age-related precautions noted in children.
• The elderly are more susceptible to the drug's hypotensive effect.
• In the elderly, age-related renal impairment may require dosage adjustment.

Precautions
• Use cautiously in patients with bundle-branch block, congestive heart failure (CHF), liver or renal impairment, marked AV-conduction disturbances, severe digoxin toxicity, and supraventricular tachyarrhythmias.

Administration and Handling
◀ALERT▶ Know that procainamide dosage and the interval of administration are individualized based on the patient's age, clinical response, renal function, and underlying myocardial disease. Also be aware that extended-release tablets are used for maintenance therapy.

PO
• Do not crush or break sustained-release tablets.
• **IM/IV**
◀ALERT▶ May give procainamide by IM injection, IV push, or IV infusion.
• Solution normally appears clear, colorless to light yellow.
• Discard if solution darkens or appears discolored or if precipitate forms.
• When diluted with D_5W, solution is stable for up to 24 hours at room temperature or for 7 days if refrigerated.
• For IV push, dilute with 5 to 10 ml D_5W.
• For initial loading IV infusion, add 1 g to 50 ml D_5W to provide a concentration of 20 mg/ml.
• For IV infusion, add 1 g to 250–500 ml D_5W to provide concentration of 2 to 4 mg/ml. Know that the maximum concentration is 4 g/250 ml.
• For IV push, with patient in the supine position, administer at a rate not exceeding 25 to 50 mg/min.
• For initial loading infusion, infuse 1 ml/min for up to 25 to 30 minutes.
• For IV infusion, infuse at 1 to 3 ml/min.
• Check B/P every 5 to 10 minutes during infusion. If a fall in B/P exceeds 15 mm Hg, discontinue drug and contact physician.
• Monitor EKG for cardiac changes, particularly widening of QRS and prolongation of PR and QT intervals. Notify physician of any significant interval changes.

• Continuously monitor B/P and EKG during IV administration. Continuously adjust the rate of infusion to eliminate arrhythmias.

Intervention and Evaluation

• Monitor the patient's EKG for cardiac changes, particularly widening of QRS and prolongation of PR and QT intervals.

• Assess the patient's pulse for its quality and for an irregular rate.

• Monitor the patient's intake and output, serum electrolyte levels, including chloride, potassium, and sodium.

• Evaluate the patient for GI upset, headache, dizziness, or joint pain.

• Assess the patient's pattern of daily bowel activity and stool consistency.

• Assess the patient for signs of dizziness.

• Monitor the patient's B/P for signs of hypotension.

• Assess the patient's skin for hypersensitivity reaction, especially in patients receiving high-dose therapy.

• Monitor the patient for a therapeutic serum level of 4 to 8 mcg/ml and a toxic serum level of greater than 10 mcg/ml.

Patient Teaching

• Advise the patient to evenly space drug doses around the clock.

• Warn the patient to notify the physician if he or she experiences fever, joint pain or stiffness, and signs of upper respiratory infection.

• Caution the patient against abruptly discontinuing the drug. Explain to the patient that compliance with therapy is essential to control arrhythmias.

• Explain to the patient that he or she should not take nasal decongestants or over-the-counter (OTC) cold preparations, especially those containing stimulants, without consulting the physician for approval.

• Encourage the patient to restrict his or her alcohol and salt consumption while taking procainamide.

propafenone hydrochloride
pro-**pah**-phen-own
(Rythmol)

CATEGORY AND SCHEDULE
Pregnancy Risk Category: C

MECHANISM OF ACTION
An antiarrhythmic that decreases the fast sodium current in Purkinje or myocardial cells. *Therapeutic Effect:* Decreases excitability and automaticity; prolongs conduction velocity and the refractory period.

AVAILABILITY
Tablets: 150 mg.

INDICATIONS AND DOSAGES
▸ **Treatment of documented, life-threatening ventricular arrhythmias, such as sustained ventricular tachycardia**
PO
Adults, Elderly. Initially, 150 mg q8h, may increase at 3-to 4-day intervals to 225 mg q8h, then to 300 mg q8h. Maximum: 900 mg/day.

UNLABELED USES
Treatment of supraventricular arrhythmias

CONTRAINDICATIONS
Bradycardia; bronchospastic disorders; cardiogenic shock; manifest electrolyte imbalance; sinoatrial, atrioventricular (AV),

and intraventricular impulse generation or conduction disorders, such as sick sinus syndrome or AV block, without the presence of a pacemaker; uncontrolled CHF

INTERACTIONS
Drug
Digoxin, propranolol: May increase concentrations of these drugs.
Warfarin: May increase warfarin effects.
Herbal
None known.
Food
None known.

DIAGNOSTIC TEST EFFECTS
May cause EKG changes, such as QRS widening and PR prolongation, positive ANA titers.

SIDE EFFECTS
Frequent (13%–7%)
Dizziness, nausea, vomiting, unusual taste, constipation
Occasional (6%–3%)
Headache, dyspnea, blurred vision, dyspepsia (heartburn, indigestion, epigastric pain)
Rare (less than 2%)
Rash, weakness, dry mouth, diarrhea, edema, hot flashes

SERIOUS REACTIONS
• May produce or worsen existing arrhythmias.
• Overdosage may produce hypotension, somnolence, bradycardia, and intra-atrial and intraventricular conduction disturbances.

NURSING CONSIDERATIONS
Baseline Assessment
• Expect to correct patient electrolyte imbalances before beginning propafenone therapy.

Precautions
• Use cautiously in patients with conduction disturbances, congestive heart failure (CHF), impaired liver or renal function, and recent myocardial infarction (MI).
Intervention and Evaluation
• Assess the patient's pulse for its quality and for an irregular rate.
• Monitor the patient's EKG for cardiac changes and performance, particularly widening of the QRS complex and prolongation of the PR interval.
• Assess the patient for gastrointestinal (GI) upset, headache, or visual disturbances.
• Monitor the patient's serum electrolyte levels.
• Assess the patient's pattern of daily bowel activity and stool consistency.
• Assess the patient for dizziness and unsteadiness.
• Monitor the patient's liver enzymes test results.
• Monitor the patient for the drug's therapeutic serum level, which is 0.06 to 1 mcg/ml.
Patient Teaching
• Stress to the patient that compliance with the therapy regimen is essential to control arrhythmias.
• Advise the patient that he or she may experience an unusual taste sensation while taking this drug.
• Instruct the patient to notify the physician if he or she experiences blurred vision, fever, or headache.
• Warn the patient to avoid tasks that require mental alertness or motor skills until his or her response to the drug is established.

quinidine
kwin-ih-deen
(Apo-Quinidine[CAN], Kinidin Durules[AUS], Quinate[CAN], Quinidex)
Do not confuse with clonidine or quinine.

CATEGORY AND SCHEDULE
Pregnancy Risk Category: C

MECHANISM OF ACTION
An antiarrhythmic that decreases sodium influx during depolarization, potassium efflux during repolarization, and reduces calcium transport across the myocardial cell membrane. *Therapeutic Effect:* Decreases myocardial excitability, conduction velocity, and contractility.

AVAILABILITY
Gluconate
Tablets (sustained-release): 324 mg.
Injection: 80 mg/ml (50 mg/ml quinidine).
Sulfate
Tablets: 200 mg, 300 mg.
Tablets (sustained-release): 300 mg.

INDICATIONS AND DOSAGES
▶ **Maintain normal sinus rhythm after conversion of atrial fibrillation or flutter; prevention of premature atrial, atrioventricular (AV), and ventricular contractions, paroxysmal atrial tachycardia, paroxysmal AV junctional rhythm, atrial fibrillation atrial flutter paroxysmal ventricular tachycardia not associated with complete heart block**
IV
Adults, Elderly. 200–400 mg/dose.
Children. 2–10 mg/kg/dose.
PO
Adults, Elderly. 100–600 mg/dose

q4–6h. (Long-acting): 324–972 mg q8–12h.
Children: 30 mg/kg/day in divided doses q4–6h.

UNLABELED USES
Treatment of malaria (IV only)

CONTRAINDICATIONS
Complete AV block, intraventricular conduction defects (widening of QRS complex)

INTERACTIONS
Drug
Antimyasthenics: May decrease effects of these drugs on skeletal muscle.
Digoxin: May increase digoxin serum concentration.
Other antiarrhythmics, pimozide: May increase cardiac effects.
Neuromuscular blockers, oral anticoagulants: May increase effects of these drugs.
Urinary alkalizers, such as antacids: May decrease quinidine renal excretion.
Herbal
None known.
Food
None known.

DIAGNOSTIC TEST EFFECTS
None known. Therapeutic serum level is 2–5 mcg/ml and the toxic level is greater than 5 mcg/ml.

IV INCOMPATIBILITIES
Furosemide (Lasix), heparin

IV COMPATIBILITIES
Milrinone (Primacor)

SIDE EFFECTS
Frequent
Abdominal pain and cramps, nausea, diarrhea, vomiting (can be immediate, intense)

Occasional

Mild cinchonism (ringing in ears, blurred vision, hearing loss) or severe cinchonism (headache, vertigo, diaphoresis, lightheadedness, photophobia, confusion, delirium)

Rare

Hypotension (particularly with IV administration), hypersensitivity reaction (fever, anaphylaxis, photosensitivity reaction)

SERIOUS REACTIONS

• Cardiotoxic effects occur most commonly with IV administration, particularly at high concentrations, observed as conduction changes (50% widening of QRS complex, prolonged QT interval, flattened T waves, disappearance of P wave), ventricular tachycardia or flutter, frequent premature ventricular contractions (PVCs), or complete AV block.

• Quinidine-induced syncope may occur with usual dosage.

• Severe hypotension may result from high dosages.

• Atrial flutter and fibrillation patients may experience a paradoxical, extremely rapid ventricular rate that may be prevented by prior digitalization.

• Liver toxicity with jaundice due to drug hypersensitivity may occur.

NURSING CONSIDERATIONS

Baseline Assessment

• Check the patient's blood pressure (B/P) and pulse for 1 full minute before giving quinidine unless the patient is on a continuous cardiac monitor.

• Monitor the results of the BUN, complete blood count (CBC), serum alkaline phosphatase, bilirubin, creatinine, and SGOT (AST) and SGPT (ALT) levels for patients receiving long-term therapy.

Precautions

• Use cautiously in patients with digoxin toxicity, incomplete AV block, liver or renal impairment, myasthenia gravis, myocardial depression, and sick sinus syndrome.

Administration and Handling

◄ALERT► Keep in mind that quinidine's therapeutic serum level is 2–5 mcg/ml and the toxic level is greater than 5 mcg/ml.

PO

• Ensure that the patient doesn't crush or chew sustained-release tablets.

• To reduce gastrointestinal (GI) upset, give quinidine with food.

IV

◄ALERT► Continuously monitor the patient's blood pressure (B/P) and EKG waveform during IV administration and adjust the rate of the infusion as appropriate and as ordered to minimize arrhythmias and hypotension.

• Use only clear, colorless solution.

• Solution is stable for up to 24 hours at room temperature when diluted with D_5W.

• For IV infusion, dilute 800 mg with 40 ml D_5W to provide concentration of 16 mg/ml.

• Administer with patient in supine position.

• For IV infusion, give at rate of 1 ml (16 mg)/min because a rapid rate may markedly decrease arterial pressure.

• Monitor the patient's EKG for cardiac changes, particularly prolongation of PR or QT interval and widening of the QRS complex. Notify the physician of any significant EKG changes.

Intervention and Evaluation

• Monitor the patient's complete blood count (CBC), intake and

output, liver and renal function tests, and serum potassium levels.
• Assess the patient's pattern of daily bowel activity and stool consistency.
• Monitor the patient's B/P for hypotension, especially in those receiving high-dose therapy.
• Expect to discontinue the drug if the patient develops quinidine-induced syncope.
• Notify the physician immediately if the patient experiences cardiotoxic effects.

Patient Teaching
• Warn the patient to notify the physician if he or she experiences fever, rash, ringing in the ears, unusual bleeding or bruising, or visual disturbances.
• Advise the patient that quinidine may cause a photosensitivity reaction. Urge the patient to avoid contact with direct sunlight or artificial light.

tocainide hydrochloride
toe-**kay**-nied
(Tonocard)

CATEGORY AND SCHEDULE
Pregnancy Risk Category: C

MECHANISM OF ACTION
An amide-type local anesthetic that shortens the action potential duration and decreases the effective refractory period and automaticity in the His-Purkinje system of the myocardium by blocking sodium transport across myocardial cell membranes. *Therapeutic Effect:* Suppresses ventricular arrhythmias.

AVAILABILITY
Tablets: 400 mg, 600 mg.

INDICATIONS AND DOSAGES
▸ **Suppression and prevention of ventricular arrhythmias**
PO
Adults, Elderly. Initially, 400 mg q8h. Maintenance: 1.2–1.8 g/day in divided doses q8h. Maximum: 2,400 mg/day.

CONTRAINDICATIONS
Hypersensitivity to local anesthetics, second- or third-degree atrioventricular (AV) block

INTERACTIONS
Drug
Beta-adrenergic blockers: May increase pulmonary wedge pressure and decrease cardiac index. *Other antiarrhythmics:* May increase risk of adverse cardiac effects.
Herbal
None known.
Food
None known.

DIAGNOSTIC TEST EFFECTS
None known.

SIDE EFFECTS
Expected
Generally well tolerated.
Frequent (10%–3%)
Minor, transient lightheadedness, dizziness, nausea, paresthesia, rash, tremor
Occasional (3%–1%)
Clammy skin, night sweats, joint pain
Rare (less than 1%)
Restlessness, nervousness, disorientation, mood changes, ataxia (muscular incoordination), visual disturbances

SERIOUS REACTIONS
• High dosage may produce brady-cardia or tachycardia, hypotension, palpitations, increased ventricular arrhythmias, premature ventricular contractions (PVCs), chest pain, and exacerbation of congestive heart failure (CHF).

NURSING CONSIDERATIONS

Baseline Assessment
• Assess the patient's baseline EKG and pulse for its quality and for an irregular rate.

Precautions
• Use cautiously in patients with bone marrow failure, CHF, liver or renal impairment, and preexisting arrhythmias.

Administration and Handling
◀ALERT▶ When giving tocainide in those receiving IV lidocaine, give single 600-mg dose 6 hours before cessation of lidocaine and repeat in 6 hours, as prescribed. Then give standard tocainide maintenance doses.

◀ALERT▶ Know that tocainide's therapeutic serum level is 4 to 10 mcg/ml and toxic has not been established.

Intervention and Evaluation
• Monitor the patient's EKG for changes, particularly shortening of the QT interval. Notify the physician of any significant interval changes.
• Monitor the patient's fluid status and serum electrolyte levels.

• Assess the patient's hand move-ment for tremors, which is usually the first clinical sign that the maxi-mum dose is being reached.
• Evaluate the sleeping patient for night sweats.
• Determine if the patient is experi-encing numbness or tingling in the feet or hands.
• Assess the patient's skin for clamminess and rash.
• Observe the patient for central nervous system (CNS) disturbances, including disorientation, incoordina-tion, mood changes, and restless-ness.
• Assess the patient for signs and symptoms of CHF including dis-tended neck veins, dyspnea (particu-larly on exertion or lying down), night cough, and peripheral edema.
• Monitor the patient's intake and output and note that an increase in weight or decrease in urine output may indicate CHF.
• Monitor blood tests for a thera-peutic serum level between 4 and 10 mcg/ml.

Patient Teaching
• Advise the patient to avoid tasks that require mental alertness or motor skills until his or her re-sponse to the drug is established.
• Warn the patient to notify the physician if he or she experiences breathing difficulties, chills, cough, fever, palpitations, sore throat, tremor, or unusual bleeding.
• Explain to the patient that tocai-nide may be taken with food.

24 Antihyperlipidemics

atorvastatin
cholestyramine resin
colesevelam
ezetimibe
fenofibrate
fluvastatin
gemfibrozil
lovastatin
niacin, nicotinic acid
pravastatin
rosuvastatin calcium
simvastatin

Uses: Antihyperlipidemics are used to lower abnormally high blood levels of cholesterol and triglycerides, which are linked with the development and progression of atherosclerosis. Effective management of cholesterol and triglycerides includes dietary modification along with pharmacologic treatment.

Action: Five subclasses of antihyperlipidemics act in different ways. *Bile acid sequestrants,* such as cholestyramine and colesevelam, bind with bile acids in the intestine, preventing their active transport and reabsorption and enhancing their excretion. By depleting hepatic bile acid, these agents increase the conversion of cholesterol to bile acids.

HMG-CoA reductase inhibitors (statins), such as atorvastatin and lovastatin, inhibit HMG-CoA reductase, an enzyme required for the last regulated step in cholesterol synthesis. This action reduces cholesterol synthesis in the liver.

Niacin (nicotinic acid) reduces hepatic synthesis of triglycerides and the secretion of very low-density lipoproteins by inhibiting the mobilization of free fatty acids from peripheral tissues.

Fibric acids, such as fenofibrate, increase fatty acid oxidation in the liver, resulting in reduced secretion of triglyceride-rich lipoprotein. They also increase lipoprotein lipase activity and fatty acid uptake.

Cholesterol absorption inhibitors, such as ezetimibe, act in the gut wall to prevent cholesterol absorption through the intestinal villi.

COMBINATION PRODUCTS

PRAVIGARD: pravastatin/aspirin (an antiplatelet) 20 mg/81 mg; 20 mg/325 mg; 40 mg/81 mg; 40 mg/325 mg; 80 mg/81 mg; 80 mg/325 mg.

atorvastatin
ah-tore-**vah**-stah-tin
(Lipitor)
Do not confuse with Levatol.

CATEGORY AND SCHEDULE
Pregnancy Risk Category: X

MECHANISM OF ACTION
Inhibits HMG-CoA reductase, the enzyme that catalyzes the early step in cholesterol synthesis. *Therapeutic Effect:* Decreases LDL cholesterol, VLDL cholesterol, and plasma triglycerides; increases HDL cholesterol.

PHARMACOKINETICS
Poorly absorbed from the gastrointestinal (GI) tract. Protein binding: greater than 98%. Metabolized in liver. Minimally eliminated in urine. Plasma levels markedly increased with chronic alcoholic liver disease, unaffected by renal disease. **Half-life:** 14 hrs.

AVAILABILITY
Tablets: 10 mg, 20 mg, 40 mg, 80 mg.

INDICATIONS AND DOSAGES
▸ **Hyperlipidemia**
PO
Adults, Elderly. Initially, 10–40 mg a day given as a single dose. Dose Range: Increase at 2- to 4-wk intervals up to maximum of 80 mg/day.

CONTRAINDICATIONS
Active liver disease, lactation, pregnancy, unexplained elevated liver function tests

INTERACTIONS
Drug
Antacids, colestipol, propranolol: Decreases atorvastatin activity.
Cyclosporine, erythromycin, gemfibrozil, nicotinic acid: Increases the risk of acute renal failure and rhabdomyolysis with these drugs.
Digoxin, itraconazole levels, oral contraceptives, warfarin: May increase atorvastatin blood concentration, producing severe muscle inflammation, pain, and weakness.

Herbal
None known.
Food
None known.

DIAGNOSTIC TEST EFFECTS
May increase serum creatine kinase and transaminase concentrations.

SIDE EFFECTS
Generally well tolerated. Side effects are usually mild and transient.
Frequent (16%)
Headache
Occasional (5%–2%)
Myalgia, rash or pruritus, allergy
Rare
Flatulence, dyspepsia

SERIOUS REACTIONS
• There is a potential for developing cataracts and photosensitivity.

NURSING CONSIDERATIONS
Baseline Assessment
• Determine if the patient is pregnant before beginning atorvastatin therapy. Atorvastatin is pregnancy category X.
• Assess the patient's baseline lab results and document serum cholesterol, triglyceride levels, and liver function test results.
Lifespan Considerations
• Be aware that atorvastatin is distributed in breast milk and contraindicated during pregnancy because it may produce skeletal malformation.
• Be aware that the safety and efficacy of atorvastatin have not been established in children.
• There are no age-related precautions noted in the elderly.
Precautions
• Use cautiously in patients with a history of liver disease, hypotension, major surgery, severe acute

infection, substantial alcohol consumption, and trauma, and those receiving anticoagulant therapy, or who have severe acute infection, severe endocrine, electrolyte, or metabolic disorders, trauma, or uncontrolled seizures.

Administration and Handling
PO
• May be given without regard to food.
• Do not break film-coated tablets.

Intervention and Evaluation
• Monitor the patient for headache.
• Assess the patient for malaise, pruritus, and rash.
• Monitor the patient's cholesterol and triglyceride values for therapeutic response.

Patient Teaching
• Instruct the patient to follow his or her prescribed diet. Explain that diet is an important part of treatment.
• Advise the patient that periodic lab tests are an essential part of therapy.
• Warn the patient not to take other medications without notifying the physician.

---

cholestyramine resin
coal es-**tie**-rah-mean
(Novo-Cholamine[CAN], Prevalite, Questran[CAN], Questran Lite[AUS])
Do not confuse with Quarzan.

CATEGORY AND SCHEDULE
Pregnancy Risk Category: B

MECHANISM OF ACTION
An antihyperlipoproteinemic that binds with bile acids in the intestine, forming an insoluble complex. Binding results in partial removal of bile acid from enterohepatic circulation. *Therapeutic Effect:* Removes low-density lipoproteins (LDL) and cholesterol from plasma.

PHARMACOKINETICS
Not absorbed from the gastrointestinal (GI) tract. Decreases in LDL apparent in 5–7 days and serum cholesterol in 1 mo. Serum cholesterol returns to baseline levels about 1 mo after discontinuing drug.

AVAILABILITY
Powder: 4 g.

INDICATIONS AND DOSAGES
▶ **Primary hypercholesterolemia**
PO
Adults, Elderly. 3–4 g 3–4 times/day. Maximum: 16–32 g/day in 2–4 divided doses.
Children older than 10 yrs. 2 g/day up to 8 g/day.
Children 10 yrs and younger. Initially, 2 g/day. Range: 1–4 g/day.

UNLABELED USES
Treatment of diarrhea (due to bile acids); hyperoxaluria

CONTRAINDICATIONS
Complete biliary obstruction, hypersensitivity to cholestyramine or tartrazine (frequently seen in aspirin hypersensitivity)

INTERACTIONS
Drug
Anticoagulants: May increase effects of these drugs by decreasing vitamin K.
Digoxin, folic acid, penicillins, propranolol, tetracyclines, thiazides, thyroid hormones, and other medications: May bind and decrease absorption of these drugs.
Oral vancomycin: Binds and de-

creases the effects of oral vancomycin.
Warfarin: May decrease warfarin absorption.
Herbal
None known.
Food
None known.

DIAGNOSTIC TEST EFFECTS

May increase serum alkaline phosphatase, serum magnesium, SGOT (AST), and SGPT (ALT) levels. May decrease serum calcium, potassium, and sodium levels. May prolong prothrombin time.

SIDE EFFECTS

Frequent
Constipation (may lead to fecal impaction), nausea, vomiting, stomach pain, indigestion
Occasional
Diarrhea, belching, bloating, headache, dizziness
Rare
Gallstones, peptic ulcer, malabsorption syndrome

SERIOUS REACTIONS

• GI tract obstruction, hyperchloremic acidosis, and osteoporosis secondary to calcium excretion may occur.
• High dosage may interfere with fat absorption, resulting in steatorrhea.

NURSING CONSIDERATIONS

Baseline Assessment
• Determine the patient's history of hypersensitivity to aspirin, cholestyramine, and tartrazine before beginning drug therapy.
• Check the patient's baseline electrolytes and serum cholesterol and triglyceride levels.

Lifespan Considerations
• Be aware that cholestyramine is not systemically absorbed and may interfere with maternal absorption of fat-soluble vitamins.
• There are no age-related precautions noted in children. Cholestyramine use is limited in pediatric patients younger than 10 years of age.
• The elderly are at an increased risk of experiencing adverse nutritional effects and GI side effects.
Precautions
• Use cautiously in patients with bleeding disorders, GI dysfunction (especially constipation), hemorrhoids, and osteoporosis.
Administration and Handling
PO
• Give other drugs at least 1 hour before or 4 to 6 hours after cholestyramine because this drug is capable of binding drugs in the GI tract.
• Don't give cholestyramine in its dry form because it is highly irritating. Mix with 3 to 6 oz fruit juice, milk, soup, or water.
• Place powder on the surface of the liquid for 1 to 2 minutes to prevent lumping, then mix thoroughly.
• When mixing the powder with carbonated beverages, use an extra large glass and stir the liquid slowly to avoid excessive foaming.
• Administer before meals.
Intervention and Evaluation
• Assess the patient's pattern of daily bowel activity and stool consistency.
• Evaluate the patient's abdominal discomfort, flatulence, and food tolerance.
• Monitor the patient's blood chemistry test results.
• Encourage the patient to drink

several glasses of water between meals.

Patient Teaching

• Advise the patient to complete a full course of therapy. Caution the patient against omitting or changing drug doses.

• Instruct the patient to take other drugs at least 1 hour before or 4 to 6 hours after cholestyramine.

• Warn the patient never to take cholestyramine in its dry form.

• Teach the patient to mix the powder with 3 to 6 oz fruit juice, milk, soup, or water. Explain to the patient that he or she should place the powder on the surface of a liquid for 1 to 2 minutes to prevent lumping and then mix the powder into liquid. When mixing the powder with carbonated beverages, advise the patient to use an extra large glass and to stir the liquid slowly to avoid excessive foaming.

• Instruct the patient to take cholestyramine before meals and to drink several glasses of water between meals.

• Encourage the patient to eat high-fiber foods such as fruits, whole grain cereals, and vegetables to reduce the risk of constipation.

coleyesevelam
ko-leh-**sev**-eh-lam
(Welchol)

CATEGORY AND SCHEDULE
Pregnancy Risk Category: B

MECHANISM OF ACTION
A bile acid sequestrant and non-systemic polymer that binds with bile acids in the intestines, pre-venting their reabsorption and removing them from the body. *Therapeutic Effect:* Decreases low-density lipoprotein (LDL) cholesterol.

AVAILABILITY
Tablets: 625 mg.

INDICATIONS AND DOSAGES
Decrease elevated LDL cholesterol in primary hypercholesterolemia (Fredrickson type IIa)
PO
Adults, Elderly. 3 tablets with meals 2 times/day or 6 tablets once daily with meal. May increase daily dose to 7 tablets/day.

CONTRAINDICATIONS
Complete biliary obstruction, hypersensitivity to colesevelam

INTERACTIONS
Drug
Aspirin, clindamycin, digoxin, furosemide, glipizide, hydrocortisone, imipramine, NSAIDs, phenytoin, propranolol, tetracyclines, thiazide diuretics, and vitamin A, D, E, K: May decrease the absorption of these drugs.
Herbal
None known.
Food
None known.

DIAGNOSTIC TEST EFFECTS
None known.

SIDE EFFECTS
Frequent (12%–8%)
Flatulence, constipation, infection, dyspepsia (heartburn, epigastric distress)

SERIOUS REACTIONS
• Gastrointestinal (GI) tract obstruction may be noted.

NURSING CONSIDERATIONS

Baseline Assessment
• Assess the patient's baseline lab results for cholesterol and triglyceride levels and liver function.

Lifespan Considerations
• Be aware that colesevelam is not absorbed systemically and may decrease proper maternal vitamin absorption and may have effect on breast-feeding infants.
• Be aware that the safety and efficacy of colesevelam have not been established in children.
• There are no age-related precautions noted in the elderly.

Precautions
• Use cautiously in patients with dysphagia and severe GI motility disorders.
• Use cautiously in patients who've had major GI tract surgery and those susceptible to fat-soluble vitamin deficiency.

Intervention and Evaluation
• Monitor the patient's cholesterol and triglyceride levels for therapeutic response.
• Assess the patient's pattern of daily bowel activity and stool consistency.

Patient Teaching
• Advise the patient to follow the prescribed diet and explain that the diet is an important part of treatment.
• Stress to the patient that periodic lab tests are an essential part of therapy.
• Explain to the patient that he or she should not take any medications, including over-the-counter (OTC) drugs, without consulting the physician.

ezetimibe
eh-**zeh**-tih-myb
Zetia

CATEGORY AND SCHEDULE
Pregnancy Risk Category: C

MECHANISM OF ACTION
An antihyperlipidemic that inhibits cholesterol absorption in the small intestine, leading to a decrease in the delivery of intestinal cholesterol to the liver. *Therapeutic Effect:* Reduces total cholesterol and LDL cholesterol and triglycerides and increases HDL cholesterol.

PHARMACOKINETICS
Well absorbed following oral administration. Protein binding: greater than 90%. Metabolized in the small intestine and liver. Excreted by the kidneys and bile.
Half-life: 22 hrs.

AVAILABILITY
Tablets: 10 mg.

INDICATIONS AND DOSAGES
▶ **Hypercholesterolemia**
PO
Adults, Elderly. Initially, 10 mg once a day, given with or without food. For patients also receiving a bile acid sequestrant, give ezetimibe at least 2 hrs before or at least 4 hrs after the administration of a bile acid sequestrant.

CONTRAINDICATIONS
Concurrent use of an HMG-CoA reductase inhibitor (atorvastatin, cerivastatin, fluvastatin, lovastatin, pravastatin, or simvastatin) in patients with active liver disease or unexplained persistent elevations in

serum transaminases, moderate or severe liver insufficiency

INTERACTIONS
Drug
Aluminum and magnesium-containing antacids, cyclosporine, fenofibrate, gemfibrozil: Increase ezetimibe plasma concentration.
Cholestyramine: Decreases drug effectiveness.
Herbal
None known.
Food
None known.

DIAGNOSTIC TEST EFFECTS
May increase serum alkaline phosphatase, serum bilirubin, SGOT (AST), and SGPT (ALT) levels.

SIDE EFFECTS
Occasional (4%–3%)
Back pain, diarrhea, arthralgia, sinusitis, abdominal pain
Rare (2%)
Cough, pharyngitis, fatigue

SERIOUS REACTIONS
• None known.

NURSING CONSIDERATIONS
Baseline Assessment
• Assess the results of the patient's blood counts, lipid cholesterol and triglyceride levels, and liver function tests, including serum ALT, during initial therapy and periodically during treatment. Discontinue treatment if the patient's liver enzyme levels persist greater than 3 times the normal limit.
Lifespan Considerations
• Be aware that it is unknown if ezetimibe crosses the placenta or is distributed in breast milk.
• The safety and efficacy of ezetimibe have not been established

in children younger than 10 years of age.
• In the elderly, age-related mild liver impairment requires dosage adjustment. This drug is not recommended for use in elderly patients with moderate or severe liver impairment.
Precautions
• Use cautiously in patients with chronic renal failure, diabetes, hypothyroidism, liver function impairment, and obstructive liver disease.
Administration and Handling
• Give ezetimibe without regard to food.
Intervention and Evaluation
• Assess the patient's pattern of daily bowel activity and stool consistency.
• Evaluate the patient for signs and symptoms of abdominal disturbances and back pain.
• Monitor the patient's cholesterol and triglyceride concentrations for a therapeutic response.
Patient Teaching:
• Stress to the patient that periodic lab tests are an essential part of therapy.
• Caution the patient against discontinuing the medication without consulting the physician.

fenofibrate
fen-oh-**figh**-brate
(Apo-Fenofibrate[CAN], Tricor)

CATEGORY AND SCHEDULE
Pregnancy Risk Category: C

MECHANISM OF ACTION
An antihyperlipidemic that enhances synthesis of lipoprotein lipase and reduces triglyceride-rich lipopro-

teins, very low-density lipoproteins (VLDL). *Therapeutic Effect:* Increases VLDL catabolism, reduces total plasma triglycerides.

PHARMACOKINETICS

Well absorbed from the gastrointestinal (GI) tract. Absorption increased when given with food. Protein binding: 99%. Rapidly metabolized in liver to active metabolite. Excreted primarily in urine, lesser amount in feces. Not removed by hemodialysis. **Half-life:** 20 hrs.

AVAILABILITY

Capsules: 67 mg, 134 mg, 200 mg.
Tablets: 54 mg, 160 mg.

INDICATIONS AND DOSAGES

▸ **Reduce very high elevations of serum triglyceride levels in patients at risk for pancreatitis**
PO
Adults, Elderly. For the capsule form, initially, 67 mg/day and may increase to 200 mg/day. For the tablet form, initially, 54 mg/day and may increase to 160 mg/day.
▸ **Hypercholesterolemia**
PO
Adults, Elderly. For the capsule form, 200 mg/day with meals. For the tablet form, 160 mg/day with meals.

CONTRAINDICATIONS

Gallbladder disease, hypersensitivity to fenofibrate, severe renal or hepatic dysfunction (including primary biliary cirrhosis, unexplained persistent liver function abnormality)

INTERACTIONS

Drug
Anticoagulants: Potentiates effects of these drugs.

Bile acid sequestrants: May impede fenofibrate absorption.
Cyclosporine: Increases risk of nephrotoxicity.
HMG-CoA reductase inhibitors: Increases risk of severe myopathy, rhabdomyolysis, and acute renal failure.
Herb
None known.
Food
Food: Increases drug absorption.

DIAGNOSTIC TESTS

May increase blood urea, serum creatine kinase (CK), serum transaminase (SGOT [AST], and SGPT [ALT]), levels. May decrease blood Hgb and Hct levels, serum uric acid levels, and WBC count.

SIDE EFFECTS

Frequent (8%–4%)
Pain, rash, headache, asthenia or fatigue, flu syndrome, dyspepsia, nausea or vomiting, rhinitis
Occasional (3%–2%)
Diarrhea, abdominal pain, constipation, flatulence, arthralgia, decreased libido, dizziness, pruritus
Rare (less than 2%)
Increased appetite, insomnia, polyuria, cough, blurred vision, eye floaters, earache

SERIOUS REACTIONS

• May increase cholesterol excretion into bile, leading to cholelithiasis.
• Pancreatitis, hepatitis, thrombocytopenia, and agranulocytosis occur rarely.

NURSING CONSIDERATIONS

Baseline Assessment
• Check the results of the patient's blood counts, serum lipid cholesterol and triglyceride levels, and liver function tests, including serum

SGPT [ALT], if ordered, during initial therapy and periodically during treatment. Expect to discontinue treatment if the patient's liver enzyme levels persist at greater than 3 times the normal limit.

Lifespan Considerations
• Be aware that the safety of fenofibrate use during pregnancy is not established and that use of the drug should be avoided in breast-feeding women.
• Be aware that the safety and efficacy of fenofibrate have not been established in children.
• There are no age-related precautions noted in the elderly.

Precautions
• Use cautiously in patients receiving anticoagulant therapy, with a history of liver disease, and who consume substantial amounts of alcohol.

Administration and Handling
PO
• Give fenofibrate with meals.
• Administer fenofibrate 1 hr before or 4 to 6 hrs after giving a bile acid sequestrant.

Intervention and Evaluation
• Monitor patients also receiving HMG-CoA reductase inhibitors for signs and symptoms of myopathy, including muscle pain and weakness.
• Monitor the patient's serum creatine kinase, cholesterol, and triglyceride levels for a therapeutic response.

Patient Teaching
• Instruct the patient to take fenofibrate with food.
• Advise the patient to notify the physician if constipation, diarrhea, or nausea becomes severe.
• Warn the patient to notify the physician if he or she experiences dizziness, insomnia, muscle pain, skin rash or irritation, or tremors.

fluvastatin
flu-vah-**stah**-tin
(Lescol, Lescol XL, Vastin[AUS])
Do not confuse with fluoxetine.

CATEGORY AND SCHEDULE
Pregnancy Risk Category: X

MECHANISM OF ACTION
An antihyperlipidemic that inhibits HMG-CoA reductase, the enzyme that catalyzes the early step in cholesterol synthesis. *Therapeutic Effect:* Decreases LDL cholesterol, VLDL, and plasma triglycerides. Increases HDL cholesterol concentration slightly.

PHARMACOKINETICS
Well absorbed from the gastrointestinal (GI) tract and is unaffected by food. Does not cross blood-brain barrier. Protein binding: greater than 98%. Primarily eliminated in feces. **Half-life:** 1.2 hrs.

AVAILABILITY
Capsules: 20 mg, 40 mg.
Tablets (extended-release): 80 mg.

INDICATIONS AND DOSAGES
▸ **Hyperlipoproteinemia**
PO
Adults, Elderly. Initially, 20 mg/day in the evening. May increase up to 40 mg/day. Maintenance: 20–40 mg/day in single or divided doses. *Patients requiring more than a 25% decrease in LDL-C.* 40 mg 1–2 times/day or 80 mg tablet once a day.

CONTRAINDICATIONS
Active liver disease, unexplained increased serum transaminase

INTERACTIONS
Drug
Cyclosporine, erythromycin, gemfibrozil, immunosuppressants, niacin:
Increase the risk of acute renal failure and rhabdomyolysis with these drugs.
Herbal
None known.
Food
None known.

DIAGNOSTIC TEST EFFECTS
May increase creatine kinase (CK) levels, serum transaminase concentrations

SIDE EFFECTS
Frequent (8%–5%)
Headache, dyspepsia, back pain, myalgia, arthralgia, diarrhea, abdominal cramping, rhinitis
Occasional (4%–2%)
Nausea, vomiting, insomnia, constipation, flatulence, rash, fatigue, cough, dizziness

SERIOUS REACTIONS
• Myositis, inflammation of voluntary muscle, with or without increased CK, and muscle weakness, occurs rarely. May progress to frank rhabdomyolysis and renal impairment.

NURSING CONSIDERATIONS

Baseline Assessment
• Determine if the patient is pregnant before beginning fluvastatin therapy.
• Assess the patient's baseline serum cholesterol and triglyceride levels and liver function test results.
Lifespan Considerations
• Be aware that fluvastatin use is contraindicated in pregnancy, because the suppression of cholesterol biosynthesis may cause fetal toxicity, and also during lactation.

• Be aware that it is unknown whether fluvastatin is distributed in breast milk.
• Be aware that the safety and efficacy of fluvastatin have not been established in children.
• There are no age-related precautions noted in the elderly.
Precautions
• Use cautiously in patients on anticoagulant therapy, with a history of liver disease, and who consume substantial amounts of alcohol.
• Use cautiously in patients experiencing hypotension, major surgery, severe acute infection, severe electrolyte, endocrine, or metabolic disorders, renal failure secondary to rhabdomyolysis, and uncontrolled seizures. Expect to discontinue or withhold fluvastatin if these conditions appear.
Administration and Handling
PO
• Give fluvastatin without regard to food.
Intervention and Evaluation
• Assess the patient's pattern of daily bowel activity and stool consistency.
• Evaluate the patient for blurred vision, dizziness, and headache.
• Assess the patient for pruritus and rash.
• Monitor the patient's serum cholesterol and triglyceride levels for therapeutic response.
• Assess the patient for malaise and muscle cramping or weakness.
Patient Teaching
• Advise the patient to follow the prescribed diet and explain that the diet is an important part of treatment.
• Stress to the patient that periodic lab tests are an essential part of therapy.
• Warn the patient to notify the physician if he or she experiences

any muscle pain or weakness, especially if accompanied by fever or malaise.

gemfibrozil
gem-**fie**-bro-zill
(Apo-Gemfibrozil[CAN], Ausgem[AUS], Gemfibromax[AUS], Jezil[AUS], Lipazil [AUS], Lopid, Novo-Gemfibrozil[CAN])

CATEGORY AND SCHEDULE
Pregnancy Risk Category: C

MECHANISM OF ACTION
A fibric acid derivative that inhibits lipolysis of fat in adipose tissue; decreases liver uptake of free fatty acids and reduces hepatic triglyceride production. Inhibits synthesis of VLDL carrier apolipoprotein B. *Therapeutic Effect:* Lowers serum cholesterol and triglycerides (decreases VLDL, LDL; increases HDL).

PHARMACOKINETICS
Well absorbed from the gastrointestinal (GI) tract. Protein binding: 99%. Metabolized in liver. Primarily excreted in urine. Not removed by hemodialysis. **Half-life:** 1.5 hrs.

AVAILABILITY
Tablets: 600 mg.
Capsules: 300 mg.

INDICATIONS AND DOSAGES
▸ **Hyperlipidemia**
PO
Adults, Elderly. 900 mg to 1.5 g/day in 2 divided doses.

CONTRAINDICATIONS
Liver dysfunction (including primary biliary cirrhosis), preexisting gallbladder disease, severe renal dysfunction

INTERACTIONS
Drug
Lovastatin: May cause rhabdomyolysis, leading to acute renal failure. *Repaglinide, warfarin:* May increase the effect of these drugs.
Herbal
None known.
Food
None known.

DIAGNOSTIC TEST EFFECTS
May increase serum alkaline phosphatase, serum bilirubin, serum creatinine kinase, serum LDH concentrations, and SGOT (AST) and SGPT (ALT) levels. May decrease blood Hgb and Hct levels, leukocyte counts, and serum potassium levels.

SIDE EFFECTS
Frequent (20%)
Dyspepsia
Occasional (10%–2%)
Abdominal pain, diarrhea, nausea, vomiting, fatigue
Rare (less than 2%)
Constipation, acute appendicitis, vertigo, headache, rash, altered taste

SERIOUS REACTIONS
• Cholelithiasis, cholecystitis, acute appendicitis, pancreatitis, and malignancy occur rarely.

NURSING CONSIDERATIONS
Baseline Assessment
• Assess the patient's baseline lab results for blood glucose levels, complete blood count (CBC), serum alkaline phosphatase, bilirubin, cholesterol and triglyceride levels, and SGOT (AST) and SGPT (ALT) levels.
Lifespan Considerations
• Be aware that it is unknown if

gemfibrozil crosses the placenta or is distributed in breast milk. Also know that the decision to discontinue breast-feeding or gemfibrozil should be based on the potential for serious adverse effects to the infant.
• Be aware that gemfibrozil use is not recommended in children younger than 2 years of age because cholesterol is necessary for normal development in this age group.
• In the elderly, age-related renal impairment may require dosage adjustment.

Precautions
• Use cautiously in patients with diabetes mellitus, receiving estrogen or anticoagulant therapy, and with hypothyroidism.

Administration and Handling
PO
• Give gemfibrozil 30 minutes before morning and evening meals.

Intervention and Evaluation
• Assess the patient's pattern of daily bowel activity and stool consistency.
• Monitor the patient's serum LDL, VLDL, triglyceride, and cholesterol levels for a therapeutic response.
• Monitor the patient's hematology and liver function test results.
• Assess the patient for pruritus and rash.
• Evaluate the patient for blurred vision, dizziness, and headache.
• Assess the patient for pain, especially in the right upper quadrant of the abdomen, because epigastric pain may indicate cholecystitis or cholelithiasis.
• Monitor the blood glucose of patients receiving insulin or oral antihyperglycemics.

Patient Teaching
• Advise the patient to follow the prescribed diet and explain that the diet is an important part of treatment.

• Instruct the patient to take gemfibrozil before meals.
• Stress to the patient that periodic laboratory tests are an essential part of therapy.
• Warn the patient to notify the physician if he or she experiences abdominal pain, blurred vision, diarrhea, dizziness, nausea, or vomiting.

lovastatin
low-vah-**stah**-tin
(Altocor, Mevacor)
Do not confuse with Leustatin, Livostin, or Mivacron.

CATEGORY AND SCHEDULE
Pregnancy Risk Category: X

MECHANISM OF ACTION
An antihyperlipidemic that inhibits HMG-CoA reductase, the enzyme that catalyzes the early step in cholesterol synthesis. *Therapeutic Effect:* Decreases LDL cholesterol, VLDL cholesterol, plasma triglycerides; increases HDL cholesterol.

PHARMACOKINETICS

Route	Onset	Peak	Duration
PO	3 days	4–6 wks	N/A

Incompletely absorbed from the gastrointestinal (GI) tract (increased on empty stomach). Protein binding: greater than 95%. Hydrolyzed in liver to active metabolite. Primarily eliminated in feces. Not removed by hemodialysis. **Half-life:** 1.1–1.7 hrs.

AVAILABILITY
Tablets: 10 mg, 20 mg, 40 mg.

Tablets (extended-release): 20 mg, 40 mg, 60 mg.

INDICATIONS AND DOSAGES
▸ **Hyperlipoproteinemia**
·PO
Adults, Elderly. Initially, 20–40 mg/day with evening meal. Increase at 4-wk intervals up to maximum of 80 mg/day. Maintenance: 20–80 mg/day in single or divided doses.
PO (extended release)
Adults, Elderly. Initially, 20 mg/day. May increase at 4 week intervals up to 60 mg/day.
Children 10–17 yrs. 10–40 mg/day with evening meal.

CONTRAINDICATIONS
Active liver disease, pregnancy, unexplained elevated liver function tests

INTERACTIONS
Drug
Cyclosporine, erythromycin, gemfibrozil, immunosuppressants, niacin: Increases the risk of acute renal failure and rhabdomyolysis.
Erythromycin, itraconazole, ketoconazole: May increase lovastatin blood concentration causing severe muscle inflammation, pain, and weakness.
Herbal
None known.
Food
Grapefruit juice: Large amounts of grapefruit juice may increase risk of side effects, such as muscle pain and weakness.

DIAGNOSTIC TEST EFFECTS
May increase serum creatine kinase and serum transaminase concentrations.

SIDE EFFECTS
Generally well tolerated. Side effects usually mild and transient.

Frequent (9%–5%)
Headache, flatulence, diarrhea, abdominal pain or cramps, rash and pruritus
Occasional (4%–3%)
Nausea, vomiting, constipation, dyspepsia
Rare (2%–1%)
Dizziness, heartburn, myalgia, blurred vision, eye irritation

SERIOUS REACTIONS
• There is a potential for cataract development.

NURSING CONSIDERATIONS
Baseline Assessment
• Determine if the female patient is pregnant before beginning lovastatin therapy.
• Assess the patient's baseline laboratory test results including serum cholesterol and triglycerides and liver function tests.
Lifespan Considerations
• Be aware that lovastatin use is contraindicated in pregnancy, because the suppression of cholesterol biosynthesis may cause fetal toxicity, and lactation.
• Be aware that it is unknown if lovastatin is distributed in breast milk.
• Be aware that the safety and efficacy of lovastatin have not been established in children.
• There are no age-related precautions noted in the elderly.
Precautions
• Use cautiously in patients who also use cyclosporine, fibrates, and niacin.
• Use cautiously in patients with a history of heavy alcohol use and renal impairment
Administration and Handling
PO
• Give lovastatin with meals.

Intervention and Evaluation
• Assess the patient's daily pattern of bowel activity.
• Evaluate the patient for blurred vision, dizziness, and headache.
• Assess the patient for pruritus and rash.
• Monitor the patient's serum cholesterol and triglyceride levels for a therapeutic response.
• Be alert for the onset of malaise, muscle cramping, or weakness.

Patient Teaching
• Instruct the patient to take lovastatin with meals.
• Encourage the patient to follow the prescribed diet.
• Stress to the patient that the prescribed diet and periodic laboratory tests are essential parts of therapy.
• Urge the patient to avoid consuming grapefruit juice during lovastatin therapy.
• Warn the patient to notify the physician if her or she experiences changes in the color of his or her stool or urine, muscle pain or weakness, severe gastric upset, unusual bruising, vision changes, and yellowing of eyes or skin.

niacin, nicotinic acid
(Niacor, Niaspan, Nico-400, Nicotinex)
Do not confuse with Nitro-Bid.
OTC

CATEGORY AND SCHEDULE
Pregnancy Risk Category: A (C if used at dosages above the recommended daily allowance [RDA])

MECHANISM OF ACTION
An antihyperlipidemic, water-soluble vitamin that is a component of 2 coenzymes needed for tissue respiration, lipid metabolism, glycogenolysis. Inhibits synthesis of very-low-density lipoproteins (VLDLs). *Therapeutic Effect:* Reduces total and LDL cholesterol, triglycerides, increases HDL cholesterol. Necessary for lipid metabolism, tissue respiration, and glycogenolysis. Lowers serum cholesterol and triglycerides (decreases LDL, VLDL, increases HDL).

PHARMACOKINETICS
Readily absorbed from the gastrointestinal (GI) tract. Widely distributed. Metabolized in liver. Primarily excreted in urine. **Half-life:** 45 min.

AVAILABILITY
Tablets: 50 mg, 100 mg, 250 mg, 500 mg.
Tablets (time-release): 500 mg, 750 mg, 1,000 mg.
Capsules (time-release): 125 mg, 250 mg, 400 mg, 500 mg.
Elixir: 50 mg/5 ml.

INDICATIONS AND DOSAGES
▶ **Hyperlipidemia**
PO (immediate-release)
Adults, Elderly. Initially, 50–100 mg 2 times/day for 7 days. Increase gradually by doubling dose qwk up to 1–1.5 g/day in 2–3 doses. Maximum: 3 g/day.
Children. Initially, 100–250 mg/day (Maximum: 10 mg/kg/day) in 3 divided doses. May increase by 100 mg/wk or 250 mg q2–3wks. Maximum: 2,250 mg/day.
PO (extended-release)
Adults, Elderly. Initially, 500 mg/day in divided doses 2 times/day for 1 wk; then increase to 500 mg 2 times/day. Maintenance: 2 g/day.

▶ **Nutritional supplement**
PO
Adults, Elderly. 10–20 mg/day.

CONTRAINDICATIONS

Active peptic ulcer, arterial hemorrhaging, hypersensitivity to niacin or tartrazine (frequently seen in patients sensitive to aspirin), liver dysfunction, severe hypotension

INTERACTIONS
Drug
Lovastatin, pravastatin, simvastatin: May increase the risk of acute renal failure and rhabdomyolysis.
Herbal
None known.
Food
None known.

DIAGNOSTIC TEST EFFECTS
May increase serum uric acid levels.

SIDE EFFECTS
Frequent
Flushing (especially of face and neck) occurring within 20 min of administration and lasting for 30–60 min, GI upset, pruritus
Occasional
Dizziness, hypotension, headache, blurred vision, burning or tingling of skin, flatulence, nausea, vomiting, diarrhea
Rare
Hyperglycemia, glycosuria, rash, hyperpigmentation, dry skin

SERIOUS REACTIONS
• Arrhythmias occur rarely.

NURSING CONSIDERATIONS
Baseline Assessment
• Determine if the patient has a history of hypersensitivity to aspirin, niacin, or tartrazine before beginning drug therapy.

• Assess the patient's baseline blood glucose level, serum cholesterol and triglyceride levels, and liver function tests.
Lifespan Considerations
• Be aware that niacin is not recommended for use during pregnancy and lactation.
• Be aware that niacin is distributed in breast milk.
• There are no age-related precautions noted in children or the elderly.
• Niacin use is not recommended in children younger than 2 years of age.
Precautions
• Use cautiously in patients with diabetes mellitus, gallbladder disease, gout, and a history of liver disease or jaundice.
Administration and Handling
PO
• Give niacin without regard to meals.
• Administer the drug at bedtime.
Intervention and Evaluation
• Assess the patient's degree of discomfort and flushing.
• Evaluate the patient for blurred vision, dizziness, and headache.
• Assess the patient's pattern of daily bowel activity and stool consistency.
• Monitor the patient's blood glucose levels, serum alkaline phosphatase, bilirubin, cholesterol and triglyceride levels, uric acid levels, and SGOT (AST) and SGPT (ALT) levels.
• Monitor the blood glucose levels frequently, as ordered, in patients on insulin or oral antihyperglycemics.
• Assess the patient's skin for dryness.
Patient Teaching
• Advise the patient to take the drug at bedtime and to avoid alcohol consumption.
• Advise the patient that itching, flushing of the skin, sensation of warmth, and tingling may occur.

• Warn the patient to notify the physician if he or she experiences dark urine, dizziness, loss of appetite, nausea, vomiting, weakness, or yellowing of the skin.
• Suggest to the patient to avoid sudden changes in posture to help prevent bouts of dizziness.

pravastatin
pra-vah-sta-tin
(Pravachol)
Do not confuse with Prevacid or propranolol.

CATEGORY AND SCHEDULE
Pregnancy Risk Category: X

MECHANISM OF ACTION
A HMG-CoA reductase inhibitor that interferes with cholesterol biosynthesis by preventing the conversion of HMG-CoA reductase to mevalonate, a precursor to cholesterol. *Therapeutic Effect:* Lowers LDL cholesterol, VLDL, plasma triglycerides; increases HDL concentration.

PHARMACOKINETICS
Poorly absorbed from the gastrointestinal (GI) tract. Protein binding: 50%. Metabolized in liver (minimal active metabolites). Primarily excreted in feces via biliary system. Not removed by hemodialysis.
Half-life: 2.7 hrs.

AVAILABILITY
Tablets: 10 mg, 20 mg, 40 mg, 80 mg.

INDICATIONS AND DOSAGES
▸ **Treatment of hypercholesterolemia by reducing total and LDL cholesterol, apo B, triglycerides,** increasing HDL cholesterol; preventive therapy to reduce risks of the following in patients with previous myocardial infarction (MI) and normal cholesterol levels: recurrent MI, undergoing myocardial revascularization procedures, stroke or transient ischemic attack (TIA); prevention of cardiovascular events in patients with elevated cholesterol levels.
PO
Adults, Elderly. Initially, 40 mg/day. Titrate to desired response. Range: 10–80 mg/day.
Children 14–18 yrs. 40 mg/day.
Children 8–13 yrs. 20 mg/day.
▸ **Dosage in liver and renal impairment**
Adults. Initially, 10 mg/day. Titrate to desired response.

CONTRAINDICATIONS
Active liver disease or unexplained, persistent elevations of liver function tests

INTERACTIONS
Drug
Cyclosporine, erythromycin, gemfibrozil, immunosuppressants, niacin: Increases the risk of acute renal failure and rhabdomyolysis.
Herbal
None known.
Food
None known.

DIAGNOSTIC TEST EFFECTS
May increase serum creatinine kinase and transaminase concentrations.

SIDE EFFECTS
Generally well tolerated. Side effects usually mild and transient.
Occasional (7%–4%)
Nausea, vomiting, diarrhea, consti-

pation, abdominal pain, headache, rhinitis, rash, pruritus
Rare (3%–2%)
Heartburn, myalgia, dizziness, cough, fatigue, flu-like symptoms

SERIOUS REACTIONS
• There is a potential for malignancy and cataracts.
• Hypersensitivity occurs rarely.

NURSING CONSIDERATIONS
Baseline Assessment
• Determine if the patient is pregnant before beginning pravastatin therapy.
• Assess the patient's baseline lab results including serum cholesterol and triglycerides levels and liver function tests.
Lifespan Considerations
• Be aware that pravastatin use is contraindicated in pregnancy because suppression of cholesterol biosynthesis may cause fetal toxicity and is also contraindicated during lactation.
• Be aware that it is unknown if pravastatin is distributed in breast milk, but there is risk of serious adverse reactions in breast-feeding infants.
• Be aware that the safety and efficacy of this drug have not been established in children.
• There are no age-related precautions noted in the elderly.
Precautions
• Use cautiously in patients with a history of liver disease, severe electrolyte, endocrine, or metabolic disorders, and who consume a substantial amount of alcohol.
• Withholding or discontinuing pravastatin may be necessary when the patient is at risk for renal failure secondary to rhabdomyolysis.

Administration and Handling
◀**ALERT**▶ Before beginning pravastatin therapy, know that the patient should be on a standard cholesterol-lowering diet for minimum of 3 to 6 months. The patient should continue the diet throughout pravastatin therapy.
PO
• Give pravastatin without regard to meals.
• Administer in the evening.
Intervention and Evaluation
• Monitor the patient's serum cholesterol and triglyceride lab results for a therapeutic response.
• Monitor the patient's serum alkaline phosphatase, bilirubin, SGOT (AST) and SGPT (ALT) levels to assess liver function.
• Assess the patient's pattern of daily bowel activity and stool consistency.
• Evaluate the patient for dizziness and headache. Help the patient with ambulation if he or she experiences dizziness.
• Assess the patient for pruritus and rash.
• Assess the patient for malaise and muscle cramping or weakness. If these conditions occur and are accompanied by fever, expect that pravastatin may be discontinued.
Patient Teaching
• Advise the patient to follow the prescribed diet and explain that the diet is an important part of treatment.
• Stress to the patient that periodic lab tests are an essential part of therapy.
• Warn the patient to notify the physician if he or she experiences muscle pain or weakness, especially if accompanied by fever or malaise.
• Advise the patient to avoid tasks that require mental alertness or motor skills if he or she experiences dizziness.

• Urge the patient to use nonhormonal contraception while taking pravastatin. Explain to the patient that pravastatin is pregnancy risk category X.

rosuvastatin calcium
ross-uh-vah-**stah**-tin
(Crestor)

CATEGORY AND SCHEDULE
Pregnancy Risk Category: X

MECHANISM OF ACTION
An antihyperlipidemic that interferes with cholesterol biosynthesis by inhibiting the conversion of the enzyme HMG-CoA to mevalonate, a precursor to cholesterol. *Therapeutic Effect:* Decreases LDL cholesterol, VLDL, plasma triglycerides, increases HDL concentration.

PHARMACOKINETICS
Protein binding: 88%. Minimal hepatic metabolism. Primarily eliminated in the feces. **Half-life:** 19 hrs (half-life is increased in patients with severe renal dysfunction).

AVAILABILITY
Tablets: 5 mg, 10 mg, 20 mg, 40 mg.

INDICATIONS AND DOSAGES
▸ **Hyperlipidemia, dyslipidemia**
PO
Adults, Elderly. 5 to 40 mg/day. Usual starting dosage is 10 mg/day, with adjustments based on lipid levels, monitored q2-4 weeks until desired level is achieved.

▸ **Renal impairment**
PO
Adults, Elderly. 5 mg/day; do not exceed 10 mg/day.
▸ **Concurrent cyclosporine use**
PO
Adults, Elderly. 5 mg/day.
▸ **Concurrent lipid-lowering therapy**
PO
Adults, Elderly. 10 mg/day.

CONTRAINDICATIONS
Active liver disease, breast-feeding, pregnancy, and unexplained, persistent elevations of serum transaminase

INTERACTIONS
Drug
Cyclosporine, gemfibrozil, niacin: Increases the risk of myopathy with cyclosporine, gemfibrozil, and niacin.
Erythromycin: Reduces the plasma concentration of erythromycin.
Ethinylestradiol, norgestrel: Increases the plasma concentrations of ethinylestradiol and norgestrel.
Warfarin: Enhances anticoagulant effect.
Herbal
None known.
Food
None known.

DIAGNOSTIC TEST EFFECTS
May increase serum creatinine kinase and transaminase concentrations. May produce hematuria and proteinuria.

SIDE EFFECTS
Generally well tolerated. Side effects usually mild and transient.
Occasional (9%–3%)
Pharyngitis, headache, diarrhea, dyspepsia, including heartburn and epigastric distress, nausea

Rare (less than 3%)
Myalgia, asthenia or unusual fatigue
and weakness, back pain

SERIOUS REACTIONS
• There is potential for lens opacities.
• Hypersensitivity reaction and hepatitis occur rarely.

NURSING CONSIDERATIONS

Baseline Assessment
• Determine if the female patient is pregnant before beginning rosuvastatin therapy.
• Assess the patient's baseline lab results for cholesterol and triglycerides levels and liver function tests.
• Know that prior to initiating therapy, patient should be on standard cholesterol-lowering diet for minimum of 3-6 mos. Continue diet throughout rosuvastatin therapy.

Lifespan Considerations
• Be aware that rosuvastatin use is contraindicated in pregnancy and lactation. The suppression of cholesterol biosynthesis may cause fetal toxicity.
• Be aware that rosuvastatin carries the risk of serious adverse reactions in nursing infants.
• Be aware that the safety and efficacy of rosuvastatin have not been established in children.
• There are no age-related precautions noted in the elderly.

Precautions
• Use cautiously in patients with a history of liver disease, hypotension, severe acute infection, severe electrolyte, endocrine, or metabolic disorders, trauma, and uncontrolled seizures.
• Use cautiously in patients on anticoagulant therapy, patients who consume a substantial amount of alcohol, or those who have had recent major surgery.

Administration and Handling
PO
• Give rosuvastatin without regard to meals.
• Administer in the evening.

Intervention and Evaluation
• Monitor the patient's cholesterol and triglyceride lab results for therapeutic response.
• Monitor the patient's liver function test results, including serum alkaline phosphatase, bilirubin, SGOT (AST) and SGPT (ALT) levels.
• Assess the patient's daily pattern of bowel activity and stool consistency.
• Evaluate the patient for headache and sore throat.
• Be alert for signs and symptoms of patient muscle aches and weakness.

Patient Teaching
• Tell the patient to use appropriate contraceptive measures during rosuvastatin therapy. Explain to the patient that rosuvastatin is pregnancy risk category X.
• Stress to the patient that periodic lab tests are an essential part of therapy.
• Instruct the patient to continue following a cholesterol-lowering diet. Explain that the diet is an important part of treatment.

simvastatin
sim-vah-**stay**-tin
(Lipex[AUS], Zocor)
Do not confuse with Cozaar.

CATEGORY AND SCHEDULE
Pregnancy Risk Category: X

MECHANISM OF ACTION
A HMG-CoA reductase inhibitor that interferes with cholesterol biosynthesis by inhibiting the conversion of the enzyme HMG-CoA to mevalonate. *Therapeutic Effect:* Decreases LDL, cholesterol, VLDL, plasma triglycerides; slightly increases HDL concentration.

PHARMACOKINETICS

Route	Onset	Peak	Duration
PO to reduce cholesterol	greater than 3 days	14 days	N/A

Well absorbed from the gastrointestinal (GI) tract. Protein binding: 95%. Undergoes extensive first-pass metabolism. Hydrolyzed to active metabolite. Primarily eliminated in feces. Unknown if removed by hemodialysis.

AVAILABILITY
Tablets: 5 mg, 10 mg, 20 mg, 40 mg, 80 mg.

INDICATIONS AND DOSAGES
▸ **Decrease elevated total and LDL cholesterol in hypercholesterolemia (types IIa and IIb), lower triglyceride levels, and increase HDL levels; reduce risk of death and prevent MI in patients with heart disease and elevated cholesterol; reduce risk of revascularization procedures; decrease risk of stroke or TIA.**
PO
Adults. Initially, 10–40 mg/day in evening. Dosage adjustment at 4-wk intervals.
Elderly. Initially, 10 mg/day. May increase by 5–10 mg/day q4wks.

Range: 5–80 mg/day. Maximum: 80 mg/day.

CONTRAINDICATIONS
Active liver disease or unexplained, persistent elevations of liver function tests, age less than 18 yrs, pregnancy

INTERACTIONS
Drug
Cyclosporine, erythromycin, gemfibrozil, immunosuppressants, niacin: Increases the risk of acute renal failure and rhabdomyolysis.
Erythromycin, itraconazole, ketoconazole: May increase simvastatin blood concentration and cause muscle inflammation, pain, or weakness.
Herbal
None known.
Food
None known.

DIAGNOSTIC TEST EFFECTS
May increase serum creatine kinase and serum transaminase concentrations.

SIDE EFFECTS
Generally well tolerated. Side effects usually mild and transient.
Occasional (3%–2%)
Headache, abdominal pain or cramps, constipation, upper respiratory infection
Rare (less than 2%)
Diarrhea, flatulence, asthenia (loss of strength and energy), nausea or vomiting

SERIOUS REACTIONS
• There is a potential for lens opacities.
• Hypersensitivity reaction and hepatitis occur rarely.

NURSING CONSIDERATIONS

Baseline Assessment

• Determine if the patient is pregnant or has a history of hypersensitivity to simvastatin before beginning drug therapy.

• Assess the patient's baseline lab results, including cholesterol and triglyceride levels and liver function tests.

Lifespan Considerations

• Be aware that simvastatin use is contraindicated in lactation and also pregnancy because suppression of cholesterol biosynthesis may cause fetal toxicity. Also know that there is a risk of serious adverse reactions in breast-feeding infants.

• Be aware that the safety and efficacy of simvastatin have not been established in children.

• There are no age-related precautions noted in the elderly.

Precautions

• Use cautiously in patients with a history of liver disease, severe electrolyte, endocrine, or metabolic disorders, and who consume substantial amounts of alcohol.

• Withholding or discontinuing simvastatin may be necessary when the patient is at risk for renal failure secondary to rhabdomyolysis.

Administration and Handling

◀ALERT▶ Be aware that before beginning simvastatin therapy, the patient should be placed on a standard cholesterol-lowering diet for a minimum of 3 to 6 months. Also know that the patient should continue the diet throughout simvastatin therapy.

PO

• Give simvastatin without regard to meals and administer in the evening.

Intervention and Evaluation

• Monitor the patient's serum cholesterol and triglyceride levels and liver function test results, including serum alkaline phosphatase, bilirubin, SGOT (AST) and SGPT (ALT) levels, for a therapeutic response.

• Assess the patient's pattern of daily bowel activity and stool consistency.

• Evaluate the patient for headache.

Patient Teaching

• Advise the patient to use appropriate contraceptive measures while taking simvastatin. Explain that the drug is pregnancy risk category X.

• Stress to the patient that periodic lab tests are an essential part of therapy.

25 Beta-Adrenergic Blocking Agents

acebutolol
atenolol
betaxolol
bisoprolol fumarate
carvedilol
esmolol hydrochloride
labetalol
  hydrochloride
metoprolol tartrate
nadolol
propranolol
  hydrochloride
sotalol hydrochloride
timolol maleate

Uses: Beta-adrenergic blockers are used to manage hypertension, angina pectoris, arrhythmias, hypertrophic subaortic stenosis, migraine headaches, and glaucoma. They're also used to prevent myocardial infarction.

Action: Beta-adrenergic blockers competitively block $beta_1$-adrenergic receptors, located primarily in the myocardium, and $beta_2$-adrenergic receptors, located primarily in bronchial and vascular smooth muscle. By occupying beta-receptor sites, these agents prevent endogenous or administered epinephrine and norepinephrine from exerting their effects. The results are basically opposite to those of sympathetic stimulation.

Effects of $beta_1$-blockade include slowing the heart rate and decreasing cardiac output and contractility. Effects of $beta_2$-blockade include bronchoconstriction and increased airway resistance in patients with asthma or chronic obstructive pulmonary disease. Beta-adrenergic blockers can affect cardiac rhythm and automaticity, decreasing the sinus rate and sinoatrial and atrioventricular (AV) conduction and increasing the refractory period in the AV node.

These agents decrease systolic and diastolic blood pressure. Although this effect's exact mechanism of action is unknown, it may result from peripheral receptor blockade, decreased sympathetic outflow from the central nervous system, or decreased renin release from the kidneys.

All beta-adrenergic blockers mask the tachycardia that occurs with hypoglycemia. When applied to the eyes, they reduce intraocular pressure and aqueous production.

COMBINATION PRODUCTS

CORZIDE: nadolol/bendroflumethiazide (a diuretic) 40 mg/5 mg; 80 mg/5 mg.
COSOPT: timolol/dorzolamide (a carbonic anhydrase inhibitor) 0.5%/2%.
INDERIDE: propranolol/hydrochlorothiazide (a diuretic) 40 mg/25 mg; 80 mg/25 mg.
INDERIDE LA: propranolol/hydrochlorothiazide (a diuretic) 80 mg/50 mg; 120 mg/50 mg; 160 mg/50 mg.

LOPRESSOR HCT: metoprolol/
hydrochlorothiazide (a diuretic)
50 mg/25 mg; 100 mg/25 mg;
100 mg/50 mg.
NORMOZIDE: labetalol/
hydrochlorothiazide (a diuretic)
100 mg/25 mg; 200 mg/25 mg;
300 mg/25 mg.
TENORETIC: atenolol/chlorthalidone
(a diuretic) 50 mg/25 mg;
100 mg/25 mg.
TIMOLIDE: timolol/hydrochloro-
thiazide (a diuretic) 10 mg/
25 mg.
ZIAC: bisoprolol/hydrochlorothiazide
(a diuretic) 2.5 mg/6.25 mg; 5 mg/
6.25 mg; 10 mg/6.25 mg.

acebutolol
ah-see-**beaut**-oh-lol
(Monitan[CAN], Novo-
Acebutolol[CAN], Rhotral[CAN],
Sectral)
**Do not confuse with Factrel or
Septra.**

CATEGORY AND SCHEDULE
Pregnancy Risk Category: B
(D if used in second or third
trimester)

MECHANISM OF ACTION
A beta$_1$-adrenergic blocker
that competitively blocks beta$_1$-
adrenergic receptors in cardiac
tissue Reduces the rate of spontaneous firing of the sinus pacemaker
and atrioventricular (AV) conduction. *Therapeutic Effect:* Slows
heart rate, decreases cardiac output, decreases blood pressure
(B/P), exhibits antiarrhythmic
activity.

PHARMACOKINETICS

Route	Onset	Peak	Duration
PO (hypo-tensive)	1–1.5 hrs	2–8 hrs	24 hrs
PO (antiar-rhyth-mic)	1 hr	4–6 hrs	10 hrs

Well absorbed from the gastrointestinal (GI) tract. Protein binding:
26%. Undergoes extensive first-pass
liver metabolism to active metabolite. Eliminated via bile, secreted
into GI tract via intestine, excreted
in urine. Removed by hemodialysis.
Half-life: 3–4 hrs; metabolite: 8–13
hrs.

AVAILABILITY
Capsules: 200 mg, 400 mg.

INDICATIONS AND DOSAGES
▶ **Mild to moderate hypertension**
PO
• *Adults.* Initially, 400 mg/day in 12
divided doses. Range: Up to 1,200
mg/day in 2 divided doses.
Maintenance: 400–800 mg/day.
▶ **Ventricular arrhythmias**
PO
Adults. Initially, 200 mg q12h.
Increase gradually up to 600–1,200
mg/day in 2 divided doses.
Elderly. Initially, 200–400 mg/day.
Maximum: 800 mg/day.
▶ **Dosage in Renal Impairment**

Creatinine Clearance	% of Normal Dosage
less than 50 ml/min	50
less than 25 ml/min	25

UNLABELED USES
Treatment of anxiety, chronic angina pectoris, hypertrophic cardiomyopathy, myocardial infarction,
pheochromocytoma, syndrome of

mitral valve prolapse, thyrotoxicosis, and tremors

CONTRAINDICATIONS
Cardiogenic shock, heart block greater than first degree, overt heart failure, and severe bradycardia

INTERACTIONS
Drug
Diuretics, other hypotensives: May increase hypotensive effect of acebutolol.
Sympathomimetics, xanthines: May mutually inhibit effects of acebutolol; may mask symptoms of hypoglycemia, prolong hypoglycemic effect of insulin and oral hypoglycemics.
Herbal
None known.
Food
None known.

DIAGNOSTIC TEST EFFECTS
May increase serum alkaline phosphatase, ANA titer, serum bilirubin, BUN, serum creatinine, LDH, lipoproteins, serum potassium, SGOT (AST), SGPT (ALT), triglycerides, and uric acid.

SIDE EFFECTS
Frequent
Hypotension manifested as dizziness, nausea, diaphoresis, headache, cold extremities, fatigue, constipation, or diarrhea
Occasional
Insomnia, urinary frequency, impotence or decreased libido
Rare
Rash, arthralgia, myalgia, confusion (especially in the elderly), change in taste

SERIOUS REACTIONS
• Overdosage may produce profound bradycardia and hypotension.

• Abrupt withdrawal may result in sweating, palpitations, headache, and tremulousness.
• May precipitate congestive heart failure (CHF) or myocardial infarction (MI) in patients with heart disease; thyroid storm in those with thyrotoxicosis; or peripheral ischemia in those with existing peripheral vascular disease.
• Hypoglycemia may occur in previously controlled diabetics.
• Signs of thrombocytopenia, such as unusual bleeding or bruising, occur rarely.

NURSING CONSIDERATIONS
Baseline Assessment
• Assess apical pulse and B/P immediately before drug is administered. If pulse is 60/minute or lower or systolic B/P is less than 90 mm Hg, withhold medication and notify the physician.
Lifespan Considerations
• Acebutolol readily crosses the placenta and is distributed in breast milk.
• During delivery, acebutolol may produce apnea, bradycardia, hypoglycemia, and hypothermia as well as low-birth-weight infants.
• Be aware that, for children, there are no age-related precautions and dosages have not been established.
• Use cautiously in the elderly who may have age-related peripheral vascular disease.
Precautions
• Use cautiously in patients with bronchospastic disease, diabetes, hyperthyroidism, impaired renal or liver function, inadequate cardiac function, or peripheral vascular disease.

Administration and Handling
PO
* May be given without regard to meals.

Intervention and Evaluation
* Monitor B/P for hypotension and assess respiratory status for shortness of breath.
* Assess pulse for quality, rate, and rhythm.
* Monitor electrocardiogram (EKG) for arrhythmias, shortening of QT interval or prolongation of PR interval.
* Assess the frequency and consistency of the patient's stools.
* Assess for signs and symptoms CHF such as decreased urine output, distended neck veins, dyspnea (particularly on exertion or lying down), night cough, peripheral edema, and weight gain.
* Assess for diaphoresis, fatigue, headache, and nausea.

Patient Teaching
* Caution the patient against abruptly discontinuing the drug. Advise the patient that compliance with the therapy regimen is essential to control hypertension and arrhythmias.
* Instruct the patient to report excessive fatigue, headache, prolonged dizziness, shortness of breath, or weight gain.
* Explain to the patient not to use nasal decongestants or over-the-counter (OTC) cold preparations (stimulants) without physician approval.
* Suggest to the patient that he or she restrict salt and alcohol intake.

atenolol
ay-**ten**-oh-lol
(Apo-Atenol[CAN], AteHexal[AUS], Noten[AUS], Tenolin[CAN], Tenormin, Tensig[AUS])
Do not confuse with albuterol.

CATEGORY AND SCHEDULE
Pregnancy Risk Category: D

MECHANISM OF ACTION
A beta$_1$-adrenergic blocker that acts as an antianginal, antiarrhythmic, and antihypertensive agent by blocking beta$_1$-adrenergic receptors in cardiac tissue. *Therapeutic Effect:* Slows sinus node heart rate, decreasing cardiac output and blood pressure (B/P). Decreases myocardial oxygen (O$_2$) demand.

PHARMACOKINETICS

Route	Onset	Peak	Duration
PO	1 hr	2–4 hrs	24 hrs

Incompletely absorbed from the gastrointestinal (GI) tract. Protein binding: 6%–16%. Minimal liver metabolism. Primarily excreted unchanged in urine. Removed by hemodialysis. **Half-life:** 6–7 hrs (half-life increased in impaired renal function).

AVAILABILITY
Tablets: 25 mg, 50 mg, 100 mg.
Injection: 5 mg/10 ml.

INDICATIONS AND DOSAGES
▸ **Hypertension**
PO
Adults. Initially, 25–50 mg once a day. May increase dose up to 100 mg once a day.

Elderly. Usual initial dose, 25 mg a day.
Children. Initially, 0.8–1 mg/kg/dose.

▸ **Angina pectoris**
PO
Adults, Initially, 50 mg once a day. May increase dose up to 200 mg once a day.
Elderly. Usual initial dose, 25 mg a day.

▸ **Acute myocardial infarction**
IV
Adults. Give 5 mg over 5 min, and may repeat in 10 min. In those who tolerate full 10-mg IV dose, begin 50-mg tablets 10 min after last IV dose followed by another 50-mg oral dose 12 hrs later. Thereafter, give 100 mg once a day or 50 mg twice a day for 6–9 days. Alternatively, for those who do not tolerate full IV dose, give 50 mg orally 2 times a day or 100 mg once a day for at least 7 days.

▸ **Dosage in renal impairment**

Creatinine Clearance	Dosage
15–35 ml/min	50 mg a day
less than 15 ml/min	50 mg every other day

UNLABELED USES
Improves survival in diabetics with heart disease. Treatment of hypertrophic cardiomyopathy, pheochromocytoma, and syndrome of mitral valve prolapse, prophylaxis of migraine, thyrotoxicosis, and tremors

CONTRAINDICATIONS
Cardiogenic shock, overt heart failure, second- or third-degree heart block, severe bradycardia

INTERACTIONS
Drug
Cimetidine: May increase blood atenolol concentration.
Diuretics, other hypotensives: May increase hypotensive effect of atenolol.
Insulin, oral hypoglycemics: May mask symptoms of hypoglycemia and prolong hypoglycemic effect of insulin and oral hypoglycemics.
NSAIDs: May decrease antihypertensive effect of atenolol.
Sympathomimetics, xanthines: May mutually inhibit effects.
Herbal
None known.
Food
None known.

DIAGNOSTIC TEST EFFECTS
May increase serum ANA titer, BUN, and serum creatinine, potassium, lipoproteins, triglycerides, and uric acid levels.

IV INCOMPATIBILITIES
Amphotericin complex (Abelcet, AmBisome, Amphotec)

SIDE EFFECTS
Generally well tolerated, with mild and transient side effects.
Frequent
Hypotension manifested as cold extremities, constipation or diarrhea, diaphoresis, dizziness, fatigue, headache, and nausea
Occasional
Insomnia, flatulence, urinary frequency, impotence or decreased libido
Rare
Rash, arthralgia, myalgia, confusion (especially in elderly), change in taste

SERIOUS REACTIONS
• Overdosage may produce profound bradycardia and hypotension.

• Abrupt atenolol withdrawal may result in sweating, palpitations, headache, and tremulousness.

• Atenolol administration may precipitate congestive heart failure (CHF) or myocardial infarction (MI) in those with cardiac disease; thyroid storm in those with thyrotoxicosis; and peripheral ischemia in those with existing peripheral vascular disease.

• Hypoglycemia may occur in previously controlled diabetics.

• Thrombocytopenia, manifested as unusual bruising or bleeding, occurs rarely.

NURSING CONSIDERATIONS

Baseline Assessment

• Assess the patient's apical pulse rate and B/P immediately before giving atenolol. If the pulse is 60 beats a minute or less or if the systolic B/P is less than 90 mm Hg, withhold the medication and notify the physician.

• If atenolol is being given as an antianginal, record the onset, type (such as dull, sharp, or squeezing), radiation, location, intensity, and duration, of anginal pain. Also, document the precipitating factors, such as emotional stress or exertion.

• Obtain the patient's baseline renal and liver function test results.

Lifespan Considerations

• Be aware that atenolol readily crosses the placenta and is distributed in breast milk.

• Know that atenolol use should be avoided in pregnant women during the first trimester because the drug may produce apnea, bradycardia, hypoglycemia, or hypothermia during childbirth as well as low-birth-weight infants.

• There are no age-related precautions noted in children.

• Use cautiously in the elderly, who may have age-related peripheral vascular disease and impaired renal function.

Precautions

• Use cautiously in patients with bronchospastic disease, diabetes, hyperthyroidism, impaired renal or liver function, inadequate cardiac function, or peripheral vascular disease.

Administration and Handling

PO

• May give without regard to meals.

• Crush tablets if necessary.

IV

• Store at room temperature.

• After reconstitution, store parenteral form for up to 48 hours at room temperature.

• Give undiluted or dilute in 10–50 ml 0.9% NaCl or D_5W.

• Give IV push over 5 minutes and IV infusion over 15 minutes.

Intervention and Evaluation

• Monitor the patient's B/P for hypotension, pulse for bradycardia, and respirations for difficulty breathing.

• Assess the patient's pattern of daily bowel activity and stool consistency.

• Examine the patient for evidence of CHF, including distended neck veins, dyspnea, particularly on exertion or lying down, night cough, and peripheral edema.

• Monitor the patient's intake and output and weights. An increase in weight or decrease in urine output may indicate CHF.

• Assess the patient's extremities for coldness.

• Assist the patient with ambulation if dizziness occurs.

Patient Teaching

• Warn the patient not to abruptly discontinue atenolol.

• Explain to the patient that compliance with therapy is essential to control angina or hypertension.

• To reduce the drug's orthostatic effects, instruct the patient to rise slowly from lying to sitting position and permit legs to dangle from bed momentarily before standing.

• Warn the patient to avoid tasks that require alertness or motor skills until his or her response to the drug established.

• Advise the patient to report confusion, depression, dizziness, rash, or unusual bruising or bleeding to the physician.

• Teach outpatients the correct technique to monitor their B/P and pulse before taking atenolol.

• Urge the patient to restrict his or her alcohol and salt intake.

• Advise the patient that the therapeutic antihypertensive effect of atenolol should be noted within 1 to 2 weeks.

betaxolol
beh-**tax**-oh-lol
(Betoptic-S, Betoquin[AUS], Kerlone)
Do not confuse with bethanechol.

CATEGORY AND SCHEDULE
Pregnancy Risk Category: C
(D if used in second or third trimesters)

MECHANISM OF ACTION
An antihypertensive and antiglaucoma agent that blocks beta$_1$-adrenergic receptors in cardiac tissue. Reduces aqueous humor production. *Therapeutic Effect:* Slows sinus heart rate, decreases blood pressure (B/P). Reduces intraocular pressure (IOP).

AVAILABILITY
Tablets: 10 mg, 20 mg.
Ophthalmic Solution: 0.5%.
Ophthalmic Suspension: 0.25%.

INDICATIONS AND DOSAGES
▸ **Hypertension**
PO
Adults. Initially, 10 mg/day alone or added to diuretic therapy. Dose may be doubled if no response in 7–14 days. If used alone, addition of another antihypertensive to be considered.
Elderly. Initially, 5 mg/day.
▸ **Chronic open-angle glaucoma and ocular hypertension**
Eye drops
Adults, Elderly. 1 drop 2 times/day.
▸ **Dosage in renal impairment (dialysis)**
Adults, Elderly. Initially, 5 mg/day, increase by 5 mg/day q2wks. Maximum: 20 mg/day.

UNLABELED USES
Treatment of angle-closure glaucoma during or after iridectomy, malignant glaucoma, secondary glaucoma; with miotics, decreases intraocular pressure (IOP) in acute and chronic angle-closure glaucoma

CONTRAINDICATIONS
Cardiogenic shock, overt cardiac failure, second- or third-degree heart block, sinus bradycardia

INTERACTIONS
Drug
Cimetidine: May increase betaxolol blood concentration.
Diuretics, other hypotensives: May increase hypotensive effect.
Insulin, oral hypoglycemics: May prolong hypoglycemic effect of these drugs.
NSAIDs: May decrease antihypertensive effect.

Sympathomimetics, xanthines: May mutually inhibit hypotensive effects and may mask symptoms of hypoglycemia.

Herbal

None known.

Food

None known.

DIAGNOSTIC TEST EFFECTS

May increase ANA titer, BUN and serum lipoproteins, creatinine, potassium, uric acid, and triglyceride levels.

SIDE EFFECTS

Generally well tolerated, with mild and transient side effects.

Frequent

Systemic: Hypotension manifested as dizziness, nausea, diaphoresis, headache, fatigue, constipation or diarrhea, shortness of breath

Ophthalmic: Eye irritation, visual disturbances

Occasional

Systemic: Insomnia, flatulence, urinary frequency, impotence or decreased libido

Ophthalmic: Increased light sensitivity, watering of eye

Rare

Systemic: Rash, arrhythmias, arthralgia, myalgia, confusion, change in taste, increased urination

Ophthalmic: Dry eye, conjunctivitis, eye pain

SERIOUS REACTIONS

• Oral form may produce profound bradycardia, hypotension, and bronchospasm.

• Abrupt withdrawal may result in sweating, palpitations, headache, and tremulousness.

• May precipitate congestive heart failure (CHF) or myocardial infarction (MI) in those with cardiac disease, thyroid storm in patients with thyrotoxicosis, and peripheral ischemia in patients with existing peripheral vascular disease.

• Hypoglycemia may occur in previously controlled diabetics.

• Ophthalmic overdosage may produce bradycardia, hypotension, bronchospasm, and acute cardiac failure.

NURSING CONSIDERATIONS

Baseline Assessment

• Assess the patient's baseline liver and renal function tests.

• Assess the patient's apical pulse rate and B/P immediately before giving the drug. If the patient's pulse rate is 60/min or less or systolic B/P is less than 90 mm Hg, withhold betaxolol and notify the physician.

Precautions

• Use cautiously in patients with diabetes, hyperthyroidism, impaired liver or renal function, inadequate cardiac function, and peripheral vascular disease.

Intervention and Evaluation

• Monitor the patient's B/P for signs of hypotension.

• Assess the patient's pulse for its rate and quality and monitor for bradycardia and an irregular rate.

• Assess the patient's pattern of daily bowel activity and stool consistency.

• Assist the patient with ambulation if he or she experiences dizziness.

• Evaluate the patient for signs and symptoms of CHF including decrease in urine output, distended neck veins, dyspnea, particularly on exertion or lying down, increase in weight, night cough, and peripheral edema.

• Assess the patient for diaphoresis, fatigue, headache, and nausea.

Patient Teaching
- Caution the patient against abruptly discontinuing the drug.
- Advise the patient that compliance with the therapy regimen is essential to control glaucoma and hypertension.
- To avoid betaxolol's orthostatic effects, teach the patient to rise slowly from lying to sitting position and wait momentarily before standing.
- Advise the patient to avoid tasks that require mental alertness or motor skills until his or her response to the drug is established.
- Warn the patient to notify the physician if he or she experiences excessive fatigue, headache, prolonged dizziness, or shortness of breathing.
- Explain to the patient that he or she should not use nasal decongestants or over-the-counter (OTC) cold preparations, especially stimulants, without physician approval.
- Urge the patient to limit his or her alcohol and salt intake.

bisoprolol fumarate
bye-**sew**-prow-lol
(Zebeta)
Do not confuse with DiaBeta.

CATEGORY AND SCHEDULE
Pregnancy Risk Category: C (D if used in second or third trimester)

MECHANISM OF ACTION
An antihypertensive that blocks beta$_1$-adrenergic receptors in cardiac tissue. *Therapeutic Effect:* Slows sinus heart rate, decreases blood pressure (B/P).

PHARMACOKINETICS
Well absorbed from the gastrointestinal (GI) tract. Protein binding: 26%–33%. Metabolized in liver. Primarily excreted in urine. Not removed by hemodialysis. **Half-life:** 9–12 hrs (half-life is increased in impaired renal function).

AVAILABILITY
Tablets: 5 mg, 10 mg.

INDICATIONS AND DOSAGES
▸ **Hypertension**
PO
Adults. Initially, 5 mg/day. May increase up to 20 mg/day.
Elderly. Initially, 2.5–5 mg/day. May increase by 2.5–5 mg/day. Maximum: 20 mg/day.
▸ **Creatinine clearance (less than 40 ml/min), liver impairment (cirrhosis, hepatitis)**
PO
Adults, Elderly. Initially, 2.5 mg.

UNLABELED USES
Angina pectoris, premature ventricular contractions (PVCs), supraventricular arrhythmias,

CONTRAINDICATIONS
Cardiogenic shock, overt cardiac failure, second- or third-degree heart block

INTERACTIONS
Drug
Cimetidine: May increase bisoprolol blood concentration.
Diuretics, other hypotensives: May increase the hypotensive effect of bisoprolol.
Insulin, oral hypoglycemics: May mask symptoms of hypoglycemia and prolong the hypoglycemic effect of these drugs.
NSAIDs: May decrease antihypertensive effect.

Sympathomimetics, xanthines: May mutually inhibit effects.

Herbal

None known.

Food

None known.

DIAGNOSTIC TEST EFFECTS

May increase ANA titer, BUN and serum lipoproteins, creatinine, potassium, uric acid, and triglyceride levels.

SIDE EFFECTS

Frequent

Hypotension manifested as dizziness, nausea, diaphoresis, headache, cold extremities, fatigue, constipation or diarrhea

Occasional

Insomnia, flatulence, urinary frequency, impotence or decreased libido

Rare

Rash, arthralgia, myalgia, confusion (especially in the elderly), change in taste

SERIOUS REACTIONS

• Overdosage may produce profound bradycardia and hypotension.

• Abrupt withdrawal may result in sweating, palpitations, headache, and tremulousness.

• May precipitate congestive heart failure (CHF) and myocardial infarction (MI) in patients with heart disease; thyroid storm in patients with thyrotoxicosis; and peripheral ischemia in patients with existing peripheral vascular disease.

• Hypoglycemia may occur in previously controlled diabetics.

• Thrombocytopenia, including unusual bruising and bleeding, occurs rarely.

NURSING CONSIDERATIONS

Baseline Assessment

• Assess the patient's baseline liver and renal function test results.

• Assess the patient's apical pulse rate and B/P immediately before giving bisoprolol. If the patient's pulse rate is 60/min or less or systolic B/P is less than 90 mm Hg, withhold the medication and contact the physician.

Lifespan Considerations

• Be aware that bisoprolol readily crosses the placenta and is distributed in breast milk and that its use should be avoided during the first trimester of pregnancy. Know that bisoprolol use may produce apnea, bradycardia, hypoglycemia, hypothermia during delivery, and low birth-weight infants.

• Be aware that the safety and efficacy of bisoprolol have not been established in children.

• In the elderly, age-related peripheral vascular disease may increase risk of decreased peripheral circulation.

Precautions

• Use cautiously in patients with bronchospastic disease, diabetes, hyperthyroidism, impaired liver or renal function, inadequate cardiac function, and peripheral vascular disease.

Administration and Handling

PO

• May give bisoprolol without regard to food.

• If necessary, crush scored tablet.

Intervention and Evaluation

• Assess the patient's pulse for an irregular rate, for its quality, and for bradycardia.

• Assist the patient with ambulation if dizziness occurs.

• Assess the patient for peripheral edema of the feet and hands. For

ambulatory patients, check behind the medial malleolus and for bedridden patients, check the sacral area.
• Assess the patient's pattern of daily bowel activity and stool consistency.

Patient Teaching
• Caution the patient against abruptly discontinuing the drug.
• Advise the patient that compliance with the therapy regimen is essential to control hypertension.
• Instruct the patient that if he or she experiences dizziness, to sit or lie down immediately.
• Warn the patient to avoid tasks that require mental alertness or motor skills until his or her response to the drug is established.
• Teach the patient how to properly take his or her pulse before each dose and to report to the physician if he or she experiences dizziness, excessively slow pulse rates (less than 60 beats/min), or peripheral numbness.
• Explain to the patient that he or she should not use nasal decongestants and over-the-counter (OTC) cold preparations, especially those containing stimulants, without physician approval.
• Urge the patient to limit his or her alcohol and salt intake.

carvedilol
car-**veh**-dih-lol
(Coreg, Dilatrend[AUS])
Do not confuse with carteolol.

CATEGORY AND SCHEDULE
Pregnancy Risk Category: C
(D if used in the second or third trimester)

MECHANISM OF ACTION
An antihypertensive that possesses nonselective beta-blocking and alpha-adrenergic blocking activity. Causes vasodilation. *Therapeutic Effect:* Reduces cardiac output, exercise-induced tachycardia, and reflex orthostatic tachycardia; reduces peripheral vascular resistance.

PHARMACOKINETICS

Route	Onset	Peak	Duration
PO	30 min	1–2 hrs	24 hrs

Rapidly and extensively absorbed from the gastrointestinal (GI) tract. Protein binding: 98%. Metabolized in liver. Excreted primarily via bile into feces. Minimally removed by hemodialysis. **Half-life:** 7–10 hrs. Food delays rate of absorption.

AVAILABILITY
Tablets: 3.125 mg, 6.25 mg, 12.5 mg, 25 mg.

INDICATIONS AND DOSAGES
▸ **Hypertension; reduce cardiovascular mortality**
PO
Adults, Elderly. Initially, 6.25 mg twice a day. May double at 7-to 14-day intervals to highest tolerated dosage. Maximum: 50 mg/day.
▸ **Congestive heart failure (CHF)**
PO
Adults, Elderly. Initially, 3.125 mg twice a day. May double at 2-wk intervals to highest tolerated dosage. Maximum: For patients weighing less than 85 kg, give 25 mg twice a day; and for those weighing more than 85 kg, give 50 mg twice a day.

UNLABELED USES
Treatment of angina pectoris, idiopathic cardiomyopathy

CONTRAINDICATIONS

Bronchial asthma or related bronchospastic conditions, cardiogenic shock, pulmonary edema, second- or third-degree atrioventricular (AV) block, severe bradycardia

INTERACTIONS
Drug

Calcium blockers: Increase risk of conduction disturbances.
Catapres: May potentiate blood pressure (B/P) effects.
Cimetidine: May increase carvedilol blood concentration.
Digoxin: Increases concentrations of this drug.
Diuretics, other hypotensives: May increase hypotensive effect.
Insulin, oral hypoglycemics: May mask symptoms of hypoglycemia and prolong hypoglycemic effect of these drugs.
Rifampin: Decreases carvedilol blood concentration.
Herbal
None known.
Food
None known.

DIAGNOSTIC TEST EFFECTS

None known.

SIDE EFFECTS

Generally well tolerated, with mild and transient side effects.
Frequent (6%–4%)
Fatigue, dizziness
Occasional (2%)
Diarrhea, bradycardia, rhinitis, back pain
Rare (less than 2%)
Postural hypotension, somnolence, urinary tract infection, viral infection

SERIOUS REACTIONS

• Overdosage may produce profound bradycardia, hypotension, bronchospasm, cardiac insufficiency, cardiogenic shock, and cardiac arrest.
• Abrupt withdrawal may result in sweating, palpitations, headache, and tremulousness.
• May precipitate CHF and myocardial infarction (MI) in patients with heart disease, thyroid storm in patients with thyrotoxicosis, and peripheral ischemia in patients with existing peripheral vascular disease.
• Hypoglycemia may occur in patients with previously controlled diabetes.

NURSING CONSIDERATIONS

Baseline Assessment
• Assess the patient's apical pulse rate and B/P immediately before giving carvedilol. If the patient's pulse rate is 60/min or less or systolic B/P is less than 90 mm Hg, withhold the medication and contact the physician.
Lifespan Considerations
• Be aware that it is unknown if carvedilol crosses the placenta or is distributed in breast milk. Know that carvedilol use may produce apnea, bradycardia, hypoglycemia, hypothermia during delivery, and low-birth-weight infants.
• Be aware that the safety and efficacy of carvedilol have not been established in children.
• In the elderly, the incidence of dizziness may be increased.
Precautions
• Use cautiously in patients undergoing anesthesia, CHF controlled with angiotensin-converting enzyme inhibitor, digoxin or diuretics, diabetes mellitus, hypoglycemia, impaired liver function, peripheral vascular disease, and thyrotoxicosis.

Administration and Handling
PO
• Give with food, which slows the rate of absorption and reduces the risk of orthostatic hypotension.
• To assess the patient's tolerance of the drug, assess a standing systolic B/P 1 hour after giving carvedilol.

Intervention and Evaluation
• Monitor the patient's B/P for hypotension and respiratory status for breathlessness.
• Assess the patient's pulse for an irregular rate, for its quality, and for bradycardia.
• Monitor the patient's EKG for arrhythmias.
• Assist the patient with ambulation if he or she experiences dizziness.
• Evaluate the patient for signs and symptoms of CHF, including distended neck veins, dyspnea (particularly on exertion or lying down), night cough, and peripheral edema
• Monitor the patient's intake and output and weights. Keep in mind that an increase in weight or a decrease in urine output may indicate CHF.

Patient Teaching
• Explain to the patient that the full antihypertensive effect of carvedilol will be noted in 1 to 2 weeks.
• Advise patients who are contact lens wearers that they may experience decreased tearing.
• Teach the patient to take carvedilol with food.
• Caution the patient against abruptly discontinuing carvedilol. Advise the patient that compliance with the therapy regimen is essential to control hypertension.
• Advise the patient to avoid tasks that require mental alertness or motor skills until his or her response to the drug is established.
• Warn the patient to notify the physician if he or she experiences excessive fatigue or prolonged dizziness.
• Explain to the patient that he or she should not take nasal decongestants and over-the-counter (OTC) cold preparations, especially those containing stimulants, without physician approval.
• Instruct the patient to check his or her pulse rate and B/P before taking the medication.
• Urge the patient to limit his or her alcohol and salt intake.

esmolol hydrochloride
ez-moe-lol
(Brevibloc)

CATEGORY AND SCHEDULE
Pregnancy Risk Category: C

MECHANISM OF ACTION
An antiarrhythmic that selectively blocks beta$_1$-adrenergic receptors. *Therapeutic Effect:* Slows sinus heart rate, decreases cardiac output, decreasing blood pressure (B/P).

AVAILABILITY
Injection: 10 mg/ml, 250 mg/ml.

INDICATIONS AND DOSAGES
▸ **Rapid, short-term control of ventricular rate in those with supraventricular arrhythmias, including sinus tachycardia, intraoperative and postoperative control of tachycardia and hypertension**
IV
Adults, Elderly. Initially, loading dose of 500 mcg/kg/min for 1 min, followed by 50 mcg/kg/min for 4 min. If optimum response is not attained in 5 min, give second loading dose of 500 mcg/kg/min for

1 min, followed by infusion of 100 mcg/kg/min for 4 min. Additional loading doses can be given and infusion increased by 50 mcg/kg/min, up to 200 mcg/kg/min, for 4 min. Once desired response is attained, cease loading dose and increase infusion by no more than 25 mcg/kg/min. Interval between doses may be increased to 10 min. Infusion usually administered over 24–48 hrs in most patients. Range: 50–200 mcg/kg/min with average dose of 100 mcg/kg/min.

CONTRAINDICATIONS
Cardiogenic shock, overt cardiac failure, second- and third-degree heart block, sinus bradycardia

INTERACTIONS
Drug
Insulin, oral hypoglycemics: May mask symptoms of hypoglycemia and prolong hypoglycemic effect of these drugs.
MAOIs: May cause significant hypertension.
Sympathomimetics, xanthines: May mutually inhibit effects.
Herbal
None known.
Food
None known.

DIAGNOSTIC TEST EFFECTS
None known.

IV INCOMPATIBILITIES
Amphotericin B complex (Abelcet, AmBisome, Amphotec), furosemide (Lasix)

IV COMPATIBILITIES
Amiodarone (Cordarone), diltiazem (Cardizem), dopamine (Intropin), heparin, magnesium, midazolam (Versed), potassium chloride, propofol (Diprivan)

SIDE EFFECTS
Generally well tolerated, with transient and mild side effects.
Frequent
Hypotension (systolic B/P less than 90 mm Hg) manifested as dizziness, nausea, diaphoresis, headache, cold extremities, fatigue
Occasional
Anxiety, drowsiness, flushed skin, vomiting, confusion, inflammation at injection site, fever

SERIOUS REACTIONS
• Excessive dosage may produce profound hypotension, bradycardia, dizziness, syncope, drowsiness, breathing difficulty, bluish fingernails or palms of hands, and seizures.
• May potentiate insulin-induced hypoglycemia in diabetic patients.

NURSING CONSIDERATIONS
Baseline Assessment
• Assess the patient's apical pulse and B/P immediately before giving esmolol. If the patient's pulse is 60/min or less or systolic B/P is less than 90 mm Hg, withhold the medication and contact physician.
Precautions
• Use cautiously inpatients with bronchial asthma, bronchitis, CHF, diabetes, emphysema, history of allergy, and impaired renal function.
Administration and Handling
◀ALERT▶ Give esmolol by IV infusion. Avoid using butterfly needles and very small veins.
IV
• Use only clear and colorless to light yellow solution.
• After dilution, solution is stable for 24 hours.
• Discard solution if it is discolored or if precipitate forms.
• To prevent vein irritation, dilute

the 250 mg/ml ampoule to a final concentration not to exceed 10 mg/ml. Don't administer the drug by direct IV injection.

• For IV infusion, remove 20 ml from 500-ml container of D_5W, D_5W/Ringer's, D_5W/lactated Ringer's, D_5W/0.9% NaCl, D_5W/0.45% NaCl, 0.9% NaCl, lactated Ringer's or 0.45% NaCl and dilute 5-g vial esmolol to remaining 480 ml of solution to provide concentration of 10 mg/ml. Maximum concentration: 10 g/250 ml (40 mg/ml).

• Administer by controlled infusion device and titrate according to the patient's tolerance and response.

• Infuse IV loading dose over 1 to 2 minutes.

• Monitor the patient for hypotension, a systolic B/P of less than 90 mm Hg, which is greatest during first 30 minutes of IV infusion.

Intervention and Evaluation

• Monitor the patient's B/P for hypotension, EKG, and heart and respiratory rates.

• Monitor the patient for diaphoresis or dizziness, the first signs of impending hypotension.

• Assess the patient's pulse for its quality, an irregular rate, and for bradycardia.

• Assess the patient's extremities for coldness.

• Assist the patient with ambulation if he or she experiences dizziness.

• Evaluate the patient for diaphoresis, fatigue, headache, and nausea.

Patient Teaching

• Explain to the patient that his or her blood pressure and heart will be continuously monitored during esmolol therapy.

• Urge patient to immediately report if he or she experiences cold extremities, dizziness, faintness, or nausea.

labetalol hydrochloride

lah-**bet**-ah-lol
(Normodyne, Presolol[AUS], Trandate)
Do not confuse with Trental.

CATEGORY AND SCHEDULE

Pregnancy Risk Category: C (D if used in second or third trimester)

MECHANISM OF ACTION

An antihypertensive that blocks $alpha_1$-, $beta_1$-, $beta_2$-(large doses) adrenergic receptor sites. *Therapeutic Effect:* Slows sinus heart rate; decreases peripheral vascular resistance, cardiac output, blood pressure (B/P). Large doses increase airway resistance.

PHARMACOKINETICS

Route	Onset	Peak	Duration
PO	0.5–2 hrs	2–4 hrs	8–12 hrs
IV	2–5 min	5–15 min	2–4 hrs

Completely absorbed from the gastrointestinal (GI) tract. Protein binding: 50%. Undergoes first-pass metabolism. Metabolized in liver. Primarily excreted in urine. Not removed by hemodialysis. **Half-life:** PO: 6–8 hrs; IV: 5.5 hrs.

AVAILABILITY

Tablets: 100 mg, 200 mg, 300 mg.
Injection: 5 mg/ml.

INDICATIONS AND DOSAGES

▶ **Hypertension**
PO
Adults. Initially, 100 mg 2 times/day adjusted in increments of 100 mg 2 times/day q2–3 days.

Maintenance: 200–400 mg 2 times/ day. Maximum: 2.4 g/day.
Elderly. Initially, 100 mg 1–2 times/ day. May increase as needed.
▸ **Severe hypertension, hypertensive emergency**
IV
Adults. Initially, 20 mg. Additional doses of 20–80 mg may be given at 10-min intervals, up to total dose of 300 mg.
IV infusion
Adults. Initially, 2 mg/min up to total dose of 300 mg.
PO (after IV therapy)
Adults. Initially, 200 mg; then, 200–400 mg in 6–12 hrs. Increase dose at 1-day intervals to desired level.

UNLABELED USES
To control hypotension during surgery, treatment of chronic angina pectoris

CONTRAINDICATIONS
Bronchial asthma, cardiogenic shock, second- or third-degree heart block, severe bradycardia, uncontrolled congestive heart failure (CHF)

INTERACTIONS
Drug
Diuretics, other hypotensives: May increase hypotensive effect.
Insulin, oral hypoglycemics: May mask symptoms of hypoglycemia and prolong hypoglycemic effect of these drugs.
MAOIs: May produce hypertension.
Sympathomimetics, xanthines: May mutually inhibit effects.
Herbal
None known.
Food
None known.

DIAGNOSTIC TEST EFFECTS
May increase serum ANA titer; BUN, serum LDH, lipoprotein, alkaline phosphatase, bilirubin, creatinine, potassium, triglyceride, uric acid, SGOT (AST), and SGPT (ALT) levels.

IV INCOMPATIBILITIES
Amphotericin B complex (Abelcet, AmBisome, Amphotec), ceftriaxone (Rocephin), furosemide (Lasix), heparin, nafcillin (Nafcil), thiopental

IV COMPATIBILITIES
Aminophylline, amiodarone (Cordarone), calcium gluconate, diltiazem (Cardizem), dobutamine (Dobutrex), dopamine (Intropin), enalapril (Vasotec), fentanyl (Sublimaze), hydromorphone (Dilaudid), lidocaine, lorazepam (Ativan), magnesium sulfate, midazolam (Versed), milrinone (Primacor), morphine, nitroglycerin, norepinephrine (Levophed), potassium chloride, potassium phosphate, propofol (Diprivan)

SIDE EFFECTS
Frequent
Drowsiness, trouble sleeping, unusually tired or weak, decreased sexual ability, transient scalp tingling
Occasional
Dizziness, difficulty breathing, swelling of hands or feet, depression, anxiety, constipation, diarrhea, nasal congestion, nausea, vomiting, stomach discomfort
Rare
Altered taste, dry eyes, increased urination, numbness or tingling in fingers, toes, or scalp

SERIOUS REACTIONS
• May precipitate or aggravate CHF due to decreased myocardial stimulation.

• Abrupt withdrawal may precipitate ischemic heart disease, producing sweating, palpitations, headache, and tremor.
• Beta-blockers may mask signs, symptoms of acute hypoglycemia (tachycardia, B/P changes) in diabetic patients.

NURSING CONSIDERATIONS
Baseline Assessment
• Assess the patient's baseline liver and renal function test results.
• Assess the patient's apical pulse and B/P immediately before giving labetalol. If the patient's pulse is 60/min or less or systolic B/P is less than 90 mm Hg, withhold the medication and contact the physician.
Lifespan Considerations
• Be aware that labetalol crosses the placenta and is distributed in small amounts in breast milk.
• Be aware that the safety and efficacy of labetalol have not been established in children.
• In the elderly, age-related peripheral vascular disease may increase susceptibility to decreased peripheral circulation.
Precautions
• Use cautiously in patients with diabetes mellitus, drug-controlled CHF, impaired cardiac or liver function, nonallergic bronchospastic disease, including chronic bronchitis and emphysema, and pheochromocytoma.
Administration and Handling
PO
• Give labetalol without regard to food.
• Crush tablets if necessary.
IV
◀ALERT▶ Place patient in a supine position for IV administration and for 3 hours after receiving the medication. Expect a substantial

drop in B/P if the patient stands within 3 hours following drug administration.
• Store at room temperature.
• After dilution, IV solution is stable for 24 hours.
• Solution normally appears clear, colorless to light yellow.
• Discard if precipitate forms or discoloration occurs.
• For IV infusion, dilute 200 mg in 160 ml D_5W, 0.9% NaCl, lactated Ringer's, or any combination of these solutions to provide a concentration of 1 mg/ml.
• For IV push, give over 2 minutes at 10-minute intervals.
• For IV infusion, administer at rate of 2 mg/min (2 ml/min) initially. Adjust the rate according to the patient's B/P.
• Monitor the patient's B/P immediately before and every 5 to 10 minutes during IV administration. Know that the maximum effect occurs within 5 minutes.
Intervention and Evaluation
• Monitor the patient's B/P for signs of hypotension and EKG for arrhythmias.
• Assess the patient's pulse for bradycardia or an irregular rate.
• Assess the patient's pattern of daily bowel activity and stool consistency.
• Assist the patient with ambulation if he or she experiences dizziness.
• Evaluate the patient for signs and symptoms of CHF, including distended neck veins, dyspnea (particularly on exertion or lying down), night cough, and peripheral edema.
• Monitor the patient's intake and output and weights. Know that an increase in patient weight or a decrease in patient urine output may indicate CHF.
Patient Teaching
• Caution the patient against discontinuing the drug except upon the

advice of the physician. Explain that stopping the drug abruptly may precipitate heart failure.
• Stress to the patient that compliance with the therapy regimen is essential to control arrhythmias and hypertension.
• Advise the patient to avoid tasks that require mental alertness or motor skills until his or her response to the drug is established.
• Warn the patient to notify the physician if he or she experiences excessive fatigue, headache, prolonged dizziness, shortness of breath, and weight gain.
• Explain to the patient that he or she should not take any nasal decongestants and over-the-counter (OTC) cold preparations, especially those containing stimulants, without physician approval.

---

metoprolol tartrate
meh-**toe**-pro-lol
(Apo-Metoprolol[CAN], Betaloc[CAN], Lopressor, Metohexal[AUS], Metolol[AUS], Minax[AUS], Nu-Metop[CAN], PMS-Metoprolol [CAN], Toprol XL)
Do not confuse with metaproterenol or metolazone.

CATEGORY AND SCHEDULE
Pregnancy Risk Category: C (D if used in second or third trimester)

MECHANISM OF ACTION
An antianginal, antihypertensive, and myocardial infarction (MI) adjunct that selectively blocks beta$_1$-adrenergic receptors; high dosages may block beta$_2$-adrenergic receptors. Decreases O_2 requirements. *Therapeutic Effect:* Slows sinus node heart rate, decreases cardiac output, reduces blood pressure (B/P). Decreases myocardial ischemia severity. Increases airway resistance at high dosages.

PHARMACOKINETICS

Route	Onset	Peak	Duration
PO	10–15 min	N/A	6 hrs
PO (extended release)	N/A	6–12 hrs	24 hrs
IV	Immediate	20 min	5–8 hrs

Well absorbed from the gastrointestinal (GI) tract. Protein binding: 12%. Widely distributed. Metabolized in liver (undergoes significant first-pass metabolism). Primarily excreted in urine. Removed by hemodialysis. **Half-life:** 3–7 hrs.

AVAILABILITY
Tablets: 50 mg, 100 mg.
Tablets (extended-release): 25 mg, 50 mg, 100 mg, 200 mg.
Injection: 1 mg/ml.

INDICATIONS AND DOSAGES
▶ **Mild to moderate hypertension**
PO
Adults. Initially, 100 mg/day as single or divided dose. Increase at weekly (or longer) intervals. Maintenance: 100–450 mg/day.
Elderly. Initially, 25 mg/day. Range: 25–300 mg/day.
▶ **PO (extended-release tablets)**
Adults. 50–100 mg/day as single dose. May increase at least at weekly intervals until optimum B/P attained. Maximum: 200 mg/day.
▶ **Chronic, stable angina pectoris**
PO
Adults. Initially, 100 mg/day as

single or divided dose. Increase at weekly (or longer) intervals.
Maintenance: 100–450 mg/day.
PO (extended-release tablets)
Adults. Initially, 100 mg/day as single dose. May increase at least at weekly intervals until optimum clinical response achieved.
Maximum: 200 mg/day.
▸ **Heart failure**
PO (extended-release tablets)
Adults. Initially, 25 mg/day. May double dose q2wks. Maximum: 200 mg/day.
▸ **Early treatment of myocardial infarction (MI)**
IV
Adults. 5 mg q2min for 3 doses, followed by 50 mg orally q6h for 48 hrs. Begin oral dose 15 min after last IV dose. Alternatively, in those who do not tolerate full IV dose, give 25–50 mg orally q6h, 15 min after last IV dose.
▸ **Late treatment and maintenance after an MI**
PO
Adults. 100 mg 2 times/day for at least 3 mos.

UNLABELED USES

Increases survival rate in diabetic patients with heart disease. Treatment or prophylaxis of anxiety, cardiac arrhythmias, hypertrophic cardiomyopathy, mitral valve prolapse syndrome, pheochromocytoma, tremors, thyrotoxicosis, vascular headache

CONTRAINDICATIONS

Cardiogenic shock, myocardial infarction with a heart rate less than 45 beats/min or systolic blood pressure less than 100 mm Hg, overt heart failure, second- or third-degree heart block, sinus bradycardia

INTERACTIONS
Drug
Cimetidine: May increase metoprolol blood concentration.
Diuretics, other hypotensives: May increase hypotensive effect.
Insulin, oral hypoglycemics: May mask symptoms of hypoglycemia and prolong hypoglycemic effect of these drugs.
NSAIDs: May decrease antihypertensive effect.
Sympathomimetics, xanthines: May mutually inhibit effects.
Herbal
None known.
Food
None known.

DIAGNOSTIC TEST EFFECTS

May increase ANA titer, BUN, serum lipoprotein levels, serum LDH concentration, serum alkaline phosphatase, serum bilirubin, serum creatinine, serum potassium, serum uric acid, SGOT (AST), SGPT (ALT), and serum triglyceride levels.

IV INCOMPATIBILITIES

Amphotericin B complex (Abelcet, AmBisome, Amphotec)

IV COMPATIBILITIES

Alteplase (Activase)

SIDE EFFECTS

Generally well tolerated, with transient and mild side effects.
Frequent
Decreased sexual function, drowsiness, insomnia, unusual tiredness or weakness
Occasional
Anxiety, nervousness, diarrhea, constipation, nausea, vomiting, nasal congestion, stomach discomfort, dizziness, difficulty breathing, cold hands or feet

Rare
Altered taste, dry eyes, nightmares, numbness in fingers and feet, allergic reaction (rash, pruritus)

SERIOUS REACTIONS

• Excessive dosage may produce profound bradycardia, hypotension, and bronchospasm.
• Abrupt withdrawal may result in diaphoresis, palpitations, headache, tremulousness, exacerbation of angina, MI, and ventricular arrhythmias.
• May precipitate congestive heart failure (CHF) and MI in patients with heart disease; thyroid storm in patients with thyrotoxicosis; and peripheral ischemia in patients with existing peripheral vascular disease.
• Hypoglycemia may occur in patients with previously controlled diabetes.

NURSING CONSIDERATIONS

Baseline Assessment
• Assess the patient's baseline liver and renal function test results.
• Assess the patient's apical pulse and B/P immediately before giving metoprolol. If the patient's pulse is 60/min or less, or systolic B/P is less than 90 mm Hg, withhold the medication and contact the physician.
• In patients receiving metoprolol for treatment of angina, record the onset, type (sharp, dull, squeezing), radiation, location, intensity, duration of anginal pain and its precipitating factors, including exertion and emotional stress.

Lifespan Considerations
• Be aware that metoprolol crosses the placenta and is distributed in breast milk. Know that metoprolol use should be avoided during the first trimester and that metoprolol

use may produce apnea, bradycardia, hypoglycemia, hypothermia during delivery, and low-birth-weight infants.
• Be aware that the safety and efficacy of metoprolol have not been established in children.
• In the elderly, age-related peripheral vascular disease may increase susceptibility to decreased peripheral circulation.

Precautions
• Use cautiously in patients with bronchospastic disease, diabetes, hyperthyroidism, impaired renal function, inadequate cardiac function, and peripheral vascular disease.

Administration and Handling
PO
• Crush tablets if necessary; do not crush or break extended-release tablets.
• Give at same time each day.
• Give with or immediately after meals to enhance absorption.
IV
• Store at room temperature.
• Give undiluted as necessary.
• Administer IV injection over 1 minute.
• Monitor EKG during administration.

Intervention and Evaluation
• Measure the patient's B/P near the end of the dosing interval to determine whether the B/P is controlled throughout day.
• Monitor the patient's B/P for signs of hypotension and respirations for shortness of breath.
• Assess the patient's pulse for its quality and for bradycardia or an irregular rate.
• Evaluate the patient for signs and symptoms of CHF, including distended neck veins, dyspnea (particularly on exertion or lying down), night cough, and peripheral edema.
• Monitor the patient's intake and

output and weights. Be aware that an increase in weight or a decrease in urine output may indicate CHF.

• Expect the therapeutic response to hypertension to be noted in 1 to 2 weeks.

Patient Teaching

• Caution the patient against discontinuing the drug.

• Stress to the patient that compliance with the therapy regimen is essential to control arrhythmias and hypertension.

• Instruct the patient that if a dose is missed, he or she should take the next scheduled dose and should not double the dose.

• Teach the patient to rise slowly from a lying to a sitting position and to wait momentarily before standing to avoid the drug's hypotensive effect.

• Warn the patient to notify the physician if he or she experiences dizziness or excessive fatigue.

• Explain to the patient that he or she should not take any nasal decongestants and over-the-counter (OTC) cold preparations, especially those containing stimulants, without physician approval.

• Instruct outpatients to monitor their B/P and pulse before taking the medication.

• Urge the patient to limit alcohol and salt intake.

---

nadolol

nay-**doe**-lol

(Apo-Nadol[CAN], Corgard, Novo-Nadolol[CAN])

CATEGORY AND SCHEDULE

Pregnancy Risk Category: C (D if used in second or third trimester)

MECHANISM OF ACTION

A nonselective beta-blocker that blocks beta$_1$- and beta$_2$-adrenergic receptors. *Therapeutic Effect:* Slows sinus heart rate; decreases cardiac output and blood pressure (B/P); increases airway resistance. Decreases myocardial ischemia severity by decreasing O$_2$ requirements.

AVAILABILITY

Tablets: 20 mg, 40 mg, 80 mg, 120 mg, 160 mg.

INDICATIONS AND DOSAGES

▸ **Mild to moderate hypertension, angina**

PO

Adults. Initially, 40 mg/day. May increase by 40–80 mg at 3–7 day intervals. Maximum: 240–360 mg/day.

Elderly. Initially, 20 mg/day. May increase gradually. Range: 20–240 mg/day.

▸ **Dosage in renal impairment**

Dosage is modified based on creatinine clearance.

Creatinine Clearance	% Normal Dosage
10–50 ml/min	50
less than 10 ml/min	25

UNLABELED USES

Treatment of arrhythmias, hypertrophic cardiomyopathy, myocardial infarction (MI), pheochromocytoma, vascular headaches, tremors, thyrotoxicosis, mitral valve prolapse syndrome, neuroleptic-induced akathisia

CONTRAINDICATIONS

Bronchial asthma, cardiogenic shock, chronic obstructive pulmonary disease (COPD), congestive heart failure (CHF) secondary to tachyarrhythmias, patients receiving MAOI therapy, second- or third-degree heart block, sinus bradycardia, uncontrolled cardiac failure

INTERACTIONS
Drug
Cimetidine: May increase nadolol blood concentration.
Diuretics, other hypotensives: May increase hypotensive effect.
Insulin, oral hypoglycemics: May mask symptoms of hypoglycemia and prolong the hypoglycemic effect of insulin and oral hypoglycemics.
NSAIDs: May decrease antihypertensive effect.
Sympathomimetics, xanthines: May mutually inhibit effects.
Herbal
None known.
Food
None known.

DIAGNOSTIC TEST EFFECTS
May increase ANA titer, BUN, serum LDH concentration, serum lipoprotein levels, serum alkaline phosphatase, serum bilirubin, serum creatinine, serum potassium, serum uric acid, SGOT (AST), SGPT (ALT), and serum triglyceride levels.

SIDE EFFECTS
Generally well tolerated, with transient and mild side effects.
Frequent
Decreased sexual ability, drowsiness, unusual tiredness or weakness
Occasional
Bradycardia, difficulty breathing, depression, cold hands or feet, diarrhea, constipation, anxiety, nasal congestion, nausea, vomiting
Rare
Altered taste, dry eyes, itching

SERIOUS REACTIONS
• Excessive dosage may produce profound bradycardia and hypotension.
• Abrupt withdrawal may result in diaphoresis, palpitations, headache, tremulousness, exacerbation of angina, MI, and ventricular arrhythmias.
• May precipitate CHF and MI in patients with cardiac disease; thyroid storm in patients with thyrotoxicosis; and peripheral ischemia in patients with existing peripheral vascular disease.
• Hypoglycemia may occur in patients with previously controlled diabetes.

NURSING CONSIDERATIONS
Baseline Assessment
• Assess the patient's baseline liver and renal function tests.
• Assess the patient's apical pulse and B/P immediately before giving nadolol. If the patient's pulse is 60/min or less, or systolic B/P is less than 90 mm Hg, withhold the medication and contact the physician.
• Record the onset, type (sharp, dull, or squeezing), radiation, location, intensity, and duration of anginal pain and its precipitating factors, such as exertion or emotional stress.
Precautions
• Use cautiously in patients with diabetes mellitus, hyperthyroidism, impaired liver or renal function, and inadequate cardiac function.
Administration and Handling
PO
• Give nadolol without regard to meals.
• Tablets may be crushed.
Intervention and Evaluation
• Monitor the patient's B/P for hypotension and respiration for shortness of breath.

• Assess the patient's pulse for its rate and quality and be alert for bradycardia and an irregular rate.

• Examine the patient's fingers for lack of color and numbness (Raynaud's disease).

• Evaluate the patient for signs and symptoms of CHF, including distended neck veins, dyspnea (particularly on exertion or lying down), night cough, and peripheral edema.

• Monitor the patient's intake and output. Be aware that an increase in patient weight or a decrease in the patient's urine output may indicate CHF.

Patient Teaching

• Caution the patient against abruptly discontinuing the drug because this action may precipitate angina.

• Warn the patient to notify the physician if he or she experiences confusion, depression, difficulty breathing, dizziness, fever, night cough, rash, slow pulse, sore throat, swelling of arms and legs, and unusual bleeding or bruising.

• Advise the patient to avoid tasks that require mental alertness or motor skills until his or her response to the drug is established.

propranolol hydrochloride
pro-**pran**-oh-lol
(Apo-Propranolol[CAN], Deralin[AUS], Inderal, Inno-Pran XL)
Do not confuse with Adderall, Isordil, or Pravachol.

CATEGORY AND SCHEDULE
Pregnancy Risk Category: C (D if used in second or third trimester)

MECHANISM OF ACTION
An antihypertensive, antianginal, antiarrhythmic, and antimigraine agent that blocks beta$_1$- and beta$_2$-adrenergic receptors. Decreases O_2 requirements. Slows AV conduction and increases refractory period in atrioventricular (AV) node. *Therapeutic Effect:* Slows sinus heart rate, decreases cardiac output, and decreases blood pressure (B/P). Increases airway resistance. Decreases myocardial ischemia severity. Exhibits antiarrhythmic activity.

PHARMACOKINETICS

Route	Onset	Peak	Duration
PO	1–2 hrs	N/A	6 hrs

Well absorbed from the gastrointestinal (GI) tract. Protein binding: 93%. Widely distributed. Metabolized in liver. Primarily excreted in urine. Not removed by hemodialysis. **Half-life:** 3–5 hrs.

AVAILABILITY
Tablets: 10 mg, 20 mg, 40 mg, 60 mg, 80 mg.
Capsules (sustained-release): 60 mg, 80 mg, 120 mg, 160 mg.
Oral Solution: 4 mg/ml, 8 mg/ml.
Solution (concentrate): 80 mg/ml.
Injection: 1 mg/ml.

INDICATIONS AND DOSAGES
▶ **Hypertension**
PO
Adults, Elderly. Initially, 40 mg 2 times/day. May increase dose q3-7 days. Range: Up to 320 mg/day in divided doses. Maximum: 640 mg/day.
Children. Initially, 0.5–1 mg/kg/day in divided doses q6-12h. May increase at 3–5 day intervals. Usual

dose: 1–5 mg/kg/day. Maximum: 8 mg/kg/day.

▸ **Angina**
PO
Adults, Elderly. 80–320 mg/day in divided doses. (long acting): Initially, 80 mg/day. Maximum: 320 mg/day.

▸ **Arrhythmias**
IV
Adults, Elderly. 1 mg/dose. May repeat q5min. Maximum: 5 mg total dose.
Children. 0.01–0.1 mg/kg. Maximum (infants): 1 mg; (children): 3 mg.
PO
Adults, Elderly. Initially, 10–20 mg q6-8h. May gradually increase dose. Range: 40–320 mg/day.
Children. Initially, 0.5–1 mg/kg/day in divided doses q6-8h. May increase q3-5 days. Usual dosage: 2–4 mg/kg/day. Maximum: 16 mg/kg/day or 60 mg/day.

▸ **Life-threatening arrhythmias**
IV
Adults, Elderly. 0.5–3 mg. Repeat once in 2 min. Give additional doses at intervals of at least 4 hrs.
Children. 0.01–0.1 mg/kg.

▸ **Hypertrophic subaortic stenosis**
PO
Adults, Elderly. 20–40 mg in 3–4 divided doses or 80–160 mg/day as extended-release capsule.

▸ **Adjunct to alpha-blocking agents to treat pheochromocytoma**
PO
Adults, Elderly. 60 mg/day in divided doses with alpha-blocker for 3 days before surgery. Maintenance (inoperable tumor): 30 mg/day with alpha-blocker.

▸ **Migraine headache**
PO
Adults, Elderly. 80 mg/day in divided doses or 80 mg once daily as extended-release capsule. Increase

up to 160–240 mg/day in divided doses.
Children. 0.6–1.5 mg/kg/day in divided doses q8h. Maximum: 4 mg/kg/day.

▸ **Reduce cardiovascular mortality and reinfarction in patients with previous myocardial infarction (MI)**
PO
Adults, Elderly. 180–240 mg/day in divided doses.

▸ **Essential tremor**
PO
Adults, Elderly. Initially, 40 mg 2 times/day increased up to 120–320 mg/day in 3 divided doses.

UNLABELED USES
Treatment of adjunct anxiety, mitral valve prolapse syndrome, thyrotoxicosis

CONTRAINDICATIONS
Asthma, bradycardia, cardiogenic shock, chronic obstructive pulmonary disease (COPD), heart block, Raynaud's syndrome, uncompensated congestive heart failure (CHF)

INTERACTIONS
Drug
Diuretics, other hypotensives: May increase hypotensive effect.
Insulin, oral hypoglycemics: May mask symptoms of hypoglycemia and prolong the hypoglycemic effect of insulin and oral hypoglycemics.
IV phenytoin: May increase cardiac depressant effect.
NSAIDs: May decrease antihypertensive effect.
Sympathomimetics, xanthines: May mutually inhibit effects.
Herbal
None known.
Food
None known.

DIAGNOSTIC TEST EFFECTS

May increase ANA titer, BUN, serum LDH concentration, serum lipoprotein levels, serum alkaline phosphatase, serum bilirubin, serum creatinine, serum potassium, serum uric acid, SGOT (AST), SGPT (ALT), and serum triglyceride levels.

IV INCOMPATIBILITIES

Amphotericin B complex (Abelcet, AmBisome, Amphotec)

IV COMPATIBILITIES

Alteplase (Activase), heparin, milrinone (Primacor), potassium chloride, propofol (Diprivan)

SIDE EFFECTS

Frequent
Decreased sexual ability, drowsiness, difficulty sleeping, unusual tiredness or weakness
Occasional
Bradycardia, depression, cold hands or feet, diarrhea, constipation, anxiety, nasal congestion, nausea, vomiting
Rare
Altered taste; dry eyes; itching; numbness of fingers, toes, scalp

SERIOUS REACTIONS

• May produce profound bradycardia and hypotension.
• Abrupt withdrawal may result in sweating, palpitations, headache, and tremulousness.
• May precipitate CHF and MI in patients with cardiac disease; thyroid storm in patients with thyrotoxicosis; and peripheral ischemia in patients with existing peripheral vascular disease.
• Hypoglycemia may occur in patients with previously controlled diabetes.

NURSING CONSIDERATIONS

Baseline Assessment

• Assess the patient's baseline liver and renal function tests.
• Assess the patient's apical pulse and B/P immediately before giving propranolol. If the patient's pulse rate is 60/min or less or systolic B/P is less than 90 mm Hg, withhold the medication and contact the physician.
• Document the onset, type (sharp, dull, or squeezing), radiation, location, intensity, and duration of the patient's anginal pain and its precipitating factors, such as exertion and emotional stress.

Lifespan Considerations

• Be aware that propranolol crosses the placenta and is distributed in breast milk and that propranolol use should be avoided during the first trimester of pregnancy. Know that propranolol use can produce apnea, bradycardia, hypoglycemia, hypothermia during delivery, and low-birth-weight infants.
• There are no age-related precautions noted in children.
• In the elderly, age-related peripheral vascular disease may increase susceptibility to decreased peripheral circulation.

Precautions

• Use cautiously in patients who are also receiving calcium channel blockers, especially when giving propranolol IV.
• Use cautiously in patients with diabetes and liver or renal impairment.

Administration and Handling

PO
• Crush scored tablets if necessary.
• Give at same time each day.
IV
• Store at room temperature.
• Give undiluted for IV push.

• For IV infusion, may dilute each 1 mg in 10 ml D_5W.
• Do not exceed 1 mg/min injection rate.
• For IV infusion, give 1 mg over 10 to 15 minutes.

Intervention and Evaluation
• Assess the patient's pulse for bradycardia and an irregular rate.
• Monitor the patient's EKG for arrhythmias.
• Examine the patient's fingers for lack of color and numbness, which may indicate Raynaud's syndrome.
• Evaluate the patient for signs and symptoms of CHF, including distended neck veins, dyspnea (particularly on exertion or lying down), night cough, and peripheral edema.
• Monitor the patient's intake and output. Be aware that an increase in patient weight or a decrease in patient urine output may indicate CHF.
• Assess the patient for behavioral changes, fatigue, and rash.
• Know the therapeutic response ranges from a few days to several weeks.
• Measure the patient's B/P near the end of the dosing interval to determine if B/P is controlled throughout day.

Patient Teaching
• Caution the patient against discontinuing the drug.
• Stress to the patient that compliance with the therapy regimen is essential to control anginal pain, arrhythmias, and hypertension.
• Instruct the patient that if a dose is missed, he or she should take the next scheduled dose and should not double the dose.
• Teach the patient to rise slowly from lying to sitting position, wait momentarily before standing to avoid the drug's hypotensive effect.

• Explain to the patient that he or she should not take any nasal decongestants and over-the-counter (OTC) cold preparations, especially those containing stimulants, without physician approval.
• Urge the patient to limit alcohol and salt intake.
• Advise the patient to avoid tasks that require mental alertness or motor skills until his or her response to the drug is established.
• Warn the patient to report if he or she experiences dizziness, excessively slow pulse rate (less than 60 beats/min), or peripheral numbness.

sotalol hydrochloride
sew-tah-lol
(Betapace, Cardol[AUS], Sotacor[CAN], Solavert[AUS], Sotab[AUS], Sotahexal[AUS])
Do not confuse with Stadol.

CATEGORY AND SCHEDULE
Pregnancy Risk Category: B (D if used in second or third trimester)

MECHANISM OF ACTION
A beta-adrenergic blocking agent that prolongs action potential, effective refractory period, and QT interval. Decreases heart rate and atrioventricular (AV) nodal conduction; increases AV nodal refractoriness. *Therapeutic Effect:* Produces antiarrhythmic activity.

PHARMACOKINETICS
Well absorbed from the gastrointestinal (GI) tract. Protein binding: None. Widely distributed. Primarily excreted unchanged in urine. Removed by hemodialysis. **Half-life:**

12 hrs (half-life is increased in the elderly and patients with impaired renal function).

AVAILABILITY
Tablets: 80 mg, 120 mg, 160 mg, 240 mg.

INDICATIONS AND DOSAGES
▶ **To treat documented, life-threatening arrhythmias**
PO
Adults, Elderly. Initially, 80 mg 2 times/day. May increase gradually at 2-to 3-day intervals. Range: 240–320 mg/day.
▶ **Dosage in renal impairment**

Creatinine Clearance	Dosage Interval
30–60 ml/min	24 hrs
10–30 ml/min	36–48 hrs
less than 10 ml/min	Individualized

UNLABELED USES
Maintenance of normal heart rhythm in chronic or recurring atrial fibrillation or flutter; treatment of anxiety, chronic angina pectoris, hypertension, hypertrophic cardio-myopathy, mitral valve prolapse syndrome, myocardial infarction (MI), pheochromocytoma, thyrotoxi-cosis, tremors

CONTRAINDICATIONS
Bronchial asthma, cardiogenic shock, prolonged QT syndrome (unless functioning pacemaker is present), second- and third-degree heart block, sinus bradycardia, uncontrolled cardiac failure

INTERACTIONS
Drug
Antiarrhythmics, phenothiazine, tricyclic antidepressants: May increase prolonged QT interval.

Calcium channel blockers: May increase effect on AV conduction and blood pressure (B/P).
Clonidine: May potentiate rebound hypertension after clonidine is discontinued.
Digoxin: May increase risk of proarrhythmias.
Insulin, oral hypoglycemics: May mask signs of hypoglycemia and prolong the effects of insulin and oral hypoglycemics.
Sympathomimetics: May inhibit the effects of sympathomimetics.
Herbal
None known.
Food
None known.

DIAGNOSTIC TEST EFFECTS
May increase blood glucose, serum alkaline phosphatase, serum LDH, serum lipoprotein, SGOT (AST), SGPT (ALT), and serum triglyceride levels.

SIDE EFFECTS
Frequent
Decreased sexual function, drowsiness, insomnia, unusual tiredness or weakness
Occasional
Depression, cold hands or feet, diarrhea, constipation, anxiety, nasal congestion, nausea, vomiting
Rare
Altered taste, dry eyes, itching, numbness of fingers, toes, scalp

SERIOUS REACTIONS
• Bradycardia, congestive heart failure (CHF), hypotension, bronchospasm, hypoglycemia, prolonged QT interval, torsades de pointes, ventricular tachycardia, and premature ventricular complexes (PVCs) may occur.

NURSING CONSIDERATIONS

Baseline Assessment
• As ordered, institute continuous cardiac monitoring when beginning sotalol therapy. If the patient's pulse rate is 60 beats/min or less, consult with the physician before beginning sotalol therapy.

Lifespan Considerations
• Be aware that sotalol crosses the placenta and is excreted in breast milk.
• Be aware that the safety and efficacy of sotalol have not been established in children.
• In the elderly, age-related peripheral vascular disease may increase susceptibility to decreased peripheral circulation.

Precautions
• Use cautiously in patients with cardiomegaly, CHF, diabetes mellitus, excessive QT-interval prolongation, history of ventricular tachycardia, hypokalemia, hypomagnesemia, severe and prolonged diarrhea, sick sinus syndrome, and ventricular fibrillation.
• Use cautiously in patients at risk of developing thyrotoxicosis.

Administration and Handling
◀ALERT▶ Know that some patients may require 480–640 mg/day. Also be aware that the drug has a long half life and dosing more than 2 times a day is usually not necessary. Avoid abrupt withdrawal of sotalol.
PO
• Give sotalol without regard to food.

Intervention and Evaluation
• Diligently monitor the patient for arrhythmias.
• Assess the patient's B/P for hypotension and pulse for bradycardia.
• Evaluate the patient for signs and symptoms of CHF, including decreased urine output, distended neck veins, dyspnea, jugular vein distention, peripheral edema, rales in lungs, and weight gain.

Patient Teaching
• Caution the patient against abruptly discontinuing the drug without physician approval.
• Warn the patient to avoid tasks that require mental alertness or motor skills because sotalol may cause drowsiness.
• Explain to the patient that periodic lab tests and EKGs are a necessary part of therapy.

timolol maleate
tim-oh-lol
(Apo-Timol[CAN], Apo-Timop[CAN], Betimol, Blocadren, Gen-Timolol[CAN], Novo-Timol [CAN], Optimol[AUS], Tenopt[AUS], Timoptic, Timoptic XE, Timoptol[AUS])
Do not confuse with atenolol or Viroptic.

CATEGORY AND SCHEDULE
Pregnancy Risk Category: C (D if used in second or third trimester)

MECHANISM OF ACTION
An antihypertensive, antimigraine, and antiglaucoma agent that blocks beta$_1$- and beta$_2$-adrenergic receptors. *Therapeutic Effect:* Reduces intraocular pressure by reducing aqueous humor production, reduces blood pressure (B/P), and produces negative chronotropic and inotropic activity.

PHARMACOKINETICS

Route	Onset	Peak	Duration
Eyedrops	30 min	1–2 hrs	12–24 hrs

Well absorbed from the gastrointestinal (GI) tract. Protein binding: less than 10%. Minimal absorption after ophthalmic administration. Metabolized in liver. Primarily excreted in urine. Not removed by hemodialysis. **Half-life:** 4 hrs. Ophthalmic: Systemic absorption may occur.

AVAILABILITY
Tablets: 5 mg, 10 mg, 20 mg.
Ophthalmic Solution: 0.25%, 0.5%.
Ophthalmic Gel: 0.25%, 0.5%.

INDICATIONS AND DOSAGES
▸ **Mild to moderate hypertension**
PO
Adults, Elderly. Initially, 10 mg 2 times/day, alone or in combination with other therapy. Gradually increase at intervals of not less than 1 wk. Maintenance: 20–60 mg/day in 2 divided doses.
▸ **Reduce cardiovascular mortality in definite or suspected acute myocardial infarction (MI)**
PO
Adults, Elderly. 10 mg 2 times/day, beginning within 1–4 wks after infarction.
▸ **Migraine prophylaxis**
PO
Adults, Elderly. Initially, 10 mg 2 times/day. Range: 10–30 mg/day.
▸ **Reduce intraocular pressure (IOP) in open-angle glaucoma, aphakic glaucoma, ocular hypertension, and secondary glaucoma**
Ophthalmic
Adults, Elderly, Children. 1 drop of 0.25% solution in affected eye(s) 2 times/day. May be increased to 1 drop of 0.5% solution in affected eye(s) 2 times/day. When intraocular pressure (IOP) is controlled, dosage may be reduced to 1 drop 1 time/day. If patient is switched to timolol from another antiglaucoma agent, administer concurrently for

1 day. Discontinue other agent on following day.
▸ **Ophthalmic (Timoptic XE)**
Adults, Elderly. 1 drop/day.

UNLABELED USES
Systemic: Treatment of anxiety, cardiac arrhythmias, chronic angina pectoris, hypertrophic cardiomyopathy, migraines, pheochromocytoma, thyrotoxicosis, tremors
Ophthalmic: With miotics decreases IOP in acute or chronic angle-closure glaucoma, treatment of angle-closure glaucoma during and after iridectomy, malignant glaucoma, secondary glaucoma

CONTRAINDICATIONS
Bronchial asthma, cardiogenic shock, chronic obstructive pulmonary disease (COPD), congestive heart failure (CHF) unless secondary to tachyarrhythmias, patients receiving MAOI therapy, second- or third-degree heart block, sinus bradycardia, uncontrolled cardiac failure

INTERACTIONS
Drug
Diuretics, other hypotensives: May increase hypotensive effect.
Insulin, oral hypoglycemics: May mask symptoms of hypoglycemia and prolong hypoglycemic effects of these drugs.
NSAIDs: May decrease antihypertensive effect.
Sympathomimetics, xanthines: May mutually inhibit effects.
Herbal
None known.
Food
None known.

DIAGNOSTIC TEST EFFECTS
May increase ANA titer, BUN, serum LDH, serum lipoprotein,

serum alkaline phosphatase, serum bilirubin, serum creatinine, serum potassium, serum uric acid, SGOT (AST), SGPT (ALT), and serum triglyceride levels.

SIDE EFFECTS

Frequent
Decreased sexual function, drowsiness, difficulty sleeping, unusual tiredness or weakness
Ophthalmic: Eye irritation, visual disturbances
Occasional
Depression, cold hands or feet, diarrhea, constipation, anxiety, nasal congestion, nausea, vomiting
Rare
Altered taste, dry eyes, itching, numbness of fingers, toes, scalp

SERIOUS REACTIONS

• Oral form may produce profound bradycardia, hypotension, and bronchospasm.
• Abrupt withdrawal may result in diaphoresis, palpitations, headache, and tremulousness.
• May precipitate CHF and MI in patients with cardiac disease; thyroid storm in patients with thyrotoxicosis; and peripheral ischemia in patients with existing peripheral vascular disease.
• Hypoglycemia may occur in patients with previously controlled diabetes.
• Ophthalmic overdosage may produce bradycardia, hypotension, bronchospasm, and acute cardiac failure.

NURSING CONSIDERATIONS

Baseline Assessment
• Assess the patient's apical pulse and B/P immediately before giving timolol. If the patient's pulse is 60/min or less or systolic B/P is

less than 90 mm Hg, withhold the medication and contact the physician.

Lifespan Considerations
• Be aware that timolol is distributed in breast milk and is not for use in breast-feeding women because of the potential for serious adverse effects on the breast-fed infant. Know that timolol use should be avoided during the first trimester of pregnancy and that the drug may produce apnea, bradycardia, hypoglycemia, hypothermia during delivery, and low-birth-weight infants.
• Be aware that the safety and efficacy of timolol have not been established in children.
• In the elderly, age-related peripheral vascular disease increases susceptibility to decreased peripheral circulation.

Precautions
• Use cautiously in patients with hyperthyroidism, impaired liver or renal function, and inadequate cardiac function. Precautions also apply to oral and ophthalmic administration due to systemic absorption of ophthalmic timolol.

Administration and Handling
PO
• Give timolol without regard to meals.
• Tablets may be crushed.
Ophthalmic
◀ALERT▶ When using gel, invert container and shake once before each use.
• Place a gloved finger on the patient's lower eyelid and pull it out until pocket is formed between the eye and lower lid.
• Hold the dropper above the pocket and place the prescribed number of drops or amount of prescribed gel into pocket. Instruct the patient to

close eyes gently so that medication will not be squeezed out of the sac.
• Apply gentle digital pressure to the patient's lacrimal sac at the inner canthus for 1 minute after installation to lessen the risk of systemic absorption.

Intervention and Evaluation
• Assess the patient's pulse for quality and assess for bradycardia or an irregular rate.
• Monitor the patient's EKG for arrhythmias, particularly premature ventricular contractions (PVCs).
• Assess the patient's pattern of daily bowel activity and stool consistency.
• Monitor the patient's B/P, heart rate, IOP (ophthalmic preparation), and liver and renal function test results.

Patient Teaching
• Caution the patient against abruptly discontinuing timolol.
• Stress to the patient that compliance with the therapy regimen is essential to control angina, arrhythmias, glaucoma, and hypertension.

• Advise the patient to avoid tasks that require mental alertness or motor skills until his or her response to the drug is established.
• Warn the patient to notify the physician if he or she experiences excessive fatigue, prolonged dizziness or headache, or shortness of breath.
• Explain to the patient that he or she should not use nasal decongestants and over-the-counter (OTC) cold preparations, especially those containing stimulants, without physician approval.
• Urge the patient to limit alcohol and salt intake.
• Teach the patient receiving the ophthalmic form of timolol the correct way to instill drops and obtain his or her pulse.
• Advise the patient receiving the ophthalmic form of timolol that he or she may experience transient discomfort or stinging upon instillation.

26 Calcium Channel Blockers

amlodipine
diltiazem
  hydrochloride
felodipine
isradipine
nicardipine
  hydrochloride
nifedipine
nimodipine
verapamil
  hydrochloride

Uses: Calcium channel blockers are used to treat essential hypertension, to prevent and treat angina pectoris (including vasospastic, chronic stable, and unstable forms), to prevent and control supraventricular tachyarrhythmias, and to prevent neurologic damage caused by subarachnoid hemorrhage.

Action: Calcium channel blockers inhibit the flow of extracellular calcium ions across cell membranes in cardiac and vascular tissue. They relax arterial smooth muscle, depress the rate of firing in the sinus node (the heart's normal pacemaker), slow atrioventricular conduction, and decrease the heart rate. Although they also produce negative inotropic effects, these effects are rarely seen clinically because of the reflex response. Calcium channel blockers decrease coronary vascular resistance, increase coronary blood flow, and reduce myocardial oxygen demand. The degree of action varies with the specific drug.

COMBINATION PRODUCTS
LEXXEL: felodipine/enalapril (an ACE inhibitor) 2.5 mg/5 mg; 5 mg/5 mg.
LOTREL: amlodipine/benazepril (an ACE inhibitor) 2.5 mg/10 mg; 5 mg/10 mg; 5 mg/20 mg; 10 mg/20 mg.
TARKA: verapamil/trandolapril (an ACE inhibitor) 240 mg/1 mg; 180 mg/2 mg; 240 mg/2 mg; 240 mg/4 mg.
TECZEM: diltiazem/enalapril (an ACE inhibitor) 180 mg/5 mg.

amlodipine
am-**low**-dih-peen
(Norvasc)
Do not confuse with Navane or Vascor.

CATEGORY AND SCHEDULE
Pregnancy Risk Category: C

MECHANISM OF ACTION
A calcium channel blocker that inhibits calcium movement across cardiac and vascular smooth muscle cell membranes. *Therapeutic Effect:* Dilates coronary arteries, peripheral arteries, and arterioles. Decreases total peripheral vascular resistance by vasodilation.

PHARMACOKINETICS

Route	Onset	Peak	Duration
PO	0.5–1 hr	6–12 hrs	24 hrs

Slowly absorbed from the gastrointestinal (GI) tract. Protein binding: 93%. Undergoes first-pass metabolism in liver. Excreted primarily in urine. Not removed by hemodialysis. **Half-life:** 30–50 hrs (half-life increased in elderly and those with liver cirrhosis).

AVAILABILITY
Tablets: 2.5 mg, 5 mg, 10 mg.

INDICATIONS AND DOSAGES
▶ **Hypertension**
PO
Adults. Initially, 5 mg/day as a single dose. Maximum: 10 mg/day.
Small-Frame, Fragile, Elderly. Initially, 2.5 mg/day as a single dose.
▶ **Angina (chronic stable or vasospastic)**
PO
Adults. 5–10 mg/day as a single dose.
Elderly, Liver Insufficiency: 5 mg/day as a single dose.
▶ **Dosage in renal impairment**
PO
Adults, Elderly. 2.5 mg/day.

CONTRAINDICATIONS
Severe hypotension

INTERACTIONS
Drug
None known.
Herbal
None known.
Food
Grapefruit and grapefruit juice: May increase amlodipine blood concentration and hypotensive effects.

DIAGNOSTIC TEST EFFECTS
None known.

SIDE EFFECTS
Frequent (greater than 5%)
Peripheral edema, headache, flushing
Occasional (less than 5%)
Dizziness, palpitations, nausea, unusual tiredness or weakness (asthenia)
Rare (less than 1%)
Chest pain, bradycardia, orthostatic hypotension

SERIOUS REACTIONS
• Overdosage may produce excessive peripheral vasodilation and marked hypotension with reflex tachycardia.

NURSING CONSIDERATIONS
Baseline Assessment
• Assess the patient's baseline apical pulse, blood pressure (B/P), and renal and liver function blood chemistry test results.
Lifespan Considerations
• Be aware that it is unknown if amlodipine crosses the placenta or is distributed in breast milk.
• Be aware that the safety and efficacy of amlodipine have not been established in children.
• The elderly are more sensitive to amlodipine's hypotensive effects and the half-life may be increased.
Precautions
• Use cautiously in patients with aortic stenosis, congestive heart failure (CHF), and impaired liver function.
Administration and Handling
PO
◀**ALERT**▶ Expect to increase the drug dosage slowly over 7 to 14 days based on the patient's response.

• May give without regard to food.
• Avoid giving with grapefruit juice, which may increase amlodipine blood concentration.

Intervention and Evaluation

• Determine the patient's blood pressure (B/P). Withhold the medication and notify the physician if the patient's systolic B/P is less than 90 mm Hg.
• Assess the patient's skin for flushing and peripheral edema, especially behind the medial malleolus and the sacral area.
• Determine if the patient is experiencing asthenia or headache.

Patient Teaching

• Caution the patient against abruptly discontinuing the drug. Explain that compliance with therapy is essential to control hypertension.
• Warn the patient to avoid tasks that require alertness and motor skills until his or her response to the drug is established.
• Urge the patient to avoid drinking grapefruit juice while taking this drug.

---

diltiazem hydrochloride

dill-**tie**-ah-zem
(Apo-Diltiaz[CAN], Auscard[AUS], Cardcal[AUS], Cardizem, Cardizem CD, Cartia, Cardizem LA, Coras [AUS], Dilacor XR, Diltahexal[AUS], Diltiamax[AUS], Dilzem[AUS], Novo-Diltiazem[CAN], Tiazac)
Do not confuse with Cardene or Ziac.

CATEGORY AND SCHEDULE

Pregnancy Risk Category: C

MECHANISM OF ACTION

An antianginal, antihypertensive, and antiarrhythmic agent that inhibits calcium movement across cardiac and vascular smooth muscle cell membranes. This action causes the dilation of coronary arteries, peripheral arteries and arterioles. *Therapeutic Effect:* Decreases heart rate, myocardial contractility, slows sinoatrial (SA) and atrioventricular (AV) conduction. Decreases total peripheral vascular resistance by vasodilation.

PHARMACOKINETICS

Route	Onset	Peak	Duration
PO	0.5–1 hr	N/A	N/A
Extended-release	2–3 hrs	N/A	N/A
IV	3 min	N/A	N/A

Well absorbed from the gastrointestinal (GI) tract. Protein binding: 70%–80%. Undergoes first-pass metabolism in liver. Metabolized in liver to active metabolite. Primarily excreted in urine. Not removed by hemodialysis. **Half-life:** 3–8 hrs.

AVAILABILITY

Tablets: 30 mg, 60 mg, 90 mg, 120 mg.
Capsules (sustained-release): 60 mg, 90 mg, 120 mg, 180 mg, 240 mg, 300 mg, 360 mg, 420 mg.
Injection (Ready-to-Hang Infusion): 1 mg/ml.

INDICATIONS AND DOSAGES

▸ **Angina related to coronary artery spasm (Prinzmetal's variant), chronic stable angina (effort-associated)**
PO
Adults, Elderly. Initially, 30 mg 4 times/day. Increase up to 180–360

mg/day in 3–4 divided doses at
1- to 2-day intervals.
Adults, Elderly (Cardizem CD).
Initially, 120–180 mg/day; titrate
over 7–14 days. Range: Up to 480
mg/day.

▸ **Essential hypertension**
PO
Adults, Elderly (extended-release).
Initially, 60–120 mg 2 times/day.
Adults, Elderly (Cardizem CD).
Initially, 180–240 mg/day. Range:
240–360 mg in 2 divided doses.
Adults, Elderly (Dilacor XR). Ini-
tially, 180–240 mg/day. Range:
180–480 mg/day.

▸ **Temporary control of rapid ventricular rate in atrial fibrillation or
flutter, rapid conversion of PSVT to
normal sinus rhythm.**
IV push
Adults, Elderly. Initially, 0.25
mg/kg actual body weight over 2
min. May repeat in 15 min at dose
of 0.35 mg/kg actual body weight.
Subsequent doses individualized.
IV infusion
Adults, Elderly. After initial bolus
injection, 5–10 mg/hr, may increase
at 5 mg/hr up to 15 mg/hr. Maintain over 24 hrs.

CONTRAINDICATIONS
Acute myocardial infarction (MI),
pulmonary congestion, severe hypotension (less than 90 mm Hg, systolic), sick sinus syndrome and
second- or third-degree AV block
(except in the presence of a pacemaker)

INTERACTIONS
Drug
Beta-blockers: May have additive
effect.
*Carbamazepine, quinidine,
theophylline:* May increase diltiazem blood concentration and risk of
toxicity.

Digoxin: May increase serum digoxin concentration.
Procainamide, quinidine: May
increase risk of QT-interval prolongation.
Herbal
None known.
Food
None known.

DIAGNOSTIC TEST EFFECTS
PR interval may be increased.

IV INCOMPATIBILITIES
Acetazolamide (Diamox), acyclovir
(Zovirax), aminophylline, ampicillin, ampicillin/sulbactam (Unasyn),
cefoperazone (Cefobid), diazepam
(Valium), furosemide (Lasix), heparin, insulin, nafcillin, phenytoin
(Dilantin), rifampin (Rifadin),
sodium bicarbonate

IV COMPATIBILITIES
Albumin, aztreonam (Azactam),
bumetanide (Bumex), cefazolin
(Ancef), cefotaxime (Claforan),
ceftazidime (Fortaz), ceftriaxone
(Rocephin), cefuroxime (Zinacef),
cimetidine (Tagamet), ciprofloxacin
(Cipro), clindamycin (Cleocin),
digoxin (Lanoxin), dobutamine
(Dobutrex), dopamine (Intropin),
gentamicin (Garamycin), hydromorphone (Dilaudid), lidocaine, lorazepam (Ativan), metoclopramide
(Reglan), metronidazole (Flagyl),
midazolam (Versed), morphine,
multivitamins, nitroglycerin, norepinephrine (Levophed), potassium
chloride, potassium phosphate,
tobramycin (Nebcin), vancomycin
(Vancocin)

SIDE EFFECTS
Frequent (10%–5%)
Peripheral edema, dizziness, lightheadedness, headache, bradycardia,
asthenia (loss of strength, weakness)

Occasional (5%–2%)
Nausea, constipation, flushing, altered EKG
Rare (less than 2%)
Rash, micturition disorder (polyuria, nocturia, dysuria, frequency of urination), abdominal discomfort, somnolence

SERIOUS REACTIONS
• Abrupt withdrawal may increase frequency or duration of angina.
• Congestive heart failure (CHF) and second- and third-degree AV block occur rarely.
• Overdosage produces nausea, drowsiness, confusion, slurred speech, and profound bradycardia.

NURSING CONSIDERATIONS
Baseline Assessment
• Concurrent sublingual nitroglycerin therapy may be used for relief of anginal pain.
• Document the onset, type (sharp, dull, or squeezing), radiation, location, intensity, and duration of anginal pain and its precipitating factors, such as exertion or emotional stress.
• Assess the patient's baseline liver and renal function blood chemistry test results.
• Assess the patient's apical pulse and blood pressure (B/P) immediately before diltiazem is administered.
Lifespan Considerations
• Be aware that diltiazem is distributed in breast milk.
• There are no age-related precautions noted in children.
• In the elderly, age-related renal impairment may require caution.
Precautions
• Use cautiously in patients with CHF and impaired liver or renal function.

Administration and Handling
PO
• Give diltiazem before meals and at bedtime.
• Crush tablets as needed.
• Do not crush or open sustained-release capsules.
IV
◄ALERT► Refer to manufacturer's information for dose concentration and infusion rates.
• Refrigerate vials.
• After dilution, solution is stable for 24 hours.
• Add 125 mg to 100 ml D_5W, 0.9% NaCl to provide a concentration of 1 mg/ml. Add 250 mg to 250 or 500 ml diluent to provide a concentration of 0.83 mg/ml or 0.45 mg/ml, respectively. The maximum concentration is 1.25 g/250 ml or 5 mg/ml.
• Infuse per dilution or rate chart provided by manufacturer.
Intervention and Evaluation
• Assist the patient with ambulation if he or she experiences dizziness.
• Assess the patient for peripheral edema behind the medial malleolus or in the sacral area in bedridden patients.
• Monitor the patient's pulse rate for bradycardia.
• For patients receiving IV diltiazem, assess B/P, EKG, and liver and renal function test results.
• Assess the patient for signs or symptoms of asthenia or headache.
Patient Teaching
• Caution the patient against abruptly discontinuing the medication.
• Stress to the patient that compliance with the treatment regimen is essential to control anginal pain.
• Instruct the patient to rise slowly from a lying to a sitting position and wait momentarily before stand-

ing to avoid diltiazem's hypotensive effect.

• Warn the patient to avoid tasks that require mental alertness or motor skills until his or her response to the drug is established.

• Warn the patient to notify the physician if he or she experiences constipation, irregular heartbeat, nausea, pronounced dizziness, or shortness of breath.

felodipine

feh-**low**-dih-peen
(AGON SR[AUS], Felodur[AUS], Plendil, Renedil[CAN])
Do not confuse with pindolol, Pletal, or Prinivil.

CATEGORY AND SCHEDULE
Pregnancy Risk Category: C

MECHANISM OF ACTION
An antihypertensive and antianginal agent that inhibits calcium movement across cardiac and vascular smooth muscle cell membranes. Potent peripheral vasodilator (does not depress sinoatrial [SA] or atrioventricular [AV] nodes). *Therapeutic Effect:* Increases myocardial contractility, heart rate, and cardiac output; decreases peripheral vascular resistance and blood pressure (B/P).

PHARMACOKINETICS

Route	Onset	Peak	Duration
PO	2–5 hrs	N/A	N/A

Rapidly, completely absorbed from the gastrointestinal (GI) tract. Protein binding: Greater than 99%. Undergoes first-pass metabolism in liver. Metabolized in liver. Primarily excreted in urine. Not removed by hemodialysis. **Half-life:** 11–16 hrs.

AVAILABILITY
Tablets (extended-release): 2.5 mg, 5 mg, 10 mg.

INDICATIONS AND DOSAGES
▶ **Hypertension**
PO
Adults. Initially, 5 mg/day as single dose.
Elderly, patients with impaired liver function. Initially, 2.5 mg/day. Adjust dosage at no less than 2-wk intervals. Maintenance: 2.5–10 mg/day.

UNLABELED USES
Treatment of chronic angina pectoris, congestive heart failure (CHF), Raynaud's phenomena

CONTRAINDICATIONS
None known

INTERACTIONS
Drug
Beta-blockers: May have additive effect.
Digoxin: May increase digoxin blood concentration.
Erythromycin: May increase felodipine blood concentration and risk of toxicity.
Hypokalemia-producing agents: May increase risk of arrhythmias.
Procainamide, quinidine: May increase risk of QT-interval prolongation.
Herbal
DHEA: May increase felodipine blood concentrations.
Food
Grapefruit and grapefruit juice: May increase the absorption and blood concentrations of felodipine.

DIAGNOSTIC TEST EFFECTS
None known.

SIDE EFFECTS
Frequent (22%–18%)
Headache, peripheral edema
Occasional (6%–4%)
Flushing, respiratory infection,
dizziness, lightheadedness, asthenia
(loss of strength, weakness)
Rare (less than 3%)
Paresthesia, abdominal discomfort,
nervousness, muscle cramping,
cough, diarrhea, constipation

SERIOUS REACTIONS
• Overdosage produces nausea,
drowsiness, confusion, slurred
speech, hypotension, and bradycardia.

NURSING CONSIDERATIONS

Baseline Assessment
• Assess the patient's apical pulse
and B/P immediately before beginning felodipine administration. If
the patient's pulse rate is 60/min or
less or systolic B/P is less than 90
mm Hg, withhold the medication
and contact the physician.

Lifespan Considerations
• Be aware that it is unknown if
felodipine crosses the placenta or is
distributed in breast milk.
• Be aware that the safety and
efficacy of this drug have not been
established in children.
• The elderly may experience a
greater hypotensive response.
• Constipation may be more problematic in the elderly.

Precautions
• Use cautiously in patients with
CHF, concomitant administration
with beta-blockers or digoxin,
edema, hypertrophic cardiomyopathy, liver or renal impairment, and
severe left ventricular dysfunction.

Administration and Handling
PO
• Give felodipine without regard to
food.
• Do not crush or break tablets.

Intervention and Evaluation
• Assist the patient with ambulation
if he or she experiences dizziness or
lightheadedness.
• Assess for peripheral edema
behind media malleolus in ambulatory patients or the sacral area in
bedridden patients.
• Monitor the patient's hepatic
blood chemistry test results and
pulse rate for bradycardia.
• Examine the patient's skin for
flushing.
• Evaluate the patient for asthenia
and headache.

Patient Teaching
• Caution the patient against
abruptly discontinuing the drug.
• Stress to the patient that compliance with the therapy regimen is
essential to control hypertension.
• Instruct the patient to rise slowly
from a lying to a sitting position
and wait momentarily before standing to avoid felodipine's hypotensive effect.
• Advise the patient to avoid tasks
that require mental alertness or
motor skills until his or her response to the drug is established.
• Warn the patient to notify the
physician if he or she experiences
an irregular heartbeat, nausea,
prolonged dizziness, or shortness of
breath.
• Teach the patient to swallow
felodipine tablets whole. Explain to
the patient the he or she should not
crush or chew felodipine tablets.
• Urge the patient to avoid grapefruit and grapefruit juice because
these foods increase the blood
concentration and effects of felodipine.

isradipine
iss-**rah**-dih-peen
(DynaCirc, DynaCirc CR)
Do not confuse with Dynabac or Dynacin.

CATEGORY AND SCHEDULE
Pregnancy Risk Category: C

MECHANISM OF ACTION
An antihypertensive that inhibits calcium movement across cardiac and vascular smooth muscle cell membranes. Potent peripheral vasodilator that does not depress sinoatrial [SA] or atrioventricular [AV] nodes. *Therapeutic Effect:* Produces relaxation of coronary vascular smooth muscle and coronary vasodilation. Increases myocardial oxygen delivery to those with vasospastic angina.

PHARMACOKINETICS

Route	Onset	Peak	Duration
PO	2–3 hrs	2–4 wks	N/A

Well absorbed from the gastrointestinal (GI) tract. Protein binding: 95%. Metabolized in liver (undergoes first-pass effect). Primarily excreted in urine. Not removed by hemodialysis. **Half-life:** 8 hrs.

AVAILABILITY
Capsules: 2.5 mg, 5 mg.
Capsules (extended-release): 5 mg, 10 mg.

INDICATIONS AND DOSAGES
▶ **Hypertension**
PO
Adults, Elderly. Initially 2.5 mg 2 times/day. May increase by 2.5 mg at 2- to 4-wk intervals. Range: 5–20 mg/day

UNLABELED USES
Treatment of chronic angina pectoris, Raynaud's phenomenon

CONTRAINDICATIONS
Cardiogenic shock, congestive heart failure (CHF), heart block, hypotension, sinus bradycardia, ventricular tachycardia

INTERACTIONS
Drug
Beta-blockers: May have additive effect.
Herbal
None known.
Food
Grapefruit and grapefruit juice: May increase the absorption of isradipine.

DIAGNOSTIC TEST EFFECTS
None known.

SIDE EFFECTS
Frequent (7%–4%)
Peripheral edema, palpitations (higher frequency in females)
Occasional (3%)
Facial flushing, cough
Rare (2%–1%)
Angina, tachycardia, rash, pruritus

SERIOUS REACTIONS
• CHF occurs rarely.
• Overdosage produces nausea, drowsiness, confusion, and slurred speech.

NURSING CONSIDERATIONS
Baseline Assessment
• Assess the patient's baseline liver and renal function blood chemistry test results.
• Assess the patient's apical pulse and B/P immediately before giving isradipine. If the patient's pulse rate

is 60/min or less or systolic B/P is less than 90 mm Hg, withhold the medication and contact the physician.

Lifespan Considerations
• Be aware that it is unknown if isradipine crosses the placenta or is distributed in breast milk.
• Be aware that the safety and efficacy of isradipine have not been established in children.
• In the elderly, age-related renal impairment may require cautious use.

Precautions
• Use cautiously in patients with edema, liver disease, severe left ventricular dysfunction, and sick sinus syndrome.
• Use cautiously in patients on concurrent therapy with beta-blockers or digoxin.

Administration and Handling
PO
• Do not crush, open, or break capsule.

Intervention and Evaluation
• Assess for peripheral edema behind medial malleolus in ambulatory patients or in the sacral area in bedridden patients.
• Monitor the patient's pulse rate for bradycardia.
• Monitor the patient's B/P.
• Observe the patient for signs and symptoms of CHF.
• Examine the patient's skin for flushing.

Patient Teaching
• Caution the patient against abruptly discontinuing the drug.
• Stress to the patient that compliance with the treatment regimen is essential to control hypertension.
• Instruct the patient to rise slowly from a lying to sitting position and wait momentarily before standing to avoid isradipine's hypotensive effect.

• Warn the patient to notify the physician if he or she experiences an irregular heartbeat, nausea, pronounced dizziness, or shortness of breath.
• Urge the patient to avoid grapefruit and grapefruit juice because these foods may increase the absorption of isradipine.

nicardipine hydrochloride
nigh-**car**-dih-peen
(Cardene, Cardene IV, Cardene SR)
Do not confuse with Cardizem SR, codeine, or nifedipine.

CATEGORY AND SCHEDULE
Pregnancy Risk Category: C

MECHANISM OF ACTION
An antianginal and antihypertensive agent that inhibits calcium ion movement across cell membrane, depressing contraction of cardiac and vascular smooth muscle. *Therapeutic Effect:* Increases heart rate and cardiac output. Decreases systemic vascular resistance and blood pressure (B/P).

PHARMACOKINETICS

Route	Onset	Peak	Duration
PO	N/A	1–2 hrs	8 hrs

Rapidly, completely absorbed from the gastrointestinal (GI) tract. Protein binding: greater than 95%. Undergoes first-pass metabolism in liver. Primarily excreted in urine. Not removed by hemodialysis.
Half-life: 2–4 hrs.

AVAILABILITY
Capsules: 20 mg, 30 mg.
Capsules (sustained-release):
30 mg, 45 mg, 60 mg.
Injection: 2.5 mg/ml.

INDICATIONS AND DOSAGES
▸ **Chronic stable (effort-associated) angina**
PO
Adults, Elderly. Initially, 20 mg 3 times/day. Range: 20–40 mg 3 times/day.
▸ **Essential hypertension**
PO
Adults, Elderly. Initially, 20 mg 3 times/day. Range: 20–40 mg 3 times/day.
PO (sustained-release)
Adults, Elderly. Initially, 30 mg 2 times/day. Range: 30–60 mg 2 times/day.
▸ **Short-term treatment of hypertension when oral therapy not feasible or desirable (substitute for oral nicardipine)**
IV
Adults, Elderly. 0.5 mg/hr (20 mg q8h), 1.2 mg/hr (30 mg q8h), 2.2 mg/hr (40 mg q8h).
▸ **Drug-free patient**
IV
Adults, Elderly (gradual B/P decrease). Initially, 5 mg/hr. May increase by 2.5 mg/hr q15min. After B/P goal is achieved, decrease rate to 3 mg/hr.
Adults, Elderly (rapid B/P decrease). Initially, 5 mg/hr. May increase by 2.5 mg/hr q5min. Maximum: 15 mg/hr until desired B/P attained. After B/P goal achieved, decrease rate to 3 mg/hr.
▸ **Changing to oral antihypertensive therapy**
Adults, Elderly. Begin 1 hr after IV discontinued; for nicardipine, give first dose 1 hr before discontinuing IV.

▸ **Dosage in liver impairment**
Adults, Elderly. Initially, 20 mg 2 times/day, then titrate.
▸ **Dosage in renal impairment**
Adults, Elderly. Initially, 20 mg q8h (30 mg 2 times/day sustained-release), then titrate.

UNLABELED USES
Treatment of associated neurologic deficits, Raynaud's phenomena, subarachnoid hemorrhage, vasospastic angina

CONTRAINDICATIONS
Atrial fibrillation or flutter associated with accessory conduction pathways, cardiogenic shock, congestive heart failure (CHF), second- or third-degree heart block, severe hypotension, sinus bradycardia, ventricular tachycardia, within several hours of IV beta-blocker therapy

INTERACTIONS
Drug
Beta-blockers: May have additive effect.
Digoxin: May increase blood concentration of this drug.
Hypokalemia-producing agents: May increase risk of arrhythmias.
Procainamide, quinidine: May increase risk of QT-interval prolongation.
Herbal
None known.
Food
Grapefruit and grapefruit juice: May alter absorption of nicardipine.

DIAGNOSTIC TEST EFFECTS
None known.

IV INCOMPATIBILITIES
Furosemide (Lasix), heparin, thiopental (Pentothal)

IV COMPATIBILITIES

Diltiazem (Cardizem), dobutamine (Dobutrex), dopamine (Intropin), epinephrine, hydromorphone (Dilaudid), labetalol (Trandate), lorazepam (Ativan), midazolam (Versed), milrinone (Primacor), morphine, nitroglycerin, norepinephrine (Levophed)

SIDE EFFECTS

Frequent (10%–7%)
Headache, facial flushing, peripheral edema, lightheadedness, dizziness
Occasional (6%–3%)
Asthenia (loss of strength, energy), palpitations, angina, tachycardia
Rare (less than 2%)
Nausea, abdominal cramps, dyspepsia, dry mouth, rash

SERIOUS REACTIONS

• Overdosage is manifested as confusion, slurred speech, drowsiness, marked hypotension, and bradycardia.

NURSING CONSIDERATIONS

Baseline Assessment
• Know that concurrent therapy of sublingual nitroglycerin may be used for relief of anginal pain.
• Record the onset, type (sharp, dull, or squeezing), radiation, location, intensity, and duration of anginal pain and its precipitating factors, such as exertion or emotional stress.

Lifespan Considerations
• Be aware that it is unknown if nicardipine is distributed in breast milk.
• Be aware that the safety and efficacy of nicardipine have not been established in children.
• In the elderly, age-related renal impairment may require cautious use.

Precautions
• Use cautiously in patients with cardiomyopathy, concomitant beta-blocker or digoxin therapy, edema, liver or renal impairment, severe left ventricular dysfunction, and sick sinus syndrome.

Administration and Handling
PO
• Do not crush, open, or break oral, sustained-release capsules.
• Give nicardipine without regard to food.
IV
• Store at room temperature.
• Store diluted IV solution for up to 24 hours at room temperature.
• Dilute each 25-mg ampoule with 250 ml D_5W, 0.9% NaCl, 0.45% NaCl, or any combination thereof to provide a concentration of 1 mg/10 ml.
• Give by slow IV infusion.
• Change IV site every 12 hours if administered by a peripheral rather than a central venous catheter line.

Intervention and Evaluation
• Monitor the patient's B/P during and following the IV infusion.
• Assess for peripheral edema behind the medial malleolus in ambulatory patients and in the sacral area in bedridden patients.
• Examine the patient's skin for dermatitis, facial flushing, and rash.
• Evaluate the patient for asthenia and headache.
• Monitor the patient's hepatic blood chemistry test results.
• Assess the patient for palpitations and the EKG and pulse for tachycardia.

Patient Teaching
• Instruct the patient to take nicardipine's sustained-release form with food and not to crush or open the capsules.
• Urge the patient to avoid alcohol and limit caffeine while taking nicardipine.

• Warn the patient to notify the physician if he or she experiences angina pain not relieved by the medication, constipation, dizziness, hypotension, irregular heartbeat, nausea, shortness of breath, or swelling.

nifedipine
nye-**fed**-ih-peen
(Adalat CC, Adalat FT, Adalat, PA, Adalat Oros[AUS], Apo-Nifed[CAN], Nifedicol XL, Nifehexal[AUS], Novonifedin[CAN], Nyefax[AUS], Procardia)
Do not confuse with nicardipine.

CATEGORY AND SCHEDULE
Pregnancy Risk Category: C

MECHANISM OF ACTION
An antianginal and antihypertensive agent that inhibits calcium ion movement across cell membrane, depressing contraction of cardiac and vascular smooth muscle. *Therapeutic Effect:* Increases heart rate and cardiac output. Decreases systemic vascular resistance and blood pressure (B/P).

PHARMACOKINETICS

Route	Onset	Peak	Duration
Sublingual	1–5 min	N/A	N/A
PO	20–30 min	N/A	4–8 hrs
PO (extended release)	2 hrs	N/A	24 hrs

Rapidly, completely absorbed from the gastrointestinal (GI) tract. Protein binding: 92%–98%. Undergoes first-pass metabolism in liver. Primarily excreted in urine. Not removed by hemodialysis. **Half-life:** 2–5 hrs.

AVAILABILITY
Capsules: 10 mg, 20 mg.
Tablets (extended-release): 30 mg, 60 mg, 90 mg.

INDICATIONS AND DOSAGES
▸ **Prinzmetal's variant angina, chronic stable (effort-associated) angina**
PO
Adults, Elderly. Initially, 10 mg 3 times/day. Increase at 7- to 14-day intervals. Maintenance: 10 mg 3 times/day up to 30 mg 4 times/day.
PO (extended-release)
Adults, Elderly. Initially, 30–60 mg/day. Maintenance: Up to 120 mg/day.
▸ **Essential hypertension**
PO (extended-release)
Adults, Elderly. Initially, 30–60 mg/day. Maintenance: Up to 120 mg/day.

UNLABELED USES
Treatment of Raynaud's phenomena

CONTRAINDICATIONS
Advanced aortic stenosis, severe hypotension

INTERACTIONS
Drug
Beta-blockers: May have additive effect.
Digoxin: May increase digoxin blood concentration.
Hypokalemia-producing agents: May increase risk of arrhythmias.
Herbal
None known.
Food
Grapefruit and grapefruit juice: May increase nifedipine plasma concentration.

DIAGNOSTIC TEST EFFECTS
May cause positive ANA, direct Coombs' test.

SIDE EFFECTS
Frequent (30%–11%)
Peripheral edema, headache, flushed skin, dizziness
Occasional (12%–6%)
Nausea, shakiness, muscle cramps and pain, drowsiness, palpitations, nasal congestion, cough, dyspnea, wheezing
Rare (5%–3%)
Hypotension, rash, pruritus, urticaria, constipation, abdominal discomfort, flatulence, sexual difficulties

SERIOUS REACTIONS
• May precipitate congestive heart failure (CHF) and myocardial infarction (MI) in patients with cardiac disease and peripheral ischemia.
• Overdose produces nausea, drowsiness, confusion, and slurred speech.

NURSING CONSIDERATIONS

Baseline Assessment
• Know that concurrent therapy of sublingual nitroglycerin may be used for relief of anginal pain.
• Record the onset, type (sharp, dull, or squeezing), radiation, location, intensity, and duration of anginal pain and its precipitating factors, such as exertion or emotional stress,
• Check the patient's B/P for hypotension immediately before giving nifedipine.

Lifespan Considerations
• Be aware that an insignificant amount of nifedipine is distributed in breast milk.
• Be aware that the safety and efficacy of nifedipine have not been established in children.
• In the elderly, age-related renal impairment may require cautious use.

Precautions
• Use cautiously in patients with impaired liver or renal function.

Administration and Handling
◀ ALERT ▶ May give 10–20 mg sublingual as needed for acute attack of angina.

PO
• Do not crush or break film-coated tablet or sustained-release capsule.
• Give nifedipine without regard to meals.
• Grapefruit juice may alter absorption.

Sublingual
• Capsule must be punctured, chewed, and squeezed to express liquid into mouth.

Intervention and Evaluation
• Assist the patient with ambulation if he or she experiences dizziness or lightheadedness.
• Assess for peripheral edema behind the medial malleolus in ambulatory patients and in the sacral area in bedridden patients.
• Examine the patient's skin for flushing.
• Monitor the patient's hepatic blood chemistry test results.

Patient Teaching
• Instruct the patient to rise slowly from lying to sitting position and to permit legs to dangle from bed momentarily before standing to reduce nifedipine's hypotensive effect.
• Warn the patient to notify the physician if he or she experiences irregular heartbeat, prolonged dizziness, nausea, or shortness of breath.
• Urge the patient to avoid alcohol, grapefruit, and grapefruit juice.

nimodipine
nih-**moad**-ih-peen
(Nimotop)

CATEGORY AND SCHEDULE
Pregnancy Risk Category: C

MECHANISM OF ACTION
A cerebral vasospasm agent that inhibits movement of calcium ions across vascular smooth muscle cell membranes. *Therapeutic Effect:* Produces favorable effect on severity of neurologic deficits due to cerebral vasospasm. Greatest effect on cerebral arteries; may prevent cerebral spasm.

PHARMACOKINETICS
Rapidly absorbed from the gastrointestinal (GI) tract. Protein binding: greater than 95%. Metabolized in liver. Excreted in urine, eliminated in feces. Not removed by hemodialysis. **Half-life:** (terminal): 3 hrs.

AVAILABILITY
Capsules: 30 mg.

INDICATIONS AND DOSAGES
▸ **Improve neurologic deficits after subarachnoid hemorrhage from ruptured congenital aneurysms**
PO
Adults, Elderly. 60 mg q4h for 21 days. Begin within 96 hrs of subarachnoid hemorrhage.

UNLABELED USES
Treatment of chronic and classic migraine, chronic cluster headaches

CONTRAINDICATIONS
Atrial fibrillation or flutter, cardiogenic shock, congestive heart failure (CHF), heart block, sinus bradycardia, ventricular tachycardia, within several hours of IV beta-blocker therapy

INTERACTIONS
Drug
Beta-blockers: May prolong sinoatrial (SA) and atrioventricular (AV) conduction, which may lead to severe hypotension, bradycardia and cardiac failure.
Erythromycin, itraconazole, ketoconazole, protease inhibitors: May inhibit the metabolism of nimodipine.
Rifabutin, rifampin: May increase the metabolism of nimodipine.
Herbal
Garlic: May increase antihypertensive effect.
Ginseng, yohimbe: May worsen hypertension.
Food
Grapefruit juice: May increase nimodipine blood concentration and risk of toxicity.

DIAGNOSTIC TEST EFFECTS
None known.

SIDE EFFECTS
Occasional (6%–2%)
Hypotension, peripheral edema, diarrhea, headache
Rare (less than 2%)
Allergic reaction (rash, hives), tachycardia, flushing of skin

SERIOUS REACTIONS
• Overdosage produces nausea, weakness, dizziness, drowsiness, confusion, and slurred speech.

NURSING CONSIDERATIONS
Baseline Assessment
• Assess the patient's level of consciousness (LOC) and neurologic response, initially and throughout nimodipine therapy.

• Monitor the patient's baseline hepatic blood chemistry test results.
• Assess the patient's apical pulse and blood pressure (B/P) immediately before giving nimodipine. If the patient's pulse rate is 60/min or less or systolic B/P is less than 90 mm Hg, withhold the medication and contact physician.

Lifespan Considerations
• Be aware that it is unknown if nimodipine crosses the placenta or is distributed in breast milk.
• Be aware that the safety and efficacy of nimodipine have not been established in children.
• In the elderly, age-related renal impairment may require cautious use.
• The elderly may experience greater hypotensive response and constipation.

Precautions
• Use cautiously in patients with impaired liver or renal function.

Administration and Handling
PO
• If the patient is unable to swallow, place a hole in both ends of capsule with 18-gauge needle to extract contents into syringe.
• Empty into a nasogastric (NG) tube; flush tube with 30 ml normal saline.

Intervention and Evaluation
• Monitor the patient's B/P, central nervous system (CNS) response, and heart rate for signs and symptoms of CHF and hypotension.

Patient Teaching
• Instruct the patient not to crush or chew capsules.
• Warn the patient to notify the physician if he or she experiences constipation, dizziness, irregular heartbeats, nausea, shortness of breath, and swelling.

verapamil hydrochloride
ver-**ap**-ah-mill
(Anpec[AUS], Apo-Verap[CAN], Calan, Chronovera[CAN], Cordilox[AUS], Covera-HS, Isoptin, Novoveramil[CAN], Veracaps SR[AUS], Verahexal[AUS], Verelan, Verelan PM)
Do not confuse with Intropin, Virilon, Vivarin, or Voltaren.

CATEGORY AND SCHEDULE
Pregnancy Risk Category: C

MECHANISM OF ACTION
A calcium channel blocker and antianginal, antiarrhythmic, and antihypertensive agent that inhibits calcium ion entry across cardiac and vascular smooth muscle cell membranes. This action causes the dilation of coronary arteries, peripheral arteries, and arterioles. *Therapeutic Effect*: Decreases heart rate and myocardial contractility and slows sinoatrial (SA) and atrioventricular (AV) conduction. Decreases total peripheral vascular resistance by vasodilation.

PHARMACOKINETICS

Route	Onset	Peak	Duration
PO	30 min	1–2 hrs	6–8 hrs
PO (extended-release)	30 min	N/A	N/A
IV	1–2 min	3–5 min	10–60 min

Well absorbed from the gastrointestinal (GI) tract. Protein binding: 90%, (60% in neonates.) Undergoes first-pass metabolism in liver. Metabolized in liver to active metabolite. Primarily excreted in urine. Not

Calcium Channel Blockers 543

removed by hemodialysis. **Half-life:**
2–8 hrs.

AVAILABILITY
Tablets: 40 mg, 80 mg, 120 mg,
120 mg (sustained-release), 180 mg
(sustained-release), 240 mg
(sustained-release).
Capsules (sustained-release): 100
mg (Verelan PM), 120 mg, 180 mg,
200 mg (Verelan PM), 240 mg,
300 mg (Verelan PM), 360 mg.
Injection: 5 mg/2 ml.

INDICATIONS AND DOSAGES
‣ **Supraventricular tachyarrhythmias, temporary control of rapid
ventricular rate with atrial fibrillation or flutter**
IV
Adults, Elderly. Initially, 5–10 mg,
repeat in 30 min with 10-mg dose.
Children 1 to 15 yrs. 0.1 mg/kg.
May repeat in 30 min up to a maximum second dose of 10 mg. Not
recommended in children younger
than 1 yr.
‣ **Arrhythmias, including prevention
of recurrent PSVT and control of
ventricular resting rate in chronic
atrial fibrillation or flutter (with
digoxin)**
PO
Adults, Elderly. 240–480 mg/day in
3–4 divided doses.
‣ **Vasospastic angina (Prinzmetal's
variant), unstable (crescendo or
preinfarction) angina, chronic
stable (effort-associated) angina**
PO
Adults, Elderly. Initially, 80–120 mg
3 times/day. For elderly patients and
those with liver dysfunction, 40 mg
3 times/day. Titrate to optimal dose.
Maintenance: 240–480 mg/day in
3–4 divided doses.
PO (Covera-HS)
Adults, Elderly. 180–480 mg/day at
bedtime.

‣ **Hypertension**
PO
Adults, Elderly. Initially, 40–80 mg
3 times/day. Maintenance: 480 mg
or less a day.
PO (Covera-HS)
Adults, Elderly. 180–480 mg/day at
bedtime.
PO (extended-release)
Adults, Elderly. 120–240 mg/day.
May give 480 mg or less a day in
2 divided doses.
PO (Verelan PM)
Adults, Elderly. 100–300 mg/day.

UNLABELED USES
Treatment of hypertrophic
cardiomyopathy, vascular headaches

CONTRAINDICATIONS
Atrial fibrillation or flutter and an
accessory bypass tract, cardiogenic
shock, heart block, sinus bradycardia, ventricular tachycardia

INTERACTIONS
Drug
Beta-blockers: May have additive
effect.
*Carbamazepine, quinidine, theo-
phylline:* May increase verapamil
blood concentration and risk of
toxicity.
Digoxin: May increase digoxin
blood concentration.
Disopyramide: May increase nega-
tive inotropic effect.
Procainamide, quinidine: May
increase risk of QT-interval prolon-
gation.
Herbal
None known.
Food
Grapefruit and grapefruit juice:
May increase verapamil blood
concentration.

DIAGNOSTIC TEST EFFECTS

EKG waveform may show increased PR interval. Therapeutic blood level is 0.08–0.3 mcg/ml.

IV INCOMPATIBILITIES

Amphotericin B complex (Abelcet, AmBisome, Amphotec), nafcillin (Nafcil), propofol (Diprivan), sodium bicarbonate

IV COMPATIBILITIES

Amiodarone (Cordarone), calcium chloride, calcium gluconate, dexamethasone (Decadron), digoxin (Lanoxin), dobutamine (Dobutrex), dopamine (Intropin), furosemide (Lasix), heparin, hydromorphone (Dilaudid), lidocaine, magnesium sulfate, metoclopramide (Reglan), milrinone (Primacor), morphine, multivitamins, nitroglycerin, norepinephrine (Levophed), potassium chloride, potassium phosphate, procainamide (Pronestyl), propranolol (Inderal)

SIDE EFFECTS

Frequent (7%)
Constipation
Occasional (4%–2%)
Dizziness, lightheadedness, headache, asthenia (loss of strength, energy), nausea, peripheral edema, hypotension
Rare (less than 1%)
Bradycardia, dermatitis or rash

SERIOUS REACTIONS

• Rapid ventricular rate in atrial flutter or fibrillation, marked hypotension, extreme bradycardia, congestive heart failure (CHF), asystole, and second- and third-degree AV block occur rarely.

NURSING CONSIDERATIONS

Baseline Assessment
• Assess and document the onset, type (such as sharp, dull, or squeezing), radiation, location, intensity, and duration of the patient's anginal pain. Also, assess and record precipitating factors, including exertion and emotional stress.
• Before giving verapamil, assess the patient's blood pressure (B/P) for signs of hypotension and pulse rate for signs of bradycardia.
Lifespan Considerations
• Be aware that verapamil crosses the placenta, is distributed in breast milk, and that breast-feeding is not recommended for patients taking this drug.
• Know that there are no age-related precautions for children.
• In the elderly, be aware that age-related renal impairment may require cautious use of this drug.
Precautions
• Use cautiously in patients with CHF, liver or renal impairment, and sick sinus syndrome.
• Use cautiously in patients also receiving beta-blocker or digoxin therapy.
Administration and Handling
PO
• Do not give with grapefruit juice.
• Give tablets that are not sustained-release with or without food.
• Have patient swallow extended-release or sustained-released preparations whole and without chewing or crushing.
• If needed, open sustained-release capsules and sprinkle contents on applesauce. Have the patient swallow the applesauce immediately without chewing.
IV
• Store vials at room temperature.

- Give undiluted, if desired.
- Administer IV push over more than 2 minutes for adults and children and over more than 3 minutes for the elderly.
- Know that continuous EKG monitoring during IV injection is required for children and recommended for adults.
- Monitor the patient's EKG for asystole, extreme bradycardia, heart block, PR-interval prolongation, and rapid ventricular rates. Notify the physician of significant EKG changes.
- Monitor the patient's B/P every 5–10 minutes, or as ordered.
- Keep patient in a recumbent position for at least 1 hour after IV administration.

Intervention and Evaluation

- Assess the patient's pulse for irregular rate and rhythm and quality.
- ◀ALERT▶ Monitor the patient's EKG for changes, particularly PR-interval prolongation. Notify physician of significant PR-interval or other EKG changes.
- Assist the patient with ambulation if he or she experiences dizziness.
- Assess for peripheral edema behind the medial malleolus in ambulatory patients, and in the sacral area in bedridden patients.

- For patients taking the oral form of verapamil, assess stool consistency and frequency.
- Keep in mind that the therapeutic serum level for verapamil is 0.08 to 0.3 mcg/ml.

Patient Teaching

- Caution the patient against abruptly discontinuing the drug.
- Stress that compliance with the treatment regimen is essential to control anginal pain.
- To avoid the orthostatic effects of verapamil, instruct the patient to rise slowly from a lying to sitting position and to wait momentarily before standing.
- Advise the patient to avoid tasks that require mental alertness or motor skills until his or her response to the drug is established.
- Urge the patient to avoid consuming grapefruit or grapefruit juice and to limit caffeine intake while taking verapamil.
- Warn the patient to notify the physician if he or she experiences anginal pain not reduced by the drug, constipation, dizziness, irregular heartbeats, nausea, shortness of breath, and swelling of the hands and feet.

27 Cardiac Glycosides

digoxin
milrinone lactate

Uses: Cardiac glycosides are used to treat congestive heart failure, atrial fibrillation, paroxysmal atrial tachycardia, and cardiogenic shock with pulmonary edema.

Action: Cardiac glycosides act directly on the myocardium to increase the force of contraction, which leads to increased stroke volume and cardiac output. These agents also depress the firing of the sinoatrial node, decrease conduction time through the atrioventricular node, and decrease electrical impulses caused by a slow heart rate from vagal stimulation. Their ability to increase myocardial contractility may result from the improved transport of calcium, sodium, and potassium ions across cell membranes.

digoxin
di-**jox**-in
(Lanoxicaps, Lanoxin)
Do not confuse with Desoxyn, doxepin, Levsinex, or Lonox.

CATEGORY AND SCHEDULE
Pregnancy Risk Category: C

MECHANISM OF ACTION
A cardiac glycoside that increases the influx of calcium from extracellular to intracellular cytoplasm. *Therapeutic Effect:* Potentiates the activity of the contractile cardiac muscle fibers and increases the force of myocardial contraction. Decreases conduction through the sinoatrial (SA) and atrioventricular (AV) nodes.

PHARMACOKINETICS

Route	Onset	Peak	Duration
PO	0.5–2 hrs	28 hrs	3–4 days
IV	5–30 min	1–4 hrs	3–4 days

Readily absorbed from the gastrointestinal (GI) tract. Widely distributed. Protein binding: 30%. Partially metabolized in liver. Primarily excreted in urine. Minimally removed by hemodialysis. **Half-life:** 36–48 hrs (half-life is increased with impaired renal function and in the elderly).

AVAILABILITY
Tablets: 0.125 mg, 0.25 mg, 0.5 mg.
Capsules: 0.05 mg, 0.1 mg, 0.2 mg.
Elixir: 0.05 mg/ml.
Injection: 0.25 mg/ml, 0.1 mg/ml.

INDICATIONS AND DOSAGES
▶ **Rapid loading dose for the prophylactic management and treatment of congestive heart failure (CHF); control of ventricular rate in patients with atrial fibrillation; treatment and prevention of recurrent paroxysmal atrial tachycardia**
IV
Adults, Elderly. 0.6–1 mg.
Children older than 10 yrs. 8–12 mcg/kg.

Children 5–10 yrs. 15–30 mcg/kg.
Children 2–5 yrs. 25–35 mcg/kg.
Children 1–24 mos. 30–50 mcg/kg.
Neonates, full-term. 20–30 mcg/kg.
Neonates, premature. 15–25 mcg/kg.
PO
Adults, Elderly. Initially, 0.5–0.75 mg, additional doses of 0.125–0.375 mg at 6- to 8-hr intervals. Range: 0.75–1.25 mg.
Children older than 10 yrs. 10–15 mcg/kg.
Children 5–10 yrs. 20–35 mcg/kg.
Children 2–5 yrs. 30–40 mcg/kg.
Children 1–24 mos. 35–60 mcg/kg.
Neonate, full-term. 25–35 mcg/kg.
Neonate, premature. 20–30 mcg/kg.
▸ **Maintenance dosage for CHF; control of ventricular rate in patients with atrial fibrillation; treatment and prevention of recurrent paroxysmal atrial tachycardia**
PO/IV
Adults, Elderly. 0.125–0.375 mg/day.
Children. 25%–35% loading dose (20%–30% for premature neonates)
▸ **Dosage in renal impairment**
Total digitalizing dose: decrease by 50%, in end stage renal disease.

Creatinine Clearance	Dosage
10–50 ml/min	25%–75% normal
less than 10 ml/min	10%–25% normal

CONTRAINDICATIONS
Ventricular fibrillation, ventricular tachycardia unrelated to CHF

INTERACTIONS
Drug
Amiodarone: May increase digoxin blood concentration and risk of toxicity and have an additive effect on the sinoatrial (SA) and atrioventricular (AV) nodes.
Amphotericin, glucocorticoids, potassium-depleting diuretics: May increase risk of toxicity due to hypokalemia.
Antiarrhythmics, parenteral calcium, sympathomimetics: May increase risk of arrhythmias. Antidiarrheals, cholestyramine, colestipol, sucralfate: May decrease absorption of digoxin.
Diltiazem, fluoxetine, quinidine, verapamil: May increase digoxin blood concentration.
Parenteral magnesium: May cause cardiac conduction changes and heart block.
Herbal
Siberian ginseng: May increase serum digoxin levels.
Food
None known.

DIAGNOSTIC TEST EFFECTS
None known.

IV INCOMPATIBILITIES
Amphotericin B complex (Abelcet, Amphotec, AmBisome), fluconazole (Diflucan), foscarnet (Foscavir), propofol (Diprivan)

IV COMPATIBILITIES
Cimetidine (Tagamet), diltiazem (Cardizem), furosemide (Lasix), heparin, insulin (regular), lidocaine, midazolam (Versed), milrinone (Primacor), morphine, potassium chloride, propofol (Diprivan)

SIDE EFFECTS
None known. However, there is a very narrow margin of safety between a therapeutic and toxic result. Chronic therapy may produce mammary gland enlargement in women but is reversible when drug is withdrawn.

SERIOUS REACTIONS

• The most common early manifestations of toxicity are GI disturbances (anorexia, nausea, vomiting) and neurologic abnormalities (fatigue, headache, depression, weakness, drowsiness, confusion, nightmares).

• Facial pain, personality change, and ocular disturbances (photophobia, light flashes, halos around bright objects, yellow or green color perception) may be noted.

NURSING CONSIDERATIONS

Baseline Assessment

• Assess the patient's apical pulse for 60 seconds, or 30 seconds if receiving maintenance therapy. If pulse is 60/min or less in adults or 70/min or less for children, withhold the drug and contact the physician.

• Expect to obtain blood samples for digoxin level 6 to 8 hours after digoxin dose or just before next digoxin dose.

Lifespan Considerations

• Be aware that digoxin crosses the placenta and is distributed in breast milk.

• Be aware that premature infants are more susceptible to toxicity.

• In the elderly, age-related liver or renal function impairment may require adjusted dosage.

• In the elderly, there is an increased risk of loss of appetite.

Precautions

• Use cautiously in patients with acute MI, advanced cardiac disease, cor pulmonale, hypokalemia, hypothyroidism, impaired liver or renal function, incomplete atrioventricular (AV) block, and pulmonary disease.

Administration and Handling

◀ALERT▶ Avoid giving the drug by the IM route because the drug may cause severe local irritation and has erratic absorption. If no other route is possible, give deep into the muscle followed by massage. Give no more than 2 ml at any one site.

◀ALERT▶ Expect to adjust the digoxin dosage in elderly patients and those with renal dysfunction. Know that larger digoxin doses are often required for adequate control of ventricular rate in patients with atrial fibrillation or flutter. Administer digoxin loading dosage in several doses at 4- to 8-hour intervals.

PO

• May give without regard to meals.

• Crush tablets if necessary.

IV

• Give undiluted or dilute with at least a 4-fold volume of Sterile Water for Injection, or D_5W because less than this may cause a precipitate to form. Use immediately.

• Give IV slowly over at least 5 minutes.

Intervention and Evaluation

• Monitor the patient's pulse for bradycardia and EKG for arrhythmias for 1 to 2 hours after giving digoxin. Excessive slowing of the patient's pulse may be the first sign of toxicity.

• Assess the patient for signs and symptoms of digoxin toxicity, including GI disturbances and neurologic abnormalities, every 2 to 4 hours during digitalization and daily during maintenance therapy.

• Monitor the patient's serum potassium and magnesium levels. Know that the therapeutic serum level is 0.8 to 2 ng/ml and toxic blood serum level is greater than 2 ng/ml.

Patient Teaching

• Stress to the patient the importance of follow-up visits and tests.

• Teach the patient to take the

apical pulse correctly and to notify the physician of a pulse rate of 60/min or less or a rate as indicated by the physician.

• Instruct the patient to recognize the signs and symptoms of toxicity and to notify physician if he or she experiences them.

• Advise the patient to carry or wear identification that he or she is receiving digoxin and to inform dentists or other physicians about digoxin therapy.

• Caution the patient not to increase or skip digoxin doses.

• Explain to the patient that he or she should not take over-the-counter (OTC) medications without first consulting the physician.

• Warn the patient to notify the physician if he or she experiences decreased appetite, diarrhea, nausea, visual changes, or vomiting.

milrinone lactate
mill-rih-known
(Primacor)

CATEGORY AND SCHEDULE
Pregnancy Risk Category: C

MECHANISM OF ACTION
This cardiac inotropic agent inhibits phosphodiesterase, which increases cAMP and potentiates the delivery of calcium to myocardial contractile systems. *Therapeutic Effect:* Relaxes vascular muscle, causes vasodilation. Increases cardiac output, decreases pulmonary capillary wedge pressure, vascular resistance.

PHARMACOKINETICS

Route	Onset	Peak	Duration
IV	5–15 min	N/A	N/A

Protein binding: 70%. Primarily excreted unchanged in urine. **Half-life:** 2.4 hrs.

AVAILABILITY
Injection: 1 mg/ml.
Injection (premix): 200 mcg/ml.

INDICATIONS AND DOSAGES
▸ **Short-term management of congestive heart failure (CHF)**
IV
Adults. Initially, 50 mcg/kg over 10 min. Continue with maintenance infusion rate of 0.375–0.75 mcg/kg/min based on hemodynamic and clinical response. Total daily dose: 0.59–1.13 mg/kg. Reduce dose to 0.2–0.43 mcg/kg/min for severe renal impairment.

CONTRAINDICATIONS
None known

INTERACTIONS
Drug
Cardiac glycosides: Produces additive inotropic effects with these drugs.
Herbal
None known.
Food
None known.

DIAGNOSTIC TEST EFFECTS
None known.

IV INCOMPATIBILITIES
Furosemide (Lasix)

IV COMPATIBILITIES
Calcium gluconate, digoxin (Lanoxin), diltiazem (Cardizem), dobutamine (Dobutrex), dopamine (Intropin), heparin, lidocaine, magnesium, midazolam (Versed), nitroglycerin, potassium, propofol (Diprivan)

SIDE EFFECTS
Occasional (3%–1%)
Headache, hypotension
Rare (less than 1%)
Angina, chest pain

SERIOUS REACTIONS
• Supraventricular and ventricular arrhythmias (12%), nonsustained ventricular tachycardia (2%), and sustained ventricular tachycardia (1%) occur.

NURSING CONSIDERATIONS

Baseline Assessment
• Offer the patient emotional support, especially if he or she has become anxious as a result of experiencing difficulty breathing.
• Assess the patient's apical pulse and blood pressure (B/P) before beginning treatment and during IV therapy.
• Assess the patient's lung sounds for rales and rhonchi and check the patient's skin for edema.

Lifespan Considerations
• Be aware that it is unknown if milrinone crosses the placenta or is distributed in breast milk.
• Be aware that the safety and efficacy of milrinone have not been established in children.
• In the elderly, age-related renal impairment may require dosage adjustment.

Precautions
• Use cautiously in patients with atrial fibrillation or flutter, history of ventricular arrhythmias, impaired renal function, and severe obstructive aortic or pulmonic valvular disease.

Administration and Handling
IV
• Store at room temperature.
• For IV infusion, dilute 20-mg (20-ml) vial with 80 or 180 ml diluent (0.9% NaCl, D_5W) to provide concentration of 200 or 100 mcg/ml, respectively. Maximum concentration: 100 mg/250 ml.
• For a loading dose IV injection, administer the drug undiluted slowly over 10 minutes.
• Monitor the patient for arrhythmias and hypotension during IV therapy. Reduce or temporarily discontinue infusion until condition stabilizes.

Intervention and Evaluation
• Monitor the patient's B/P, cardiac output, EKG, heart rate, renal function, serum potassium levels.
• Monitor the patient for signs and symptoms of CHF.

Patient Teaching
• Warn patient to immediately report palpitations or chest pain.
• Explain to patient that milrinone is not a cure for CHF and will help relieve symptoms.

28 Sympatholytics

clonidine
doxazosin mesylate
methyldopa
prazosin
  hydrochloride
terazosin
  hydrochloride

Uses: Sympatholytics, also called adrenergic inhibitors, are used to treat mild to severe hypertension. Because these agents effectively control blood pressure, they help prevent the development and progression of serious cardiovascular complications.

Action: Sympatholytics can act centrally or peripherally. (See illustration, *Sites of Action: Sympatholytics,* page 552.) Central-acting agents, such as clonidine and methyldopa, stimulate alpha$_2$-adrenergic receptors in the cardiovascular centers of the central nervous system, reducing sympathetic outflow and producing antihypertensive effects. *Peripheral-acting agents,* such as doxazosin and prazosin, block alpha$_1$-adrenergic receptors in arterioles and veins, inhibiting vasoconstriction and decreasing peripheral vascular resistance, which reduces blood pressure.

COMBINATION PRODUCTS

ALDORIL: methyldopa/hydrochlorothiazide (a diuretic) 250 mg/15 mg; 250 mg/25 mg; 500 mg/30 mg; 500 mg/50 mg.
COMBIPRES: clonidine/chlorthalidone (a diuretic) 0.1 mg/15 mg; 0.2 mg/15 mg; 0.3 mg/15 mg.
MINIZIDE: prazosin/polythiazide (a diuretic) 1 mg/0.5 mg; 2 mg/0.5 mg; 5 mg/0.5 mg.

clonidine

klon-ih-deen
(Catapres, Catapres TTS, Dixarit[CAN], Duraclon)
Do not confuse with Cetapred, clomiphene, Klonopin, or quinidine.

CATEGORY AND SCHEDULE

Pregnancy Risk Category: C

MECHANISM OF ACTION

An antiadrenergic, sympatholytic agent that prevents pain signal transmission to the brain and produces analgesia at pre- and post-alpha adrenergic receptors in the spinal cord. *Therapeutic Effect:* Reduces peripheral resistance; decreases blood pressure (B/P) and heart rate.

PHARMACOKINETICS

Route	Onset	Peak	Duration
PO	0.5–1 hr	2–4 hrs	Up to 8 hrs

Well absorbed from the gastrointestinal (GI) tract. Transdermal best absorbed from chest, upper arm; least absorbed from thigh. Protein binding: 20%–40%. Metabolized in liver. Primarily excreted in urine. Minimal removal by hemodialysis.
Half-life: 12–16 hrs (half-life is

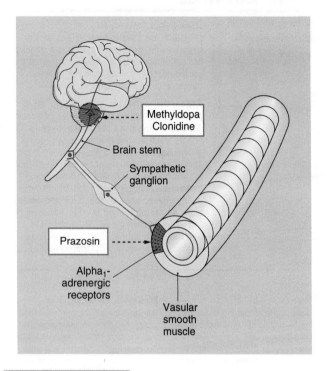

Sites of Action: Sympatholytics

Sympatholytics inhibit sympathetic nervous system (SNS) activity, which plays a major role in regulating blood pressure. Normally when the SNS is stimulated, nerve impulses travel from the cardiovascular center of the central nervous system (CNS) to the sympathetic ganglia. From there, the impulses travel along postganglionic fibers to specific effector organs, such as the heart and blood vessels. SNS stimulation also triggers the release of norepinephrine, which acts primarily at alpha-adrenergic receptors.

Sympatholytics fall into two subclasses: central-acting $alpha_2$ agonists and peripheral-acting $alpha_1$-adrenergic antagonists. Central-acting $alpha_2$ agonists, such as methyldopa and clonidine, stimulate $alpha_2$-adrenergic receptors in the cardiovascular center of the CNS and reduce activity in the vasomotor center of the brain, interfering with sympathetic stimulation of the heart and blood vessels. This causes blood vessel dilation and decreased cardiac output, which leads to reduced blood pressure.

Peripheral-acting $alpha_1$-adrenergic antagonists, such as prazosin, inhibit the stimulation of $alpha_1$-adrenergic receptors by norepinephrine in vascular smooth muscle, interfering with SNS-induced vasoconstriction. As a result, the blood vessels dilate, reducing peripheral vascular resistance and venous return to the heart. These effects, in turn, lead to decreased blood pressure.

increased with impaired renal function).

AVAILABILITY
Tablets: 0.1 mg, 0.2 mg, 0.3 mg.
Transdermal Patch: 2.5 mg (release at 0.1 mg/24 hrs), 5 mg (release at 0.2 mg/24 hrs), 7.5 mg (release at 0.3 mg/24 hrs).
Injection: 100 mcg/ml, 500 mcg/ml.

INDICATIONS AND DOSAGES
▶ **Hypertension**
PO
Adults. Initially, 0.1 mg 2 times/day. Increase by 0.1–0.2 mg q2–4 days. Maintenance: 0.2–1.2 mg/day in 2–4 divided doses up to maximum of 2.4 mg/day.
Children. 5–25 mcg/kg/day in divided doses q6h; increase at 5- to 7-day intervals. Maximum: 0.9 mg/day.
Elderly. Initially, 0.1 mg at bedtime. May increase gradually.
Transdermal
Adults, Elderly. System delivering 0.1 mg/24 hrs up to 0.6 mg/24 hrs q7 days.
▶ **Attention deficit hyperactivity disorder (ADHD)**
PO
Children. Initially, 0.05 mg/day. May increase by 0.05 mg/day q3–7 days. Maximum: 0.3–0.4 mg/day.
▶ **Severe pain**
Epidural
Adults, Elderly. 30–40 mcg/hr.
Children. Initially, 0.5 mcg/kg/hr, not to exceed adult dose.

UNLABELED USES
Attention deficit hyperactivity disorder (ADHD), diagnosis of pheochromocytoma, opioid withdrawal, prevention of migraine headaches, treatment of dysmenorrhea or menopausal flushing

CONTRAINDICATIONS
Epidural contraindicated in those with bleeding diathesis or infection at the injection site, those receiving anticoagulation therapy

INTERACTIONS
Drug
Beta-blockers (used concurrently): Discontinuing these drugs may increase risk of clonidine-withdrawal hypertensive crisis.
Tricyclic antidepressants: May decrease effect of clonidine.
Herbal
None known.
Food
None known.

DIAGNOSTIC TEST EFFECTS
None known.

IV INCOMPATIBILITIES
No known drug incompatibilities.

IV COMPATIBILITIES
Bupivacaine (Marcaine, Sensorcaine), fentanyl (Sublimaze), heparin, ketamine (Ketalar), lidocaine, lorazepam (Ativan)

SIDE EFFECTS
Frequent
Dry mouth (40%), drowsiness (33%), dizziness (16%), sedation, constipation (10%)
Occasional (5%–1%)
Depression, swelling of feet, loss of appetite, decreased sexual ability, itching eyes, dizziness, nausea, vomiting, nervousness
Transdermal: Itching, red skin, darkening of skin
Rare (less than 1%)
Nightmares, vivid dreams, cold feeling in fingers and toes

SERIOUS REACTIONS
• Overdosage produces profound hypotension, irritability, bradycardia, respiratory depression, hypothermia, miosis (pupillary constriction), arrhythmias, and apnea.
• Abrupt withdrawal may result in rebound hypertension associated with nervousness, agitation, anxiety, insomnia, hand tingling, tremor, flushing, and sweating.

NURSING CONSIDERATIONS
Baseline Assessment
• Obtain the patient's B/P immediately before giving each dose, in addition to regular monitoring. Be alert for B/P fluctuations.
Lifespan Considerations
• Be aware that clonidine crosses the placenta and is distributed in breast milk.
• Be aware that children are more sensitive to clonidine's effects. Use clonidine with caution in children.
• The elderly may be more sensitive to the hypotensive effect of clonidine.
• In the elderly, age-related renal impairment may require dosage adjustment.
Precautions
• Use cautiously in patients with cerebrovascular disease, chronic renal failure, Raynaud's disease, recent myocardial infarction (MI), severe coronary insufficiency, and thromboangiitis obliterans.
Administration and Handling
PO
• Give clonidine without regard to food.
• Tablets may be crushed.
• Give last oral dose just before bedtime.
Transdermal
• Apply transdermal system to dry,

hairless area of intact skin on upper arm or chest.
• Rotate sites to prevent skin irritation.
• Do not trim patch to adjust dose.
Intervention and Evaluation
• Assess the patient's pattern of daily bowel activity and stool consistency.
• Expect to discontinue concurrent beta-blocker therapy several days before discontinuing clonidine therapy to prevent clonidine withdrawal hypertensive crisis. Also, expect to slowly reduce clonidine dosage over 2 to 4 days.
Patient Teaching
• Recommend sips of tepid water and sugarless gum to the patient to help relieve dry mouth.
• Instruct the patient to rise slowly from lying to sitting position and permit legs to dangle momentarily before standing to avoid clonidine's hypotensive effect.
• Warn the patient that skipping doses or voluntarily discontinuing clonidine may produce severe, rebound hypertension.
• Advise the patient that clonidine's side effects tend to diminish during therapy.

doxazosin mesylate
docks-ah-**zoe**-sin
(Cardura)
Do not confuse with Cardene, Cordarone, Coumadin, doxapram, doxepin, doxorubicin, K-Dur, or Ridaura.

CATEGORY AND SCHEDULE
Pregnancy Risk Category: C

MECHANISM OF ACTION
An antihypertensive that selectively blocks alpha$_1$-adrenergic receptors, decreasing peripheral vascular resistance. *Therapeutic Effect:* Results in peripheral vasodilation and lowering of blood pressure (B/P). Also relaxes smooth muscle of bladder and prostate.

PHARMACOKINETICS

Route	Onset	Peak	Duration
PO	N/A	2–6 hrs	24 hrs

Well absorbed from the gastrointestinal (GI) tract. Protein binding: 98%–99%. Metabolized in liver. Primarily eliminated in feces. Not removed by hemodialysis. **Half-life:** 19–22 hrs.

AVAILABILITY
Tablets: 1 mg, 2 mg, 4 mg, 8 mg.

INDICATIONS AND DOSAGES
▸ **Mild to moderate hypertension**
PO
Adults. Initially, 1 mg once a day. May increase up to 16 mg/day.
Elderly. Initially, 0.5 mg once a day.
▸ **Benign prostatic hyperplasia**
PO
Adults, Elderly. Initially, 1 mg/day. May increase q1–2 wks. Maximum: 8 mg/day.

CONTRAINDICATIONS
None known.

INTERACTIONS
Drug
Estrogen, NSAIDs: May decrease the effects of doxazosin.
Hypotension-producing medications: May increase the effect of doxazosin.

Herbal
None known.
Food
None known.

DIAGNOSTIC TEST EFFECTS
None known.

SIDE EFFECTS
Frequent (20%–10%)
Dizziness, asthenia, headache, edema
Occasional (9%–3%)
Nausea, pharyngitis, rhinitis, pain in extremities, somnolence
Rare (3%–1%)
Palpitations, diarrhea, constipation, dyspnea, muscle pain, altered vision, dizziness, nervousness

SERIOUS REACTIONS
• First-dose syncope, hypotension with sudden loss of consciousness, generally occurs 30 to 90 minutes following initial dose of 2 mg or greater, a too rapid increase in dose, or addition of another antihypertensive agent to therapy. First-dose syncope may be preceded by tachycardia (pulse rate of 120–160 beats/min).

NURSING CONSIDERATIONS
Baseline Assessment
• Give first doxazosin dose at bedtime. If the initial dose is given during the daytime, keep the patient recumbent for 3 to 4 hours.
• Assess the patient's B/P and pulse immediately before each dose, and every 15 to 30 minutes until B/P is stabilized. Be alert for fluctuations in B/P.
Lifespan Considerations
• Be aware that it is unknown if doxazosin crosses the placenta or is distributed in breast milk.

• Be aware that the safety and efficacy of doxazosin have not been established in children.
• The elderly may be more sensitive to the hypotensive effects of doxazosin.

Precautions
• Use cautiously in patients with chronic renal failure and impaired liver function.

Administration and Handling
PO
• Give doxazosin without regard to food.

Intervention and Evaluation
• Monitor the patient's pulse frequently because first-dose syncope may be preceded by a rapid pulse rate.
• Assess the patient for signs and symptoms of edema and headache.
• Assist the patient with ambulation if he or she experiences dizziness or lightheadedness.

Patient Teaching
• Advise the patient that the full therapeutic effect of doxazosin may not appear for 3 to 4 weeks.
• Explain to the patient that doxazosin use may cause fainting or syncope.
• Caution the patient to avoid driving for 12 to 24 hours after the first doxazosin dose or after any increase in doxazosin dosage.
• Warn the patient to be extremely cautious when driving, operating heavy machinery, or rising from a sitting or lying position.

methyldopa
meth-ill-**doe**-pah
(Aldomet, Apo-Methyldopa[CAN], Hydopa[AUS], Novomedopa[CAN], Nudopa[AUS])
Do not confuse with Anzemet.

CATEGORY AND SCHEDULE
Pregnancy Risk Category: B

MECHANISM OF ACTION
An antihypertensive that stimulates central inhibitory alpha-adrenergic receptors and lowers arterial pressure and reduces plasma renin activity. *Therapeutic Effect*: Reduces standing and supine blood pressure (B/P).

AVAILABILITY
Tablets: 125 mg, 250 mg, 500 mg.
Oral Suspension: 250 mg/5 ml.
Injection: 250 mg/5 ml.

INDICATIONS AND DOSAGES
▶ **Moderate to severe hypertension**
PO
Adults. Initially, 250 mg 2–3 times/day for 2 days. Adjust dosage at intervals of 2 days (minimum).
Elderly. Initially, 125 mg 1–2 times/day. May increase by 125 mg q2–3 days. Maintenance: 500 mg to 2 g/day in 2–4 divided doses.
Children. Initially, 10 mg/kg/day in 2–4 divided doses. Adjust dosage at intervals of 2 days (minimum). Maximum: 65 mg/kg/day or 3 g/day, whichever is less.
IV
Adults. 250–1000 mg q6-8h. Maximum: 4 g/day.
Children. Initially, 2–4 mg/kg/dose. May increase to 5-10 mg/kg/dose in 4-6h if no response. Maximum: 65 mg/kg/day or 3 g/day, whichever is less.

CONTRAINDICATIONS

Liver disease, pheochromocytoma

INTERACTIONS

Drug

Hypotensive-producing medications: May increase the effects of methyldopa.

Lithium: May increase risk of toxicity of lithium.

MAOIs: May cause hyperexcitability.

NSAIDs, tricyclic antidepressants: May decrease the effects of methyldopa.

Sympathomimetics: May decrease the effects of sympathomimetics.

Herbal

None known.

Food

None known.

DIAGNOSTIC TEST EFFECTS

May increase BUN, serum prolactin, alkaline phosphatase, bilirubin, creatinine, potassium, sodium, uric acid, SGOT (AST), and SGPT (ALT) levels. May produce false-positive Coombs' test and prolong prothrombin time.

SIDE EFFECTS

Frequent
Peripheral edema, drowsiness, headache, dry mouth

Occasional
Mental changes (e.g., anxiety, depression), decreased sexual function or interest, diarrhea, swelling of breasts, nausea, vomiting, lightheadedness, numbness in hands or feet, rhinitis

SERIOUS REACTIONS

• Liver toxicity (abnormal liver function tests, jaundice, hepatitis), hemolytic anemia, unexplained fever and flu-like symptoms may occur. If these conditions appear,

discontinue the medication and contact the physician.

NURSING CONSIDERATIONS

Baseline Assessment
• Obtain the patient's baseline B/P, pulse, and weight.

Precautions
• Use cautiously in patients with renal impairment.

Intervention and Evaluation
• Assess the patient's B/P and pulse closely every 30 minutes until stabilized.
• Monitor the patient's weight daily during initial therapy.
• Monitor the patient's liver function tests, including serum alkaline phosphatase, bilirubin, SGOT (AST), and SGPT (ALT) levels.
• Assess the patient for peripheral edema. Be aware that the first area of low extremity swelling is usually behind medial malleolus in ambulatory patients and in the sacral area in bedridden patients.

Patient Teaching
• Urge the patient to avoid consuming alcohol while taking methyldopa.
• Warn the patient to avoid tasks requiring mental alertness and motor skills until his or her response to the drug is established.

prazosin hydrochloride

pray-zoe-sin
(Minipress, Prasig[AUS], Pratisol[AUS], Pressin[AUS])

CATEGORY AND SCHEDULE

Pregnancy Risk Category: C

MECHANISM OF ACTION
An antidote, antihypertensive, and vasodilator agent that selectively blocks alpha$_1$-adrenergic receptors, decreasing peripheral vascular resistance. *Therapeutic Effect:* Produces vasodilation of veins and arterioles; decreases total peripheral resistance; relaxes smooth muscle in bladder neck, and prostate.

AVAILABILITY
Capsules: 1 mg, 2 mg, 5 mg.

INDICATIONS AND DOSAGES
▸ **Mild to moderate hypertension**
PO
Adults, Elderly. Initially, 1 mg 2–3 times/day. Maintenance: 3–15 mg/day in divided doses. Maximum: 20 mg/day.
Children. 5 mcg/kg/dose q6h. Gradually increase up to 25 mcg/kg/dose. Maximum: 15 mg or 400 mcg/kg/day.

UNLABELED USES
Treatment of benign prostate hypertrophy, congestive heart failure (CHF), ergot alkaloid toxicity, pheochromocytoma, Raynaud's phenomena

CONTRAINDICATIONS
None known

INTERACTIONS
Drug
Estrogen, NSAIDs, sympathomimetics: May decrease the effects of prazosin.
Hypotension-producing medications: May increase antihypertensive effect.
Herbal
Licorice: Causes sodium and water retention and potassium loss.
Food
None known.

DIAGNOSTIC TEST EFFECTS
None known.

SIDE EFFECTS
Frequent (10%–7%)
Dizziness, drowsiness, headache, asthenia (loss of strength, energy)
Occasional (5%–4%)
Palpitations, nausea, dry mouth, nervousness
Rare (less than 1%)
Angina, urinary urgency

SERIOUS REACTIONS
• First-dose syncope, hypotension with sudden loss of consciousness, generally occurs 30 to 90 minutes after giving initial prazosin dose of 2 mg or more, instituting a too rapid increase in dosage, or adding another hypotensive agent to therapy. First-dose syncope may be preceded by tachycardia (pulse rate of 120–160 beats/min).

NURSING CONSIDERATIONS
Baseline Assessment
• Give the first prazosin dose at bedtime. If the initial drug dose is given during the daytime, keep the patient recumbent for 3 to 4 hours.
• Assess the patient's B/P and pulse immediately before each dose and every 15 to 30 minutes until stabilized. Be alert for B/P fluctuations.
Precautions
• Use cautiously in patients with chronic renal failure and impaired liver function.
Administration and Handling
PO
• Give prazosin without regard to food.
• Administer first dose at bedtime to minimize the risk of fainting from first-dose syncope.

Intervention and Evaluation
• Monitor the patient's B/P and pulse frequently because first-dose syncope may be preceded by tachycardia.
• Assess the patient's pattern of daily bowel activity and stool consistency.
• Assist the patient with ambulation if he or she experiences dizziness.

Patient Teaching
• Warn the patient to avoid asks that require mental alertness or motor skills for 12 to 24 hours after the first dose or any increase in dosage.
• Warn the patient to use caution when driving or operating machinery and when rising from sitting or lying position.
• Advise the patient to notify the physician if dizziness or palpitations become bothersome.

terazosin hydrochloride
tear-**aye**-zoe-sin
(Apo-Terazosin[CAN], Hytrin)

CATEGORY AND SCHEDULE
Pregnancy Risk Category: C

MECHANISM OF ACTION
An antihypertensive and benign prostatic hyperplasia agent that blocks alpha-adrenergic receptors. Produces vasodilation, decreases peripheral resistance, and targets receptors around bladder neck and prostate. *Therapeutic Effect:* In hypertension, causes a decrease in blood pressure (B/P). In benign prostatic hyperplasia, causes relaxation of smooth muscle and improves urine flow.

PHARMACOKINETICS

Route	Onset	Peak	Duration
PO	15 min	1–2 hrs	12–24 hrs

Rapidly, completely absorbed from the gastrointestinal (GI) tract. Protein binding: 90%–94%. Metabolized in liver to active metabolite. Primarily eliminated in feces via biliary system; excreted in urine. Not removed by hemodialysis.
Half-life: 12 hrs.

AVAILABILITY
Capsules: 1 mg, 2 mg, 5 mg, 10 mg.
Tablets: 2 mg, 5 mg, 10 mg.

INDICATIONS AND DOSAGES
▸ **Mild to moderate hypertension**
PO
Adults, Elderly. Initially, 1 mg at bedtime. Slowly increase dosage to desired levels. Range: 1–5 mg/day as single or 2 divided doses. Maximum: 20 mg.
▸ **Benign prostatic hyperplasia**
PO
Adults, Elderly. Initially, 1 mg at bedtime. May increase up to 10 mg/day. Maximum: 20 mg/day.

CONTRAINDICATIONS
None known

INTERACTIONS
Drug
Estrogen, NSAIDs, sympathomimetics: May decrease the effects of terazosin.
Hypotension-producing medications: May increase antihypertensive effect.
Herbal
Dong quai, ginseng, garlic, yohimbe: May decrease antihypertensive effect.

Food
None known.

DIAGNOSTIC TEST EFFECTS
May decrease blood Hgb and Hct levels, serum albumin levels, total serum protein levels, and white blood cell (WBC) count.

SIDE EFFECTS
Frequent (9%–5%)
Dizziness, headache, unusual tiredness
Rare (less than 2%)
Peripheral edema, orthostatic hypotension, back or joint pain, blurred vision, nausea, vomiting, nasal congestion, drowsiness

SERIOUS REACTIONS
• First-dose syncope, hypotension with sudden loss of consciousness (LOC) generally occurs 30 to 90 minutes after giving initial terazosin dose of 2 mg or more, instituting a too rapid increase in dose, or adding another hypotensive agent to therapy. First-dose syncope may be preceded by tachycardia (pulse rate of 120–160 beats/min).

NURSING CONSIDERATIONS

Baseline Assessment
• Give first terazosin dose at bedtime. If the initial drug dose is given during the daytime, keep the patient recumbent for 3 to 4 hours.
• Assess the patient's blood pressure (B/P) and pulse immediately before each terazosin dose and every 15 to 30 minutes until stabilized. Be alert for B/P fluctuations.

Lifespan Considerations
• Be aware that it is unknown if terazosin crosses the placenta or is distributed in breast milk.

• Be aware that the safety and efficacy of terazosin have not been established in children.
• There are no age-related precautions noted in the elderly, but this age group may be more sensitive to the drug's hypotensive effects.

Precautions
• Use cautiously in patients with confirmed or suspected coronary artery disease.

Administration and Handling
◀ALERT▶ If terazosin is discontinued for several days, expect to restart therapy with a 1-mg dose at bedtime.
PO
• Give terazosin without regard to food.
• Tablets may be crushed.
• Administer first dose at bedtime to minimize the risk of fainting due to first-dose syncope.

Intervention and Evaluation
• Monitor the patient's pulse frequently because first-dose syncope may be preceded by tachycardia.
• Assist the patient with ambulation if he or she experiences dizziness.
• Assess for peripheral edema. Know that the first area swelling is typically behind the medial malleolus in ambulatory patients and in the sacral area in bedridden patients.
• Monitor the patient's B/P and genitourinary (GU) symptoms.

Patient Teaching
• Suggest to the patient that consuming dry toast, non-cola carbonated beverages, and unsalted crackers may relieve nausea.
• Inform the patient that nasal congestion may occur.
• Advise the patient that the full

therapeutic effect of terazosin may not occur for 3 to 4 weeks.

• Explain to the patient that he or she should use caution when driving, performing tasks requiring mental alertness, and when rising from a sitting or lying position.

• Warn the patient to notify the physician if he or she experiences dizziness or palpitations.

29 Vasodilators

bosentan
epoprostenol sodium,
  PG$_2$, PGX,
  prostacyclin
fenoldopam
hydralazine
  hydrochloride
isosorbide dinitrate,
  isosorbide
  mononitrate
minoxidil
nesiritide
nitroglycerin
nitroprusside sodium

Uses: Vasodilators are used primarily to treat essential hypertension, angina pectoris, heart failure, and myocardial infarction. Some of these agents are also used to manage peripheral vascular disease and to produce controlled hypotension during surgery. In addition, minoxidil is used as a hair growth stimulant.

Action: For vasodilators, the exact mechanism of action isn't known. These agents directly relax smooth muscle, which reduces vascular resistance. Some of them act primarily on arterioles, others affect veins, and still others work on both types of vessels.

COMBINATION PRODUCTS

APRESAZIDE: hydralazine/
hydrochlorothiazide (a diuretic)
25 mg/25 mg; 50 mg/50 mg;
100 mg/50 mg.

bosentan
baws-en-tan
(Tracleer)

CATEGORY AND SCHEDULE
Pregnancy Risk Category: X

MECHANISM OF ACTION
An endothelin receptor antagonist that blocks endothelin-1, the neurohormone that constricts pulmonary arteries. *Therapeutic Effect:* Improves exercise ability and decreases rate of clinical worsening of pulmonary arterial hypertension.

PHARMACOKINETICS
Highly bound to plasma proteins, mainly albumin. Metabolized in the liver. Eliminated by biliary excretion. **Half-life:** Approx. 5 hrs.

AVAILABILITY
Tablets: 62.5 mg, 125 mg.

INDICATIONS AND DOSAGES
▸ **Pulmonary arterial hypertension (PAH) in those with World Health Organization Class III or IV symptoms**
PO
Adults, Elderly. 62.5 mg twice a day for 4 wks, then increase to maintenance dose of 125 mg twice daily.
Children weighing less than 40 kg but older than 12 yrs. 62.5 mg twice a day.

CONTRAINDICATIONS
Coadministration with cyclosporine or glyburide, pregnancy

INTERACTIONS
Drug
Atorvastatin, glyburide, hormonal contraceptives (including oral,

injectable, and implantable), lovastatin, simvastatin, warfarin: May decrease the plasma concentrations of these drugs.
Cyclosporine, ketoconazole: May increase plasma concentration of bosentan.

Herbal
None known.

Food
None known.

DIAGNOSTIC TEST EFFECTS

May increase serum bilirubin, SGOT (AST), and SGPT (ALT) levels. May decrease blood Hgb and Hct levels.

SIDE EFFECTS

Occasional
Headache, nasopharyngitis, flushing
Rare
Dyspepsia (heartburn, epigastric distress), fatigue, pruritus, hypotension

SERIOUS REACTIONS

• Abnormal liver function, lower extremity edema, and palpitations occur rarely.

NURSING CONSIDERATIONS

Baseline Assessment
• Determine if the patient is pregnant before beginning bosentan therapy. Know that pregnancy must be prevented during bosentan therapy. Be aware that a negative result from a urine or serum pregnancy test performed during the first 5 days of a normal menstrual period and at least 11 days after the last act of sexual intercourse must be obtained before beginning drug therapy. Expect the patient to undergo monthly pregnancy tests during bosentan therapy.

Lifespan Considerations
• Be aware that bosentan may induce atrophy of seminiferous tubules of the testes, cause male infertility, or reduce sperm count.
• Be aware that bosentan causes fetal harm and has teratogenic effects on the fetus, including malformations of face, head, large vessels, and mouth. Also, know that breast-feeding is not recommended in this patient population.
• Be aware that the safety and efficacy of bosentan have not been established in children.
• Use caution in dosing the elderly due to the higher frequency of decreased cardiac, liver, and renal function.

Precautions
• Use extremely cautiously in patients with moderate to severe liver function impairment.
• Use cautiously in patients with mild liver impairment.

Administration and Handling
• Give bosentan in the morning and evening, with or without food.
• Do not break or crush film-coated tablets. Have the patient swallow the film-coated tablets whole and avoid chewing them.

Intervention and Evaluation
• Assess the patient's hepatic enzyme levels [aminotransferase serum alkaline phosphatase, bilirubin, SGOT (AST), and SGPT (ALT)] before beginning bosentan therapy and monthly thereafter. Expect to initiate changes in monitoring and treatment if an elevation in hepatic enzymes occurs. Expect to stop treatment if clinical symptoms of liver injury, including abdominal pain, fatigue, jaundice, nausea, and vomiting, occur or if the patient's bilirubin level increases.
• Monitor the patient's blood Hgb

levels at 1 and 3 months during treatment, then every 3 months.
• Monitor the patient's blood Hct and Hgb levels. A decrease signifies anemia.

Patient Teaching
• Discuss with the patient the importance of pregnancy testing and the avoidance of pregnancy while taking bosentan. Teach the patient about the various methods of effective contraception.

epoprostenol sodium, PG₂, PGX, prostacyclin
ep-oh-**pros**-ten-awl
(Flolan)

CATEGORY AND SCHEDULE
Pregnancy Risk Category: B

MECHANISM OF ACTION
An antihypertensive that directly vasodilates pulmonary and systemic arterial vascular beds and inhibits platelet aggregation. *Therapeutic Effect:* Reduces right and left ventricular afterload; increases cardiac output and stroke volume.

AVAILABILITY
Powder for Reconstitution: 0.5 mg, 1.5 mg.

INDICATIONS AND DOSAGES
▶ **Long-term treatment of New York Heart Association Class III and IV primary pulmonary hypertension**
IV infusion
Adults, Elderly. Acute dose-ranging procedure: Initially, 2 ng/kg/min increased in increments of 2 ng/kg/min q15min until dose-limiting adverse effects occur. Chronic infusion: Start at 4 ng/kg/min less

than the maximum dose rate tolerated during acute dose ranging (or one half of the maximum rate if rate was less than 5 ng/kg/min).

UNLABELED USES
Cardiopulmonary bypass surgery; hemodialysis, pulmonary hypertension associated with acute respiratory distress syndrome (ARDS), systemic lupus erythematosus, or congenital heart disease, neonatal pulmonary hypertension, refractory congestive heart failure (CHF), severe community-acquired pneumonia

CONTRAINDICATIONS
Chronic use in those with CHF (severe ventricular systolic dysfunction)

INTERACTIONS
Drug
Acetate in dialysis fluids, other vasodilators: May increase hypotensive effects.
Anticoagulants, antiplatelets: May increase the risk of bleeding.
Vasoconstrictors: May decrease effects of epoprostenol.
Herbal
None known.
Food
None known.

DIAGNOSTIC TEST EFFECTS
None known.

IV INCOMPATIBILITIES
Do not mix with any other medications.

SIDE EFFECTS
Frequent
Acute phase: Flushing (58%), headache (49%), nausea (32%), vomiting (32%), hypotension (16%), anxiety

(11%), chest pain (11%), dizziness (8%)

Chronic phase (greater than 20%): Dyspnea, asthenia, dizziness, headache, chest pain, nausea, vomiting, palpitations, edema, jaw pain, tachycardia, flushing, myalgia, nonspecific muscle pain, paresthesia, diarrhea, anxiety, chills, fever, or flu-like symptoms

Occasional

Acute phase (5%–2%): Bradycardia, abdominal pain, muscle pain, dyspnea, back pain

Chronic phase (20%–10%): Rash, depression, hypotension, pallor, syncope, bradycardia, ascites

Rare

Chronic phase (less than 2%): Diaphoresis, dyspepsia, paresthesia, tachycardia

SERIOUS REACTIONS

• Overdose may cause hyperglycemia or ketoacidosis manifested as increased urination, thirst, and fruitlike breath.

• Angina, myocardial infarction (MI), and thrombocytopenia occur rarely.

• Abrupt withdrawal, including a large reduction in dosage or interruption in drug delivery, may produce rebound pulmonary hypertension as evidenced by dyspnea, dizziness, and asthenia.

NURSING CONSIDERATIONS

Precautions

• Use cautiously in elderly patients.

Administration and Handling

◀ALERT▶ Infuse epoprostenol continuously through an indwelling central venous catheter using an infusion pump. If necessary and on a temporary basis, infuse through a peripheral vein.

IV

• Store unopened vial at room temperature.

• Do not freeze.

• Reconstituted solutions are stable for up to 48 hours if refrigerated.

◀ALERT▶ Use only the diluent provided by the manufacturer.

• Follow instructions of manufacturer for dilution to specific concentrations.

• Give as pump infusion only.

Intervention and Evaluation

• Monitor the patient's standing and supine blood pressure (B/P) for several hours after any dosage adjustment.

• Assess the patient for a therapeutic response as evidenced by decreased chest pain, dyspnea on exertion, fatigue, pulmonary arterial pressure, pulmonary vascular resistance, syncope, and an improvement in pulmonary function.

Patient Teaching

• Teach the patient how to reconstitute and administer epoprostenol. Educate the patient on the care of the permanent central venous catheter.

• Advise the patient that brief interruptions in drug delivery may result in rapid, deteriorating symptoms.

• Explain to the patient that epoprostenol therapy will be necessary for a prolonged period, possibly years.

fenoldopam

phen-**ole**-doe-pam
(Corlopam)

CATEGORY AND SCHEDULE

Pregnancy Risk Category: B

MECHANISM OF ACTION

A rapid-acting vasodilator. An agonist for D_1-like dopamine receptors and produces vasodilation in coronary, renal, mesenteric, and peripheral arteries. *Therapeutic Effect:* Reduces systolic and diastolic blood pressure (B/P) and increases heart rate.

PHARMACOKINETICS

After IV administration, metabolized in the liver. Primarily excreted in urine. Unknown if removed by hemodialysis. **Half-life:** Approx. 5 min.

AVAILABILITY

Injection: 10 mg/ml.

INDICATIONS AND DOSAGES

▸ **Short-term management of severe hypertension when rapid, but quickly reversible emergency reduction of B/P is clinically indicated, including malignant hypertension with deteriorating end-organ function**
IV infusion (continuous)
Adults. Initially, 0.1 mcg/kg/min. Maximum: 1.7 mcg/kg/min. Titrate dose up or down in increments of 0.05–0.1 mcg/kg/min no more frequently than q15min. May discontinue gradually or abruptly.

CONTRAINDICATIONS

None known

INTERACTIONS

Drug
Beta-blockers (used concurrently): May produce excessive hypotension.
Herbal
None known.
Food
None known.

DIAGNOSTIC TEST EFFECTS

May elevate BUN, blood glucose levels, serum LDH concentrations, and serum transaminase levels. May decrease serum potassium levels.

IV INCOMPATIBILITIES

Do not mix with any other medication. Specific IV incompatibilities not available.

SIDE EFFECTS

Expected
Beta-blockers may cause unexpected hypotension.
Occasional
Headache (7%), flushing (3%), nausea (4%), hypotension (2%)
Rare (2% or less)
Nervousness or anxiety, vomiting, constipation, nasal congestion, diaphoresis, back pain

SERIOUS REACTIONS

• Excessive hypotension occurs occasionally. Monitor B/P diligently during infusion.
• Substantial tachycardia may lead to ischemic cardiac events or worsened heart failure.
• Allergic-type reactions, including anaphylaxis and life-threatening asthmatic exacerbation may occur in patients with sulfite sensitivity.

NURSING CONSIDERATIONS

Baseline Assessment
• Obtain the patient's baseline apical pulse and B/P before beginning therapy. Diligently monitor the patient's B/P and EKG during the fenoldopam infusion to assess for signs of hypotension and to avoid a too rapid decrease in B/P.
• Assess the patient's medication

history, especially for beta-blocker use.
• Obtain the patient's baseline serum electrolytes, particularly potassium, as ordered, and periodically monitor the patient's electrolytes thereafter during the fenoldopam infusion.
• Determine if asthmatic patients have a history of sulfite sensitivity.
• Be sure to check with the physician for the desired B/P range level for each patient.

Lifespan Considerations
• Be aware that it is unknown if fenoldopam is distributed in breast milk.
• The safety and efficacy of fenoldopam have not been established in children.
• There are no age-related precautions noted in the elderly.

Precautions
• Use cautiously in patients with glaucoma, hypokalemia, hypotension, intraocular hypertension, sulfite sensitivity, and tachycardia.

Administration and Handling
◄ALERT► Give fenoldopam only by continuous IV infusion and not as a bolus injection.
IV
• Store ampoules at room temperature.
• Diluted solution is stable for 24 hours. Discard any solution not used within 24 hours.
• Each 10 mg (1 ml) must be diluted with 250 ml 0.9% NaCl or D_5W to provide a concentration of 40 mcg/ml.
• Use an infusion pump and administer as an IV infusion at an initial rate of 0.1 mcg/kg/min.

Intervention and Evaluation
• Monitor the rate of the fenoldopam infusion frequently.
• Monitor the patient's EKG for tachycardia (which may lead to

angina, ischemic heart disease, myocardial infarction [MI], extrasystoles, or worsening heart failure).
• Observe the patient closely for symptomatic hypotension.

hydralazine hydrochloride
hy-**dral**-ah-zeen
(Alphapress[AUS], Apresoline, Novohylazin[CAN])
Do not confuse with hydroxyzine.

CATEGORY AND SCHEDULE
Pregnancy Risk Category: C

MECHANISM OF ACTION
An antihypertensive with direct vasodilating effects on the arterioles. *Therapeutic Effect:* Decreases blood pressure (B/P) and systemic resistance.

PHARMACOKINETICS

Route	Onset	Peak	Duration
PO	20–30 min	N/A	2–4 hrs
IV	5–20 min	N/A	2–6 hrs

Well absorbed from the gastrointestinal (GI) tract. Widely distributed. Protein binding: 85%–90%. Metabolized in liver to active metabolite. Primarily excreted in urine. Not removed by hemodialysis. **Half-life:** 3–7 hrs (half-life increased with impaired renal function).

AVAILABILITY
Tablets: 10 mg, 25 mg, 50 mg, 100 mg.
Injection: 20 mg/ml.

INDICATIONS AND DOSAGES
▸ **Moderate to severe hypertension**
PO
Adults. Initially, 10 mg 4 times/day.
May increase by 10–25 mg/dose
q2–5 days. Maximum: 300 mg/day.
Children. Initially, 0.75–1 mg/kg/
day in 2–4 divided doses, not
to exceed 25 mg/dose. May increase over 3–4 wks. Maximum:
7.5 mg/kg/day (5 mg/kg/day in
infants).
IM/IV
Adults, Elderly. Initially, 10–20 mg/
dose q4–6h. May increase to 40 mg/
dose.
Children. Initially, 0.1–0.2 mg/kg/
dose (Maximum 20 mg) q4–6h as
needed up to 1.7–3.5 mg/kg/day in
divided doses q4–6h.
▸ **Dosage in renal impairment**

Creatinine Clearance	Dosage Interval
10–50 ml/min	q8h
less than 10 ml/min	q8–24h

UNLABELED USES
Treatment of congestive heart
failure (CHF), hypertension secondary to eclampsia and preeclamp-
sia, primary pulmonary hypertension.

CONTRAINDICATIONS
Coronary artery disease, lupus
erythematosus, rheumatic heart
disease

INTERACTIONS
Drug
Diuretics, other hypotensives: May
increase hypotensive effect.
Herbal
None known.
Food
None known.

DIAGNOSTIC TEST EFFECTS
May produce positive direct
Coombs' test.

IV INCOMPATIBILITIES
Aminophylline, ampicillin (Polycillin), furosemide (Lasix)

IV COMPATIBILITIES
Dobutamine (Dobutrex), heparin,
hydrocortisone (Solu-Cortef), nitroglycerin, potassium

SIDE EFFECTS
Frequent
Headache, palpitations, tachycardia
(generally disappears in 7–10 days)
Occasional
GI disturbance (nausea, vomiting,
diarrhea), paresthesia, fluid retention, peripheral edema, dizziness,
flushed face, nasal congestion

SERIOUS REACTIONS
• High dosage may produce lupus
erythematosus–like reaction, including fever, facial rash, muscle and
joint aches, and splenomegaly.
• Severe orthostatic hypotension,
skin flushing, severe headache,
myocardial ischemia, and cardiac
arrhythmias may develop.
• Profound shock may occur in
cases of severe overdosage.

NURSING CONSIDERATIONS
Baseline Assessment
• Obtain the patient's blood pressure
(B/P) and pulse immediately before
each hydralazine dose, in addition
to regular B/P monitoring. Be alert
for B/P fluctuations.
Lifespan Considerations
• Be aware that hydralazine crosses
the placenta and it is unknown if
hydralazine is distributed in breast
milk.
• Be aware that hematomas, leuko-

penia, petechial bleeding, and
thrombocytopenia have occurred in
newborns and that these conditions
resolve within 1 to 3 weeks.
• There are no age-related precautions noted in children.
• The elderly are more sensitive to
the drug's hypotensive effects.
• In the elderly, age-related renal
impairment may require dosage
adjustment.

Precautions
• Use cautiously in patients with
cerebrovascular disease and impaired renal function.

Administration and Handling
PO
• Hydralazine is best given with
food or regularly spaced meals.
• Crush tablets if necessary.
IV
• Store at room temperature.
• Give undiluted if necessary.
• Give single dose over 1 minute.

Intervention and Evaluation
• Monitor the patient for headache,
palpitations, and tachycardia.
• Assess for peripheral edema of
feet and hands. Usually the first
area of lower extremity swelling is
behind the medial malleolus in
ambulatory patients and in the
sacral area in bedridden patients.
• Assess the patient's pattern of
daily bowel activity and stool consistency.

Patient Teaching
• Instruct the patient to rise slowly
from lying to a sitting position and
permit legs to dangle from the bed
momentarily before standing to
reduce the hypotensive effect of
hydralazine.
• Suggest to the patient that consuming dry toast or unsalted crackers may relieve nausea.
• Warn high-dose therapy patients
to notify the physician if they
experience fever (lupus-like reac-

tion) or report joint and muscle
aches.

---

isosorbide dinitrate
eye-sew-**sore**-bide
(Apo-ISDN[CAN], Cedocard[CAN],
Dilatrate, Isogen[AUS], Isordil,
Sorbidin[AUS])

isosorbide mononitrate
(Duride[AUS], Imdur, Imtrate[AUS],
ISMO, Monodur Durules[AUS],
Monoket)
**Do not confuse with Inderal,
Isuprel, K-Dur, or Plendil.**

CATEGORY AND SCHEDULE
Pregnancy Risk Category: C

MECHANISM OF ACTION
A nitrate that stimulates intracellular
cyclic guanosine monophosphate
(GMP.) *Therapeutic Effect:* Relaxes
vascular smooth muscle of both
arterial and venous vasculature.
Decreases preload and afterload.

PHARMACOKINETICS

Route	Onset	Peak	Duration
Sublingual	2–10 min	N/A	1–2 hrs
Chewable	3 min	N/A	0.5–2 hrs
PO	45–60 min	N/A	4–6 hrs
Sustained release	30 min	N/A	6–12 hrs

Mononitrate well absorbed after PO
administration. Dinitrate poorly
absorbed and metabolized in the
liver to its activate metabolite
isosorbide mononitrate. Excreted in
urine and feces. **Half-life:** Dinitrate
is 1–4 hrs and mononitrate is 4 hrs.

AVAILABILITY
Tablets: 5 mg (Dinitrate), 10 mg

(Dinitrate and Mononitrate), 20 mg
(Dinitrate and Mononitrate), 30 mg
(Dinitrate), 40 mg (Dinitrate).
Tablets (sublingual): 10 mg.
Capsules (sustained-release):
40 mg.
Tablets (extended-release): 30 mg,
60 mg, 120 mg.

INDICATIONS AND DOSAGES
▸ **Acute angina, prophylactic management in situations likely to provoke attack**
Sublingual
Adults, Elderly. Initially, 2.5–5 mg.
Repeat at 5–10 min intervals. No
more than 3 doses in 15–30 min
period.
▸ **Acute prophylactic management of angina**
Sublingual
Adults, Elderly. 5–10 mg q2–3h.
▸ **Long-term prophylaxis of angina**
PO
Adults, Elderly. Initially, 5–20 mg
3–4 times/day. Maintenance: 10–40
mg q6h. Consider 2–3 times/day,
last dose no later than 7 pm to
minimize intolerance.
PO (Mononitrate)
Adults, Elderly. 20 mg 2 times/day,
7 hrs apart. First dose upon awakening in morning.
PO (extended-release)
Adults, Elderly. Initially, 40 mg.
Maintenance: 40–80 mg 2–3 times/
day. Consider 1–2 times/day, last
dose at 2 pm to minimize intolerance.
PO (Imdur)
Adults, Elderly. 60–120 mg/day as
single dose.

UNLABELED USES
Congestive heart failure (CHF),
dysphagia, pain relief, relief of
esophageal spasm with gastroesophageal (GE) reflux

CONTRAINDICATIONS
Closed-angle glaucoma, gastrointestinal (GI) hypermotility or malabsorption (extended-release tablets),
head trauma, hypersensitivity to
nitrates, increased intracranial pressure, postural hypotension, severe
anemia (extended-release tablets)

INTERACTIONS
Drug
*Alcohol, antihypertensives,
vasodilators:* May increase risk of
orthostatic hypotension.
Herbal
None known.
Food
None known.

DIAGNOSTIC TEST EFFECTS
May increase urine catecholamines,
urine VMA (vanillylmandelic acid).

SIDE EFFECTS
Frequent
Burning and tingling at oral point of
dissolution (sublingual), headache
(may be severe) occurs mostly in
early therapy, diminishes rapidly in
intensity, usually disappears during
continued treatment; transient flushing of face and neck, dizziness
(especially if patient is standing
immobile or is in a warm environment), weakness, postural hypotension, nausea, vomiting, restlessness
Occasional
GI upset, blurred vision, dry mouth

SERIOUS REACTIONS
• Blurred vision or dry mouth may
occur (drug should be discontinued).
• Severe postural hypotension manifested by fainting, pulselessness,
cold or clammy skin, and diaphoresis may occur.
• Tolerance may occur with repeated, prolonged therapy (minor

tolerance with intermittent use of sublingual tablets). Tolerance may not occur with extended-release form.
• High dose tends to produce severe headache.

NURSING CONSIDERATIONS

Baseline Assessment
• Record the onset, type (sharp, dull, or squeezing), radiation, location, intensity, and duration of anginal pain and its precipitating factors, such as exertion or emotional stress.

Lifespan Considerations
• Be aware that it is unknown if isosorbide crosses the placenta or is distributed in breast milk.
• Be aware that the safety and efficacy of isosorbide have not been established in children.
• The elderly may be more sensitive to the drug's hypotensive effects.
• In the elderly, age-related decreased renal function may require cautious use.

Precautions
• Use cautiously in patients with acute myocardial infarction (MI), blood volume depletion from therapy, glaucoma (contraindicated in closed-angle glaucoma), liver or renal disease, and systolic B/P less than 90 mm Hg.

Administration and Handling
PO
• Best if taken on an empty stomach; however, administer isosorbide with meals if the patient experiences a headache.
• Oral tablets may be crushed.
• Do not crush or break sublingual or extended-release form.
• Do not crush chewable form before administering.
Sublingual

• Do not crush or have patient chew sublingual tablets.
• Have patient dissolve tablets under tongue without swallowing.

Intervention and Evaluation
• Assist the patient with ambulation if he or she experiences dizziness or lightheadedness.
• Assess the patient for facial or neck flushing.
• Monitor and document the number of anginal episodes and the patient's orthostatic B/P.

Patient Teaching
• Teach the patient to take sublingual tablets while sitting down. Explain to the patient that he or she should not chew or crush sublingual or sustained-release forms. Instruct the patient to dissolve sublingual tablets under the tongue and not to swallow them.
• Instruct the patient to take isosorbide at the first sign or symptom of angina. Explain to the patient that if angina is not relieved within 5 minutes that he or she can dissolve a second tablet under the tongue and repeat dosage in another 5 minutes if he or she feels no relief. Warn patient to seek immediate emergency assistance if anginal pain persists.
• Advise the patient that after anginal pain is completely relieved, he or she should expel any remaining sublingual tablet from under the tongue.
• Instruct the patient to rise slowly from lying to sitting position and dangle legs momentarily before standing.
• Teach the patient to take the oral form of isosorbide on an empty stomach unless headache occurs during management therapy. Advise the patient that if he or she experiences headache, to take the oral form with meals.

• Caution the patient against changing from one brand of drug to another.
• Urge the patient to avoid alcohol during isosorbide therapy as alcohol intensifies the drug's hypotensive effect. Explain to the patient that if alcohol is ingested soon after taking nitrates, he or she may experience an acute hypotensive episode marked by a drop in B/P, pallor, and vertigo.

minoxidil
min-**ox**-ih-dill
(Apo-Gain, Loniten, Milnox, Regaine[AUS], Rogaine, Rogaine Extra Strength)
Do not confuse with Lotensin.

CATEGORY AND SCHEDULE
Pregnancy Risk Category: C
OTC (topical solution)

MECHANISM OF ACTION
An antihypertensive and hair growth stimulant that has direct action on vascular smooth muscle, producing vasodilation of arterioles. *Therapeutic Effect:* Decreases peripheral vascular resistance, blood pressure (B/P); increases cutaneous blood flow; stimulates hair follicle epithelium and hair follicle growth.

PHARMACOKINETICS

Route	Onset	Peak	Duration
PO	0.5 hr	2–8 hrs	2–5 days

Well absorbed from the gastrointestinal (GI) tract, minimal absorption after topical application. Protein binding: None. Widely distributed.

Metabolized in liver to active metabolite. Primarily excreted in urine. Removed by hemodialysis. **Half-life:** 4.2 hrs.

AVAILABILITY
Tablets: 2.5 mg, 10 mg.
Topical Solution: 2% (20 mg/ml), 5% (50 mg/ml).

INDICATIONS AND DOSAGES
‣ **Severe symptomatic hypertension, hypertension associated with organ damage, hypertension that has failed to respond to maximal therapeutic dosages of a diuretic or two other antihypertensive agents**
PO
Adults. Initially, 5 mg/day. Increase with at least 3-day intervals to 10 mg, 20 mg, up to 40 mg/day in 1–2 doses.
Elderly. Initially, 2.5 mg/day. May increase gradually. Maintenance: 10–40 mg/day. Maximum: 100 mg/day.
Children. Initially, 0.1–0.2 mg/kg (5 mg maximum) daily. Gradually increase at minimum 3-day intervals of 0.1–2 mg/kg. Maintenance: 0.25–1 mg/kg/day in 1–2 doses. Maximum: 50 mg/day.
‣ **Hair regrowth**
Topical
Adults. 1 ml to total affected areas of scalp 2 times/day. Total daily dose not to exceed 2 ml.

CONTRAINDICATIONS
Pheochromocytoma

INTERACTIONS
Drug
Parenteral antihypertensives: May increase hypotensive effect.
NSAIDs: May decrease the effects of minoxidil.

Herbal
None known.
Food
None known.

DIAGNOSTIC TEST EFFECTS

May increase BUN, plasma renin activity, serum alkaline phosphatase, serum creatinine, and serum sodium. May decrease blood Hgb and Hct levels and erythrocyte count.

SIDE EFFECTS

Frequent
PO: Edema with concurrent weight gain, hypertrichosis (elongation, thickening, increased pigmentation of fine body hair) develops in 80% of patients within 3–6 wks after beginning therapy
Occasional
PO: T-wave changes but usually revert to pretreatment state with continued therapy or drug withdrawal.
Topical: Itching, skin rash, dry or flaking skin, erythema.
Rare
PO: Rash, pruritus, breast tenderness in male and female, headache, photosensitivity reaction
Topical: Allergic reaction, alopecia, burning scalp, soreness at hair root, headache, visual disturbances

SERIOUS REACTIONS

• Tachycardia and angina pectoris may occur because of increased oxygen (O_2) demands associated with increased heart rate and cardiac output.
• Fluid and electrolyte imbalance and congestive heart failure (CHF) may be observed, especially if a diuretic is not given concurrently with minoxidil.
• Too rapid reduction in B/P may result in syncope, cerebrovascular accident, myocardial infarction

(MI), and ischemia of sense organs (vision, hearing).
• Pericardial effusion and tamponade may be seen in those with impaired renal function not on dialysis.

NURSING CONSIDERATIONS

Baseline Assessment
• Assess the patient's B/P on both arms and take the patient's pulse for 1 full minute immediately before giving the medication. If the patient's pulse increases 20 beats/min or more over baseline, or systolic or diastolic B/P decreases less than 20 mm Hg, withhold minoxidil and contact physician.
Lifespan Considerations
• Be aware that minoxidil crosses the placenta and is distributed in breast milk.
• There are no age-related precautions noted in children.
• The elderly are more sensitive to the drug's hypotensive effects.
• In the elderly, age-related renal impairment may require dosage adjustment.
Precautions
• Use cautiously in patients with chronic CHF, coronary artery disease, recent MI (within 1 month), and severe renal impairment.
Administration and Handling
PO
• Give without regard to food (with food if GI upset occurs).
• Crush tablets if necessary.
Topical
• Shampoo and dry patient's hair before applying medication.
• Wash hands immediately after application.
• Do not use hair dryer after application (reduces effectiveness).
Intervention and Evaluation
• Monitor the patient's B/P, body

weight, and serum electrolyte levels.
• Assess for peripheral edema of feet and hands. Usually the first area of low extremity swelling is behind medial malleolus in ambulatory patients and in the sacral area in bedridden patients.
• Assess the patient for signs and symptoms of CHF, including cool extremities, cough, dyspnea on exertion, and rales at the base of the lungs.
• Evaluate the patient for distant or muffled heart sounds by auscultation, which may indicate pericardial effusion or tamponade.

Patient Teaching
• Advise the patient that the maximum B/P response occurs 3 to 7 days and reversible growth of fine body hair may begin 3 to 6 weeks after minoxidil treatment is initiated.
• Explain to the patient that when minoxidil is used topically for stimulation of hair growth, minoxidil treatment must continue on a permanent basis and that any cessation of treatment will begin reversal of new hair growth.
• Warn the patient to avoid exposure to sunlight and artificial light sources.

---

nesiritide
ness-**ear**-ih-tide
(Natrecor)

CATEGORY AND SCHEDULE
Pregnancy Risk Category: C

MECHANISM OF ACTION
This brain natriuretic peptide facilitates cardiovascular homeostasis and fluid status through counterregulation of the renin-angiotensin-aldosterone system, stimulating cyclic guanosine monophosphate, leading to smooth muscle cell relaxation. *Therapeutic Effect:* Promotes vasodilation, natriuresis, and diuresis, correcting congestive heart failure (CHF).

PHARMACOKINETICS

Route	Onset	Peak	Duration
IV	15–30 min	1–2 hrs	4 hrs

Excreted primarily in the heart by the left ventricle. Metabolized by the natriuretic neutral endopeptidase enzymes on the vascular luminal surface. **Half-life:** 18–23 min.

AVAILABILITY
Injection: 1.5 mg/5 ml vial.

INDICATIONS AND DOSAGES
▸ **Treatment of acutely decompensated CHF in patients with dyspnea at rest or with minimal activity**
IV bolus
Adults, Elderly. 2 mcg/kg followed by a continuous IV infusion of 0.01 mcg/kg/min. May be incrementally increased q3h to a maximum of 0.03 mcg/kg/min.

CONTRAINDICATIONS
Cardiogenic shock, systolic blood pressure (B/P) less than 90 mm Hg

INTERACTIONS
Drug
Angiotensin-converting enzyme (ACE) inhibitors, IV nitroglycerin, milrinone, nitroprusside: May increase risk of hypotension.
Herbal
None known.
Food
None known.

DIAGNOSTIC TEST EFFECTS

None known.

IV INCOMPATIBILITIES

Sodium metabisulfite, bumetanide (Bumex), enalapril (Vasotec), ethacrynic acid (Edecrin), furosemide (Lasix), heparin, hydralazine (Apresoline), insulin

SIDE EFFECTS

Frequent (11%)
Hypotension
Occasional (8%–2%)
Headache, nausea, bradycardia
Rare (1% or less)
Confusion, paresthesia, somnolence, tremor

SERIOUS REACTIONS

• Ventricular arrhythmias, including ventricular tachycardia, atrial fibrillation, atrioventricular node conduction abnormalities, and angina pectoris occur rarely.

NURSING CONSIDERATIONS

Baseline Assessment
• Obtain the patient's B/P immediately before each nesiritide dose, in addition to regular monitoring. Be alert to B/P fluctuations. Place the patient in the supine position with legs elevated if he or she experiences an excessive reduction in B/P.

Lifespan Considerations
• Be aware that it is unknown if nesiritide crosses the placenta or is distributed in breast milk.
• Be aware that the safety and efficacy of nesiritide have not been established in children.
• There are no age-related precautions noted in the elderly.

Precautions
• Use cautiously in patients with atrial conduction defects, constrictive pericarditis, hypotension, liver impairment, pericardial tamponade, renal impairment, restrictive or obstructive cardiomyopathy, significant valvular stenosis, suspected low cardiac filling pressures, and ventricular conduction defects.

Administration and Handling
◀ALERT▶ Do not mix with other injections or infusions. Do not give IM.
IV
• Store vial at room temperature. Once reconstituted, use within 24 hours at room temperature or if refrigerated.
• Reconstitute one 1.5-mg vial with 5 ml D_5W or 0.9% NaCl, 0.2% NaCl or any combination thereof. Swirl or rock gently, and add to 250-ml bag D_5W or 0.9% NaCl, 0.2% NaCl, or any combination thereof yielding a solution of 6 mcg/ml.
• Give as an IV bolus over approximately 60 seconds initially followed by continuous IV infusion.

Intervention and Evaluation
• Frequently monitor the patient's B/P for hypotension and pulse rate for abnormalities during nesiritide therapy.
• Establish parameters for adjusting rate or stopping infusion with the physician.
• Maintain accurate patient intake and output records and assess the patient's urine output frequently.
• Immediately notify the physician of cardiac arrhythmias, decreased urine output, or a significant decrease in B/P or heart rate.

Patient Teaching
• Explain to patient that nesiritide is not a cure for CHF and that it will help relieve symptoms.
• Caution the patient to immediately report if he or she experiences chest pain or palpitations.

nitroglycerin

nigh-trow-**glih**-sir-in
(Anginine[AUS], Minitran,
Nitradisc[AUS], Nitrek, Nitro-Bid,
Nitro-Dur, Nitrogard,
Nitroject[CAN], Nitrolingual,
Nitrong-SR, NitroQuick,
Nitrostat, Nitro-Tab,
Rectogesic[AUS], Tansiderm
Nitro[AUS], Trinipatch[CAN])
**Do not confuse with Hyperstat,
Nicobid, Nicoderm, Nilstat,
nitroprusside, Nizoral, or
Nystatin.**

CATEGORY AND SCHEDULE
Pregnancy Risk Category: B

MECHANISM OF ACTION
A nitrate that decreases myocardial
oxygen (O_2) demand. Reduces left
ventricular preload and afterload.
Therapeutic Effect: Dilates coronary
arteries, improves collateral blood
flow to ischemic areas within myocardium. IV form produces peripheral vasodilation.

PHARMACOKINETICS

Route	Onset	Peak	Duration
Sublingual	2–5 min	4–8 min	30–60 min
Transmuco-sal Tablet	2–5 min	4–10 min	3–5 hrs
Extended-release	20–45 min	N/A	3–8 hrs
Topical	15–60 min	0.5–2 hrs	3–8 hrs
Patch	30–60 min	1–3 hrs	8–12 hrs
IV	1–2 min	N/A	3–5 min

Well absorbed after PO, sublingual,
topical administration. Undergoes
extensive first-pass metabolism.
Metabolized in liver and by enzymes in bloodstream. Primarily
excreted in urine. Not removed by
hemodialysis. **Half-life:** 1–4 min.

AVAILABILITY
Tablets (sublingual): 0.3 mg,
0.4 mg, 0.6 mg.
Spray: 0.4 mg/dose.
Tablets (buccal, controlled-release):
3 mg.
Capsules (sustained-release):
2.5 mg, 6.5 mg, 9 mg.
Transdermal: 0.1 mg/hr, 0.2 mg/hr,
0.3 mg/hr, 0.4 mg/hr, 0.6 mg/hr.
Topical Ointment: 2%.
Injection: 5 mg/ml.
Injection Solution: 100 mcg/ml,
200 mcg/ml.

INDICATIONS AND DOSAGES
▸ **Acute relief of angina pectoris,
acute prophylaxis**
Lingual spray
Adults, Elderly. 1 spray onto or
under tongue q3–5min until relief is
noted (no more than 3 sprays in
15-min period).
Sublingual
Adults, Elderly. 0.4 mg q5min until
relief is noted (no more than 3
doses in 15-min period). Use prophylactically 5–10 min before
activities that may cause an acute
attack.
▸ **Long-term prophylaxis of angina**
PO (extended-release)
Adults, Elderly. 2.5–9 mg q8–12h.
Topical
Adults, Elderly. Initially, ½ inch
q8h. Increase by ½ inch with each
application. Range: 1–2 inches q8h
up to 4–5 inches q4h.
Transdermal patch
Adults, Elderly. Initially, 0.2–0.4
mg/hr. Maintenance: 0.4–0.8 mg/hr.
Consider patch on 12–14 hrs, patch
off 10–12 hrs (prevents tolerance).
▸ **Treatment of congestive heart
failure (CHF) associated with acute
myocardial infarction (MI)**

IV
Adults, Elderly. Initially, 5 mcg/
min via infusion pump. Increase in
5 mcg/min increments at 3- to
5-min intervals until B/P response is
noted or until dosage reaches 20
mcg/min; then increase as needed
by 10 mcg/min. Dosage may be
further titrated according to patient,
therapeutic response up to 200
mcg/min.
Children. Initially, 0.25–0.5 mcg/
kg/min; titrate by 0.5–1 mcg/kg/
min up to 20 mcg/kg/min.

CONTRAINDICATIONS
Allergy to adhesives (transdermal),
closed-angle glaucoma, constrictive
pericarditis (IV), early MI (sublingual), gastrointestinal (GI) hypermotility or malabsorption (extended-
release), head trauma, hypersensitivity to nitrates, hypotension (IV),
inadequate cerebral circulation (IV),
increased intracranial pressure,
pericardial tamponade (IV), postural
hypotension, severe anemia, uncorrected hypovolemia (IV)

INTERACTIONS
Drug
*Alcohol, antihypertensives,
vasodilators:* May increase risk of
orthostatic hypotension.
Herbal
None known.
Food
None known.

DIAGNOSTIC TEST EFFECTS
May increase blood methemo-
globin concentrations, urine
catecholamines, and urine vanillylmandelic acid (VMA) concentrations.

IV INCOMPATIBILITIES
Alteplase (Activase)

IV COMPATIBILITIES
Amiodarone (Cordarone), diltiazem
(Cardizem), dobutamine (Dobutrex),
dopamine (Intropin), epinephrine,
famotidine (Pepcid), fentanyl (Sublimaze), furosemide (Lasix), heparin, hydromorphone (Dilaudid),
insulin, labetalol (Trandate), lidocaine, lorazepam (Ativan), midazolam (Versed), milrinone (Primacor), morphine, nicardipine
(Cardene), nitroprusside (Nipride),
norepinephrine (Levophed), propofol (Diprivan)

SIDE EFFECTS
Frequent
Headache (may be severe) occurs
mostly in early therapy, diminishes
rapidly in intensity, usually disappears during continued treatment;
transient flushing of face and neck;
dizziness (especially if patient is
standing immobile or is in a warm
environment); weakness; postural
hypotension
Sublingual: Burning, tingling sensation at oral point of dissolution
Ointment: Erythema, pruritus
Occasional
GI upset
Transdermal: Contact dermatitis

SERIOUS REACTIONS
• Nitroglycerin should be discontinued if blurred vision or dry mouth
occurs.
• Severe postural hypotension manifested by fainting, pulselessness,
cold or clammy skin, and profuse
sweating may occur.
• Tolerance may occur with repeated, prolonged therapy (minor
tolerance with intermittent use of
sublingual tablets).
• High dose tends to produce severe
headache.

NURSING CONSIDERATIONS

Baseline Assessment
• Document the onset, type (sharp, dull, or squeezing), radiation, location, intensity, and duration of anginal pain, and its precipitating factors, such as exertion and emotional stress.
• Assess the patient's apical pulse and B/P before administration and periodically after nitroglycerin dose.
• Continuously monitor the patient's EKG during IV administration.

Lifespan Considerations
• Be aware that it is unknown if nitroglycerin crosses the placenta or is distributed in breast milk.
• Be aware that the safety and efficacy of nitroglycerin have not been established in children.
• The elderly are more susceptible to the hypotensive effects of nitroglycerin.
• In the elderly, age-related renal impairment may require cautious use.

Precautions
• Use cautiously in patients with acute MI, blood volume depletion from diuretic therapy, glaucoma (contraindicated in closed-angle glaucoma), liver or renal disease, and systolic B/P less than 90 mm Hg.

Administration and Handling
PO
• Instruct the patient to swallow extended-release form whole. Capsule should not be chewed or crushed.
• Do not shake oral aerosol canister before lingual spraying.
Sublingual
• Have the patient dissolve the sublingual form under the tongue and avoid swallowing.
• Administer while the patient is seated.

• To lessen the burning sensation under the tongue, place the tablet in the buccal pouch.
• Keep sublingual tablets in original container.
Topical
• Spread thin layer on clean, dry, hairless skin of upper arm or body, not below the knee or elbow, using applicator or dose-measuring papers. Do not use fingers; do not rub or massage into skin.
Transdermal
• Apply patch on clean, dry, hairless skin of upper arm or body and not below the knee or elbow.
IV
• Store at room temperature.
• Know that the IV form is available in ready-to-use injectable containers.
• Dilute vials in 250 or 500 ml D_5W or 0.9% NaCl to a maximum concentration of 250 mg/250 ml.
• Use microdrop or infusion pump.

Intervention and Evaluation
◀ALERT▶ Remove the transdermal dosage form before cardioversion or defibrillation because the electrical current may cause arcing which can burn the patient and damage the paddles.
• Monitor the patient's B/P and heart rate.
• Examine the patient for facial or neck flushing.

Patient Teaching
• Teach the patient to take oral nitroglycerin on an empty stomach. Advise the patient to take the medication with meals if he or she experiences headache during therapy.
• Teach the patient to use inhalant nitroglycerin only when lying down.
• Teach the patient to dissolve sublingual nitroglycerin tablets under the tongue. Stress to the patient that he or she should not swallow sublingual tablets.

• Instruct the patient to take sublingual tablets at the first sign of angina. Explain that if anginal pain is not relieved within 5 minutes of the first dose, that he or she may dissolve a second tablet under the tongue. Then, advise the patient that if the second dose does not relive his or her anginal pain within 5 minutes, he or she may dissolve a third tablet under the tongue. Warn the patient that if anginal pain continues with no relief from the third tablet, that he or she should immediately notify the physician or seek emergency medical help.

• Teach the patient using nitroglycerin lingual aerosol to spray it on or under the tongue. Explain that the patient should avoid inhaling or swallowing the lingual aerosol.

• Teach the patient to place transmucosal tablets under the upper lip or buccal pouch, which is between the cheek and gum. Advise the patient to avoid chewing or swallowing transmucosal tablets.

• Instruct the patient to expel any remaining intrabuccal, lingual, or sublingual tablets after the anginal pain is completely relieved.

• Teach the patient to keep the drug container away from heat and moisture.

• Caution the patient against changing brands of the nitroglycerin.

• Instruct the patient to rise slowly from a lying to a sitting position and dangle legs momentarily before standing to avoid the drug's hypotensive effect.

• Urge the patient to avoid alcohol during nitroglycerin therapy. Explain that alcohol intensifies the drug's hypotensive effect. Warn the patient that alcohol ingested soon after taking nitroglycerin can cause an acute hypotensive episode noted by a marked drop in B/P, vertigo, and pallor.

---

nitroprusside sodium
nigh-troe-**pruss**-eyd
(Nipride, Nitropress)
Do not confuse with nitroglycerin.

CATEGORY AND SCHEDULE
Pregnancy Risk Category: C

MECHANISM OF ACTION
Potent vasodilator used to treat emergent hypertensive conditions; acts directly on arterial and venous smooth muscle. Decreases peripheral vascular resistance, preload, afterload; improves cardiac output. *Therapeutic Effect:* Dilates coronary arteries, decreases oxygen (O_2) consumption, relieves persistent chest pain.

PHARMACOKINETICS

Route	Onset	Peak	Duration
IV	1–10 min	Dependent on infusion rate	Dissipates rapidly after stopping IV

Reacts with Hgb in erythrocytes, producing cyanmethemoglobin, cyanide ions. Primarily excreted in urine. **Half-life:** less than 10 min.

AVAILABILITY
Powder for Injection: 50 mg.
Injection: 25 mg/ml.

INDICATIONS AND DOSAGES
▸ **Immediate reduction of blood pressure (B/P) in hypertensive**

crisis; produce controlled hypotension in surgical procedures to reduce bleeding; treatment of acute congestive heart failure (CHF)

IV

Adults, Elderly, Children. Initially, 0.3 mcg/kg/min. Range: 0.5–10 mcg/kg/min. Do not exceed 10 mcg/kg/min (risk of precipitous drop in B/P).

UNLABELED USES

Control paroxysmal hypertension before and during surgery for pheochromocytoma, peripheral vasospasm caused by ergot alkaloid overdose, treatment adjunct for myocardial infarction (MI), valvular regurgitation

CONTRAINDICATIONS

Compensatory hypertension (atrioventricular [AV] shunt or coarctation of aorta), inadequate cerebral circulation, moribund patients

INTERACTIONS

Drug

Dobutamine: May increase cardiac output and decrease pulmonary wedge pressure.

Hypotensive-producing medications: May increase hypotensive effect.

Herbal

None known.

Food

None known.

DIAGNOSTIC TEST EFFECTS

None known.

IV INCOMPATIBILITIES

Cisatracurium (Nimbex)

IV COMPATIBILITIES

Diltiazem (Cardizem), dobutamine (Dobutrex), dopamine (Intropin), enalapril (Vasotec), heparin, insulin, labetalol (Normodyne, Trandate), lidocaine, midazolam (Versed), milrinone (Primacor), nitroglycerin, propofol (Diprivan)

SIDE EFFECTS

Occasional

Flushing of skin, increased intracranial pressure, rash, pain or redness at injection site

SERIOUS REACTIONS

• A too rapid IV rate reduces B/P too quickly.

• Nausea, retching, diaphoresis, apprehension, headache, restlessness, muscle twitching, dizziness, palpitations, retrosternal pain, and abdominal pain may occur. Symptoms disappear rapidly if rate of administration is slowed or temporarily discontinued.

• Overdosage produces metabolic acidosis and tolerance to therapeutic effect.

NURSING CONSIDERATIONS

Baseline Assessment

• Continuously monitor the patient's B/P and EKG.

• Determine, with the physician, the desired B/P level. Know that the B/P is normally maintained about 30% to 40% below pretreatment levels.

• Expect to discontinue nitroprusside if the therapeutic response is not achieved within 10 minutes after IV infusion at 10 mcg/kg/min is initiated.

Lifespan Considerations

• Be aware that it is unknown if nitroprusside crosses the placenta or is distributed in breast milk.

• Be aware that the safety and efficacy of nitroprusside have not been established in children.

• The elderly are more sensitive to the drug's hypotensive effect.

• In the elderly, age-related renal impairment may require cautious use.

Precautions

• Use cautiously in patients with hyponatremia, hypothyroidism, and severe liver or renal impairment.

• Use cautiously in elderly patients.

Administration and Handling

IV

• Protect solution from light.

• Inspect solution, which normally appears very faint brown. Be aware that a color change from brown to blue, green, or dark red indicates drug deterioration.

• Use only freshly prepared solution. Once prepared, do not keep or use longer than 24 hours.

• Discard unused portion.

• Reconstitute 50-mg vial with 2–3 ml D_5W or Sterile Water for Injection without preservative.

• Further dilute with 250 to 1,000 ml D_5W to provide concentration of 200 mcg to 50 mcg/ml, respectively, up to a maximum concentration of 200 mg/250 ml.

• Wrap infusion bottle in aluminum foil immediately after mixing.

• Give by IV infusion only using infusion rate chart provided by manufacturer or protocol.

• Administer using IV infusion pump or microdrip (60 gtt/ml).

• Be alert for extravasation, which produces severe pain and sloughing.

Intervention and Evaluation

• Monitor the patient's rate of infusion frequently.

• Monitor the patient's blood acid-base balance, electrolytes, intake and output, and laboratory results.

• Assess the patient for signs and symptoms of metabolic acidosis, including disorientation, headache, hyperventilation, nausea, vomiting, and weakness.

• Assess the patient for therapeutic response to medication.

• Monitor the patient's B/P for potential rebound hypertension after infusion is discontinued.

Patient Teaching

• Advise the patient to immediately report if he or she experiences dizziness, headache, nausea, palpitations, or other unusual signs or symptoms.

• Warn the patient to immediately report if he or she experiences pain, redness, or swelling at the IV insertion site.

30 Vasopressors

dobutamine hydrochloride
dopamine hydrochloride
epinephrine
midodrine
norepinephrine bitartrate
phenylephrine hydrochloride

Uses: Different groups of vasopressors are used for different effects. *Alpha₁-receptor stimulators,* such as midodrine and phenylephrine, are used to induce vasoconstriction primarily in the skin and mucous membranes, to provide nasal decongestion, and to delay local anesthetic absorption. They're also used to increase blood pressure in certain hypotensive states and to produce mydriasis, facilitating eye examinations and ocular surgery.

Many vasopressors, however, produce their effects by working on a combination of adrenergic receptors. In most cases, the site of action depends on the drug dose. For example, at low doses, dopamine stimulates dopaminergic receptors, dilating renal arteries. But at much higher doses, the drug stimulates alpha₁ receptors, causing vasoconstriction. The chart below shows how vasopressors stimulate particular receptors and produce the corresponding therapeutic effects.

Name	Receptor Specificity	Uses	Dosage Range
Dobutamine	Beta$_1$, beta$_2$, alpha$_1$	Inotropic support in cardiac decompensation	2.5–10 mcg/kg/min IV
Dopamine	Beta$_1$, alpha$_1$, dopaminergic	Vasopressor, cardiac stimulant	Dopaminergic: 0.5–3 mcg/kg/min IV Beta$_1$: 2–10 mcg/kg/min IV Alpha$_1$: greater than 10 mcg/kg/min IV
Epinephrine	Beta$_1$, beta$_2$, alpha$_1$	Cardiac arrest, anaphylactic shock	Vasopressor: 1–10 mcg/min IV Cardiac arrest: 1 mg q3–5 min IV during resuscitation
Midodrine	Alpha$_1$	Vasopressor, orthostatic hypotension	10 mg PO, 3 times daily
Norepinephrine	Beta$_1$, alpha$_1$	Vasopressor	0.5–1 mcg/min up to 2–12 mcg/min IV
Phenylephrine	Alpha$_1$	Vasopressor	Initially, 10–180 mcg/min, then 40–60 mcg/min IV

Action: The sympathetic nervous system (SNS) maintains homeostasis, including the regulation of heart rate, cardiac contractility, blood pressure, bronchial airway tone, and carbohydrate and fatty acid metabolism. The SNS is mediated by neurotransmitters (primarily norepinephrine, epinephrine, and dopamine) that act on adrenergic receptors, which include $alpha_1$, $alpha_2$, $beta_1$, $beta_2$, and dopaminergic receptors. Vasopressors differ widely in their actions based on their specificity for these receptors:
• $Alpha_1$-receptor stimulation causes constriction of arterioles and veins.
• $Beta_1$-receptor stimulation increases the rate, force of contraction, and conduction velocity of the heart and releases renin from the kidneys.
• $Beta_2$-receptor stimulation dilates arterioles.
• Dopamine-receptor stimulation dilates renal vessels.

COMBINATION PRODUCTS

AC GEL: epinephrine/cocaine (an anesthetic).

LIDOCAINE WITH EPINEPHRINE: lidocaine (an anesthetic)/epinephrine 2%/1:50,000; 1%/1:100,000; 1%/1:200,000; 0.5%/1:2000,000.

PHENERGAN VC: phenylephrine/promethazine (an antihistamine) 5 mg/5 mg.

PHENERGAN VC WITH CODEINE: phenylephrine/promethazine (an antihistamine)/codeine (an analgesic) 6.25 mg/5 mg/10 mg.

TAC: epinephrine/tetracaine (an anesthetic)/cocaine (an anesthetic).

dobutamine hydrochloride
do-**byew**-ta-meen
(Dobutrex)
Do not confuse with Dopamine.

CATEGORY AND SCHEDULE
Pregnancy Risk Category: B

MECHANISM OF ACTION
A direct-acting inotropic agent acting primarily on $beta_1$-adrenergic receptors. *Therapeutic Effect:* Decreases preload and afterload, enhances myocardial contractility, stroke volume, and cardiac output. Improves renal blood flow and urine output.

PHARMACOKINETICS

Route	Onset	Peak	Duration
IV	1–2 min	10 min	Length of infusion

Metabolized in liver. Primarily excreted in urine. Not removed by hemodialysis. **Half-life:** 2 min.

AVAILABILITY
Injection: 12.5 mg/ml vial.
Infusion (ready-to-use): 1 mg/ml, 2 mg/ml, 4 mg/ml.

INDICATIONS AND DOSAGES
▸ **Short-term management of cardiac decompensation**
IV infusion
Adults, Elderly, Children. 2.5–15 mcg/kg/min. Rarely, infusion rate up to 40 mcg/kg/min to increase cardiac output.
Neonates. 2–15 mcg/kg/min.

CONTRAINDICATIONS
Hypovolemic patients, idiopathic hypertrophic subaortic stenosis, sulfite sensitivity

INTERACTIONS
Drug
Beta-blockers: May antagonize the effects of dobutamine.
Digoxin: May increase the risk of arrhythmias, and provide additional inotropic effect.
MAOIs, oxytocics, tricyclic antidepressants: May increase the adverse effects of dobutamine, such as arrhythmias and hypertension.
Herbal
None known.
Food
None known.

DIAGNOSTIC TEST EFFECTS
Decreases serum potassium levels

IV INCOMPATIBILITIES
Acyclovir (Zovirax), alteplase (Activase), amphotericin B complex (Abelcet, AmBisome, Amphotec), bumetanide (Bumex), cefepime (Maxipime), foscarnet (Foscavir), furosemide (Lasix), heparin, piperacillin/tazobactam (Zosyn)

IV COMPATIBILITIES
Amiodarone (Cordarone), calcium chloride, calcium gluconate, diltiazem (Cardizem), dopamine (Intropin), enalapril (Vasotec), famotidine (Pepcid), hydromorphone (Dilaudid), insulin (regular), lidocaine, lorazepam (Ativan), magnesium sulfate, midazolam (Versed), milrinone (Primacor), morphine, nitroglycerin, norepinephrine (Levophed), potassium chloride, propofol (Diprivan)

SIDE EFFECTS
Frequent (greater than 5%)
Increased heart rate, blood pressure
Occasional (5%–3%)
Pain at injection site
Rare (3%–1%)
Nausea, headache, anginal pain, shortness of breath, fever

SERIOUS REACTIONS
• Overdosage may produce marked increase in heart rate, 30 beats/min or higher, marked increase in systolic blood pressure (B/P), 50 mm Hg or higher, anginal pain, and premature ventricular beats.

NURSING CONSIDERATIONS

Baseline Assessment
• Perform continuous cardiac monitoring of the patient to check for arrhythmias.
• Determine the patient's body weight in kilograms for dosage calculation.
• Obtain the patient's initial B/P, heart rate, and respirations.
• Correct hypovolemia before beginning dobutamine therapy.

Lifespan Considerations
• Be aware that it is unknown if dobutamine crosses the placenta or is distributed in breast milk, so it is not administered to pregnant women.
• There are no age-related precautions noted in children or the elderly.
Precautions
• Use cautiously in patients with atrial fibrillation and hypertension.
Administration and Handling
◀ALERT▶ Dobutamine dosage is determined by the patient's response to the drug.
◀ALERT▶ Plan to correct hypovolemia with volume expanders before dobutamine infusion. Expect to treat patients with atrial fibrillation with digoxin prior to infusion. Administer by IV infusion only.
IV
• Store at room temperature because freezing produces crystallization.
• Pink discoloration of solution, caused by oxidation, does not indicate loss of potency if used within recommended time period.
• Further diluted solution for infusion must be used within 24 hours.
• Dilute 250-mg ampoule with 10 ml sterile water for injection or D_5W for injection; the resulting solution is 25 mg/ml. Add additional 10 ml of diluent if not completely dissolved; the resulting solution is 12.5 mg/ml.
• Further dilute 250-mg vial with D_5W or 0.9% NaCl. Maximum concentration is 3.125 g/250 ml, or 12.5 mg/ml.
• Use infusion pump to control flow rate.
• Titrate dosage to individual response, as prescribed.
• Be aware that infiltration of the IV solution causes local inflammatory changes, and may cause dermal necrosis.
Intervention and Evaluation
• Continuously monitor the patient for arrhythmias or changes in the heart rate.
• Establish parameters with the physician for adjusting the drug rate or stopping infusion.
• Maintain accurate intake and output records. Measure the patient's urine output frequently.
• Assess the patient's serum potassium levels and dobutamine plasma levels. Keep in mind that the therapeutic range is 40 to 190 ng/ml.
• Continuously monitor the patient's B/P. Keep in mind that high blood pressure is a greater risk in patients with preexisting hypertension.
• Check the patient's cardiac output and pulmonary wedge pressure or central venous pressure frequently.
• Immediately notify the physician if the patient experiences cardiac arrhythmias, decreased urine output, or a significant increase or decrease in the B/P or heart rate.
Patient Teaching
• Tell the patient to let you know if he or she develops pain or burning at the IV site.
• Urge your patient to let you know if he or she experiences chest pain or palpitations during the infusion.

dopamine hydrochloride
dope-a-meen
(Intropin)
Do not confuse with dobutamine, Dopram, or Isoptin.

CATEGORY AND SCHEDULE
Pregnancy Risk Category: C

MECHANISM OF ACTION

A sympathomimetic (adrenergic agonist) that stimulates adrenergic receptors; effects are dose dependent. Low Dosages (1–5 mcg/kg/min): Stimulates dopaminergic receptors causing renal vasodilation. *Therapeutic Effect:* Increases renal blood flow, urine flow, sodium excretion. Low to Moderate Dosages (5–15 mcg/kg/min): Positive inotropic effect by direct action, release of norepinephrine. *Therapeutic Effect:* Increases myocardial contractility, stroke volume, cardiac output. High Dosages (greater than 15 mcg/kg/min): Stimulates alpha-receptors. *Therapeutic Effect:* Increases peripheral resistance, renal vasoconstriction, increases systolic and diastolic blood pressure (B/P).

PHARMACOKINETICS

Route	Onset	Peak	Duration
IV	1–2 min	–	<10 min

Widely distributed. Does not cross blood-brain barrier. Metabolized in liver, kidney, plasma. Primarily excreted in urine. Not removed by hemodialysis. **Half-life:** 2 min.

AVAILABILITY

Injection: 40 mg/ml, 80 mg/ml, 160 mg/ml.
Injection (premix with dextrose): 80 mg/100 ml, 160 mg/100 ml, 320 mg/100 ml.

INDICATIONS AND DOSAGES

▸ **Prophylaxis and treatment of acute hypotension, shock that's associated with cardiac decompensation, myocardial infarction (MI), open heart surgery, renal failure, trauma, treatment of low cardiac output, congestive heart failure (CHF)**
IV
Adults, Elderly. 1 mcg/kg/min up to 50 mcg/kg/min titrated to desired response.
Children. 1–20 mcg/kg/min. Maximum: 50 mcg/kg/min.
Neonates. 1–20 mcg/kg/min.

CONTRAINDICATIONS

Pheochromocytoma, sulfite sensitivity, uncorrected tachyarrhythmias, ventricular fibrillation

INTERACTIONS

Drug
Beta-blockers: May decrease the effects of dopamine.
Digoxin: May increase the risk of arrhythmias.
Ergot alkaloids: May increase vasoconstriction.
MAOIs: May increase cardiac stimulation and vasopressor effects.
Tricyclic antidepressants: May increase cardiovascular effects.
Herbal
None known.
Food
None known.

DIAGNOSTIC TEST EFFECTS

None known.

IV INCOMPATIBILITIES

Acyclovir (Zovirax), amphotericin B complex (Abelcet, AmBisome, Amphotec), cefepime (Maxipime), furosemide (Lasix), insulin

IV COMPATIBILITIES

Amiodarone (Cordarone), calcium chloride, diltiazem (Cardizem), dobutamine (Dobutrex), enalapril (Vasotec), heparin, hydromorphone (Dilaudid), labetalol (Trandate), levofloxacin (Levaquin), lidocaine, lorazepam (Ativan), methylprednisolone (Solu-Medrol), midazolam (Versed), milrinone (Primacor), morphine, nicardipine (Cardene), nitroglycerin, norepinephrine (Levophed), piperacillin tazobactam (Zosyn), potassium chloride, propofol (Diprivan)

SIDE EFFECTS
Frequent
Headache, ectopic beats, tachycardia, anginal pain, palpitations, vasoconstriction, hypotension, nausea, vomiting, dyspnea
Occasional
Piloerection or goose bumps, bradycardia, widening of QRS complex.

SERIOUS REACTIONS
• High dosages may produce ventricular arrhythmias.
• Patients with occlusive vascular disease are high-risk candidates for further compromise of circulation to extremities, which may result in gangrene.
• Tissue necrosis with sloughing may occur with extravasation of IV solution.

NURSING CONSIDERATIONS

Baseline Assessment
• Determine if the patient has been on MAOI therapy within last 2 to 3 wks because it requires dopamine dosage reduction.
• Expect to place the patient on a continuous cardiac monitor to assess for arrhythmias.
• Determine the patient's weight for dosage calculation.
• Obtain the patient's initial B/P, heart rate, and respirations.
Lifespan Considerations
• Be aware that it is unknown if dopamine crosses the placenta or is distributed in breast milk.

• Closely monitor pediatric patients because gangrene due to extravasation has been reported.
• There are no age-related precautions noted in the elderly.
Precautions
• Use cautiously in patients with ischemic heart disease and occlusive vascular disease.
Administration and Handling
◀ALERT▶ Expect to correct blood volume depletion before administering dopamine. Blood volume replacement may occur simultaneously with dopamine infusion.
IV
• Do not use solutions darker than slightly yellow or discolored to yellow, brown, or pink to purple because it indicates decomposition of drug.
• Know that the drug is stable for 24 hours after dilution.
• Dilute each 5-ml (200-mg) ampoule in 250–500 ml 0.9% NaCl, $D_5W/0.45$ NaCl, $D_5W/0.45$ NaCl, D_5W/lactated Ringer's or lactated Ringer's. Keep in mind the concentration is dependent on the dosage and the patient's fluid requirements. Remember that a 250 ml solution yields 800 mcg/ml, and a 500 ml solution yields 400 mcg/ml. The maximum concentration is 3.2 g/250 ml or 12.8 mg/ml. Know that the drug is available prediluted in 250 or 500 ml D_5W.
• Administer into large vein, such as the antecubital or subclavian vein, to prevent drug extravasation.
• Use an infusion pump to control rate of flow.
• Titrate dosage to the desired hemodynamic values or optimum urine flow, as prescribed.
Intervention and Evaluation
• Continuously monitor the patient for cardiac arrhythmias.

• Measure the patient's urine output frequently.

• If extravasation occurs, immediately infiltrate the affected tissue with 10 to 15 ml 0.9% NaCl solution containing 5 to 10 mg phentolamine mesylate, as ordered.

• Monitor the patient's B/P, heart rate, and respirations at least every 15 minutes during dopamine administration.

• Assess the patient's cardiac output and pulmonary wedge pressure or central venous pressure frequently.

• Examine the patient's peripheral circulation by palpating pulses and noting the color and temperature of extremities.

• Immediately notify the physician if the patient experiences cardiac arrhythmias, decreased peripheral circulation, marked by cold, pale, or mottled extremities, decreased urine output, and significant changes in B/P or heart rate, or failure to respond to increase or decrease in infusion rate.

• Taper off the dopamine dosage before discontinuing the drug because abrupt cessation of dopamine therapy may result in marked hypotension.

• Be alert to excessive vasoconstriction as evidenced by decreased urine output, disproportionate increase in diastolic B/P, and increased arrhythmias or heart rate. Slow or temporarily stop the dopamine infusion and notify the physician if excessive vasoconstriction occurs.

Patient Teaching

• Tell the patient to let you know if he or she develops pain or burning at the IV site.

• Urge your patient to let you know if he or she experiences chest pain or palpitations during the infusion.

epinephrine
eh-pih-**nef**-rin
(Adrenalin, Adrenaline Injection[AUS], EpiPen, Primatene)
Do not confuse with ephedrine.

CATEGORY AND SCHEDULE
Pregnancy Risk Category: C

MECHANISM OF ACTION
A sympathomimetic, adrenergic agonist that stimulates alpha-adrenergic receptors causing vasoconstriction and pressor effects, beta$_1$-adrenergic receptors, resulting in cardiac stimulation, and beta$_2$-adrenergic receptors, resulting in bronchial dilation and vasodilation. *Therapeutic Effect:* Relaxes smooth muscle of the bronchial tree, produces cardiac stimulation, dilates skeletal muscle vasculature. Ophthalmic: Increases outflow of aqueous humor from anterior eye chamber. *Therapeutic Effect:* Dilates pupils and constricts conjunctival blood vessels.

PHARMACOKINETICS

Route	Onset	Peak	Duration
Subcutaneous	5–10 min	20 min	1–4 hrs
IM	5–10 min	20 min	1–4 hrs
Inhalation	3–5 min	20 min	1–3 hrs
Ophthalmic	1 hr	4–8 hrs	12–24 hrs

Minimal absorption after inhalation, well absorbed after parenteral administration. Metabolized in liver, other tissues, sympathetic nerve endings. Excreted in urine. Ophthalmic: May have systemic absorption from drainage into nasal pharyngeal passages. Mydriasis occurs within several minutes, persists several hours; vasoconstriction occurs within 5 min, lasts less than 1 hr.

AVAILABILITY
Injection in Prefilled Injector: 0.3 mg/0.3 ml, 0.15 mg/0.3 ml.
• *Injection:* 0.1 mg/ml, 1 mg/ml.
• *Solution for Oral Inhalation:* 2.25%, 1.125%.
• *Ophthalmic Solution:* 0.5%, 1%, 2%.

INDICATIONS AND DOSAGES
▶ **Asystole**
IV
Adults, Elderly. 1 mg q3–5min up to 0.1 mg/kg q3–5min.
Children. 0.01 mg/kg (0.1 ml/kg of 1:10,000 solution). May repeat q3–5min. Subsequent doses 0.1 mg/kg (0.1 ml/kg) of a 1:1000 solution q3–5min.
▶ **Bradycardia**
IV infusion
Adults, Elderly. 1–10 mcg/min titrated to desired effect.
IV
Children. 0.01 mg/kg (0.1 mg/kg of 1:10,000 solution) q3–5min.
Maximum: 1 mg/10 ml.
▶ **Bronchodilator**
IM/Subcutaneous
Adults, Elderly. 0.1–0.5 mg (1:1000) q10–15min to 4 hrs.
Subcutaneous
Children. 10 mcg/kg (0.01 ml/kg of 1:1000) Maximum: 0.5 mg or suspension (1:200) 0.005 ml/kg/dose (0.025 mg/kg/dose) to a maximum of 0.15 ml (0.75 mg for single dose) q8–12h.
▶ **Hypersensitivity reaction**
IM/Subcutaneous
Adults, Elderly. 0.3–0.5 mg q15–20min.
Subcutaneous
Children. 0.01 mg/kg q15min for 2

doses, then q4h. Maximum single dose: 0.5 mg.
Inhalation
Adults, Elderly, Children older than 4 yrs. 1 inhalation, may repeat in at least 1 min; subsequent doses no sooner than 3 hrs.
Nebulizer
Adults, Elderly, Children older than 4 yrs. 1–3 deep inhalations; subsequent doses no sooner than 3 hrs.
▶ **Glaucoma**
Ophthalmic
Adults, Elderly. 1–2 drops 1–2 times/day.

UNLABELED USES
Systemic: Treatment of gingival or pulpal hemorrhage, priapism
Ophthalmic: Treatment of conjunctival congestion during surgery, secondary glaucoma

CONTRAINDICATIONS
Cardiac arrhythmias, cerebrovascular insufficiency, hypertension, hyperthyroidism, ischemic heart disease, narrow-angle glaucoma, shock

INTERACTIONS
Drug
Beta-blockers: May decrease the effects of beta blockers.
Digoxin, sympathomimetics: May increase risk of arrhythmias.
Ergonovine, methergine, oxytocin: May increase vasoconstriction.
MAOIs, tricyclic antidepressants: May increase cardiovascular effects.
Herbal
None known.
Food
None known.

DIAGNOSTIC TEST EFFECTS
May decrease serum potassium levels.

IV INCOMPATIBILITIES
Ampicillin (Omnipen, Polycillin)

IV COMPATIBILITIES
Calcium chloride, calcium gluconate, diltiazem (Cardizem), dobutamine (Dobutrex), dopamine (Intropin), fentanyl (Sublimaze), heparin, hydromorphone (Dilaudid), lorazepam (Ativan), midazolam (Versed), milrinone (Primacor), morphine, nitroglycerin, norepinephrine (Levophed), potassium chloride, propofol (Diprivan)

SIDE EFFECTS
Frequent
Systemic: Tachycardia, palpitations, nervousness
Ophthalmic: Headache, stinging, burning or other eye irritation, watering of eyes
Occasional
Systemic: Dizziness, lightheadedness, facial flushing, headache, diaphoresis, increased B/P, nausea, trembling, insomnia, vomiting, weakness
Ophthalmic: Blurred or decreased vision, eye pain
Rare
Systemic: Chest discomfort/pain, arrhythmias, bronchospasm, dry mouth or throat

SERIOUS REACTIONS
• Excessive doses may cause acute hypertension or arrhythmias.
• Prolonged or excessive use may result in metabolic acidosis due to increased serum lactic acid concentrations.
• Observe for disorientation, weakness, hyperventilation, headache, nausea, vomiting, and diarrhea.

Baseline Assessment
• Obtain baseline vital signs, especially heart rate and blood pressure.
• Obtain a baseline EKG to monitor for arrhythmias.
Lifespan Considerations
• Be aware that epinephrine crosses the placenta and is distributed in breast milk.
• There are no age-related precautions noted in children or the elderly.
Precautions
• Use cautiously in patients with angina pectoris, diabetes mellitus, hypoxia, myocardial infarction (MI), psychoneurotic disorders, tachycardia, and severe liver or renal impairment.
• Use cautiously in elderly patients.
Administration and Handling
Subcutaneous
• Shake ampoule thoroughly.
• Use tuberculin syringe for subcutaneous injection into lateral deltoid region.
• Massage injection site to minimize vasoconstriction effect.
IV
• Store parenteral forms at room temperature.
• Do not use if solution appears discolored or contains a precipitate.
• For injection, dilute each 1 mg of 1:1,000 solution with 10 ml 0.9 NaCl to provide 1:10,000 solution, and inject each 1 mg or fraction thereof over greater than 1 minute.
• For infusion, further dilute with 250 to 500 D_5W. Maximum concentration is 64 mg/250 ml.
• For IV infusion, give at 1 to 10 mcg/min, and titrate to desired response.

Intervention and Evaluation
• Monitor the patient for changes in vital signs.
• Assess the patient's lung sounds for crackles, rhonchi, and wheezing.
• Monitor the patient's arterial blood gases (ABGs).
• Monitor the B/P, EKG, and pulse, especially in the cardiac arrest patient.

Patient Teaching
• Urge the patient to avoid consuming an excessive amount of caffeine derivatives such as chocolate, cocoa, coffee, cola, or tea.
• Explain to the patient receiving the ophthalmic solution that he or she will feel a slight burning or stinging when the drug is initially administered.
• Warn the patient receiving the ophthalmic solution to immediately report any new symptoms such as dizziness, shortness of breath, or tachycardia because they may be a sign of systemic absorption.

midodrine
my-doe-dreen
(Amatine, ProAmatine)
Do not confuse with protamine.

CATEGORY AND SCHEDULE
Pregnancy Risk Category: C

MECHANISM OF ACTION
A vasopressor that forms the active metabolite desglymidodrine, which is an alpha$_1$-agonist, activating alpha receptors of arteriolar and venous vasculature. *Therapeutic Effect:* Increases vascular tone, blood pressure (B/P).

AVAILABILITY
Tablets: 2.5 mg, 5 mg, 10 mg.

INDICATIONS AND DOSAGES
▸ **Orthostatic hypotension**
PO
Adults, Elderly. 10 mg 3 times/day. Give during day when patient is upright, such as upon arising, midday, and late afternoon—not later than 6 p.m.
▸ **Dosage in renal impairment**
Adults, Elderly. 2.5 mg 3 times/day increase gradually, as tolerated.

CONTRAINDICATIONS
Acute renal function impairment, persistent hypertension, pheochromocytoma, severe cardiac disease, thyrotoxicosis, urine retention

INTERACTIONS
Drug
Digoxin: May have additive bradycardia effects.
Sodium-retaining steroids (e.g., fludrocortisone): May increase sodium retention.
Vasoconstrictors: May have an additive effect.
Herbal
None known.
Food
None known.

DIAGNOSTIC TEST EFFECTS
None known.

SIDE EFFECTS
Frequent (20%–7%)
Paresthesia, piloerection, pruritus, dysuria, supine hypertension
Occasional (less than 7%–1%)
Pain, rash, chills, headache, facial flushing, confusion, dry mouth, anxiety

SERIOUS REACTIONS
• None known.

NURSING CONSIDERATIONS
Baseline Assessment
• Assess the patient's hypersensitivity to midodrine, and determine if he or she is taking other medications, especially digoxin, sodium-retaining steroids, and vasoconstrictors.
• Assess the patient's medical problems, including acute renal function impairment, severe hypertension, and cardiac disease.
Precautions
• Use cautiously in patients with a history of vision problems and renal or liver impairment.
Intervention and Evaluation
• Monitor the patient's blood pressure (B/P) and liver or renal function blood chemistry test results.
Patient Teaching
• Instruct the patient to not take the last dose of the day after evening meal or less than 4 hours before to bedtime. Do not give if the patient will be supine.
• Use caution with OTC medications that may affect B/P, such as cough and cold, diet medications.

norepinephrine bitartrate
nor-eh-pih-**nef**-rin
(Levophed)

CATEGORY AND SCHEDULE
Pregnancy Risk Category: C

MECHANISM OF ACTION
A sympathomimetic that stimulates beta$_1$-adrenergic receptors, alpha-adrenergic receptors, increasing peripheral resistance. *Therapeutic Effect:* Enhances contractile myocardial force, increases cardiac output. Constricts resistance and capacitance vessels. Increases systemic blood pressure (B/P), coronary blood flow.

PHARMACOKINETICS

Route	Onset	Peak	Duration
IV	Rapid	1–2 min	N/A

Localized in sympathetic tissue. Metabolized in liver. Primarily excreted in urine.

AVAILABILITY
Injection: 1 mg/ml ampoules.

INDICATIONS AND DOSAGES
▸ **Acute hypotension unresponsive to fluid volume replacement**
IV
Adults, Elderly. Initially, administer at 0.5–1 mcg/min. Adjust rate of flow to establish, maintain desired B/P that's 40 mm Hg below preexisting systolic pressure. Average maintenance dose: 8–12 mcg/min. *Children.* Initially, 0.05–0.1 mcg/kg/min; titrate to desired effect. Maximum: 1–2 mcg/kg/min. Range: 0.5–3 mcg/min.

CONTRAINDICATIONS
Hypovolemic states—unless as an emergency measure, mesenteric or peripheral vascular thrombosis, profound hypoxia

INTERACTIONS
Drug
Beta-blockers: May have mutually inhibitory effects.
Digoxin: May increase risk of arrhythmias.
Ergonovine, oxytocin: May increase vasoconstriction.
Maprotiline, tricyclic antidepressants: May increase cardiovascular effects.

Methyldopa: May decrease the effects of methyldopa.

Herbal
None known.

Food
None known.

DIAGNOSTIC TEST EFFECTS
None known.

IV INCOMPATIBILITIES
Regular Insulin

IV COMPATIBILITIES
Amiodarone (Cordarone), calcium gluconate, diltiazem (Cardizem), dobutamine (Dobutrex), dopamine (Intropin), epinephrine, esmolol (Brevibloc), fentanyl (Sublimaze), furosemide (Lasix), haloperidol (Haldol), heparin, hydromorphone (Dilaudid), labetalol (Trandate), lorazepam (Ativan), magnesium, midazolam (Versed), milrinone (Primacor), morphine, nicardipine (Cardene), nitroglycerin, potassium chloride, propofol (Diprivan)

SIDE EFFECTS
Norepinephrine produces less pronounced and less frequent side effects than epinephrine.
Occasional (5%–3%)
Anxiety; bradycardia; awareness of slow, forceful heartbeat
Rare (2%–1%)
Nausea, anginal pain, shortness of breath, fever

SERIOUS REACTIONS
• Extravasation may produce tissue necrosis and sloughing.
• Overdosage is manifested as severe hypertension with violent headache, which may be the first clinical sign of overdosage, arrhythmias, photophobia, retrosternal or pharyngeal pain, pallor, excessive sweating, and vomiting.

• Prolonged therapy may result in plasma volume depletion.
• Hypotension may recur if plasma volume is not restored.

NURSING CONSIDERATIONS

Baseline Assessment
• Assess the patient's B/P and EKG continuously. Be alert to precipitous drops in B/P.
• Don't leave the patient alone during a norepinephrine IV infusion.
• Be alert to any patient complaint of headache.

Lifespan Considerations
• Be aware that norepinephrine readily crosses the placenta. Know that norepinephrine may produce fetal anoxia due to constriction of uterine blood vessels and uterine contraction.
• There are no age-related precautions noted in children or the elderly.

Precautions
• Use cautiously in patients with hypertension, hypothyroidism, and severe cardiac disease.
• Use cautiously in patients on concurrent MAOI therapy.

Administration and Handling
◀ALERT▶ Expect to restore blood and fluid volume before administering norepinephrine.
IV
• Do not use if solution is brown or contains precipitate.
• Store ampoules at room temperature.
• Add 4 ml (4 mg) to 250 ml (16 mcg/ml). Maximum concentration: 32 ml (32 mg) to 250 ml (128 mcg/ml).
• If available, administer infusion through a central venous catheter to avoid extravasation.
• Closely monitor the IV infusion flow rate with a microdrip or infusion pump.

• Monitor the patient's B/P every 2 minutes during IV infusion until desired therapeutic response is achieved, then every 5 minutes during remaining IV infusion.
• Never leave the patient unattended during IV infusion.
• Plan to maintain the patient's B/P at 80 to 100 mm Hg in previously normotensive patients, and 30 to 40 mm Hg below preexisting B/P in previously hypertensive patients.
• Reduce IV infusion gradually, as prescribed. Avoid abrupt withdrawal.
• Check the peripherally inserted catheter IV site frequently for blanching, coldness, and hardness, and pallor to extremity, signs of extravasation.

Intervention and Evaluation
• Monitor the patient's IV flow rate diligently.
• Assess the patient for extravasation characterized by blanching of skin over vein, and mottling and coolness of the IV site extremity. If extravasation occurs, expect to infiltrate the affected area with 10 to 15 ml sterile saline containing 5 to 10 mg phentolamine. Know that phentolamine does not alter pressor effects of norepinephrine.
• Assess the patient's capillary refill, and the strength of his or her peripheral pulses, to monitor circulation.
• Monitor the patient's intake and output hourly, or as ordered. In patients with a urine output of less than 30 ml per hour, expect to stop the infusion unless the systolic B/P falls below 70 to 80 mm Hg.

Patient Teaching
• Instruct the patient to notify the nurse on duty immediately if he or she experiences burning, pain, or coolness at the IV site.

phenylephrine hydrochloride
fen-ill-**eh**-frin
(AK-Dilate, Isopto Frin [AUS], Neo-Synephrine, Prefrin)

CATEGORY AND SCHEDULE
Pregnancy Risk Category: C
OTC (nasal solution, nasal spray, ophthalmic solution)

MECHANISM OF ACTION
A sympathomimetic, alpha receptor stimulant that acts on the alpha-adrenergic receptors of vascular smooth muscle. *Therapeutic Effect:* Causes vasoconstriction of arterioles of nasal mucosa or conjunctiva, activates dilator muscle of the pupil to cause contraction, produces systemic arterial vasoconstriction.

PHARMACOKINETICS

Route	Onset	Peak	Duration
Subcuta-neous	10–15 min	N/A	1 hr
IM	10–15 min	N/A	0.5–2 hrs
IV	Immediate	N/A	15–20 min

Minimal absorption after intranasal, ophthalmic administration. Metabolized in liver, gastrointestinal (GI) tract. Primarily excreted in urine. **Half-life:** 2.5 hrs.

AVAILABILITY
Injection: 1% (10 mg/ml).
Nasal Solution: 0.25%, 0.5%.
Nasal Spray: 0.25%, 0.5%, 1%.
Ophthalmic Solution: 0.12%, 2.5%, 10%.

INDICATIONS AND DOSAGES
▸ **Nasal decongestant**
PO
Adults, Elderly, Children older than

12 yrs. 2–3 drops, 1–2 sprays of 0.25%–0.5% solution into each nostril.
Children 6–12 yrs. 2–3 drops or 1–2 sprays of 0.25% solution in each nostril.
Children younger than 6 yrs. 2–3 drops of 0.125% solution in each nostril. Repeat q4h as needed. Do not use for more than 3 days.

▸ **Conjunctival congestion, itching, and minor irritation, whitening of sclera**

Ophthalmic
Adults, Elderly, Children older than 12 yrs. 1–2 drops of 0.125% solution q3–4h.

▸ **Hypotension, shock**

IM/Subcutaneous
Adults, Elderly. 2–5 mg/dose q1–2h.
Children. 0.1 mg/kg/dose q1–2h.
IV bolus
Adults, Elderly. 0.1–0.5 mg/dose q10–15min as needed.
Children. 5–20 mcg/kg/dose q10–15min.
IV infusion
Adults, Elderly. 100–180 mcg/min.
Children. 0.1–0.5 mcg/kg/min. Titrate to desired effect.

CONTRAINDICATIONS

Acute pancreatitis, heart disease, hepatitis, narrow-angle glaucoma, pheochromocytoma, severe hypertension, thrombosis, ventricular tachycardia

INTERACTIONS
Drug

Beta-blockers: May have mutually inhibitory effects with beta-blockers.
Digoxin: May increase risk of arrhythmias with digoxin.
Ergonovine, oxytocin: May increase vasoconstriction.
MAOIs: May increase vasopressor effects.

Maprotiline, tricyclic antidepressants: May increase cardiovascular effects.
Methyldopa: May decrease effects of methyldopa.
Herbal
None known.
Food
None known.

DIAGNOSTIC TEST EFFECTS
None known.

IV INCOMPATIBILITIES
Thiopentothal (Pentothal)

IV COMPATIBILITIES
Amiodarone (Cordarone), dobutamine (Dobutrex), lidocaine, potassium chloride, propofol (Diprivan)

SIDE EFFECTS
Frequent
Nasal: Rebound nasal congestion due to overuse, especially when used longer than 3 days
Occasional
Mild CNS stimulation, such as restlessness, nervousness, tremors, headache, insomnia, particularly in those hypersensitive to sympathomimetics, such as elderly patients
Nasal: Stinging, burning, drying of nasal mucosa
Ophthalmic: Transient burning or stinging, brow ache, blurred vision

SERIOUS REACTIONS
• Large doses may produce tachycardia, palpitations, particularly in those with cardiac disease, lightheadedness, nausea, and vomiting.
• Overdosage in those older than

60 yrs may result in hallucinations, CNS depression, and seizures.
• Prolonged nasal use may produce chronic swelling of nasal mucosa and rhinitis.

NURSING CONSIDERATIONS
Baseline Assessment
• Be sure to obtain baseline vital signs, including apical heart rate and blood pressure.
• Check to see if the patient has irritation of nasal mucosa before administering nasal preparation.
Lifespan Considerations
• Be aware that phenylephrine crosses the placenta and is distributed in breast milk.
• Be aware that children may exhibit increased absorption and toxicity with nasal preparation.
• Know that there are no age-related precautions noted with systemic use in children.
• The elderly are more likely to experience adverse effects.
Precautions
• Use cautiously in patients with bradycardia, heart block, hyperthyroidism, and severe arteriosclerosis.
• If phenylephrine 10% ophthalmic is instilled into denuded or damaged corneal epithelium, know that corneal clouding may result.
Administration and Handling
Nasal
• Instruct the patient to blow his or her nose before giving the medication. Tilt back the patient's head and instill nasal solution drops in one nostril, as prescribed. Have the patient remain in the same position and wait 5 minutes before applying drops in other nostril.
• Administer nasal spray into each nostril with the patient's head erect.

Instruct the patient to sniff briskly while squeezing container, then wait 3 to 5 minutes before blowing nose gently.
• Rinse tip of spray bottle.
Ophthalmic
• Instruct patient to tilt head backward and look up.
• With a gloved finger, gently pull the patient's lower eyelid down to form a pouch and instill medication.
• Do not touch tip of applicator to eyelids or any surface.
• When lower eyelid is released, have patient keep eye open without blinking for at least 30 seconds.
• Apply gentle finger pressure to lacrimal sac, which is located at the bridge of the nose, inside corner of the eye, for 1 to 2 minutes.
• Remove excess solution around eye with tissue. Wash hands immediately to remove medication on hands.
IV
• Store vials at room temperature.
• For IV push, dilute 1 ml of 10 mg/ml solution with 9 ml sterile water for injection to provide a concentration of 1 mg/ml. Give over 20 to 30 seconds
• For IV infusion, dilute 10-mg vial with 500 ml D_5W or 0.9% NaCl to provide a concentration of 2 mcg/ml. Maximum concentration: 500 mg/250 ml. Titrate as prescribed
Intervention and Evaluation
• Monitor the patient's blood pressure (B/P) and heart rate.
Patient Teaching
• Tell the patient to discontinue the drug if adverse reactions occur.
• Instruct the patient not to use the drug for nasal decongestion longer than 3 to 5 days due to the risk of rebound congestion.

• Warn the patient to discontinue the drug if he or she experiences dizziness, feeling of irregular heartbeat, insomnia, tremor, or weakness.

• Tell the patient of the drug's common side effects with all preparations of the drug.

• Warn the patient to discontinue ophthalmic medication and notify the physician, if he or she experiences redness or swelling of eyelids or itching.

31 Miscellaneous Cardiovascular Agents

alfuzosin
  hydrochloride
alprostadil
  (prostaglandin E_1,
  PGE_1)
digoxin immune FAB
eplerenone
sodium polystyrene
  sulfonate
tamsulosin
  hydrochloride

Uses: Several miscellaneous agents are used primarily for their cardiovascular therapeutic effects. Although *alfuzosin and tamsulosin* are chemically related to other cardiovascular agents, they're used to improve urine flow and relieve symptoms of benign prostatic hypertrophy. *Alprostadil* is used to maintain patency of the ductus arteriosus until surgery can be performed; it's also used to treat erectile dysfunction. *Digoxin immune FAB* is used as an antidote for digoxin intoxication. *Eplerenone* may be used alone or with other antihypertensives to control hypertension. *Sodium polystyrene sulfonate* is used to correct hyperkalemia, which can cause serious or life-threatening arrhythmias.

Action: Each of the cardiovascular agents in this section acts in a different way. *Alfuzosin and tamsulosin* block $alpha_1$-adrenergic receptors in the lower urinary tract, causing relaxation of smooth muscle in the bladder neck and prostate. As a prostaglandin, *alprostadil* directly affects vascular and ductus arteriosus smooth muscle and relaxes trabecular smooth muscle. *Digoxin immune FAB* binds with digoxin molecules, preventing them from binding at their sites of action. *Eplerenone* binds to mineralocorticoid receptors in the kidneys, heart, blood vessels, and brain, blocking the binding of aldosterone. Because *sodium polystyrene sulfonate* is a cation exchange resin, it releases sodium ions in exchange primarily for potassium ions and promotes potassium excretion from the body; this action prevents serious complications, such as life-threatening arrhythmias.

alfuzosin hydrochloride
ale-few-**zoe**-sin
(Uroxatrel)

CATEGORY AND SCHEDULE
Pregnancy Risk Category: This drug is not indicated for use in women.

MECHANISM OF ACTION
An alpha$_1$ antagonist that targets receptors around bladder neck and prostate capsule. *Therapeutic Effect:* Results in relaxation of smooth muscle, improvement in urinary flow, symptoms of prostate hyperplasia.

PHARMACOKINETICS
Rapidly absorbed following PO administration. Widely distributed. Protein binding: 90%. Extensively metabolized in liver. Primarily excreted in urine. **Half-life:** 3–9 hrs.

AVAILABILITY
Tablets, extended-release: 10 mg

INDICATIONS AND DOSAGES
▸ **Benign prostatic hypertrophy**
PO
Adults. 10 mg once a day, approximately 30 min after same meal each day.

CONTRAINDICATIONS
History of hypersensitivity to alfuzosin

INTERACTIONS
Drug
Cimetidine: May increase alfuzosin blood concentration.
Other alpha blocking agents, such as doxazosin, prazosin, tamsulosin, and terazosin: May have additive effects.

Herbal
None known.
Food
None known.

DIAGNOSTIC TEST EFFECTS
None known.

SIDE EFFECTS
Frequent (7%–6%)
Dizziness, headache, malaise
Occasional (4%)
Dry mouth
Rare (3%–2%)
Nausea, dyspepsia, such as heartburn, and epigastric discomfort, diarrhea, orthostatic hypotension, tachycardia, drowsiness

SERIOUS REACTIONS
• Ischemia-related chest pain may occur rarely (2%).

NURSING CONSIDERATIONS
Baseline Assessment
• Determine the patient's sensitivity to alfuzosin and use of other alpha-blocking agents, including doxazosin, prazosin, tamsulosin, and terazosin.
Lifespan Considerations
• Be aware that alfuzosin is not indicated for use in women and children.
• There are no age-related precautions noted in the elderly.
Precautions
• Use cautiously in patients with coronary artery disease, hepatic impairment, and orthostatic hypotension.
• Use cautiously in patients under general anesthesia.
Administration and Handling
PO
• Give after the same meal each day. Do not chew or crush extended-release tablet.

Intervention and Evaluation
• Assist the patient with ambulation if he experiences dizziness.
• Warn the patient to notify the physician if he experiences headache.

Patient Teaching
• Instruct the patient to take alfuzosin after the same meal each day.
• Warn the patient to avoid performing tasks that require mental alertness or motor skills until his or her response to the drug is established.
• Teach the patient not to chew or crush extended-release tablets.

---

alprostadil (prostaglandin E₁; PGE₁)

ale-**pros**-tah-dill
(Caverject, Edex, Muse, Prostin VR Pediatric)

CATEGORY AND SCHEDULE
Pregnancy Risk Category: C

MECHANISM OF ACTION
A prostaglandin that directly effects vascular and ductus arteriosus smooth muscle and relaxes trabecular smooth muscle. *Therapeutic Effect:* Causes vasodilation; dilates cavernosal arteries, allowing blood flow to and entrapment in the lacunar spaces of the penis.

AVAILABILITY
Injection: 500 mcg/ml.
Powder for Injection: 10 mcg, 20 mcg, 40 mcg.
Urethral Pellet (Muse): 125 mcg, 250 mcg, 500 mcg, 1,000 mcg.

INDICATIONS AND DOSAGES
▸ **Maintain patency of ductus arteriosus**
IV infusion
Neonates. Initially, 0.05–0.1 mcg/kg/min. After therapeutic response achieved, use lowest dosage to maintain response. Maximum: 0.4 mcg/kg/min.
▸ **Impotence**
Pellet, Intracavernosal
Individualized.

UNLABELED USES
Treatment of atherosclerosis, gangrene, pain due to severe peripheral arterial occlusive disease

CONTRAINDICATIONS
Conditions predisposing to anatomic deformation of penis, hyaline membrane disease, penile implants, priapism, respiratory distress syndrome

INTERACTIONS
Drug
Anticoagulants, including heparin, thrombolytics: May increase risk of bleeding.
Sympathomimetics: May decrease effect of alprostadil.
Vasodilators: May increase risk of hypotension.
Herbal
None known.
Food
None known.

DIAGNOSTIC TEST EFFECTS
May increase blood bilirubin levels. May decrease glucose, serum calcium, and serum potassium.

IV INCOMPATIBILITIES
No information available via Y-site administration.

SIDE EFFECTS

Frequent

Intracavernosal (4%–1%): Penile pain (37%), prolonged erection, hypertension, local pain, penile fibrosis, injection site hematoma or ecchymosis, headache, respiratory infection, flu-like symptoms

Intraurethral (3%): Penile pain (36%), urethral pain or burning, testicular pain, urethral bleeding, headache, dizziness, respiratory infection, flu-like symptoms

Systemic (greater than 1%): Fever, seizures, flushing, bradycardia, hypotension, tachycardia, apnea, diarrhea, sepsis

Occasional

Intracavernosal (less than 1%): Hypotension, pelvic pain, back pain, dizziness, cough, nasal congestion

Intraurethral (less than 3%): Fainting, sinusitis, back and pelvic pain

Systemic (less than 1%): Jitteriness, lethargy, stiffness, arrhythmias, respiratory depression, anemia, bleeding, thrombocytopenia, hematuria

SERIOUS REACTIONS

• Overdosage occurs and is manifested as apnea, flushing of the face and arms, and bradycardia.

• Cardiac arrest and sepsis occur rarely.

NURSING CONSIDERATIONS

Precautions

• Use cautiously in patients with coagulation defects, leukemia, multiple myeloma, polycythemia, severe liver disease, sickle cell disease, or thrombocythemia.

Administration and Handling

◀ALERT▶ Doses greater than 40 mcg (Edex) or 60 mcg (Caverject) are not recommended.

• Urethral pellet

• Refrigerate pellet unless used within 14 days.

IV

◀ALERT▶ Give by continuous IV infusion or through umbilical artery catheter placed at ductal opening.

• Store the parenteral form in refrigerator.

• Dilute drug prior to administration. Prepare fresh dose every 24 hours and discard unused portions.

• Prepare continuous IV infusion by diluting 1 ml of alprostadil, containing 500-mcg, with D_5W or 0.9% NaCl to yield a solution containing 2 to 20 mcg/ml. Diluting volumes can range from 25 ml to 250 ml, depending on the patient and the available infusion device

• Infuse the lowest possible dose over the shortest possible time.

• Decrease the infusion rate immediately if a significant decrease in arterial pressure is noted via auscultation, Doppler transducer, or umbilical artery catheter.

• Discontinue the infusion immediately if signs and symptoms of overdosage, such as apnea or bradycardia, occur.

Intervention and Evaluation

• For patients with patent ductus arteriosus, monitor arterial pressure by auscultation, Doppler transducer, or umbilical artery catheter. Decrease the infusion rate immediately if a significant decrease in arterial pressure occurs. Expect to maintain continuous cardiac monitoring. Also, frequently assess the patient's heart sounds, femoral pulse (to monitor lower extremity circulation), and respiratory status.

• For patients with patent ductus arteriosus, monitor the patient for signs and symptoms of hypotension, assess blood pressure (B/P), arterial blood gas values, and temperature. If apnea or bradycardia occurs, discontinue infusion immediately and notify the physician.

Patient Teaching

• For patients with patent ductus arteriosus, explain to his or her parents the purpose of this palliative therapy.

• For patients with impotence, inform the patient that his erection should occur within 2 to 5 minutes of administration.

• For the patient with impotence, warn the patient not to use this drug if his female sexual partner is pregnant, unless the couple is using a condom barrier.

• For the patient with impotence, advise the patient to notify the physician if his erection lasts more than 4 hours or becomes painful.

digoxin immune FAB
(Digibind, DigiFab)

CATEGORY AND SCHEDULE
Pregnancy Risk Category: C

MECHANISM OF ACTION
An antidote that binds molecularly to digoxin in the extracellular space. *Therapeutic Effect:* Makes digoxin unavailable for binding at its site of action on cells in the body.

PHARMACOKINETICS

Route	Onset	Peak	Duration
IV	30 min	N/A	3–4 days

Widely distributed into extracellular space. Excreted in urine. **Half-life:** 15–20 hrs.

AVAILABILITY
Powder for Injection: 38-mg vial, 40 mg vial (DigiFab).

INDICATIONS AND DOSAGES
▸ **Treatment of potentially life-threatening digoxin overdose**
Dosage varies according to amount of digoxin to be neutralized. Refer to manufacturer's dosing guidelines.

CONTRAINDICATIONS
None known

INTERACTIONS
Drug
None known.
Herbal
None known.
Food
None known.

DIAGNOSTIC TEST EFFECTS
May alter serum potassium levels. Serum digoxin concentration may increase precipitously and persist for up to 1 wk until FAB/digoxin complex is eliminated from body.

IV INCOMPATIBILITIES
None known.

SIDE EFFECTS
None known

SERIOUS REACTIONS
• As result of digitalis toxicity, hyperkalemia may occur. Look for signs of diarrhea, paresthesia of extremities, heaviness of legs, decreased blood pressure (B/P), cold skin, grayish pallor, hypotension, mental confusion, irritability, flaccid paralysis, tented T waves, widening QRS, and ST depression.
• When effect of digitalis is reversed, hypokalemia may develop rapidly. Look for muscle cramping, nausea, vomiting, hypoactive bowel

sounds, abdominal distention, difficulty breathing, and postural hypotension.
• Rarely, low cardiac output and congestive heart failure (CHF) may occur.

NURSING CONSIDERATIONS

Baseline Assessment
• Obtain the patient's serum digoxin level before administering the drug. If the serum digoxin level was drawn less than 6 hours before the last digoxin dose, the serum digoxin level may be unreliable.
• Know that those with impaired renal function may require longer than 1 week before serum digoxin assay is reliable.
• Assess the patient's mental status and muscle strength.

Lifespan Considerations
• Be aware that it is unknown if digoxin immune FAB crosses the placenta or is distributed in breast milk.
• There are no age-related precautions noted in children.
• In the elderly, age-related renal impairment may require caution.

Precautions
• Use cautiously in patients with impaired cardiac or renal function.

Administration and Handling
IV
• Refrigerate vials.
• After reconstitution, solution is stable for 4 hours if refrigerated.
• Use immediately after reconstitution.
• Reconstitute each 38-mg vial with 4 ml sterile water for injection to provide a concentration of 9.5 mg/ml.
• Further dilute with 50 ml 0.9% NaCl.
• Infuse over 30 minutes. It is

recommended that the solution be infused through a 0.22-micron filter.
• If cardiac arrest is imminent, may give IV push.

Intervention and Evaluation
• Closely monitor the patient's B/P, electrocardiogram (EKG), serum potassium, and temperature during and after the drug is administered.
• Observe the patient for changes from the initial assessment. Hypokalemia may result in cardiac arrhythmias, changes in mental status, muscle cramps, muscle strength changes, or tremor. Hyponatremia may result in cold and clammy skin, confusion, and thirst.
• Assess for signs and symptoms of an arrhythmia, such as palpitations, or heart failure, such as dyspnea and edema, if the digoxin level falls below the therapeutic level.

Patient Teaching
• Before discharge, review the digoxin dosages carefully with the patient, and make sure he or she knows how to take the drug as prescribed.
• Instruct the patient about any follow-up care, including serum digoxin levels.
• Make sure the patient knows the signs and symptoms of digoxin toxicity, including anorexia, nausea, and vomiting, as well as visual changes.

eplerenone
eh-**pleh**-reh-known
(Inspra)

CATEGORY AND SCHEDULE
Pregnancy Risk Category: B

MECHANISM OF ACTION
An aldosterone receptor antagonist that binds to the mineralocorticoid

receptors in the kidney, heart, blood vessels, brain, blocking the binding of aldosterone. *Therapeutic Effect:* Reduces blood pressure (B/P).

PHARMACOKINETICS

Absorption unaffected by food. Protein binding: 50%. No active metabolites. Not removed by hemodialysis. Excreted in the urine with a lesser amount eliminated in the feces. **Half-life:** 4–6 hrs.

AVAILABILITY

Tablets: 25 mg, 50 mg, 100 mg.

INDICATIONS AND DOSAGES

▸ **Hypertension**
PO
Adults, Elderly. 50 mg once a day. If 50 mg once a day presents an inadequate B/P response, may increase dosage to 50 mg twice a day. If patient is on concurrent erythromycin, saquinavir, verapamil, or fluconazole, reduce initial dose to 25 mg once a day.

CONTRAINDICATIONS

Patients with concurrent use of potassium supplements or potassium-sparing diuretics, such as amiloride, spironolactone, triamterene, or strong inhibitors of the cytochrome P450 3A4 enzyme system, including ketoconazole and itraconazole, creatinine clearance less than 50 ml/min, serum creatinine greater than 2 mg/dL in males or greater than 1.8 mg/dL in females, serum potassium greater than 5.5 mEq/L, type 2 diabetes mellitus with microalbuminuria

INTERACTIONS

Drug
Angiotensin II antagonists, angiotensin-converting enzyme (ACE) inhibitors, erythromycin,
fluconazole, saquinavir, verapamil: Increases risk of hyperkalemia.
Herbal
St. John's wort: Decreases eplerenone effectiveness.
Food
Grapefruit juice: Produces small increase in potassium level.

DIAGNOSTIC TEST EFFECTS

May increase serum potassium levels. May decrease serum sodium levels.

SIDE EFFECTS

Rare (3%–1%)
Dizziness, diarrhea, cough, fatigue, influenza-like symptoms, abdominal pain

SERIOUS REACTIONS

• Hyperkalemia may occur, particularly in patients with type 2 diabetes mellitus and microalbuminuria.

NURSING CONSIDERATIONS

Baseline Assessment
• Obtain the patient's apical heart rate and B/P immediately before each dose, in addition to regular monitoring. Be alert to B/P fluctuations. If an excessive reduction in B/P occurs, place the patient in the supine position with feet slightly elevated, and notify the physician.
Lifespan Considerations
• Be aware that it is unknown if eplerenone crosses the placenta or is distributed in breast milk.
• Be aware that the safety and efficacy of eplerenone have not been established in children.
• There are no age-related precautions noted in the elderly.
Precautions
• Use cautiously in patients with hyperkalemia and liver function impairment.

Administration and Handling
Do not break, crush, or chew film-coated tablets.
Intervention and Evaluation
• Assist the patient with ambulation, if he or she experiences dizziness.
• Monitor the patient's serum potassium and sodium levels.
• Assess the patient's B/P for hypertension or hypotension.
• Assess the patient's pattern of daily bowel activity and stool consistency.
• Evaluate the patient for evidence of flu-like symptoms.
Patient Teaching
• Warn the patient to avoid tasks that require mental alertness or motor skills until his or her response to the drug is established.
• Explain to the patient that he or she will need to take eplerenone for lifelong control.
• Tell the patient not to break, crush, or chew film-coated tablets
• Caution the patient against exercising outside during hot weather because of the risks of dehydration and hypotension.

sodium polystyrene sulfonate
(Kayexalate, Resonium A[AUS], SPS)

CATEGORY AND SCHEDULE
Pregnancy Risk Category: C

MECHANISM OF ACTION
An ion exchange resin that releases sodium ions in exchange primarily for potassium ions. *Therapeutic Effect:* Removes potassium from the blood and into the intestine so it can be expelled from the body.

AVAILABILITY
Suspension: 15 g/60 ml.
Powder.

INDICATIONS AND DOSAGES
▸ **Hyperkalemia**
PO
Adults, Elderly. 60 ml (15 g) 1–4 times/day.
Children. 1 g/kg/dose q6h.
Rectal
Adults, Elderly. 30–50 g as needed q6h.
Children. 1 g/kg/dose q2–6h.

CONTRAINDICATIONS
Hypernatremia, intestinal obstruction or perforation

INTERACTIONS
Drug
Cation-donating antacids, laxatives (e.g., magnesium hydroxide): May decrease effect of sodium polystyrene sulfonate, and cause systemic alkalosis in patients with renal impairment.
Herbal
None known.
Food
None known.

DIAGNOSTIC TEST EFFECTS
May decrease serum calcium and magnesium levels.

SIDE EFFECTS
Frequent
High dosage: Anorexia, nausea, vomiting, constipation
High dosage in elderly: Fecal impaction, characterized by severe stomach pain with nausea or vomiting
Occasional
Diarrhea, sodium retention, marked by decreased urination, peripheral edema, and increased weight

SERIOUS REACTIONS

• Serious potassium deficiency may occur. Early signs of hypokalemia include confusion, delayed thought processes, extreme weakness, irritability, and EKG changes, including prolonged QT interval, widening, flattening, or inversion of T wave, and prominent U waves.

• Hypocalcemia, manifested by abdominal or muscle cramps, occurs occasionally.

• Arrhythmias and severe muscle weakness may be noted.

NURSING CONSIDERATIONS

Baseline Assessment

• Keep in mind that sodium polystyrene sulfonate does not rapidly correct severe hyperkalemia; it may take hours to days. Consider other measures, such as dialysis, IV glucose and insulin, IV calcium, and IV sodium bicarbonate to correct severe hyperkalemia in a medical emergency.

Lifespan Considerations

• Be aware that it is unknown if sodium polystyrene sulfonate crosses the placenta or is distributed in breast milk.

• Know that there are no age-related precautions noted in children.

• The elderly may be at increased risk of fecal impaction.

Precautions

• Use cautiously in patients with edema, hypertension, and severe congestive heart failure (CHF).

Administration and Handling

PO

• Give with 20 to 100 ml sorbitol to aid in potassium removal, facilitate passage of resin through intestinal tract, and prevent constipation.

• Do not mix this drug with foods, liquids containing potassium.

Rectal

• After initial cleansing enema, insert large rubber tube well into sigmoid colon and tape in place.

• Introduce suspension with 100 ml sorbitol by gravity.

• Flush with 50 to 100 ml fluid and clamp.

• Retain for several hours, if possible.

• Irrigate colon with a non–sodium-containing solution to remove resin.

Intervention and Evaluation

• Monitor the patient's potassium levels frequently.

• Assess the patient's clinical condition and EKG, which is valuable in determining when treatment should be discontinued.

• In addition to checking serum potassium levels, monitor serum calcium and magnesium levels.

• Assess the patient's pattern of daily bowel activity and stool consistency. Remember that fecal impaction may occur in patients receiving high dosages of sodium polystyrene sulfonate, particularly the elderly.

Patient Teaching

• Instruct the patient to drink the entire amount of the resin for best results.

• Explain that if the resin is given rectally, he or she should try to avoid expelling the solution, and to try retain the solution for several hours, if possible.

• Instruct the patient about which foods are rich in potassium. Plan to consult a dietician to provide dietary counseling.

tamsulosin hydrochloride

tam-sul-**owe**-sin
(Flomax)
Do not confuse with Fosamax or Volmax.

CATEGORY AND SCHEDULE
Pregnancy Risk Category: B (Not indicated for use in women.)

MECHANISM OF ACTION
An alpha$_1$ antagonist that targets receptors around bladder neck and prostate capsule. *Therapeutic Effect:* Results in relaxation of smooth muscle with improvement in urinary flow, symptoms of prostate hyperplasia.

PHARMACOKINETICS
Well absorbed after PO administration. Protein binding: 94%–99%. Widely distributed. Metabolized in liver. Primarily excreted in urine. Unknown if removed by hemodialysis. **Half-life:** 9–13 hrs.

AVAILABILITY
Capsules: 0.4 mg.

INDICATIONS AND DOSAGES
▶ **Treat symptoms of benign prostatic hyperplasia**
PO
Adults. 0.4 mg once a day, approximately 30 min after same meal each day. May increase dosage if inadequate response in 2–4 wks.

CONTRAINDICATIONS
History of sensitivity to tamsulosin

INTERACTIONS
Drug
Other alpha-adrenergic blocking agents (i.e. cimetidine, doxazosin,
prazosin, terazosin): May have additive effects.
Warfarin: May alter the effects of warfarin.
Herbal
None known.
Food
None known.

DIAGNOSTIC TEST EFFECTS
None known.

SIDE EFFECTS
Frequent (9%–7%)
Dizziness, drowsiness
Occasional (5%–3%)
Headache, anxiety, insomnia, postural hypotension
Rare (less than 2%)
Nasal congestion, pharyngitis, rhinitis, nausea, vertigo, impotence

SERIOUS REACTIONS
• First-dose syncope, hypotension with sudden loss of consciousness (LOC) may occur within 30 to 90 minutes after giving the initial drug dose. First-dose syncope may be preceded by tachycardia (pulse rate 120–160 beats/min).

NURSING CONSIDERATIONS
Baseline Assessment
• Determine if the patient is hypersensitive to tamsulosin and uses other alpha-adrenergic blocking agents or warfarin.
Lifespan Considerations
• Be aware that tamsulosin is not indicated for use in women or children.
• There are no age-related precautions noted in the elderly.
Precautions
• Use cautiously in patients with renal function impairment.
Administration and Handling
PO

• Give at the same time each day, 30 minutes after the same meal.
• Do not crush or open capsule unless directed by physician.

Intervention and Evaluation
• Assist the patient with ambulation if he experiences dizziness.
• Monitor the patient's B/P and renal function.

Patient Teaching
• Instruct the patient to take tamsulosin at the same time each day, 30 minutes after the same meal. Teach the patient not to chew, crush, or open the capsules.
• Advise the patient to use caution when getting up from a sitting or lying position.
• Warn the patient to avoid tasks that require mental alertness or motor skills until his response to the drug is established.

32 Antianxiety Agents

alprazolam
buspirone
  hydrochloride
chlordiazepoxide
clorazepate
  dipotassium
diazepam
doxepin hydrochloride
hydroxyzine
lorazepam
midazolam
  hydrochloride
oxazepam

Uses: Antianxiety agents are used to treat anxiety. In addition, some benzodiazepines are used as hypnotics to induce sleep, as anticonvulsants to prevent delirium tremors during alcohol withdrawal, and as adjunctive therapy for relaxation of skeletal muscle spasms. Midazolam, a short-acting benzodiazepine, is used for preoperative sedation and relief of anxiety in short diagnostic endoscopic procedures.

Action: Although the exact mechanism of action is unknown, antianxiety agents may increase the inhibiting effect of gamma-aminobutyric acid (GABA), an inhibitory neurotransmitter. Benzodiazepines, the largest and most frequently prescribed group of antianxiety agents, may inhibit nerve impulse transmission by binding to specific benzodiazepine receptors in various areas of the central nervous system. (See illustration, *Mechanism of Action: Benzodiazepines*, page 610.)

COMBINATION PRODUCTS
LIBRAX: chlordiazepoxide/clidinium (an anticholinergic) 5 mg/2.5 mg.
LIMBITROL: chlordiazepoxide/amitriptyline (an antidepressant) 5 mg/12.5 mg; 10 mg/25 mg.

alprazolam
ale-**praz**-oh-lam
(Apo-Alpraz[CAN], Kalma[AUS], Novo-Alprazol[CAN], Xanax, Xanax XR)
Do not confuse with lorazepam, Tenex, or Zantac.

CATEGORY AND SCHEDULE
Pregnancy Risk Category: D
Controlled Substance: Schedule IV

MECHANISM OF ACTION
A benzodiazepine that acts as an antianxiety agent by enhancing the action of inhibitory neurotransmitters in the brain. *Therapeutic Effect*: Produces anxiolytic effect from its central nervous system (CNS) depressant action.

PHARMACOKINETICS
Well absorbed from gastrointestinal (GI) tract. Protein binding: 80%. Metabolized in liver. Primarily excreted in urine. Minimal removal by hemodialysis. **Half-life:** 11–16 hrs.

AVAILABILITY
Tablets: 0.25 mg, 0.5 mg, 1 mg, 2 mg.
Tablets (extended release): 0.5 mg, 1 mg, 2 mg, 3 mg.
Oral Solution: 1 mg/ml.

INDICATIONS AND DOSAGES
▶ Anxiety disorders
PO
Adults (older than 18 yrs). Initially,

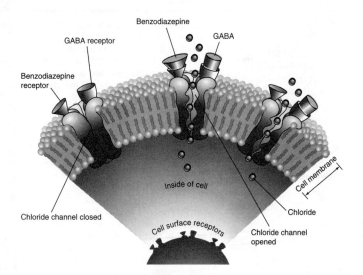

Benzodiazepines reduce anxiety by stimulating the action of the inhibitory neurotransmitter, gamma-aminobutyric acid (GABA), in the limbic system. The limbic system plays an important role in the regulation of human behavior. Dysfunction of GABA neurotransmission in the limbic system may be linked to the development of certain anxiety disorders.

The limbic system contains a highly dense area of benzodiazepine receptors that may be linked to the antianxiety effects of benzodiazepines. These benzodiazepine receptors are located on the surface of neuronal cell membranes and are adjacent to receptors for GABA. The binding of a benzodiazepine to its receptor enhances the affinity of a GABA receptor for GABA. In the absence of a benzodiazepine, the binding of GABA to its receptor causes the chloride channel in the cell membrane to open, which increases the influx of chloride into the cell. This influx of chloride results in hyperpolarization of the neuronal cell membrane and reduces the neuron's ability to fire, which is why GABA is considered an inhibitory neurotransmitter. A benzodiazepine acts only in the presence of GABA and when it binds to a benzodiazepine receptor, the time the chloride channel remains open is prolonged. This results in greater depression of neuronal function and a reduction in anxiety.

0.25–0.5 mg 3 times/day. Titrate to maximum of 4 mg/day in divided doses.
Elderly, debilitated, liver disease, low serum albumin. Initially, 0.25 mg 2–3 times/day. Gradually increase to optimum therapeutic response.

▸ **Panic disorder**
PO
Adults. Initially, 0.5 mg 3 times/day. May increase at 3- to 4-day intervals at no more than 1 mg/day. Range: 1–10 mg/day.
Elderly. Initially, 0.125–0.25 mg 2 times/day; may increase in

0.125-mg increments until desired
effect attained.
▸ **Panic attack (extended release)**
PO
Adults, Elderly. 0.5–1 mg once a
day. May increase every 3–4 days
up to a maximum of 10 mg/day.
▸ **Premenstrual syndrome**
PO
Adults. 0.25 mg 3 times/day.

UNLABELED USES
Improves mood, prevents insomnia,
and relieves cramps related to
premenstrual syndrome; management of irritable bowel syndrome

CONTRAINDICATIONS
Acute alcohol intoxication with
depressed vital signs, acute narrow-
angle glaucoma, concurrent use of
itraconazole or ketoconazole, myasthenia gravis, severe chronic obstructive pulmonary disease (COPD)

INTERACTIONS
Drug
*Central nervous system (CNS)
depressants, including alcohol:*
Potentiates effects of alprazolam.
*Fluvoxamine, ketoconazole,
nefazodone:* May inhibit liver me-
tabolism and increase alprazolam
blood serum concentrations.
Herbal
Kava kava, valerian: May increase
CNS depressant effect of alpra-
zolam.
Food
Grapefruit juice: May inhibit alpra-
zolam's metabolism.

DIAGNOSTIC TEST EFFECTS
None known.

SIDE EFFECTS
Frequent
Muscular incoordination (ataxia),
lightheadedness, transient mild

drowsiness, slurred speech (particularly in elderly or debilitated patients)
Occasional
Confusion, depression, blurred
vision, constipation, diarrhea, dry
mouth, headache, nausea
Rare
Behavioral problems such as anger,
impaired memory, paradoxical
reactions such as insomnia, nervousness, or irritability

SERIOUS REACTIONS
• Abrupt or too rapid withdrawal
may result in pronounced restlessness, irritability, insomnia, hand
tremors, abdominal and muscle
cramps, sweating, vomiting, and
seizures.
• Overdosage results in somnolence,
confusion, diminished reflexes, and
coma.
• Blood dyscrasias have been reported rarely.

NURSING CONSIDERATIONS
Baseline Assessment
• Offer emotional support to the
anxious patient.
• Assess the patient's motor responses to note any agitation, tension, or trembling and check autonomic responses to detect cold or
clammy hands and sweating.
Lifespan Considerations
• Be aware that alprazolam crosses
the placenta and is distributed in
breast milk.
• Chronic ingestion of alprazolam
during pregnancy may produce
withdrawal symptoms in women
and CNS depression in neonates.
• Be aware that the safety and
efficacy of alprazolam have not
been established in children.
• In the elderly, use small initial
doses and gradually increase them

to avoid excessive sedation or ataxia as evidenced by muscular incoordination.

Precautions
• Use cautiously in patients with impaired renal or liver function.

Administration and Handling
PO
• May be given without regard to meals.
• Tablets may be crushed.

Intervention and Evaluation
• Expect to perform blood tests periodically to assess hepatic and renal function in those patients receiving long-term therapy.
• Assess the patient for a paradoxical reaction, particularly during early therapy.
• Evaluate the patient to determine if medication administration has resulted in the desired therapeutic response manifested as a calm facial expression, decreased insomnia, and decreased restlessness.

Patient Teaching
• Advise the patient that the drowsiness caused by the drug usually disappears during continued therapy.
• Instruct the patient that if dizziness occurs, to change positions slowly from horizontal, to sitting, then standing.
• Warn the patient to avoid tasks that require mental alertness or motor skills until his or her response to the drug is established.
• Encourage the patient to stop smoking and explain that smoking reduces alprazolam's effectiveness.
• Inform the patient that sour hard candy, gum, or sips of tepid water may relieve dry mouth.
• Caution the patient not to abruptly withdraw medication after long-term therapy.
• Urge the patient to avoid alcohol.
• Explain to the patient not to take other medications, including over-the-counter (OTC) drugs, without consulting the physician.

buspirone hydrochloride
byew-spear-own
(BuSpar, Buspirex[CAN], Bustab[CAN])
Do not confuse with bupropion.

CATEGORY AND SCHEDULE
Pregnancy Risk Category: B

MECHANISM OF ACTION
Although the exact mechanism of action is unknown, this nonbarbiturate is thought to bind to serotonin and dopamine receptors in the central nervous system (CNS). The drug may also increase norepinephrine metabolism in the locus ceruleus. *Therapeutic Effect:* Produces antianxiety effect.

PHARMACOKINETICS
Rapidly, completely absorbed from the gastrointestinal (GI) tract. Protein binding: 95%. Undergoes extensive first-pass metabolism. Metabolized in liver to active metabolite. Primarily excreted in urine. Not removed by hemodialysis. **Half-life:** 2–3 hrs.

AVAILABILITY
Tablets: 5 mg, 7.5 mg, 10 mg, 15 mg, 30 mg.

INDICATIONS AND DOSAGES
▶ **Short-term management, up to 4 wks of anxiety disorders**
PO
Adults. 5 mg 2–3 times a day or 7.5 mg 2 times/day. May increase in 5-mg increments/day at intervals of 2–4 days. Maintenance: 15–30

mg/day in 2–3 divided doses. Do not exceed 60 mg/day.
Elderly. Initially, 5 mg 2 times/day. May increase by 5 mg q2–3 days. Maximum: 60 mg.
Children. Initially, 5 mg/day. May increase by 5 mg/day at weekly intervals. Maximum: 60 mg/day.

UNLABELED USES
Management of panic attack, symptoms of premenstrual syndrome (PMS), including aches, pain, fatigue, irritability.

CONTRAINDICATIONS
MAOI therapy, severe liver or renal impairment

INTERACTIONS
Drug
Alcohol, CNS depressants: May increase sedation.
Erythromycin, itraconazole: May increase buspirone blood concentration and risk of toxicity.
MAOIs: May increase blood pressure (B/P).
Herbal
Kava kava: May increase sedation.
Food
Grapefruit and grapefruit juice: May increase buspirone blood concentration and risk of toxicity.

DIAGNOSTIC TEST EFFECTS
None known.

SIDE EFFECTS
Frequent (12%–6%)
Dizziness, drowsiness, nausea, headache
Occasional (5%–2%)
Nervousness, fatigue, insomnia, dry mouth, lightheadedness, mood swings, blurred vision, poor concentration, diarrhea, numbness in hands and feet

Rare
Muscle pain and stiffness, nightmares, chest pain, involuntary movements

SERIOUS REACTIONS
• There is no evidence of tolerance or psychological and physical dependence or withdrawal syndrome.
• Overdosage may produce severe nausea, vomiting, dizziness, drowsiness, abdominal distention, and excessive pupil contraction.

NURSING CONSIDERATIONS
Baseline Assessment
• Offer emotional support to the anxious patient.
• Assess the patient's autonomic responses, such as cold, clammy hands; sweating and motor responses, including agitation, trembling, tension.
Lifespan Considerations
• Be aware that it is unknown if buspirone crosses the placenta or is distributed in breast milk.
• Be aware that the safety and efficacy of buspirone have not been established in children.
• There are no age-related precautions noted in the elderly.
Precautions
• Use cautiously in patients with liver or renal impairment.
Administration and Handling
PO
• Give buspirone without regard to meals.
• Crush tablets as needed.
Intervention and Evaluation
• Plan to perform blood tests periodically to assess hepatic and renal function in patients on long-term therapy.
• Assist the patient with ambulation if he or she experiences drowsiness or lightheadedness.

• Evaluate the patient for a therapeutic response, including a calm facial expression and decreased restlessness and insomnia.

Patient Teaching

• Explain to the patient that improvement may be noted in 7–10 days, but optimum therapeutic effect generally takes 3–4 weeks to appear.
• Tell the patient that drowsiness usually disappears during continued therapy.
• Instruct the patient to change position slowly from recumbent to sitting position before standing to avoid dizziness.
• Warn the patient to avoid tasks that require mental alertness and motor skills until his or her response to buspirone is established.
• Caution the patient not to take the drug with grapefruit juice. Explain that grapefruit may increase carbamazepine absorption and blood concentration.

chlordiazepoxide

klor-dye-az-eh-**pox**-eyd
(Apo-Chlordiazepoxide[CAN], Librium, Lipoxide, Libritabs, Novopoxide[CAN])

CATEGORY AND SCHEDULE
Pregnancy Risk Category: D

MECHANISM OF ACTION
A benzodiazepine that enhances action of gamma aminobutyric acid (GABA) neurotransmission in the central nervous system (CNS). *Therapeutic Effect:* Produces anxiolytic effect.

AVAILABILITY
Capsules: 5 mg, 10 mg, 25 mg.
Tablets: 25 mg.

INDICATIONS AND DOSAGES
▶ **Alcohol withdrawal symptoms**
PO
Adults, Elderly. 50–100 mg. May repeat q2–4h. Maximum: 300 mg/24 hrs.
▶ **Anxiety**
PO
Adults. 15–100 mg/day in 3–4 divided doses.
Elderly. 5 mg 2–4 times/day.

UNLABELED USES
Treatment of panic disorder, tension headache, tremors

CONTRAINDICATIONS
Acute alcohol intoxication, acute narrow-angle glaucoma

INTERACTIONS
Drug
Alcohol, CNS depressants: May increase CNS depressant effect.
Herbal
Kava kava, valerian: May increase CNS depression.
Food
None known.

DIAGNOSTIC TEST EFFECTS
None known. Therapeutic serum level is 1–3 mcg/ml; toxic serum level is greater than 5 mcg/ml.

SIDE EFFECTS
Frequent
Pain with IM injection; drowsiness, ataxia, dizziness, confusion with oral dose, particularly in elderly, debilitated
Occasional
Rash, peripheral edema, gastrointestinal (GI) disturbances
Rare
Paradoxical CNS hyperactivity or nervousness in children, excitement/restlessness in elderly (generally noted during first 2 wks of therapy,

particularly noted in presence of uncontrolled pain)

SERIOUS REACTIONS
• IV route may produce pain, swelling, thrombophlebitis, and carpal tunnel syndrome.
• Abrupt or too rapid withdrawal may result in pronounced restlessness, irritability, insomnia, hand tremors, abdominal or muscle cramps, sweating, vomiting, and seizures.
• Overdosage results in somnolence, confusion, diminished reflexes, and coma.

NURSING CONSIDERATIONS
Baseline Assessment
• Assess the patient's B/P, pulse, and respirations immediately before giving chlordiazepoxide.
• Expect the patient to remain recumbent for up to 3 hrs after parenteral administration to reduce the drug's hypotensive effect.
Precautions
• Use cautiously in patients with impaired liver or kidney function.
Administration and Handling
◀ALERT▶ Expect to use the smallest effective chlordiazepoxide dosage in elderly or debilitated and patients with liver disease or low serum albumin.
Intervention and Evaluation
• Assess the patient's autonomic responses, such as cold or clammy hands, sweating, and motor responses, including agitation, trembling, and tension.
• Examine pediatric and elderly patients for paradoxical reaction, particularly during early therapy.
• Assist the patient with ambulation if he or she experiences ataxia or drowsiness.

• Know that the therapeutic serum level for chlordiazepoxide is 1–3 mcg/ml, and the toxic serum level of chlordiazepoxide is greater than 5 mcg/ml.
Patient Teaching
• Tell the patient that he or she may experience discomfort with IM injection.
• Explain to the patient that drowsiness usually disappears during continued therapy.
• Instruct the patient to change positions slowly from recumbent to sitting before standing if the patient experiences dizziness.
• Urge the patient to stop smoking tobacco products. Explain to the patient that smoking reduces the drug's effectiveness.
• Warn the patient to avoid alcohol consumption while taking this drug.
• Caution the patient not to abruptly discontinue the medication after long-term therapy.

clorazepate dipotassium
klor-**az**-eh-payt
(Novoclopate[CAN], Tranxene)
Do not confuse with clofibrate.

CATEGORY AND SCHEDULE
Pregnancy Risk Category: D

MECHANISM OF ACTION
A benzodiazepine that depresses all levels of the CNS, including limbic and reticular formation, by binding to benzodiazepine site on the GABA receptor complex. Modulates GABA, which is a major inhibitory neurotransmitter in the brain. *Therapeutic Effect:* Produces anxiolytic effect, suppresses seizure activity.

AVAILABILITY
Capsules: 3.75 mg, 7.5 mg, 15 mg.
Tablets: 3.75 mg, 7.5 mg, 15 mg.
Tablets (single dose): 11.5 mg, 22.5 mg.

INDICATIONS AND DOSAGES
▶ **Anxiety**
PO
Adults. 30 mg a day in divided doses or single dose at bedtime.
Elderly, debilitated. 7.5–15 mg in divided doses or single bedtime dose. Daily dose range: 15–60 mg.
▶ **Partial seizures**
PO
Adults, Children older than 12 yrs. Initially, up to 7.5 mg 3 times a day. Do not increase dosage more than 7.5 mg/wk or exceed 90 mg/day.
Children 9–12 yrs. 3.75–7.5 mg/dose 2 times/day. Maximum: 60 mg/day in 2–3 divided doses.
▶ **Alcohol withdrawal**
PO
Adults, Elderly. Initially, 30 mg, then 15 mg 2–4 times/day on first day. Maximum: 90 mg/day. Gradually decrease dosage over subsequent days.

CONTRAINDICATIONS
Acute narrow-angle glaucoma

INTERACTIONS
Drug
Alcohol, central nervous system (CNS) depressants: May increase CNS depressant effect.
Herbal
Kava kava, valerian: May increase CNS depression.
Food
None known.

DIAGNOSTIC TEST EFFECTS
None known. Therapeutic serum level is Peak: 0.12–1.5 mcg/ml; toxic serum level is greater than 5 mcg/ml.

SIDE EFFECTS
Frequent
Drowsiness
Occasional
Dizziness, gastrointestinal (GI) disturbances, nervousness, blurred vision, dry mouth, headache, confusion, ataxia, rash, irritability, slurred speech
Rare
Paradoxical CNS hyperactivity or nervousness in children, excitement or restlessness in the elderly or debilitated. Symptoms are generally noted during first 2 wks of therapy, particularly in presence of uncontrolled pain.

SERIOUS REACTIONS
• Abrupt or too rapid withdrawal may result in pronounced restlessness, irritability, insomnia, hand tremors, abdominal or muscle cramps, sweating, vomiting, and seizures.
• Overdosage results in somnolence, confusion, diminished reflexes, and coma.

NURSING CONSIDERATIONS
Baseline Assessment
• In anxiety patients, assess autonomic response, such as cold or clammy hands, sweating, and motor response, including agitation, trembling, and tension.
• Offer emotional support to the anxious patient.
• In the seizure patient, review the patient's history of seizure disorder, including the duration, intensity, frequency, and his or her level of consciousness (LOC).
• Observe the patient frequently for

recurrence of seizure activity. Initiate seizure precautions.

Precautions

• Use cautiously in patients with acute alcohol intoxication and impaired liver or renal function.

Administration and Handling

◀ALERT▶ When replacement by another anticonvulsant is necessary, plan to decrease clorazepate gradually as therapy begins with low-replacement dosage.

Intervention and Evaluation

• Assess the patient for paradoxical reaction, particularly during early therapy.

• Assist the patient with ambulation if he or she experiences dizziness and drowsiness.

• Evaluate the patient for therapeutic response. Keep in mind that in anxious patients, the therapeutic response is a calm facial expression and decreased restlessness. In patients with seizure disorder, the therapeutic response is a decrease in intensity or frequency of seizures.

• Monitor the patient's serum level of the drug. Peak therapeutic serum level is 0.12–1.5 mcg/ml; toxic serum level is greater than 5 mcg/ml.

Patient Teaching

• Caution the patient against abruptly withdrawing the medication after long-term use as this may precipitate seizures.

• Explain to the patient that strict maintenance of drug therapy is essential for seizure control.

• Tell the patient that drowsiness usually disappears during continued therapy.

• Warn the patient to avoid tasks that require mental alertness or motor skills until his or her response to the drug is established.

• Instruct the patient to change positions slowly from recumbent to sitting position before standing, if the patient experiences dizziness.

• Urge the patient to stop smoking tobacco products and to avoid alcohol during clorazepate therapy. Explain to the patient that smoking reduces the drug's effectiveness.

diazepam
dye-**az**-eh-pam
(Antenex[AUS], Apo-Diazepam[CAN], Diastat, Diazemuls[CAN], Dizac, Ducene[AUS],Valium, Valpam[AUS], Vivol [CAN])
Do not confuse with diazoxide, Ditropan, or Valcyte.

CATEGORY AND SCHEDULE
Pregnancy Risk Category: D
Controlled Substance: Schedule IV

MECHANISM OF ACTION
A benzodiazepine that depresses all levels of the central nervous system (CNS) by binding to the benzodiazepine receptor on the GABA receptor complex, a major inhibitory neurotransmitter in the brain. *Therapeutic Effect:* Produces anxiolytic effect, elevates seizure threshold, produces skeletal muscle relaxation.

PHARMACOKINETICS

Route	Onset	Peak	Duration
PO	30 min	1–2 hrs	2–3 hrs
IM	15 min	30–90 min	30–90 min
IV	1–5 min	15 min	15–60 min

Well absorbed from the gastrointestinal (GI) tract. Widely distributed. Protein binding: 98%. Metabolized in liver to active metabolite. Excreted in urine. Minimally removed by hemodialysis. **Half-life**: 20–70 hrs, half-life is increased in elderly, liver dysfunction.

AVAILABILITY
Tablets: 2 mg, 5 mg, 10 mg.
Capsules (sustained-release): 15 mg.
Oral Solution: 5 mg/5 ml.
Injection: 5 mg/ml.
Injectable Emulsion: 5 mg/ml.
Rectal Gel: 2.5 mg, 10 mg, 15 mg, 20 mg.

INDICATIONS AND DOSAGES
▸ **Anxiety, skeletal muscle relaxant**
PO
Adults. 2–10 mg 2–4 times/day.
Elderly. 2.5 mg 2 times/day.
Children. 0.12–0.8 mg/kg/day in divided doses q6–8h.
IM/IV
Adults. 2–10 mg; repeat in 3–4 hrs.
Children. 0.04–0.3 mg/kg/dose q2–4h. Maximum: 0.5 mg/kg in an 8-hr period.
▸ **Preanesthesia**
IV
Adults, Elderly. 5–15 mg 5–10 min before procedure.
Children. 0.2–0.3 mg/kg.
Maximum: 10 mg.
▸ **Alcohol withdrawal**
PO
Adults, Elderly. 10 mg 3–4 times during first 24 hrs, then reduce to 5–10 mg 3–4 times/day as needed.
IM/IV
Adults, Elderly. Initially, 10 mg, followed by 5–10 mg q3–4h.
▸ **Status epilepticus**
IV
Adults, Elderly. 5–10 mg q10–15min up to 30 mg/8 hrs.
Children 5 yrs and older. 0.05–0.3 mg/kg/dose q15–30min. Maximum total dose: 10 mg.
Children older than 1 mo to younger than 5 yrs. 0.05–0.3 mg/kg/

dose q15–30min. Maximum total dose: 5 mg.
▸ **Control of increased seizure activity in refractory epilepsy in those on stable regimens**
Rectal gel
Adults, Children 12 yrs and older. 0.2 mg/kg.
Children 6–11 yrs. 0.3 mg/kg.
Children 2–5 yrs. 0.5 mg/kg. Dose may be repeated in 4–12 hrs.

UNLABELED USES
Treatment of panic disorders, tension headache, tremors

CONTRAINDICATIONS
Comatose patient, narrow-angle glaucoma, preexisting CNS depression, respiratory depression, severe uncontrolled pain

INTERACTIONS
Drug
Alcohol, CNS depressants: May increase CNS depressant effect.
Herbal
Kava kava, valerian: May increase CNS depressant effects.
Food
None known.

DIAGNOSTIC TEST EFFECTS
May produce abnormal renal function tests and elevate serum LDH concentration, serum alkaline phosphatase, serum bilirubin, SGOT (AST), and SGPT (ALT) levels. Therapeutic serum level is 0.5–2 mcg/ml; toxic serum level is greater than 3 mcg/ml.

IV INCOMPATIBILITIES
Amphotericin B complex (AmBisome, Amphotec, Abelcet), cefepime (Maxipime), diltiazem (Cardizem), fluconazole (Diflucan), foscarnet (Foscavir), heparin, hydrocortisone (Solu-Cortef), hydromor-

phone (Dilaudid), meropenem
(Merrem IV), potassium chloride,
propofol (Diprivan), vitamins

IV COMPATIBILITIES
Dobutamine (Dobutrex), fentanyl,
morphine

SIDE EFFECTS
Frequent
Pain with IM injection, drowsiness,
fatigue, ataxia or muscular incoordination
Occasional
Slurred speech, orthostatic hypotension, headache, hypoactivity, constipation, nausea, blurred vision
Rare
Paradoxical CNS hyperactivity or
nervousness in children, excitement
or restlessness in elderly or debilitated, generally noted during first 2
wks of therapy, particularly noted in
presence of uncontrolled pain

SERIOUS REACTIONS
• IV route may produce pain, swelling, thrombophlebitis, and carpal
tunnel syndrome.
• Abrupt or too rapid withdrawal
may result in pronounced restlessness, irritability, insomnia, hand
tremors, abdominal or muscle
cramps, diaphoresis, vomiting, and
seizures.
• Abrupt withdrawal in patients
with epilepsy may produce an
increase in the frequency or severity
of seizures.
• Overdosage results in somnolence,
confusion, diminished reflexes, CNS
depression, and coma.

NURSING CONSIDERATIONS

Baseline Assessment
• Assess the patient's blood pressure
(B/P), pulse, and respirations imme-
diately before giving diazepam.

• Know that the patient must remain
recumbent for up to 3 hours after
parenteral administration to reduce
the drug's hypotensive effect.
• Assess autonomic response, including cold, clammy hands, sweating and motor response, such as
agitation, trembling, and tension for
antianxiety patients.
• For patients with musculoskeletal
spasm, record the duration, location,
onset, and type of pain.
• Check the patient for immobility,
stiffness, and swelling.
• Review the history of the seizure
disorder, including duration, frequency, intensity, and length, as
well as his or her level of consciousness (LOC) in patients with
seizure disorder.
• Observe the patient frequently for
recurrence of seizure activity, and
initiate seizure precautions.

Lifespan Considerations
• Be aware that diazepam crosses
the placenta and is distributed in
breast milk. Diazepam may increase
the risk of fetal abnormalities if
administered during the first trimester of pregnancy.
• Chronic diazepam ingestion during pregnancy may produce withdrawal symptoms and CNS depression in neonates.
• Plan to use small initial doses
with gradual increases to avoid
ataxia or excessive sedation in
children and the elderly.

Precautions
• Use cautiously in patients with
hypoalbuminemia or liver or renal
impairment and who are taking
other CNS depressants.

Administration and Handling
Rectal
◀ALERT▶ Do not administer more
than 5 times a month or more than
once every 5 days.

PO
• Give diazepam without regard to meals.
• Dilute oral concentrate with carbonated beverages, juice, or water; may also be mixed in semisolid food, such as applesauce or pudding.
• Crush tablets as needed.
• Do not crush or break capsules.
IM
• Injection may be painful. Give IM injection deeply into deltoid muscle.
IV
• Store at room temperature.
• Give by IV push into tubing of a flowing IV solution as close to the vein insertion point as possible.
• Administer directly into a large vein to reduce the risk of phlebitis and thrombosis. Do not use small veins, such as wrist or dorsum of hand.
• Administer IV at rate not exceeding 5 mg/min. For children, give over a 3-minute period, a too rapid IV may result in hypotension, respiratory depression.
• Monitor respirations every 5–15 minutes for 2 hours.

Intervention and Evaluation
• Monitor the patient's B/P, heart rate, and respiratory rate.
• Assess pediatric and elderly patients for paradoxical reaction, particularly during early therapy.
• Evaluate the patient for therapeutic response. In patients with seizure disorder, the therapeutic response is a decrease in the frequency or intensity of seizures. In antianxiety patients, the therapeutic response is a calm facial expression, decreased intensity of skeletal muscle pain, and decreased restlessness.
• Know the therapeutic serum level for diazepam is 0.5–2 mcg/ml, and the toxic serum level for diazepam is greater than 3 mcg/ml.

Patient Teaching
• Urge the patient to avoid consuming alcohol, and to limit his or her caffeine intake during diazepam therapy.
• Tell the patient that diazepam may cause drowsiness and impair his or her ability to perform activities requiring mental alertness or motor skills.
• Explain to the patient that diazepam may be habit forming.
• Warn the patient to avoid abruptly discontinuing the drug after prolonged use.
• Tell the patient not to take the rectal form of the drug more than 5 times a month, or more than once every 5 days.

doxepin hydrochloride
dox-eh-pin
(Deptran[AUS], Novo-Doxepin[CAN], Prudoxin, Sinequan, Zonalon)
Do not confuse with doxapram, doxazosin, Doxidan, or saquinavir.

CATEGORY AND SCHEDULE
Pregnancy Risk Category: C
(B for topical preparation)

MECHANISM OF ACTION
A tricyclic antidepressant, antianxiety, antineuralgic, antiulcer, and antipruritic agent that increases synaptic concentrations of norepinephrine and serotonin. *Therapeutic Effect:* Produces antidepressant, anxiolytic effect.

PHARMACOKINETICS
Rapidly, well absorbed from the gastrointestinal (GI) tract. Protein

binding: 80%–85%. Metabolized in liver to active metabolite. Primarily excreted in urine. Not removed by hemodialysis. **Half-life:** 6–8 hrs. Topical: Absorbed through skin, distributed to body tissues, metabolized to active metabolite, eliminated renally.

AVAILABILITY
Capsules: 10 mg, 25 mg, 50 mg, 75 mg, 100 mg, 150 mg.
Oral Concentrate: 10 mg/ml.
Cream: 5%.

INDICATIONS AND DOSAGES
▸ **Depression, anxiety**
PO
Adults. 30–150 mg/day at bedtime or in 2–3 divided doses. May increase to 300 mg/day.
Adolescents. Initially, 25–50 mg/day as single or divided doses. May increase to 100 mg/day.
Children younger than 12 yrs. 1–3 mg/kg/day.
Elderly. Initially, 10–25 mg at bedtime. May increase by 10–25 mg/day q3–7 days. Maximum: 75 mg/day.
▸ **Treatment of pruritus associated with eczema**
Topical
Adults, Elderly. Apply a thin layer 4 times/day.

UNLABELED USES
Treatment of neurogenic pain, panic disorder, prophylaxis for vascular headache, pruritus in idiopathic urticaria

CONTRAINDICATIONS
Hypersensitivity to other tricyclic antidepressants, narrow-angle glaucoma, urinary retention

INTERACTIONS
Drug
Alcohol, CNS depressants: May increase central nervous system (CNS) and respiratory depression, and have hypotensive effects.
Antithyroid agents: May increase risk of agranulocytosis.
Cimetidine: May increase doxepin blood concentration and risk of toxicity.
Clonidine, guanadrel: May decrease the effects of clonidine and guanadrel.
MAOIs: May increase the risk of hypertensive crisis, hyperthermia, and seizures.
Phenothiazines: May increase anticholinergic, sedative effects.
Sympathomimetics: May increase cardiac effects with sympathomimetics.
Herbal
None known.
Food
None known.

DIAGNOSTIC TEST EFFECTS
May alter EKG readings, and blood glucose levels. Therapeutic serum level is 110–250 ng/ml; toxic serum level is greater than 300 ng/ml.

SIDE EFFECTS
Frequent
PO: Orthostatic hypotension, drowsiness, dry mouth, headache, increased appetite or weight, nausea, unusual tiredness, unpleasant taste
Topical: Edema at application site, increased itching or eczema, burning, stinging of skin, altered taste, dizziness, drowsiness, dry skin, dry mouth, fatigue, headache, thirst
Occasional
PO: Blurred vision, confusion, constipation, hallucinations, difficult urination, eye pain, irregular heartbeat, fine muscle tremors, nervousness, impaired sexual function, diarrhea, increased sweating, heartburn, insomnia

Topical: Anxiety, skin irritation or cracking, nausea
Rare
Allergic reaction, alopecia, tinnitus, breast enlargement
Topical: Fever

SERIOUS REACTIONS

• High dosage may produce confusion, seizures, severe drowsiness, arrhythmias, fever, hallucinations, agitation, shortness of breath, vomiting, and unusual tiredness or weakness.

• Abrupt withdrawal from prolonged therapy may produce headache, malaise, nausea, vomiting, and vivid dreams.

NURSING CONSIDERATIONS

Baseline Assessment

• Assess the patient's blood pressure (B/P) and pulse.

• Assess EKGs in patients with a history of cardiovascular disease.

Lifespan Considerations

• Be aware that doxepin crosses the placenta and is distributed in breast milk.

• Be aware that the safety and efficacy of doxepin have not been established in children.

• In the elderly, there is an increased risk of toxicity (lower dosages recommended).

Precautions

• Use cautiously in patients with cardiac disease, diabetes mellitus, glaucoma, hiatal hernia, history of seizures, history of urinary obstruction or retention, hyperthyroidism, increased intraocular pressure (IOP), liver disease, prostatic hypertrophy, renal disease, and schizophrenia.

Administration and Handling

PO

• Give doxepin with food or milk if gastrointestinal (GI) distress occurs.

• Dilute concentrate in 8-oz glass of grapefruit, orange, pineapple, prune, or tomato juice, milk, or water. Avoid carbonated drinks because they are incompatible with the drug.

Intervention and Evaluation

• Monitor the patient's B/P, pulse, and weight.

• Closely supervise suicidal-risk patients during early therapy. As depression lessens, be aware that the patient's energy level generally improves, which increases the suicide potential. Assess the patient's appearance, behavior, level of interest, mood, and speech pattern.

• Monitor the patient's serum drug level. The therapeutic serum level for doxepin is 110–250 ng/ml, and the toxic serum level for doxepin is greater than 300 ng/ml.

Patient Teaching

• Tell the patient that doxepin may cause drowsiness and dry mouth.

• Warn the patient to avoid tasks requiring mental alertness or motor skills until his or her response to the drug is established.

• Urge the patient to avoid alcohol and limit his or her caffeine intake while taking doxepin as these items may increase his or her appetite.

• Stress to the patient that he or she should avoid exposure to sunlight or artificial light sources while on doxepin therapy.

• Explain to the patient that the therapeutic effect of doxepin may be noted within 2 to 5 days with the maximum effect appearing within 2–3 weeks.

hydroxyzine
high-**drox**-ih-zeen
(Apo-Hydroxyzine[CAN], Atarax,
Novohydroxyzin[CAN], Vistaril)
**Do not confuse with
hydralazine or hydroxyurea.**

CATEGORY AND SCHEDULE
Pregnancy Risk Category: C

MECHANISM OF ACTION
A piperazine derivative that competes with histamine for receptor sites in the gastrointestinal (GI) tract, blood vessels, and respiratory tract. Diminishes vestibular stimulation, depresses labyrinthine function. *Therapeutic Effect:* Produces anticholinergic, antihistaminic, analgesic effects; relaxes skeletal muscle. Controls nausea, vomiting.

PHARMACOKINETICS

Route	Onset	Peak	Duration
PO	15–30 min	N/A	4–6 hrs

Well absorbed from GI tract, parenteral administration. Metabolized in liver. Primarily excreted in urine. Not removed by hemodialysis. **Half-life:** 20–25 hrs (half-life is increased in elderly).

AVAILABILITY
Tablets: 10 mg, 25 mg, 50 mg, 100 mg.
Capsules: 25 mg, 50 mg, 100 mg.
Oral Suspension: 25 mg/5 ml.
Injection: 25 mg/ml, 50 mg/ml.

INDICATIONS AND DOSAGES
▶ **Antiemetic**
IM
Adults, Elderly. 25–100 mg/dose q4–6h.

▶ **Usual pediatric dosage**
IM
Children. 0.5–1 mg/kg/dose q4–6h.
PO
Children. 2 mg/kg/day in divided doses q6–8h.
▶ **Anxiety**
PO
Adults, Elderly. 25–100 mg 4 times/ day. Maximum: 600 mg/day.
▶ **Pruritus**
PO
Adults, Elderly. 25 mg 3–4 times/ day.

CONTRAINDICATIONS
None known

INTERACTIONS
Drug
Alcohol, central nervous system (CNS) depressants: May increase CNS depressant effects.
MAOIs: May increase anticholinergic and CNS depressant effects.
Herbal
None known.
Food
None known.

DIAGNOSTIC TEST EFFECTS
May cause false positives with urine 17-hydroxy corticosteroid determinations.

SIDE EFFECTS
Side effects are generally mild and transient.
Frequent
Drowsiness, dry mouth, marked discomfort with IM injection
Occasional
Dizziness, ataxia or muscular incoordination, weakness, slurred speech, headache, agitation, increased anxiety
Rare
Paradoxical CNS hyperactivity or nervousness in children, excitement

or restlessness in elderly or debilitated patients that's generally noted during first 2 wks of therapy, particularly in presence of uncontrolled pain

SERIOUS REACTIONS
• Hypersensitivity reaction, including wheezing, dyspnea, and chest tightness, may occur.

NURSING CONSIDERATIONS

Baseline Assessment
• Offer emotional support to the anxious patient.
• Assess the anxious patient for autonomic responses, including cold or clammy hands, sweating and motor responses, such as agitation, trembling, and tension.
• Assess the patient for signs and symptoms of dehydration, including dry mucous membranes, longitudinal furrows in the tongue, and poor skin turgor, if he or she experiences excessive vomiting.

Lifespan Considerations
• Be aware that it is unknown if hydroxyzine crosses the placenta or is distributed in breast milk.
• Keep in mind that hydroxyzine use is not recommended in newborns and premature infants due to an increased risk of anticholinergic effects.
• Be aware that paradoxical excitement may occur in pediatric patients.
• In the elderly there is an increased risk of confusion, dizziness, and sedation.
• Hypotension and hyperexcitability may occur in the elderly.

Precautions
• Use cautiously in patients with asthma, bladder neck obstruction, chronic obstructive pulmonary disease (COPD), narrow-angle glaucoma, and prostatic hypertrophy.

Administration and Handling
PO
• Shake oral suspension thoroughly.
• Crushed scored tablets as needed, but do not crush or break capsules.
IM
◀ALERT▶ Don't give drug by the subcutaneous, intra-arterial, or IV route because it can cause significant tissue damage, thrombosis, and gangrene.
• Give drug undiluted IM.
• Inject deep IM into gluteus maximus or midlateral thigh in adults, midlateral thigh in children. Use the Z-track technique of injection to prevent subcutaneous infiltration.

Intervention and Evaluation
• Plan to perform complete blood counts and blood serum chemistry tests periodically for those patients on long-term therapy.
• Monitor the patient's lung sounds for signs of hypersensitivity reaction, such as wheezing.
• Monitor serum electrolytes in patients with severe vomiting.
• Assess the patient for paradoxical reaction, particularly during early therapy.
• Assist the patient with ambulation if he or she experiences drowsiness or lightheadedness.

Patient Teaching
• Tell the patient that marked discomfort may occur with IM injection.
• Recommend taking sips of tepid water and chewing sugarless gum to help relieve dry mouth.
• Tell the patient that drowsiness usually diminishes with continued therapy.
• Warn the patient to avoid tasks that require mental alertness and

motor skills until his or her response to the drug is established.

lorazepam

low-**raz**-ah-pam
(Apo-Lorazepam[CAN], Ativan, Novolorazepam[CAN])
Do not confuse with Alprazolam.

CATEGORY AND SCHEDULE
Pregnancy Risk Category: D
Controlled Substance: Schedule IV

MECHANISM OF ACTION
A benzodiazepine that enhances inhibitory neurotransmitter gamma-aminobutyric acid (GABA) neurotransmission at the central nervous system (CNS), affecting memory, motor, sensory, and cognitive functions. *Therapeutic Effect:* Produces anxiolytic, muscle relaxation, anticonvulsant, sedative, antiemetic effect.

PHARMACOKINETICS

Route	Onset	Peak	Duration
PO	60 min	N/A	8–12 hrs
IM	30–60 min	N/A	8–12 hrs
IV	15–30 min	N/A	8–12 hrs

Well absorbed after PO, IM administration. Protein binding: 85%. Widely distributed. Metabolized in liver. Primarily excreted in urine. Not removed by hemodialysis. **Half-life:** 10–20 hrs.

AVAILABILITY
Tablets: 0.5 mg, 1 mg, 2 mg.
Injection: 2 mg/ml, 4 mg/ml.

INDICATIONS AND DOSAGES
▸ **Anxiety**
PO

Adults. 1–10 mg/day in 2–3 divided doses. Average: 2–6 mg/day.
Elderly. Initially, 0.5–1 mg/day. May increase gradually.
IV
Adults, Elderly. Titrate to desired effect.
PO/IV
Children. 0.05 mg/kg/dose q4–8h. Range: 0.02–0.1 mg/kg. Maximum: 2 mg/dose.
▸ **Insomnia due to anxiety**
PO
Adults. 2–4 mg at bedtime.
Elderly. 0.5–1 mg at bedtime.
▸ **Preoperative**
IM
Adults, Elderly. 0.05 mg/kg given 2 hrs before procedure. Do not exceed 4 mg.
IV
Adults, Elderly. 0.044 mg/kg, up to 2 mg total, 15–20 min before surgery.
▸ **Status epilepticus**
IV
Adults, Elderly. 4 mg/dose over 2–5 min. May repeat in 10–15 min, 8 mg maximum in 12-hr period.
Children. 0.1 mg/kg over 2–5 min. Maximum: 4 mg. May repeat second dose of 0.05 mg/kg in 15–20 min.
Neonate. 0.05 mg/kg. May repeat in 10–15 min.

UNLABELED USES
Treatment of alcohol withdrawal, adjunct to endoscopic procedures —helps to diminishes patient recall, panic disorders, skeletal muscle spasms, cancer chemotherapy–induced nausea or vomiting, tension headache, tremors

CONTRAINDICATIONS
Preexisting CNS depression, narrow-angle glaucoma, severe

hypotension, severe uncontrolled pain

INTERACTIONS
Drug
Alcohol, CNS depressants: May increase CNS depressant effect.
Herbal
Kava kava, valerian: May increase CNS depression.
Food
None known.

DIAGNOSTIC TEST EFFECTS
None known. Therapeutic serum level is 50–240 ng/ml; toxic serum level is unknown.

IV INCOMPATIBILITIES
Aldesleukin (Proleukin), aztreonam (Azactam), idarubicin (Idamycin), ondansetron (Zofran), sufentanil (Sufenta)

IV COMPATIBILITIES
Bumetanide (Bumex), cefepime (Maxipime), diltiazem (Cardizem), dobutamine (Dobutrex), dopamine (Intropin), heparin, labetalol (Normodyne, Trandate), milrinone (Primacor), norepinephrine (Levophed), piperacillin/tazobactam (Zosyn), potassium, propofol (Diprivan)

SIDE EFFECTS
Frequent
Drowsiness, ataxia or incoordination, confusion. Morning drowsiness may occur initially.
Occasional
Blurred vision, slurred speech, hypotension, headache
Rare
Paradoxical CNS restlessness, excitement in elderly or debilitated

SERIOUS REACTIONS
• Abrupt or too rapid withdrawal may result in pronounced restlessness, irritability, insomnia, hand tremors, abdominal or muscle cramps, diaphoresis, vomiting, and seizures.
• Overdosage results in somnolence, confusion, diminished reflexes, and coma.

NURSING CONSIDERATIONS
Baseline Assessment
• Offer emotional support to the anxious patient.
• Know the patient must remain recumbent for up to 8 hours after parenteral administration to reduce the drug's hypotensive effect.
• Assess the patient's autonomic responses, including cold and clammy hands and diaphoresis, and motor responses, such as agitation, trembling, tension.
Lifespan Considerations
• Be aware that lorazepam may cross the placenta and be distributed in breast milk.
• Lorazepam may increase the risk of fetal abnormalities if administered during first trimester of pregnancy.
• Chronic lorazepam ingestion during pregnancy may produce CNS depression in neonates, fetal toxicity, and withdrawal symptoms.
• Be aware that the safety and efficacy of this drug have not been established in children younger than 12 yrs.
• Use small initial doses with gradual increases to avoid ataxia or excessive sedation in the elderly.
Precautions
• Use cautiously in neonates and patients with concomitant CNS depressant use, compromised pulmonary function, and liver or renal impairment.
Administration/Handling
PO
• Give with food.

• Crush tablets, as needed.

IM

• Give deep IM into large muscle mass, such as gluteus maximus.

IV

• Refrigerate parenteral form, but avoid freezing.

• Do not use if precipitate forms, or solution appears discolored.

• Dilute with equal volume of Sterile Water for Injection, 0.9% NaCl, or D_5W. To dilute prefilled syringe, remove air from half-filled syringe, aspirate equal volume of diluent, pull plunger back slightly to allow for mixing, and gently invert syringe several times, but do not shake vigorously.

• Give by IV push into tubing of free-flowing IV infusion (0.9% NaCl, D_5W) at rate not to exceed 2 mg/min.

Intervention and Evaluation

• Monitor the patient's blood pressure (B/P), complete blood count (CBC), and blood serum chemistry tests to assess heart rate, liver and renal function, and respiratory rate, especially during long-term therapy.

• Assess the patient for paradoxical reaction, particularly during early therapy.

• Evaluate the patient for therapeutic response, a calm facial expression, decreased restlessness and insomnia.

• Monitor the patient's drug serum levels. The therapeutic blood serum level for lorazepam is 50–240 ng/ml and the toxic blood serum level of lorazepam is unknown.

Patient Teaching

• Tell the patient that drowsiness usually disappears during continued therapy.

• Warn the patient to avoid tasks that require mental alertness or motor skills until his or her re-

sponse to the drug is established.

• Urge the patient to stop smoking tobacco products and to avoid alcohol and other CNS depressants. Explain to the patient that smoking reduces the effectiveness of lorazepam.

• Caution the patient against abruptly withdrawing the medication after long-term therapy.

• Stress to the patient that contraception is recommended for patients on long-term therapy. Teach the patient about various methods of contraception.

• Warn the patient to notify the physician immediately if pregnancy is suspected.

midazolam hydrochloride

my-**day**-zoe-lam
(Hypnovel[AUS], Versed)
Do not confuse with VePesid.

CATEGORY AND SCHEDULE

Pregnancy Risk Category: D
Controlled substance: Schedule IV

MECHANISM OF ACTION

A benzodiazepine that enhances action of inhibitory neurotransmitter gamma-aminobutyric acid (GABA), one of the major inhibitory transmitters in the brain. *Therapeutic Effect:* Produces anxiolytic, hypnotic, anticonvulsant, muscle relaxant, and amnestic effects.

PHARMACOKINETICS

Route	Onset	Peak	Duration
PO	10–20 min	N/A	N/A
IM	5–15 min	15–60 min	2–6 hrs
IV	1–5 min	5–7 min	20–30 min

Well absorbed after IM administration. Protein binding: 97%. Metabolized in liver to active metabolite. Primarily excreted in urine. Not removed by hemodialysis. **Half-life:** 1–5 hrs.

AVAILABILITY
Injection: 1 mg/ml, 5 mg/ml.
Syrup: 2 mg/ml.

INDICATIONS AND DOSAGES
▶ **Preop sedation**
IM
Adults, Elderly. 0.07–0.08 mg/kg 30–60 min prior to surgery.
Children. 0.1–0.15 mg/kg 30–60 min prior to surgery. Maximum total dose: 10 mg.
IV
Children 6–12 yrs. 0.025–0.05 mg/kg.
Children 6 mos–5 yrs. 0.05–0.1 mg/kg.
PO
Children. 0.25–0.5 mg/kg. Maximum: 20 mg.
▶ **Conscious sedation for procedures**
IV
Adults, Elderly. 1–2.5 mg over 2 min. Titrate as needed. Total dose: 2.5–5 mg.
▶ **Conscious sedation during mechanical ventilation**
IV
Adults, Elderly. 0.01–0.05 mg/kg; may repeat at 10- to 15-min intervals until adequately sedated, then continuous infusion: initially, 0.02–0.1 mg/kg/hr (1–7 mg/hr).
Children older than 32 wks. Initially, 1 mcg/kg/min as continuous infusion.
Children 32 wks and younger. Initially, 0.5 mcg/kg/min as continuous infusion.

▶ **Status epilepticus**
IV
Children older than 2 mos. Loading dose of 0.15 mg/kg followed by continuous infusion of 1 mcg/kg/min. Titrate. Range: 1–18 mcg/kg/min.

CONTRAINDICATIONS
Acute alcohol intoxication, acute narrow-angle glaucoma, coma, shock

INTERACTIONS
Drug
Alcohol, CNS depressants: May increase CNS and respiratory depression and hypotensive effects of midazolam.
Hypotension-producing medications: May increase hypotensive effects of midazolam.
Herbal
Kava kava, valerian: May increase CNS depression.
Food
Grapefruit juice: Increases oral absorption.

DIAGNOSTIC TEST EFFECTS
None known.

IV INCOMPATIBILITIES
Albumin, ampicillin/sulbactam (Unasyn), amphotericin B complex (Abelcet, AmBisome, Amphotec), ampicillin (Polycillin), bumetanide (Bumex), dexamethasone (Decadron), fosphenytoin (Cerebyx), furosemide (Lasix), hydrocortisone (Solu-Cortef), methotrexate, nafcillin (Nafcil), sodium bicarbonate, sodium pentothal (Thiopental), sulfamethoxazole-trimethoprim (Bactrim)

IV COMPATIBILITIES
Amiodarone (Cordarone), calcium gluconate, diltiazem (Cardizem),

dobutamine (Dobutrex), dopamine (Intropin), etomidate (Amidate), fentanyl (Sublimaze), heparin, hydromorphone (Dilaudid), insulin, lorazepam (Ativan), milrinone (Primacor), morphine, nitroglycerin, norepinephrine (Levophed), potassium chloride, propofol (Diprivan)

SIDE EFFECTS
Frequent (10%–4%)
Decreased respiratory rate, tenderness at IM/IV injection site, pain during injection, desaturation, hiccups
Occasional (3%–2%)
Pain at IM injection site, hypotension, paradoxical reaction
Rare (less than 2%)
Nausea, vomiting, headache, coughing, hypotensive episodes

SERIOUS REACTIONS
• Too much or too little dosage or improper administration may result in cerebral hypoxia, agitation, involuntary movements, hyperactivity, and combativeness.
• Underventilation or apnea may produce hypoxia and cardiac arrest.
• A too rapid IV rate, excessive doses, or a single large dose increases risk of respiratory depression or arrest.

NURSING CONSIDERATIONS
Baseline Assessment
• Ensure that resuscitative equipment, such as endotracheal tubes, suction, and oxygen (O_2) are readily available.
• Obtain the patient's vital signs before drug administration.
Lifespan Considerations
• Be aware that midazolam crosses the placenta, and it is unknown if midazolam is distributed in breast milk.

• Know that neonates are more likely to experience respiratory depression.
• In the elderly, age-related renal impairment may require dosage adjustment.
Precautions
• Use cautiously in patients with acute illness, a congestive heart, liver impairment, pulmonary impairment, renal impairment, severe fluid and electrolyte imbalance, and treated open-angle glaucoma.
Administration and Handling
◀ALERT▶ Plan to individualize midazolam dosage based on the patient's age, underlying disease, medications, and desired effect.
IM
• Give deep IM into large muscle mass, such as the gluteus maximus.
IV
• Store vials at room temperature.
• May give undiluted or as infusion.
• Make sure resuscitative equipment, such as O_2 is readily available before IV is administered.
• Administer by slow IV injection, in incremental dosages. Give each incremental dose over at least 2 minutes, and at intervals of at least 2 minutes apart.
• Reduce IV rate in patients older than 60 years of age who are debilitated, or have chronic diseases and impaired pulmonary function.
• A too rapid IV rate, excessive doses, or a single large dose increases risk of respiratory depression or arrest.
Intervention and Evaluation
• Monitor the patient's respiratory rate and oxygen saturation continuously during parenteral administration for apnea and underventilation.
• Monitor the patient's level of sedation every 3 to 5 minutes and vital signs during recovery period.

Patient Teaching
• When giving before a procedure, let the patient know that the drug produces an amnesic effect.

oxazepam
ox-**az**-eh-pam
(Alepam[AUS], Apo-Oxazepam[CAN], Murelax[AUS], Serax. Serepax[AUS])
Do not confuse with Eurax, oxaprozin, or Xerac.

CATEGORY AND SCHEDULE
Pregnancy Risk Category: D
Controlled substance: Schedule IV

MECHANISM OF ACTION
A benzodiazepine that potentiates effects of GABA and other inhibitory neurotransmitters by binding to specific receptors in CNS. *Therapeutic Effect:* Produces anxiolytic effect, skeletal muscle relaxation.

PHARMACOKINETICS
Well absorbed from GI tract. Protein binding: greater than 97%. Metabolized in liver. Primarily excreted in urine. Not removed by hemodialysis. **Half-life:** 5–20 hrs.

AVAILABILITY
Capsules: 10 mg, 15 mg, 30 mg.

INDICATIONS AND DOSAGES
▸ **Mild to moderate anxiety**
PO
Adults. 10–15 mg 3–4 times/day.
▸ **Severe anxiety**
PO
Adults. 15–30 mg 3–4 times/day.
▸ **Alcohol withdrawal**
PO
Adults. 15–30 mg 3–4 times/day.

Elderly. Initially, 10–20 mg 3 times/day. May gradually increase up to 30–45 mg/day.

CONTRAINDICATIONS
Narrow-angle glaucoma, preexisting CNS depression, severe uncontrolled pain

INTERACTIONS
Drug
Other central nervous system (CNS) depressant, including alcohol: Potentiates effects when used with CNS depressants.
Herbal
Kava kava, valerian: May increase CNS depression.
Food
None known.

DIAGNOSTIC TEST EFFECTS
May produce abnormal renal function tests, elevate LDH concentrations, serum alkaline phosphatase, bilirubin, SGOT (AST), and SGPT (ALT) levels. Therapeutic serum level is 0.2–1.4 mcg/ml; toxic blood serum level is not established.

SIDE EFFECTS
Frequent
Mild, transient drowsiness at beginning of therapy.
Occasional
Dizziness, headache
Rare
Paradoxical CNS hyperactivity or nervousness in children, excitement or restlessness in elderly or debilitated, generally noted during first 2 weeks of therapy.

SERIOUS REACTIONS
• Abrupt or too rapid withdrawal may result in pronounced restlessness, irritability, insomnia, hand tremors, abdominal or muscle

cramps, sweating, vomiting, and seizures.
• Overdose results in somnolence, confusion, diminished reflexes, and coma.

NURSING CONSIDERATIONS

Baseline Assessment
• Offer emotional support to the anxious patient.
• Assess the patient's autonomic responses, including cold or clammy hands, sweating, and motor responses, such as agitation, trembling, tension.

Precautions
• Use cautiously in patients with a history of drug dependence.

Administration and Handling
◀ALERT▶ Plan to use smallest effective dosage in elderly, debilitated, those with liver disease or low serum albumin.

Intervention and Evaluation
• Plan to perform a complete blood count and blood serum chemistry tests to assess liver and renal function periodically on patients on long-term therapy.
• Assess the patient for paradoxical reaction, particularly during early therapy.
• Assist the patient with ambulation if he or she experiences drowsiness or lightheadedness.
• Evaluate the patient for therapeutic response, a calm facial expression and decreased restlessness and insomnia.
• Monitor the patient's drug serum levels. The therapeutic serum level for oxazepam is 0.2–1.4 mcg/ml, and the toxic serum level for oxazepam is not established.

Patient Teaching
• Urge the patient to avoid alcohol and other CNS depressants while taking oxazepam.
• Tell the patient that oxazepam may cause drowsiness. Warn the patient to avoid tasks requiring mental alertness.
• Caution the patient to avoid abruptly discontinuing the drug.

33 Anticonvulsants

carbamazepine
clonazepam
clorazepate
  dipotassium
diazepam
fosphenytoin
gabapentin
lamotrigine
levetiracetam
oxcarbazepine
phenobarbital
phenytoin, phenytoin
  sodium
primidone
tiagabine
topiramate
valproic acid,
  valproate sodium,
  divalproex sodium
zonisamide

Uses: Anticonvulsants are used to treat seizure disorders. Seizures can be divided into two broad categories: partial seizures and generalized seizures. Partial seizures begin focally in the cerebral cortex and spread to limited areas. Simple partial seizures don't involve loss of consciousness (unless they evolve into generalized seizures) and typically last less than 1 minute. Complex partial seizures involve an alteration in consciousness and usually last longer than 1 minute. Generalized seizures may be convulsive or nonconvulsive and usually produce immediate loss of consciousness.

Action: Anticonvulsants can prevent or reduce excessive discharge by neurons with seizure foci or decrease the spread of excitation from seizure foci to normal neurons. Although their exact mechanism is unknown, these agents may act by suppressing sodium influx, suppressing calcium influx, or increasing the action of gamma-aminobutyric acid (GABA), which inhibits neurotransmitters in the brain.

COMBINATION PRODUCTS
BELLERGAL-S: phenobarbital/
ergotamine (an antimigraine)/
belladonna (an anticholinergic)
40 mg/0.6 mg/0.2 mg.
DILANTIN WITH PB: phenytoin/
phenobarbital (an anticonvulsant)
100 mg/15 mg; 100 mg/30 mg.

carbamazepine
car-bah-**may**-zeh-peen
(Apo-Carbamazepine[CAN],
Carbatrol, Epitol, Tegretol,
Tegretol CR[AUS], Tegretol XR,
Teril[AUS]) ·
**Do not confuse with Toradol or
Trental.**

CATEGORY AND SCHEDULE
Pregnancy Risk Category: D

MECHANISM OF ACTION
An iminostilbene derivative that
decreases sodium, calcium ion
influx into neuronal membranes,
reducing posttetanic potentiation at

synapse. *Therapeutic Effect:* Produces anticonvulsant effect.

PHARMACOKINETICS

Slowly, completely absorbed from the gastrointestinal (GI) tract. Protein binding: 75%. Metabolized in liver to active metabolite. Primarily excreted in urine. Not removed by hemodialysis. **Half-life:** 25–65 hrs; half-life is decreased with chronic use.

AVAILABILITY

Capsules (controlled-release): 200 mg (Carbatrol), 300 mg (Carbatrol).
Suspension: 100 mg/5 ml.
Tablets (chewable): 100 mg, 200 mg.
Tablets: 200 mg.
Tablets (controlled-release): 100 mg, 400 mg.

INDICATIONS AND DOSAGES
▸ **Seizure control**
PO
Adults, children older than 12 yrs. Initially, 200 mg 2 times/day. Increase dosage up to 200 mg/day at weekly intervals until response is attained. Maintenance: 800–1,200 mg/day. Do not exceed 1,000 mg/day in children 12–15 yrs, 1,200 mg/day in patients older than 15 yrs.
Children 6–12 yrs. Initially, 100 mg 2 times/day. Increase by 100 mg/day until response is attained. Maintenance: 400–800 mg/day. Give dosages of 200 mg/day or more in 3–4 equally divided doses.
Elderly. Initially, 100 mg 1–2 times/day. May increase by 100 mg at weekly intervals. Range: 400–1,000 mg/day.
Suspension
Children 6–12 yrs. Initially, 50 mg 4 times/day. Increase dosage slowly (reduces sedation risk).
Children younger than 6 yrs. 10–20 mg/kg/day in 2–4 divided doses. Maximum: 35 mg/kg/day.
▸ **Trigeminal neuralgia**
PO
Adults, Elderly. 100 mg 2 times/day on day 1. Increase by 100 mg q12h until pain is relieved. Maintenance: 200–1,200 mg/day. Do not exceed 1,200 mg/day.

UNLABELED USES
Treatment of alcohol withdrawal, bipolar disorder, diabetes insipidus, neurogenic pain, psychotic disorders

CONTRAINDICATIONS
Concomitant use of MAOIs, history of bone marrow depression, history of hypersensitivity to tricyclic antidepressants

INTERACTIONS
Drug
Anticoagulants, steroids: May decrease the effects of anticoagulants and steroids.
Anticonvulsants, barbiturates, benzodiazepines, valproic acid: May increase the metabolism of anticonvulsants, barbiturates, benzodiazepines, and valproic acid.
Antipsychotics, haloperidol, tricyclic antidepressants: May increase central nervous system (CNS) depressant effects.
Cimetidine: May increase carbamazepine blood concentration and risk of toxicity.
Clarithromycin, diltiazem, erythromycin, estrogens, propoxyphene, quinidine: May decrease the effects of clarithromycin, diltiazem, erythromycin, estrogens, propoxyphene, and quinidine.
Isoniazid: May increase metabolism of this drug, carbamazepine blood concentration, and risk of toxicity.
MAOIs: May cause convulsions and hypertensive crises.

Verapamil: May increase the toxicity of carbamazepine.

Herbal

None known.

Food

Grapefruit: May increase the absorption and blood concentration of carbamazepine.

DIAGNOSTIC TEST EFFECTS

May increase BUN, blood glucose levels, cholesterol levels, HDL levels, protein levels, serum alkaline phosphatase, bilirubin, SGOT (AST), SGPT (ALT), and triglyceride levels. May decrease serum calcium, and T_3, T_4, T_4 index. Therapeutic serum level is 4–12 mcg/ml; toxic serum level is greater than 12 mcg/ml.

SIDE EFFECTS

Frequent

Drowsiness, dizziness, nausea, vomiting

Occasional

Visual abnormalities, such as spots before eyes, difficulty focusing, blurred vision, dry mouth or pharynx, tongue irritation, headache, water retention, increased sweating, constipation or diarrhea

SERIOUS REACTIONS

• Toxic reactions appear as blood dyscrasias, including aplastic anemia, agranulocytosis, thrombocytopenia, leukopenia, leukocytosis, eosinophilia, cardiovascular disturbances, such as congestive heart failure (CHF), hypotension or hypertension, thrombophlebitis, arrhythmias, and dermatologic effects, such as rash, urticaria, pruritus, photosensitivity.

• Abrupt withdrawal may precipitate status epilepticus.

NURSING CONSIDERATIONS

Baseline Assessment

• Review the history of the seizure disorder, including the duration, frequency, intensity, and of seizures, as well as his or her level of consciousness (LOC). Initiate seizure precautions.

• Provide the patient with a quiet, dark environment and safety precautions.

• Expect to perform BUN, complete blood count (CBC), serum iron determination, and urinalysis before beginning carbamazepine therapy and periodically during therapy.

Lifespan Considerations

• Be aware that carbamazepine crosses the placenta and is distributed in breast milk. Carbamazepine accumulates in fetal tissue.

• Know that behavioral changes are more likely to occur in pediatric patients taking carbamazepine.

• The elderly are more susceptible to agitation, atrioventricular (AV) block, bradycardia, confusion, and syndrome of inappropriate antidiuretic hormone (SIADH).

Precautions

• Use cautiously in patients with impaired cardiac, liver, or renal function.

Administration and Handling

◄ALERT► When replacement by another anticonvulsant is necessary, plan to decrease carbamazepine gradually as therapy begins with a low replacement dose. When transferring from tablets to suspension, expect to divide total tablet daily dose into smaller, more frequent doses of suspension. Also plan to administer extended-release tablets in 2 divided doses.

PO

• Store oral suspension, tablets at room temperature.

• Give with meals to reduce risk of gastrointestinal (GI) distress.
• Shake oral suspension well. Do not administer simultaneously with other liquid medicine.
• Do not crush extended-release tablets.

Intervention and Evaluation
• Observe the seizure patient frequently for recurrence of seizure activity.
• Monitor the patient for therapeutic serum levels.
• Assess the seizure patient for clinical improvement, a decrease in the frequency and intensity of seizures.
• Assess the patient for clinical evidence of early toxic signs, such as easy bruising, fever, joint pain, mouth ulcerations, sore throat, and unusual bleeding.
• Avoid cold food or liquids, draft, hot food or liquids, jarring bed, talking, warm food or liquids, washing face in neuralgia patients because it could trigger tic douloureux.
• Know the therapeutic serum level for carbamazepine in neuralgia patients is 4–12 mcg/ml and the toxic serum level for carbamazepine in neuralgia patients is greater than 12 mcg/ml.

Patient Teaching
• Caution the patient against abruptly withdrawing the medication after long-term use as this may precipitate seizures.
• Stress to the patient that strict maintenance of drug therapy is essential for seizure control.
• Tell the patient that drowsiness usually disappears during continued therapy.
• Warn the patient to avoid tasks that require mental alertness and motor skills until his or her response to the drug is established.
• Instruct the patient to notify the physician if he or she experiences visual abnormalities.
• Explain to the patient that blood tests should be repeated frequently during first 3 months of therapy and at monthly intervals thereafter for 2–3 years.
• Teach the patient not to take the oral suspension of carbamazepine simultaneously with other liquid medicine.
• Caution the patient not to take the drug with grapefruit juice. Explain that grapefruit may increase carbamazepine absorption and blood concentration.

clonazepam
klon-**nah**-zih-pam
(Apo-Clonazepam[CAN], Clonapam[CAN], Klonopin, Paxam[AUS], Rivotril[CAN])
Do not confuse with clonidine or lorazepam.

CATEGORY AND SCHEDULE
Pregnancy Risk Category: D

MECHANISM OF ACTION
A benzodiazepine that depresses all levels of the central nervous system (CNS). Depresses nerve transmission in the motor cortex. *Therapeutic Effect:* Suppresses abnormal discharge in petite mal seizures. Produces anxiolytic effect.

PHARMACOKINETICS
Well absorbed from the gastrointestinal (GI) tract. Protein binding: 85%. Metabolized in liver. Excreted in urine. Not removed by hemodialysis. **Half-life:** 18–50 hrs.

AVAILABILITY
Tablets: 0.5 mg, 1 mg, 2 mg.
Tablets (disintegrating): 0.125 mg, 0.25 mg, 0.5 mg, 1 mg, 2 mg.

INDICATIONS AND DOSAGES
▶ **Anticonvulsant**
PO
Adults, Elderly. 1.5 mg/day. Dosage may be increased in 0.5- to 1-mg increments at 3-day intervals until seizures are controlled. Do not exceed maintenance dosage of 20 mg/day.
Infants, children younger than 10 yrs or weighing less than 30 kg. 0.01–0.03 mg/kg/day in 2–3 divided doses. Dosage may be increased in up to 0.5-mg increments at 3-day intervals until seizures are controlled. Do not exceed maintenance dosage of 0.2 mg/kg/day.
▶ **Panic disorder**
PO
Adults, Elderly. Initially, 0.25 mg 2 times/day. Increase in increments of 0.125–0.25 mg 2 times/day at 3-day intervals. Maximum: 4 mg/day.

UNLABELED USES
Adjunct treatment of seizures, tonic-clonic seizures, treatment of simple and complex partial seizures

CONTRAINDICATIONS
Narrow-angle glaucoma, significant liver disease

INTERACTIONS
Drug
Alcohol, central nervous system (CNS) depressants: May increase CNS depressant effect.
Herbal
Kava kava: May increase CNS sedation.
Food
None known.

DIAGNOSTIC TEST EFFECTS
None known.

SIDE EFFECTS
Frequent
Mild, transient drowsiness; ataxia; behavioral disturbances, especially in children manifested as aggression, irritability, agitation
Occasional
Rash, ankle or facial edema, nocturia, dysuria, change in appetite or weight, dry mouth, sore gums, nausea, blurred vision
Rare
Paradoxical reaction, including hyperactivity or nervousness in children, excitement or restlessness in elderly—particularly noted in presence of uncontrolled pain.

SERIOUS REACTIONS
• Abrupt withdrawal may result in pronounced restlessness, irritability, insomnia, hand tremors, abdominal or muscle cramps, sweating, vomiting, and status epilepticus.
• Overdosage results in somnolence, confusion, diminished reflexes, and coma.

NURSING CONSIDERATIONS
Baseline Assessment
• Review the seizure patient's history of seizure disorder, including the duration, frequency, intensity, of seizures, as well as level of consciousness (LOC). Initiate seizure precautions.
• Assess the panic attack patient's autonomic responses, including cold or clammy hands, diaphoresis, and motor responses, such as agitation, trembling, tension.
Lifespan Considerations
• Be aware that clonazepam crosses the placenta and may be distributed in breast milk.
• Be aware that chronic clonazepam

ingestion during pregnancy may produce withdrawal symptoms and CNS depression in neonates.

• Know that long-term clonazepam use may adversely affect the mental and physical development of children.

• Usually the elderly are more sensitive to the clonazepam's CNS effects, such as ataxia, dizziness, and oversedation. Expect to use a low clonazepam dosage, increasing it gradually.

Precautions

• Use cautiously in patients with chronic respiratory disease and impaired kidney and liver function.

Administration and Handling

◀ALERT▶ When replacement by another anticonvulsant is necessary, plan to decrease clonazepam dose gradually as therapy begins with low replacement dosage.

PO

• Give clonazepam without regard to meals.

• Crush tablets, as needed.

Intervention and Evaluation

• Assess pediatric and elderly patients for paradoxical reaction, particularly during early therapy.

• Implement safety measures, and observe frequently for recurrence of seizure activity in seizure patients.

• Assist the patient with ambulation if he or she experiences ataxia or drowsiness.

• Perform complete blood counts and blood serum chemistry tests to assess liver and renal function periodically for patients on long-term clonazepam therapy.

• Evaluate the patient for therapeutic response to the drug, in seizure patients, a decrease in the frequency or intensity of seizures, or if used in panic attack, calm facial expression and decreased restlessness.

Patient Teaching

• Tell the patient that drowsiness usually diminishes with continued therapy.

• Warn the patient to avoid tasks that require mental alertness or motor skills until his or her response to the drug is established.

• Urge the patient to stop smoking and to avoid alcohol. Explain to the patient that smoking reduces the drug's effectiveness.

• Caution the patient against abruptly withdrawing the medication after long-term therapy.

• Stress to the patient that strict maintenance of drug therapy is essential for seizure control.

---

clorazepate (Tranxene)

See antianxiety agents

---

diazepam

See antianxiety agents

---

fosphenytoin
fos-**phen**-ih-twon
(Cerebyx)
Do not confuse with Celebrex.

CATEGORY AND SCHEDULE
Pregnancy Risk Category: D

MECHANISM OF ACTION

A hydantoin that stabilizes neuronal membranes, limits spread of seizure activity. Decreases sodium and calcium, ion influx in neurons. Decreases posttetanic potentiation and repetitive afterdischarge. *Therapeutic Effect:* Decreases seizure activity.

PHARMACOKINETICS

Completely absorbed after IM administration. Protein binding: 95%–99%. After IM or IV administration, rapidly and completely hydrolyzed to phenytoin. Time of complete conversion to phenytoin: IM: 4 hrs after injection; IV: 2 hrs after the end of infusion. **Half-life** for conversion to phenytoin: 8–15 min.

AVAILABILITY

Injection: 75 mg/ml, equivalent to 50 mg/ml phenytoin, or 50 mg phenytoin equivalent/ml

INDICATIONS AND DOSAGES

▸ **Status epilepticus**
IV
Adults. Loading dose: 15–20 mg PE/kg infused at rate of 100–150 mg PE/min.
▸ **Nonemergent seizures**
IV
Adults. Loading dose: 10–20 mg PE/kg. Maintenance: 4–6 mg PE/kg/day.

CONTRAINDICATIONS

Adams-Stokes syndrome, hypersensitivity to fosphenytoin or phenytoin, second- or third-degree atrioventricular (AV) block, severe bradycardia, sinoatrial (SA) block

INTERACTIONS

Drug
Alcohol, central nervous system (CNS) depressants: May increase CNS depression.
Amiodarone, anticoagulants, cimetidine, disulfiram, fluoxetine, isoniazid, sulfonamides: May increase fosphenytoin blood concentration, effects, and risk of toxicity.
Antacids: May decrease the absorption of fosphenytoin.
Fluconazole, ketoconazole, miconazole: May increase fosphenytoin blood concentration.
Glucocorticoids: May decrease effect of glucocorticoids.
Lidocaine, propranolol: May increase cardiac depressant effects.
Valproic acid: May increase fosphenytoin blood concentration and decrease the metabolism of fosphenytoin.
Xanthine: May increase the metabolism of xanthine.
Herbal
None known.
Food
None known.

DIAGNOSTIC TEST EFFECTS

May increase blood glucose levels, serum GGT levels, and serum alkaline phosphatase.

IV INCOMPATIBILITIES

Midazolam (Versed)

IV COMPATIBILITIES

Lorazepam (Ativan), phenobarbital, potassium chloride

SIDE EFFECTS

Frequent
Dizziness, paresthesia, tinnitus, pruritus, headache, somnolence
Occasional
Morbilliform rash

SERIOUS REACTIONS

• A too high fosphenytoin blood concentration may produce ataxia, muscular incoordination, nystagmus, or rhythmic oscillation of eyes, double vision, lethargy, slurred speech, nausea, vomiting, and hypotension. As level increases, extreme lethargy to comatose states occur.

NURSING CONSIDERATIONS

Baseline Assessment
• Review the patient's history of seizure disorder, including the duration, frequency, and intensity of seizures, as well as his or her level of consciousness (LOC). Initiate seizure precautions.
• Obtain the patient's medication history, especially the use of phenytoin or other anticonvulsants, and vital signs.

Lifespan Considerations
• Be aware that fosphenytoin may increase the frequency of seizures during pregnancy, and that its use increases the risk of congenital malformations of the fetus.
• Be aware that it is unknown if fosphenytoin is excreted in breast milk.
• Be aware that the safety of this drug has not been established in children.
• A lower fosphenytoin dosage is recommended in the elderly.

Precautions
• Use cautiously in patients with hypoalbuminemia, hypotension, liver disease, porphyria, renal disease, and severe myocardial insufficiency.

Administration and Handling
◄ALERT► Know that 150 mg fosphenytoin yields 100 mg phenytoin, and that the dose, concentration solution, and infusion rate of fosphenytoin are expressed in terms of phenytoin equivalent (PE). Keep in mind that lower, less frequent dosing in the elderly may be required, and that the drug is not approved for pediatric use.

IV
• Refrigerate and do not store at room temperature longer than 48 hours. After dilution, keep in mind the solution is stable for 8 hours at room temperature, or 24 hours if refrigerated.
• Dilute in D_5W or 0.9% NaCl to a concentration ranging from 1.5 to 25 mg PE/ml.
• Administer at rate of 150 mg PE/min or less to decrease the risk of hypotension.

Intervention and Evaluation
• Measure the patient's blood pressure (B/P), cardiac function, EKG, and respiratory function during and immediately following fosphenytoin infusion for approximately 10–20 minutes.
• Discontinue fosphenytoin infusion, as ordered, if the patient develops a skin rash.
• Expect to interrupt or decrease the infusion rate if the patient experiences arrhythmias or hypotension.
• Assess the patient postinfusion. The patient may feel ataxic, dizzy, or drowsy.
• Assess the patient's blood levels of fosphenytoin 2 hours post IV infusion, or 4 hours post IM injection.

Patient Teaching
• Teach the patient about his or her seizure condition. Explain to the patient his or her role in seizure management.
• Discuss with the patient and resolve any reasons for noncompliance with drug therapy, especially if therapy noncompliance is an issue in causing acute seizures.

gabapentin
gah-bah-**pen**-tin
(Gantin[AUS], Neurontin)
Do not confuse with Noroxin.

CATEGORY AND SCHEDULE
Pregnancy Risk Category: C

MECHANISM OF ACTION

An anticonvulsant and antineuralgic agent whose exact mechanism unknown. May be due to increased gamma-aminobutyric acid (GABA) synthesis rate, increased GABA accumulation, or binding to as yet undefined receptor sites in brain tissue. *Therapeutic Effect:* Produces anticonvulsant activity, reduces neuropathic pain.

PHARMACOKINETICS

Well absorbed from the gastrointestinal (GI) tract (not affected by food). Protein binding: less than 5%. Widely distributed. Crosses blood-brain barrier. Primarily excreted unchanged in urine. Removed by hemodialysis. **Half-life:** 5–7 hrs (half-life is increased with impaired renal function, elderly).

AVAILABILITY

Capsules: 100 mg, 300 mg, 400 mg.
Oral Solution: 250 mg/5 ml.
Tablets: 600 mg, 800 mg.

INDICATIONS AND DOSAGES

▶ **Adjunct Therapy for Seizure Control**
PO
Adults, Elderly, Children older than 12 yrs. Initially, 300 mg 3 times/day. May titrate. Range: 900–1800 mg/day in 3 divided doses. Maximum: 3600 mg/day.
Children 3–12 yrs. Initially, 10–15 mg/kg/day in 3 divided doses. May titrate up to 25–35 mg/kg/day (children 5–12 yrs) and 40 mg/kg/day (children 3–4 yrs) Maximum: 50 mg/kg/day.
▶ **Adjunct therapy for neuropathic pain**
PO
Adults, Elderly. Initially, 100 mg 3 times/day; may increase by 300 mg/day at weekly intervals. Maximum: up to 3600 mg/day in 3 divided doses.
Children. Initially 5 mg/kg/dose at bedtime, then 5 mg/kg/dose for 2 doses on day 2, then 5 mg/kg/dose for 3 doses on day 3. Range: 8–35 mg/kg/day in 3 divided doses.
▶ **Postherpetic neuralgia**
PO
Adults, Elderly. 300 mg day 1, 300 mg 2 times/day on day 2, 300 mg 3 times/day on day 3. Titrate up to 1800 mg/day.
▶ **Dosage in renal function impairment**
Based on creatinine clearance:

Creatinine Clearance	Dosage
greater than 60 ml/min	400 mg q8h
30–60 ml/min	300 mg q12h
15–30 ml/min	300 mg daily
less than 15 ml/min	300 mg every other day
Hemodialysis	200–300 mg after each 4-hr hemodialysis

UNLABELED USES

Treatment of essential tremors, hot flashes, hyperhidrosis, migraines, psychiatric disorders

CONTRAINDICATIONS

None known

INTERACTIONS

Drug
None known.
Herbal
None known.
Food
None known.

DIAGNOSTIC TEST EFFECTS

May decrease serum white blood cell (WBC) count.

SIDE EFFECTS
Frequent (19%–10%)
Fatigue, somnolence, dizziness, ataxia
Occasional (8%–3%)
Nystagmus (rapid eye movements), tremor, diplopia (double vision), rhinitis, weight gain
Rare (less than 2%)
Nervousness, dysarthria (speech difficulty), memory loss, dyspepsia, pharyngitis, myalgia

SERIOUS REACTIONS
• Abrupt withdrawal may increase seizure frequency.
• Overdosage may result in double vision, slurred speech, drowsiness, lethargy, and diarrhea.

NURSING CONSIDERATIONS
Baseline Assessment
• Review the seizure patient's history of seizure disorder, including the onset, duration, frequency, intensity, and type of seizures, as well as his or her level of consciousness (LOC). Initiate seizure precautions.
• Know that routine laboratory monitoring of serum levels of gabapentin is not necessary for the drug's safe use.
Lifespan Considerations
• Be aware that it is unknown whether gabapentin is distributed in breast milk.
• Be aware that the safety and efficacy of this drug have not been established in pediatric patients less than 3 years of age.
• In the elderly, age-related renal impairment may require dosage adjustment.
Precautions
• Use cautiously in patients with renal impairment.
Administration and Handling
◄ALERT► Keep in mind that the

maximum time between drug doses should not exceed 12 hours.
PO
• Give gabapentin without regard to meals; may give with food to avoid or reduce gastrointestinal (GI) upset.
• If treatment is discontinued or anticonvulsant therapy is added, expect to make changes gradually over at least 1 week to reduce the risk of loss of seizure control.
Intervention and Evaluation
• Provide the patient with safety measures as needed.
• Monitor the patient's behavior, especially with children, as well as body weight, renal function, and seizure duration and frequency.
Patient Teaching
• Instruct the patient to take gabapentin only as prescribed.
• Caution the patient against abruptly discontinuing the drug as this may increase seizure frequency.
• Warn the patient to avoid tasks requiring mental alertness or motor skills because of the potential for dizziness and somnolence.
• Urge the patient to avoid alcohol while taking gabapentin.
• Tell the patient to always carry an identification card or wear an identification bracelet that displays his or her seizure disorder and anticonvulsant therapy.

lamotrigine
lam-**oh**-trih-geen
(Lamictal)
Do not confuse with lamivudine.

CATEGORY AND SCHEDULE
Pregnancy Risk Category: C

MECHANISM OF ACTION

An anticonvulsant whose exact mechanism is unknown. May be due to inhibition of voltage-sensitive sodium channels, stabilizing neuronal membranes, and regulating presynaptic transmitter release of excitatory amino acids. *Therapeutic Effect:* Produces anticonvulsant activity.

AVAILABILITY

Tablets: 25 mg, 100 mg, 150 mg, 200 mg.
Tablets (chewable): 5 mg, 25 mg.

INDICATIONS AND DOSAGES

▸ **Seizure control in patients receiving enzyme-inducing antiepileptic drug (EIAEDs), but not valproate**
PO
Adults, Elderly, Children older than 12 yrs. Recommended as add-on therapy: 50 mg once/day for 2 wks, followed by 100 mg/day in 2 divided doses for 2 wks.
Maintenance: Dosage may be increased by 100 mg/day every week, up to 300–500 mg/day in 2 divided doses.
Children 2–12 yrs. 0.6 mg/kg/day in 2 divided doses for 2 wks, then 1.2 mg/kg/day in 2 divided doses for wks 3 and 4. Maintenance: 5–15 mg/kg/day. Maximum: 400 mg/day.
▸ **Seizure control in patients receiving combination therapy of valproic acid and EIAEDs**
PO
Adults, Elderly, Children older than 12 yrs. 25 mg every other day for 2 wks, followed by 25 mg once/day for 2 wks. Maintenance: Dosage may be increased by 25–50 mg/day q1–2wks, up to 150 mg/day in 2 divided doses.
Children 2–12 yrs. 0.15 mg/kg/day in 2 divided doses for 2 wks, then 0.3 mg/kg/day in 2 divided doses

for wks 3 and 4. Maintenance: 1–5 mg/kg/day in 2 divided doses. Maximum: 200 mg/day.
▸ **Conversion to monotherapy**
PO
Adults, Children older than 12 yrs. Add lamotrigine 50 mg/day for 2 wks; then 100 mg/day during wks 3 and 4. Increase by 100 mg/day q1–2wks until maintenance dosage achieved (300–500 mg/day in 2 divided doses/day). Gradually discontinue other EIAEDs over 4 wks once maintenance dose achieved.
▸ **Bipolar disorder**
PO
Adults, Elderly. Initially, 25 mg/day. May double dose after wks 2, 4, and 5. Target dose: 200 mg/day.
▸ **Renal function impairment**
Adults, Children older than 12 yrs.: Same dosage as combination therapy.
▸ **Discontinuation therapy**
Adults, Children older than 12 yrs. A reduction in dosage over at least 2 wks, approximately 50% per week, is recommended.

CONTRAINDICATIONS

None known

INTERACTIONS

Drug
Carbamazepine, phenobarbital, phenytoin, primidone, valproic acid: Decreases lamotrigine blood concentration.
Carbamazepine, valproic acid: May increase serum levels of carbamazepine and valproic acid.
Herbal
None known.
Food
None known.

DIAGNOSTIC TEST EFFECTS

None known.

SIDE EFFECTS

Frequent

Dizziness (38%), double vision (28%), headache (29%), ataxia (muscular incoordination) (22%), nausea (19%), blurred vision (16%), somnolence, rhinitis (14%)

Occasional (10%–5%)

Rash, pharyngitis, vomiting, cough, flu syndrome, diarrhea, dysmenorrhea, fever, insomnia, dyspepsia

Rare

Constipation, tremor, anxiety, pruritus, vaginitis, sensitivity reaction

SERIOUS REACTIONS

• Abrupt withdrawal may increase seizure frequency.

NURSING CONSIDERATIONS

Baseline Assessment

• Review the patient's drug history, including other anticonvulsants, history of seizure disorder, along with the duration, frequency, intensity, onset, and type of seizure, and level of consciousness (LOC), and other medical conditions, such as renal function impairment.

• Provide the patient with a quiet, dark environment and safety precautions.

Precautions

• Use cautiously in patients with cardiac, liver, and renal function impairment.

Administration and Handling

◀ALERT▶ If the patient is currently taking valproic acid, expect to reduce lamotrigine dosage to less than half the normal dosage.

PO

• Give lamotrigine without regard to food.

Intervention and Evaluation

• Notify the physician promptly if the patient experiences a rash, and expect to discontinue the drug.

• Assist the patient with ambulation, if he or she experiences ataxia or dizziness.

• Assess the patient for clinical improvement, including a decrease in the frequency and intensity of seizures.

• Assess the patient for headache and visual abnormalities.

Patient Teaching

• Instruct the patient to take lamotrigine only as prescribed. Caution the patient not to abruptly withdraw the medication after long-term therapy.

• Warn the patient to avoid alcohol and tasks that require mental alertness and motor skills until his or her response to the drug is established.

• Tell the patient to carry an identification card or wear an identification bracelet to note anticonvulsant therapy.

• Stress to the patient that strict maintenance of drug therapy is essential for seizure control.

• Warn the patient to notify the physician of the first sign of fever, rash, and swelling of glands.

• Explain to the patient that lamotrigine may cause a photosensitivity reaction. Instruct the patient to avoid exposure to sunlight and artificial light.

levetiracetam

leave-ty-rah-**see**-tam
(Keppra)
Do not confuse with Kaletra.

CATEGORY AND SCHEDULE

Pregnancy Risk Category: C

MECHANISM OF ACTION

An anticonvulsant that inhibits burst firing without affecting normal neuronal excitability. *Therapeutic Effect:* Prevents seizure activity.

AVAILABILITY
Tablets: 250 mg, 500 mg, 750 mg.
Liquid: 100 mg/ml.

INDICATIONS AND DOSAGES
▶ **Partial-onset seizures**
PO
Adults, Elderly. Initially, 500 mg q12h. May increase by 1,000 mg/day q2wks. Maximum: 3,000 mg/day.
▶ **Dosage in renal impairment**

Creatinine Clearance (ml/min)	Dosage
80	500–1500 mg q12h
50–80	500–1000 mg q12h
30–50	250–750 mg q12h
less than 30	250–500 mg q12h
ESRD using dialysis	500–1000 mg q12h, following dialysis, a 250- to 500-mg supplemental dose is recommended.

CONTRAINDICATIONS
Hypersensitivity reaction

INTERACTIONS
Drug
None known.
Herbal
None known.
Food
None significant.

DIAGNOSTIC TEST EFFECTS
May increase blood Hgb, Hct, red blood cell (RBC) and white blood cell (WBC) counts.

SIDE EFFECTS
Frequent (15%–10%)
Somnolence, asthenia (loss of strength, energy), headache, infection

Occasional (9%–3%)
Dizziness, pharyngitis, pain, depression, nervousness, vertigo, rhinitis, anorexia
Rare (less than 3%)
Amnesia, anxiety, emotional lability, cough, sinusitis, anorexia, diplopia

SERIOUS REACTIONS
• None known.

NURSING CONSIDERATIONS
Baseline Assessment
• Review with the patient the history of the seizure disorder, including the duration, frequency, intensity, and level of consciousness (LOC) of seizures. Initiate seizure precautions.
• Assess the patient for hypersensitivity to levetiracetam.
• Obtain the patient's BUN and creatinine laboratory test results to assess renal function.
Precautions
• Use cautiously in patients with renal function impairment.
Intervention and Evaluation
• Observe the patient for recurrence of seizure activity.
• Assess the patient for clinical improvement, a decrease in the frequency or intensity of seizures.
• Monitor the patient's renal function test results.
• Assist the patient with ambulation if he or she experiences dizziness.
Patient Teaching
• Warn the patient to avoid tasks that require mental alertness or motor skills until his or her response to the drug is established.
• Caution the patient against abruptly discontinuing therapy as this may precipitate seizures.
• Advise the patient that dizziness or somnolence usually diminishes with continued therapy.

• Stress to the patient that strict maintenance of drug therapy is essential for seizure control.

oxcarbazepine
ox car-**bah**-zeh-peen
(Trileptal)

CATEGORY AND SCHEDULE
Pregnancy Risk Category: C

MECHANISM OF ACTION
An anticonvulsant that produces blockade of sodium channels, resulting in stabilization of hyperexcited neural membranes, inhibiting repetitive neuronal firing, diminishing synaptic impulses. *Therapeutic Effect:* Prevents seizures.

PHARMACOKINETICS
Completely absorbed and extensively metabolized to active metabolite in the liver. Protein binding: 40%. Primarily excreted in urine. **Half-life:** 2 hrs (metabolite: 6–10 hrs).

AVAILABILITY
Tablets: 150 mg, 300 mg, 600 mg.
Oral Suspension: 300 mg/5 ml.

INDICATIONS AND DOSAGES
▸ **Adjunctive therapy**
PO
Adults, Elderly. Initially, 600 mg/day in 2 divided doses. May increase by a maximum of 600 mg/day at weekly intervals. Maximum: 2,400 mg/day.
Children 4–16 yrs. 8–10 mg/kg. Maximum: 600 mg/day. Achieve maintenance dose over 2 wks based on patient's weight.
Children weighing 20–29 kg. 900 mg/day.

Children weighing 29.1–39 kg. 1,200 mg/day.
Children weighing more than 39 kg. 1,800 mg/day.
▸ **Conversion to monotherapy**
PO
Adults, Elderly. 600 mg/day in 2 divided doses, while decreasing concomitant antiepilepsy drug over 3–6 wks, increasing up to 2,400 mg/day over 2–4 wks. See previous for guideline to increasing dosage.
▸ **Initiation of monotherapy**
PO
Adults, Elderly. 600 mg/day in 2 divided doses. May increase by 300 mg/day q3 days up to 1,200 mg/day.
▸ **Dosage in renal impairment**
Creatinine clearance less than 30 ml/min. Give 50% of normal starting dose, then titrate slowly to desired dose.

UNLABELED USES
Atypical panic disorder

CONTRAINDICATIONS
None known

INTERACTIONS
Drug
Carbamazepine, phenobarbital, phenytoin, valproic acid, verapamil: May decrease the concentration and effect of oxcarbazepine.
Felodipine, oral contraceptives: May decrease the concentration and effect of these drugs.
Phenobarbital, phenytoin: May increase the concentration and risk of toxicity of phenobarbital, phenytoin.
Herbal
None known.
Food
None known.

DIAGNOSTIC TEST EFFECTS
May increase gamma G-T and liver function tests. May increase or decrease blood glucose levels. May decrease serum calcium, potassium, and sodium levels.

SIDE EFFECTS
Frequent (22%–13%)
Dizziness, nausea, headache
Occasional (7%–5%)
Vomiting, diarrhea, ataxia (muscular incoordination), nervousness, dyspepsia, characterized by heartburn, indigestion, epigastric pain, constipation
Rare (4%)
Tremor, rash, back pain, nosebleed, sinusitis, diplopia or double vision

SERIOUS REACTIONS
• May produce clinically significant hyponatremia.

NURSING CONSIDERATIONS

Baseline Assessment
• Review the patient's drug history, especially other anticonvulsants, and history of seizure disorder, including duration, frequency, intensity, onset and type of seizures, as well as his or her level of consciousness (LOC). Initiate seizure precautions.
• Provide the patient with a quiet, dark environment and safety precautions.
Lifespan Considerations
• Be aware that oxcarbazepine crosses the placenta and is distributed in breast milk.
• Know that there are no age-related precautions in children older than 4 years of age.
• In the elderly, age-related renal impairment may require dosage adjustment.
Precautions
• Use cautiously in patients with renal function impairment and sensitivity to carbamazepine.
Administration and Handling
◀ALERT▶ Plan to give all doses in a twice a day regimen.
PO
• Give oxcarbazepine without regard to food.
Intervention and Evaluation
• Assist the patient with ambulation if he or she experiences ataxia or dizziness.
• Assess the patient for headache and visual abnormalities.
• Monitor the patient's serum sodium levels. Assess the patient for signs and symptoms of hyponatremia including confusion, headache, lethargy, malaise, and nausea.
• Assess the patient for clinical improvement, a decrease in the frequency or intensity of seizures.
Patient Teaching
• Caution the patient against abruptly discontinuing the drug as this may increase seizure activity.
• Warn the patient to notify the physician if he or she experiences dizziness, headache, nausea, and rash.
• Tell the patient that he or she may need periodic blood tests.

phenobarbital
feen-oh-**bar**-bih-tall
(Luminal, Phenobarbitone[AUS])

CATEGORY AND SCHEDULE
Pregnancy Risk Category: D
Controlled substance: Schedule IV

MECHANISM OF ACTION
A barbiturate that binds at GABA receptor complex, enhancing GABA activity. *Therapeutic Effect:* Depresses central nervous system

(CNS) activity, reticular activating system.

PHARMACOKINETICS

Route	Onset	Peak	Duration
PO	20–60 min	N/A	6–10 hrs
IV	5 min	30 min	4–10 hrs

Well absorbed after PO, parenteral administration. Protein binding: 35%–50%. Rapidly, widely distributed. Metabolized in liver. Primarily excreted in urine. Removed by hemodialysis. **Half-life:** 53–118 hrs.

AVAILABILITY

Tablets: 30 mg, 100 mg.
Elixir: 20 mg/5 ml.
Injection: 60 mg/ml, 130 mg/ml.

INDICATIONS AND DOSAGES

▸ **Status epilepticus**
IV
Adults, Elderly, Children, Neonates. (Loading dose): 15–20 mg/kg as single dose or in divided doses.
▸ **Anticonvulsant**
IV/PO
Adults, Elderly, Children older than 12 yrs. 1–3 mg/kg/day.
Children 6–12 yrs. 4–6 mg/kg/day.
Children 1–5 yrs. 6–8 mg/kg/day.
Children less than 1 yr. 5–6 mg/kg/day.
Neonates. 3–4 mg/kg/day.
▸ **Sedation**
PO/IM
Adults, Elderly. 30–120 mg/day in 2–3 divided doses.
Children. 2 mg/kg 3 times/day.
▸ **Hypnotic**
PO/IM/IV/Subcutaneous
Adults, Elderly. 100–320 mg at bedtime.
Children. 3–5 mg/kg.

UNLABELED USES

Prophylaxis and treatment of hyperbilirubinemia

CONTRAINDICATIONS

Porphyria, preexisting central nervous system (CNS) depression, severe pain, severe respiratory disease

INTERACTIONS

Drug
Alcohol, CNS depressants: May increase the effects of phenobarbital.
Carbamazepine: May increase the metabolism of carbamazepine.
Digoxin, glucocorticoids, metronidazole, oral anticoagulants, quinidine, tricyclic antidepressants: May decrease the effects of digoxin, glucocorticoids, metronidazole, oral anticoagulants, quinidine, tricyclic antidepressants.
Valproic acid: Decreases the metabolism and increases the concentration and risk of toxicity of phenobarbital.
Herbal
None known.
Food
None known.

DIAGNOSTIC TEST EFFECTS

May decrease serum bilirubin levels. Therapeutic serum level is 10–40 mcg/ml; toxic serum level is greater than 40 mcg/ml.

IV INCOMPATIBILITIES

Amphotericin B complex (Abelcet, AmBisome, Amphotec), hydrocortisone (Solu-Cortef), hydromorphone (Dilaudid), insulin

IV COMPATIBILITIES

Calcium gluconate, enalapril (Vasotec), fentanyl (Sublimaze), fosphenytoin (Cerebyx), morphine, propofol (Diprivan)

SIDE EFFECTS

Occasional (3%–1%)
Somnolence
Rare (less than 1%)
Confusion, paradoxical CNS hyperactivity or nervousness in children, excitement or restlessness in elderly, generally noted during first 2 wks of therapy, particularly noted in presence of uncontrolled pain

SERIOUS REACTIONS

• Abrupt withdrawal after prolonged therapy may produce effects ranging from markedly increased dreaming, nightmares or insomnia, tremor, sweating, vomiting, to hallucinations, delirium, seizures, and status epilepticus.
• Skin eruptions appear as hypersensitivity reaction.
• Blood dyscrasias, liver disease, and hypocalcemia occur rarely.
• Overdosage produces cold or clammy skin, hypothermia, severe CNS depression, cyanosis, rapid pulse, and Cheyne-Stokes respirations.
• Toxicity may result in severe renal impairment.

NURSING CONSIDERATIONS

Baseline Assessment
• Assess the patient's blood pressure (B/P), pulse, and respirations immediately before giving phenobarbital.
• Provide the patient using the drug as a hypnotic with an environment conducive to sleep, such as low lighting and a quiet environment. As a safety precaution, raise the bed rails.
• Review the seizure patient's history of seizure disorder, including duration of seizures. Observe

the patient frequently for recurrence of seizure activity. Initiate seizure precautions.

Lifespan Considerations
• Be aware that phenobarbital readily crosses the placenta and is distributed in breast milk.
• Keep in mind that phenobarbital lowers serum bilirubin concentrations in neonates, produces respiratory depression in neonates during labor, and may cause postpartum hemorrhage or hemorrhagic disease in newborn.
• Be aware that withdrawal symptoms may appear in neonates born to women receiving barbiturates during last trimester of pregnancy.
• Be aware that phenobarbital use may cause paradoxical excitement in children.
• Know that elderly patient taking phenobarbital may exhibit confusion, excitement, and mental depression.

Precautions
• Use cautiously in patients with liver or renal impairment.

Administration and Handling
◀ALERT▶ Expect to administer maintenance dose 12 hours after loading dose.
PO
• Give phenobarbital without regard to meals.
• Crush tablets as needed.
• Elixir may be mixed with fruit juice, milk, or water.
IM
• Do not inject more than 5 ml in any one IM injection site because it produces tissue irritation.
• Inject IM deeply into the gluteus maximus or lateral aspect of thigh.
IV
• Store vials at room temperature.
• May give undiluted, or may dilute with NaCl, D_5W, lactated Ringer's.
• Expect to adequately hydrate the

patient before and immediately after infusion to decrease the risk of adverse renal effects.

• Do not inject IV faster than 1 mg/kg/min, or more than 30 mg/min for children and 60 mg/min for adults. Injecting too rapidly may produce marked respiratory depression and severe hypotension.

• Beware that inadvertent intra-arterial injection may result in arterial spasm with severe pain and tissue necrosis. Also know that extravasation in subcutaneous tissue may produce redness, tenderness, and tissue necrosis. If either occurs, treat the patient with 0.5% procaine solution into the affected area and apply moist heat, as ordered.

Intervention and Evaluation

• Monitor the patient's B/P, CNS status, heart rate, liver function, renal function, respiratory rate, and seizure activity.

• Monitor the patient for therapeutic serum levels (10–30 mcg/ml) of phenobarbital. The therapeutic blood serum level of phenobarbital is 10–40 mcg/ml and the toxic blood serum level is greater than 40 mcg/ml.

Patient Teaching

• Urge the patient to avoid alcohol consumption and to limit caffeine intake while taking phenobarbital.

• Tell the patient that phenobarbital may be habit-forming.

• Caution the patient against abruptly discontinuing the drug.

• Warn the patient to avoid tasks that require mental alertness or motor skills as this drug may cause dizziness and drowsiness.

phenytoin
phen-ih-toyn
(Dilantin, Epamin)
Do not confuse with Dilaudid or mephenytoin.

phenytoin sodium
(Dilantin)

CATEGORY AND SCHEDULE
Pregnancy Risk Category: D

MECHANISM OF ACTION
An anticonvulsant and antiarrhythmic agent that stabilizes neuronal membranes in motor cortex, and decreases abnormal ventricular automaticity. *Therapeutic Effect:* Limits spread of seizure activity. Stabilizes threshold against hyperexcitability. Decreases posttetanic potentiation and repetitive discharge. Shortens refractory period, QT interval, and action potential duration.

PHARMACOKINETICS
Slowly, variably absorbed after PO administration; slow but completely absorbed after IM administration. Protein binding: 90%–95%. Widely distributed. Metabolized in liver. Primarily excreted in urine. Not removed by hemodialysis. **Half-life:** 22 hrs.

AVAILABILITY
Capsules: 30 mg, 100 mg.
Tablets (chewable): 50 mg.
Oral Suspension: 125 mg/5 ml.
Injection: 50 mg/ml.

INDICATIONS AND DOSAGES
▶ **Status epilepticus**
IV
Adults, Elderly, Children. Loading dose: 15–18 mg/kg. Maintenance

dose: 300 mg/day in 2–3 divided doses.

Children 10–16 yrs. Loading dose: 15–18 mg/kg. Maintenance dose: 6–7 mg/kg/day.

Children 7–9 yrs. Loading dose: 15–18 mg/kg. Maintenance dose 7–8 mg/kg/day.

Children 4–6 yrs. Loading dose: 15–18 mg/kg. Maintenance dose: 7.5–9 mg/kg/day

Children 6 mos–3 yrs. Loading dose 15–18 mg/kg. Maintenance dose: 8–10 mg/kg/day.

Neonates. Loading dose: 15–20 mg/kg. Maintenance dose: 5–8 mg/kg/day.

▸ **Anticonvulsant**
PO
Adults, Elderly, Children. Loading dose: 15–20 mg/kg in 3 divided doses 2–4 hrs apart. Maintenance dose: Same as above.

▸ **Arrhythmias**
IV
Adults, Elderly, Children. Loading dose: 1.25 mg/kg q5min. May repeat up to total dose of 15 mg/kg.
PO
Adults, Elderly. Maintenance Dose: 250 mg 4 times/day for 1 day, then 250 mg 2 times/day for 2 days, then 300–400 mg/day in divided doses 1–4 times/day.
PO/IV
Children. Maintenance dose: 5–10 mg/kg/day in 2–3 divided doses.

UNLABELED USES
Adjunct in treatment of tricyclic antidepressant toxicity, muscle relaxant in treatment of muscle hyperirritability, treatment of digoxin-induced arrhythmias and trigeminal neuralgia

CONTRAINDICATIONS
Hydantoin hypersensitivity, seizures due to hypoglycemia

IV: Adam-Stokes syndrome, second- and third-degree heart block, sino-atrial block, sinus bradycardia

INTERACTIONS
Drug
Alcohol, central nervous system (CNS) depressants: May increase CNS depression.
Amiodarone, anticoagulants, cimetidine, disulfiram, fluoxetine, isoniazid, sulfonamides: May increase phenytoin blood concentration, effects, and risk of toxicity.
Antacids: May decrease the absorption of phenytoin.
Fluconazole, ketoconazole, miconazole: May increase phenytoin blood concentration.
Glucocorticoids: May decrease the effects of glucocorticoids.
Lidocaine, propranolol: May increase cardiac depressant effects.
Valproic acid: May increase phenytoin blood concentration and decrease the metabolism of phenytoin.
Xanthine: May increase the metabolism of xanthine.
Herbal
None known.
Food
None known.

DIAGNOSTIC TEST EFFECTS
May increase blood glucose levels, serum gamma glutamyl transferase (GGT) levels, and serum alkaline phosphatase levels. Therapeutic serum level is 10–20 mcg/ml; toxic serum level is greater than 20 mcg/ml.

IV INCOMPATIBILITIES
Diltiazem (Cardizem), dobutamine (Dobutrex), enalapril (Vasotec), heparin, hydromorphone (Dilaudid), insulin, lidocaine, morphine, nitroglycerin, norepinephrine

(Levophed), potassium chloride, propofol (Diprivan)

SIDE EFFECTS

Frequent
Drowsiness, lethargy, confusion, slurred speech, irritability, gingival hyperplasia, hypersensitivity reaction, including fever, rash, and lymphadenopathy, constipation, dizziness, nausea
Occasional
Headache, hair growth, insomnia, muscle twitching

SERIOUS REACTIONS

• Abrupt withdrawal may precipitate status epilepticus.
• Blood dyscrasias, lymphadenopathy, and osteomalacia, caused by interference of vitamin D metabolism, may occur.
• Toxic phenytoin blood concentration of 25 mcg/ml may produce ataxia, characterized by muscular incoordination, nystagmus or rhythmic oscillation of eyes, and double vision. As level increases, extreme lethargy to comatose states occur.

NURSING CONSIDERATIONS

Baseline Assessment

• Review the anticonvulsant patient's history of seizure disorder, including the duration, frequency, intensity, and level of consciousness (LOC) of seizures. Initiate seizure precautions.
• Perform a complete blood count (CBC) and blood serum chemistry tests to assess liver function before beginning phenytoin therapy and periodically during therapy. Repeat the CBC 2 weeks after beginning phenytoin therapy, and 2 weeks after the phenytoin maintenance dose is given.

Lifespan Considerations

• Be aware that phenytoin crosses the placenta and is distributed in small amounts in breast milk. Know that fetal hydantoin syndrome, marked by craniofacial abnormalities, digital or nail hypoplasia, prenatal growth deficiency, has been reported.
• Be aware that there is an increased frequency of seizures in pregnant women due to altered absorption and metabolism of phenytoin.
• Keep in mind that phenytoin use may increase the risk of hemorrhage in neonates and maternal bleeding during delivery.
• Be aware that children are more susceptible to coarsening of facial features, excess body hair, and gingival hyperplasia.
• There are no age-related precautions noted but lower dosages are recommended in the elderly.

Precautions

• Use IV phenytoin extremely cautiously in patients with congestive heart failure (CHF), damaged myocardium, myocardial infarction (MI), and respiratory depression.
• Use cautiously in patients with hyperglycemia, hypotension, impaired liver or renal function, and severe myocardial insufficiency.
• Look for signs of IV phenytoin toxicity, such as cardiovascular collapse and CNS depression.

Administration and Handling

◀ALERT▶ Remember that the maintenance dose is usually given 12 hours after the loading dose.
PO
• Give phenytoin with food if gastrointestinal (GI) distress occurs.
• Do not chew, open, or break capsules. Tablets may be chewed.
• Shake oral suspension well before using.

IV

◀ **ALERT** ▶ Give by IV push.

• Keep in mind that precipitate may form if parenteral form is refrigerated, but precipitate will dissolve at room temperature.

• Do not use if solution is not clear or if precipitate is present. Keep in mind that slight yellow discoloration of parenteral form does not affect potency.

• May give undiluted or may dilute with 0.9% NaCl.

• Administer 50 mg over 2 to 3 minutes for elderly patients. In neonates, administer at rate not exceeding 1–3 mg/kg/min.

• Don't give the IV injection faster than 50 mg/min for adults to avoid cardiovascular collapse and severe hypotension.

• To minimize pain from chemical irritation of the vein, flush the catheter with sterile saline solution after each bolus of phenytoin.

Intervention and Evaluation

• Observe the patient frequently for recurrence of seizure activity.

• Assess the patient for clinical improvement, a decrease in the frequency or intensity of seizures.

• Monitor the patient's blood pressure (B/P) with IV use, as well as CBC, and liver or renal function tests.

• Assist the patient with ambulation if he or she experiences drowsiness or lethargy.

• Monitor the patient for therapeutic serum levels, 10–20 mcg/ml. The therapeutic serum level for phenytoin is 10–20 mcg/ml, and the toxic serum level for phenytoin is greater than 20 mcg/ml.

Patient Teaching

• Warn the patient that he or she may experience pain with IV injection.

• Encourage the patient to maintain good oral hygiene care with gum massage and regular dental visits to prevent gingival hyperplasia, marked by bleeding, swelling, and tenderness of gums.

• Stress to the patient that a CBC should be performed every month for 1 year after the maintenance dose is established and every 3 months thereafter.

• Explain to the patient that his or her urine may appear pink, red, or red-brown and that drowsiness usually diminishes with continued therapy.

• Warn the patient to notify the physician if he or she experiences fever, glandular swelling, skin reaction, signs of hematologic toxicity, or sore throat.

• Caution the patient against abruptly withdrawing the medication after long-term use because it may precipitate seizures.

• Explain to the patient that strict maintenance of drug therapy is essential for arrhythmia and seizure control.

• Warn the patient to avoid tasks that require mental alertness or motor skills until his or her response to the drug is established.

• Urge the patient to avoid alcohol while taking phenytoin.

primidone
prih-mih-doan
(Apo-Primidone[CAN], Mysoline)
Do not confuse with prednisone.

CATEGORY AND SCHEDULE
Pregnancy Risk Category: D

MECHANISM OF ACTION
A barbiturate that decreases motor activity to electrical and chemical

stimulation, stabilizes threshold against hyperexcitability. *Therapeutic Effect:* Produces anticonvulsant effect.

AVAILABILITY
Tablets: 50 mg, 250 mg.

INDICATIONS AND DOSAGES
▸ **Anticonvulsant**
PO
Adults, Elderly, Children 8 yrs and older. 125–150 mg/day at bedtime. May increase by 125–250 mg/day q3–7 days. Maximum: 2 g/day.
Children younger than 8 yrs.: Initially, 50–125 mg/day at bedtime. May increase by 50–125 mg/day q3–7 days. Usual dose: 10–25 mg/kg/day in divided doses.
Neonates. 12–20 mg/kg/day in divided doses.

UNLABELED USES
Treatment of essential tremor

CONTRAINDICATIONS
History of bronchopneumonia, porphyria

INTERACTIONS
Drug
Alcohol, central nervous system (CNS) depressants: May increase the effects of primidone.
Carbamazepine: May increase the metabolism of carbamazepine.
Digoxin, glucocorticoids, metronidazole, oral anticoagulants, quinidine, tricyclic antidepressants: May decrease the effects of digoxin, glucocorticoids, metronidazole, oral anticoagulants, quinidine, tricyclic antidepressants.
Valproic acid: Decreases the metabolism, increases the concentration, and risk of toxicity of primidone.

Herbal
None known.
Food
None known.

DIAGNOSTIC TEST EFFECTS
May decrease bilirubin. Therapeutic serum level is 4–12 mcg/ml; toxic serum level is greater than 12 mcg/ml.

SIDE EFFECTS
Frequent
Ataxia, dizziness
Occasional
Loss of appetite, drowsiness, mental changes, nausea, vomiting, paradoxical excitement
Rare
Skin rash

SERIOUS REACTIONS
• Abrupt withdrawal after prolonged therapy may produce effects ranging from markedly increased dreaming, nightmares and insomnia, tremor, sweating, and vomiting to hallucinations, delirium, seizures, and status epilepticus.
• Skin eruptions may appear as hypersensitivity reaction.
• Blood dyscrasias, liver disease, and hypocalcemia occur rarely.
• Overdosage produces cold or clammy skin, hypothermia, and severe CNS depression followed by high fever and coma.

NURSING CONSIDERATIONS
Baseline Assessment
• Review the patient's history of seizure disorder, including duration, frequency, and intensity of seizures, as well as his or her level of consciousness (LOC). Initiate seizure precautions.
• Observe the patient frequently for recurrence of seizure activity.

Precautions
• Use cautiously in patients with liver or renal impairment.

Intervention and Evaluation
• Monitor the patient's complete blood count (CBC), neurologic status, including duration, frequency, and severity of seizures, and serum concentrations of primidone.
• Monitor the patient for therapeutic serum levels. The therapeutic serum level for primidone is 4–12 mcg/ml, and the toxic serum level for primidone is greater than 12 mcg/ml.

Patient Teaching
• Caution the patient against abruptly withdrawing the medication after long-term use as this may precipitate seizures.
• Stress to the patient that strict maintenance of drug therapy is essential for seizure control.
• Tell the patient that drowsiness usually disappears during continued therapy.
• Instruct the patient to change positions slowly from recumbent to sitting position before standing if he or she experiences dizziness.
• Warn the patient to avoid tasks that require mental alertness or motor skills until his or her response to the drug is established.
• Urge the patient to avoid alcohol while taking primidone.

tiagabine
tie-**ag**-ah-bean
(Gabitril)

CATEGORY AND SCHEDULE
Pregnancy Risk Category: C

MECHANISM OF ACTION
An anticonvulsant that blocks the reuptake of gamma aminobutyric acid (GABA) in the presynaptic neurons, the major inhibitory neurotransmitter in the central nervous system (CNS), increasing GABA levels at postsynaptic neurons.
Therapeutic Effect: Inhibits seizures.

AVAILABILITY
Tablets: 2 mg, 4 mg, 12 mg, 16 mg.

INDICATIONS AND DOSAGES
‣ **Adjunctive therapy for the treatment of partial seizures**
PO
Adults, Elderly. Initially, 4 mg once a day. May increase by 4–8 mg/day at weekly intervals. Maximum: 56 mg/day.
Children 12–18 yrs. Initially, 4 mg once a day, may increase by 4 mg at week 2 and by 4–8 mg/wk thereafter. Maximum: 32 mg/day.

CONTRAINDICATIONS
None known.

INTERACTIONS
Drug
Carbamazepine, phenobarbital, phenytoin: May increase tiagabine clearance.
Valproate: May alter the effects of valproate.
Herbal
None known.
Food
None known.

DIAGNOSTIC TEST EFFECTS
None known.

SIDE EFFECTS
Frequent (34%–20%)
Dizziness, asthenia or loss of strength and energy, somnolence, nervousness, confusion, headache, infection, tremor

Occasional
Nausea, diarrhea, stomach pain, difficulty concentrating, weakness

SERIOUS REACTIONS
• Overdosage is characterized by agitation, confusion, hostility, and weakness. Full recovery occurs within 24 hrs.

NURSING CONSIDERATIONS
Baseline Assessment
• Review the patient's history of seizure disorder, including duration, frequency, and intensity, of seizures, as well as his or her level of consciousness (LOC). Initiate seizure precautions.
• Observe the patient frequently for recurrence of seizure activity.
Precautions
• Use cautiously in patients with liver function impairment and who concurrently use alcohol or other CNS depressants.
Intervention and Evaluation
• Plan to perform complete blood count (CBC) and blood serum chemistry tests to assess liver and renal function periodically for patients on long-term therapy.
• Assist the patient with ambulation if he or she experiences dizziness.
• Assess the patient for signs of clinical improvement, manifested by a decrease in frequency or intensity of seizures.
Patient Teaching
• Instruct the patient to change positions slowly from recumbent to sitting position before standing, if he or she experiences dizziness.
• Warn the patient to avoid tasks that require mental alertness or motor skills until his or her response to the drug is established.
• Urge the patient to avoid alcohol while taking tiagabine.

topiramate
toe-**pie**-rah-mate
(Topamax)

CATEGORY AND SCHEDULE
Pregnancy Risk Category: C

MECHANISM OF ACTION
An anticonvulsant that blocks repetitive, sustained firing of neurons by enhancing the ability of gamma-aminobutyric acid (GABA) to induce a flux of chloride ions into the neurons; may block sodium channels. *Therapeutic Effect:* Decreases spread of seizure activity.

PHARMACOKINETICS
Rapidly absorbed after PO administration. Protein binding: 13%–17%. Not extensively metabolized. Primarily excreted unchanged in the urine. Removed by hemodialysis.
Half-life: 21 hrs.

AVAILABILITY
Tablets: 25 mg, 100 mg, 200 mg.
Sprinkle Capsules: 15 mg, 25 mg.

INDICATIONS AND DOSAGES
▸ **Adjunctive therapy for the treatment of partial seizures**
PO
Adults, Elderly, Children older than 17 yrs. Initially, 25–50 mg for 1 wk. May increase by 25–50 mg/day at weekly intervals. Maximum: 1,600 mg/day.
Children 2–16 yrs. Initially, 1–3 mg/kg/day. Maximum: 25 mg. May increase by 1–3 mg/kg/day at weekly intervals. Maintenance: 5–9 mg/kg/day in 2 divided doses.
▸ **Tonic-clonic seizures**
PO
Adults, Elderly, Children. Individual and titrated.

UNLABELED USES
Prevention of migraine headaches

CONTRAINDICATIONS
None known.

INTERACTIONS
Drug
Alcohol, central nervous system (CND) depressants: May increase CNS depression.
Carbamazepine, phenytoin, valproic acid: May decrease topiramate blood concentration.
Carbonic anhydrase inhibitors: May increase the risk of renal calculi.
Oral contraceptives: May decrease the effectiveness of oral contraceptives.
Herbal
None known.
Food
None known.

DIAGNOSTIC TEST EFFECTS
None known.

SIDE EFFECTS
Frequent (30%–10%)
Somnolence, dizziness, ataxia, nervousness, nystagmus or involuntary eye movement, diplopia or double vision, paresthesia, nausea, tremor
Occasional (9%–3%)
Confusion, breast pain, dysmenorrhea, dyspepsia, depression, asthenia or loss of strength, pharyngitis, weight loss, anorexia, rash, back or abdominal or leg pain, difficulty with coordination, sinusitis, agitation, flu-like symptoms
Rare (3%–2%)
Mood disturbances, such as irritability and depression, dry mouth, aggressive reaction

SERIOUS REACTIONS
• Psychomotor slowing, difficulty with concentration, language problems, including word-finding difficulties, and memory disturbances occur occasionally. These reactions are generally mild to moderate, but may be severe enough to require withdrawal from drug therapy.

NURSING CONSIDERATIONS
Baseline Assessment
• Review the patient's history of seizure disorder, including duration, frequency, and intensity of seizures, as well as his or her level of consciousness (LOC). Initiate seizure precautions.
• Provide the patient with a quiet, dark environment and safety precautions.
• Determine if the patient is pregnant, sensitive to topiramate, or using other anticonvulsant medication, especially carbamazepine, carbonic anhydrase inhibitors, phenytoin, and valproic acid.
• Obtain the patient's BUN and serum creatinine levels to assess renal function.
• Instruct the patient to use additional or alternative means of contraception if she uses oral contraceptives. Explain to the patient that topiramate decreases the effectiveness of oral contraceptives.
Lifespan Considerations
• Be aware that it is unknown if topiramate is distributed in breast milk.
• Know that there are no age-related precautions noted in children older than 2 years of age.
• In the elderly, age-related renal impairment may require dosage adjustment.
Precautions
• Use cautiously in patients with impaired liver or renal function, predisposition to renal calculi, and sensitivity to topiramate.

Administration and Handling
◀**ALERT**▶ Expect to reduce drug dosage by 50% if creatinine clearance is less than 70 ml/min in tonic-clonic seizure patients.

PO
• Do not break tablets because it produces a bitter taste.
• Give topiramate without regard to meals.
• Capsules may be swallowed whole or contents sprinkled on a teaspoonful of soft food and swallowed immediately. Do not chew.

Intervention and Evaluation
• Observe the patient frequently for recurrence of seizure activity.
• Institute seizure safety precautions.
• Assess the patient for clinical improvement, a decrease in the frequency and intensity of seizures.
• Monitor the patient's renal function tests, including BUN and serum creatinine levels.
• Assist the patient with ambulation if he or she experiences dizziness.

Patient Teaching
• Warn the patient to avoid tasks that require mental alertness or motor skills until his or her response to the drug is established. Keep in mind that topiramate may cause dizziness, drowsiness, or impaired thinking.
• Urge the patient to avoid alcohol and taking other CNS depressants while on topiramate therapy.
• Caution the patient against abruptly discontinuing the drug as this may precipitate seizures.
• Stress to the patient that strict maintenance of drug therapy is essential for seizure control.
• Tell the patient that drowsiness usually diminishes with continued therapy.
• Instruct the patient not to break tablets to avoid their bitter taste.

• Urge the patient to maintain adequate fluid intake to decrease the risk of renal stone formation.
• Warn the patient to notify the physician if he or she experiences blurred vision or eye pain.

valproic acid
val-**pro**-ick
(Depakene)
valproate sodium
(Depakene syrup, Epilim[AUS], Valpro[AUS])
divalproex sodium
(Depacon, Depakote, Epival[CAN])

CATEGORY AND SCHEDULE
Pregnancy Risk Category: D

MECHANISM OF ACTION
An anticonvulsant, antimanic, and antimigraine agent that directly increases concentration of the inhibitory neurotransmitter gamma-aminobutyric acid (GABA). *Therapeutic Effect:* Produces anticonvulsant effect.

PHARMACOKINETICS
Well absorbed from the gastrointestinal (GI) tract. Protein binding: 80%–90%. Metabolized in liver. Primarily excreted in urine. Not removed by hemodialysis. **Half-life:** 6–16 hrs, half-life may be increased with impaired liver function, elderly, children younger than 18 mos.

AVAILABILITY
Capsules: 250 mg (valproic acid).
Syrup: 250 mg/5 ml (valproic acid).
Tablets (delayed-release): 125 mg, 250 mg, 500 mg (divalproex).

Tablets (extended-release): 250 mg, 500 mg.
Capsules (sprinkle): 125 mg (divalproex).
Injection: 100 mg/ml.

INDICATIONS AND DOSAGES
▸ **Seizures**
PO
Adults, Elderly, Children older than 10 yrs. Initially, 10–15 mg/kg/day in 1–3 divided doses. May increase by 5–10 mg/kg/day at weekly intervals up to 30–60 mg/kg/day (usual adult dosage: 1,000–2,500 mg/day).
IV
Adults, Elderly, Children. IV dose equal to oral dose but given at a frequency of q6h.
▸ **Manic episodes**
PO
Adults, Elderly. Initially, 750 mg/day in divided doses. Maximum: 60 mg/kg/day.
▸ **Migraine prophylaxis**
PO (extended-release tablets)
Adults, Elderly. Initially, 500 mg/day for 7 days. May increase up to 1000 mg/day.
PO (delayed-release tablets)
Adults, Elderly. Initially, 250 mg 2 times/day. May increase up to 1,000 mg/day.

UNLABELED USES
Treatment of myoclonic, simple partial, tonic-clonic seizures

CONTRAINDICATIONS
Active liver disease

INTERACTIONS
Drug
Alcohol, central nervous system (CNS) depressants: May increase CNS depressant effects.
Amitriptyline, primidone: May increase the concentration of amitriptyline and primidone.
Anticoagulants, heparin, platelet aggregation inhibitors, thrombolytics: May increase the risk of bleeding.
Carbamazepine: May decrease valproic acid blood concentration.
Liver toxic medications: May increase risk of liver toxicity.
Phenytoin: May alter phenytoin protein binding, increasing the risk of toxicity. Phenytoin may decrease the effects of valproic acid.
Herbal
None known.
Food
None known.

DIAGNOSTIC TEST EFFECTS
May increase LDH concentrations, serum bilirubin, SGOT (AST), and SGPT (ALT) levels. Therapeutic serum level is 50–100 mcg/ml; toxic serum level is greater than 100 mcg/ml.

IV INCOMPATIBILITIES
Do not mix with any other medications.

SIDE EFFECTS
Frequent
Epilepsy: Abdominal pain, irregular menses, diarrhea, transient alopecia, indigestion, nausea, vomiting, trembling, weight change
Mania (22%–19%): Nausea, somnolence
Occasional
Epilepsy: Constipation, dizziness, drowsiness, headache, skin rash, unusual excitement, restlessness
Mania (12%–6%): Asthenia, abdominal pain, dyspepsia (heartburn, indigestion, epigastric distress), rash
Rare
Epilepsy: Mood changes, double

vision, nystagmus, spots before eyes, unusual bleeding or bruising

SERIOUS REACTIONS
• Liver toxicity may occur, particularly in the first 6 months of valproic acid therapy. Liver toxicity may not be preceded by abnormal liver function tests but may be noted as loss of seizure control, malaise, weakness, lethargy, anorexia, and vomiting.
• Blood dyscrasias may occur.

NURSING CONSIDERATIONS

Baseline Assessment
• Review the patient's history of seizure disorder, including duration, frequency, and intensity, of seizures, as well as his or her level of consciousness (LOC). Initiate seizure precautions.
• Maintain safety measures, and provide the patient with a dark, quiet environment.
• Perform a complete blood count (CBC) with platelet count before beginning and 2 weeks after valproic acid therapy and 2 weeks after the valproic acid maintenance dose is given in seizure patients.
• Assess the appearance, behavior, emotional status, response to environment, speech pattern, and thought content in manic patients.
• Determine the duration, location, and onset of migraine headache and its precipitating symptoms in migraine patients.

Lifespan Considerations
• Be aware that valproic acid crosses the placenta and is distributed in breast milk.
• Be aware that there is an increased risk of liver toxicity in children younger than 2 years of age.
• There are no age-related precau-

tions, but lower dosages are recommended in the elderly.

Precautions
• Use cautiously in patients with bleeding abnormalities and a history of liver disease.

Administration and Handling
◀ ALERT ▶ Regular release and delayed-release formulations of valproic acid are given in 2–4 divided doses per day, extended-release formulation of valproic acid is given once a day.

PO
• May give with or without regard to food. Do not administer with carbonated drinks.
• May sprinkle capsule contents on applesauce and give immediately, but do not break, chew, or crush sprinkle beads.
• Delayed-release or extended-release tablets should be given whole.

IV
• Store vials at room temperature.
• Diluted solutions are stable for 24 hours.
• Discard unused portion.
• Dilute each single dose with at least 50 ml D_5W, 0.9% NaCl, or lactated Ringer's.
• Infuse over 5–10 minutes.
• Do not exceed rate of 3 mg/kg/min (5-min infusion) or 1.5 mg/kg/min (10-min infusion). Too rapid an infusion rate increases the likelihood of side effects.

Intervention and Evaluation
• Monitor the patient's complete blood count (CBC), serum alkaline phosphatase, ammonia, bilirubin, SGOT (AST), and SGPT (ALT) levels.
• Observe seizure patients frequently for recurrence of seizure activity.
• Assess the seizure patient's skin for bruising and petechiae.
• Monitor the seizure patient for

clinical improvement, a decrease in the frequency or intensity of seizures.
• Assess the manic patient for therapeutic response, such as an increased ability to concentrate, interest in his or her surroundings, and a relaxed facial expression.
• Evaluate migraine patients for relief of migraine headache and resulting nausea, phonophobia, photophobia, and vomiting.
• Monitor the patient's valproic acid blood serum level. The therapeutic serum level for valproic acid is 50–100 mcg/ml, and the toxic serum level for valproic acid is greater than 100 mcg/ml.

Patient Teaching
• Caution the patient against abruptly withdrawing the medication after long-term use as this may precipitate seizures.
• Stress to the patient that strict maintenance of drug therapy is essential for seizure control.
• Explain to the patient that drowsiness usually disappears during continued therapy.
• Warn the patient to avoid tasks that require mental alertness or motor skills until his or her response to the drug is established.
• Urge the patient to avoid alcohol while taking valproic acid.
• Recommend to the patient that he or she carry an identification card or wear an identification bracelet to note anticonvulsant therapy.
• Warn the patient to notify the physician if he or she experiences abdominal pain, altered mental status, bleeding, easy bruising, lethargy, loss of appetite, nausea, vomiting, weakness, or yellowing of skin.

zonisamide
zoe-**niss**-ah-mide
(Zonegran)

CATEGORY AND SCHEDULE
Pregnancy Risk Category: C

MECHANISM OF ACTION
A succinimide that may stabilize neuronal membranes and suppress neuronal hypersynchronization by action at sodium and calcium channels. *Therapeutic Effect:* Produces anticonvulsant effect.

PHARMACOKINETICS
Well absorbed after PO administration. Extensively bound to erythrocytes. Protein binding: 40%. Primarily excreted in urine. **Half-life:** 63 hrs (plasma), 105 hrs (RBCs).

AVAILABILITY
Capsules: 25 mg, 50 mg, 100 mg.

INDICATIONS AND DOSAGES
▶ **Partial seizures**
PO
Adults, Children older than 16 yrs.
Initially, 100 mg/day for 2 wks. May increase by 100 mg/day at intervals of 2 wks or longer. Maximum: 400 mg/day.

CONTRAINDICATIONS
Allergy to sulfonamides

INTERACTIONS
Drug
Carbamazepine, phenobarbital, phenytoin, valproic acid: May increase the metabolism and decrease the effect of zonisamide.
Herbal
None known.
Food
None known.

DIAGNOSTIC TEST EFFECTS
May increase BUN and serum creatinine levels.

SIDE EFFECTS
Frequent (17%–9%)
Somnolence, dizziness, anorexia, headache, agitation, irritability, nausea
Occasional (8%–5%)
Fatigue, ataxia, confusion, depression, memory or concentration impairment, insomnia, abdominal pain, double vision, diarrhea, speech difficulty
Rare (4%–3%)
Paresthesia, nystagmus or involuntary movement of eyeball, anxiety, rash, dyspepsia, including heartburn, indigestion, and epigastric distress, weight loss

SERIOUS REACTIONS
• Overdosage is characterized by bradycardia, hypotension, respiratory depression, and comatose state.
• Leukopenia, anemia, and thrombocytopenia occur rarely.

NURSING CONSIDERATIONS

Baseline Assessment
• Review the patient's history of seizure disorder, including duration, frequency, and intensity, of seizures, as well as his or her level of consciousness (LOC). Initiate seizure precautions.
• Plan to perform a complete blood count (CBC) and blood serum chemistry tests to assess renal and liver function before beginning and periodically during therapy.

Lifespan Considerations
• Be aware that it is unknown if zonisamide is distributed in breast milk.
• Be aware that the safety and efficacy of this drug have not been established in children younger than 16 years of age.
• There are no age-related precautions noted, but lower dosages are recommended in the elderly.
Precautions
• Use cautiously in patients with renal function impairment.
Administration and Handling
PO
• May take with or without food.
• Swallow capsules whole.
• Do not give to patients allergic to sulfonamides.
Intervention and Evaluation
• Observe the patient frequently for recurrence of seizure activity.
• Assess the patient for clinical improvement, a decrease in the frequency or intensity of seizures.
• Assist the patient with ambulation if he or she experiences dizziness.
Patient Teaching
• Stress to the patient that strict maintenance of drug therapy is essential for seizure control.
• Warn the patient to avoid tasks that require mental alertness or motor skills until his or her response to the drug is established.
• Urge the patient to avoid alcohol while taking zonisamide.
• Warn the patient to notify the physician if he or she experiences abdominal or back pain, blood in urine, easy bruising, fever, rash, sore throat, or ulcers in the mouth.

amitriptyline hydrochloride

bupropion

citalopram hydrobromide

clomipramine hydrochloride

desipramine hydrochloride

doxepin hydrochloride

escitalopram

fluoxetine hydrochloride

imipramine

mirtazapine

nefazodone hydrochloride

nortriptyline hydrochloride

paroxetine hydrochloride

phenelzine sulfate

sertraline hydrochloride

tranylcypromine sulfate

trazodone hydrochloride

venlafaxine

Uses: Antidepressants are used primarily to treat depression. In addition, imipramine is used for childhood enuresis. Clomipramine is used only for obsessive-compulsive disorder. Monoamine oxidase inhibitors (MAOIs) are rarely prescribed as initial therapy, except for patients who don't respond to, or who have contraindications for, other antidepressants.

Action: Antidepressants are classified as tricyclic antidepressants, MAOIs, or second-generation antidepressants, which include selective serotonin reuptake inhibitors (SSRIs) and atypical antidepressants. Depression may result from decreased amounts (or effects at the receptor sites) of monoamine neurotransmitters, such as norepinephrine, serotonin, and dopamine, in the central nervous system.

Antidepressants block the metabolism of monoamine neurotransmitters, increasing their levels and effects at receptor sites. These agents also change the responsiveness and sensitivity of presynaptic and postsynaptic receptor sites. (See illustration, *Mechanisms of Action: Antidepressants,* page 663.)

COMBINATION PRODUCTS

ETRAFON: amitriptyline/perphenazine (an antipsychotic) 10 mg/2 mg; 25 mg/2 mg; 10 mg/4 mg; 25 mg/4 mg.

LIMBITROL: amitriptyline/chlordiazepoxide (an antianxiety agent) 12.5 mg/5 mg; 25 mg/10 mg.

TRIAVIL: amitriptyline/perphenazine (an antipsychotic) 10 mg/2 mg; 25 mg/2 mg; 10 mg/4 mg; 25 mg/4 mg.

amitriptyline hydrochloride

a-me-**trip**-tih-leen

(Apo-Amitriptyline[CAN], Elavil, Endep[AUS], Levate[CAN], Novo-Triptyn[CAN], Tryptanol[AUS])

Do not confuse with Mellaril or nortriptyline.

CATEGORY AND SCHEDULE

Pregnancy Risk Category: C

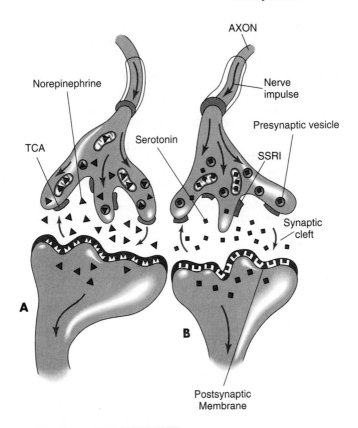

Mechanisms of Action: Antidepressants

Depression is thought to occur when levels of neurotransmitters, such as norepineph-rine and serotonin, are reduced at postsynaptic receptor sites. These neurotransmit-ters affect a wide array of functions, including mood, obsessions, appetite, and anxi-ety. Antidepressants work by increasing the availability of these neurotransmitters at postsynaptic membranes and by enhancing and prolonging their effects. As a result, these agents improve mood, reduce anxiety, and minimize obsessions.

Antidepressants typically are classified as tricyclic antidepressants (TCAs), mono-amine oxidase inhibitors (not shown), selective serotonin reuptake inhibitors (SSRIs), and atypical antidepressants (not shown). TCAs, such as amitriptyline and desipramine, primarily block norepinephrine reuptake at presynaptic membranes, thereby increasing the norepinephrine concentration at synapses and making more available at postsyn-aptic receptors (A).

SSRIs, such as fluoxetine and paroxetine, selectively inhibit serotonin uptake at presynaptic membranes. This action leads to increased serotonin availability at post-synaptic receptors (B).

MECHANISM OF ACTION

This tricyclic antidepressant has strong anticholinergic activity and acts by blocking the reuptake of neurotransmitters, including norepinephrine and serotonin, at presynaptic membranes, thus increasing synaptic concentration at postsynaptic receptor sites. *Therapeutic Effect:* Results in antidepressant effect.

PHARMACOKINETICS

Rapid, well absorbed from gastrointestinal (GI) tract. Protein binding: 90%. Metabolized in liver, undergoes first-pass metabolism. Primarily excreted in urine. Minimal removal by hemodialysis. **Half-life:** 10–26 hrs.

AVAILABILITY

Tablets: 10 mg, 25 mg, 50 mg, 75 mg, 100 mg, 150 mg.
Injection: 10 mg/ml.

INDICATIONS AND DOSAGES

▸ **Depression**
PO
Adults. 30–100 mg/day as a single dose at bedtime or in divided doses. May gradually increase up to 300 mg/day. Titrate to lowest effective dosage.
Elderly. Initially, 10–25 mg at bedtime. May increase by 10–25 mg/wk at weekly intervals. Range: 25–150 mg/day.
Children 6–12 yrs. 1–5 mg/kg/day in 2 divided doses.
IM
Adults. 20–30 mg 4 times/day.
▸ **Pain management**
PO
Adults, Elderly. 25–100 mg at bedtime.

UNLABELED USES

Relieves neuropathic pain, such as that experienced by patients with diabetic neuropathy and postherpetic neuralgia, as well as those being treated for bulimia nervosa

CONTRAINDICATIONS

Acute recovery period after myocardial infarction (MI), within 14 days of monoamine oxidase inhibitor (MAOI) ingestion

INTERACTIONS

Drug
Antithyroid agents: May increase the risk of agranulocytosis.
Cimetidine, valproic acid: May increase amitriptyline blood concentration and risk for amitriptyline toxicity.
Clonidine, guanadrel: May decrease effects of clonidine and guanadrel.
CNS depressants, including alcohol, anticonvulsants, barbiturates, phenothiazines, and sedative-hypnotics: May increase the hypotensive effects, respiratory depression, and sedation caused by amitriptyline.
MAOIs: May increase the risk of hypertensive crisis, as evidenced by seizures, and a hyperpyrexis with these drugs.
Phenothiazines: May increase sedative and anticholinergic effects of amitriptyline.
Sympathomimetics: May increase cardiac effects with sympathomimetics.
Herbal
None known.
Food
None known.

DIAGNOSTIC TEST EFFECTS

May alter electrocardiogram (EKG) readings (flattens T wave) or increase or decrease blood glucose levels. Therapeutic serum level: Peak ranges 120–250 ng/ml; toxic serum level is greater than 500 ng/ml.

SIDE EFFECTS

Frequent

Dizziness, drowsiness, dry mouth, orthostatic hypotension, headache, increased appetite or weight, nausea, unusual tiredness, unpleasant taste

Occasional

Blurred vision, confusion, constipation, hallucinations, delayed micturition, eye pain, arrhythmias, fine muscle tremors, parkinsonian syndrome, nervousness, diarrhea, increased sweating, heartburn, insomnia

Rare

Hypersensitivity, alopecia, tinnitus, breast enlargement

SERIOUS REACTIONS

• High amitriptyline dosage may produce confusion, seizures, severe drowsiness, irregular heartbeat, fever, hallucinations, agitation, shortness of breath, vomiting, and unusual tiredness or weakness.

• Abrupt withdrawal from prolonged therapy may produce headache, malaise, nausea, vomiting, and vivid dreams.

• Blood dyscrasias and cholestatic jaundice occur rarely.

NURSING CONSIDERATIONS

Baseline Assessment

• Assess the patient's psychological status by observing and documenting his or her appearance, behavior, interest in the environment, level of contentment, and sleep patterns.

• Expect to periodically obtain a complete blood count as well as blood serum chemistry profile for patients receiving long-term therapy.

Lifespan Considerations

• Be aware that amitriptyline crosses the placenta and is minimally distributed in breast milk.

• Be aware that children are more sensitive to an increased drug dosage and have a higher risk for amitriptyline toxicity.

• In the elderly, there is an increased risk of amitriptyline toxicity and increased sensitivity to anticholinergic effects.

Precautions

• Use cautiously in patients with cardiovascular disease, diabetes mellitus, glaucoma, hiatal hernia, history of seizures, history of urinary retention or obstruction, hyperthyroidism, increased intraocular pressure, liver disease, prostatic hypertrophy, renal disease, and schizophrenia.

Administration and Handling

PO

• Give with food or milk if gastrointestinal (GI) distress occurs.

IM

• Give by IM injection only if PO administration is not feasible.

• If crystals form in the ampoule, immerse it in hot water for 1 minute.

• Give deep IM slowly.

Intervention and Evaluation

• Closely supervise patients at risk for committing suicide during early therapy. As the patient's depression lessens, his or her energy level will improve, thereby increasing the likelihood of suicide attempts.

• Assess the patient's appearance, behavior, level of interest, mood, and speech pattern to determine the therapeutic effect of the drug.

• Expect to monitor the patient's blood pressure (B/P) and pulse to watch for the occurrence of arrhythmias and hypotension.

Patient Teaching

• Caution the patient not to abruptly discontinue the drug.

• Advise the patient to change positions slowly to avoid the drug's hypotensive effect.

• Explain to the patient that he or she will develop a tolerance to the

postural hypotensive, sedative, and anticholinergic effects of amitriptyline during early therapy.
• Tell the patient that the maximum therapeutic effect may be noted in 2 to 4 weeks.
• Advise the patient that he or she may develop sensitivity to sunlight.
• Urge the patient to report any visual disturbances.
• Warn the patient to avoid tasks that require alertness or motor skills until his or her response to the drug is established.
• Suggest to the patient that sips of tepid water and chewing sugarless gum may relieve dry mouth.

bupropion
byew-**pro**-peon
(Wellbutrin, Wellbutrin SR, Wellbutrin XL, Zyban, Zyban sustained release[aus])
Do not confuse with buspirone, Wellcovorin, Wellferon, or Zagam.

CATEGORY AND SCHEDULE
Pregnancy Risk Category: B

MECHANISM OF ACTION
An aminoketone that blocks the reuptake of neurotransmitters, including serotonin, norepinephrine at central nervous system (CNS) presynaptic membranes, increasing their availability at postsynaptic receptor sites. Reduces firing rate of noradrenergic neurons. *Therapeutic Effect:* Resulting enhancement of synaptic activity produces antidepressant effect. Eliminates nicotine withdrawal symptoms.

PHARMACOKINETICS
Rapidly absorbed from the gastrointestinal (GI) tract. Crosses blood-brain barrier. Protein binding: 84%. Extensive first-pass metabolism in liver to active metabolite. Primarily excreted in urine. **Half-life:** 14 hrs.

AVAILABILITY
Tablets: 75 mg, 100 mg.
Tablets (sustained-release): 100 mg, 150 mg, 200 mg.
Tablets (extended-release): 150 mg, 300 mg.

INDICATIONS AND DOSAGES
▶ **Depression**
PO
Adults. Immediate-release: Initially, 100 mg 2 times/day, may increase to 100 mg 3 times/day no sooner than 3 days after beginning therapy. Maximum: 450 mg/day. Sustained-release: Initially, 150 mg/day as single dose in the morning. May increase to 300 mg/day at 150 mg 2 times/day as early as day 4 of dosing. Maximum: 400 mg/day. Extended-release: 150 mg once a day. May increase to 300 mg once a day.
Elderly. 37.5 mg 2 times/day. May increase by 37.5 mg q3–4 days. Maintenance: Lowest effective dosage. Sustained-release: 50–100 mg/day. May increase by 50–100 mg/day q3–4 days. Maintenance: Lowest effective dosage.
▶ **Smoking cessation**
PO
Adults. Initially, 150 mg a day for 3 days; then 150 mg 2 times/day. Continue for 7–12 wks.

UNLABELED USES
Attention deficit hyperactivity disorder in adults, children

CONTRAINDICATIONS
Current or prior diagnosis of anorexia nervosa or bulimia, concurrent use of MAOI, seizure disorder.

INTERACTIONS
Drug
Alcohol, lithium, ritonavir, trazodone, tricyclic antidepressants: May increase risk of seizures.
MAOIs: May increase risk of acute bupropion toxicity.
Herbal
None known.
Food
None known.

DIAGNOSTIC TEST EFFECTS
May decrease serum white blood cell (WBC) count.

SIDE EFFECTS
Frequent (32%–18%)
Constipation, weight gain or loss, nausea, vomiting, anorexia, dry mouth, headache, increased sweating, tremor, sedation, insomnia, dizziness, agitation
Occasional (10%–5%)
Diarrhea, akinesia, blurred vision, tachycardia, confusion, hostility, fatigue

SERIOUS REACTIONS
• There is an increased risk of seizures with an increase in bupropion dosage greater than 150 mg/dose, in patients with a history of bulimia or seizure disorders, and in patients discontinuing agents that may lower seizure threshold.

NURSING CONSIDERATIONS
Baseline Assessment
• Expect to obtain blood serum chemistry levels to assess liver and renal function periodically for patients receiving long-term therapy.
Lifespan Considerations
• Be aware that it is unknown if bupropion crosses the placenta or is distributed in breast milk.
• Be aware that the safety and

efficacy of bupropion have not been established in children younger than 18 years of age.
• The elderly are more sensitive to the anticholinergic, cardiovascular, and sedative effects of bupropion.
• In the elderly, age-related impaired renal function may require dosage adjustment.
Precautions
• Use cautiously in patients with a history of cranial trauma or seizure, impaired liver or renal function, or who are currently taking antidepressants or antipsychotics.
Administration and Handling
◀ALERT▶ Expect to gradually increase bupropion dosage to minimize agitation, insomnia, and motor restlessness.
• Be aware that fewer side effects are noted with the sustained-release form of bupropion.
PO
• Take with food to reduce GI irritation.
• Expect to space the dosages 4 hours apart for immediate onset tablets, and 8 hours apart for sustained-release tablet to avoid seizures.
• Avoid bedtime dosage to decrease the risk of insomnia.
• Do not crush sustained-release preparations.
Intervention and Evaluation
• Closely supervise suicidal-risk patients during early therapy. As depression lessens, be aware that the patient's energy level generally improves, which increases the suicide potential.
• Assess the patient's appearance, behavior, level of interest, mood, and speech pattern.
Patient Teaching
• Advise the patient that the full therapeutic effect of bupropion may be noted in 4 weeks.

• Warn the patient to avoid tasks that require mental alertness or motor skills until his or her response to the drug is established.
• Suggest to the patient that sips of tepid water or chewing sugarless gum may help relieve dry mouth.

citalopram hydrobromide

sigh-**tail**-oh-pram high-dro-**broh**-mide
(Celexa, Cipramil[AUS])
Do not confuse with Celebrex, Zyprexa, or Cerebyx.

CATEGORY AND SCHEDULE
Pregnancy Risk Category: C

MECHANISM OF ACTION
A serotonin reuptake inhibitor that blocks the uptake of the neurotransmitter serotonin at central nervous system (CNS) neuronal presynaptic membranes, increasing its availability at postsynaptic receptor sites. *Therapeutic Effect:* Produces antidepressant effect.

PHARMACOKINETICS
Well absorbed after PO administration. Protein binding: 80%. Primarily metabolized in the liver. Primarily excreted in the feces with a lesser amount eliminated in the urine. **Half-life:** 35 hrs.

AVAILABILITY
Tablets: 10 mg, 20 mg, 40 mg.
Oral Solution: 10 mg/5 ml.

INDICATIONS AND DOSAGES
▸ **Antidepressant**
PO
Adults. Initially, 20 mg once a day in the morning or evening. Dosage may be increased in 20-mg incre-

ments at intervals of no less than 1 wk. Maximum: 60 mg/day.
Elderly, impaired liver function. 20 mg/day. May titrate to 40 mg/day only for nonresponding patients.

UNLABELED USES
Treatment of alcohol abuse, dementia, diabetic neuropathy, obsessive-compulsive disorder, smoking cessation

CONTRAINDICATIONS
Concurrent use of MAOIs, sensitivity to citalopram

INTERACTIONS
Drug
Antifungals, cimetidine, macrolide antibiotics: May increase citalopram plasma levels.
Carbamazepine: May decrease citalopram plasma levels.
MAOIs: May cause serotonergic syndrome, marked by autonomic hyperactivity, coma, diaphoresis, excitement, hyperthermia, rigidity.
Metoprolol: Increases the plasma levels of metoprolol.
Herbal
None known.
Food
None known.

DIAGNOSTIC TEST EFFECTS
May reduce serum sodium levels.

SIDE EFFECTS
Frequent (21%–11%)
Nausea, dry mouth, somnolence, insomnia, excessive sweating
Occasional (8%–4%)
Tremor, diarrhea or loose stools, abnormal ejaculation, dyspepsia, fatigue, anxiety, vomiting, anorexia
Rare (3%–2%)
Sinusitis, sexual dysfunction, menstrual disorder, abdominal pain, agitation, decreased libido

SERIOUS REACTIONS
• Overdosage is manifested as dizziness, drowsiness, tachycardia, severe somnolence, confusion, and seizures.

NURSING CONSIDERATIONS

Baseline Assessment
• As ordered, obtain a complete blood count and serum blood chemistry profile tests periodically for patients on long-term therapy.
• Observe and record patient behavior.
• Assess the patient's appearance, interest in environment, psychological status, sleep pattern, and thought content.

Lifespan Considerations
• Be aware that citalopram is distributed in breast milk.
• Be aware that citalopram use in children may cause increased anticholinergic effects or hyperexcitability.
• The elderly are more sensitive to the drug's anticholinergic effects, such as dry mouth, and are more likely to experience confusion, dizziness, hyperexcitability, hypotension, and sedation.

Precautions
• Use cautiously in patients with a history of hypomania, mania, or seizures and with liver or renal impairment.

Administration and Handling
PO
• Give citalopram without regard to food.
• Crush scored tablets if necessary

Intervention and Evaluation
• Supervise the suicidal-risk patient closely during early therapy because as the patient's depression lessens and his or her energy level improves, the risk for suicide increases.

• Assess the patient's appearance, behavior, level of interest, mood, and speech pattern.

Patient Teaching
• Caution the patient against discontinuing the medication or increasing the dosage.
• Urge the patient to avoid alcohol while taking citalopram.
• Warn the patient to avoid tasks that require mental alertness or motor skills until his or her response to the drug is established.
• Suggest to the patient that sips of tepid water and chewing sugarless gum may help relieve dry mouth.

clomipramine hydrochloride
klow-**mih**-prah-meen
(Anafranil, Apo-Clomipramine[CAN], Clopram[AUS], Novo-Clopamine[CAN], Placil[AUS])
Do not confuse with alfentanil, chlorpromazine, clomiphene, enalapril, or nafarelin.

CATEGORY AND SCHEDULE
Pregnancy Risk Category: C

MECHANISM OF ACTION
A tricyclic antidepressant that blocks the reuptake of neurotransmitters, such as norepinephrine and serotonin, at central nervous system (CNS) presynaptic membranes, increasing their availability at postsynaptic receptor sites. *Therapeutic Effect:* Reduces obsessive-compulsive behavior.

AVAILABILITY
Capsules: 25 mg, 50 mg, 75 mg.

INDICATIONS AND DOSAGES
▸ **Obsessive-compulsive disorder**
PO
Adults, Elderly. Initially, 25 mg/day.
May gradually increase to 100
mg/day in the first 2 wks.
Maximum: 250 mg/day.
Children 10 yrs and older. Initially,
25 mg/day. May gradually increase
up to maximum of 200 mg/day.

UNLABELED USES
Treatment of bulimia, cataplexy
associated with narcolepsy, mental
depression, neurogenic pain, panic
disorder

CONTRAINDICATIONS
Acute recovery period following
myocardial infarction (MI), within
14 days of MAOI ingestion

INTERACTIONS
Drug
Alcohol, CNS depressants: May
increase CNS and respiratory depression and clomipramine's hypotensive effects.
Antithyroid agents: May increase
the risk of agranulocytosis.
Cimetidine: May increase clomipramine blood concentration and
risk of toxicity.
Clonidine, guanadrel: May decrease
the effects of clonidine and guanadrel
MAOIs: May increase the risk of
convulsions, hyperpyresis, and
hypertensive crisis.
Phenothiazines: May increase the
anticholinergic and sedative effects
of clomipramine.
Sympathomimetics: May increase
cardiac effects.
Herbal
None known.
Food
None known.

DIAGNOSTIC TEST EFFECTS
May alter blood glucose levels and
EKG readings.

SIDE EFFECTS
Frequent
Drowsiness, fatigue, dry mouth,
blurred vision, constipation, sexual
dysfunction (42%), ejaculatory
failure (20%), impotence, weight
gain (18%), delayed micturition,
postural hypotension, excessive
sweating, disturbed concentration,
increased appetite, urinary retention
Occasional
Gastrointestinal (GI) disturbances,
such as nausea, GI distress, and
metallic taste, asthenia, aggressiveness, muscle weakness
Rare
Paradoxical reactions (agitation,
restlessness, nightmares, insomnia,
extrapyramidal symptoms, particularly fine hand tremor), laryngitis,
seizures

SERIOUS REACTIONS
• High dosage may produce cardiovascular effects, including severe
postural hypotension, dizziness,
tachycardia, palpitations, and arrhythmias, and seizures. High dosage may also result in altered temperature regulation, such as
hyperpyrexia or hypothermia.
• Abrupt withdrawal from prolonged therapy may produce headache, malaise, nausea, vomiting, and
vivid dreams.
• Anemia has been noted.

NURSING CONSIDERATIONS
Precautions
• Use cautiously in patients with
cardiac disease, diabetes mellitus,
glaucoma, hiatal hernia, history of
seizures, history of urinary obstruction or retention, hyperthyroidism,

increased intraocular pressure (IOP), liver disease, prostatic hypertrophy, renal disease, and schizophrenia.

Intervention and Evaluation

• Closely supervise suicidal-risk patients during early therapy. As depression lessens, the patient's energy level improves, which increases the suicide potential.

• Assess the patient's appearance, behavior, level of interest, mood, and speech pattern.

• Monitor complete blood count results to assess for signs of anemia and agranulocytosis.

• Monitor EKG tracings for arrhythmias.

Patient Teaching

• Advise the patient that clomipramine may cause blurred vision, constipation, and dry mouth.

• Warn the patient to change positions slowly, especially in the beginning of therapy, to avoid or lessen postural hypotension.

• Advise the patient that he or she will develop a tolerance to the drug's anticholinergic effect, postural hypotension, and sedative effects during early therapy.

• Explain to the patient that the maximum therapeutic effect of clomipramine may be noted in 2 to 4 weeks.

• Caution the patient against abruptly discontinuing the medication.

• Warn the patient to avoid tasks that require mental alertness or motor skills until his or her response to the drug is established.

• Urge the patient to avoid alcohol while taking clomipramine.

desipramine hydrochloride

deh-**sip**-rah-meen
(Apo-Desipramine[CAN], Norpramin, Novo-Desipramine[CAN], Pertofran[AUS])
Do not confuse with disopyramide or imipramine.

CATEGORY AND SCHEDULE
Pregnancy Risk Category: C

MECHANISM OF ACTION
A tricyclic antidepressant that increases synaptic concentration of norepinephrine and/or serotonin by inhibiting their reuptake by presynaptic membranes. Strong anticholinergic activity. *Therapeutic Effect:* Produces antidepressant effect.

PHARMACOKINETICS
Rapidly, well absorbed from the gastrointestinal (GI) tract. Protein binding: 90%. Metabolized in liver. Primarily excreted in urine. Minimally removed by hemodialysis. **Half-life:** 12–27 hrs.

AVAILABILITY
Tablets: 10 mg, 25 mg, 50 mg, 75 mg, 100 mg, 150 mg.

INDICATIONS AND DOSAGES
▸ **Depression**
PO
Adults. 75 mg/day. May gradually increase to 150–200 mg/day. Maximum: 300 mg/day.
Elderly. Initially, 10–25 mg/day. May gradually increase to 75–100 mg/day. Maximum: 300 mg/day.
Children older than 12 yrs.: Initially, 25–50 mg/day. May gradually increase to 100 mg/day. Maximum: 150 mg/day.

Children 6–12 yrs. 1–3 mg/kg/day.
Maximum: 5 mg/kg/day.

UNLABELED USES
Treatment of attention deficit hyperactivity disorder (ADHD), bulimia nervosa, cataplexy associated with narcolepsy, cocaine withdrawal, neurogenic pain, panic disorder

CONTRAINDICATIONS
Narrow-angle glaucoma, use of MAOIs within 14 days

INTERACTIONS
Drug
Alcohol, central nervous system (CNS) depressants: May increase CNS and respiratory depression and the hypotensive effects of desipramine.
Antithyroid agents: May increase risk of agranulocytosis.
Cimetidine: May increase desipramine blood concentration and risk of toxicity.
Clonidine, guanadrel: May decrease the effects of clonidine and guanadrel.
MAOIs: May increase the risk of hyperpyrexia, hypertensive crisis, and seizures.
Phenothiazines: May increase the anticholinergic and sedative effects of desipramine.
Phenytoin: May decrease desipramine blood concentration.
Sympathomimetics: May increase the cardiac effects.
Herbal
St. John's wort: May have additive effects.
Food
None known.

DIAGNOSTIC TEST EFFECTS
May alter blood glucose levels and EKG readings. Therapeutic serum level is 115–300 ng/ml; toxic serum level is greater than 400 ng/ml.

SIDE EFFECTS
Frequent
Drowsiness, fatigue, dry mouth, blurred vision, constipation, delayed micturition, postural hypotension, diaphoresis, disturbed concentration, increased appetite, urinary retention
Occasional
Gastrointestinal (GI) disturbances, such as nausea, GI distress, metallic taste sensation
Rare
Paradoxical reaction, marked by agitation, restlessness, nightmares, insomnia, extrapyramidal symptoms, particularly fine hand tremor

SERIOUS REACTION
High dosage may produce confusion, seizures, severe drowsiness, arrhythmias, fever, hallucinations, agitation, shortness of breath, vomiting, and unusual tiredness or weakness.
Abrupt withdrawal from prolonged therapy may produce severe headache, malaise, nausea, vomiting, and vivid dreams.

NURSING CONSIDERATIONS
Baseline Assessment
• Plan to perform a complete blood count and blood serum chemistry tests to assess liver and renal function periodically for patients on long-term therapy.
Lifespan Considerations
• Be aware that desipramine crosses the placenta and is minimally distributed in breast milk.
• Be aware that desipramine use is not recommended in children younger than 6 years of age.
• Expect to use lower dosages in the elderly. Higher dosages are not tolerated well, and increase the risk of toxicity in the elderly.

Precautions
• Use cautiously in patients with cardiac conduction disturbances, cardiovascular disease, hyperthyroidism, seizure disorders, and urinary retention, and in patients who are taking thyroid replacement therapy.

Administration and Handling
PO
• Give with food or milk if GI distress occurs.

Intervention and Evaluation
• Supervise the suicidal-risk patient closely during early therapy because as the patient's depression lessens and his or her energy level improves, the risk for suicide increases.
• Assess the patient's appearance, behavior, level of interest, mood, and speech pattern.
• Monitor the patient for therapeutic desipramine serum levels. Know that the therapeutic serum level for desipramine is 115 to 300 ng/ml, and the toxic serum level for desipramine is greater than 400 ng/ml.
• Expect to perform and monitor EKGs if the patient has a history of arrhythmias.

Patient Teaching
• Instruct the patient to change positions slowly to avoid the drug's hypotensive effect.
• Explain to the patient that a tolerance to the drug's anticholinergic and sedative effects as well as postural hypotension usually develops during early therapy.
• Advise the patient that the drug's maximum therapeutic effect may be noted in 2 to 4 weeks.
• Caution the patient against abruptly discontinuing the medication.

doxepin hydrochloride
dox-eh-pin
(Deptran[AUS], Novo-Doxepin[CAN], Prudoxin, Sinequan, Zonalon)
Do not confuse with doxapram, doxazosin, Doxidan, or saquinavir.

CATEGORY AND SCHEDULE
Pregnancy Risk Category: C
(B topical)

MECHANISM OF ACTION
A tricyclic antidepressant, antianxiety, antineuralgic, antipruritic, and antiulcer agent that increases synaptic concentrations of norepinephrine and serotonin. *Therapeutic Effect:* Produces antidepressant, anxiolytic effect.

PHARMACOKINETICS
Rapidly, well absorbed from the gastrointestinal (GI) tract. Protein binding: 80%–85%. Metabolized in liver to active metabolite. Primarily excreted in urine. Not removed by hemodialysis. **Half-life:** 6–8 hrs. Topical: Absorbed through skin, distributed to body tissues, metabolized to active metabolite, eliminated renally.

AVAILABILITY
Capsules: 10 mg, 25 mg, 50 mg, 75 mg, 100 mg, 150 mg.
Oral Concentrate: 10 mg/ml.
Cream: 5%.

INDICATIONS AND DOSAGES
▸ **Depression or anxiety**
PO
Adults. 30–150 mg/day at bedtime or in 2–3 divided doses. May increase to 300 mg/day.

Adolescents. Initially, 25–50 mg/day as single or divided doses. May increase to 100 mg/day.
Children younger than 12 yrs. 1–3 mg/kg/day.
Elderly. Initially, 10–25 mg at bedtime. May increase by 10–25 mg/day q3–7 days. Maximum: 75 mg/day.

▶ **Treatment of pruritus associated with eczema**
Topical
Adults, Elderly. Apply thin film 4 times/day.

UNLABELED USES
Treatment of neurogenic pain, panic disorder, prophylaxis vascular headache, pruritus in idiopathic cold urticaria

CONTRAINDICATIONS
Narrow-angle glaucoma, hypersensitivity to other tricyclic antidepressants, urine retention

INTERACTIONS
Drug
Alcohol, central nervous system (CNS) depressants: May increase CNS and respiratory depression and the hypotensive effects of doxepin.
Antithyroid agents: May increase the risk of agranulocytosis.
Cimetidine: May increase doxepin blood concentration and risk of toxicity.
Clonidine, guanadrel: May decrease the effects of clonidine and guanadrel.
MAOIs: May increase the risk of convulsions, hyperpyrexia, and hypertensive crisis.
Phenothiazines: May increase the anticholinergic and sedative effects of doxepin.
Sympathomimetics: May increase cardiac effects.

Herbal
None known.
Food
None known.

DIAGNOSTIC TEST EFFECTS
May alter blood glucose levels and EKG readings. Therapeutic serum level is 110–250 ng/ml; toxic serum level is greater than 300 ng/ml.

SIDE EFFECTS
Frequent
PO: Orthostatic hypotension, drowsiness, dry mouth, headache, increased appetite or weight, nausea, unusual tiredness, unpleasant taste
Topical: Edema at application site, increased itching or eczema, burning, stinging of skin, altered taste, dizziness, drowsiness, dry skin, dry mouth, fatigue, headache, thirst
Occasional
PO: Blurred vision, confusion, constipation, hallucinations, difficult urination, eye pain, irregular heartbeat, fine muscle tremors, nervousness, impaired sexual function, diarrhea, increased sweating, heartburn, insomnia
Topical: Anxiety, skin irritation or cracking, nausea
Rare
Allergic reaction, alopecia, tinnitus, breast enlargement
Topical: Fever

SERIOUS REACTIONS
• High dosage may produce confusion, seizures, severe drowsiness, fast or slow irregular heartbeat, fever, hallucinations, agitation, shortness of breath, vomiting, and unusual tiredness or weakness.
• Abrupt withdrawal from prolonged therapy may produce headache, malaise, nausea, vomiting, and vivid dreams.

NURSING CONSIDERATIONS

Baseline Assessment
• Assess the patient's blood pressure (B/P), and pulse.
• In patients with a history of cardiovascular disease, monitor the EKG.

Lifespan Considerations
• Be aware that doxepin crosses the placenta and is distributed in breast milk.
• Be aware that the safety and efficacy of this drug have not been established in children.
• The elderly are at an increased risk of toxicity. Lower doxepin dosages are recommended in the elderly.

Precautions
• Use cautiously in patients with cardiac disease, diabetes mellitus, glaucoma, hiatal hernia, history of seizures, history of urinary obstruction or retention, hyperthyroidism, increased intraocular pressure (IOP), liver disease, prostatic hypertrophy, renal disease, and schizophrenia.

Administration and Handling
PO
• Give with food or milk, if GI distress occurs.
• Dilute concentrate in 8-oz glass of fruit juice, such as grapefruit, orange, pineapple, or prune, milk, or water. Avoid diluting in carbonated drinks because they are incompatible with doxepin.

Intervention and Evaluation
• Monitor the patient's B/P, pulse, and weight.
• Closely supervise suicidal-risk patients during early therapy. As depression lessens, be aware that the patient's energy level generally improves, which increases the suicide potential.
• Assess the patient's appearance, behavior, level of interest, mood, and speech pattern.
• Monitor the patient for therapeutic serum levels. Know that the therapeutic serum level for doxepin is 110 to 250 ng/ml and the toxic serum level for doxepin is greater than 300 ng/ml.

Patient Teaching
• Advise the patient that doxepin may cause drowsiness or decrease his or her ability to perform tasks requiring mental alertness or physical coordination. Warn the patient to avoid tasks that require mental alertness and motor skills until his or her response to the drug is established.
• Warn the patient to change positions slowly, especially early in therapy, to avoid postural hypotension.
• Advise the patient that doxepin may cause dry mouth and increased appetite.
• Urge the patient to avoid alcohol and limit caffeine intake while taking doxepin.
• Caution the patient to avoid exposure to sunlight or artificial light sources.
• Explain to the patient that the therapeutic effect of doxepin may be noted within 2 to 5 days with the maximum effect noted within 2 to 3 weeks.

escitalopram
es-sih-**tail**-oh-pram
(Lexapro)

CATEGORY AND SCHEDULE
Pregnancy Risk Category: C

MECHANISM OF ACTION
An antidepressant that blocks the uptake of the neurotransmitter

serotonin at central nervous system (CNS) neuronal presynaptic membranes, increasing its availability at postsynaptic receptor sites. *Therapeutic Effect:* Antidepressant effect.

PHARMACOKINETICS
Well absorbed after PO administration. Primarily metabolized in the liver. Primarily excreted in the feces with a lesser amount eliminated in the urine. **Half-life:** 35 hrs.

AVAILABILITY
Tablets: 5 mg, 10 mg, 20 mg.
Oral Solution: 5 mg/5 ml.

INDICATIONS AND DOSAGES
▸ **Antidepressant**
PO
Adults. Initially, 10 mg once a day in the morning or evening. May increase to 20 mg, after a minimum of 1 wk.
Elderly, impaired liver function. 10 mg/day.

CONTRAINDICATIONS
Breast-feeding, concurrent use of MAOIs

INTERACTIONS
Drug
Antifungals, cimetidine, macrolide antibiotics: May increase plasma levels of escitalopram.
Carbamazepine: May decrease plasma levels of escitalopram.
MAOIs: May cause serotonergic syndrome, including autonomic hyperactivity, coma, diaphoresis, excitement, hyperthermia, and rigidity.
Metoprolol: Increases plasma levels of metoprolol.
Herbal
None known.
Food
None known.

DIAGNOSTIC TEST EFFECTS
May reduce serum sodium levels.

SIDE EFFECTS
Frequent (21%–11%)
Nausea, dry mouth, somnolence, insomnia, excessive sweating
Occasional (8%–4%)
Tremor, diarrhea or loose stools, abnormal ejaculation, dyspepsia, fatigue, anxiety, vomiting, anorexia
Rare (3%–2%)
Sinusitis, sexual dysfunction, menstrual disorder, abdominal pain, agitation, decreased libido

SERIOUS REACTIONS
• Overdosage is manifested as dizziness, drowsiness, tachycardia, severe somnolence, confusion, and seizures.

NURSING CONSIDERATIONS
Baseline Assessment
• As ordered, perform complete blood counts and liver and renal function tests periodically for patients on long-term therapy.
• Observe and record the patient's behavior, as well as his or her appearance, interest in the environment, psychological status, sleep pattern, and thought content.
Lifespan Considerations
• Be aware that escitalopram is distributed in breast milk.
• Be aware that escitalopram use may cause increased anticholinergic effects or hyperexcitability in children.
• The elderly are more sensitive to the drug's anticholinergic effects (e.g., dry mouth) and are more likely to experience confusion, dizziness, hyperexcitability, hypotension, and sedation.

Precautions
• Use cautiously in patients concurrently using CNS depressants.
• Use cautiously in patients with history of hypomania, mania, or seizures, and liver or renal impairment.

Administration and Handling
PO
• Give escitalopram without regard to food.
• Do not crush film-coated tablets.

Intervention and Evaluation
• Closely supervise suicidal-risk patients during early therapy. As depression lessens, be aware that the patient's energy level generally improves, which increases the suicide potential.
• Assess the patient's appearance, behavior, level of interest, mood, and speech pattern.

Patient Teaching
• Caution the patient against discontinuing the medication or increasing its dosage.
• Urge the patient to avoid alcohol while taking escitalopram.
• Warn the patient to avoid tasks that require mental alertness and motor skills until his or her response to the drug is established.

---

fluoxetine hydrochloride
flew-**ox**-eh-teen
(Lovan[AUS], Novo-Fluoxetine[CAN], Prozac, Prozac Weekly, Sarafem, Zactin[AUS])
Do not confuse with fluvastatin, Prilosec, Proscar, ProSom, or Serophene.

CATEGORY AND SCHEDULE
Pregnancy Risk Category: C

MECHANISM OF ACTION
A psychotherapeutic agent that selectively inhibits serotonin uptake in the central nervous system (CNS), enhancing serotonergic function. *Therapeutic Effect:* Resulting enhancement of synaptic activity produces antidepressant, antiobsessional, antibulimic effect.

PHARMACOKINETICS
Well absorbed from the gastrointestinal (GI) tract. Crosses blood-brain barrier. Protein binding: 94%. Metabolized in liver to active metabolite. Primarily excreted in urine. Not removed by hemodialysis.
Half-life: 2–3 days; metabolite: 7–9 days.

AVAILABILITY
Capsules: 10 mg, 20 mg, 40 mg, 90 mg.
Liquid: 20 mg/5 ml.
Tablets: 10 mg, 20 mg.

INDICATIONS AND DOSAGES
▶ **Depression, obsessive-compulsive disorder (OCD)**
PO
Adults. Initially, 20 mg each morning. If therapeutic improvement does not occur after 2 wks, gradually increase dose to maximum 80 mg/day in 2 equally divided doses in morning, noon. Prozac Weekly: 90 mg/wk, begin 7 days after last dose of 20 mg.
Elderly. Initially, 10 mg/day. May increase by 10–20 mg q2wks. Avoid administration at night.
Children 7–17 yrs. Initially, 5–10 mg/day. Titrate upward as needed (20 mg/day usual dosage).
▶ **Bulimia**
PO
Adults. 60 mg once a day in morning.

▸ **Premenstrual dysphoric disorder**
PO
Adults. 20 mg/day.

UNLABELED USES
Treatment of hot flashes

CONTRAINDICATIONS
Avoid giving within 14 days of MAOI ingestion

INTERACTIONS
Drug
Alcohol, CNS depressants: Antagonize CNS depressant effect.
Highly protein-bound medications, including oral anticoagulants: May displace highly protein-bound drugs from protein-binding sites.
MAOIs: May produce serotonin syndrome.
Phenytoin: May increase blood concentration and risk of toxicity of phenytoin.
Herbal
St. John's wort: May have additive effect.
Food
None known.

DIAGNOSTIC TEST EFFECTS
None known.

SIDE EFFECTS
Frequent (more than 10%)
Headache, asthenia (loss of strength), inability to sleep, anxiety, nervousness, drowsiness, nausea, diarrhea, decreased appetite
Occasional (9%–2%)
Dizziness, tremor, fatigue, vomiting, constipation, dry mouth, abdominal pain, nasal congestion, diaphoresis
Rare (less than 2%)
Flushed skin, lightheadedness, decreased ability to concentrate

SERIOUS REACTIONS
• Overdosage may produce seizures, nausea, vomiting, excessive agitation, and restlessness.

NURSING CONSIDERATIONS
Baseline Assessment
• Expect to perform baseline and periodic complete blood counts and liver and renal function tests for patients on long-term therapy.
Lifespan Considerations
• Be aware that it is unknown if fluoxetine crosses the placenta or is distributed in breast milk.
• Be aware that children may be more sensitive to the drug's behavioral side effects, such as insomnia and restlessness.
• There are no age-related precautions noted in the elderly.
Precautions
• Use cautiously in patients with cardiac dysfunction, diabetes, and seizure disorder.
• Use cautiously in patients at high risk for suicide.
Administration and Handling
◀ALERT▶ Expect to use lower or less frequent doses in patients with liver or renal impairment, who are elderly, have concurrent disease, or are on multiple medications.
PO
• Give fluoxetine with food or milk if GI distress occurs.
Intervention and Evaluation
• Closely supervise suicidal-risk patients during early therapy. As depression lessens, the patient's energy level improves, which increases the suicide potential.
• Assess the patient's appearance, behavior, level of interest, mood, and speech pattern.
• Assess the patient's pattern of daily bowel activity and stool consistency.

• Assess the patient's skin for the appearance of rash.
• Monitor the patient's blood glucose levels, and serum alkaline phosphatase, bilirubin, sodium, SGOT (AST), and SGPT (ALT) levels.

Patient Teaching
• Explain to the patient that the drug's maximum therapeutic response may require 4 weeks or more of therapy.
• Caution the patient against abruptly discontinuing the medication.
• Warn the patient to avoid tasks that require mental alertness or motor skills until his or her response to the drug is established.
• Urge the patient to avoid alcohol while taking fluoxetine.
• Instruct the patient to take the last dose of the drug before 4 p.m. to avoid insomnia.

imipramine
ih-**mih**-prah-meen
(Apo-Imipramine[CAN], Melipramine[AUS], Tofranil, Tofranil-PM)
Do not confuse with desipramine.

CATEGORY AND SCHEDULE
Pregnancy Risk Category: D

MECHANISM OF ACTION
A tricyclic antibulimic, anticataplectic, antidepressant, antinarcoleptic, antineuralgic, antineuritic, and antipanic agent that blocks the reuptake of neurotransmitters, such as norepinephrine and serotonin, at presynaptic membranes, increasing their concentration at postsynaptic receptor sites. *Therapeutic Effect:* Results in antidepressant effect. Anticholinergic effect controls nocturnal enuresis.

AVAILABILITY
Tablets: 10 mg, 25 mg, 50 mg.
Capsules: 75 mg, 100 mg, 125 mg, 150 mg.

INDICATIONS AND DOSAGES
▸ **Depression**
PO
Adults. Initially, 75–100 mg a day. Dosage may be gradually increased to 300 mg a day for hospitalized patients, 200 mg for outpatients, then reduce dosage to effective maintenance level, 50–150 mg a day.
Elderly. Initially, 10–25 mg/day at bedtime. May increase by 10–25 mg q3–7 days. Range: 50–150 mg.
Children. 1.5 mg/kg/day. May increase 1 mg/kg q3–4 days. Maximum: 5 mg/kg/day.
▸ **Childhood enuresis**
PO
Children older than 6 yrs.: Initially, 10–25 mg at bedtime. May increase by 25 mg/day. Maximum 6–12 yrs: 50 mg. Maximum older than 12 yrs: 75 mg.

UNLABELED USES
Treatment of attention-deficit hyperactivity disorder (ADHD), cataplexy associated with narcolepsy, neurogenic pain, panic disorder

CONTRAINDICATIONS
Acute recovery period after myocardial infarction (MI), within 14 days of MAOI ingestion

INTERACTIONS
Drug
Alcohol, central nervous system (CNS) depressants: May increase CNS and respiratory depression and the hypotensive effects of imipramine.
Antithyroid agents: May increase the risk of agranulocytosis.

Cimetidine: May increase imipramine blood concentration and risk of toxicity.

Clonidine, guanadrel: May decrease the effects of *clonidine and guanadrel.*

MAOIs: May increase the risk of hyperpyrexia, hypertensive crisis, and seizures.

Phenothiazines: May increase anticholinergic and sedative effects of imipramine.

Phenytoin: May decrease imipramine blood concentration.

Sympathomimetics: May increase the cardiac effects.

Herbal

Ginkgo biloba: May decrease seizure threshold.

St. John's wort: May have additive effect.

Food

None known.

DIAGNOSTIC TEST EFFECTS

May alter blood glucose levels and EKG readings. Therapeutic serum level is 225–300 ng/ml; toxic serum level is greater than 500 ng/ml.

SIDE EFFECTS

Frequent

Drowsiness, fatigue, dry mouth, blurred vision, constipation, delayed micturition, postural hypotension, diaphoresis, disturbed concentration, increased appetite, urinary retention, photosensitivity.

Occasional

Gastrointestinal (GI) disturbances, such as nausea, and a metallic taste sensation.

Rare

Paradoxical reaction, marked by agitation, restlessness, nightmares, insomnia, extrapyramidal symptoms, particularly fine hand tremors.

SERIOUS REACTIONS

• High dosage may produce cardiovascular effects, such as severe postural hypotension, dizziness, tachycardia, palpitations, arrhythmias and seizures. High dosage may also result in altered temperature regulation, including hyperpyrexia or hypothermia.

• Abrupt withdrawal from prolonged therapy may produce headache, malaise, nausea, vomiting, and vivid dreams.

NURSING CONSIDERATIONS

Baseline Assessment

• Expect to perform a complete blood count and blood serum chemistry tests to assess blood glucose level, liver, and renal function periodically for patients on long-term therapy.

• Plan to perform a baseline EKG, if the patient is at risk for arrhythmias.

Precautions

• Use cautiously in patients with cardiac disease, diabetes mellitus, glaucoma, hiatal hernia, history of seizures, history or urinary obstruction or retention, hyperthyroidism, increased intraocular pressure (IOP), liver disease, prostatic hypertrophy, renal disease, and schizophrenia.

Administration and Handling

PO

• Give with food or milk if GI distress occurs.

• Do not crush or break film-coated tablets.

Intervention and Evaluation

• Closely supervise suicidal-risk patients during early therapy. As depression lessens, be aware that the patient's energy level generally improves, which increases the suicide potential.

• Assess the patient's appearance, behavior, level of interest, mood, and speech pattern.

• Assess the patient's pattern of daily bowel activity and stool consistency.
• Monitor the patient's blood pressure (B/P) for hypotension and the pulse for irregularities that may represent an arrhythmia.
• Palpate the patient's bladder for evidence of urinary retention.
• Monitor the patient's therapeutic serum levels of imipramine. Know that the therapeutic serum level for imipramine is 225 to 300 ng/ml, and the toxic serum level of imipramine is greater than 500 ng/ml.

Patient Teaching
• Instruct the patient to change positions slowly to avoid the drug's hypotensive effect.
• Explain to the patient that a tolerance to anticholinergic effects, postural hypotension, and sedative effects usually develops during early therapy.
• Tell the patient that the drug's therapeutic effect may be noted within 2 to 5 days with maximum effect noted within 2 to 3 weeks.
• Suggest to the patient that taking sips of tepid water and chewing sugarless gum may relieve dry mouth.
• Caution the patient against abruptly discontinuing the medication.
• Warn the patient to avoid tasks that require mental alertness or motor skills until his or her response to the drug is established.

mirtazapine
murr-**taz**-ah-peen
(Avanza[AUS], Remeron, Remeron Soltab)
Do not confuse with Premarin.

CATEGORY AND SCHEDULE
Pregnancy Risk Category: C

MECHANISM OF ACTION
A tetracyclic compound that acts as antagonist at presynaptic alpha$_2$-adrenergic receptors, increasing both norepinephrine and serotonin neurotransmission. *Therapeutic Effect*: Produces antidepressant effect, with prominent sedative effects and low anticholinergic activity.

PHARMACOKINETICS
Rapidly, completely absorbed after PO administration, and not affected by food. Protein binding: 85%. Metabolized in liver. Primarily excreted in urine. Unknown if removed by hemodialysis. **Half-life:** 20–40 hrs, longer in males than females (37 hrs vs. 26 hrs).

AVAILABILITY
Tablets: 15 mg, 30 mg, 45 mg.
Disintegrating Tablets: 15 mg, 30 mg, 45 mg.

INDICATIONS AND DOSAGES
▸ **Depression**
PO
Adults. Initially, 15 mg at bedtime. May increase by 15 mg/day q1–2wks. Maximum: 45 mg/day.
Elderly. Initially, 7.5 mg at bedtime. May increase by 7.5–15 mg/day q1–2wks. Maximum: 45 mg/day.

CONTRAINDICATIONS
Within 14 days of MAOI ingestion

INTERACTIONS
Drug
Alcohol, diazepam: May increase impairment of cognition and motor skills.
MAOIs: May increase risk of hypertensive crisis and severe convulsions.
Herbal
None known.

Food
None known.

DIAGNOSTIC TEST EFFECTS
May increase serum cholesterol and triglyceride levels, as well as SGOT (ALT) and SGPT (AST).

SIDE EFFECTS
Frequent
Somnolence (54%), dry mouth (25%), increase in appetite (17%), constipation (13%), weight gain (12%)
Occasional
Asthenia (8%), dizziness (7%), flu syndrome (5%), abnormal dreams (4%)
Rare
Abdominal discomfort, vasodilation, paresthesia, acne, dry skin, thirst, arthralgia

SERIOUS REACTIONS
• Higher incidence of seizures than with tricyclic antidepressants, especially in those with no previous history of seizures.
• High dosage may produce cardiovascular effects, such as severe postural hypotension, dizziness, tachycardia, palpitations, and arrhythmias.
• Abrupt withdrawal from prolonged therapy may produce headache, malaise, nausea, vomiting, and vivid dreams.
• Agranulocytosis occurs rarely.

NURSING CONSIDERATIONS
Baseline Assessment
• Plan to perform a complete blood count and obtain serum alkaline phosphatase, bilirubin, SGOT (AST), and SGPT (ALT) levels to assess liver and renal function periodically for patients on long-term therapy. Expect to perform a baseline EKG, if the patient is at risk for an arrhythmia.

Lifespan Considerations
• Be aware that it is unknown if mirtazapine is distributed in breast milk.
• Be aware that the safety and efficacy of this drug have not been established in children.
• In the elderly, age-related renal impairment may require cautious use.

Precautions
• Use cautiously in patients with cardiovascular disorders, GI disorders, narrow-angle glaucoma, liver impairment, prostatic hyperplasia, renal impairment, and urine retention.

Administration and Handling
◀ALERT▶ Make sure at least 14 days elapse between discontinuing MAOIs and instituting mirtazapine therapy. Also, plan to allow at least 14 days to pass after discontinuing mirtazapine and instituting MAOI therapy.
PO
• Give mirtazapine without regard to food.
• May crush or break scored tablets.

Intervention and Evaluation
• Closely supervise suicidal-risk patients during early therapy. As depression lessens, the patient's energy level improves, which increases the suicide potential.
• Assess the patient's appearance, behavior, level of interest, mood, and speech pattern.
• Monitor the patient's blood pressure (B/P) for hypotension, and pulse for irregularities that could represent an arrhythmia.

Patient Teaching
• Instruct the patient to take mirtazapine as a single bedtime dose.
• Urge the patient to avoid alcohol and other sedating medications.
• Warn the patient that mirtazapine

use may impair his or her ability to perform activities requiring mental alertness or physical coordination, such as driving.

nefazodone hydrochloride
nef-**ah**-zoh-doan
(Serzone)

CATEGORY AND SCHEDULE
Pregnancy Risk Category: C

MECHANISM OF ACTION
An antidepressant whose exact mechanism is unknown. Appears to inhibit neuronal uptake of serotonin and norepinephrine and antagonize alpha$_1$-adrenergic receptors. *Therapeutic Effect:* Produces antidepressant effect.

PHARMACOKINETICS
Rapidly, completely absorbed from the gastrointestinal (GI) tract. Protein binding: greater than 99%. Food delays absorption. Widely distributed in body tissues, including central nervous system (CNS). Extensively metabolized to active metabolites. Excreted in urine and eliminated in feces. Unknown if removed by hemodialysis. **Half-life:** 2–4 hrs.

AVAILABILITY
Tablets: 50 mg, 100 mg, 150 mg, 200 mg, 250 mg.

INDICATIONS AND DOSAGES
▶ **Depression, prevention of relapse of acute depressive episode**
PO
Adults. Initially, 200 mg/day, given in 2 divided doses. Gradually increase dose in increments of 100–200 mg/day on a twice a day schedule, at intervals of at least 1 wk. Range: 300–600 mg/day.
Elderly. Initially, 100 mg/day on a twice a day schedule. Adjust the rate of subsequent dose titration based on clinical response. Range: 200–400 mg/day.
Children. 300–400 mg/day.

CONTRAINDICATIONS
Within 14 days of MAOI ingestion

INTERACTIONS
Drug
Alprazolam, triazolam: May increase the blood concentration and risk of toxicity of alprazolam, and triazolam, so plan to reduce their dosage.
MAOIs: May produce severe reactions. At least 14 days should elapse between discontinuing MAOIs and initiating of nefazodone therapy. At least 7 days should elapse after discontinuing nefazodone and initiating MAOI therapy.
Herbal
St. John's wort: May increase the risk of adverse effects.
Food
None known.

DIAGNOSTIC TEST EFFECTS
None known.

SIDE EFFECTS
Elderly and the debilitated experience increased susceptibility to side effects.
Frequent
Headache (36%); dry mouth, somnolence (25%); nausea (22%); dizziness (17%); constipation (14%); insomnia, asthenia (loss of strength, energy), lightheadedness (10%)
Occasional
Dyspepsia, blurred vision (9%);

diarrhea, infection (8%); confusion, abnormal vision (7%); pharyngitis (6%); increased appetite (5%); postural hypotension, vasodilation, including flushing and feeling of warmth (4%); peripheral edema, cough, flu syndrome (3%).

SERIOUS REACTIONS

• Serious reactions, such as hyperthermia, rigidity, myoclonus, extreme agitation, delirium, or coma will occur if there is concurrent MAOI administration, or if the time frame between discontinuation and initiation of drug therapy is not followed.

NURSING CONSIDERATIONS

Baseline Assessment

• Determine if the patient has a history of sensitivity to nefazodone, trazodone, or other medication, especially alprazolam, MAOIs, terfenadine, and triazolam.

• Obtain a careful patient history, looking for the presence of cardiovascular or cerebrovascular disease, hypomania, mania, or seizures.

Lifespan Considerations

• Be aware that it is unknown if nefazodone crosses the placenta or is distributed in breast milk.

• Be aware that the safety and efficacy of this drug have not been established in children.

• There are no age-related precautions noted, but lower dosages are recommended in the elderly.

Precautions

• Use cautiously in patients with cerebrovascular disease, dehydration, heart disease, history of hypomania or mania, history of seizures, hypovolemia, liver cirrhosis, recent myocardial infarction (MI), and unstable heart disease.

Administration and Handling

◀ALERT▶ Plan to allow at least 14 days to elapse between discontinuing MAOIs and initiating nefazodone therapy, and at least 7 days after discontinuing nefazodone and initiating MAOI therapy.

PO

• Give nefazodone without regard to meals.

Intervention and Evaluation

• Monitor the patient's blood pressure (B/P) and pulse.

• Closely supervise suicidal-risk patients during early therapy. As depression lessens, be aware that the patient's energy level generally improves, which increases the suicide potential.

• Assess the patient's appearance, behavior, level of interest, mood, and speech pattern.

• Assist the patient with ambulation if he or she experiences dizziness or lightheadedness.

• Assess the patient's daily pattern of bowel activity and stool consistency.

Patient Teaching

• Tell the patient that the drug's maximum therapeutic response may require several weeks of nefazodone therapy.

• Suggest to the patient that taking sips of tepid water and chewing sugarless gum may help relieve dry mouth.

• Warn the patient to notify the physician if he or she experiences headache, nausea, or visual disturbances.

• Explain to the patient that nefazodone may cause dizziness.

• Warn the patient to avoid tasks that require mental alertness or motor skills, until his or her response to the drug is established.

• Urge the patient to avoid alcohol while taking nefazodone.

nortriptyline hydrochloride

nor-**trip**-teh-leen
(Allegron[AUS], Aventyl,
Norventyl, Pamelor)
**Do not confuse with Ambenyl,
amitriptyline, or Bentyl.**

CATEGORY AND SCHEDULE
Pregnancy Risk Category: D

MECHANISM OF ACTION
A tricyclic compound that blocks
reuptake of neurotransmitters (norepinephrine, serotonin) at neuronal
presynaptic membranes, increasing
availability at postsynaptic receptor
sites. *Therapeutic Effect:* Resulting
enhancements of synaptic activity
produces antidepressant effect.

AVAILABILITY
Capsules: 10 mg, 25 mg, 50 mg,
75 mg.
Oral Solution: 10 mg/5 ml.

INDICATIONS AND DOSAGES
▶ **Depression**
PO
Adults. 75–100 mg/day in 1–4
divided doses until therapeutic
response achieved. Reduce dosage
gradually to effective maintenance
level.
Elderly. Initially, 10–25 mg at
bedtime. May increase by 25 mg
q3–7 days. Maximum: 150 mg/day.
Children older than 12 yrs. 30–50
mg/day in 3–4 divided doses.
Children 6–12 yrs. 10–20 mg/day in
3–4 divided doses.
▶ **Enuresis**
PO
Children older than 11 yrs. 25–35
mg/day.
Children 8–11 yrs. 10–20 mg/day.
Children 6–7 yrs. 10 mg/day.

UNLABELED USES
Treatment of neurogenic pain, panic
disorder, prophylaxis of migraine
headache

CONTRAINDICATIONS
Acute recovery period following
myocardial infarction (MI), within
14 days of MAOI ingestion

INTERACTIONS
Drug
*Alcohol, central nervous system
(CNS) depressants:* May increase
CNS and respiratory depression and
hypotensive effects.
Antithyroid agents: May increase
the risk of agranulocytosis.
Cimetidine: May increase the blood
concentration and risk of toxicity
with nortriptyline.
Clonidine, guanadrel: May decrease
the effects of clonidine and guana-
drel
MAOIs: May increase the risk of
convulsions, hyperpyrexia, and
hypertensive crisis.
Phenothiazines: May increase the
anticholinergic and sedative effects
of nortriptyline.
Sympathomimetics: May increase
cardiac effects.
Herbal
None known.
Food
None known.

DIAGNOSTIC TEST EFFECTS
May alter blood glucose levels and
EKG readings. Peak therapeutic
serum level is 6–10 mcg/ml; trough
is 0.5–2 mcg/ml. Peak toxic serum
level is greater than 12 mcg/ml;
trough is greater than 2 mcg/ml.

SIDE EFFECTS
Frequent
Drowsiness, fatigue, dry mouth,
blurred vision, constipation, delayed

micturition, postural hypotension, excessive sweating, disturbed concentration, increased appetite, urine retention

Occasional

Gastrointestinal (GI) disturbances, including nausea, GI distress, metallic taste sensation, photosensitivity

Rare

Paradoxical reaction (agitation, restlessness, nightmares, insomnia), extrapyramidal symptoms, particularly fine hand tremors

SERIOUS REACTIONS

• High dosage may produce cardiovascular effects, such as severe postural hypotension, dizziness, tachycardia, palpitations, arrhythmias and seizures. High dosage may also result in altered temperature regulation, such as hyperpyrexia or hypothermia.

• Abrupt withdrawal from prolonged therapy may produce headache, malaise, nausea, vomiting, and vivid dreams.

NURSING CONSIDERATIONS

Baseline Assessment

• Plan to perform a complete blood count and blood serum chemistry tests to assess glucose levels, liver, and renal function periodically for patients on long-term therapy.

• Assess the patient's EKG for arrhythmias

Precautions

• Use cautiously in patients with cardiac disease, diabetes mellitus, glaucoma, hiatal hernia, history of seizures, history of urinary obstruction and retention, hyperthyroidism, increased intraocular pressure (IOP), liver disease, prostatic hypertrophy, renal disease, and schizophrenia.

Administration and Handling

PO

• Give nortriptyline with food or milk, if GI distress occurs.

Intervention and Evaluation

• Closely supervise suicidal-risk patients during early therapy. As depression lessens, the patient's energy level improves, which increases the suicide potential.

• Assess the patient's appearance, behavior, level of interest, mood, and speech pattern.

• Assess the patient's pattern of daily bowel activity and stool consistency. Help the patient to avoid constipation by stressing the consumption of high fiber foods and fluids.

• Monitor the patient's blood pressure (B/P) for hypotension and pulse for irregularities that could indicate an arrhythmia.

• Palpate the patient's bladder for signs of urine retention, and monitor his or her urine output.

• Monitor the patient's therapeutic serum levels of nortriptyline. Know that nortriptyline's peak therapeutic serum level is 6–10 mcg/ml; the trough is 0.5–2 mcg/ml. Nortriptyline's peak toxic serum level is greater than 12 mcg/ml; the trough is greater than 2 mcg/ml.

Patient Teaching

• Instruct the patient to change positions slowly to avoid the hypotensive effect of nortriptyline.

• Advise the patient that a tolerance to anticholinergic effects, postural hypotension, and sedative effects usually develops during early therapy.

• Tell the patient that nortriptyline's therapeutic effect may be noted in 2 weeks or longer.

• Caution the patient that photosensitivity to sunlight may occur.

Encourage the patient to use sunscreens and wear protective clothing.
• Suggest to the patient that taking sips of tepid water and chewing sugarless gum may relieve dry mouth.
• Warn the patient to notify the physician if he or she experiences visual disturbances.
• Caution the patient against abruptly discontinuing the medication.
• Warn the patient to avoid tasks that require mental alertness or motor skills until his or her response to the drug is established.

paroxetine hydrochloride
pear-ox-eh-teen
(Aropax 20[AUS], Asimia, Paxeva, Paxil, Paxil CR, Paxtine[AUS])
Do not confuse with Doxil, pyridoxine, or Taxol.

CATEGORY AND SCHEDULE
Pregnancy Risk Category: C

MECHANISM OF ACTION
An antianxiety, antidepressant, and antiobsessive-compulsive agent that selectively blocks uptake of the neurotransmitter serotonin at central nervous system (CNS) neuronal presynaptic membranes, thereby increasing availability at postsynaptic neuronal receptor sites. Results in enhancement of synaptic activity. *Therapeutic Effect:* Produces antidepressant effect, reduces obsessive-compulsive behavior, decreases anxiety.

PHARMACOKINETICS
Well absorbed from the gastrointestinal (GI) tract. Protein binding: 95%. Widely distributed. Metabolized in liver; excreted in urine. Not removed by hemodialysis. **Half-life:** 24 hrs.

AVAILABILITY
Tablets: 10 mg, 20 mg, 30 mg, 40 mg.
Tablets (controlled-release): 12.5 mg, 25 mg, 37.5 mg.
Oral Suspension: 10 mg/5 ml.

INDICATIONS AND DOSAGES
▸ **Depression**
PO
Adults. Initially, 20 mg/day. May increase by 10 mg/day by 1 wk or longer intervals. Maximum: 50 mg/day.
PO (controlled-release)
Adults. Initially, 25 mg/day. May increase by 12.5 mg/day by 1 wk or longer intervals. Maximum: 62.5 mg/day.
▸ **Generalized anxiety disorder (GAD)**
PO
Adults. Initially, 20 mg/day. May increase by 10 mg/day by 1 wk or longer intervals. Range: 20–50 mg/day.
▸ **Obsessive compulsive disorder (OCD)**
PO
Adults. Initially, 20 mg/day. May increase by 10 mg/day by 1 wk or longer intervals. Range: 20–60 mg/day.
▸ **Panic disorder**
PO
Adults. Initially, 10–20 mg/day. May increase by 10 mg/day by 1 wk or longer intervals. Range: 10–60 mg/day.
▸ **Social anxiety disorder (SAD)**
PO
Adults. Initially 20 mg/day. Range: 20–60 mg/day.
▸ **Premenstrual dysphoric disorder (PMDD)**
PO
Adults. Initially, 20 mg/day. May

increase by 10 mg/day by 1 wk or longer intervals. Range: 20–50 mg/day.

▸ **Usual elderly dosage**
PO
Elderly. Initially, 10 mg/day. May increase by 10 mg/day by 1 wk or longer intervals. Maximum: 40 mg/day.
PO (controlled-release)
Elderly. Initially, 12.5 mg/day. May increase by 12.5 mg/day by 1 wk or longer intervals. Maximum: 50 mg/day.

CONTRAINDICATIONS
Within 14 days of MAOI therapy

INTERACTIONS
Drug
Cimetidine: May increase paroxetine blood concentrations.
MAOIs: May cause serotonergic syndrome, marked by excitement, diaphoresis, rigidity, hyperthermia, autonomic hyperactivity, and coma.
Phenytoin: May decrease paroxetine blood concentrations.
Risperidone: Paroxetine can increase blood concentrations of this drug enough to cause extrapyramidal symptoms.
Herbal
St. John's wort: May increase adverse effects.
Food
None known.

DIAGNOSTIC TEST EFFECTS
May increase liver enzymes. May decrease blood Hgb and Hct levels and white blood cell (WBC) count.

SIDE EFFECTS
Frequent
Nausea (26%); somnolence (23%); headache, dry mouth (18%); weakness (15%); constipation (15%); dizziness, insomnia (13%); diarrhea (12%); excessive sweating (11%); tremor (8%)
Occasional
Decreased appetite, respiratory disturbance (6%); anxiety, nervousness (5%); flatulence, paresthesia, yawning (4%); decreased libido, sexual dysfunction, abdominal discomfort (3%)
Rare
Palpitations, vomiting, blurred vision, taste change, confusion

SERIOUS REACTIONS
• None known.

NURSING CONSIDERATIONS
Baseline Assessment
• Assess the patient's appearance, behavior, level of interest, mood, and speech pattern.
• Monitor the patient's liver enzymes, Hgb, Hct and white blood cell (WBC) count.
Lifespan Considerations
• Be aware that paroxetine use may impair reproductive function and that paroxetine is not distributed in breast milk.
• Be aware that the safety and efficacy of this drug have not been established in children.
• In the elderly, age-related renal impairment may require dosage adjustment.
Precautions
• Use cautiously in patients with cardiac disease, history of seizures, impaired platelet aggregation, liver impairment, mania, and renal impairment.
• Use cautiously in patients with suicidal tendencies or who are volume depleted or using diuretics.
Administration and Handling
◂ **ALERT** ▸ Expect to reduce paroxetine drug dosage in the elderly and patients with severe liver or renal

impairment. Keep in mind that the dose changes should occur at 1-wk intervals.
PO
• Give paroxetine with food or milk if GI distress occurs.
• May crush or break scored tablets.
• Plan to give as a single morning dose.

Intervention and Evaluation
• Perform complete blood counts and liver and renal function tests periodically, as ordered, for patients on long-term therapy.
• Closely supervise suicidal-risk patients during early therapy. As depression lessens, the patient's energy level improves, which increases the suicide potential.
• Assess the patient's appearance, behavior, level of interest, mood, and speech pattern.

Patient Teaching
• Advise the patient that paroxetine use may cause dry mouth.
• Urge the patient to avoid alcohol and St. John's wort while taking paroxetine.
• Tell the patient that the therapeutic effect of paroxetine may be noted within 1 to 4 weeks.
• Caution the patient against abruptly discontinuing the medication.
• Warn the patient to avoid tasks that require mental alertness or motor skills until his or her response to the drug is established.
• Explain to the patient that she must notify the physician if she suspects pregnancy, or intends to become pregnant.

phenelzine sulfate
fen-ell-zeen
(Nardil)

CATEGORY AND SCHEDULE
Pregnancy Risk Category: C

MECHANISM OF ACTION
An antidepressant that inhibits MAO enzyme system at central nervous system (CNS) storage sites. The reduced MAO activity causes an increased concentration in epinephrine, norepinephrine, serotonin, dopamine at neuron receptor sites. *Therapeutic Effect:* Produces antidepressant effect.

AVAILABILITY
Tablets: 15 mg.

INDICATIONS AND DOSAGES
▸ **Depression refractory to other antidepressants or electroconvulsive therapy**
PO
Adults. 15 mg 3 times/day. May increase to 60–90 mg/day.
Elderly. Initially, 7.5 mg/day. May increase by 7.5–15 mg/day q3–4wks up to 60 mg/day in divided doses.

UNLABELED USES
Treatment of panic disorder, vascular or tension headaches

CONTRAINDICATIONS
Cardiovascular disease, cerebrovascular disease, liver impairment, pheochromocytoma, liver impairment

INTERACTIONS
Drug
Alcohol, CNS depressants: May increase CNS depressant effects.

Buspirone: May increase blood pressure (B/P).

Caffeine-containing medications: May increase cardiac arrhythmias and hypertension.

Carbamazepine, cyclobenzaprine, maprotiline, other MAOIs: May precipitate hypertensive crises.

Fluoxetine, trazodone, tricyclic antidepressants: May cause serotonin syndrome.

Insulin, oral hypoglycemics: May increase the effects insulin and oral hypoglycemics.

Meperidine, other opioid analgesics: May produce coma, convulsions, death, diaphoresis, immediate excitation, rigidity, severe hypertension or hypotension, severe respiratory distress, or vascular collapse.

Methylphenidate: May increase the CNS stimulant effects of methylphenidate.

Sympathomimetics: May increase the cardiac stimulant and vasopressor effects of phenelzine.

Tyramine: May cause severe, sudden hypertension.

Herbal

None known.

Food

Caffeine, chocolate, dopamine, tryptophan, and tyramine-containing foods, such as aged cheese: May increase blood pressure (B/P).

DIAGNOSTIC TEST EFFECTS

None known.

SIDE EFFECTS

Frequent

Postural hypotension, restlessness, gastrointestinal (GI) upset, insomnia, dizziness, headache, lethargy, weakness, dry mouth, peripheral edema

Occasional

Flushing, increased perspiration, rash, urinary frequency, increased appetite, transient impotence

Rare

Visual disturbances

SERIOUS REACTIONS

• Hypertensive crisis, marked by severe hypertension, occipital headache radiating frontally, neck stiffness or soreness, vomiting, sweating, fever or chilliness, clammy skin, dilated pupils, palpitations, tachycardia or bradycardia, and constricting chest pain.

NURSING CONSIDERATIONS

Baseline Assessment

• Plan to perform liver function tests [serum alkaline phosphatase, bilirubin, SGOT (AST), and SGPT (ALT) levels] periodically in patients requiring high dosage or who are undergoing prolonged therapy.

Precautions

• Use cautiously in patients who ingest tyramine-containing foods.

Intervention and Evaluation

• Assess the patient's appearance, behavior, level of interest, mood, and speech pattern.

• Closely supervise suicidal-risk patients during early therapy. As depression lessens, the patient's energy level improves, which increases the suicide potential.

• Monitor the patient for occipital headache radiating frontally and neck stiffness or soreness which may be the first sign of impending hypertensive crisis.

• Monitor the patient's B/P, diet, change in mood, heart rate, and weight.

• To treat hypertensive crisis, administer phentolamine 5–10 mg IV, as prescribed.

Patient Teaching

• Tell the patient that antidepressant relief may be noted during the first

week of therapy with phenelzine's maximum benefit noted in 2 to 6 weeks.
• Warn the patient to immediately notify the physician if he or she experiences headache or neck soreness or stiffness.
• Urge the patient to avoid foods that require bacteria or molds for their preparation or preservation, or containing tyramine, including avocados, bananas, beer, broad beans, cheese, figs, meat tenderizers, papaya, raisins, sour cream, soy sauce, wine, yeast extracts, yogurt, or excessive amounts of caffeine, such as chocolate, coffee, and tea.
• Tell the patient to avoid using over-the-counter (OTC) preparations for colds, hayfever, and weight reduction.

sertraline hydrochloride
sir-trah-leen
(Zoloft)
Do not confuse with Serentil.

CATEGORY AND SCHEDULE
Pregnancy Risk Category: B

MECHANISM OF ACTION
An antidepressant, antipanic, and obsessive-compulsive adjunct agent that blocks the reuptake of the neurotransmitter serotonin at central nervous system (CNS) neuronal presynaptic membranes, increasing its availability at postsynaptic receptor sites. *Therapeutic Effect:* Produces antidepressant effect, reduces obsessive-compulsive behavior, decreases anxiety.

PHARMACOKINETICS
Incompletely, slowly absorbed from the gastrointestinal (GI) tract; food increases absorption. Protein binding: 98%. Widely distributed. Undergoes extensive first-pass metabolism in liver to active compound. Excreted in urine, eliminated in feces. Not removed by hemodialysis. **Half-life:** 26 hrs.

AVAILABILITY
Tablets: 25 mg, 50 mg, 100 mg.
Oral Concentrate: 20 mg/ml.

INDICATIONS AND DOSAGES
▸ **Antidepressant, obsessive-compulsive disorder (OCD)**
PO
Adults, Children 13-17 yrs. Initially, 50 mg/day with morning or evening meal. May increase by 50 mg/day at 7-day intervals.
Elderly, Children 6-12 yrs. Initially, 25 mg/day. May increase by 25–50 mg/day at 7-day intervals.
Maximum: 200 mg/day.
▸ **Panic disorder, posttraumatic stress disorder, social anxiety disorder**
PO
Adults, Elderly. Initially, 25 mg/day. May increase by 50 mg/day at 7-day intervals. Range: 50–200 mg/day. Maximum: 200 mg/day.
▸ **Premenstrual dysphoric disorder (PMDD)**
PO
Adults. Initially, 50 mg/day. May increase up to 150 mg/day in 50-mg increments.

CONTRAINDICATIONS
During or within 14 days of MAOI antidepressant therapy

INTERACTIONS
Drug
Highly protein-bound medications (e.g., digoxin, warfarin): May increase the blood concentration and risk of toxicity with highly protein-bound medications.
MAOIs: May cause agitation, confusion, hyperpyretic convulsions, and serotonin syndrome, marked by diaphoresis, diarrhea, fever, mental changes, restlessness, shivering.
Herbal
St. John's wort: May increase the risk of adverse effects.
Food
None known.

DIAGNOSTIC TEST EFFECTS
May increase SGOT (AST), SGPT (ALT), and serum total cholesterol and triglyceride levels. May decrease serum uric acid levels.

SIDE EFFECTS
Frequent (26%–12%)
Headache, nausea, diarrhea, insomnia, drowsiness, dizziness, fatigue, rash, dry mouth
Occasional (6%–4%)
Anxiety, nervousness, agitation, tremor, dyspepsia, excessive sweating, vomiting, constipation, abnormal ejaculation, change in vision, change in taste
Rare (less than 3%)
Flatulence, urinary frequency, paresthesia, hot flashes, chills

SERIOUS REACTIONS
• None known.

NURSING CONSIDERATIONS
Baseline Assessment
• Plan to perform complete blood counts and liver and renal function tests periodically for patients on long-term therapy.

Lifespan Considerations
• Be aware that it is unknown if sertraline crosses the placenta or is distributed in breast milk.
• There are no age-related precautions in children older than 6 years of age.
• There are no age-related precautions noted, but lower initial sertraline dosages are recommended in the elderly.
Precautions
• Use cautiously in patients with cardiac disease, liver impairment, and seizure disorders.
• Use cautiously in patients who have had a recent myocardial infarction (MI) and in suicidal patients.
Administration and Handling
PO
• Give sertraline with food or milk if GI distress occurs.
Intervention and Evaluation
• Closely supervise suicidal-risk patients during early therapy. As depression lessens, the patient's energy level improves, which increases the suicide potential.
• Assess the patient's appearance, behavior, level of interest, mood, and speech pattern.
• Monitor the patient's pattern of daily bowel activity and stool consistency.
• Assist the patient with ambulation if he or she experiences dizziness.
Patient Teaching
• Suggest to the patient that taking sips of tepid water and chewing sugarless gum may relieve dry mouth.
• Warn the patient to notify the physician if he or she becomes pregnant or experiences fatigue, headache, sexual dysfunction, or tremor.
• Tell the patient to avoid tasks that require mental alertness or motor

skills until his or her response to the drug is established.
- Explain to the patient to take the drug with food if he or she experiences nausea.
- Urge the patient to avoid alcohol while taking sertraline.
- Explain to the patient not to take over-the-counter (OTC) medications without consulting the physician.

tranylcypromine sulfate
tran-ill-**sip**-roe-meen
(Parnate)

CATEGORY AND SCHEDULE
Pregnancy Risk Category: C

MECHANISM OF ACTION
An antidepressant that inhibits MAO enzymes by assisting in the metabolism of sympathomimetic amines at central nervous system (CNS) storage sites. Levels of epinephrine, norepinephrine, serotonin, dopamine are increased at neuron receptor sites. *Therapeutic Effect:* Produces antidepressant effect.

AVAILABILITY
Tablets: 10 mg.

INDICATIONS AND DOSAGES
▶ **Treatment of depressed patients refractory to or intolerant to other therapy**
PO
Adults, Elderly. Initially, 10 mg 2 times/day. May increase by 10 mg/day at 1- to 3-wk intervals up to 60 mg/day in divided doses.

CONTRAINDICATIONS
Congestive heart failure (CHF), patients younger than 16 yrs of age, pheochromocytoma, severe liver or renal impairment, uncontrolled hypertension

INTERACTIONS
Drug
Alcohol, CNS depressants: May increase CNS depressant effects.
Buspirone: May increase blood pressure (B/P) with buspirone.
Caffeine-containing medications: May increase cardiac arrhythmias and hypertension.
Carbamazepine, cyclobenzaprine, maprotiline, other MAOIs: May precipitate hypertensive crises carbamazepine, cyclobenzaprine, maprotiline, and other MAOIs.
Fluoxetine, trazodone, tricyclic antidepressants: May cause serotonin syndrome.
Insulin, oral hypoglycemics: May increase the effects of insulin and oral hypoglycemics.
Meperidine, other opioid analgesics: May produce coma, convulsions, death, diaphoresis, immediate excitation, rigidity, severe hypertension or hypotension, severe respiratory distress, or vascular collapse.
Tyramine: May cause severe, sudden hypertension.
Herbal
None known.
Food
Caffeine, chocolate, dopamine, tryptophan, and tyramine-containing foods, such as aged cheese: May cause sudden hypertension.

DIAGNOSTIC TEST EFFECTS
None known.

SIDE EFFECTS
Frequent
Postural hypotension, restlessness, gastrointestinal (GI) upset, insom-

nia, dizziness, lethargy, weakness, dry mouth, peripheral edema
Occasional
Flushing, increased perspiration, rash, urinary frequency, increased appetite, transient impotence
Rare
Visual disturbances

SERIOUS REACTIONS
• Hypertensive crisis marked by hypertension, occipital headache radiating frontally, neck stiffness or soreness, nausea, vomiting, diaphoresis, fever or chilliness, clammy skin, dilated pupils, and palpitations may be noted. Tachycardia or bradycardia and constricting chest pain may also be present.

NURSING CONSIDERATIONS

Baseline Assessment
• Plan to perform baseline and periodic liver function tests [serum alkaline phosphatase, bilirubin, SGOT (AST), and SGPT (ALT) levels] in patients requiring high dosages or who are undergoing prolonged therapy.
• Expect to discontinue MAOI therapy 7 to 14 days before beginning therapy.
Precautions
• Use cautiously within several hours of ingestion of contraindicated substance, such as tyramine-containing food.
Intervention and Evaluation
• Assess the patient's appearance, behavior, level of interest, mood, and speech pattern.
• Closely supervise suicidal-risk patients during early therapy. As depression lessens, the patient's energy level improves, which increases the suicide potential.
• Evaluate the patient for occipital headache radiating frontally, and

neck stiffness or soreness, which may be the first sign of impending hypertensive crisis.
• Monitor the patient's B/P diligently for hypertension.
• Treat hypertensive crisis, as prescribed, with phentolamine 5 to 10 mg IV.
• Assess the patient's skin temperature for fever.
• Expect to discontinue the medication immediately if the patient experiences frequent headaches or palpitations.
• Monitor the patient's weight.
Patient Teaching
• Instruct the patient to take the second daily dose no later than 4 p.m. to avoid insomnia.
• Tell the patient that antidepressant relief may be noted during first week of therapy and the maximum benefit will be noted within 3 weeks.
• Warn the patient to notify the physician immediately if he or she experiences headache and neck soreness or stiffness.
• Instruct the patient to change from lying to sitting position slowly, and to dangle his or her legs momentarily before standing to avoid orthostatic hypotension.
• Urge the patient to avoid foods that require bacteria or molds for their preparation or preservation or contain tyramine, such as avocados, bananas, beer, broad beans, cheese, figs, liver, meat tenderizers, papaya, pickled herring, raisins, sour cream, soy sauce, wine, yeast extracts, and yogurt, or excessive amounts of caffeine, including chocolate, coffee, and tea.
• Urge the patient to avoid over-the-counter (OTC) preparations for colds, hayfever, and weight reduction.

trazodone hydrochloride

tra-zoh-doan
(Desyrel)
Do not confuse with Delsym or Zestril.

CATEGORY AND SCHEDULE
Pregnancy Risk Category: C

MECHANISM OF ACTION
An antidepressant that blocks the reuptake of serotonin by central nervous system (CNS) presynaptic neuronal membranes, increasing its availability at postsynaptic neuronal receptor sites. *Therapeutic Effect:* Produces antidepressant effect.

PHARMACOKINETICS
Well absorbed from the gastrointestinal (GI) tract. Protein binding: 85%–95%. Metabolized in liver. Primarily excreted in urine. Unknown if removed by hemodialysis. **Half-life:** 5–9 hrs.

AVAILABILITY
Tablets: 50 mg, 100 mg, 150 mg, 300 mg.

INDICATIONS AND DOSAGES
▸ **Antidepressant**
PO
Adults. Initially, 150 mg a day in equally divided doses. Increase by 50 mg/day at 3-to 4-day intervals until therapeutic response is achieved. Maximum: 600 mg/day.
Children 6–18 yrs. Initially, 1.5–2 mg/kg/day in divided doses. May increase gradually to 6 mg/kg/day in 3 divided doses.
Elderly. Initially, 25–50 mg at bedtime. May increase by 25–50 mg q3–7 days. Range: 75–150 mg/day.

UNLABELED USES
Treatment of neurogenic pain

CONTRAINDICATIONS
None known

INTERACTIONS
Drug
Alcohol, CNS depressant–producing medications: May increase CNS depression.
Antihypertensives: May increase effects antihypertensives.
Digoxin, phenytoin: May increase blood concentration of digoxin and phenytoin.
Herbal
St. John's wort: May increase the adverse effects of trazodone.
Food
None known.

DIAGNOSTIC TEST EFFECTS
May decrease serum leukocyte and neutrophil counts.

SIDE EFFECTS
Frequent (9%–3%)
Drowsiness, dry mouth, lightheadedness or dizziness, headache, blurred vision, nausea or vomiting
Occasional (3%–1%)
Nervousness, fatigue, constipation, generalized aches and pains, mild hypotension

SERIOUS REACTIONS
• Priapism, marked by painful, prolonged penile erection, decreased or increased libido, retrograde ejaculation, and impotence have been noted rarely.
• Trazodone appears to be less cardiotoxic than other antidepressants, although arrhythmias may occur in patients with preexisting cardiac disease.

NURSING CONSIDERATIONS

Baseline Assessment
• Plan to perform complete blood counts and liver and renal function tests periodically for patients on long-term therapy.

Lifespan Considerations
• Be aware that trazodone crosses the placenta and is minimally distributed in breast milk.
• Be aware that the safety and efficacy of trazodone have not been established in children younger than 6 years of age.
• The elderly are more likely to experience hypotensive or sedative. Lower dosages are recommended in the elderly.

Precautions
• Use cautiously in patients with arrhythmias and cardiac disease.

Administration and Handling
PO
• Give trazodone shortly after a meal or snack to reduces the risk of dizziness or lightheadedness.
• Crush tablets, as needed.

Intervention and Evaluation
• Closely supervise suicidal-risk patients during early therapy. As depression lessens, be aware that the patient's energy level generally improves, which increases the suicide potential.
• Assess the patient's appearance, behavior, level of interest, mood, and speech pattern.
• Monitor the patient's serum neutrophil and white blood cell (WBC) counts. Stop administering the drug, as ordered, if these levels fall below normal.
• Assist the patient with ambulation if he or she experiences dizziness or lightheadedness.
• Assess EKG for arrhythmias.

Patient Teaching
• Teach the patient that he or she may take trazodone after a meal or snack to try to avoid feeling dizzy or lightheaded.
• Teach the patient that he or she may take trazodone at bedtime if he or she experiences drowsiness while taking the drug.
• Warn the patient to immediately notify the physician if he experiences painful, prolonged penile erections.
• Instruct the patient to change positions slowly to avoid the drug's hypotensive effect.
• Tell the patient that a tolerance to the anticholinergic and sedative effects of the drug usually develops during early therapy.
• Explain to the patient that he or she may develop a photosensitivity to sunlight during trazodone therapy.
• Suggest to the patient that taking sips of tepid water and chewing sugarless gum may relieve dry mouth.
• Warn the patient to notify the physician if he or she experiences visual disturbances.
• Caution the patient against abruptly discontinuing the medication.
• Warn the patient to avoid tasks that require mental alertness or motor skills until his or her response to the drug is established.
• Urge the patient to avoid alcohol while taking trazodone.

venlafaxine
ven-lah-**facks**-een
(Effexor, Effexor XR)

CATEGORY AND SCHEDULE
Pregnancy Risk Category: C

MECHANISM OF ACTION

A phenethylamine derivative that potentiates central nervous system (CNS) neurotransmitter activity by inhibiting the reuptake of serotonin, norepinephrine, and to a lesser degree, dopamine. *Therapeutic Effect:* Produces antidepressant activity.

PHARMACOKINETICS

Well absorbed from the gastrointestinal (GI) tract. Protein binding: 25%–30%. Metabolized in liver to active metabolite. Primarily excreted in urine. Not removed by hemodialysis. **Half-life:** 3–7 hrs; metabolite: 9–13 hrs, half-life increased impaired liver or renal disease.

AVAILABILITY

Tablets: 25 mg, 37.5 mg, 37.5 mg (Effexor XR), 50 mg, 75 mg, 75 mg (Effexor XR), 100 mg, 150 mg (Effexor XR)

INDICATIONS AND DOSAGES

▶ **Depression**
PO
Adults, Elderly. Initially, 75 mg/day in 2–3 divided doses with food. May increase by 75 mg/day no sooner than 4-day intervals. Maximum: 375 mg/day in 3 divided doses.
▶ **Treatment of generalized anxiety disorder (Effexor XR extended release)**
Adults, Elderly. 75 mg/day as single dose. May increase by 75 mg/day at intervals of 4 days or longer. Maximum: 225 mg/day.
▶ **Anxiety disorder**
PO
Adults. 37.5–225 mg/day.

UNLABELED USES

Prevention of recurrent or relapses of depression, attention-deficit hyperactivity disorder (ADHD), autism, chronic fatigue syndrome, obsessive-compulsive disorder

CONTRAINDICATIONS

Use of MAOIs within 14 days

INTERACTIONS
Drug

MAOIs: May cause autonomic instability, including rapid fluctuations of vital signs, coma, extreme agitation, hyperthermia, mental status changes, myoclonus, and rigidity with these drugs. May cause neuroleptic malignant syndrome, so wait 14 days after discontinuing MAOIs to start venlafaxine or wait 7 days after discontinuing venlafaxine before starting MAOIs.
Herbal
St. John's wort: May increase the sedative-hypnotic effect of venlafaxine.
Food
None known.

DIAGNOSTIC TEST EFFECTS

May increase BUN, serum alkaline phosphatase, serum bilirubin, serum cholesterol, serum uric acid, SGOT (AST), and SGPT (ALT) levels. May decrease serum phosphate and sodium levels. May alter blood glucose and serum potassium levels.

SIDE EFFECTS

Frequent (greater than 20%)
Nausea, somnolence, headache, dry mouth
Occasional (20%–10%)
Dizziness, insomnia, constipation, diaphoresis, nervousness, asthenia or loss of strength or energy, ejaculatory disturbance, anorexia
Rare (less than 10%)
Anxiety, blurred vision, diarrhea,

vomiting, tremor, abnormal dreams, impotence

SERIOUS REACTIONS
• A sustained increase in diastolic blood pressure (B/P) by 10–15 mm Hg occurs occasionally.

NURSING CONSIDERATIONS
Baseline Assessment
• Obtain the patient's baseline B/P and initial weight.
• Assess the patient's appearance, behavior, level of interest, mood, and speech pattern.
Lifespan Considerations
• Be aware that it is unknown if venlafaxine is excreted in breast milk.
• Be aware that the safety and efficacy of venlafaxine have not been established in children.
• There are no age-related precautions noted in the elderly.
Precautions
• Use cautiously in patients with abnormal platelet function, congestive heart failure (CHF), hyperthyroidism, liver impairment, mania, narrow-angle glaucoma, renal impairment, and seizure disorder.
• Use cautiously in patients who are suicidal or volume depleted.
Administration and Handling
◀ALERT▶ Expect to decrease venlafaxine dosage by 50% in patients with moderate liver impairment, 25% in patients with mild to moderate renal impairment, and 50% in patients on dialysis, withholding dose until completion of dialysis. When discontinuing the medication, plan to taper the drug slowly over 2 weeks.

PO
• Give venlafaxine without regard to food. May give with food or milk if the patient experiences gastrointestinal (GI) distress.
• Crush scored tablets, if needed.
• Do not break, open, or crush extended-release capsules.
Intervention and Evaluation
• Monitor the patient's B/P and weight.
• Monitor the patient for signs and symptoms of depression.
• Assess the patient's sleep pattern for evidence of insomnia.
• Observe the patient during his or her waking hours for anxiety, dizziness, or somnolence and provide assistance as necessary.
• Supervise the suicidal-risk patient closely during early therapy. As the patient's depression lessens, his or her energy level improves, increasing suicide potential.
• Assess the appearance, behavior, level of interest, mood, and speech patterns for therapeutic response.
Patient Teaching
• Instruct the patient to take venlafaxine with food to minimize GI distress.
• Caution the patient against abruptly discontinuing the medication or decreasing or increasing the drug dose.
• Warn the patient to avoid tasks that require mental alertness or motor skills until his or her response to the drug is established.
• Tell the patient to notify the physician if she is breast-feeding, pregnant, or planning to become pregnant.
• Urge the patient to avoid alcohol while taking venlafaxine.

aprepitant
chlorpromazine
dimenhydrinate
dolasetron
dronabinol
granisetron
meclizine
metoclopramide
ondansetron
  hydrochloride
palonosetron
  hydrochloride
prochlorperazine
scopolamine
trimethobenzamide
  hydrochloride

Uses: Antiemetics are used to suppress vomiting (emesis). Resulting from chemotherapy, motion sickness, and other causes, emesis is a complex reflex caused by activation of the vomiting center in the medulla oblongata.

Action: Each subclass of antiemetics has a different mechanism of action. *Serotonin antagonists,* such as ondansetron, block serotonin receptors peripherally on vagal nerve terminals and centrally in the chemoreceptor trigger zone (CTZ). *Dopamine antagonists,* such as chlorpromazine, block dopamine receptors in the CTZ. *Cannabinoids,* such as dronabinol, act by an unknown mechanism. *Anticholinergics,* such as scopolamine, block muscarinic receptors in the pathway from the inner ear to the vomiting center. *Antihistamines,* such as dimenhydrinate, block histamine (H_1) and muscarinic receptors in the pathway from the inner ear to the vomiting center. In addition, *aprepitant* antagonizes neurokinin receptors in the CTZ; *palonosetron* antagonizes $5HT_3$ receptors in the CTZ and peripherally.

aprepitant
ah-**prep**-ih-tant
(Emend)

CATEGORY AND SCHEDULE
Pregnancy Risk Category: B

MECHANISM OF ACTION
A selective human substance P and neurokinin 1 (NK_1) receptor antagonist that inhibits chemotherapy-induced nausea or vomiting centrally in the chemoreceptor trigger zone. *Therapeutic Effect:* Prevents the acute and delayed phases of chemotherapy-induced emesis, including vomiting caused by high-dose cisplatin.

PHARMACOKINETICS
Crosses the blood-brain barrier. Extensively metabolized in liver. Eliminated primarily by metabolism (not excreted renally). **Half-life:** 9–13 hrs.

AVAILABILITY
Capsules: 80 mg, 125 mg.

INDICATIONS AND DOSAGES
▶ **Prevention of chemotherapy-induced nausea and vomiting**
PO
Adults, Elderly: 125 mg 1 hr before chemotherapy on day 1 and 80 mg once a day in the morning on days 2 and 3.

CONTRAINDICATIONS
Breast-feeding, concurrent use with pimozide (Orap)

INTERACTIONS
Drug
Alprazolam, docetaxel, etoposide, ifosfamide, imatinib, irinotecan, midazolam, paclitaxel, triazolam, vinblastine, vincristine, vinorelbine: Aprepitant may increase the plasma concentrations of these drugs.
Antifungals, clarithromycin, diltiazem, nefazodone, nelfinavir, ritonavir: Increases aprepitant plasma concentration.
Carbamazepine, phenytoin, rifampin: Reduces aprepitant plasma concentration.
Contraceptives: May decrease the effectiveness of contraceptives.
Paroxetine: May decrease the effectiveness of either drug.
Steroids: Increases exposure to steroids. IV steroid dose should be reduced by 25%, oral dose by 50%.
Warfarin: May decrease the effectiveness of warfarin.
Herbal
None known.
Food
None known.

DIAGNOSTIC TEST EFFECTS
May increase BUN, serum creatinine, SGOT (AST), and SGPT (ALT) levels. May produce proteinuria.

SIDE EFFECTS
Frequent (17%–10%)
Fatigue, nausea, hiccups, diarrhea, constipation, anorexia
Occasional (8%–4%)
Headache, vomiting, dizziness, dehydration, heartburn
Rare (3%–less than 2%)
Abdominal pain, epigastric discomfort, gastritis, tinnitus, insomnia

SERIOUS REACTIONS
• Neutropenia and mucous membrane disorder occur rarely.

NURSING CONSIDERATIONS
Baseline Assessment
• Assess the patient for signs and symptoms of dehydration, including dry mucous membranes, longitudinal furrow in the tongue, and poor skin turgor, if he or she experiences excessive vomiting.
Lifespan Considerations
• Be aware that it is unknown if aprepitant crosses the placenta or is distributed in breast milk.
• Be aware that the safety and efficacy of aprepitant have not been established in children.
• There are no age-related precautions noted in the elderly.
Administration and Handling
◀ALERT▶ As prescribed, give aprepitant with 12 mg dexamethasone PO and 32 mg ondansetron IV on day 1, and 8 mg dexamethasone PO on days 2 to 4.
PO
• Give aprepitant without regard to food.
Intervention and Evaluation
• Assist the patient with ambulation if he or she experiences dizziness.
• Assess the patient's bowel sounds for peristalsis, as well as his or her pattern of daily bowel activity and stool consistency and record time of evacuation.
• Offer the patient emotional support.
Patient Teaching
• Advise the patient that he or she should experience relief from nausea or vomiting shortly after drug administration.
• Warn the patient to notify the

physician if he or she experiences headache or persistent vomiting.

chlorpromazine

klor-**pro**-mah-zeen
(Chlorpromanyl[CAN],
Largactil[CAN], Thorazine)
Do not confuse with chlorpropamide, thiamide, or thioridazine.

CATEGORY AND SCHEDULE
Pregnancy Risk Category: C

MECHANISM OF ACTION
A phenothiazine that blocks dopamine neurotransmission at postsynaptic dopamine receptor sites. Possesses strong anticholinergic, sedative, antiemetic effects; moderate extrapyramidal effects; slight antihistamine action. *Therapeutic Effect:* Reduces psychosis; relieves nausea and vomiting; controls intractable hiccups, porphyria.

AVAILABILITY
Injection: 25 mg/ml.
Liquid: 100 mg/ml, 30 mg/ml.
Suppository: 100 mg.
Syrup: 10 mg/5 ml.
Tablets: 10 mg, 25 mg, 50 mg, 100 mg

INDICATIONS AND DOSAGES
▶ **Psychosis**
IM/IV
Adults, Elderly. Initially, 25 mg; may repeat in 1–4 hrs. May gradually increase to 400 mg q4–6h. Maximum: 300–800 mg/day.
Children older than 6 mos. 0.5–1 mg/kg q6–8h. Maximum (in children younger than 5 yrs): 40 mg/day. Maximum (in children 5–12 yrs): 75 mg/day.

PO
Adults, Elderly. 30–800 mg/day in 1–4 divided doses.
Children older than 6 mos. 0.5–1 mg/kg q4–6h.
▶ **Severe nausea or vomiting**
IM/IV
Adults, Elderly. 25–50 mg q4–6h.
Children. 0.5–1 mg/kg q6–8h.
PO
Adults, Elderly. 10–25 mg q4–6h.
Children. 0.5–1 mg/kg q4–6h.
Rectal
Adults, Elderly. 50–100 mg q6–8h.
Children. 1 mg/kg q6–8h.
▶ **Intractable hiccups**
PO
Adults. 25–50 mg 3 times/day. May give IM/IV.

UNLABELED USES
Treatment of choreiform movement of Huntington's disease

CONTRAINDICATIONS
Bone marrow depression, comatose states, severe cardiovascular disease, severe central nervous system (CNS) depression, subcortical brain damage

INTERACTIONS
Drug
Alcohol, CNS depressants: May increase respiratory depression and the hypotensive effects of chlorpromazine.
Antithyroid agents: May increase the risk of agranulocytosis.
Extrapyramidal symptom-producing medications: Increased risk of extrapyramidal symptoms (EPS).
Hypotensives: May increase hypotension.
Levodopa: May decrease the effects of levodopa.
Lithium: May decrease the absorption of chlorpromazine and produce adverse neurologic effects.

MAOIs, tricyclic antidepressants:
May increase the anticholinergic
and sedative effects of chlorproma-
zine.
Herbal
None known.
Food
None known.

DIAGNOSTIC TEST EFFECTS
May produce false-positive pregnancy test and phenylketonuria
(PKU). EKG changes may occur,
including Q and T wave disturbances. Therapeutic serum level is
50–300 mcg/ml; toxic serum level
is greater than 750 mcg/ml.

SIDE EFFECTS
Frequent
Drowsiness, blurred vision, hypotension, abnormal color vision,
difficulty in night vision, dizziness,
decreased sweating, constipation,
dry mouth, nasal congestion
Occasional
Difficulty urinating, increased skin
sensitivity to sun, skin rash, decreased sexual function, swelling or
pain in breasts, weight gain, nausea,
vomiting, stomach pain, tremors

SERIOUS REACTIONS
• Extrapyramidal symptoms appear
to be dose related, particularly with
high dosages, and are divided into 3
categories: akathisia, including
inability to sit still, tapping of feet,
urge to move around, parkinsonian
symptoms, such as masklike face,
tremors, shuffling gait, hypersalivation, and acute dystonias, including,
torticollis or neck muscle spasm,
opisthotonos or rigidity of back
muscles, and oculogyric crisis or
rolling back of eyes.
• Dystonic reaction may also produce profuse sweating and pallor.
• Tardive dyskinesia, including

protrusion of tongue, puffing of
cheeks, and chewing or puckering
of the mouth, occurs rarely and may
be irreversible.
• Abrupt withdrawal after long-term
therapy may precipitate nausea,
vomiting, gastritis, dizziness, and
tremors.
• Blood dyscrasias, particularly
agranulocytosis, mild leukopenia,
may occur. Blood dyscrasias may
lower seizure threshold.

NURSING CONSIDERATIONS
Baseline Assessment
• Avoid skin contact with solution
to prevent contact dermatitis.
• Assess the patient for signs and
symptoms of dehydration including
dry mucous membranes, longitudinal furrows in the tongue, and poor
skin turgor.
• Assess the patient's appearance,
behavior, emotional status, response
to environment, speech pattern, and
thought content.
Precautions
• Use cautiously in patients with
alcohol withdrawal, glaucoma,
history of seizures, hypocalcemia
(increases susceptibility to dystonias), impaired cardiac, liver, renal
or respiratory function, prostatic
hypertrophy, and urinary retention.
Intervention and Evaluation
• Monitor the patient's blood pressure (B/P) for hypotension.
• Assess the patient for extrapyramidal symptoms.
• Monitor the patient for signs of
tardive dyskinesia, such as tongue
protrusion.
• Regularly check the patient's
complete blood count (CBC), as
ordered, for blood dyscrasias.
• Monitor serum calcium levels
to determine if hypocalcemia is
present.

• Supervise the suicidal-risk patient closely during early therapy because as the patient's depression lessens and his or her energy level improves, the risk for suicide increases.

• Assess the patient for therapeutic response, including increased ability to concentrate, improvement in self care, an interest in surroundings, and a relaxed facial expression.

• Monitor the patient's therapeutic serum level. Know that the therapeutic serum level for chlorpromazine is 50 to 300 mcg/ml and the toxic serum level is greater than 750 mcg/ml.

Patient Teaching

• Explain to the patient that full therapeutic response may take up to 6 weeks to appear.

• Advise the patient that his or her urine may darken.

• Caution the patient against abruptly withdrawing from long-term drug therapy.

• Warn the patient to notify the physician if he or she experiences visual disturbances.

• Advise the patient that drowsiness generally subsides during continued therapy.

• Warn the patient to avoid tasks that require mental alertness or motor skills until his or her response to the drug is established.

• Urge the patient to avoid alcohol while taking chlorpromazine.

• Instruct the patient to avoid exposure to sunlight.

dimenhydrinate
die-men-**high**-drin-ate
(Dramamine)

CATEGORY AND SCHEDULE
Pregnancy Risk Category: B

MECHANISM OF ACTION
An antihistamine and anticholinergic that competes for H_1 receptor sites on effector cells of the gastrointestinal (GI) tract, blood vessels, respiratory tract. The anticholinergic action diminishes vestibular stimulation and depresses labyrinthine function. *Therapeutic Effect:* Prevents symptoms of motion sickness.

AVAILABILITY
Chewable Tablets: 50 mg.
Tablets: 50 mg.

INDICATIONS AND DOSAGES
▸ **Motion sickness**
PO
Adults, Elderly, Children older than 12 yrs. 50–100 mg q4–6h. Maximum: 400 mg/day.
Children 6–12 yrs. 25–50 mg q6–8h. Maximum: 150 mg/day.
Children 2–5 yrs. 12.5–25 mg q6–8h. Maximum: 75 mg/day.

CONTRAINDICATIONS
None significant

INTERACTIONS
Drug
Aminoglycosides: Masks signs and symptoms of ototoxicity associated with aminoglycosides.
Central nervous system (CNS) depressants: Increases sedation with CNS depressants.
Other anticholinergics: Increases anticholinergic effect with other anticholinergics.
Herbal
None known.
Food
None known.

DIAGNOSTIC TEST EFFECTS
None known.

SIDE EFFECTS
Occasional
Hypotension, palpitations, tachycardia, headache, drowsiness, dizziness, paradoxical stimulation, especially in children, anorexia, constipation, dysuria, blurred vision, ringing in the ears, wheezing, chest tightness
Rare
Photosensitivity, rash, urticaria

SERIOUS REACTIONS
• None significant.

NURSING CONSIDERATIONS

Baseline Assessment
• Assess the patient's other medical conditions, such as asthma, glaucoma, prostatic hypertrophy, and seizures.
• Establish the patient's medication history especially concurrent use of other anticholinergics and CNS depressants.
Precautions
• Use cautiously in patients with asthma, bladder neck obstruction, history of seizures, narrow angle glaucoma, and prostatic hypertrophy.
Administration and Handling
PO
• Give with water.
Intervention and Evaluation
• Monitor the patient's blood pressure (B/P), and for paradoxical reaction, especially in children, and signs and symptoms of motion sickness.
Patient Teaching
• Warn the patient to avoid tasks requiring mental alertness or motor skills until his or her response to the drug is established.
• Tell the patient that dimenhydrinate may cause drowsiness and dry mouth.

• Urge the patient to avoid alcohol during dimenhydrinate therapy.
• Caution the patient to avoid prolonged sun exposure as this may cause a photosensitivity reaction.

dolasetron
dole-**ah**-seh-tron
(Anzemet)
Do not confuse with Aldomet.

CATEGORY AND SCHEDULE
Pregnancy Risk Category: B

MECHANISM OF ACTION
An antiemetic that exhibits selective $5\text{-}HT_3$ receptor antagonism. Action may occur centrally in the chemotherapeutic zone (CTZ) or peripherally on the vagal nerve terminals.
Therapeutic Effect: Prevents nausea and vomiting.

PHARMACOKINETICS
Oral form readily absorbed from the gastrointestinal (GI) tract. Protein binding: 69%–77%. Metabolized in liver. Primarily excreted in urine. Unknown if removed by hemodialysis. **Half-life:** 5–10 hrs.

AVAILABILITY
Tablets: 50 mg, 100 mg.
Injection: 20 mg/ml.

INDICATIONS AND DOSAGES
▶ **Prevention of chemotherapy-induced nausea and vomiting**
IV
Adults, Children 1–16 yrs. 1.8 mg/kg as a single dose 30 min before chemotherapy.
Maximum:100 mg.
PO
Adults. 100 mg within 1 hr of chemotherapy.

Children 2–16 yrs. 1.8 mg/kg within 1 hr of chemotherapy. Maximum: 100 mg.

▸ **Treatment and prevention of postoperative nausea or vomiting**
IV
Adults. 12.5 mg.
Children 2–16 yrs. 0.35 mg/kg. Maximum: 12.5 mg. Give approximately 15 min before cessation of anesthesia or as soon as nausea presents.
PO
Adults. 100 mg.
Children 2–16 yrs. 1.2 mg/kg. Maximum: 100 mg within 2 hrs of surgery.

UNLABELED USES
Radiation therapy–induced nausea and vomiting

CONTRAINDICATIONS
None known

INTERACTIONS
Drug
None known.
Herbal
None known.
Food
None known.

DIAGNOSTIC TEST EFFECTS
May alter liver function tests.

IV INCOMPATIBILITIES
No information available via Y-site administration.

SIDE EFFECTS
Frequent (10%–5%)
Headache, diarrhea, fatigue
Occasional (5%–1%)
Fever, dizziness, tachycardia, dyspepsia

SERIOUS REACTIONS
• Overdose may produce combination of CNS stimulation and depressant effects.

NURSING CONSIDERATIONS
Baseline Assessment
• Assess the patient for signs and symptoms of dehydration, including dry mucous membranes, longitudinal furrows in the tongue, and poor skin turgor, if he or she experiences excessive vomiting.
Lifespan Considerations
• Be aware that it is unknown if dolasetron is distributed in breast milk.
• Be aware that the safety and efficacy of this drug have not been established in children younger than 2 years.
• There are no age-related precautions noted in the elderly.
Precautions
• Use cautiously in patients with congenital QT syndrome, hypokalemia, hypomagnesemia, and prolongation of cardiac conduction intervals.
• Use cautiously in patients taking diuretics with the potential for inducing electrolyte disturbances and antiarrhythmics that may lead to QT prolongation, and on cumulative high-dose anthracycline therapy.
Administration and Handling
PO
• Do not cut, break, or chew film-coated tablets.
• For children 2–16 years, mix injection form in apple or apple-grape juice, if needed, for oral dosing at 1.8 mg/kg up to a maximum of 100 mg.
IV
• Store vials at room temperature.
• After dilution, store solution for up to 24 hours at room temperature or up to 48 hours if refrigerated.
• May dilute in 0.9% NaCl, D_5W,

D_5W with 0.45% NaCl, D_5W with lactated Ringer's, lactated Ringer's, or 10% mannitol injection to 50 ml.
• Can be given as IV push as rapidly as 100 mg/30 sec.
• Give intermittent IV infusion or piggyback over 15 minutes.
Intervention and Evaluation
• Monitor the patient for therapeutic relief from nausea or vomiting.
• Monitor the EKG for high-risk patients.
• Maintain a quiet, supportive atmosphere.
• Offer the patient emotional support.
Patient Teaching
• Tell postoperative patient to report nausea as soon as it occurs. Know that prompt administration of the drug increases its effectiveness.
• Warn the patient not to cut, break, or chew film-coated tablets.
• Teach the patient other methods of reducing nausea, such as lying quietly, and avoiding strong odors.

---

dronabinol
drow-**nab**-in-all
(Marinol)
Do not confuse with droperidol.

CATEGORY AND SCHEDULE
Pregnancy Risk Category: C
Controlled substance: Schedule III

MECHANISM OF ACTION
An antiemetic, antinausea, and appetite stimulant agent that inhibits vomiting control mechanisms in the medulla oblongata. *Therapeutic Effect:* Inhibits vomiting.

AVAILABILITY
Capsules, gelatin: 2.5 mg, 5 mg, 10 mg.

INDICATIONS AND DOSAGES
▶ **Nausea, vomiting**
PO
Adults, Children. Initially, 5 mg/m^2, 1–3 hrs before chemotherapy, then q2–4h after chemotherapy for total of 4–6 doses/day. May increase by 2.5 mg/m^2 up to 15 mg/m^2 dose.
▶ **Appetite stimulant**
PO
Adults. Initially, 2.5 mg 2 times/day (before lunch, dinner). Range: 2.5–20 mg/day.

CONTRAINDICATIONS
Nausea, vomiting other than due to chemotherapy

INTERACTIONS
Drug
Central nervous system (CNS) depressants: May enhance sedative effects.
Herbal
None known.
Food
None known.

DIAGNOSTIC TEST EFFECTS
None known.

SIDE EFFECTS
Frequent (24%–3%)
Euphoria, dizziness, paranoid reaction, somnolence
Occasional (3%–1%)
Asthenia, ataxia, confusion, abnormal thinking, depersonalization
Rare (less than 1%)
Diarrhea, depression, nightmares,

speech difficulties, headache, anxiety, ringing in ears, flushed skin

SERIOUS REACTIONS
• Mild intoxication may produce increased sensory awareness, including taste, smell, and sound, altered time perception, reddened conjunctiva, dry mouth, and tachycardia.
• Moderate intoxication may produce memory impairment and urinary retention.
• Severe intoxication may produce lethargy, decreased motor coordination, slurred speech, and postural hypotension.

NURSING CONSIDERATIONS
Baseline Assessment
• Assess the patient for signs and symptoms of dehydration, including dry mucous membranes, low urine output, and poor skin turgor, if he or she experiences excessive vomiting.
Precautions
• Use cautiously in patients with depression, heart disease, hypertension, mania, and schizophrenia.
• Keep in mind that dronabinol use is not recommended in children.
Intervention and Evaluation
• Supervise the patient closely for serious behavior and mood responses.
• Monitor the patient's blood pressure (B/P) and heart rate.
Patient Teaching
• Warn the patient to notify the physician if he or she experiences visual disturbances.
• Explain to the patient that relief from nausea or vomiting generally occurs within 15 minutes of drug administration.

• Urge the patient to avoid alcohol and barbiturates while taking dronabinol.
• Warn the patient to avoid tasks that require mental alertness or motor skills until his or her response to the drug is established.
• Instruct the patient to take dronabinol before lunch and dinner to stimulate appetite.

granisetron
gran-**is**-eh-tron
(Kytril)

CATEGORY AND SCHEDULE
Pregnancy Risk Category: B

MECHANISM OF ACTION
An antiemetic that selectively blocks serotonin stimulation at receptor sites on abdominal vagal afferent nerve and chemoreceptor trigger zone. *Therapeutic Effect:* Prevents nausea, vomiting.

PHARMACOKINETICS

Route	Onset	Peak	Duration
IV	1–3 min	N/A	24 hrs

Rapidly, widely distributed to tissues. Protein binding: 65%. Metabolized in liver to active metabolite. Excreted in urine, eliminated in feces. **Half-life:** 10–12 hrs (half-life is increased in elderly).

AVAILABILITY
Tablets: 1 mg.
Injection: 1 mg/ml.
Oral Solution: 1 mg/5 ml.

INDICATIONS AND DOSAGES
▸ **Prophylaxis of chemotherapy-induced nausea and vomiting**
IV
Adults, Elderly, Children 2 yrs and older. 10 mcg/kg/dose (or 1 mg/dose) given within 30 min of chemotherapy.
PO
Adults, Elderly. 2 mg once a day up to 1 hr prior to chemotherapy or 1 mg 2 times/day.
▸ **Prophylaxis of radiation-induced nausea/vomiting**
PO
Adults, Elderly. 2 mg once a day given 1 hr prior to radiation therapy.
▸ **Postoperative nausea or vomiting**
IV
Adults, Elderly. 1 mg as a single dose.
PO
Adults, Elderly, Children 4 years and older. 20–40 mcg/kg as a single postoperative dose.

UNLABELED USES
Prophylaxis of nausea or vomiting associated with cancer radiotherapy and radiation therapy

CONTRAINDICATIONS
None known.

INTERACTIONS
Drug
Liver enzyme inducers: May decrease the effects of granisetron.
Herbal
None known.
Food
None known.

DIAGNOSTIC TEST EFFECTS
May increase SGOT (AST) and SGPT (ALT) levels.

IV INCOMPATIBILITIES
Amphotericin B (Fungizone)

IV COMPATIBILITIES
Allopurinol (Aloprim), bumetanide (Bumex), calcium gluconate, carboplatin (Paraplatin), cisplatin (Platinol), cyclophosphamide (Cytoxan), cytarabine (ARA-C), dacarbazine (DTIC), dexamethasone (Decadron), diphenhydramine (Benadryl), docetaxel (Taxotere), doxorubicin (Adriamycin), etoposide (VePesid), gemcitabine (Gemzar), magnesium, mitoxantrone (Novantrone), paclitaxel (Taxol), potassium

SIDE EFFECTS
Frequent (21%–14%)
Headache, constipation, asthenia (loss of strength)
Occasional (8%–6%)
Diarrhea, abdominal pain
Rare (less than 2%)
Altered taste, hypersensitivity reaction

SERIOUS REACTIONS
• None known.

NURSING CONSIDERATIONS
Baseline Assessment
• Ensure that granisetron is given to the patient within 30 minutes of the start of chemotherapy.
Lifespan Considerations
• Be aware that it is unknown if granisetron is distributed in breast milk.
• Be aware that the safety and efficacy of granisetron have not been established in children younger than 2 years of age.
• There are no age-related precautions noted in the elderly.
Precautions
• Use cautiously in patients younger than 2 years of age.

Administration and Handling
◀ALERT▶ Administer only on days of chemotherapy, as prescribed.
IV
• Solution normally appears clear and colorless. Inspect for particulates and discoloration.
• Store at room temperature.
• After dilution, solution is stable for at least 24 hours at room temperature.
• Give undiluted or dilute with 20 to 50 ml 0.9% NaCl or D$_5$W. Do not mix with other medications.
• Give undiluted as IV push over 30 seconds.
• For IV piggyback, infuse over 5 to 20 minutes depending on volume of diluent used.

Intervention and Evaluation
• Monitor the patient for therapeutic effect.
• Assess the patient for headache.
• Assess the patient's daily pattern of bowel activity and stool consistency.

Patient Teaching
• Tell the patient that granisetron is effective shortly after administration and that the drug prevents nausea and vomiting.
• Explain to the patient that a transitory taste disorder may occur.
• Help the patient use other methods of reducing nausea and vomiting, such as lying quietly and avoiding strong odors.

meclizine
mek-lih-zeen
(Antivert, Bonamine[CAN], Bonine)

CATEGORY AND SCHEDULE
Pregnancy Risk Category: B

MECHANISM OF ACTION
An anticholinergic that reduces labyrinth excitability and diminishes vestibular stimulation of labyrinth, affecting chemoreceptor trigger zone (CTZ). Possesses anticholinergic activity. *Therapeutic Effect:* Reduces nausea, vomiting, vertigo.

PHARMACOKINETICS

Route	Onset	Peak	Duration
PO	30–60 min	N/A	12–24 hrs

Well absorbed from the gastrointestinal (GI) tract. Widely distributed. Metabolized in liver. Primarily excreted in urine. **Half-life:** 6 hrs.

AVAILABILITY
Tablets: 12.5 mg, 25 mg, 50 mg.
Tablets (chewable): 25 mg.

INDICATIONS AND DOSAGES
▶ **Motion sickness**
PO
Adults, Elderly, Children 12 yrs and older. 12.5–25 mg 1 hr before travel. May repeat q12–24h. May require a dose of 50 mg.
▶ **Vertigo**
PO
Adults, Elderly, Children 12 yrs and older. 25–100 mg/day in divided doses, as needed.

CONTRAINDICATIONS
None known

INTERACTIONS
Drug
Alcohol, central nervous system (CNS) depression-producing medications: May increase CNS depressant effect.
Herbal
None known.

Food
None known.

DIAGNOSTIC TEST EFFECTS
May suppress wheal, flare reactions to antigen skin testing, unless meclizine discontinued 4 days before testing.

SIDE EFFECTS
Frequent
Drowsiness
Occasional
Blurred vision, dry mouth, nose, or throat

SERIOUS REACTIONS
• Children may experience dominant paradoxical reaction, including restlessness, insomnia, euphoria, nervousness, and tremors.
• Overdosage in children may result in hallucinations, convulsions, and death.
• Hypersensitivity reaction, marked by eczema, pruritus, rash, cardiac disturbances, and photosensitivity, may occur.
• Overdosage may vary from CNS depression, such as sedation, apnea, cardiovascular collapse, or death, to severe paradoxical reaction, including hallucinations, tremor, or seizures.

NURSING CONSIDERATIONS
Lifespan Considerations
• Be aware that it is unknown if meclizine crosses the placenta or is distributed in breast milk: Keep in mind that meclizine use may produce irritability in breast-feeding infants.
• Be aware that children and the elderly may be more sensitive to the drug's anticholinergic effects, such as dry mouth.

Precautions
• Use cautiously in patients with narrow-angle glaucoma and obstructive diseases of the gastrointestinal (GI) or genitourinary (GU) tract.
Administration and Handling
◀ALERT▶ Elderly patients older than 60 years of age tend to develop agitation, disorientation, dizziness, hypotension, mental confusion, psychotic-like symptoms, and sedation.
PO
• Give meclizine without regard to meals.
• Crush scored tablets as needed.
• Do not crush, open, or break capsule form.
Intervention and Evaluation
• Monitor the patient's blood pressure (B/P), especially in the elderly who are at increased risk of hypotension.
• Monitor pediatric patients closely for paradoxical reaction.
• Monitor the serum electrolytes in patients experiencing severe vomiting.
• Assess the patient's mucous membranes and skin turgor to evaluate his or her hydration status.
Patient Teaching
• Explain to the patient that a tolerance to the drug's sedative effect may occur.
• Warn the patient to avoid tasks that require mental alertness or motor skills until his or her response to the drug is established.
• Explain to the patient that he or she should expect dizziness, drowsiness, and dry mouth as responses of the drug.
• Warn the patient to avoid alcohol during meclizine therapy.
• Suggest taking sips of tepid water and chewing sugarless gum to the patient to help relieve dry mouth.

• Tell the patient that coffee or tea may help reduce drowsiness.

metoclopramide
meh-tah-**klo**-prah-myd
(Apo-Metoclop[CAN],
Pramin[AUS], Reglan)
Do not confuse with Renagel.

CATEGORY AND SCHEDULE
Pregnancy Risk Category: B

MECHANISM OF ACTION
A dopamine receptor antagonist that stimulates motility of the upper gastrointestinal (GI) tract. Decreases reflux into esophagus. Raises threshold activity of chemoreceptor trigger zone. *Therapeutic Effect:* Accelerates intestinal transit and gastric emptying. Produces antiemetic activity.

PHARMACOKINETICS

Route	Onset	Peak	Duration
PO	30–60 min	N/A	N/A
IM	10–15 min	N/A	N/A
IV	1–3 min	N/A	N/A

Well absorbed from GI tract. Metabolized in liver. Protein binding: 30%. Primarily excreted in urine. Not removed by hemodialysis.
Half-life: 4–6 hrs.

AVAILABILITY
Tablets: 5 mg, 10 mg.
Syrup: 5 mg/5 ml.
Injection: 5 mg/ml.

INDICATIONS AND DOSAGES
▸ **Diabetic gastroparesis**
PO/IV
Adults. 10 mg before meals and at bedtime for 2–8 wks.

PO
Elderly. Initially, 5 mg before meals and at bedtime. May increase to 10 mg.
IV
Elderly. 5 mg over 1–2 min. May increase to 10 mg.
▸ **Symptomatic gastroesophageal reflux**
PO
Adults. 10–15 mg up to 4 times/day; single doses up to 20 mg as needed.
Elderly. Initially, 5 mg 4 times/day. May increase to 10 mg.
Children. 0.4–0.8 mg/kg/day in 4 divided doses.
▸ **Prevention of cancer chemotherapy–induced nausea and vomiting**
IV
Adults, Elderly, Children. 1–2 mg/kg 30 min prior to chemotherapy; repeat q2h for 2 doses, then q3h as needed.
▸ **To facilitate small bowel intubation (single dose)**
IV
Adults, Elderly. 10 mg.
Children 6–14 yrs. 2.5–5 mg.
Children younger than 6 yrs. 0.1 mg/kg.
▸ **Postoperative nausea and vomiting**
IV
Adults, Elderly, Children older than 14 yrs. 10 mg; repeat q6–8h as needed.
Children 14 yrs and younger. 0.1–0.2 mg/kg/dose; repeat q6–8h as needed.
▸ **Dosage in renal impairment**

Creatinine Clearance	% of normal dose
40–50 ml/min	75%
10–40 ml/min	50%
less than 10 ml/min	25%–50%

UNLABELED USES
Prophylaxis of aspiration pneumonia, treatment of drug-related postop nausea and vomiting, persistent hiccups, slow gastric emptying, vascular headaches

CONTRAINDICATIONS
Concurrent use of medications likely to produce extrapyramidal reactions, GI hemorrhage, GI obstruction or perforation, history of seizure disorders, pheochromocytoma

INTERACTIONS
Drug
Alcohol: May increase central nervous system (CNS) depressant effect.
CNS depressants: May increase sedative effect.
Herbal
None known.
Food
None known.

DIAGNOSTIC TEST EFFECTS
May increase aldosterone, prolactin concentrations

IV INCOMPATIBILITIES
Allopurinol (Aloprim), cefepime (Maxipime), doxorubicin liposome (Doxil), furosemide (Lasix), propofol (Diprivan)

IV COMPATIBILITIES
Dexamethasone, diltiazem (Cardizem), diphenhydramine (Benadryl), fentanyl (Sublimaze), heparin, hydromorphone (Dilaudid), morphine, potassium chloride

SIDE EFFECTS
Frequent (10%)
Drowsiness, restlessness, fatigue, lassitude

Occasional (3%)
Dizziness, anxiety, headache, insomnia, breast tenderness, altered menstruation, constipation, rash, dry mouth, galactorrhea, gynecomastia
Rare (less than 3%)
Hypotension or hypertension, tachycardia

SERIOUS REACTIONS
• Extrapyramidal reactions occur most frequently in children and young adults (18–30 yrs) receiving large doses (2 mg/kg) during cancer chemotherapy and is usually limited to akathisia or motor restlessness, involuntary limb movement, and facial grimacing.

NURSING CONSIDERATIONS
Baseline Assessment
• Assess the patient taking metoclopramide as an antiemetic for signs of dehydration, such as dry mucous membranes, longitudinal furrows in tongue, and poor skin turgor.
Lifespan Considerations
• Be aware that metoclopramide crosses the placenta and is distributed in breast milk.
• Be aware that children are more susceptible to having dystonia reactions.
• Be aware that the elderly are more likely to have parkinsonism and tardive dyskinesias after long-term therapy.
Precautions
• Use cautiously in patients with cirrhosis, congestive heart failure (CHF), and impaired renal function.
Administration and Handling
◀ALERT▶ May give PO, IM, IV push, IV infusion.
◀ALERT▶ Know that doses of 2 mg/kg or more or an increase in length of therapy may result in a greater incidence of side effects.

PO
• Give 30 minutes before meals and at bedtime.
• Crush tablets as needed.
IV
• Store vials at room temperature.
• After dilution, IV piggyback infusion is stable for 48 hours.
• Dilute doses greater than 10 mg in 50 ml D_5W, 0.9% NaCl, or lactated Ringer's.
• Infuse over at least 15 minutes.
• May give slow IV push at rate of 10 mg over 1 to 2 minutes.
• A too rapid IV injection may produce intense feelings of anxiety or restlessness, followed by drowsiness.

Intervention and Evaluation
• Monitor the patient for anxiety, extrapyramidal symptoms, and restlessness during IV administration.
• Assess the patient's pattern of daily bowel activity and stool consistency.
• Assess the patient for periorbital edema.
• Assess the patient's skin for rash and urticaria.
• Evaluate the patient for therapeutic response from gastroparesis, such as relief from nausea, persistent fullness after meals, and vomiting.
• Monitor the patient's BUN, blood pressure (B/P), heart rate, and serum creatinine to assess renal function.

Patient Teaching
• Warn the patient to avoid tasks that require mental alertness or motor skills until his or her response to the drug is established.
• Tell the patient to notify the physician if he or she experiences involuntary eye, facial, or limb movement, signs of an extrapyramidal reaction.

• Urge the patient to avoid alcohol during metoclopramide therapy.

ondansetron hydrochloride
on-**dan**-sah-tron
(Zofran)
Do not confuse with Zantac and Zosyn.

CATEGORY AND SCHEDULE
Pregnancy Risk Category: B

MECHANISM OF ACTION
An antiemetic and antinausea agent that blocks serotonin, both peripherally on vagal nerve terminals and centrally in the chemoreceptor trigger zone. *Therapeutic Effect:* Prevents nausea, vomiting.

PHARMACOKINETICS
Readily absorbed from the gastrointestinal (GI) tract. Protein binding: 70%–76%. Metabolized in liver. Primarily excreted in urine. Unknown if removed by hemodialysis.
Half-life: 4 hrs.

AVAILABILITY
Tablets: 4 mg, 8 mg, 24 mg.
Oral Disintegrating Tablets: 4 mg, 8 mg.
Oral Solution: 4 mg/5 ml.
Injection: 2 mg/ml.
Injection (Premix): 32 mg/50 ml.

INDICATIONS AND DOSAGES
▶ **Prevention of chemotherapy-induced nausea and vomiting**
IV
Adults, Elderly, Children 4–18 yrs.
Single 32 mg dose or 0.15 mg/kg/dose given 30 min before chemotherapy, then 4 and 8 hrs following chemotherapy.

PO
*Adults, Elderly, Children older than
11 yrs.* 24 mg as a single dose 30
min prior to starting chemotherapy
or 8 mg q8h (first dose 30 min prior
to chemotherapy) then q12h for 1–2
days.
Children 4–11 yrs. 4 mg 30 min
prior to chemotherapy and 4 and 8
hrs following chemotherapy, then 4
mg q8h for 1–2 days.
▸ **Prevention of postoperative nausea, vomiting**
IM/IV
Adults, Elderly. 4 mg undiluted over
2–5 min.
Children weighing less than 40 kg.
0.1 mg/kg.
Children weighing 10 kg and more.
4 mg.
▸ **Prevention of nausea, vomiting
caused by radiation therapy**
PO
Adults, Elderly. 8 mg 3 times/day.

UNLABELED USES
Treatment of postop nausea, vomiting

CONTRAINDICATIONS
None known

INTERACTIONS
Drug
None known.
Herbal
None known.
Food
None known.

DIAGNOSTIC TEST EFFECTS
May transiently increase serum
bilirubin, SGOT (AST), and SGPT
(ALT) levels.

IV INCOMPATIBILITIES
Acyclovir (Zovirax), allopurinol
(Aloprim), aminophylline, amphotericin B (Fungizone), amphotericin
B complex (Abelcet, AmBisome,
Amphotec), ampicillin (Polycillin),
ampicillin/sulbactam (Unasyn),
cefepime (Maxipime), cefoperazone
(Cefobid), fluorouracil, lorazepam
(Ativan), meropenem (Merrem IV),
methylprednisolone (Solu-Medrol)

IV COMPATIBILITIES
Carboplatin (Paraplatin), cisplatin
(Platinol), cyclophosphamide (Cytoxan), cytarabine (Cytosar), dacarbazine (DTIC-Dome), daunorubicin
(Cerubidine), dexamethasone
(Decadron), diphenhydramine
(Benadryl), docetaxel (Taxotere),
dopamine (Intropin), etoposide
(VePesid), gemcitabine (Gemzar),
heparin, hydromorphone (Dilaudid),
ifosfamide (Ifex), magnesium,
mannitol, mesna (Mesnex), methotrexate, metoclopramide(Reglan),
mitomycin (Mutamycin), mitoxantrone (Novantrone), morphine,
paclitaxel (Taxol), potassium chloride, teniposide (Vumon), topotecan
(Hycamtin), vinblastine (Velban),
vincristine (Oncovin), vinorelbine
(Navelbine)

SIDE EFFECTS
Frequent (13%–5%)
Anxiety, dizziness, drowsiness,
headache, fatigue, constipation,
diarrhea, hypoxia, urinary retention
Occasional (4%–2%)
Abdominal pain, xerostomia or
diminished saliva secretion, fever,
feeling of cold, redness and pain at
injection site, paresthesia, weakness
Rare (less than 1%)
Hypersensitivity reaction, including
rash and itching, blurred vision

SERIOUS REACTIONS
• Overdose may produce combination of central nervous system
(CNS) stimulation and depressant
effects.

NURSING CONSIDERATIONS

Baseline Assessment
• Assess the patient for signs and symptoms of dehydration, including dry mucous membranes, longitudinal furrows in the tongue, and poor skin turgor, if he or she experiences excessive vomiting.
• Monitor serum bilirubin, SGOT (AST), and SGPT (ALT) levels.

Lifespan Considerations
• Be aware that it is unknown if ondansetron crosses the placenta or is distributed in breast milk.
• Be aware that the safety and efficacy of ondansetron have not been established in children.
• There are no age-related precautions noted in the elderly.

Administration and Handling
◄ALERT► Give all oral doses 30 minutes before chemotherapy and repeat at 8-hour intervals, as prescribed.
PO
• Give ondansetron without regard to food.
IM
• Inject into large muscle mass, such as the gluteus maximus.
IV
• Store at room temperature.
• Solution is stable for 48 hours after dilution.
• May give undiluted as an IV push.
• For IV infusion, dilute with 50 ml D_5W or 0.9% NaCl before administration.
• Give IV push over 2 to 5 minutes.
• Give IV infusion over 15 minutes.

Intervention and Evaluation
• Offer the patient emotional support.
• Assess and record the patient's bowel sounds for peristalsis, and his or her daily pattern of bowel activity and stool consistency.
• Evaluate the patient's mental status.

Patient Teaching
• Explain to the patient that the patient that relief from nausea and vomiting generally occurs shortly after drug administration.
• Urge the patient to avoid alcohol and barbiturates while taking ondansetron.
• Warn the patient to notify the physician if he or she experiences persistent vomiting.
• Advise the patient that ondansetron may cause dizziness or drowsiness.
• Teach the patient other methods of reducing nausea and vomiting, including lying quietly and avoiding strong odors.

palonosetron hydrochloride
pal-oh-**noe**-seh-tron
(Aloxi)

CATEGORY AND SCHEDULE
Pregnancy Risk Category: B

MECHANISM OF ACTION
A $5HT_3$ receptor antagonist located centrally (CTZ) and peripherally at the vagus nerve terminal. *Therapeutic Effect:* Prevents nausea, vomiting associated with cancer chemotherapy.

PHARMACOKINETICS
Protein binding: 52%. Eliminated in the urine. **Half-life:** 40 hrs.

AVAILABILITY
Injection: 0.25 mg/5 ml.

INDICATIONS AND DOSAGES
▶ **Nausea, vomiting related to chemotherapy**
IV
Adults, Elderly. 0.25 mg given as a
single dose 30 min prior to starting
chemotherapy.

CONTRAINDICATIONS
None known

INTERACTIONS
Drug
None known.
Herbal
None known.
Food
None known.

DIAGNOSTIC TEST EFFECTS
May transiently increase serum
bilirubin, SGOT (AST), and SGPT
(ALT) levels.

IV INCOMPATIBILITIES
Do not mix with any other drugs.

SIDE EFFECTS
Occasional (9%–5%)
Headache, constipation
Rare (less than 1%)
Diarrhea, dizziness, fatigue, abdom-
inal pain, insomnia

SERIOUS REACTIONS
• Overdose may produce combination of central nervous system
(CNS) stimulation and depressant
effects.

NURSING CONSIDERATIONS
Baseline Assessment
• Assess the patient for dehydration
if he or she experiences excessive
vomiting. Examine the patient for
dry mucous membranes, longitudinal furrows in the tongue, and poor
skin turgor.

• Provide emotional support to the
patient.
Lifespan Considerations
• Be aware that it is unknown if
palonosetron is excreted in breast
milk.
• Be aware that the safety and
efficacy of palonosetron have not
been established in children.
• There are no age-related precautions noted in the elderly.
Precautions
• Use cautiously in patients with a
history of cardiovascular disease.
Administration and Handling
IV
• Store at room temperature.
• Solution normally appears clear,
colorless. Discard if precipitate is
present or if solution appears
cloudy.
• Give undiluted as an IV push over
30 seconds. Flush infusion line with
0.9% NaCl before and after administration.
Intervention and Evaluation
• Provide the patient with supportive measures.
• Evaluate the patient's mental
status.
• Assess the patient's daily pattern
of daily bowel activity and stool
consistency and record time of
evacuation.
Patient Teaching
• Advise the patient that he or she
may expect relief from nausea and
vomiting shortly after drug administration.
• Urge the patient to consuming
alcohol and taking barbiturates
during palonosetron therapy.
• Warn the patient to notify the
physician if he or she experiences
persistent vomiting.
• Teach the patient other methods of
reducing nausea and vomiting,

including lying quietly and avoiding strong odors.

prochlorperazine
pro-klor-**pear**-ah-zeen
(Compazine, Stemetil[CAN], Stemzine[AUS])
Do not confuse with chlorpromazine or Copaxone.

CATEGORY AND SCHEDULE
Pregnancy Risk Category: C

MECHANISM OF ACTION
A phenothiazine that acts centrally to inhibit or block dopamine receptors in the chemoreceptor trigger zone, and peripherally to block the vagus nerve in the gastrointestinal (GI) tract. *Therapeutic Effect:* Relieves nausea and vomiting.

PHARMACOKINETICS

Route	(Antiemetic) Onset	Peak	Duration
Tablets, syrup	30–40 min	N/A	3–4 hrs
Extended-release	30–40 min	N/A	10–12 hrs
Rectal	60 min	N/A	3–4 hrs

Variably absorbed following PO administration. Widely distributed. Metabolized in liver, GI mucosa. Primarily excreted in urine. Unknown if removed by hemodialysis. **Half-life:** 23 hrs.

AVAILABILITY
Tablets: 5 mg, 10 mg.
Capsules (sustained-release): 10 mg, 15 mg.
Suppository: 2.5 mg, 5 mg, 25 mg.

INDICATIONS AND DOSAGES
▸ **Antiemetic**
PO
Adults, Elderly. 5–10 mg 3–4 times/day.
Children. 0.4 mg/kg/day in 3–4 divided doses.
PO (extended-release)
Adults, Elderly. 10 mg 2 times/day or 15 mg once/day.
Rectal
Adults, Elderly. 25 mg 2 times/day.
Children. 0.4 mg/kg/day in 3–4 divided doses.
▸ **Psychosis**
PO
Adults, Elderly. 5–10 mg 3–4 times/day. Maximum: 150 mg/day.
Children. 2.5 mg 2–3 times/day. Maximum 2–5 yrs: 20 mg. Maximum 6–12 yrs: 25 mg.

CONTRAINDICATIONS
Bone marrow suppression, central nervous system (CNS) depression, coma, narrow-angle glaucoma, severe hypotension or hypertension, severe liver or cardiac impairment.

INTERACTIONS
Drug
Alcohol, CNS depressants: May increase CNS and respiratory depression and hypotensive effects of prochlorperazine.
Antihypertensives: May increase hypotension.
Antithyroid agents: May increase the risk of agranulocytosis.
Extrapyramidal symptoms (EPS)-producing medications: May increase EPS.
Levodopa: May decrease the effects of levodopa.
Lithium: May decrease the absorption of prochlorperazine and produce adverse neurologic effects.
MAOIs, tricyclic antidepressants: May increase the anticholinergic

and sedative effects of prochlorperazine.

Herbal
None known.

Food
None known.

DIAGNOSTIC TEST EFFECTS
None known.

SIDE EFFECTS
Frequent
Drowsiness, hypotension, dizziness, fainting occur frequently after first dose, occasionally after subsequent dosing, and rarely with oral dosage
Occasional
Dry mouth, blurred vision, lethargy, constipation/diarrhea, muscular aches, nasal congestion, peripheral edema, urinary retention

SERIOUS REACTIONS
• Extrapyramidal symptoms appear dose-related, particularly with high dosage, and are divided into three categories: akathisia, marked by the inability to sit still, tapping of feet, urge to move around, parkinsonian symptoms, including masklike face, tremors, shuffling gait, hypersalivation, and acute dystonias, such as torticollis or neck muscle spasm, opisthotonos or rigidity of back muscles, and oculogyric crisis or rolling back of eyes. Dystonic reaction may also produce profuse sweating or pallor.
• Tardive dyskinesia, manifested by protrusion of tongue, puffing of cheeks, and chewing or puckering of the mouth occurs rarely and may be irreversible.
• Abrupt withdrawal after long-term therapy may precipitate nausea, vomiting, gastritis, dizziness, and tremors.
• Blood dyscrasias, particularly agranulocytosis, mild leukopenia,

sore mouth, gums, or throat, may occur.
• Prochlorperazine use may lower seizure threshold.

NURSING CONSIDERATIONS
Baseline Assessment
• Avoid skin contact with prochlorperazine solution because it may cause contact dermatitis.
• Assess the nausea and vomiting patient for signs and symptoms of dehydration including dry mucous membranes, longitudinal furrows in the tongue, and poor skin turgor.
• Assess the psychotic patient's appearance, behavior, emotional status, response to environment, speech pattern, and thought content.

Lifespan Considerations
• Be aware that prochlorperazine crosses the placenta and is distributed in breast milk.
• Be aware that the safety and efficacy of this drug have not been established in children younger than 2 years of age or weighing less than 9 kg.
• The elderly are more susceptible to anticholinergic effects, such as dry mouth, extrapyramidal symptoms (EPS), orthostatic hypotension, and sedative effects, so a lower prochlorperazine dosage is recommended.

Precautions
• Use cautiously in patients with Parkinson's disease and seizures and in patients younger than 2 years of age.

Administration and Handling
PO
• Give prochlorperazine without regard to meals.
Parenteral
• Note that the patient must remain recumbent for 30 to 60 minutes following drug administration, with his or her head in a low position

with legs raised to minimize the drug's hypotensive effect.
Rectal
• Moisten suppository with cold water before inserting well into rectum.
Intervention and Evaluation
• Monitor the patient's B/P for hypotension.
• Assess the patient for extrapyramidal symptoms.
• Monitor the patient's complete blood count (CBC) for blood dyscrasias.
• Evaluate the patient's fine tongue movement because it may be early sign of tardive dyskinesia.
• Closely supervise suicidal-risk patients during early therapy. As depression lessens, be aware that the patient's energy level generally improves, which increases the suicide potential.
• Assess the patient for therapeutic response, improvement in self-care, increased ability to concentrate, interest in surroundings, and a relaxed facial expression.
Patient Teaching
• Urge the patient to avoid alcohol and limit caffeine intake while taking prochlorperazine.
• Advise the patient that prochlorperazine may impair his or her ability to perform tasks requiring mental alertness or physical coordination, such as driving.

scopolamine
sko-**poll**-ah-meen
(Trans-Derm Scop, Transderm-V)

CATEGORY AND SCHEDULE
Pregnancy Risk Category: C

MECHANISM OF ACTION
An anticholinergic that reduces excitability of labyrinthine receptors, depressing conduction in vestibular cerebellar pathway. *Therapeutic Effect:* Prevents nausea or vomiting induced by motion.

AVAILABILITY
Transdermal System: 1.5 mg.

INDICATIONS AND DOSAGES
▸ **Prevention of motion sickness**
Transdermal
Adults. 1 system q72h.

CONTRAINDICATIONS
Gastrointestinal or genitourinary obstruction, myasthenia gravis, narrow-angle glaucoma, paralytic ileus, tachycardia, thyrotoxicosis

INTERACTIONS
Drug
Antihistamines, tricyclic antidepressants: May increase the anticholinergic effects of scopolamine.
Central nervous system (CNS) depressants: May increase CNS depression.
Herbal
None known.
Food
None known.

DIAGNOSTIC TEST EFFECTS
May interfere with gastric secretion test.

SIDE EFFECTS
Frequent (greater than 15%)
Dry mouth, drowsiness, blurred vision
Rare (5%–1%)
Dizziness, restlessness, hallucinations, confusion, difficulty urinating, rash

SERIOUS REACTIONS
• None known.

NURSING CONSIDERATIONS

Baseline Assessment
• Determine if the patient has a history of narrow-angle glaucoma, and plan to use other CNS depressants or drugs with anticholinergic action.

Precautions
• Use cautiously in patients with cardiac disease, liver impairment, psychoses, renal impairment, and seizures.

Administration and Handling
Transdermal
• Apply patch to hairless area behind one ear.
• If dislodged or has been applied over 72 hours, replace with fresh patch.

Intervention and Evaluation
• Monitor the patient's liver and renal function by assessing the patient's BUN, blood serum chemistry test results, and serum alkaline phosphatase, bilirubin, creatinine, SGOT (AST), and SGPT (ALT) levels.

Patient Teaching
• Warn the patient to avoid tasks requiring mental alertness or motor skills until his or her response to the drug is established.
• Instruct the patient in the proper application of the patch. Teach the patient to use only 1 patch at a time and that the patch should not be cut.
• Tell the patient to wash his or her hands after patch administration.

---

trimethobenzamide hydrochloride
try-meth-oh-**benz**-ah-mide
(Tigan)

CATEGORY AND SCHEDULE
Pregnancy Risk Category: C

MECHANISM OF ACTION
An anticholinergic that acts at the chemoreceptor trigger zone in the medulla oblongata in the central nervous system (CNS). *Therapeutic Effect:* Relieves nausea and vomiting.

PHARMACOKINETICS

Route	Onset	Peak	Duration
PO	10–40 min	N/A	3–4 hrs
IM	15–30 min	N/A	2–3 hrs

Partially absorbed from the gastrointestinal (GI) tract. Distributed primarily to liver. Metabolic fate unknown. Excreted in urine. **Half-life:** 7–9 hrs.

AVAILABILITY
Capsules: 100 mg, 250 mg.
Suppositories: 100 mg, 200 mg.
Injection: 100 mg/ml.

INDICATIONS AND DOSAGES
▸ **Control of nausea, vomiting**
PO
Adults, Elderly. 250 mg 3–4 times/day.
Children weighing 30–100 lbs. 100–200 mg 3–4 times/day.
IM
Adults, Elderly. 200 mg 3–4 times/day.
Rectal
Adults, Elderly. 200 mg 3–4 times/day.
Children weighing 30–100 lbs. 100–200 mg 3–4 times/day.
Children weighing less than 30 lbs. 100 mg 3–4 times/day. Do not use in premature or newborn infants.

CONTRAINDICATIONS
Hypersensitivity to benzocaine or similar local anesthetics; parenteral form in children, supposito-

ries in premature infants or
neonates

INTERACTIONS
Drug
*Central nervous system (CNS)
depression–producing medications:*
May increase CNS depression.
Herbal
None known.
Food
None known.

DIAGNOSTIC TEST EFFECTS
None known.

SIDE EFFECTS
Frequent
Drowsiness
Occasional
Blurred vision, diarrhea, dizziness,
headache, muscle cramps
Rare
Skin rash, seizures, depression,
opisthotonus, Parkinson's syndrome,
Reye's syndrome, marked by vomit-
ing, seizures

SERIOUS REACTIONS
• Hypersensitivity reaction manifested as extrapyramidal symptoms,
including muscle rigidity, and allergic skin reactions occurs rarely.
• Children may experience dominant paradoxical reaction, marked
by restlessness, insomnia, euphoria,
nervousness, or tremors.
• Overdosage may vary from CNS
depression, manifested by sedation,
apnea, cardiovascular collapse,
death to severe paradoxical reaction,
characterized by hallucinations,
tremor, and seizures.

NURSING CONSIDERATIONS
Baseline Assessment
• Assess the patient for signs and
symptoms of dehydration, including

dry mucous membranes, longitudinal furrows in the tongue, and poor
skin turgor, if he or she experiences
excessive vomiting.
Lifespan Considerations
• Be aware that it is unknown if
trimethobenzamide crosses the
placenta or is distributed in breast
milk.
• There are no age-related precautions noted in children or the elderly.
• Avoid the parenteral form in
children and suppositories in neonates.
Precautions
• Use cautiously in patients with
dehydration, electrolyte imbalance,
or high fever.
• Use cautiously in debilitated or
elderly patients.
Administration and Handling
◀ALERT▶ Know that elderly patients
older than 60 years of age tend to
develop agitation, disorientation,
mental confusion, and psychotic-
like symptoms.
◀ALERT▶ Do not use IV route because it produces severe hypotension.
PO
• Give trimethobenzamide without
regard to meals.
• Do not crush, open, or break
capsule form.
IM
• Give deep IM into large muscle
mass, preferably upper outer gluteus
maximus.
Rectal
• If suppository is too soft, chill for
30 minutes in the refrigerator or run
cold water over foil wrapper.
• Moisten suppository with cold
water before inserting well into
rectum.
Intervention and Evaluation
• Monitor the patient's blood pressure (B/P), especially in elderly

patients who are at an increased risk of hypotension.
• Assess pediatric patients closely for signs of a paradoxical reaction.
• Monitor serum electrolytes in patients with severe vomiting.
• Measure the patient's intake and output; assess any emesis.
• Assess the patient's mucous membranes and skin turgor to evaluate hydration status.
• Observe the patient for extrapyramidal symptoms, such as hypersensitivity.

Patient Teaching
• Tell the patient that trimethobenzamide use causes drowsiness. Warn the patient to avoid tasks requiring mental alertness or physical coordination.

• Warn the patient to notify the physician if he or she experiences headache or visual disturbances.
• Instruct the patient that dry mouth is an expected response to the medication. Suggest to the patient that taking sips of tepid water or chewing sugarless gum to the patient may relieve dry mouth.
• Teach the patient other methods of reducing nausea and vomiting, including lying quietly and avoiding strong odors.
• Tell the patient that relief from nausea or vomiting generally occurs within 30 minutes of drug administration.

almotriptan malate
dihydroergotamine
eletriptan
ergotamine tartrate
frovatriptan
naratriptan
rizatriptan benzoate
sumatriptan
zolmitriptan

Uses: Antimigraine agents are used to treat migraine headaches with aura (also called classic migraine) or without aura (also called common migraine) in patients age 18 or older. The goal of treatment includes the relief of headache and accompanying symptoms and a return to baseline functioning. Antimigraine agents are commonly used with non-drug measures, such as lifestyle modification and avoidance of headache triggers.

Action: Two groups of antimigraine agents work by different mechanisms. *Triptans,* such as sumatriptan and zolmitriptan, selectively stimulate serotonin (5-HT) receptors that inhibit neuropeptide release and vasodilation. As a result, cerebral inflammation is reduced and blood vessels constrict. Both actions are believed to reduce the pain associated with vascular headaches. *Ergot alkaloids,* such as ergotamine and dihydroergotamine, interact with neurotransmitter receptors, including serotonergic, dopaminergic, and alpha-adrenergic receptors. More specifically, they may stimulate specific subtypes of serotonin receptors. However, their exact mechanism of action is unknown.

COMBINATION PRODUCTS
BELLERGAL-S: ergotamine/belladonna (an anticholinergic)/phenobarbital (a sedative-hypnotic) 0.6 mg/0.2 mg/40 mg.

almotriptan malate
ale-moe-**trip-tan**
(Axert)

CATEGORY AND SCHEDULE
Pregnancy Risk Category: C

MECHANISM OF ACTION
A serotonin receptor agonist that binds selectively to vascular receptors, producing a vasoconstrictive effect on cranial blood vessels. *Therapeutic Effect:* Produces relief of migraine headache.

PHARMACOKINETICS
Well absorbed following PO administration. Metabolized by the liver, excreted in urine.

AVAILABILITY
Tablets: 6.5 mg, 12.5 mg.

INDICATIONS AND DOSAGES
▶ **Migraine headache**
PO
Adults, Elderly. 6.25–12.5 mg. If headache returns, dose may be

repeated after 2 hrs. Maximum: No more than 2 doses within 24 hrs.

▸ **Dosage in renal impairment**

PO

Adults, Elderly. Initially, 6.25 mg. Maximum daily dose of 12.5 mg.

CONTRAINDICATIONS

Arrhythmias associated with cardiac conduction pathways disorders, concurrent use—or within 24 hrs of ergotamine-containing preparations, concurrent use—or within 2 wks—of MAO therapy, coronary artery disease, hemiplegic or basilar migraine—within 24 hrs of another serotonin receptor agonist, ischemic heart disease, including angina pectoris, history of myocardial infarction (MI), and silent ischemia, Prinzmetal's angina, uncontrolled hypertension, Wolff-Parkinson-White syndrome

INTERACTIONS
Drug

Ergotamine-containing drugs: May produce vasospastic reaction.
Erythromycin, itraconazole, ketoconazole, ritonavir: Avoid taking erythromycin, itraconazole, ketoconazole, and ritonavir during the last 7 days of almotriptan therapy.
Fluoxetine, fluvoxamine, paroxetine, sertraline: Combined use may produce weakness, hyperreflexia, incoordination.
MAOIs: May increase almotriptan blood concentration.

Herbal
None known.

Food
None known.

DIAGNOSTIC TEST EFFECTS
None known.

SIDE EFFECTS
Frequent

Nausea, dry mouth, paresthesia, flushing
Occasional
Sensation of warm or hot, weakness, dizziness

SERIOUS REACTIONS

• Excessive dosage may produce tremor, redness of extremities, reduced respirations, cyanosis, seizures, and chest pain.
• Serious arrhythmias occur rarely, but particularly in patients with hypertension, obesity, smokers, diabetics, and those with strong family history of coronary artery disease.

NURSING CONSIDERATIONS

Baseline Assessment
• Determine the patient's history of peripheral vascular disease.
• Determine the onset, location, and duration of migraine and possible precipitating symptoms.

Lifespan Considerations
• Be aware that it is unknown if almotriptan is distributed in breast milk.
• Be aware that the safety and efficacy of almotriptan have not been established in children younger than 12 years.
• There are no age-related precautions noted in the elderly.

Precautions
• Use cautiously in patients with controlled hypertension, history of cerebrovascular accident (CVA), mild to moderate liver or renal impairment, and a profile suggesting cardiovascular risks.

Administration and Handling
PO
• Swallow tablets whole.
• Give with a full glass of water.

Intervention and Evaluation
• Evaluate the patient for relief of migraine headache and resulting

nausea, phonophobia or sound sensitivity, photophobia or light sensitivity, and vomiting.

Patient Teaching

• Instruct the patient to take a single dose of almotriptan as soon as symptoms of a migraine appear.

• Explain to the patient that this medication is intended to relieve migraine, not to prevent or reduce the number of attacks.

• Teach the patient to lie down in a quiet, dark room for additional benefit after taking this medication.

• Warn the patient to avoid tasks that require mental alertness or motor skills until his or her response to the drug is established.

• Warn the patient to notify the physician immediately if he or she experiences palpitations, pain or tightness in chest or throat, or pain or weakness of the extremities.

---

dihydroergotamine
(Migranal)
See ergotamine.

---

eletriptan
el-eh-**trip**-tan
(Relpax)

CATEGORY AND SCHEDULE
Pregnancy Risk Category: C

MECHANISM OF ACTION
A serotonin receptor agonist that binds selectively to vascular receptors producing a vasoconstrictive effect on cranial blood vessels. *Therapeutic Effect:* Produces relief of migraine headache.

PHARMACOKINETICS
Well absorbed following oral administration. Metabolized by the liver to inactive metabolite. Eliminated in urine. **Half-life:** 4.4 hrs, half-life is increased in patients with liver impairment and who are older than 65 yrs.

AVAILABILITY
Tablets: 20 mg, 40 mg.

INDICATIONS AND DOSAGES
▶ **Treatment of acute migraine headache**
PO
Adults, Elderly. 20–40 mg. If headache improves but then returns, a repeat dose may be given at least 2 hrs after the initial dose. Maximum daily dose: 80 mg.

CONTRAINDICATIONS
Arrhythmias associated with cardiac conduction pathways, coronary artery disease, ischemic heart disease, severe liver impairment, uncontrolled hypertension

INTERACTIONS
Drug
Clarithromycin, itraconazole, ketoconazole, nefazodone, nelfinavir, ritonavir: Avoid taking these drugs within 72 hrs prior to beginning eletriptan therapy.
Ergotamine containing drugs: May produce vasospastic reaction.
Sibutramine: Concurrent use with this drug may produce "serotonin syndrome," marked by altered consciousness, central nervous system (CNS) irritability, motor weakness, myoclonus, and shivering.
Herbal
None known.
Food
None known.

DIAGNOSTIC TEST EFFECTS
None known.

SIDE EFFECTS
Occasional (6%–5%)
Dizziness, somnolence, asthenia or loss of strength and energy, nausea
Rare (3%–2%)
Paresthesia, headache, dry mouth, warm or hot temperature sensation, dyspepsia or heartburn and epigastric distress, dysphagia, including throat tightness, difficulty swallowing

SERIOUS REACTIONS
• Cardiac ischemia, coronary artery vasospasm, myocardial infarction (MI), noncardiac vasospasm-related reactions, such as hemorrhage or stroke, occur rarely but particularly in patients with hypertension, obesity, diabetes, strong family history of coronary artery disease, smokers, males older than 40 years of age, and postmenopausal women.

NURSING CONSIDERATIONS

Baseline Assessment
• Determine the duration, location, onset, and precipitating symptoms of the patient's migraine.
• Obtain the patient's baseline blood pressure (B/P) for evidence of uncontrolled hypertension, as this is a contraindication.

Lifespan Considerations
• Be aware that eletriptan may decrease the possibility of ovulation.
• Be aware that eletriptan is distributed in breast milk.
• Be aware that the safety and efficacy of eletriptan have not been established in patients younger than 18 years of age.
• Be aware that in the elderly patients older than 65 years of age, there is an increased risk of hypertension.

Precautions
• Use cautiously in patients with controlled hypertension, history of cerebrovascular accident, and mild to moderate liver or renal impairment.

Administration and Handling
PO
• Do not crush or break film-coated tablets.

Intervention and Evaluation
• Assess the patient for relief of migraine headache and potential for nausea, phonophobia or sound sensitivity, photophobia or light sensitivity, and vomiting.

Patient Teaching
• Instruct the patient to take a single dose of eletriptan as soon as symptoms of a migraine appear.
• Explain to the patient that eletriptan is intended to relieve migraine headaches, not to prevent or reduce the number of attacks.
• Warn the patient to avoid tasks that require mental alertness or motor skills until his or her response to the drug is established.
• Warn the patient to notify the physician immediately if he or she experiences heart throbbing, pain or tightness in chest or throat, pain or weakness of extremities occurs, or sudden or severe abdominal pain.
• Warn female patient who anticipate pregnancy that the drug may suppress ovulation.
• Teach the patient to lie down in dark, quiet room for additional benefit after taking the drug.

ergotamine tartrate
er-got-a-meen
(Ergodryl Mono[AUS], Ergomar
Medihaler Ergotamine[CAN])

dihydroergotamine
(D.H.E., Dihydergot[AUS],
Ergomar[CAN], Migranal)

CATEGORY AND SCHEDULE
Pregnancy Risk Category: X

MECHANISM OF ACTION
An ergotamine derivative, alpha-
adrenergic blocker that directly
stimulates vascular smooth muscle.
May also have antagonist effects on
serotonin. *Therapeutic Effect:* Peripheral and cerebral vasoconstriction.

PHARMACOKINETICS
Slow, incomplete absorption from
the gastrointestinal (GI) tract; rapid,
extensive absorption rectally. Protein binding: greater than 90%.
Undergoes extensive first-pass
metabolism in liver. Metabolized to
active metabolite. Eliminated in
feces via biliary system. **Half-life:**
21 hrs.

AVAILABILITY
Tablets (sublingual): 2 mg.
Injection: 1 mg/ml.
Nasal Spray: 0.5 mg/spray.
Suppository: 2 mg, with 100 mg
caffeine.

INDICATIONS AND DOSAGES
▶ **Vascular headaches (ergotamine)**
PO
Adults, Elderly. 2 mg at onset of
headache, then 1–2 mg q30min.
Maximum: 6 mg/episode; 10 mg/
wk. (Cafergot)
Sublingual
Adults, Elderly. 1 tablet at onset of
headache, then 1 tablet q30min.
Maximum: 3 tablets/24 hrs; 5 tabs/
wk. (Ergomar)
PO/sublingual
Children. 1 mg at onset of head-
ache, then 1 mg q30min. Maximum:
3 mg/episode.
Rectal
Adults, Elderly. 1 suppository at
onset of headache, then second dose
in 1 hr. Maximum: 2/episode; 5/wk.
IM/Subcutaneous (dihydroergotamine)
Adults, Elderly. 1 mg at onset of
headache; repeat hourly. Maximum:
3 mg/day; 6 mg/wk.
IV
Adults, Elderly. 1 mg at onset of
headache; repeat hourly. Maximum:
2 mg/day; 6 mg/wk.
Intranasal
Adults, Elderly. 1 spray (0.5 mg) into
each nostril; repeat in 15 min. Maximum: 4 sprays/day; 8 sprays/wk.

CONTRAINDICATIONS
Coronary artery disease, hypertension, impaired liver or renal function, malnutrition, peripheral vascular diseases, such as thromboangiitis
obliterans, syphilitic arteritis, severe
arteriosclerosis, thrombophlebitis,
Raynaud's disease, sepsis, severe
pruritus

INTERACTIONS
Drug
Beta-blockers, erythromycin: May
increase the risk of vasospasm.
*Ergot alkaloids, systemic
vasoconstrictors:* May increase
pressor effect.
Nitroglycerin: May decrease the
effect of nitroglycerin.
Herbal
None known.
Food
None known.

DIAGNOSTIC TEST EFFECTS
None known.

SIDE EFFECTS
Occasional (5%–2%)
Cough, dizziness
Rare (less than 2%)
Muscle pain, fatigue, diarrhea, upper respiratory infection, dyspepsia

SERIOUS REACTIONS
• Prolonged administration or excessive dosage may produce ergotamine poisoning manifested as nausea, vomiting, weakness of legs, pain in limb muscles, numbness and tingling of fingers or toes, precordial pain, tachycardia or bradycardia, and hypertension or hypotension.
• Localized edema and itching due to vasoconstriction of peripheral arteries and arterioles may occur.
• Feet or hands will become cold, pale, and numb.
• Muscle pain will occur when walking and later, even at rest.
• Gangrene may occur.
• Occasionally confusion, depression, drowsiness, and seizures appear.

NURSING CONSIDERATIONS

Baseline Assessment
• Determine the patient's history of peripheral vascular disease and liver or renal impairment.
• Carefully perform an assessment of the patient's peripheral circulation, including the temperature, color, and strength of pulses in the extremities.
• Determine if the patient is pregnant.
• Determine the duration, location, onset, and precipitating symptoms of the patient's migraine.

Lifespan Considerations
• Be aware that ergotamine use is contraindicated in pregnancy as it produces uterine stimulant action resulting in possible fetal death or retarded fetal growth and increases vasoconstriction of placental vascular bed.
• Be aware that ergotamine is distributed in breast milk and may prohibit lactation.
• Be aware that ergotamine use may produce diarrhea or vomiting in the neonate.
• Keep in mind that ergotamine may be used safely in children older than 6 years, but only use when the patient is unresponsive to other medication.
• In the elderly, age-related occlusive peripheral vascular disease increases risk of peripheral vasoconstriction.
• In the elderly, age-related renal impairment may require caution.

Administration and Handling
Sublingual
• Place under tongue and allow the tablet to dissolve, then swallow. Do not administer with water.

Intervention and Evaluation
• Monitor the patient closely for evidence of ergotamine overdosage as result of prolonged administration or excessive dosage.

Patient Teaching
• Instruct the patient to begin taking ergotamine at the first sign of a migraine headache.
• Tell the patient to notify the physician if the ergotamine dosage does not relieve vascular headaches, or if he or she experiences irregular heartbeat, nausea, numbness or tingling of the fingers and toes, pain or weakness of the extremities, and vomiting.
• Warn the patient to avoid pregnancy and to report any suspected

pregnancy immediately to the physician. Explain to the patient that this drug is contraindicated in pregnancy X. Teach the patient about other methods of contraception.

frovatriptan
fro-vah-**trip**-tan
(Frovan)

CATEGORY AND SCHEDULE
Pregnancy Risk Category: C

MECHANISM OF ACTION
A serotonin receptor agonist that binds selectively to vascular receptors, producing a vasoconstrictive effect on cranial blood vessels. *Therapeutic Effect:* Produces relief of migraine headache.

PHARMACOKINETICS
Well absorbed after PO administration. Metabolized by the liver to inactive metabolite. Eliminated in urine. **Half-life:** 26 hrs, half-life is increased in liver impairment.

AVAILABILITY
Tablets: 2.5 mg.

INDICATIONS AND DOSAGES
▸ **Treatment of acute migraine attack**
PO
Adults, Elderly. Initially 2.5 mg. Second dose may be given if headache recurs, provided first dose gave some relief, but not sooner than 2 hrs from the first dose. Maximum: 7.5 mg/day.

CONTRAINDICATIONS
Cerebrovascular or peripheral vascular syndromes, concurrent use—or within 24 hrs—of ergotamine-containing preparations, concurrent—or within 2 wks—of MAO therapy, coronary artery disease, hemiplegic or basilar migraine, ischemic heart disease, such as angina pectoris, history of myocardial infarction (MI), or silent ischemia, Prinzmetal's angina, severe hepatic impairment (Child-Pugh grade C), uncontrolled hypertension, within 24 hrs of another serotonin receptor agonist

INTERACTIONS
Drug
Ergotamine-containing drugs: May produce vasospastic reaction.
Fluoxetine, fluvoxamine, paroxetine, sertraline: Combined use of these drugs may produce hyperreflexia, incoordination, and weakness.
Oral contraceptives: Reduce frovatriptan clearance and volume of distribution.
Propranolol: May dramatically increase frovatriptan plasma concentration.
Herbal
None known.
Food
None known.

DIAGNOSTIC TEST EFFECTS
None known.

SIDE EFFECTS
Occasional (8%–4%)
Dizziness, paresthesia, fatigue, flushing
Rare (3%–2%)
Hot or cold sensation, dry mouth, dyspepsia, such as heartburn and epigastric distress

SERIOUS REACTIONS
• Cardiac events, including ischemia, coronary artery vasospasm, or MI, and noncardiac vasospasm-related reactions, such as hemorrhage, stroke, occur rarely but

particularly in those with hypertension, obesity, smokers, diabetics, those with strong family history of coronary artery disease, males older than 40 years, and postmenopausal women.

NURSING CONSIDERATIONS

Baseline Assessment
• Determine if the patient has a history of liver or renal impairment or peripheral vascular disease.
• Determine if the patient is pregnant or planning to become pregnant.
• Determine the duration, location, onset, and possible precipitating symptoms of the patient's migraine.

Lifespan Considerations
• Be aware that it is unknown if frovatriptan is excreted in breast milk.
• Be aware that the safety and efficacy have not been established in children.
• Be aware that frovatriptan use is not recommended in the elderly.

Precautions
• Use cautiously in patients with mild to moderate hepatic impairment and a patient profile suggesting cardiovascular risks.

Administration and Handling
PO
• Do not crush or chew film-coated tablets.

Intervention and Evaluation
• Assess the patient for relief of migraine headache and potential for nausea, phonophobia or sound sensitivity, photophobia or light sensitivity, and vomiting.

Patient Teaching
• Instruct the patient to take a single frovatriptan dose as soon as symptoms of a migraine appear. Explain that a second dose may be given if headache recurs, provided the first dose gave some relief, but no sooner than 2 hrs from the first dose.
• Explain to the patient that frovatriptan is intended to relieve migraine headaches, not to prevent or reduce the number of attacks.
• Tell the patient to avoid tasks that require mental alertness or motor skills until his or her response to the drug is established.
• Warn the patient to notify the physician immediately if he or she experiences palpitations, pain or weakness of the extremities, pain or tightness in chest or throat, or sudden or severe abdominal pain.
• Urge females of child-bearing years to use contraceptives, and to inform the physician if she suspects she is pregnant.
• Teach the patient to lie down in dark, quiet room for additional benefit after taking the drug.

naratriptan
nar-ah-**trip**-tan
(Amerge, Naramig[AUS])
Do not confuse with Amaryl.

CATEGORY AND SCHEDULE
Pregnancy Risk Category: C

MECHANISM OF ACTION
A serotonin receptor agonist that binds selectively to vascular receptors producing a vasoconstrictive effect on cranial blood vessels. *Therapeutic Effect:* Produces relief of migraine headache.

PHARMACOKINETICS
Well absorbed after PO administration. Protein binding: 28%–31%. Metabolized by the liver to inactive metabolite. Eliminated primarily in the urine with lesser amount ex-

creted in the feces. **Half-life:** 6 hrs (half-life is increased in liver or renal impairment).

AVAILABILITY
Tablets: 1 mg, 2.5 mg.

INDICATIONS AND DOSAGES
▸ **Treatment of acute migraine attack**
PO
Adults. Give 1 mg or 2.5 mg. If headache returns or pt received only a partial response to initial dose, may repeat dose once after 4 hrs. Maximum: 5 mg per 24-hr period.
▸ **Mild to moderate liver or renal impairment**
PO
Adults. Consider with low starting dosage. Do not exceed 2.5 mg over a 24-hr period.

CONTRAINDICATIONS
Basilar or hemiplegic migraine, cerebrovascular or peripheral vascular syndromes, concurrent use or within 24 hrs of ergotamine-containing preparations, concurrent use or within 2 wks of MAO therapy, coronary artery disease, ischemic heart disease, including angina pectoris, history of myocardial infarction (MI), or silent ischemia, Prinzmetal's angina, severe renal impairment with creatinine clearance less than 15 ml/min, severe liver impairment—Child-Pugh grade C, uncontrolled hypertension, within 24 hrs of another serotonin receptor agonist

INTERACTIONS
Drug
Ergotamine-containing drugs: May produce vasospastic reaction.
Fluoxetine, fluvoxamine, paroxetine, sertraline: May produce hyperre-

flexia, incoordination, and weakness.
Oral contraceptives: Reduce naratriptan's clearance and volume of distribution.
Herbal
None known.
Food
None known.

DIAGNOSTIC TEST EFFECTS
None known.

SIDE EFFECTS
Occasional (5%)
Nausea
Rare (2%)
Paresthesia, dizziness, fatigue, drowsiness, jaw, neck, or throat pressure

SERIOUS REACTIONS
• May produce corneal opacities and defects.
• Cardiac events, including ischemia, coronary artery vasospasm, and MI, and noncardiac vasospasm-related reactions, such as hemorrhage, and stroke, occur rarely but particularly in those with hypertension, obesity, smokers, diabetics, strong family history of coronary artery disease, males older than 40 years, and postmenopausal women.

NURSING CONSIDERATIONS
Baseline Assessment
• Determine the patient's history of liver or renal impairment and peripheral vascular disease.
• Determine if the patient is pregnant.
• Determine the duration, location, onset, and possible precipitating symptoms of the patient's migraine.
Lifespan Considerations
• Be aware that it is unknown if

naratriptan is excreted in human breast milk.
• Be aware that the safety and efficacy of naratriptan have not been established in children.
• Be aware that naratriptan is not recommended in the elderly.

Precautions
• Use cautiously in patients with mild to moderate liver or renal impairment and a patient profile suggesting cardiovascular risks.

Administration and Handling
PO
• Give naratriptan without regard to food.

Intervention and Evaluation
• Assess the patient for relief of migraine headache and potential for nausea, phonophobia or sound sensitivity, photophobia or light sensitivity, and vomiting.

Patient Teaching
• Teach the patient not to crush or chew tablets and to swallow tablets whole with water.
• Instruct the patient that he or she may repeat naratriptan dose after 4 hours for a maximum of 5 mg/24 hours.
• Advise the patient that naratriptan use may cause dizziness, drowsiness, or fatigue.
• Warn the patient to use caution when performing tasks that require mental alertness or motor skills.
• Warn the patient to notify the physician if he or she experiences anxiety, any chest pain, hallucinations, heart throbbing, panic, rash, or tightness in throat.
• Instruct female patients of child bearing age to use contraception, and to notify the physician immediately if she suspects she is pregnant.
• Teach the patient to lie down in dark, quiet room for additional benefit after taking the drug.

rizatriptan benzoate
rise-ah-**trip**-tan
(Maxalt, Maxalt-MLT)

CATEGORY AND SCHEDULE
Pregnancy Risk Category: C

MECHANISM OF ACTION
A serotonin receptor agonist that binds selectively to vascular receptors, producing a vasoconstrictive effect on cranial blood vessels. *Therapeutic Effect:* Produces relief of migraine headache.

PHARMACOKINETICS
Well absorbed after PO administration. Protein binding: 14%. Crosses blood-brain barrier. Metabolized by the liver to inactive metabolite. Eliminated primarily in urine with lesser amount excreted in feces. **Half-life:** 2–3 hrs.

AVAILABILITY
Tablets: 5 mg, 10 mg.
Oral Disintegrating Tablets: 5 mg, 10 mg.

INDICATIONS AND DOSAGES
▸ **Treatment of acute migraine attack**
PO
Adults older than 18 yrs, Elderly. 5–10 mg. Separate doses by at least 2 hrs. Maximum: 30 mg/24 hrs.

CONTRAINDICATIONS
Basilar or hemiplegic migraine, concurrent use or within 24 hrs of ergotamine-containing preparations, concurrent use or within 2 wks of MAO therapy, coronary artery disease, ischemic heart disease, including angina pectoris, history of myocardial infarction (MI), and

silent ischemia, Prinzmetal's angina, uncontrolled hypertension, within 24 hrs of another serotonin receptor agonist

INTERACTIONS
Drug
Ergotamine-containing drugs: May produce vasospastic reaction.
Fluoxetine, fluvoxamine, paroxetine, sertraline: Combined use of these drugs may produce hyperreflexia, incoordination, and weakness.
MAOIs, propranolol: May dramatically increase plasma concentration of rizatriptan.
Herbal
None known.
Food
Food: Delays peak drug concentrations by 1 hr.

DIAGNOSTIC TEST EFFECTS
None known.

SIDE EFFECTS
Frequent (9%–7%)
Dizziness, somnolence, tingling in extremities, fatigue
Occasional (6%–3%)
Nausea, paresthesia, sensation of chest pressure, dry mouth
Rare (2%)
Headache, neck, throat, or jaw pressure, photosensitivity

SERIOUS REACTIONS
• Cardiac events, such as ischemia, coronary artery vasospasm, and MI, and noncardiac vasospasm-related reactions, including hemorrhage, and stroke, occur rarely but particularly in those with hypertension, obesity, smokers, diabetes, strong family history of coronary artery disease, males older than 40 yrs, and postmenopausal women.

NURSING CONSIDERATIONS
Baseline Assessment
• Determine the patient's history of liver or renal impairment and peripheral vascular disease.
• Plan to perform liver and renal function tests. Assess blood serum values of alkaline phosphatase, bilirubin, BUN, creatinine, SGOT (AST), and SGPT (ALT) levels.
• Determine the duration, location, onset, and possible precipitating symptoms of the patient's migraine.
• Obtain a baseline EKG.
Lifespan Considerations
• Be aware that it is unknown if rizatriptan is distributed in breast milk.
• Be aware that the safety and efficacy of rizatriptan have not been established in children.
• There are no age-related precautions noted in the elderly.
Precautions
• Use cautiously in patients with mild to moderate liver or renal impairment and a patient profile suggesting cardiovascular risks.
Administration and Handling
PO
• Know that oral disintegrating tablet is packaged in an individual aluminum pouch.
• Open packet with dry hands and place tablet on tongue. Allow tablet to dissolve, and then swallow. Don't administer with water.
Intervention and Evaluation
• Monitor the patient for dizziness.
• Assess the patient for relief of migraine headache and potential for nausea, phonophobia or sound sensitivity, photophobia or light sensitivity, and vomiting.
Patient Teaching
• Instruct the patient to take a single rizatriptan dose as soon as symptoms of a migraine appear.

• Explain to the patient that rizatriptan is intended to relieve migraine, not to prevent or reduce the number of attacks.
• Tell the patient to avoid tasks that require mental alertness or motor skills until his or her response to the drug is established.
• Warn the patient to notify the physician immediately if he or she experiences heart palpitations, pain or tightness in chest or throat, or pain or weakness of extremities.
• Teach the patient not to remove the orally disintegrating tablet from the blister package until just before he or she intends to take it.
• Instruct the patient to use protective measures against exposure to sunlight and ultraviolet rays, such as sunscreen and protective clothing.
• Urge the patient not to smoke tobacco.
• Teach the patient to lie down in dark, quiet room for additional benefit after taking the drug.

sumatriptan

sue-mah-**trip**-tan
(Imitrex, Suvalan[AUS])
Do not confuse with somatropin.

CATEGORY AND SCHEDULE
Pregnancy Risk Category: C

MECHANISM OF ACTION
A serotonin receptor agonist that binds selectively to serotonin (5-HT_1) receptor in cranial arteries. *Therapeutic Effect:* Causes vasoconstriction, reduces inflammation, relieves migraine.

PHARMACOKINETICS

Route	Onset	Peak	Duration
Subcuta-neous	less than 10 min	less than 2 hrs	N/A
PO	1–1.5 hrs	2–4 hrs	N/A

Rapidly absorbed after subcutaneous administration. Widely distributed, protein binding: 10%–21% undergoes first-pass hepatic metabolism; excreted in urine. **Half-life:** 2 hrs.

AVAILABILITY
Tablets: 25 mg, 50 mg, 100 mg.
Injection: 6 mg/0.5 ml.
Nasal Spray: 5 mg, 20 mg.

INDICATIONS AND DOSAGES
▸ **Vascular headache**
Subcutaneous
Adults, Elderly. 6 mg. Maximum: No more than two 6-mg injections within a 24-hr period separated by at least 1 hr between injections.
PO
Adults, Elderly. 25–50 mg. Maximum single dose: 100 mg. May repeat no sooner than 2 hrs. Maximum: 200 mg/24 hrs.
Nasal
Adults, Elderly. 5–20 mg; may repeat in 2 hrs. Maximum: 40 mg/24 hrs.

CONTRAINDICATIONS
Concomitant use of ergotamine medications, MAOIs, or vasoconstrictive medications within 14 days, ischemic heart disease, Prinzmetal angina, severe liver impairment, stroke, transischemic attack (TIA), uncontrolled hypertension

INTERACTIONS
Drug
Ergotamine-containing drugs: May produce vasospastic reaction.
MAOIs: May increase sumatriptan blood concentration and half-life.
Herbal
None known.
Food
None known.

DIAGNOSTIC TEST EFFECTS
None known.

SIDE EFFECTS
Frequent
Oral (10%–5%): Tingling, nasal discomfort
Subcutaneous (greater than 10%): Injection site reactions, tingling, warm or hot sensation, dizziness, vertigo
Nasal (greater than 10%): Bad or unusual taste, nausea, vomiting
Occasional
Oral (5%–1%): Flushing, weakness, visual disturbances
Subcutaneous (10%–2%): Burning sensation, numbness, chest discomfort, drowsiness, weakness
Nasal (5%–1%): Discomfort of nasal cavity or throat, dizziness
Rare
Oral (less than 1%): Agitation, eye irritation, dysuria
Subcutaneous (less than 2%): Anxiety, fatigue, sweating, muscle cramps, muscle pain
Nasal (less than 1%): Burning sensation

SERIOUS REACTIONS
• Excessive dosage may produce tremor, redness of extremities, reduced respirations, cyanosis, convulsions, and paralysis.
• Serious arrhythmias occur rarely, but more frequently in those with hypertension, obesity, smokers, diabetics, and those with strong family history of coronary artery disease.

NURSING CONSIDERATIONS
Baseline Assessment
• Determine the patient's history of liver or renal impairment and peripheral vascular disease.
• Determine if the patient is pregnant or planning to become pregnant.
• Determine the duration, location, onset, and possible precipitating symptoms of the patient's migraine.
• Obtain a baseline EKG.
Lifespan Considerations
• Be aware that it is unknown if sumatriptan is distributed in breast milk.
• Be aware that the safety and efficacy of sumatriptan have not been established in children.
• There are no age-related precautions noted in the elderly.
Precautions
• Use cautiously in patients with epilepsy, hypersensitivity to sulfonamides and liver or renal impairment.
Administration and Handling
PO
• Swallow tablets whole with a full glass of water.
Nasal
• A unit contains only one spray—do not test before use.
• Gently blow nose to clear nasal passages.
• With head upright, close one nostril with index finger. Breathe out gently through mouth.
• Insert nozzle into open nostril about one half an inch. Do not press blue plunger yet.
• Close mouth, and while taking a breath through nose, release spray dosage by firmly pressing the blue plunger.

• Remove nozzle from nose and gently breathe in through nose and out through mouth for 10 to 20 seconds. Do not breathe in deeply.
Subcutaneous
• Follow instructions provided by manufacturer using autoinjection device.

Intervention and Evaluation
• Evaluate the patient for relief of migraine headache and resulting nausea, phonophobia or sound sensitivity, photophobia, and vomiting.

Patient Teaching
• Teach the patient how to properly load the autoinjector, inject the medication, and discard the syringe.
• Instruct the patient to inject the drug into an area with adequate subcutaneous tissue, because the needle will penetrate the skin and adipose tissue as deeply as 6 mm.
• Tell the patient not to use more than 2 subcutaneous injections during any 24-hour period and allow at least 1 hour between injections.
• Warn the patient to notify the physician immediately if he or she experiences palpitations, pain or tightness in the chest or throat, skin rash, swelling of the eyelids, face, lips, and wheezing.
• Teach the patient to lie down in dark, quiet room for additional benefit after taking the drug.

zolmitriptan
zoll-mih-**trip**-tan
(Zomig, Zomig-ZMT)

CATEGORY AND SCHEDULE
Pregnancy Risk Category: C

MECHANISM OF ACTION
A serotonin receptor agonist that binds selectively to vascular receptors, producing a vasoconstrictive effect on cranial blood vessels.
Therapeutic Effect: Produces relief of migraine headache.

PHARMACOKINETICS
Rapidly but incompletely absorbed after PO administration. Protein binding: 15%. Undergoes first-pass metabolism in the liver to active metabolite. Eliminated primarily in the urine (60%), with lesser amount excreted in the feces (30%). **Half-life:** 3 hrs.

AVAILABILITY
Tablets: 2.5 mg, 5 mg.
Oral Disintegrating Tablets: 2.5 mg, 5 mg.

INDICATIONS AND DOSAGES
▸ **Acute migraine attack**
PO
Adults, Elderly, Children older than 18 yrs. Initially, 2.5 mg or less. If headache returns, may repeat dose in 2 hrs. Maximum: 10 mg/24 hrs.
Nasal
Adults, Elderly. 5 mg. May repeat in 2 hrs.

CONTRAINDICATIONS
Arrhythmias associated with cardiac conduction pathways disorders, basilar or hemiplegic migraine, concurrent use or within 24 hrs of ergotamine-containing preparations, concurrent use or within 2 wks of MAOIs, coronary artery disease, ischemic heart disease, including angina pectoris, history of myocardial infarction (MI), and silent ischemia, Prinzmetal's angina, uncontrolled hypertension, within 24 hrs of another serotonin receptor

agonist, Wolff-Parkinson-White syndrome

INTERACTIONS
Drug
Ergotamine-containing drugs: May produce vasospastic reaction.
Fluoxetine, fluvoxamine, paroxetine, sertraline: May produce hyperreflexia, incoordination, and weakness.
MAOIs: May dramatically increase plasma concentration of zolmitriptan.
Oral contraceptives: Reduce zolmitriptan's clearance and volume of distribution.
Herbal
None known.
Food
None known.

DIAGNOSTIC TEST EFFECTS
None known.

SIDE EFFECTS
Frequent (8%–6%)
Dizziness, tingling, neck, throat, or jaw pressure, somnolence
Nasal: unusual taste, paresthesia
Occasional (5%–3%)
Sensation of warm or hot, weakness, chest pressure
Nasal: nausea, somnolence, discomfort of the nasal cavity, dizziness, asthenia, dry mouth
Rare (2%–1%)
Diaphoresis, myalgia, paresthesia

SERIOUS REACTIONS
• Cardiac events, including ischemia, coronary artery vasospasm, and MI, and noncardiac vasospasm-related reactions, such as hemorrhage and stroke, occur rarely but particularly in those with hypertension, obesity, smokers, diabetes, strong family history of coronary artery disease, males older than 40 yrs, and postmenopausal women.

NURSING CONSIDERATIONS
Baseline Assessment
• Determine if the patient has a history of liver or renal impairment, MAOI use, and peripheral coronary artery or vascular disease.
• Determine the duration, location, onset, and possible precipitating symptoms of the patient's migraine.
Lifespan Considerations
• Be aware that it is unknown if zolmitriptan is distributed in breast milk.
• Be aware that the safety and efficacy of zolmitriptan have not been established in children younger than 12 years of age.
• There are no age-related precautions noted in the elderly.
Precautions
• Use cautiously in patients with controlled hypertension, a history of cerebrovascular accident (CVA), mild to moderate liver or renal impairment, and a patient profile suggesting cardiovascular risks.
Administration and Handling
PO
• Give zolmitriptan without regard to food.
Nasal
• Instruct the patient to gently blow his or her nose to clear nasal passages.
• With the patient's head upright, close one of the patient's nostrils with an index finger. Teach the patient to breathe gently through his or her mouth.
• Insert the nozzle into the patient's open nostril about a half (1/2) inch.
• Instruct the patient to close his or her mouth, then take a breath through his or her nose while de-

pressing the plunger and releasing the spray drug dose.

• Remove the nozzle from the patient's nose and teach the patient to gently breathe in through the nose and exhale through the mouth for 15–20 seconds. The patient should not breathe in deeply.

Intervention and Evaluation

• Monitor the patient for dizziness.

• Monitor the patient's blood pressure (B/P), especially in patients with liver impairment.

• Assess the patient for relief of migraine headache and migraine potential for nausea, phonophobia or sound sensitivity, and photophobia or light sensitivity, and vomiting.

Patient Teaching

• Instruct the patient to take a single zolmitriptan dose as soon as symptoms of an actual migraine appear.

• Explain to the patient that zolmitriptan is intended to relieve migraines, not to prevent or reduce the number of attacks.

• Teach the patient to lie down in dark, quiet room for additional benefit after taking the drug.

• Advise the patient to avoid tasks that require mental alertness or motor skills until his or her response to the drug is established.

• Warn the patient to notify the physician if he or she experiences blood in urine or stool, chest pain, easy bruising, numbness or pain in the arms or legs, palpitations, swelling of the eyelids, face, or lips, or tightness in throat.

37 Antiparkinson Agents

amantadine
  hydrochloride
benztropine mesylate
bromocriptine
  mesylate
carbidopa/levodopa
entacapone
pergolide mesylate
pramipexole
ropinirole
  hydrochloride
selegiline
  hydrochloride
tolcapone

Uses: Antiparkinson agents are used to treat Parkinson's disease. They're prescribed to reduce parkinsonian signs and symptoms, to correct the disease-induced dopamine deficit, or both. In addition, some drugs in this class have other indications. For example, amantadine is used to treat respiratory infections and control extrapyramidal reactions. Bromocriptine is used for hyperprolactemia and other treatments.

Action: Because antiparkinson agents belong to four distinct subclasses, they work by different mechanisms. *Dopaminergics*, such as carbidopa-levodopa, increase dopamine synthesis. *Dopamine agonists*, such as pramipexole, directly activate dopamine receptors and promote the release of dopamine. *Monoamine oxidase (MAO)-B inhibitors*, such as selegiline, are used with levodopa or carbidopa-levodopa, and inhibit the enzymes that break down dopamine, extending the levodopa's antiparkinsonian effect. *Catechol* O-*methyltransferase (COMT) inhibitors*, such as entacapone, are given with carbidopa-levodopa and inhibit the enzyme COMT, which increases the levodopa concentration.

CENTRAL NERVOUS SYSTEM AGENTS

COMBINATION PRODUCTS

STALEVO: entacapone/carbidopa-levodopa (an antiparkinson agent) 200 mg/12.5 mg/50 mg; 200 mg/ 25 mg/100 mg; 200 mg/37.5 mg/ 150 mg.

amantadine hydrochloride
ah-**man**-tih-deen
(Endantadine [CAN], PMS-Amantadine[CAN], Symmetrel)

CATEGORY AND SCHEDULE
Pregnancy Risk Category: C

MECHANISM OF ACTION
A dopaminergic agonist that blocks the uncoating of influenza A virus, preventing penetration into the host, and inhibiting M2 protein in the assembly of progeny virions. Amantadine locks the reuptake of dopamine into presynaptic neurons and causes direct stimulation of postsynaptic receptors. *Therapeutic Effect:* Antiviral, antiparkinson activity.

PHARMACOKINETICS
Rapidly, completely absorbed from gastrointestinal (GI) tract. Protein binding: 67%. Widely distributed. Primarily excreted in urine. Minimally removed by hemodialysis.

Half-life: 11–15 hrs (half-life increased in elderly, decreased in impaired renal function).

AVAILABILITY
Liquid: 50 mg/5 ml.
Syrup: 50 mg/5 ml.
Tablets: 100 mg.

INDICATIONS AND DOSAGES
▸ **Prophylaxis, symptomatic treatment of respiratory illness due to influenza A virus**
PO
Adults older than 64 yrs. 100 mg/day.
Adults 13–64 yrs. 200 mg/day.
Children 9–12 yrs. 100 mg 2 times/day.
Children 1–8 yrs. 5 mg/kg/day (up to 150 mg/day).
▸ **Parkinson's disease, extrapyramidal symptoms**
PO
Adults, Elderly. 100 mg 2 times/day. May increase up to 300 mg/day in divided doses.
▸ **Dosage in renal impairment**
Dose and frequency are modified based on creatinine clearance (Ccr).

Creatinine Clearance	Dosage
30–50 ml/min	200 mg first day; 100 mg/day thereafter
15–29 ml/min	200 mg first day; 100 mg on alternate days
less than 15 ml/min	200 mg every 7 days

UNLABELED USES
Treatment of attention-deficit hyperactivity disorder (ADHD) and of fatigue associated with multiple sclerosis

CONTRAINDICATIONS
None known.

INTERACTIONS
Drug
Anticholinergics, antihistamines, phenothiazine, tricyclic antidepressants: May increase anticholinergic effects of amantadine.
Hydrochlorothiazide, triamterene: May increase amantadine blood concentration and risk for toxicity.
Herbal
None known.
Food
None known.

DIAGNOSTIC TEST EFFECTS
None known.

SIDE EFFECTS
Frequent (10%–5%)
Nausea, dizziness, poor concentration, insomnia, nervousness
Occasional (5%–1%)
Orthostatic hypotension, anorexia, headache, livedo reticularis evidenced by reddish blue, netlike blotching of skin, blurred vision, urinary retention, dry mouth or nose
Rare
Vomiting, depression, irritation or swelling of eyes, rash

SERIOUS REACTIONS
• Congestive heart failure (CHF), leukopenia, and neutropenia occur rarely.
• Hyperexcitability, convulsions, and ventricular arrhythmias may occur.

NURSING CONSIDERATIONS

Baseline Assessment
• When treating infections caused by influenza A virus, expect to obtain specimens for viral diagnostic tests before giving first dose. Therapy may begin before test results are known.

Lifespan Considerations

• Be aware that it is unknown if amantadine crosses the placenta or is distributed in breast milk.
• There are no age-related precautions noted in children less than 1 year of age.
• The elderly may exhibit increased sensitivity to amantadine's anticholinergic effects.
• In the elderly, age-related decreased renal function may require dosage adjustment.

Precautions

• Use cautiously in patients with cerebrovascular disease, CHF, history of seizures, liver disease, orthostatic hypotension, peripheral edema, recurrent eczema-toid dermatitis, renal dysfunction, and those receiving CNS stimulants.

Administration and Handling

PO
◄ALERT► Give as a single or in 2 divided doses.
• May give without regard to food.
• Administer nighttime dose several hours before bedtime to prevent insomnia.

Intervention and Evaluation

• Expect to monitor the patient's intake and output and renal function tests, if ordered.
• Check for peripheral edema. Assess the patient's skin for blotching or rash.
• Evaluate the patient's food tolerance and episodes of nausea or vomiting.
• Assess the patient for dizziness.
• For patients with Parkinson's disease, assess for clinical reversal of symptoms as evidenced by an improvement of the masklike facial expression, muscular rigidity, shuffling gait, and tremor of the head and hands at rest.

Patient Teaching

• Advise the patient to continue therapy for the full length of treatment and to evenly space drug doses around the clock.
• Explain to the patient that he or she should not take any medications, including over-the-counter (OTC) drugs, without first consulting the physician.
• Warn the patient to avoid alcoholic beverages.
• Caution the patient not to drive, use machinery, or engage in other activities that require mental acuity if he or she is experiencing dizziness or blurred vision.
• Teach the patient to get up slowly from a sitting or lying position.
• Stress to the patient that he or she notify the physician of new symptoms, especially any blurred vision, dizziness, nausea or vomiting, and skin blotching or rash.
• Tell the patient to take the nighttime dose several hours before bedtime to prevent insomnia.

benztropine mesylate

benz-**trow**-peen
(Apo-Benztropine[CAN], Cogentin)
Do not confuse with bromocriptine.

CATEGORY AND SCHEDULE

Pregnancy Risk Category: C

MECHANISM OF ACTION

An antiparkinson agent that selectively blocks central cholinergic receptors, assists in balancing cholinergic and dopaminergic activity. *Therapeutic Effect:* Reduces incidence, severity of akinesia, rigidity, tremor.

AVAILABILITY
Tablets: 0.5 mg, 1 mg, 2 mg.
Injection: 1 mg/ml.

INDICATIONS AND DOSAGES
▶ **Parkinsonism**
PO
Adults. 0.5–6 mg/day in 1–2 divided doses. Titrate by 0.5 mg at 5–6 day intervals.
Elderly. Initially, 0.5 mg 1–2 times/day. Titrate by 0.5 mg at 5–6 day intervals. Maximum: 4 mg/day.
▶ **Drug-induced extrapyramidal symptoms**
PO/IM
Adults. 1–4 mg 1–2 times/day.
▶ **Acute dystonic reactions**
IM/IV
Adults. 1–2 mg, then 1–2 mg PO 2 times/day to prevent recurrence.

CONTRAINDICATIONS
Angle-closure glaucoma, children younger than 3 yrs, gastrointestinal (GI) obstruction, intestinal atony, megacolon, myasthenia gravis, paralytic ileus, prostatic hypertrophy, severe ulcerative colitis

INTERACTIONS
Drug
Alcohol, central nervous system (CNS) depressants: May increase sedation.
Amantadine, anticholinergics, MAOIs: May increase the effects of benztropine.
Antacids, antidiarrheals: May decrease the absorption and effects of benztropine.
Herbal
None known.
Food
None known.

DIAGNOSTIC TEST EFFECTS
None known.

SIDE EFFECTS
Frequent
Drowsiness, dry mouth, blurred vision, constipation, decreased sweating or urination, GI upset, photosensitivity
Occasional
Headache, memory loss, muscle cramping, nervousness, peripheral paresthesia, orthostatic hypotension, abdominal cramping
Rare
Rash, confusion, eye pain

SERIOUS REACTIONS
• Overdosage may vary from severe anticholinergic effects, such as unsteadiness, severe drowsiness, severe dryness of mouth, nose, or throat, tachycardia, shortness of breath, and skin flushing.
• Also produces severe paradoxical reaction, marked by hallucinations, tremor, seizures, and toxic psychosis.

NURSING CONSIDERATIONS
Baseline Assessment
• Assess the patient's mental status for agitation, confusion, disorientation, and psychotic-like symptoms because medication frequently produces such side effects in patients older than 60 years of age.
Precautions
◀ALERT▶ Elderly patients older than 60 years of age tend to develop agitation, disorientation, mental confusion, and psychotic-like symptoms.
• Use cautiously in patients with arrhythmias, heart disease, hypertension, liver or renal impairment, obstructive diseases of the gastrointestinal (GI) or genitourinary (GU) tracts, prostatic hypertrophy, tachy-

cardia, treated open-angle glaucoma, and urinary retention.

Intervention and Evaluation

• Be alert to the patient's neurologic effects including agitation, headache, lethargy, and mental confusion.

• Assess the patient for the relief of symptoms, such as an improvement of masklike facial expression, muscular rigidity, shuffling gait, and resting tremors of hands and head.

Patient Teaching

• Warn the patient to avoid tasks that require mental alertness or motor skills until his or her response to the drug is established.

• Tell the patient that dizziness, drowsiness, and dry mouth may be expected responses to the drug. Explain that drowsiness tends to diminish or disappear with continued therapy.

• Caution the patient to avoid alcoholic beverages during benztropine therapy.

bromocriptine mesylate

brom-oh-**crip**-teen
(Apo-Bromocriptine[CAN], Bromohexal[AUS], Parlodel)
Do not confuse with benztropine, pindolol.

CATEGORY AND SCHEDULE
Pregnancy Risk Category: C

MECHANISM OF ACTION

A dopamine agonist that inhibits prolactin secretion, directly stimulates dopamine receptors in the corpus striatum. *Therapeutic Effect:* Suppresses galactorrhea, improves symptoms of parkinsonism.

PHARMACOKINETICS

Indication	Onset	Peak	Duration
Prolactin lowering	2 hrs	8 hrs	24 hrs
Antiparkinson	0.5–1.5 hrs	2 hrs	N/A
Growth hormone	1–2 hrs	4–8 wks	4–8 hrs

Minimal absorption from the gastrointestinal (GI) tract. Protein binding: 90%–96%. Metabolized in liver. Excreted in feces via biliary secretion. **Half-life:** 15 hrs.

AVAILABILITY

Tablets: 2.5 mg.
Capsules: 5 mg.

INDICATIONS AND DOSAGES

▶ **Hyperprolactinemia**
PO
Adults, Elderly. Initially, 1.25–2.5 mg/day. May increase by 2.5 mg/day at 3-to 7-day intervals. Range: 2.5 mg 2–3 times/day.

▶ **Parkinson's disease**
PO
Adults, Elderly. Initially, 1.25 mg 2 times/day. Increase by 2.5 mg/day q14–28 days.
Range: 30–90 mg/day.

▶ **Acromegaly**
PO
Adults, Elderly. Initially, 1.25–2.5 mg/day at bedtime for 3 days. May increase by 1.25–2.5 mg/day q3–7 days. Range: 20–30 mg/day. Maximum: 100 mg/day.

UNLABELED USES

Treatment of cocaine addiction, hyperprolactinemia associated with pituitary adenomas, neuroleptic malignant syndrome

CONTRAINDICATIONS

Hypersensitivity to ergot alkaloids, peripheral vascular disease, pregnancy, severe ischemic heart disease, uncontrolled hypertension

INTERACTIONS
Drug

Alcohol: Disulfiram reaction, manifested by chest pain, confusion, flushed face, nausea, vomiting.
Erythromycin, ritonavir: May increase bromocriptine blood concentration and risk of toxicity.
Estrogens, progestins: May decrease the effects of bromocriptine.
Haloperidol, MAOIs, phenothiazines: May decrease prolactin effect.
Hypotensive agents: May increase hypotension.
Levodopa: May increase the effects of bromocriptine.
Risperidone: May increase serum prolactin concentrations and interfere with the effects of bromocriptine.

Herbal
None known.

Food
None known.

DIAGNOSTIC TEST EFFECTS

May increase plasma concentration of growth hormone.

SIDE EFFECTS

Frequent
Nausea (49%), headache (19%), dizziness (17%)
Occasional (7%–3%)
Fatigue, lightheadedness, vomiting, abdominal cramps, diarrhea, constipation, nasal congestion, drowsiness, dry mouth
Rare
Muscle cramping, urinary hesitancy

SERIOUS REACTIONS

• Visual or auditory hallucinations noted in parkinsonism syndrome.
• Long-term, high-dose therapy may produce continuing rhinorrhea, fainting, GI hemorrhage, peptic ulcer, and severe abdominal or stomach pain.

NURSING CONSIDERATIONS

Baseline Assessment

• Expect to rule out pituitary gland tumor before beginning treatment for hyperprolactinemia with amenorrhea or galactorrhea and infertility.
• Plan to obtain a pregnancy test to rule out pregnancy.

Lifespan Considerations

• Be aware that bromocriptine use is not recommended during pregnancy or while breast-feeding.
• Be aware that the safety and efficacy of bromocriptine have not been established in children.
• In the elderly, central nervous system (CNS) effects may occur more frequently.

Precautions

◀ALERT▶ Know that the incidence of side effects is high, especially at the beginning of therapy or with high dosage.
• Use cautiously in patients with cardiac or liver function impairment, hypertension, and psychiatric disorders.

Administration and Handling
PO
• Make sure patient is lying down before administering first dose to avoid lightheadedness.
• Give after food intake to decreases incidence of nausea.

Intervention and Evaluation

• Assist the patient with ambulation if he or she experiences dizziness after drug administration.

• Assess the patient for therapeutic response, such as a decrease in breast engorgement or parkinsonism symptoms.
• Monitor the patient for constipation.

Patient Teaching
• Instruct the patient to rise slowly from lying to sitting position, and permit legs to dangle momentarily before standing to avoid lightheadedness. Tell the patient to avoid sudden posture changes.
• Warn the patient to avoid tasks that require mental alertness or motor skills until his or her response to the drug is established.
• Explain to the patient that she must use alternatives to oral contraceptives during treatment.
• Caution the patient to notify the physician if he or she experiences any watery nasal discharge.

carbidopa/levodopa

car-bih-dope-ah/**lev**-oh-dope-ah
(Apo-Levocarb[CAN], Sinemet, Sinemet CR)

CATEGORY AND SCHEDULE
Pregnancy Risk Category: C

MECHANISM OF ACTION
An antiparkinson agent that is converted to dopamine in basal ganglia. Increases dopamine concentration in brain, inhibiting hyperactive cholinergic activity. Carbidopa prevents peripheral breakdown of levodopa, allowing more levodopa to be available for transport into brain. *Therapeutic Effect:* Reduces tremor.

PHARMACOKINETICS
Carbidopa: Rapidly, completely absorbed from the gastrointestinal (GI) tract. Widely distributed. Excreted primarily in urine. **Half-life:** 1–2 hrs. Levodopa: Converted to dopamine. Excreted primarily in urine. **Half-life:** 1–3 hrs.

AVAILABILITY
Tablets (expressed as carbidopa/ levodopa): 10 mg/100 mg, 25 mg/ 100 mg, 25 mg/250 mg.
Tablets (extended-release): 25 mg/ 100 mg, 50 mg/200 mg.

INDICATIONS AND DOSAGES
▸ **Parkinsonism**
PO
Adults. Initially, 25/100 mg 2–4 times/day. May increase up to a maximum of 200/2,000 mg.
Elderly. Initially, 25/100 mg 2 times/day. May increase as necessary. Conversion from Sinemet, based on total daily dose of levodopa, to Sinemet CR (50/200 mg):

Sinemet	Sinemet CR
300–400 mg	1 tab 2 times/day
500–600 mg	1.5 tab 2 times/day or 1 tab 3 times/day
700–800 mg	4 tabs in 3 or more divided doses
900–1,000 mg	5 tabs in 3 or more divided doses

Intervals between Sinemet CR should be 4–8 hrs while awake.
▸ **Receiving only levodopa**
PO
Adults, 1,500 mg levodopa/day and less. 1 tablet (25/100 mg) 3–4 times/day.
Adults, over 1,500 mg levodopa/day. 1 tablet (25/250 mg) 3–4 times/day.
Sustained-release
Adults. 1 tablet 2 times/day.

▸ **Receiving carbidopa/levodopa**
Adults. Provide about 10% more levodopa; may increase up to 30% more at 4- to 8-hr dosing intervals.

CONTRAINDICATIONS
Narrow-angle glaucoma, those on MAOI therapy

INTERACTIONS
Drug
Anticonvulsants, benzodiazepines, haloperidol, phenothiazines: May decrease the effects of carbidopa/levodopa.
MAOIs: May increase risk of hypertensive crises.
Selegiline: May increase dyskinesias, nausea, orthostatic hypotension, confusion, hallucinations.
Herbal
None known.
Food
None known.

DIAGNOSTIC TEST EFFECTS
May increase BUN, LDH concentrations, serum alkaline phosphatase and bilirubin, SGOT (AST), and SGPT (ALT) levels.

SIDE EFFECTS
Frequent (90%–10%)
Uncontrolled body movements, including face, tongue, arms, upper body, nausea and vomiting (80%), anorexia (50%)
Occasional
Depression, anxiety, confusion, nervousness, difficulty urinating, irregular heartbeats, dizziness, lightheadedness, decreased appetite, blurred vision, constipation, dry mouth, flushed skin, headache, insomnia, diarrhea, unusual tiredness, darkening of urine
Rare
Hypertension, ulcer, hemolytic anemia, marked by tiredness or weakness

SERIOUS REACTIONS
• High incidence of involuntary choreiform, dystonic, and dyskinetic movements may be noted in patients on long-term therapy.
• Mental changes, such as paranoid ideation, psychotic episodes, depression, may be noted.
• Numerous mild to severe central nervous system (CNS) psychiatric disturbances may include reduced attention span, anxiety, nightmares, daytime somnolence, euphoria, fatigue, paranoia, and hallucinations.

NURSING CONSIDERATIONS
Baseline Assessment
• Instruct the patient to void before giving carbidopa/levodopa to reduce the risk of urine retention.
Lifespan Considerations
• Be aware that it is unknown if carbidopa/levodopa crosses the placenta or is distributed in breast milk. Know that carbidopa/levodopa may inhibit lactation. Do not breastfeed while taking this drug.
• Be aware that the safety and efficacy of carbidopa/levodopa have not been established in children younger than 18 years.
• The elderly are more sensitive to the effects of levodopa. Anxiety, confusion, and nervousness more common in elderly patients receiving anticholinergics.
Precautions
• Use cautiously in patients with active peptic ulcer, bronchial asthma—tartrazine sensitivity—emphysema, history of myocardial infarction (MI), severe cardiac, endocrine, liver, pulmonary, and renal impairment, and treated open-angle glaucoma.

Administration and Handling
◀ ALERT ▶ Plan to discontinue levodopa at least 8 hours prior to giving carbidopa/levodopa. Expect to initiate with dose providing at least 25% of previous levodopa dosage.
PO
• Crush scored tablets as needed.
• May be given without regard to meals.
• Do not crush sustained-release tablet; may cut in half.
Intervention and Evaluation
• Be alert to neurologic effects including agitation, headache, lethargy, and mental confusion.
• Monitor the patient for dyskinesia, characterized by difficulty with movement.
• Assess the patient for clinical reversal of symptoms, such as improvement of masklike facial expression, muscular rigidity, shuffling gait, and resting tremors of hands and head.
Patient Teaching
• Warn the patient to avoid tasks that require mental alertness or motor skills until his or her response to the drug is established.
• Caution the patient to avoid alcoholic beverages during therapy.
• Suggest to the patient that taking sips of tepid water and chewing sugarless gum may relieve dry mouth.
• Instruct the patient to take carbidopa/levodopa with food to minimize gastrointestinal (GI) upset.
• Explain to the patient that therapeutic effects may be delayed from several weeks to months
• Tell the patient that carbidopa/levodopa use may produce a dark-

ening in the color of sweat or urine, which is not harmful.
• Warn the patient to notify the physician if he or she experiences difficulty urinating, irregular heartbeats, mental changes, severe nausea or vomiting, or uncontrolled movement of arms, eyelids, face, hands, mouth, legs, or tongue.

entacapone
en-tah-cah-**pone**
(Comtan)

CATEGORY AND SCHEDULE
Pregnancy Risk Category: C

MECHANISM OF ACTION
An antiparkinson agent that inhibits the enzyme, catechol-*O*-methyltransferase (COMT), potentiating dopamine activity and increasing the duration of action of levodopa. *Therapeutic Effect:* Decreases signs and symptoms of Parkinson's disease.

PHARMACOKINETICS
Rapidly absorbed after PO administration. Protein binding: 98%. Metabolized in the liver. Primarily eliminated via biliary excretion. Not removed by hemodialysis. **Half-life:** 2.4 hrs.

AVAILABILITY
Tablets: 200 mg.

INDICATIONS AND DOSAGES
▸ **Parkinson's disease**
PO
Adults, Elderly. 200 mg concomitantly with each dose of levodopa/carbidopa to maximum of 8 times/day (1,600 mg).

CONTRAINDICATIONS

Concomitant use of MAOIs, hypersensitivity

INTERACTIONS
Drug

Ampicillin, cholestyramine, erythromycin, probenecid: May decrease the excretion of entacapone.
Bitolterol, dobutamine, dopamine, epinephrine, isoetharine, isoproterenol, epinephrine, methyldopa, norepinephrine: May increase risk of arrhythmias, changes in blood pressure (B/P).
Nonselective MAOIs, including phenelzine: May result in inhibiting pathway for normal catecholamine metabolism.
Other central nervous system (CNS) depressants: May have additive effect.
Herbal
None known.
Food
None known.

DIAGNOSTIC TEST EFFECTS

None known.

SIDE EFFECTS

Frequent (greater than 10%)
Dyskinesia or uncontrolled body movements, nausea, urine discoloration—dark yellow or orange, diarrhea
Occasional (9%–3%)
Abdominal pain, vomiting, constipation, dry mouth, fatigue, back pain
Rare (less than 2%)
Anxiety, somnolence, agitation, dyspepsia, flatulence, diaphoresis, asthenia, dyspnea

SERIOUS REACTIONS

• None known.

NURSING CONSIDERATIONS

Baseline Assessment
• Assess the patient for symptoms of Parkinson's disease such as, improvement of masklike facial expression, muscular rigidity, shuffling gait, and resting tremors of hands and head.
• Obtain baseline vital signs, including blood pressure.
Lifespan Considerations
• Be aware that it is unknown if entacapone is distributed in breast milk.
• Know that this drug is not indicated for pediatric use.
• There are no age-related precautions noted in the elderly.
Precautions
• Use cautiously in patients with liver or renal impairment.
• Know that entacapone use may exacerbate dyskinesias and increase the risk of orthostatic hypotension and syncope.
Administration and Handling
◀ALERT▶ Always administer with levodopa/carbidopa.
PO
• Give entacapone without regard to food.
Intervention and Evaluation
• Monitor the patient for dyskinesia or difficulty with movement.
• Assess the patient for relief of symptoms, including the improvement of masklike facial expression, muscular rigidity, shuffling gait, and tremor of hands and head at rest.
• Monitor the patient's B/P.
• Evaluate the patient for diarrhea and orthostatic hypotension.
Patient Teaching
• Caution the patient to avoid tasks that require mental alertness or motor skills until his or her response to the drug is established.
• Tell the patient that entacapone

use may cause a color change in his or her sweat or produce dark yellow or orange urine.
• Warn the patient to notify the physician if he or she experiences any uncontrolled movement of arms, eyelids, face, hands, legs, mouth, or tongue.
• Explain that entacapone should be taken with levodopa/carbidopa for best results.

pergolide mesylate
purr-go-lied
(Permax)
Do not confuse with Pentrax or Pernox.

CATEGORY AND SCHEDULE
Pregnancy Risk Category: B

MECHANISM OF ACTION
A centrally active dopamine agonist. *Therapeutic Effect:* Assists in reduction in tremor, improvement in akinesia or absence of movement, posture and equilibrium disorders, rigidity of parkinsonism.

PHARMACOKINETICS
Well absorbed from the gastrointestinal (GI) tract. Protein binding: 90%. Metabolized in liver—undergoes extensive first-pass effect. Primarily excreted in urine. Unknown if removed by hemodialysis.

AVAILABILITY
Tablets: 0.05 mg, 0.25 mg, 1 mg.

INDICATIONS AND DOSAGES
▸ Parkinsonism
PO
Adults, Elderly. Initially, 0.05 mg/day for 2 days. Increase by 0.1–0.15 mg/day q3 days over the following 12 days; then may increase by 0.25 mg/day q3 days. Maximum: 5 mg/day. Range: 2–3 mg/day in 3 divided doses.

CONTRAINDICATIONS
Hypersensitivity to pergolide or other ergot derivatives

INTERACTIONS
Drug
Haloperidol, loxapine, methyldopa, metoclopramide, phenothiazines: May decrease effect of pergolide. *Hypotension-producing medications:* May increase hypotensive effect.
Herbal
None known.
Food
None known.

DIAGNOSTIC TEST EFFECTS
May increase plasma growth hormone.

SIDE EFFECTS
Frequent (24%–10%)
Nausea, dizziness, hallucinations, constipation, rhinitis, dystonia or impaired muscle tone, confusion, somnolence
Occasional (9%–3%)
Postural hypotension, insomnia, dry mouth, peripheral edema, anxiety, diarrhea, dyspepsia, abdominal pain, headache, abnormal vision, anorexia, tremor, depression, rash
Rare (less than 2%)
Urinary frequency, vivid dreams, neck pain, hypotension, vomiting

SERIOUS REACTIONS
• Overdosage may require supportive measures to maintain B/P. Plan to monitor cardiac function, obtain vital signs, as well as check the results of arterial blood gases and serum electrolytes.
• Activated charcoal may be more

effective than emesis or lavage for overdose.

NURSING CONSIDERATIONS
Baseline Assessment
• Obtain a baseline EKG for patients with a history of cardiac disease.
• Monitor the patient's blood pressure (B/P) for hypotension and pulse for irregularities that could indicate an arrhythmia.

Lifespan Considerations
• Be aware that it is unknown if pergolide crosses the placenta or is distributed in breast milk. Pergolide may interfere with lactation.
• Be aware that the safety and efficacy of this drug have not been established in children.
• There are no age-related precautions noted in the elderly.

Precautions
• Use cautiously in patients with cardiac arrhythmias and history of confusion or hallucinations.

Administration and Handling
◄ALERT► Daily doses usually given in 3 divided doses.
PO
• Crush scored tablets as needed.
• Give pergolide without regard to meals.

Intervention and Evaluation
• Be alert to the drug's neurologic effects, including agitation, headache, lethargy, and mental confusion.
• Monitor the patient for dyskinesia or difficulty with movement.
• Monitor the patient's B/P and EKG.
• Assess the patient for clinical reversal of Parkinson symptoms, such as improvement of masklike facial expression, muscular rigidity, shuffling gait, and resting tremors of hands and head.

Patient Teaching
• Tell the patient that a tolerance to feeling of lightheadedness develops during therapy.
• Instruct the patient to rise slowly from lying to sitting position, and to dangle legs momentarily before standing to reduce the hypotensive effect of pergolide.
• Warn the patient to avoid tasks that require mental alertness or motor skills until his or her response to the drug is established.
• Explain to the patient that dizziness, drowsiness, and dry mouth may be expected side effects to the drug.
• Urge the patient to avoid alcoholic beverages during therapy.

---
pramipexole
pram-ih-**pecks**-all
(Mirapex)
Do not confuse with Mifeprex or MiraLax.

CATEGORY AND SCHEDULE
Pregnancy Risk Category: C

MECHANISM OF ACTION
An antiparkinson agent that stimulates dopamine receptors in the striatum. *Therapeutic Effect:* Relieves signs and symptoms of Parkinson's disease.

PHARMACOKINETICS
Rapid, extensive absorption after PO administration. Protein binding: 15%. Widely distributed. Steady-state concentrations achieved within 2 days. Primarily eliminated in urine. Not removed by hemodialysis. **Half-life:** 8 hrs (12 hrs in patients older than 65 yrs).

AVAILABILITY
Tablets: 0.125 mg, 0.25 mg, 0.5 mg, 1 mg, 1.5 mg.

INDICATIONS AND DOSAGES
▶ **Parkinson's disease**
PO
Adults, Elderly. Initially, 0.375 mg/day in 3 divided doses. Do not increase dose more frequently than q5–7 days. Maintenance: 1.5–4.5 mg/day in equally divided doses 3 times/day.
▶ **Renal function impairment**
PO
Adults, Elderly, creatinine clearance greater than 60 ml/min. Initially, 0.125 mg 3 times/day. Maximum: 1.5 mg 3 times/day.
Adults, Elderly, creatinine clearance 35–59 ml/min. Initially, 0.125 mg 2 times/day. Maximum: 1.5 mg twice a day.
Adults, Elderly, creatinine clearance 15–34 ml/min. Initially, 0.125 mg 1 time/day. Maximum: 1.5 mg once a day.

CONTRAINDICATIONS
History of hypersensitivity to medication

INTERACTIONS
Drug
Cimetidine: Increases pramipexole plasma concentration and half-life.
Cimetidine, diltiazem, quinidine, quinine, ranitidine, triamterene, verapamil: Combined use of these drugs may decrease pramipexole clearance.
Carbidopa or levodopa combinations: May increase plasma levels of carbidopa or levodopa combinations.
Herbal
None known.
Food
Time to maximum plasma levels is increased by 1 hr when taken with food, but the extent of absorption not affected.

DIAGNOSTIC TEST EFFECTS
None known.

SIDE EFFECTS
Frequent
Early Parkinson's disease (28%–10%): Nausea, asthenia or weakness, dizziness, somnolence, insomnia, constipation
Advanced Parkinson's disease (53%–17%): Postural hypotension, extrapyramidal signs, insomnia, dizziness, hallucinations
Occasional
Early Parkinson's disease (5%–2%): Edema, malaise, confusion, amnesia, akathisia (restlessness), anorexia, dysphagia, peripheral edema, altered vision, impotence
Advanced Parkinson's disease (10%–7%): Asthenia, somnolence, confusion, constipation, gait abnormality, dry mouth
Rare
Advanced Parkinson's disease (6%–2%): General edema, malaise, chest pain, amnesia, tremors, urinary frequency or incontinence, dyspnea, rhinitis, vision changes

SERIOUS REACTIONS
• None known.

NURSING CONSIDERATIONS
Baseline Assessment
• Assess the patient for symptoms of Parkinson's disease such as improvement of masklike facial expression, muscular rigidity, shuffling gait, and resting tremors of hands and head.
• Expect to perform renal function studies to guide the dose of the drug.

• Obtain baseline vital signs, including blood pressure.

Lifespan Considerations
• Be aware that it is unknown if pramipexole is distributed in breast milk.
• Be aware that the safety and efficacy of pramipexole have not been established in children.
• There is an increased risk of hallucinations in the elderly.

Precautions
• Use cautiously in patients with concomitant use of central nervous system (CNS) depressants, hallucinations, history of orthostatic hypotension, renal function impairment, and syncope.

Administration and Handling
PO
• Give pramipexole without regard to food.

Intervention and Evaluation
• Instruct the patient to rise from lying to sitting or sitting to standing position slowly to prevent risk of postural hypotension.
• Assess the patient for clinical improvement.
• Assist the patient with ambulation if he or she experiences dizziness.
• Assess the patient for constipation, a common side effect of the drug.

Patient Teaching
• Explain to the patient that he or she may experience hallucinations, and that this side effect occurs more in the elderly than in younger patients with Parkinson's disease.
• Tell the patient that postural hypotension may occur more frequently during initial therapy.
• Warn the patient to avoid tasks that require mental alertness or motor skills until his or her response to the drug is established.
• Instruct the patient that if he or

she experiences nausea, to take pramipexole with food.
• Caution the patient against abruptly discontinuing pramipexole.
• Encourage the patient to consume fiber and fluids and to exercise regularly.

ropinirole hydrochloride
roh-**pin**-ih-role
(Requip)

CATEGORY AND SCHEDULE
Pregnancy Risk Category: C

MECHANISM OF ACTION
An antiparkinson agent that stimulates dopamine receptors in the striatum. *Therapeutic Effect:* Relieves signs and symptoms of Parkinson's disease.

PHARMACOKINETICS
Rapidly absorbed after PO administration. Protein binding: 40%. Extensively distributed throughout the body. Extensively metabolized. Steady-state concentrations achieved within 2 days. Eliminated in urine. Unknown if removed by hemodialysis. **Half-life:** 6 hrs.

AVAILABILITY
Tablets: 0.25 mg, 0.5 mg, 1 mg, 2 mg, 4 mg, 5 mg.

INDICATIONS AND DOSAGES
▸ **Parkinson's disease**
PO
Adults, Elderly. Initially, 0.25 mg 3 times/day. Do not increase dosage more frequently than q7 days. After week 4, daily dosage may be increased, if needed, by 1.5–3 mg/day

per week to total daily dose of 24 mg/day.

CONTRAINDICATIONS
None known

INTERACTIONS
Drug
Butyrophenones, metoclopramide, phenothiazines, thioxanthenes: Diminish the effectiveness of ropinirole.
Central nervous system (CNS) depressants: Additive side effects with CNS depressants.
Cimetidine, diltiazem, enoxacin, erythromycin, fluvoxamine, mexiletine, norfloxacin, tacrine: Alter ropinirole blood concentration.
Ciprofloxacin: Increases ropinirole blood concentration.
Estrogens: Reduce the clearance of ropinirole.
Levodopa: Increases the blood concentration of levodopa.
Herbal
None known.
Food
Time to maximum plasma levels is increased by 2.5 hrs when taken with food, but the extent of absorption not affected.

DIAGNOSTIC TEST EFFECTS
May increase serum alkaline phosphatase.

SIDE EFFECTS
Frequent (60%–40%)
Nausea, dizziness, excessive drowsiness
Occasional (12%–5%)
Syncope, vomiting, fatigue, viral infection, dyspepsia, increased sweating, weakness, orthostatic hypotension, abdominal discomfort, pharyngitis, abnormal vision, dry mouth, hypertension, hallucinations, confusion

Rare (4% or less)
Anorexia, peripheral edema, memory loss, rhinitis, sinusitis, palpitations, impotence

SERIOUS REACTIONS
• None known.

NURSING CONSIDERATIONS
Baseline Assessment
• Assess the patient for Parkinson symptoms, such as masklike facial expression, muscular rigidity, shuffling gait, and resting tremors of hands and head.
• Obtain baseline vital signs, especially blood pressure (B/P).
• Expect to obtain baseline serum alkaline phosphatase levels.
Lifespan Considerations
• Be aware that ropinirole is distributed in breast milk and drug activity is possible in the breast-feeding infant.
• Be aware that the safety and efficacy of ropinirole have not been established in children.
• There are no age-related precautions noted in the elderly, but this patient population experiences hallucinations more frequently than other age groups.
Precautions
• Use cautiously in patients with hallucinations, especially in the elderly, history of orthostatic hypotension, and syncope.
• Use cautiously in patients who concurrently use CNS depressants.
Administration and Handling
PO
• Expect the dose schedule to increase very gradually at weekly intervals. Plan to begin with week 1 starting at 0.25 mg 3 times per day to total daily dose 0.75 mg. Week 2 expect increase to 0.5 mg 3 times per day to total daily dose 1.5 mg.

For week 3, plan to administer 0.75 mg 3 times per day to total daily dose 2.25 mg. Week 4 increase to 1 mg 3 times per day to total daily dose 3 mg, as prescribed.
• Plan to discontinue medication gradually at 7-day intervals. Expect to decrease frequency from 3 times/ day to 2 times/day for 4 days. For the remaining 3 days, decrease frequency to once a day prior to complete withdrawal, as prescribed.

Intervention and Evaluation
• Assess the patient for clinical improvement and reversal of symptoms, improvement of masklike facial expression, muscular rigidity, shuffling gait, and tremors of the hand and head at rest.
• Assist the patient with ambulation if he or she experiences dizziness.

Patient Teaching
• Explain to the patient that dizziness and drowsiness may be initial responses to the drug.
• Instruct the patient to rise from lying to sitting or sitting to standing position slowly to prevent risk of postural hypotension. Explain to the patient that postural hypotension may occur more frequently during initial therapy.
• Warn the patient to avoid tasks that require mental alertness or motor skills until his or her response to the drug is established.
• Teach the patient that if he or she experiences nausea, to take ropinirole with food.
• Tell the patient that he or she may experience hallucinations. Explain that this side effect occurs more in the elderly than in younger patients with Parkinson's disease.

selegiline hydrochloride
sell-**eh**-geh-leen
(Eldepryl, Novo-Selegiline[CAN], Selgene[AUS])
Do not confuse with enalapril or Stelazine.

CATEGORY AND SCHEDULE
Pregnancy Risk Category: C

MECHANISM OF ACTION
An antiparkinson agent that irreversibly inhibits MAO type B activity. Increases dopaminergic action. *Therapeutic Effect:* Assists in reduction in tremor, akinesia or absence of sense of movement, posture and equilibrium disorders, rigidity of parkinsonism.

PHARMACOKINETICS
Rapidly absorbed from the gastrointestinal (GI) tract. Crosses blood-brain barrier. Metabolized in liver to active metabolites. Primarily excreted in urine. **Half-life:** (amphetamine): 17 hrs, (methamphetamine): 20 hrs.

AVAILABILITY
Capsules: 5 mg.
Tablets: 5 mg.

INDICATIONS AND DOSAGES
▸ **Adjunctive therapy for Parkinsonism**
PO
Adults. 10 mg/day in divided doses, such as 5 mg at breakfast and lunch.
Elderly. Initially, 5 mg in morning. May increase up to 10 mg/day.

CONTRAINDICATIONS
None known

INTERACTIONS
Drug
Fluoxetine: May cause mania, serotonin syndrome, marked by diaphoresis, diarrhea, fever, mental changes, and restlessness.
Meperidine: May cause a potentially fatal reaction, in addition to coma, diaphoresis, excitation, hypertension or hypotension.
Herbal
None known.
Food
Tyramine-rich foods: May produce hypertensive reactions.

DIAGNOSTIC TEST EFFECTS
None known.

SIDE EFFECTS
Frequent (10%–4%)
Nausea, dizziness, lightheadedness, faintness, abdominal discomfort
Occasional (3%–2%)
Confusion, hallucinations, dry mouth, vivid dreams, dyskinesia, manifested by impairment of voluntary movement
Rare (1%)
Headache, generalized aches, anxiety, diarrhea, insomnia

SERIOUS REACTIONS
• Overdosage may vary from central nervous system (CNS) depression, characterized by sedation, apnea, cardiovascular collapse, death to severe paradoxical reaction, such as hallucinations, tremor, seizures.
• Impaired motor coordination, including loss of balance, blepharospasm or blinking, facial grimace, feeling of heavy leg or stiff neck, and involuntary movements, hallucinations, confusion, depression, nightmares, delusions, overstimulation, sleep disturbance, and anger occur in some patients.

NURSING CONSIDERATIONS
Baseline Assessment
• Assess the patient for Parkinson symptoms, such as masklike facial expression, muscular rigidity, shuffling gait, and resting tremors of hands and head.
• Obtain baseline vital signs, especially blood pressure (B/P).
Lifespan Considerations
• Be aware that it is unknown if selegiline crosses the placenta or is distributed in breast milk.
• Be aware that the safety and efficacy of selegiline have not been established in children.
• There are no age-related precautions noted in the elderly.
Precautions
• Use cautiously in patients with cardiac arrhythmias, dementia, history of peptic ulcer disease, profound tremor, psychosis, and tardive dyskinesia.
Administration and Handling
PO
• Expect to administer with levodopa/carbidopa therapy.
◀ALERT▶ Keep in mind that therapy should begin with the lowest dosage, then increase in gradually over 3 to 4 weeks.
Intervention and Evaluation
• Be alert to neurologic effects including agitation, headache, lethargy, and mental confusion.
• Monitor the patient for dyskinesia or difficulty with movement.
• Assess the patient for clinical reversal of symptoms, improvement of masklike facial expression, muscular rigidity, shuffling gait, and tremor of hands and head at rest.
Patient Teaching
• Explain to the patient that a tolerance to the feeling of lightheadedness develops during therapy.
• Instruct the patient to rise slowly

from lying to sitting position and permit legs to dangle momentarily before standing to reduce the hypotensive effect of selegiline.
• Warn the patient to avoid tasks that require mental alertness or motor skills until his or her response to the drug is established.
• Tell the patient that dizziness, drowsiness, and dry mouth may be expected responses to the drug.
• Warn the patient to avoid alcoholic beverages during therapy.
• Suggest drinking coffee or tea with caffeine to help reduce drowsiness.
• Instruct the patient to avoid tyramine rich foods, such as wine and aged cheese to prevent a hypertensive reaction.

tolcapone
toll-cah-pone
(Tasmar)

CATEGORY AND SCHEDULE
Pregnancy Risk Category: C

MECHANISM OF ACTION
An antidyskinetic that inhibits the enzyme catechol-*O*-methyltransferase (COMT), sustaining plasma levels and thereby increasing the duration of action of levodopa, resulting in greater effect. *Therapeutic Effect:* Relieves signs and symptoms of Parkinson's disease.

PHARMACOKINETICS
Rapidly absorbed after PO administration. Protein binding: 99%. Metabolized in liver. Eliminated primarily in urine (60%) and to a lesser amount (40%) in feces. Un-

known if removed by hemodialysis. **Half-life:** 2–3 hrs.

AVAILABILITY
Tablets: 100 mg, 200 mg.

INDICATIONS AND DOSAGES
▸ **Adjunctive therapy for Parkinson's disease**
PO
Adults, Elderly. Initially, 100–200 mg 3 times/day. Maximum: 600 mg/day. For those with moderate to severe cirrhosis of liver, do not increase to more than 200 mg 3 times/day.

CONTRAINDICATIONS
None known

INTERACTIONS
Drug
Levodopa: Increases the duration of action of this drug.
Herbal
None known.
Food
Food given 1 hr before or 2 hrs after tolcapone administration decreases bioavailability by 10%–20%.

DIAGNOSTIC TEST EFFECTS
May increase SGOT (AST) and SGPT (ALT) levels.

SIDE EFFECTS
◂**ALERT**▸ Frequency of occurrence increases with dosage amount. Following is based on 200-mg dose.
Frequent
Nausea (35%)
Frequent (25%–16%)
Insomnia, somnolence, anorexia, diarrhea, muscle cramps, orthostatic hypotension, excessive dreaming
Occasional (11%–4%)
Headache, vomiting, confusion, hallucinations, constipation, diapho-

resis, urine discoloration (bright yellow), dry eyes, abdominal pain, dizziness, flatulence

Rare (3%–2%)

Dyspepsia, neck pain, hypotension, fatigue, chest discomfort

SERIOUS REACTIONS

• Upper respiratory infection and urinary tract infection occur occasionally (7%–5%).

• Too rapid withdrawal from therapy may produce withdrawal emergent hyperpyrexia characterized by elevated temperature, muscular rigidity, and altered consciousness.

• An increase in dyskinesia or impaired voluntary movement or dystonia or impaired muscular tone occurs frequently.

NURSING CONSIDERATIONS

Baseline Assessment

• Monitor the patient's serum transaminase levels every 2 weeks for the first year, every 4 weeks for the next 6 months, and every 8 weeks thereafter.

• Plan to discontinue treatment if the patient's SGPT (ALT) exceeds the upper limit of normal or clinical signs of the onset of liver failure appear.

• Plan to reduce the levodopa dosage if the patient experiences hallucinations. Keep in mind that hallucinations generally are accompanied by confusion and, to a lesser extent, insomnia.

Lifespan Considerations

• Be aware that it is unknown if tolcapone is distributed in breast milk.

• Be aware that tolcapone is not used in children.

• The elderly may have increased risk of hallucinations with this drug.

Precautions

• Use cautiously in patients with baseline hypotension, history of hallucinations or orthostatic hypotension, and severe liver or renal impairment.

Administration and Handling

◀ALERT▶ Plan to combine tolcapone with either the immediate or sustained-release form of levodopa/carbidopa.

PO

• Give tolcapone without regard to food.

Intervention and Evaluation

• Instruct the patient to rise from lying to sitting or sitting to standing position slowly to prevent risk of postural hypotension.

• Assist the patient with ambulation if he or she experiences dizziness.

• Assess the patient for relief of symptoms, such as improvement of masklike facial expression, muscular rigidity, shuffling gait, and tremor of hands and head at rest.

Patient Teaching

• Tell the patient if he or she experiences nausea to take tolcapone with food.

• Explain to the patient that dizziness, drowsiness, or nausea may be initial responses to the drug but will diminish or disappear with continued treatment.

• Tell the patient that postural hypotension may occur more frequently during initial therapy.

• Warn the patient to avoid tasks that require mental alertness or motor skills until his or her response to the drug is established.

• Explain to the patient that he or she may experience hallucinations and that this side effect occurs more in elderly than in younger patients with Parkinson's disease and typically within the first 2 weeks of therapy.

- Caution the patient to notify the physician if she becomes pregnant or is planning to become pregnant.
- Tell the patient that his or her urine will turn bright yellow.
- Warn the patient to notify the physician if he or she experiences abnormal contractions of the head, neck, or trunk, dark urine, falls, fatigue, itching, loss of appetite, persistent nausea, or yellowing of the skin and sclera of the eyes.

aripiprazole
chlorpromazine
clozapine
haloperidol
mesoridazine besylate
olanzapine
quetiapine
risperidone
thioridazine
thiothixene
trifluoperazine
  hydrochloride
ziprasidone

Uses: Antipsychotics are used primarily to manage psychotic illness, especially in patients with increased psychomotor activity. They're also used to treat the manic phase of bipolar disorder, behavioral problems in children, nausea and vomiting, intractable hiccups, anxiety, and agitation. In addition, these agents are used to potentiate the effects of narcotics and, as adjuncts, to treat tetanus.

Action: Antipsychotic agents produce effects at all levels of the central nervous system (CNS). Although their exact mechanism of action is unknown, they may antagonize the action of dopamine as a neurotransmitter in the basal ganglia and limbic system. Antipsychotics may block postsynaptic dopamine receptors, inhibit dopamine release, or increase dopamine turnover.

This class of drugs can be divided into phenothiazines and nonphenothiazines. Besides their use in treating the symptoms of psychiatric illness, some have antiemetic, antinausea, antihistamine, anticholinergic, or sedative effects.

aripiprazole
air-ee-**pip**-rah-zole
(Abilify)

CATEGORY AND SCHEDULE
Pregnancy Risk Category: C

MECHANISM OF ACTION
An antipsychotic agent that provides partial agonist activity at dopamine and serotonin (5-HT$_{1A}$) receptors and antagonist activity at serotonin (5-HT$_{2A}$) receptors. *Therapeutic Effect:* Improves and achieves target goals in schizophrenia.

PHARMACOKINETICS
Well absorbed through the gastrointestinal (GI) tract. Reaches steady levels reached in 2 wks. Metabolized in liver. Protein binding: 99%, primarily albumin. Eliminated primarily in the feces with a lesser extent excreted in the urine. **Half-life:** 75 hrs. Not removed by hemodialysis.

AVAILABILITY
Tablets: 10 mg, 15 mg, 20 mg, 30 mg.

INDICATIONS AND DOSAGES
▸ **Treatment of schizophrenia**
PO
Adults, Elderly. Initially, 10–15 mg once a day. May increase up to 30 mg/day.

UNLABELED USES
Schizoaffective disorder

CONTRAINDICATIONS
None known

INTERACTIONS
Drug
Carbamazepine: May decrease the concentration of aripiprazole.
Fluoxetine, ketoconazole, quinidine, paroxetine: May increase aripiprazole blood concentration.
Herbal
None known.
Food
None known.

DIAGNOSTIC TEST EFFECTS
None known.

SIDE EFFECTS
Frequent (11%–5%)
Weight gain, headache, insomnia, vomiting
Occasional (4%–3%)
Lightheadedness, nausea, akathisia or motor restlessness, somnolence
Rare (2% or less)
Blurred vision, constipation, asthenia or loss of energy and strength, anxiety, fever, rash, cough, rhinitis, orthostatic hypotension

SERIOUS REACTIONS
• Extrapyramidal symptoms and neuroleptic malignant syndrome occur rarely.

NURSING CONSIDERATIONS

Baseline Assessment
• Assess the patient's appearance, behavior, emotional status, response to environment, speech pattern, and thought content.
• Correct dehydration and hypovolemia in the patient, if experienced.

Lifespan Considerations
• Be aware that it is unknown if aripiprazole crosses the placenta. Aripiprazole may be distributed in breast milk, female patients should avoid breast-feeding.
• Be aware that the safety and efficacy of aripiprazole have not been established in children.
• There are no age-related precautions noted in the elderly.
Precautions
• Use cautiously in patients concurrently using central nervous system (CNS) depressants, including alcohol.
• Use cautiously in patients with cardiovascular or cerebrovascular diseases because it may induce hypotension, history of conditions that may lower seizure threshold, such as Alzheimer disease or seizures, liver or renal impairment, and Parkinson's disease because of potential for exacerbation.
Administration and Handling
◀ALERT▶ Keep in mind that dosage adjustment should not be made at intervals of less than 2 weeks.
Schizophrenia
PO
• May give aripiprazole without regard to meals.

Intervention and Evaluation
• Periodically monitor the patient's weight.
• Monitor the patient for extrapyramidal symptoms and tardive dyskinesia, manifested as chewing or puckering of the mouth, puffing of the cheeks, or protrusion of tongue.
• Periodically monitor the patient's blood pressure (B/P) and pulse, particularly in patients with preexisting cardiovascular disease.
• Assess the patient for therapeutic response, greater interest in surroundings, improved self-care,

increased ability to concentrate, and relaxed facial expression.

Patient Teaching
• Urge the patient to avoid alcohol during aripiprazole therapy.
• Warn the patient to avoid tasks that require mental alertness or motor skills until his or her response to aripiprazole is established.

---

chlorpromazine
See antiemetics

---

clozapine
klow-zah-peen
(Clopine[AUS], Clozaril)
Do not confuse with Clinoril, Cloxapen, or Colazal.

CATEGORY AND SCHEDULE
Pregnancy Risk Category: B

MECHANISM OF ACTION
A dibenzodiazepine derivative that interferes with the binding of dopamine at dopamine receptor sites, binds primarily at nondopamine receptor sites. *Therapeutic Effect:* Diminishes schizophrenic behavior.

AVAILABILITY
Tablets: 25 mg, 100 mg.

INDICATIONS AND DOSAGES
▶ **Schizophrenic disorders**
PO
Adults. Initially, 25 mg 1–2 times/day. May increase by 25–50 mg/day over 2 wks until dosage of 300–450 mg/day achieved. May further increase dosage by 50–100 mg/day no more frequently than 1–2 times/wk. Range: 200–600 mg/day. Maximum: 900 mg/day.

Elderly. Initially, 25 mg/day. May increase by 25 mg/day. Maximum: 450 mg/day.

CONTRAINDICATIONS
Comatose state, concurrent administration with other drugs having potential to suppress bone marrow function, history of clozapine-induced agranulocytosis or severe granulocytopenia, myeloproliferative disorders, severe central nervous system (CNS) depression

INTERACTIONS
Drug
Alcohol, CNS depressants: May increase CNS depressant effects.
Bone marrow depressants: May increase myelosuppression.
Lithium: May increase the risk of confusion, dyskinesias, and seizures.
Phenobarbital: Decreases clozapine blood concentration.
Herbal
None known.
Food
None known.

DIAGNOSTIC TEST EFFECTS
None known.

SIDE EFFECTS
Frequent
Drowsiness (39%), salivation (31%), tachycardia (25%), dizziness (19%), constipation (14%)
Occasional
Hypotension (9%); headache (7%); tremor, syncope, sweating, dry mouth (6%); nausea, visual disturbances (5%); nightmares, restlessness, akinesia, agitation, hypertension, abdominal discomfort or heartburn, weight gain (4%)
Rare
Rigidity, confusion, fatigue, insomnia, diarrhea, rash

SERIOUS REACTIONS
• Seizures occur occasionally (3%).
• Overdosage produces CNS depression, including sedation, coma, and delirium, respiratory depression, and hypersalivation.
• Blood dyscrasias, particularly agranulocytosis, and mild leukopenia may occur.

NURSING CONSIDERATIONS
Baseline Assessment
• Obtain the patient's baseline white blood cell (WBC) count before beginning treatment and monitor the patient's WBC count every week for first 6 months of continuous therapy, then biweekly for patients with acceptable WBC counts.
• Assess the patient's appearance, behavior, emotional status, response to environment, speech pattern, and thought content.
Precautions
• Use cautiously in patients with alcohol withdrawal, cardiovascular disease, glaucoma, history of seizures, impaired liver, prostatic hypertrophy, renal or respiratory function, myocarditis, and urinary retention.
Administration and Handling
PO
• Give clozapine without regard to meals
Intervention and Evaluation
• Monitor the patient's blood pressure (B/P) for hypertension or hypotension.
• Assess the patient's heart rate for tachycardia, a common side effect.
• Monitor the patient's complete blood count (CBC) for blood dyscrasias manifested as anemia, neutropenia, pancytopenia, or thrombocytopenia.
• Closely supervise suicidal-risk patients during early therapy. As depression lessens, the patient's energy level improves, which increases the suicide potential.
• Assess the patient for therapeutic response, increased ability to concentrate, improvement in self care, interest in surroundings, and relaxed facial expression.
Patient Teaching
• Caution the patient against abruptly discontinuing clozapine.
• Tell the patient that drowsiness generally subsides during continued therapy.
• Warn the patient to avoid tasks that require mental alertness or motor skills until his or her response to the drug is established.
• Urge the patient to avoid alcohol during clozapine therapy.

haloperidol
hal-oh-**pear**-ih-dawl
(Apo-Haloperidol[CAN], Haldol, Novoperidol[CAN], Peridol[CAN], Serenace[AUS])
Do not confuse with Halcion, Halog, or Stadol.

CATEGORY AND SCHEDULE
Pregnancy Risk Category: C

MECHANISM OF ACTION
An antipsychotic, antiemetic, and antidyskinetic agent that competitively blocks postsynaptic dopamine receptors, interrupts nerve impulse movement, and increases turnover of brain dopamine. *Therapeutic Effect:* Produces tranquilizing effect. Strong extrapyramidal, antiemetic effects, weak anticholinergic, sedative effects.

PHARMACOKINETICS
Readily absorbed from the gastrointestinal (GI) tract. Protein binding:

92%. Extensively metabolized in liver. Primarily excreted in urine. Not removed by hemodialysis.
Half-life: PO: 12–37 hrs; IM: 17–25 hrs, IV: 10–19 hrs.

AVAILABILITY
Tablets: 0.5 mg, 1 mg, 2 mg, 5 mg, 10 mg, 20 mg.
Oral Concentrate: 2 mg/ml.
Injection: 5 mg/ml.
Injection (Decanoate): 50 mg/ml, 100 mg/ml.

INDICATIONS AND DOSAGES
▶ **Treatment of psychoses, Tourette's disorder, severe behavioral problems in children, emergency sedation of severely agitated or delirious patients**
PO
Adults. 0.5–5 mg 2–3 times/day. Maximum: 100 mg/day.
Elderly. Initially, 0.25–0.5 mg 1–2 times/day. May increase by 0.25–0.5 mg/day at weekly intervals.
Children 3–12 yrs, weighing 15–40 kg. Initially, 0.25–0.5 mg/day in divided doses. May increase by 0.25–0.5 mg q5–7 days. Maximum: 0.15 mg/kg/day.
IM/IV (lactate)
Adults. 2–5 mg q4–8h as needed.
Children 6–12 yrs. 1–3 mg/dose q4–8h. Maximum: 0.15 mg/kg/day.
IM (Decanoate)
Adults. 10–15 times stabilized oral dose given at 3-to 4-wk intervals.

UNLABELED USES
Treatment of Huntington's chorea, infantile autism, nausea or vomiting associated with cancer chemotherapy

CONTRAINDICATIONS
Bone marrow suppression, central nervous system (CNS) depression, narrow-angle glaucoma, parkinsonism, severe cardiac or liver disease

INTERACTIONS
Drug
Alcohol, CNS depressants: May increase CNS depression.
Epinephrine: May block alpha-adrenergic effects.
Extrapyramidal symptom (EPS)-producing medications: May increase EPS.
Lithium: May increase neurologic toxicity.
Herbal
None known.
Food
None known.

DIAGNOSTIC TEST EFFECTS
None known. Therapeutic serum level is 0.2–1 mcg/ml; toxic serum level is greater than 1 mcg/ml.

IV INCOMPATIBILITIES
Allopurinol (Aloprim), amphotericin B complex (Abelcet, AmBisome, Amphotec), cefepime (Maxipime), fluconazole (Diflucan), foscarnet (Foscavir), heparin, nitroprusside (Nipride), piperacillin-tazobactam (Zosyn)

IV COMPATIBILITIES
Dobutamine (Dobutrex), dopamine (Intropin), fentanyl (Sublimaze), hydromorphone (Dilaudid), lidocaine, lorazepam (Ativan), midazolam (Versed), morphine, nitroglycerin, norepinephrine (Levophed), propofol (Diprivan)

SIDE EFFECTS
Frequent
Blurred vision, constipation, orthostatic hypotension, dry mouth, swelling or soreness of female breasts, peripheral edema

Occasional

Allergic reaction, difficulty urinating, decreased thirst, dizziness, decreased sexual function, drowsiness, nausea, vomiting, photosensitivity, lethargy

SERIOUS REACTIONS

• Extrapyramidal symptoms appear to be dose-related and may be noted in first few days of therapy.

• Marked drowsiness and lethargy, excessive salivation, and fixed stare may be mild to severe in intensity.

• Less frequently seen are severe akathisia or motor restlessness and acute dystonias, such as torticollis or neck muscle spasm, opisthotonos or rigidity of back muscles, and oculogyric crisis or rolling back of eyes.

• Tardive dyskinesia or protrusion of tongue, puffing of cheeks, chewing or puckering of the mouth may occur during long-term administration or after drug discontinuance and may be irreversible. Risk is greater in female geriatric patients. Abrupt withdrawal after long-term therapy may provoke transient dyskinesia signs.

NURSING CONSIDERATIONS

Baseline Assessment

• Assess the patient's appearance, behavior, emotional status, response to environment, speech pattern, and thought content.

Lifespan Considerations

• Be aware that haloperidol crosses the placenta and is distributed in breast milk.

• Be aware that children are more susceptible to dystonias and haloperidol use is not recommended in children younger than 3 years.

• The elderly are more susceptible to anticholinergic effects and sedation, increased risk for extrapyramidal effects, and orthostatic hypotension. A decreased dosage is recommended in the elderly.

Precautions

• Use cautiously in patients with cardiovascular disease, history of seizures, and liver or renal dysfunction.

Administration and Handling

PO

• Give haloperidol without regard to meals.

• Crush scored tablets as needed.

IM

• Patient must remain recumbent for 30 to 60 minutes in head-low position with legs raised to minimize hypotensive effect.

• Prepare haloperidol decanoate IM injection using 21-gauge needle.

• Do not exceed maximum volume of 3 ml per IM injection site.

• Give IM injection deeply and slowly into the upper, outer quadrant of gluteus maximus.

IV

◀ ALERT ▶ Only haloperidol lactate is given IV.

• Discard if precipitate forms, discoloration occurs.

• Store at room temperature.

• Protect from light, do not freeze.

• May give undiluted for IV push.

• Flush with at least 2 ml 0.9% NaCl before and after administration.

• May add to 30 to 50 ml most solutions—D_5W preferred.

• Give IV push at rate of 5 mg/min.

• Infuse IV piggyback over 30 minutes.

• For IV infusion, up to 25 mg/hr has been used, titrated to patient response.

Intervention and Evaluation

• Closely supervise suicidal-risk patients during early therapy. As depression lessens, the patient's

energy level improves, which increases the suicide potential.
• Monitor the patient for fine tongue movement, masklike facial expression, rigidity, and tremor.
• Assess the patient for therapeutic response, including improvement in self care, increased ability to concentrate, interest in surroundings, and relaxed facial expression.
• Know that the therapeutic serum level for haloperidol is 0.2 to 1 mcg/ml, and the toxic serum level of haloperidol is greater than 1 mcg/ml.

Patient Teaching
• Tell the patient that the drug's full therapeutic effect may take up to 6 weeks to appear.
• Caution the patient against abruptly discontinuing the drug from long-term drug therapy.
• Suggest sips of tepid water and sugarless gum to patients to help relieve dry mouth.
• Tell the patient that drowsiness generally subsides during continued therapy.
• Warn the patient to avoid tasks that require mental alertness or motor skills until his or her response to the drug is established.
• Urge the patient to avoid alcohol during haloperidol therapy.
• Warn the patient to notify the physician if he or she experiences muscle stiffness.
• Explain to the patient to avoid exposure to sunlight and any conditions that may cause dehydration or be overheating because of an increased risk of heat stroke.

mesoridazine besylate
mess-oh-**rid**-ah-zeen
(Serentil)
Do not confuse with Proventil or Serevent.

CATEGORY AND SCHEDULE
Pregnancy Risk Category: C

MECHANISM OF ACTION
A phenothiazine that blocks dopamine at postsynaptic receptor sites in brain. Possesses anticholinergic, sedative effects. *Therapeutic Effect:* Suppresses behavioral response in psychosis.

AVAILABILITY
Tablets: 10 mg, 25 mg, 50 mg, 100 mg.
Oral Solutions: 25 mg/ml.
Injection: 25 mg/ml.

INDICATIONS AND DOSAGES
▶ **Schizophrenia**
PO
Adults, Elderly. 25–50 mg 3 times/day. Maximum: 400 mg/day.
IM
Adults, Elderly. Initially, 25 mg. May repeat in 30–60 min. Range: 25–200 mg.
▶ **Behavioral symptoms**
PO
Elderly. Initially, 10 mg 1–2 times/day. May increase at 4–7 day intervals. Maximum: 250 mg.
IM
Adults, Elderly. Initially, 25 mg. May repeat in 30–60 min. Range: 25–200 mg.

CONTRAINDICATIONS
Bone marrow depression, comatose states, severe cardiovascular disease, severe central nervous system

(CNS) depression, subcortical brain damage

INTERACTIONS
Drug
Alcohol, CNS depressants: May increase CNS and respiratory depression, and the hypotensive effects of mesoridazine.

Antithyroid agents: May increase the risk of agranulocytosis.

Extrapyramidal symptoms (EPS)-producing medications: May increase EPS.

Hypotensives: May increase hypotension.

Levodopa: May decrease the effects of levodopa.

Lithium: May decrease the absorption of mesoridazine and produce adverse neurologic effects.

MAOIs, tricyclic antidepressants: May increase the anticholinergic and sedative effects of mesoridazine.

Herbal
None known.

Food
None known.

DIAGNOSTIC TEST EFFECTS
May produce false-positive pregnancy test, PKU. EKG changes may occur, including QRS prolongation and T-wave disturbances.

SIDE EFFECTS
Frequent
Orthostatic hypotension, dizziness, syncope occur frequently after first injection, occasionally after subsequent injections, and rarely with oral dosage

Occasional
Drowsiness during early therapy, dry mouth, blurred vision, lethargy, constipation or diarrhea, nasal congestion, peripheral edema, urinary retention

Rare
Ocular changes, skin pigmentation for those taking high dosages for prolonged periods

SERIOUS REACTIONS
• Abrupt withdrawal following long-term therapy may precipitate nausea, vomiting, gastritis, dizziness, and tremors.
• Blood dyscrasias, particularly agranulocytosis, and mild leukopenia may occur.
• May lower seizure threshold.

NURSING CONSIDERATIONS
Baseline Assessment
• Avoid skin contact with solution because it may cause contact dermatitis.
• Assess the patient's appearance, behavior, emotional status, response to environment, speech pattern, and thought content.
• Expect to perform a baseline EKG and measure the QT interval. Calculate the QTc.
Precautions
• Use cautiously in patients with alcohol withdrawal, glaucoma, history of seizures, impaired cardiac, liver, renal or respiratory function, prostatic hypertrophy, and urinary retention.
Intervention and Evaluation
• Assess the patient for orthostatic hypotension.
• Assess the patient's daily pattern of bowel activity and stool consistency.
• Closely supervise suicidal-risk patients during early therapy. As depression lessens, the patient's energy level improves, which increases the suicide potential.
• Assess the patient for therapeutic response, improvement in self-care,

increased ability to concentrate, interest in surroundings, and relaxed facial expression.

Patient Teaching
• Explain to the patient that the drug's full therapeutic effect may take up to 6 weeks to appear.
• Tell the patient that his or her urine may become pink or reddish brown.
• Caution the patient against abruptly withdrawing from long-term drug therapy.
• Warn the patient to notify the physician if he or she experiences visual disturbances.
• Explain to the patient that drowsiness generally subsides during continued therapy.
• Urge the patient not to use alcohol or other CNS depressants during mesoridazine therapy.

olanzapine
oh-**lan**-sah-peen
(Zyprexa, Zyprexa Zydis)
Do not confuse with olsalazine or Zyrtec.

CATEGORY AND SCHEDULE
Pregnancy Risk Category: C

MECHANISM OF ACTION
A dibenzepin derivative that antagonizes alpha$_1$–adrenergic, dopamine, histamine, muscarinic, and serotonin receptors. Produces anticholinergic, histaminic, central nervous system (CNS) depressant effects. *Therapeutic Effect:* Diminishes psychotic disorders.

PHARMACOKINETICS
Well absorbed after PO administration. Protein binding: 93%. Extensively distributed throughout body. Extensively metabolized by first-pass liver metabolism. Excreted in urine, with lesser amount eliminated in feces. Not removed by dialysis. **Half-life:** 21–54 hrs.

AVAILABILITY
Tablets: 2.5 mg, 5 mg, 7.5 mg, 10 mg, 15 mg, 20 mg.
Oral Disintegrating Tablets: 5 mg, 10 mg, 15 mg, 20 mg.

INDICATIONS AND DOSAGES
▶ **Schizophrenia**
PO
Adults. Initially, 5–10 mg once daily. May increase by 10 mg/day at 5–7 day intervals, then by 5–10 mg/day at 7 day intervals. Range: 10–30 mg/day.
Elderly. Initially, 2.5 mg/day. May increase as indicated. Range: 2.5–10 mg/day.
▶ **Bipolar mania**
PO
Adults. Initially, 10–15 mg/day. May increase by 5 mg/day by intervals not less than 24 hrs. Maximum: 20 mg/day.
▶ **Debilitated, predisposition to hypotensive reactions, elderly older than 65 yrs**
PO
Adults, Elderly. Initially, 5 mg/day.

UNLABELED USES
Anorexia, maintenance of treatment response in schizophrenic patients

CONTRAINDICATIONS
None known

INTERACTIONS
Drug
Alcohol, central nervous system (CNS) depressants: May increase CNS depressant effects.
Antihypertensive agents: Increase risk of hypotensive effect.

Carbamazepine: Increases the clearance of olanzapine.
Ciprofloxacin (quinolone), fluvoxamine: May increase olanzapine blood concentrations.
Dopamine agonists, levodopa: Antagonizes the effects of dopamine agonists and levodopa.
Imipramine, theophylline: May inhibit the metabolism of imipramine and theophylline.
Herbal
None known.
Food
None known.

DIAGNOSTIC TEST EFFECTS
May significantly increase GGT, prolactin, SGOT (AST), and SGPT (ALT) levels.

SIDE EFFECTS
Frequent
Somnolence (26%), agitation (23%), insomnia (20%), headache (17%), nervousness (16%), hostility (15%), dizziness (11%), rhinitis (10%)
Occasional
Anxiety, constipation (9%); nonaggressive objectionable behavior (8%); dry mouth (7%); weight gain (6%); postural hypotension, fever, joint pain, restlessness, cough, pharyngitis, dimness of vision (5%)
Rare
Tachycardia, back, chest, or abdominal pain, tremor, extremity pain

SERIOUS REACTIONS
• Seizures occur rarely.
• Neuroleptic malignant syndrome (NMS), a potentially fatal syndrome, occurs rarely and may present as hyperpyrexia, muscle rigidity, irregular pulse or blood pressure (B/P), tachycardia, diaphoresis, and cardiac arrhythmias.
• Extrapyramidal symptoms may occur.

• Dysphagia, marked by esophageal dysmotility and aspiration, may be noted.
• Overdosage (300 mg) produces drowsiness and slurred speech.

NURSING CONSIDERATIONS
Baseline Assessment
• Obtain the patient's baseline liver function lab values before beginning olanzapine treatment, as ordered.
• Assess the patient's appearance, behavior, emotional status, response to environment, speech pattern, and thought content.
Lifespan Considerations
• Be aware that it is unknown if olanzapine crosses the placenta or is distributed in breast milk.
• Be aware that the safety and efficacy of olanzapine have not been established in children.
• There are no age-related precautions noted in the elderly.
Precautions
• Use cautiously in patients with cerebrovascular disease, conditions lowering seizure threshold, such as Alzheimer's dementia, conditions predisposing patients to hypotension, such as dehydration, hypovolemia, and antihypertensive medications, history of seizures, hypersensitivity to clozapine, known cardiovascular disease, such as conduction abnormalities, history of ischemia or myocardial infarction (MI), and heart failure, and liver function impairment.
• Use cautiously in elderly patients and patients concurrently taking potentially liver toxic drugs or who are at risk of aspiration pneumonia.
• Use cautiously in patients after a dose escalation.
• Use cautiously in patients who should avoid anticholinergics, such

as patients with benign prostatic hypertrophy.

Administration and Handling

PO

• Give olanzapine without regard to meals.

Intervention and Evaluation

• Monitor the patient's blood pressure (B/P).

• Assess the patient for abnormal movements in trunk, neck, extremities, changes in gait, target behaviors, and tremors.

• Closely supervise suicidal-risk patients during early therapy. As depression lessens, the patient's energy level improves, which increases the suicide potential.

• Assess the patient for therapeutic response, improvement in self-care, increased ability to concentrate, interest in surroundings, and relaxed facial expression.

• Assist the patient with ambulation if he or she experiences dizziness.

• Assess the patient's sleep pattern.

• Monitor the patient for extrapyramidal symptoms (EPS). Notify the physician if the patient experiences EPS.

Patient Teaching

• Tell the patient to avoid dehydration, particularly during exercise, exposure to extreme heat, concurrent use of medication causing dry mouth, or other drying effects.

• Warn the patient to notify the physician if she becomes pregnant, or intends to become pregnant during olanzapine therapy.

• Instruct the patient to take olanzapine as ordered. Caution the patient against abruptly discontinuing the drug or increasing the drug dosage.

• Suggest sips of tepid water and sugarless gum to the patient to help relieve dry mouth.

• Explain to the patient that drowsiness generally subsides during continued therapy.

• Warn the patient to avoid tasks requiring mental alertness or motor skills until his or her response to the drug is established.

• Instruct the patient to maintain a healthy diet and exercise regimen to prevent weight gain.

quetiapine
kwe-**tie**-ah-peen
(Seroquel)

CATEGORY AND SCHEDULE
Pregnancy Risk Category: C

MECHANISM OF ACTION
A dibenzepin derivative that interacts with neurotransmitter receptors, including dopamine, serotonin, histamine, and alpha$_1$-adrenergic receptors. *Therapeutic Effect:* Diminishes psychotic disorders. Produces moderate sedation, few extrapyramidal effects, no anticholinergic effects.

PHARMACOKINETICS
Well absorbed after PO administration. Protein binding: 83%. Widely distributed in tissues; central nervous system (CNS) concentration exceeds plasma concentration. Extensively metabolized by first-pass liver metabolism. Primarily excreted in the urine. **Half-life:** 6 hrs.

AVAILABILITY
Tablets: 25 mg, 100 mg, 200 mg, 300 mg.

INDICATIONS AND DOSAGES
▸ **Psychiatric disorder**
PO
Adults, Elderly. Initially, 25 mg 2 times/day, then 25–50 mg

2–3 times a day on second and third days, up to 300–400 mg/day by the fourth day, given 2–3 times a day. Further adjustments of 25–50 mg 2 times/day made at 2-day or more intervals. Maintenance (adults): 300–800 mg/day; Maintenance (elderly): 50–200 mg/day.

CONTRAINDICATIONS
None known

INTERACTIONS
Drug
Alcohol, CNS depressants: May increase CNS depression.
Antihypertensives: May increase the effects of antihypertensives.
Liver enzyme inducers, such as phenytoin: May increase drug clearance.
Herbal
None known.
Food
None known.

DIAGNOSTIC TEST EFFECTS
May produce false-positive pregnancy test. May decrease serum total and free thyroxine (T_4) levels. May increase serum cholesterol, triglycerides, and transaminase levels, including SGOT (AST), SGPT (ALT).

SIDE EFFECTS
Frequent (19%–10%)
Headache, somnolence or drowsiness, dizziness
Occasional (9%–3%)
Constipation, postural hypotension, tachycardia, dry mouth, dyspepsia, rash, weakness, abdominal pain, rhinitis
Rare (2%)
Back pain, fever, weight gain

SERIOUS REACTIONS
• Overdosage produces heart block, characterized by a slow, irregular pulse, decreased blood pressure (B/P), hypokalemia, weakness, or tachycardia.

NURSING CONSIDERATIONS
Baseline Assessment
• Assess the patient's appearance, behavior, emotional status, response to environment, speech pattern, and thought content.
• Obtain the patient's baseline complete blood count (CBC) and serum blood chemistry to assess liver function before beginning treatment and periodically thereafter, as ordered.
Lifespan Considerations
• Be aware that it is unknown if quetiapine is distributed in breast milk. Quetiapine use is not recommended for breast-feeding women.
• Be aware that the safety and efficacy of quetiapine have not been established in children.
• There are no age-related precautions noted, but lower initial and target dosages may be necessary in the elderly.
Precautions
• Use cautiously in patients with Alzheimer's dementia, cardiovascular disease, such as congestive heart failure (CHF) or history of myocardial infarction (MI), cerebrovascular disease, dehydration, history of breast cancer, history of drug abuse or dependence, hypothyroidism, hypovolemia, impaired liver function, and seizures.
Administration and Handling
PO
• Know that dosage adjustments should occur at 2-day intervals.
• Initial dose and dosage titration should occur at a lower dosage in elderly, those with liver impairment,

debilitated, or those predisposed to hypotensive reactions.
• When restarting patients who have been off quetiapine for less than 1 week, titration is not required and maintenance dose can be reinstituted.
• When restarting patients who have been off quetiapine for longer than 1 week, follow initial titration schedule, as prescribed.
• Give quetiapine without regard to food.

Intervention and Evaluation
• Assist the patient with ambulation if he or she experiences dizziness.
• Closely supervise suicidal-risk patients during early therapy. As depression lessens, the patient's energy level improves, which increases the suicide potential.
• Monitor the patient's blood pressure (B/P) for hypotension.
• Assess the patient's pulse for tachycardia, especially with rapid increase in drug dosage.
• Monitor the patient's complete blood count (CBC) for blood dyscrasias manifested as anemia, neutropenia, pancytopenia, or thrombocytopenia.
• Assess the patient's daily pattern of bowel activity and stool consistency.
• Assess the patient for therapeutic response, improved thought content, improved self-care, and increased ability to concentrate.

Patient Teaching
• Urge the patient to avoid alcohol and exposure to extreme heat.
• Tell the patient to drink fluids often, especially during physical activity.
• Instruct the patient to take quetiapine as ordered. Caution the patient against abruptly discontinuing the drug or increasing the drug dosage.

• Explain to the patient that drowsiness generally subsides during continued therapy.
• Warn the patient to avoid performing tasks that require mental alertness or motor skills until his or her response to the drug is established.
• Instruct the patient to change positions slowly to reduce the hypotensive effect of quetiapine.

risperidone
ris-**pear**-ih-doan
(Risperdal, Risperdal Consta, Risperdol M-Tabs)
Do not confuse with reserpine.

CATEGORY AND SCHEDULE
Pregnancy Risk Category: C

MECHANISM OF ACTION
A benzisoxazole derivative whose action may be due to dopamine and serotonin receptor antagonism. *Therapeutic Effect:* Suppresses behavioral response in psychosis.

PHARMACOKINETICS
Well absorbed from the gastrointestinal (GI) tract and is unaffected by food. Protein binding: 90%. Extensively metabolized in liver to active metabolite. Primarily excreted in urine. **Half-life:** 3–20 hrs; metabolite: 21–30 hrs (half-life is increased in elderly).

AVAILABILITY
Injection: 25 mg, 37.5 mg, 50 mg.
Tablets: 0.25 mg, 0.5 mg, 1 mg, 2 mg, 3 mg, 4 mg.
M-Tabs: 0.5 mg, 1 mg, 2 mg.
Oral Solution: 1 mg/ml

INDICATIONS AND DOSAGES
▶ **Psychotic disorder**
PO
Adults. Initially, 0.5–1 mg 2 times/day. May increase slowly.
Elderly. Initially, 0.25–2 mg/day in 1–2 divided doses. May increase slowly. Range: 2–6 mg/day.
IM
Adults, Elderly. 25 mg q2wks. Maximum: 50 mg q2wks.
▶ **Dosage in renal impairment**
PO
Adults, Elderly. Initially, 0.25–0.5 mg 2 times/day. Titrate slowly to desired effect.

CONTRAINDICATIONS
None known

INTERACTIONS
Drug
Alcohol, central nervous system (CNS) depressants: May increase CNS depression.
Carbamazepine: May decrease risperidone blood concentration.
Clozapine: May increase risperidone blood concentration.
Dopamine agonists, levodopa: May decrease the effects of dopamine agonists and levodopa.
Paroxetine: Can increase risperidone blood concentration and risk of extrapyramidal symptoms (EPS).
Herbal
None known.
Food
None known.

DIAGNOSTIC TEST EFFECTS
May increase prolactin, serum creatine phosphatase, uric acid, SGOT (AST), SGPT (ALT), and triglyceride levels. May decrease blood glucose levels, serum potassium, protein, and sodium levels. May cause EKG changes.

SIDE EFFECTS
Frequent (26%–13%)
Agitation, anxiety, insomnia, headache, constipation
Occasional (10%–4%)
Dyspepsia, rhinitis, drowsiness, dizziness, nausea, vomiting, rash, abdominal pain, dry skin, tachycardia
Rare (3%–2%)
Visual disturbances, fever, back pain, pharyngitis, cough, arthralgia, angina, aggressive reaction

SERIOUS REACTIONS
• Neuroleptic malignant syndrome (NMS), marked by hyperpyrexia, muscle rigidity, change in mental status, irregular pulse or blood pressure (B/P), tachycardia, diaphoresis, cardiac arrhythmias, rhabdomyolysis, and acute renal failure, and tardive dyskinesia, characterized by protrusion of tongue, puffing of cheeks, and chewing or puckering of the mouth may occur.

NURSING CONSIDERATIONS
Baseline Assessment
• Draw a blood serum chemistry value including BUN, serum alkaline phosphatase, bilirubin, creatinine, SGOT (AST), and SGPT (ALT) levels to assess liver and renal function before beginning risperidone therapy, as ordered.
• Assess the patient's appearance, behavior, emotional status, response to environment, speech pattern, and thought content.
Lifespan Considerations
• Be aware that it is unknown if risperidone crosses the placenta or is excreted in breast milk. Breastfeeding is not recommended in this patient population.
• Be aware that the safety and efficacy of this drug have not been established in children.

• The elderly are more susceptible to postural hypotension.
• In the elderly, age-related renal or liver impairment may require dosage adjustment.

Precautions
• Use cautiously in patients with cardiac disease, breast cancer, liver or renal impairment, recent myocardial infarction (MI), risk for aspiration pneumonia, seizure disorders, and suicidal patients.
• Use cautiously in patients with dementia. Risperidone use in these patients may increase the risk of stroke.

Administration and Handling
PO
• Give risperidone without regard to food.
• May mix oral solution with coffee, low-fat milk, orange juice, and water. Do not mix with cola or tea.

Intervention and Evaluation
• Monitor the patient's B/P, heart rate, liver function tests, EKG, and weight.
• Monitor the patient for fine tongue movement, which may be the first sign of irreversible tardive dyskinesia.
• Closely supervise suicidal-risk patients during early therapy. As depression lessens, the patient's energy level improves, which increases the suicide potential.
• Assess the patient for therapeutic response, greater interest in surroundings, improved self-care, increased ability to concentrate, and relaxed facial expression.
• Monitor the patient for potential neuroleptic malignant syndrome (NMS) manifested as altered mental status, fever, irregular B/P or pulse, and muscle rigidity.

Patient Teaching
• Tell the patient that risperidone may cause dizziness or drowsiness.

• Warn the patient to avoid tasks that may require mental alertness or motor skills until his or her response to the drug has been established.
• Urge the patient to avoid alcohol during risperidone therapy.
• Instruct the patient to use caution when changing position from lying or sitting to standing.
• Warn the patient to notify the physician if he or she experiences altered gait, difficulty breathing, palpitations, rash, pain or swelling in breasts, severe dizziness or fainting, trembling fingers, unusual muscle or skeletal movements, and visual changes.

thioridazine
thigh-oh-**rid**-ah-zeen
(Aldazine[AUS], Apo-Thioridazine[CAN], Mellaril, Melleril[AUS])
Do not confuse with Mebaral, thiothixene, or Thorazine.

CATEGORY AND SCHEDULE
Pregnancy Risk Category: C

MECHANISM OF ACTION
A phenothiazine that blocks dopamine at postsynaptic receptor sites. Possesses strong anticholinergic, sedative effects. *Therapeutic Effect:* Suppresses behavioral response in psychosis, reducing locomotor activity, aggressiveness and suppressing conditioned responses.

AVAILABILITY
Tablets: 10 mg, 15 mg, 100 mg, 150 mg, 200 mg.
Oral Solution (concentrate): 30 mg/ml.

INDICATIONS AND DOSAGES
▶ **Psychosis**
PO
Adults, Elderly, Children older than 12 yrs. Initially, 25–100 mg 3 times/day. Gradually increase. Maximum: 800 mg/day.
Children 2–12 yrs. Initially, 0.5 mg/kg/day in 2–3 divided doses. Maximum: 3 mg/kg/day.

UNLABELED USES
Behavioral problems in children, dementia, depressive neurosis

CONTRAINDICATIONS
Drugs that prolong QT interval, cardiac arrhythmias, severe central nervous system (CNS) depression, narrow-angle glaucoma, blood dyscrasias, liver or cardiac impairment

INTERACTIONS
Drug
Alcohol, CNS depressants: May increase respiratory depression and the hypotensive effects of thioridazine.
Antithyroid agents: May increase the risk of agranulocytosis.
Extrapyramidal symptom (EPS)-producing medications: May increase EPS.
Hypotensives: May increase hypotension.
Levodopa: May decrease the effects of levodopa.
Lithium: May decrease the absorption of thioridazine and produce adverse neurologic effects.
MAOIs, tricyclic antidepressants: May increase the anticholinergic and sedative effects of thioridazine.
Herbal
None known.
Food
None known.

DIAGNOSTIC TEST EFFECTS
May cause EKG changes. Therapeutic serum level is 0.2–2.6 mcg/ml; toxic blood serum level is not established.

SIDE EFFECTS
Generally well tolerated with only mild and transient effects
Occasional
Drowsiness during early therapy, dry mouth, blurred vision, lethargy, constipation or diarrhea, nasal congestion, peripheral edema, urinary retention
Rare
Ocular changes, skin pigmentation in those taking high dosages for prolonged periods, photosensitivity

SERIOUS REACTIONS
• Prolongation of QT interval may produce torsades de pointes, a form of ventricular tachycardia, and sudden death.

NURSING CONSIDERATIONS
Baseline Assessment
• Avoid skin contact with solution because it can cause contact dermatitis.
• Assess the patient's appearance, behavior, emotional status, response to environment, speech pattern, and thought content.
• Plan to obtain a baseline EKG, and to measure the QT interval. Calculate the QTc.
Precautions
• Use cautiously in patients with seizures.
Intervention and Evaluation
• Assess the patient for EPS.
• Monitor the patient's blood pressure (B/P), complete blood count (CBC), EKG, eye exams, liver function test results, including serum alkaline phosphatase, bilirubin, potassium, and SGOT (AST) and SGPT (ALT) levels.

• Monitor the patient for fine tongue movement, which may be early sign of tardive dyskinesia.
• Closely supervise suicidal-risk patients during early therapy. As depression lessens, the patient's energy level improves, which increases the suicide potential.
• Assess the patient for therapeutic response, improvement in self care, increased ability to concentrate, interest in surroundings, and relaxed facial expression.
• Know the therapeutic serum level for thioridazine is 0.2 to 2.6 mcg/ml, and the toxic serum level for thioridazine is not established.

Patient Teaching
• Tell the patient that the drug's full therapeutic effect may take up to 6 weeks to appear.
• Explain to the patient that his or her urine may darken.
• Caution the patient against abruptly withdrawing from long-term drug therapy.
• Warn the patient to notify the physician if he or she experiences visual disturbances.
• Suggest sips of tepid water and sugarless gum to the patient to help relieve dry mouth.
• Explain to the patient that drowsiness generally subsides during continued therapy.
• Warn the patient to avoid tasks that require mental alertness or motor skills until his or her response to the drug is established.
• Urge the patient to avoid alcohol and exposure to artificial light and sunlight during thioridazine therapy.

thiothixene
thigh-oh-**thicks**-een
(Navane)
Do not confuse with thioridazine.

CATEGORY AND SCHEDULE
Pregnancy Risk Category: C

MECHANISM OF ACTION
An antipsychotic that blocks post-synaptic dopamine receptor sites in brain. Has alpha-adrenergic blocking effects; depresses release of hypothalamic, hypophyseal hormones. *Therapeutic Effect:* Suppresses behavioral response in psychosis.

PHARMACOKINETICS
Well absorbed from the gastrointestinal (GI) tract after IM administration. Widely distributed. Metabolized in liver. Primarily excreted in urine. Unknown if removed by hemodialysis. **Half-life:** 34 hrs.

AVAILABILITY
Capsules: 1 mg, 2 mg, 5 mg, 10 mg, 20 mg.
Oral Concentrate: 5 mg/ml.

INDICATIONS AND DOSAGES
▶ **Psychosis**
PO
Adults, Elderly, Children older than 12 yrs. Initially, 2 mg 3 times/day. Maximum: 60 mg/day.

CONTRAINDICATIONS
Blood dyscrasias, central nervous system (CNS) depression, circulatory collapse, comatose states, history of seizures

INTERACTIONS
Drug
Alcohol, CNS depressants:
May increase CNS and respira-

tory depression, and increase hypotension.

Extrapyramidal symptom (EPS)–producing medications: May increase risk of EPS.

Levodopa: May inhibit the effects of levodopa.

Quinidine: May increase cardiac effects with quinidine.

Herbal
Kava kava, St. John's wort, valerian: May increase CNS depression.

Food
None known.

DIAGNOSTIC TEST EFFECTS
May decrease serum uric acid.

SIDE EFFECTS
Expected
Hypotension, dizziness, fainting occur frequently after first injection, occasionally after subsequent injections, rarely with oral dosage
Frequent
Transient drowsiness, dry mouth, constipation, blurred vision, nasal congestion
Occasional
Diarrhea, peripheral edema, urinary retention, nausea
Rare
Ocular changes, skin pigmentation alterations with those taking high dosage for prolonged periods, photosensitivity

SERIOUS REACTIONS
• Akathisia or motor restlessness and anxiety is the most frequently noted extrapyramidal symptom.
• Occurring less frequently is akinesia or rigidity, tremor, salivation, masklike facial expression, and reduced voluntary movements.
• Infrequently noted are dystonias including torticollis or neck muscle spasm, opisthotonos or rigidity of

back muscles, and oculogyric crisis or rolling back of eyes.
• Tardive dyskinesia, characterized by protrusion of tongue, puffing of cheeks, and chewing or puckering of mouth, occurs rarely but may be irreversible. Tardive dyskinesia risk is greater in female geriatric patients.
• Grand mal seizures may occur in epileptic patients, with a higher risk noted with IM administration.
• Neuroleptic malignant syndrome occurs rarely.

NURSING CONSIDERATIONS
Baseline Assessment
• Assess the patient's appearance, behavior, emotional status, response to environment, speech pattern, and thought content.
Lifespan Considerations
• Be aware that thiothixene crosses the placenta and is distributed in breast milk.
• Be aware that children may develop extrapyramidal symptoms (EPS), or neuromuscular symptoms, especially dystonias.
• The elderly are more prone to anticholinergic effects, such as dry mouth, EPS, orthostatic hypotension, and sedation symptoms.
Precautions
• Use cautiously in patients with alcohol withdrawal, exposure to extreme heat, glaucoma, prostatic hypertrophy, and severe cardiovascular disorders.
Administration and Handling
PO
• Give thiothixene without regard to meals.
• Avoid skin contact with oral solution because it can cause contact dermatitis.
Intervention and Evaluation
• Closely supervise suicidal-risk patients during early therapy. As

depression lessens, the patient's energy level improves, which increases the suicide potential.
• Monitor the patient's blood pressure (B/P) for hypotension.
• Evaluate the patient for peripheral edema.
• Assess the patient's daily pattern of bowel activity and stool consistency.
• Monitor the patient for EPS, tardive dyskinesia, and potentially fatal, rare neuroleptic malignant syndrome, such as altered mental status, fever, irregular pulse or B/P, and muscle rigidity.
• Assess the patient for therapeutic response, improvement in self-care, increased ability to concentrate, interest in surroundings, and relaxed facial expression.

Patient Teaching
• Tell the patient that the drug's full therapeutic effect may take up to 6 weeks to appear.
• Warn the patient to notify the physician if he or she experiences visual disturbances.
• Suggest sips of tepid water and sugarless gum to the patient to help relieve dry mouth.
• Explain to the patient that drowsiness generally subsides during continued therapy.
• Warn the patient to avoid tasks that require mental alertness or motor skills until his or her response to the drug is established.
• Urge the patient to avoid alcohol, exposure to artificial light or direct sunlight, and other CNS depressants during thiothixene therapy.

trifluoperazine hydrochloride
try-floo-oh-**pear**-ah-zeen
(Apo-Trifluoperazine[CAN], Stelazine)
Do not confuse with selegiline or triflupromazine.

CATEGORY AND SCHEDULE
Pregnancy Risk Category: C

MECHANISM OF ACTION
A phenothiazine derivative that blocks dopamine at postsynaptic receptor sites. Possess strong extrapyramidal, antiemetic action; weak anticholinergic, sedative effects. *Therapeutic Effect:* Suppresses behavioral response in psychosis, reducing locomotor activity or aggressiveness, suppresses conditioned responses.

AVAILABILITY
Oral Concentrate: 10 mg/ml.
Tablets: 1 mg, 2 mg, 5 mg, 10 mg.

INDICATIONS AND DOSAGES
▸ **Psychotic disorders**
PO
Adults, Elderly, Children older than 12 yrs. Initially, 2–5 mg 1–2 times/day. Range: 15–20 mg/day. Maximum: 40 mg/day.
Children 6–12 yrs. Initially, 1 mg 1–2 times/day. Maintenance: Up to 15 mg/day.

CONTRAINDICATIONS
Bone marrow suppression, circulatory collapse, narrow-angle glaucoma, severe cardiac or liver disease, severe hypertension or hypotension

INTERACTIONS
Drug
Alcohol, central nervous system (CNS) depressants: May increase CNS and respiratory depression and the hypotensive effects of trifluoperazine.

Antithyroid agents: May increase the risk of agranulocytosis.

Extrapyramidal symptom (EPS)-producing medications: May increase EPS.

Hypotensives: May increase hypotension.

Levodopa: May decrease the effects of levodopa.

Lithium: May decrease the absorption of trifluoperazine and produce adverse neurologic effects.

MAOIs, tricyclic antidepressants: May increase anticholinergic and sedative effects of trifluoperazine.
Herbal
None known.
Food
None known.

DIAGNOSTIC TEST EFFECTS
May cause EKG changes.

SIDE EFFECTS
Frequent
Hypotension, dizziness, and fainting occur frequently after first injection, occasionally after subsequent injections, and rarely with oral dosage
Occasional
Drowsiness during early therapy, dry mouth, blurred vision, lethargy, constipation or diarrhea, nasal congestion, peripheral edema, urinary retention
Rare
Ocular changes, skin pigmentation in those taking high dosages for prolonged periods

SERIOUS REACTIONS
• Extrapyramidal symptoms appear to be dose-related, particularly high dosage, and are divided into 3 categories: akathisia or inability to sit still, tapping of feet, urge to move around; parkinsonian symptoms, such as masklike face, tremors, shuffling gait, and hypersalivation; and acute dystonias: torticollis or neck muscle spasm, opisthotonos or rigidity of back muscles, and oculogyric crisis or rolling back of eyes.
• Dystonic reaction may also produce profuse diaphoresis and pallor.
• Tardive dyskinesia, marked by protrusion of tongue, puffing of cheeks, and chewing or puckering of the mouth, occurs rarely but may be irreversible.
• Abrupt withdrawal after long-term therapy may precipitate nausea, vomiting, gastritis, dizziness, and tremors.
• Blood dyscrasias, particularly agranulocytosis, and mild leukopenia may occur.
• May lower seizure threshold.

NURSING CONSIDERATIONS
Baseline Assessment
• Avoid skin contact with oral concentrate because it may cause contact dermatitis.
• Assess the patient's appearance, behavior, emotional status, response to environment, speech pattern, and thought content.
Precautions
• Use cautiously in patients with Parkinson's disease and seizure disorders.
Administration and Handling
PO
• Oral concentrate must be diluted in 2 to 4 oz of carbonated beverage, juice, pudding, or water.

• Do not take antacids within 1 hour of trifluoperazine.

Intervention and Evaluation

• Monitor the patient's blood pressure (B/P) for hypotension.

• Assess the patient for extrapyramidal symptoms (EPS).

• Monitor the patient's white blood cell (WBC) count for blood dyscrasias manifested as anemia, neutropenia, pancytopenia, or thrombocytopenia.

• Monitor the patient for abnormal movement in trunk, neck, or extremities, fine tongue movement that may be early sign of tardive dyskinesia, gait changes, or tremors.

• Supervise the suicidal-risk patient closely during early therapy. As the patient's depression lessens, his or her energy level improves, increasing suicide potential.

• Monitor the patient's target behaviors.

• Assess the patient for therapeutic response, improvement in self-care, increased ability to concentrate, interest in surroundings, and relaxed facial expression.

Patient Teaching

• Teach the patient to dilute the oral concentrate in 2 to 4 oz of carbonated beverage, juice, pudding, or water.

• Instruct the patient not to take antacids within 1 hour of trifluoperazine.

• Urge the patient to avoid alcohol and excessive exposure to artificial light and sunlight during trifluoperazine therapy.

• Tell the patient that trifluoperazine may cause drowsiness. Warn the patient to avoid tasks requiring mental alertness or motor skills until his or her response to the drug is established.

• Instruct the patient to rise slowly from lying or sitting position to prevent hypotension.

ziprasidone
zip-**rah**-zih-doan
(Geodon)

CATEGORY AND SCHEDULE
Pregnancy Risk Category: C

MECHANISM OF ACTION
A piperazine derivative that antagonizes alpha-adrenergic, dopamine, histamine, and serotonin receptors; inhibits reuptake of serotonin and norepinephrine. *Therapeutic Effect:* Diminishes schizophrenic, antidepressant symptoms.

PHARMACOKINETICS
Extensively metabolized in liver. Food increases bioavailability. Protein binding: 99%. **Half-life:** 7 hrs. Not removed by hemodialysis.

AVAILABILITY
Capsules: 20 mg, 40 mg, 60 mg, 80 mg.
Injection: 20 mg/ml.

INDICATIONS AND DOSAGES
▸ **Schizophrenia**
PO
Adults, Elderly. Initially, 20 mg twice a day with food. Titrate at intervals of no less than 2 days. Maximum: 80 mg twice a day.
IM
Adults, Elderly. 10 mg q2h or 20 mg q4h. Maximum: 40 mg/day.

CONTRAINDICATIONS
Conditions associated with a risk of prolonging the QT interval

INTERACTIONS
Drug
Alcohol, central nervous system (CNS) depressants: May increase CNS depression.

Carbamazepine: May decrease ziprasidone blood concentration.
Ketoconazole: May increase ziprasidone blood concentration.

Herbal
None known.

Food
Food: Enhances the bioavailability of ziprasidone.

DIAGNOSTIC TEST EFFECTS
May produce prolongation of QT interval.

SIDE EFFECTS
Frequent (30%–16%)
Headache, somnolence, dizziness
Occasional
Rash, orthostatic hypotension, weight gain, restlessness, constipation, dyspepsia, including heartburn and gastric upset

SERIOUS REACTIONS
• Prolongation of QT interval as seen in EKG may produce torsades de pointes, a form of ventricular tachycardia, may occur. Patients with bradycardia, hypokalemia, and hypomagnesemia are at increased risk.

NURSING CONSIDERATIONS

Baseline Assessment
• Assess the patient's appearance, behavior, emotional status, response to environment, speech pattern, and thought content.
• Obtain an EKG, as ordered, to assess for QT prolongation before beginning the medication.
• Plan to obtain the patient's blood chemistry levels to check magnesium and potassium levels before beginning therapy and routinely thereafter.

Lifespan Considerations
• Be aware that it is unknown if ziprasidone crosses the placenta or is distributed in breast milk.
• Be aware that the safety and efficacy of ziprasidone have not been established in children.
• There are no age-related precautions noted in the elderly.

Precautions
• Use cautiously in patients with bradycardia, hypokalemia, and hypomagnesemia as these patients may be at greater risk for developing torsades de pointes.

Administration and Handling
PO
• Give ziprasidone with food because it increases bioavailability.
IM
• Store vials at room temperature, protect from light.
• Reconstitute each vial with 1.2 ml sterile water for injection to provide a concentration of 20 mg/ml.
• Reconstituted solution is stable for 24 hours at room temperature or 7 days refrigerated.

Intervention and Evaluation
• Assess the patient for therapeutic response, greater interest in surroundings, improved self-care, increased ability to concentrate, and relaxed facial expression.
• Closely supervise suicidal-risk patients during early therapy. As depression lessens, the patient's energy level improves, which increases the suicide potential.
• Monitor the patient's weight.

Patient Teaching
• Warn the patient to avoid tasks requiring mental alertness or motor skills until his or her response to the drug is established.
• Instruct the patient to take the drug with food to increase its effectiveness.

donepezil hydrochloride
galantamine
memantine hydrochloride
rivastigmine tartrate
tacrine hydrochloride

Uses: Cholinesterase inhibitors are used to treat mild to moderate dementia of Alzheimer's disease and to slow the progression of the disease.

Action: Most agents in this class inhibit anticholinesterase, which normally hydrolyzes acetylcholine. By preventing acetylcholine breakdown, these agents increase the acetylcholine level at cholinergic synapses, which enhances cholinergic transmission in the central nervous system. This is helpful in Alzheimer's disease, which is thought to involve degeneration of cholinergic neuronal pathways. Memantine decreases the effects of glutamate, which is the main excitatory neurotransmitter in the brain and which may contribute to symptoms of Alzheimer's disease.

donepezil hydrochloride
doh-**neh**-peh-zil
(Aricept)
Do not confuse with Aciphex or Ascriptin.

CATEGORY AND SCHEDULE
Pregnancy Risk Category: C

MECHANISM OF ACTION
A cholinesterase inhibitor that enhances cholinergic function by increasing the concentration of acetylcholine through inhibition of the hydrolysis of acetylcholine by the enzyme acetylcholinesterase. *Therapeutic Effect:* Slows the progression of Alzheimer's disease.

PHARMACOKINETICS
Well absorbed after PO administration. Protein binding: 96%. Extensively metabolized. Eliminated in urine and feces. **Half-life:** 70 hrs.

AVAILABILITY
Tablets: 5 mg, 10 mg.

INDICATIONS AND DOSAGES
▸ **Alzheimer's disease**
PO
Adults, Elderly. 5–10 mg/day as a single dose. If initial dose is 5 mg, do not increase to 10 mg for 4–6 wks.

CONTRAINDICATIONS
History of hypersensitivity to donepezil or piperidine derivatives

INTERACTIONS
Drug
Anticholinergics: Decreases the effect of anticholinergics.
Cholinergic agonists, neuromuscular blocking agents, succinylcholine: Increases the synergistic effects of cholinergic agonists, neuromuscular blocking agents, and succinylcholine.
Ketoconazole, quinidine: Inhibits the metabolism of donepezil.

NSAIDs: Increases gastric acid secretion of NSAIDs.

Paroxetine: May decrease the metabolism and increase the blood concentration of donepezil.

Herbal
None known.

Food
None known.

DIAGNOSTIC TEST EFFECTS

May increase blood glucose levels, LDH concentrations, and serum creatine kinase. May decrease serum potassium levels.

SIDE EFFECTS

Frequent (11%–8%)
Nausea, diarrhea, headache, insomnia, nonspecific pain, dizziness
Occasional (6%–3%)
Mild muscle cramps, fatigue, vomiting, anorexia, ecchymosis
Rare (3%–2%)
Depression, abnormal dreams, weight loss, arthritis, somnolence, syncope, frequent urination

SERIOUS REACTIONS

• Overdosage may result in cholinergic crisis, characterized by severe nausea, increased salivation, diaphoresis, bradycardia, hypotension, flushed skin, stomach pain, respiratory depression, seizures, and cardiorespiratory collapse.

• Increasing muscle weakness may occur, resulting in death if respiratory muscles are involved. Antidote: 1–2 mg IV atropine sulfate with subsequent doses based on therapeutic response.

NURSING CONSIDERATIONS

Baseline Assessment
• Obtain the patient's baseline vital signs.
• Determine the patient's history of

asthma, cardiac conduction disturbances, chronic obstructive pulmonary disease (COPD), peptic ulcer disease, seizure disorder, and urinary obstruction.

Lifespan Considerations
• Be aware that it is unknown if donepezil is distributed in breast milk.
• Be aware that the safety and efficacy of donepezil have not been established.
• There are no age-related precautions noted in the elderly.

Precautions
• Use cautiously in patients with asthma, bladder outflow obstruction, COPD, history of peptic ulcer disease, seizures, and "sick sinus syndrome" or other supraventricular cardiac conduction conditions.
• Use cautiously in patients on concurrent NSAID therapy.

Administration and Handling
PO
• May be given without regard to meals or in the morning or evening. However best results may be achieved if given at bedtime.

Intervention and Evaluation
• Monitor the patient for cholinergic reaction, such as diaphoresis, dizziness, excessive salivation, feeling of facial warmth, gastrointestinal (GI) cramping or discomfort, lacrimation, pallor, and urinary urgency.
• Monitor the patient for diarrhea, headache, insomnia, and nausea.

Patient Teaching
• Warn the patient to notify the physician if he or she experiences abdominal pain, diarrhea, diaphoresis, dizziness, increased salivary secretions, nausea, severe abdominal pain, and vomiting.
• Teach the patient that donepezil may be taken without regard to food.

• Tell the patient that donepezil is not a cure for Alzheimer's disease, but may slow the progression of its symptoms.

---

galantamine
gal-**an**-tah-mine
(Reminyl)
Do not confuse with Remeron or Remicade.

CATEGORY AND SCHEDULE
Pregnancy Risk Category: B

MECHANISM OF ACTION
A cholinesterase inhibitor that elevates acetylcholine concentrations in cerebral cortex by slowing degeneration of acetylcholine released by intact cholinergic neurons. *Therapeutic Effect:* Slows progression of Alzheimer's disease.

PHARMACOKINETICS
Rapidly absorbed from the gastrointestinal (GI) tract. Protein binding: 18%. Distributed to blood cells; binds to plasma proteins, mainly albumin. Metabolized in the liver. Excreted in the urine. Plasma concentration increases in patients with moderate to severe hepatic impairment. **Half-life:** 7 hrs.

AVAILABILITY
Tablets: 4 mg, 8 mg, 12 mg.
Oral Solution: 4 mg/ml.

INDICATIONS AND DOSAGES
▸ **Alzheimer's disease**
PO
Adults, Elderly. Initially, 4 mg twice a day (8 mg/day). If well tolerated and after a minimum of 4 wks, may increase to 8 mg twice a day (16 mg/day). After a minimum of 4 wks, may increase to 12 mg twice daily (24 mg/day). Range: 16–24 mg/day in 2 divided doses.
▸ **Dosage in renal impairment**
Moderate impairment: maximum of 16 mg/day
Severe impairment: not recommended

CONTRAINDICATIONS
Severe liver or renal impairment

INTERACTIONS
Drug
Bethanechol, succinylcholine: May interfere with the effects of bethanechol, succinylcholine.
Cimetidine, erythromycin, ketoconazole, paroxetine: May increase galantamine concentration.
Herbal
None known.
Food
None known.

DIAGNOSTIC TEST EFFECTS
None known.

SIDE EFFECTS
Frequent (17%–5%)
Nausea, vomiting, diarrhea, anorexia, weight loss
Occasional (9%–4%)
Abdominal pain, insomnia, depression, headache, dizziness, fatigue, rhinitis
Rare (less than 3%)
Tremors, constipation, confusion, cough, anxiety, urinary incontinence

SERIOUS REACTIONS
• Overdose can cause cholinergic crises, including increased salivation, lacrimation, urination, defecation, bradycardia, hypotension, and increased muscle weakness. Treatment is aimed at general supportive measures and the use of anticholinergics, such as atropine.

NURSING CONSIDERATIONS

Baseline Assessment
• Assess the patient's behavioral, cognitive, and functional deficits.
• Obtain the patient's liver and renal function lab values.

Lifespan Considerations
• Be aware that it is unknown if galantamine crosses the placenta or is distributed in breast milk.
• Be aware that galantamine is not prescribed for children.
• There are no age-related precautions noted in the elderly, but use is not recommended in patients with severe liver or renal impairment with a creatinine clearance of less than 9 ml/min.

Precautions
• Use cautiously in patients with asthma, bladder outflow obstruction, chronic obstructive pulmonary disease (COPD), history of peptic ulcer disease, moderately impaired liver or renal function, and supraventricular cardiac conduction conditions.
• Use cautiously in patients on concurrent NSAID therapy.

Administration and Handling
◄ALERT► Remember, if galantamine therapy is interrupted for several days or longer, reinstitute therapy as noted.

PO
• Give galantamine with morning and evening meals.

Intervention and Evaluation
• Monitor the patient's behavioral, cognitive, and functional status.
• Assess the patient's EKG and periodic rhythm strips in patients with underlying arrhythmias.
• Monitor the patient for GI bleeding and ulcer.

Patient Teaching
• Instruct the patient to take galantamine with morning and evening meals to reduce the risk of nausea.

• Tell the patient to avoid tasks that require mental alertness or motor skills until his or her response to the drug is established.
• Warn the patient to notify the physician if he or she experiences diaphoresis, depression, dizziness, excessive fatigue, increased muscle weakness, insomnia, salivation, or tearing, and persistent GI disturbances.
• Refer the patient's family to the local chapter of the Alzheimer's Disease Association for a guide to local services available to these patients.

memantine hydrochloride
meh-**man**-teen
(Namenda)

CATEGORY AND SCHEDULE
Pregnancy Risk Category: B

MECHANISM OF ACTION
A neurotransmitter inhibitor that decreases the effects of glutamate, the principle excitatory neurotransmitter in the brain. Alzheimer's disease involves degeneration of cholinergic neuronal pathways.
Therapeutic Effect: May reduce clinical deterioration in moderate to severe Alzheimer's disease.

PHARMACOKINETICS
Rapidly and completely absorbed following PO administration. Undergoes little metabolism with the majority of the dose excreted unchanged in the urine. Protein binding: 45%. **Half-life:** 60–80 hrs.

AVAILABILITY
Tablets: 5 mg, 10 mg.

INDICATIONS AND DOSAGES
▶ **Alzheimer's disease**
PO
Adults, Elderly. 5 mg once a day, with target dose of 20 mg/day. Increase in 5 mg increments to 10 mg/day or 5 mg twice a day, 15 mg/day or 5 mg and 10 mg as separate doses, 20 mg/day or 10 mg twice daily. The recommended minimum interval between dose increases is 1 week.

CONTRAINDICATIONS
Not recommended in patients with severe renal impairment

INTERACTIONS
Drug
Carbonic anhydrase inhibitors, sodium bicarbonate: May reduce the renal elimination of memantine.
Herbal
None known.
Food
None known.

DIAGNOSTIC TEST EFFECTS
None known.

SIDE EFFECTS
Occasional (7%–4%)
Dizziness, headache, confusion, constipation, hypertension, cough
Rare (3%–2%)
Back pain, nausea, fatigue, anxiety, peripheral edema, arthralgia, insomnia

SERIOUS REACTIONS
• None known.

NURSING CONSIDERATIONS
Baseline Assessment
• Evaluate the patient's behavioral, cognitive, and functional deficits.
• Expect to obtain baseline renal function tests including BUN and serum creatinine levels.
Lifespan Considerations
• Be aware that it is unknown if memantine crosses the placenta or is distributed in breast milk.
• Be aware that memantine is not prescribed for use in children.
• There are no age-related precautions noted in the elderly, but use is not recommended in elderly patients with severe renal impairment with creatinine clearance less than 9 ml/min.
Precautions
• Use cautiously in patients with moderately impaired renal function.
Administration and Handling
PO
• Give memantine without regard to food.
Intervention and Evaluation
• Monitor the patient's behavioral, cognitive, and functional status.
• Monitor the patient's urine pH because alkaline urine may lead to an accumulation of the drug and a possible increase in side effects.
Patient Teaching
• Caution the patient against reducing the drug dosage or abruptly discontinuing memantine. Instruct the patient not to increase the drug dosage without physician direction.
• Urge the patient to maintain adequate fluid intake.
• Teach the patient that if therapy is interrupted for several days, he or she should restart the drug at the lowest dose and titrate to current dose at minimum of 1-week intervals, as prescribed.
• Inform the patient's family of local chapter of Alzheimer's Disease Association to provide a guide to services for the patient.

rivastigmine tartrate
rye-vah-**stig**-meen
(Exelon)

CATEGORY AND SCHEDULE
Pregnancy Risk Category: B

MECHANISM OF ACTION
A cholinesterase inhibitor that increases the concentration of acetylcholine through reversible inhibition of its hydrolysis by cholinesterase. *Therapeutic Effect:* Enhances cholinergic function.

PHARMACOKINETICS
Rapidly and completely absorbed. Protein binding: 60%. Widely distributed throughout the body. Rapidly and extensively metabolized. Primarily excreted in urine. **Half-life:** 1.5 hrs.

AVAILABILITY
Capsules: 1.5 mg, 3 mg, 4.5 mg, 6 mg.
Oral Solution: 2 mg/ml.

INDICATIONS AND DOSAGES
▸ **Alzheimer's disease**
PO
Adults, Elderly. Initially, 1.5 mg twice a day. May increase after minimum of 2 wks to 3 mg twice a day. Subsequent increases to 4.5 mg and 6 mg twice a day may be made after a minimum of 2 wks at the previous dose. Maximum: 6 mg twice a day.

CONTRAINDICATIONS
None known

INTERACTIONS
Drug
Anticholinergic drugs: May interfere with anticholinergic drugs.

Bethanecol: May have an additive effect with this drug.
Herbal
None known.
Food
None known.

DIAGNOSTIC TEST EFFECTS
None known.

SIDE EFFECTS
Frequent (47%–17%)
Nausea, vomiting, dizziness, diarrhea, headache, anorexia
Occasional (13%–6%)
Abdominal pain, insomnia, dyspepsia, including heartburn, indigestion, and epigastric pain, confusion, urinary tract infection, depression
Rare (5%–3%)
Anxiety, somnolence, constipation, malaise, hallucinations, tremor, flatulence, rhinitis, hypertension, flu-like symptoms, weight decrease, syncope

SERIOUS REACTIONS
• Overdosage can produce cholinergic crisis characterized by severe nausea, vomiting, salivation, diaphoresis, bradycardia, hypotension, respiratory depression, and seizures.

NURSING CONSIDERATIONS
Baseline Assessment
• Obtain the patient's baseline vital signs.
• Determine the patient's history of asthma, chronic obstructive pulmonary disease (COPD), peptic ulcer disease, and urinary obstruction.
• Assess the patient's behavioral, cognitive, and functional deficits related to Alzheimer's disease.
Lifespan Considerations
• Be aware that it is unknown if rivastigmine is distributed in breast milk.

- Keep in mind that rivastigmine use is not indicated in children.
- There are no age-related precautions noted in the elderly.

Precautions
- Use cautiously in patients with asthma, bradycardia, COPD, peptic ulcer disease, seizure disorders, sick sinus syndrome, and urinary obstruction.
- Use cautiously in patients on concurrent NSAID therapy.

Administration and Handling
PO
- Give with food in divided doses morning and evening.

Oral Solution
- Using oral syringe provided by manufacturer, withdraw prescribed amount of rivastigmine from container.
- May be swallowed directly from syringe or mixed in small glass of cold fruit juice, soda, or water. Plan to use within 4 hours of mixing.

Intervention and Evaluation
- Monitor the patient for cholinergic reaction, including diaphoresis, dizziness, excessive salivation, feeling of facial warmth, gastrointestinal (GI) cramping or discomfort, lacrimation, pallor, and urinary urgency.
- Examine the patient's eyes for pupillary constriction.
- Monitor for the patient for diarrhea, headache, insomnia, and nausea.

Patient Teaching
- Instruct the patient to take rivastigmine with meals, at breakfast and dinner.
- Teach the patient to swallow the capsule whole and not to break, chew, or crush capsules.
- Warn the patient to notify the physician if he or she experiences diarrhea, diaphoresis, dizziness, increased salivary secretions, nausea, severe abdominal pain, and vomiting.
- Refer the patient's family to the local chapter of the Alzheimer's Disease Association for a guide to local services available to these patients.

tacrine hydrochloride
tay-crin
(Cognex)

CATEGORY AND SCHEDULE
Pregnancy Risk Category: C

MECHANISM OF ACTION
A cholinesterase inhibitor that elevates acetylcholine concentrations in cerebral cortex by slowing degeneration of acetylcholine released by still intact cholinergic neurons. *Therapeutic Effect:* Slows Alzheimer's disease process.

AVAILABILITY
Capsules: 10 mg, 20 mg, 30 mg, 40 mg.

INDICATIONS AND DOSAGES
▸ **Alzheimer's disease**
PO
Adults, Elderly. Initially, 10 mg 4 times/day for 6 wks; then 20 mg 4 times/day for 6 wks; then 30 mg 4 times/day for 12 wks; then to maximum of 40 mg 4 times/day if needed.
▸ **Dosage in liver impairment**
ALT greater than 3–5 times normal. Decrease dose by 40 mg/day. Resume normal dose when ALT returns to normal.
ALT greater than 5 times normal. Stop treatment, restart when ALT returns to normal.

CONTRAINDICATIONS

Active, severe liver disease, active and untreated duodenal or gastric ulcers, breast-feeding, childbearing potential, current treatment with other cholinesterase inhibitors, hypersensitivity to cholinergics, mechanical obstruction of intestine or urinary tract, pregnancy

INTERACTIONS
Drug

Anticholinergics: May interfere with anticholinergics.
Cimetidine: May increase tacrine blood concentration.
NSAIDs: May increase the adverse effects of NSAIDS.
Theophylline: May increase the blood concentration of theophylline.
Herbal
None known.
Food
None known.

DIAGNOSTIC TEST EFFECTS

Increases SGOT (AST) and SGPT (ALT) levels. Alters blood Hgb, Hct, and serum electrolyte levels.

SIDE EFFECTS

Frequent (28%–11%)
Headache, nausea, vomiting, diarrhea, dizziness
Occasional (9%–4%)
Fatigue, chest pain, dyspepsia, anorexia, abdominal pain, flatulence, constipation, confusion, agitation, rash, depression, ataxia or muscular incoordination, insomnia, rhinitis, myalgia
Rare (less than 3%)
Weight loss, anxiety, cough, facial flushing, urinary frequency, back pain, tremor

SERIOUS REACTIONS

• Overdose can cause cholinergic crisis, marked by increased salivation, lacrimation, urination, defecation, bradycardia, hypotension, and increased muscle weakness. Treatment aimed at general supportive measures and the use of anticholinergics, such as atropine.

NURSING CONSIDERATIONS
Baseline Assessment
• Assess the patient's behavioral, cognitive, and functional deficits.
• Expect to obtain blood serum enzyme levels to assess liver function.
Precautions
• Use cautiously in patients with alcohol abuse, asthma, bradycardia, cardiac arrhythmias, chronic obstructive pulmonary disease (COPD), history of gastric or intestinal ulcers, hyperthyroidism, liver dysfunction, and seizure disorders.
Administration and Handling
◀ALERT▶ If medication is stopped for longer than 14 days, plan to reinstitute as noted above.
PO
• Give tacrine without regard to food.
Intervention and Evaluation
• Monitor the patient's behavioral, cognitive, and functional status.
• Monitor the patient's SGOT (AST) and SGPT (ALT) levels.
• Monitor the EKG and rhythm strips in patients with underlying arrhythmias.
• Assess the patients for signs of gastrointestinal (GI) bleeding and ulcer.
Patient Teaching
• Instruct the patient to take tacrine at regular intervals, between meals. Advise the patient that if he or she experiences GI upset that tacrine may be taken with meals.
• Caution the patient against abruptly discontinuing the medication or adjusting the drug dosage.

- Urge the patient to avoid smoking during tacrine therapy. Explain to the patient that smoke reduces the plasma concentration of tacrine.

- Refer the patient's family to the local chapter of the Alzheimer's Disease Association for a guide to local services available to these patients.

atomoxetine
dexmethylphenidate
  hydrochloride
dextroamphetamine
  sulfate
methylphenidate
  hydrochloride
modafinil
pemoline

Uses: Most central nervous system stimulants are used to treat attention deficit hyperactivity disorder, primarily in children age 6 and younger. In adults, several of these agents are used to treat narcolepsy. In addition, dextroamphetamine is used for short-term treatment of obesity.

Action: In this classification, specific subgroups and individual agents act by different mechanisms. *Amphetamines*, such as dextroamphetamine, promote the release and action of norepinephrine and dopamine by blocking reuptake from synapses; they also inhibit the action of monoamine oxidase. *Methylphenidate* blocks the reuptake mechanisms of dopaminergic neurons. *Modafinil's* exact mechanism of action is unknown, but the drug may bind to dopamine re-uptake carrier sites, increasing alpha activity and decreasing delta, theta, beta brain wave activity. *Pemoline* blocks the reuptake of dopamine at neurons in the cerebral cortex and subcortical structures.

atomoxetine
ah-toe-**mocks**-eh-teen
(Strattera)

CATEGORY AND SCHEDULE
Pregnancy Risk Category: C

MECHANISM OF ACTION
A norepinephrine reuptake inhibitor that enhances noradrenergic function by selective inhibition of the presynaptic norepinephrine transporter. *Therapeutic Effect:* Improves symptoms of attention-deficit hyperactivity disorder (ADHD).

PHARMACOKINETICS
Rapidly absorbed after oral administration. 98% bound to protein, primarily albumin. Eliminated primarily in the urine with less amount excreted in the feces. Not removed by hemodialysis. **Half-life:** 4–5 hrs found in the major population, 22 hrs in 7% of Caucasians and in 2% of African-Americans. Half-life is increased in moderate to severe liver insufficiency.

AVAILABILITY
Capsules: 10 mg, 18 mg, 25 mg, 40 mg, 60 mg.

INDICATIONS AND DOSAGES
▶ **Attention-deficit hyperactivity disorder (ADHD)**
PO
Adults, children weighing 70 kg and more. 40 mg once a day. May increase after a minimum of 3 days

to 80 mg as a single daily dose or in divided doses. Maximum: 100 mg.
Children weighing less than 70 kg. Initially, 0.5 mg/kg/day. May increase to 1.2 mg/kg/day after minimum of 3 days. Maximum: 1.4 mg/kg/day.

CONTRAINDICATIONS
Concurrent use of MAOIs or within 2 weeks of discontinuing an MAOI, narrow angle glaucoma

INTERACTIONS
Drug
Fluoxetine, paroxetine, quinidine: May increase atomoxetine blood concentration.
MAOIs: May increase toxic effects.
Herbal
None known.
Food
None known.

DIAGNOSTIC TEST EFFECTS
None known.

SIDE EFFECTS
Frequent
Headache, dyspepsia (epigastric distress, heartburn), nausea, vomiting, fatigue, reduced appetite, dizziness, changes in mood
Occasional
Increase in heart rate and blood pressure, weight loss, slowing of growth
Rare
Insomnia, sexual dysfunction in adults (desire, performance, satisfaction)

SERIOUS REACTIONS
• Urinary retention or urinary hesitance may occur.
• In an overdose, gastric emptying and repeated activated charcoal may prevent systemic absorption.

NURSING CONSIDERATIONS
Baseline Assessment
• Assess the patient's blood pressure (B/P) and pulse before beginning atomoxetine therapy, following dose increases, and periodically while on therapy.
Lifespan Considerations
• Be aware that it is unknown if atomoxetine is excreted in breast milk.
• Be aware that the safety and efficacy of atomoxetine have not been established in children younger than 6 yrs.
• In the elderly, age-related cardiovascular or cerebrovascular disease and decreased liver or renal impairment may increase the risk of side effects of atomoxetine.
Precautions
◀ALERT▶ Avoid concurrent use of medications that can increase heart rate or blood pressure.
• Use cautiously in patients with cardiovascular disease, hypertension, moderate or severe liver impairment, risk of urinary retention, and tachycardia.
Administration and Handling
◀ALERT▶ Reduce atomoxetine dosage to 50% in those with moderate liver impairment and to 25% in those with severe liver impairment.
PO
• Give atomoxetine without regard to meals.
Intervention and Evaluation
• Monitor the patient's urinary output. A patient complaint of inability to urinate (urinary retention) or hesitancy may be a related adverse reaction.
• Assist the patient with ambulation if he or she experiences dizziness.
• Be alert to mood changes in the patient.
• Monitor the fluid and electrolyte

status in patients experiencing significant vomiting.

Patient Teaching

• Advise the patient to avoid tasks that require mental alertness and motor skills until his or her response to the drug is established.

• Instruct the patient to take the last dose of the day early in the evening to avoid insomnia.

• Warn the patient to notify the physician if he or she experiences fever, nervousness, palpitations, skin rash, or vomiting.

---

dexmethylphenidate hydrochloride
dex-meh-thyl-**fen**-ih-date
(Focalin)

CATEGORY AND SCHEDULE
Pregnancy Risk Category: C
Controlled substance: Schedule II

MECHANISM OF ACTION
A piperidine derivative B that blocks the reuptake mechanisms of norepinephrine and dopamine into presynaptic neurons. Increases the release of these neurotransmitters into the synaptic cleft. *Therapeutic Effect:* Decreases motor restlessness, enhances attention span. Increases motor activity, mental alertness; diminishes sense of fatigue; enhances spirit.

PHARMACOKINETICS

Route	Onset	Peak	Duration
PO	N/A	N/A	4–5 hrs

Readily absorbed from the gastrointestinal (GI) tract. Plasma concentrations increase rapidly. Metabo-

lized in liver. Excreted unchanged in urine. **Half-life:** 2.2 hrs.

AVAILABILITY
Tablets: 2.5 mg, 5 mg, 10 mg.

INDICATIONS AND DOSAGES
▸ **Attention-deficit hyperactivity disorder (ADHD)**
PO
Patients new to dexmethylphenidate, methylphenidate. 2.5 mg twice a day (5 mg/day). May adjust dosage in 2.5- to 5-mg increments. Maximum: 20 mg/day.
Patients currently taking methylphenidate. Half the methylphenidate dosage. Maximum: 20 mg/day.

CONTRAINDICATIONS
Diagnosis or family history of Tourette's syndrome, glaucoma, history of marked agitation, anxiety, or tension, patients undergoing treatment with MAOIs within 14 days following discontinuation of an MAOI, patients with motor tics

INTERACTIONS
Drug
Amitriptyline, phenobarbital, phenytoin, primidone: Downward dosage adjustments of amitriptyline, phenobarbital, phenytoin, and primidone may be necessary.
Central nervous system (CNS) stimulants: May have an additive effect.
MAOIs: May increase the effects of dexmethylphenidate.
Warfarin: May inhibit the metabolism of warfarin.
Herbal
None known.
Food
None known.

DIAGNOSTIC TEST EFFECTS
None known.

SIDE EFFECTS
Frequent
Abdominal discomfort
Occasional
Anorexia, fever, nausea
Rare
Blurred vision, difficulty with accommodation, motor, vocal tics, insomnia, tachycardia

SERIOUS REACTIONS
• Withdrawal after chronic therapy may unmask symptoms of the underlying disorder.
• May lower the seizure threshold in those with history of seizures.
• Overdosage produces excessive sympathomimetic effects, including vomiting, tremors, hyperreflexia, seizures, confusion, hallucinations, and diaphoresis.
• Prolonged administration to children may produce temporary suppression of normal weight gain.

NURSING CONSIDERATIONS

Baseline Assessment
• Obtain baseline height and weight, and plan to weigh the patient regularly to monitor for growth retardation.

Lifespan Considerations
• Be aware that it is unknown if dexmethylphenidate is excreted in breast milk.
• Be aware that children are more susceptible to developing abdominal pain, anorexia, insomnia, and weight loss.
• Be aware that chronic dexmethylphenidate use may inhibit growth in children.
• Know that in psychotic children, dexmethylphenidate use may exacerbate symptoms of behavior disturbance and thought disorder.
• There are no age-related precautions noted in the elderly.

Precautions
• Use cautiously in patients with cardiovascular disease, psychosis, and seizure disorders.
• Avoid dexmethylphenidate use in those with a history of substance abuse.

Administration and Handling
PO
• Do not give drug in afternoon or evening because it can cause insomnia.
• Crush tablets, as needed.
• May give dexmethylphenidate with or without food.

Intervention and Evaluation
• Plan to perform a complete blood count (CBC) to assess white blood cell count (WBC), differential, and platelet count routinely during therapy.
• Discontinue or reduce dexmethylphenidate dose if paradoxical return of attention deficit occurs.

Patient Teaching
• Warn the patient to avoid tasks that require mental alertness or motor skills until his or her response to the drug is established.
• Tell the patient to notify the physician of any increase in seizures, fever, nervousness, palpitations, and vomiting.
• Instruct the patient to take the last dose of the day several hours before retiring to prevent insomnia.

dextroamphetamine sulfate

dex-tro-am-**fet**-ah-meen
(Dexedrine)
**Do not confuse with Dextran,
dextromethorphan, or Excedrin.**

CATEGORY AND SCHEDULE
Pregnancy Risk Category: C
Controlled substance: Schedule II

MECHANISM OF ACTION
An amphetamine that enhances
release, action of catecholamine
(dopamine, norepinephrine) by
blocking reuptake, inhibiting monoamine oxidase. *Therapeutic Effect:*
Increases motor activity, mental
alertness; decreases drowsiness,
fatigue.

AVAILABILITY
Tablets: 5 mg, 10 mg.
Capsules (sustained-release): 5 mg,
10 mg, 15 mg.

INDICATIONS AND DOSAGES
▸ **Narcolepsy**
PO
Adults, Children older than 12 yrs.
Initially, 10 mg/day. Increase by
10 mg at weekly intervals until
therapeutic response achieved.
Children 6–12 yrs. Initially, 5 mg/
day. Increase by 5 mg/day at
weekly intervals until therapeutic
response achieved. Maximum:
60 mg/day.
▸ **Attention deficit disorder (ADD)**
PO
Children 6 yrs and older. Initially,
5 mg 1–2 times/day. Increase by
5 mg/day at weekly intervals until
therapeutic response achieved.
Children 3–5 yrs. Initially, 2.5
mg/day. Increase by 2.5 mg/day at
weekly intervals until therapeutic

response achieved. Maximum:
40 mg/day.
▸ **Appetite suppressant**
PO
Adults. 5–30 mg daily in divided
doses of 5–10 mg each dose, given
30–60 min before meals. Extended-
release: 1 capsule in morning.

CONTRAINDICATIONS
Advanced arteriosclerosis, agitated
states, glaucoma, history of drug
abuse, history of hypersensitivity to
sympathomimetic amines, hyperthyroidism, moderate to severe hypertension, symptomatic cardiovascular
disease, within 14 days following
discontinuation of an MAOI

INTERACTIONS
Drug
Beta-blockers: May increase risk of
bradycardia, heart block, and hypertension.
*Central nervous system (CNS)
stimulants:* May increase the effects
of dextroamphetamine.
Digoxin: May increase the risk of
arrhythmias with this drug.
MAOIs: May prolong and intensify
the effects of dextroamphetamine.
Meperidine: May increase the risk
of hypotension, respiratory depression, seizures, and vascular collapse.
Thyroid hormones: May increase
the effects of thyroid this drug and
of dextroamphetamine.
Tricyclic antidepressants: May
increase cardiovascular effects.
Herbal
None known.
Food
None known.

DIAGNOSTIC TEST EFFECTS
May increase plasma corticosteroid
concentrations.

SIDE EFFECTS
Frequent
Irregular pulse, increased motor activity, talkativeness, nervousness, mild euphoria, insomnia
Occasional
Headache, chills, dry mouth, gastrointestinal (GI) distress, worsening depression in patients who are clinically depressed, tachycardia, palpitations, chest pain

SERIOUS REACTIONS
• Overdose may produce skin pallor or flushing, arrhythmias, and psychosis.
• Abrupt withdrawal following prolonged administration of high dosage may produce lethargy (may last for weeks).
• Prolonged administration to children with ADD may produce a temporary suppression of normal weight and height patterns.

NURSING CONSIDERATIONS
Precautions
• Use cautiously in debilitated and elderly patients and in patients who are tartrazine-sensitive.
Intervention and Evaluation
• Monitor the patient for CNS overstimulation, an increase in blood pressure (B/P), and weight loss.
Patient Teaching
• Advise the patient that normal dosage levels may produce tolerance to the drug's anorexic mood-elevating effects within a few weeks.
• Warn the patient to avoid performing tasks that require mental alertness or motor skills until his or her response to the drug is established.
• Suggest to the patient that sips of tepid water and sugarless gum may relieve dry mouth.
• Instruct the patient to take dextroamphetamine early in the day.
• Caution the patient that this drug may mask signs and symptoms of extreme fatigue.
• Warn the patient to notify the physician if he or she experiences decreased appetite, dizziness, dry mouth, or pronounced nervousness.

methylphenidate hydrochloride
meh-thyl-**fen**-ih-date
(Attenta[AUS], Concerta, Metadate, Ritalin, Ritalin LA, Ritalin SR)
Do not confuse with Rifadin.

CATEGORY AND SCHEDULE
Pregnancy Risk Category: C
Controlled Substance: Schedule II

MECHANISM OF ACTION
A piperidine derivative B that blocks reuptake mechanisms of dopaminergic neurons. *Therapeutic Effect:* Decreases motor restlessness, enhances ability to pay attention. Increases motor activity, mental alertness; diminishes sense of fatigue; enhances spirit; produces mild euphoria.

PHARMACOKINETICS

Onset	Peak	Duration
Immediate-release	2 hrs	3–5 hrs
Sustained release	4–7 hrs	3–8 hrs
Extended-release	N/A	8–12 hrs

Slowly, incompletely absorbed from the gastrointestinal (GI) tract. Protein binding: 15%. Metabolized in liver. Excreted in urine, eliminated in feces via biliary system. Unknown if removed by hemodialysis. **Half-life:** 2–4 hrs.

AVAILABILITY
Capsules (extended-release): 10 mg (Metadate CD), 20 mg (Metadate CD), 20 mg (Ritalin LA), 30 mg (Metadate CD), 30 mg (Ritalin LA), 40 mg (Ritalin LA).
Tablets: 5 mg (Ritalin), 10 mg (Ritalin), 20 mg (Ritalin).
Tablets (extended-release): 10 mg (Metadate ER, Methylin ER), 18 mg (Concerta), 20 mg (Metadate ER, Methylin ER), 27 mg (Concerta), 36 mg (Concerta), 54 mg (Concerta).
Tablets (sustained-release): 20 mg (Ritalin SR).

INDICATIONS AND DOSAGES
▸ **Attention-deficit hyperactivity disorder (ADHD)**
PO
Children older than 6 yrs. Initially, 2.5–5 mg before breakfast and lunch. May increase by 5–10 mg/day at weekly intervals. Maximum: 60 mg/day.
Concerta: Initially, 18 mg once a day; may increase by 18 mg/day at weekly intervals. Maximum: 54 mg/day.
Metadate CD: Initially, 20 mg/day. May increase by 20 mg/day at 7 day intervals. Maximum: 60 mg/day.
Ritalin LA: Initially, 20 mg/day. May increase by 10 mg/day at 7 day intervals. Maximum: 60 mg/day.
▸ **Narcolepsy**
PO
Adults, Elderly. 10 mg 2–3 times/day. Range: 10–60 mg/day.

UNLABELED USES
Treatment of secondary mental depression

CONTRAINDICATIONS
Use of MAOIs within 14 days

INTERACTIONS
Drug
Central nervous system (CNS) stimulants: May have an additive effect.
MAOIs: May increase the effects of methylphenidate.
Herbal
None known.
Food
None known.

DIAGNOSTIC TEST EFFECTS
None known.

SIDE EFFECTS
Frequent
Nervousness, insomnia, anorexia
Occasional
Dizziness, drowsiness, headache, nausea, stomach pain, fever, rash, joint pain
Rare
Blurred vision, Tourette's syndrome, marked by uncontrolled vocal outbursts, repetitive body movements, and tics

SERIOUS REACTIONS
• Prolonged administration to children with attention deficit disorder may produce a temporary suppression of normal weight gain pattern.
• Overdose may produce tachycardia, palpitations, cardiac irregularities, chest pain, psychotic episode, seizures, and coma.
• Hypersensitivity reactions and blood dyscrasias occur rarely.

NURSING CONSIDERATIONS

Baseline Assessment
• Obtain baseline height and weight, and plan to weigh the patient regularly to monitor for growth retardation.

Lifespan Considerations
• Be aware that it is unknown if methylphenidate crosses the placenta or is distributed in breast milk.
• Be aware that children may be more susceptible to develop abdominal pain, anorexia, decreased weight, and insomnia. Chronic methylphenidate use may inhibit growth in children.
• There are no age-related precautions noted in the elderly.

Precautions
• Use cautiously in patients with acute stress reaction, emotional instability, history of drug dependence, hypertension, and seizures.

Administration and Handling
◀ALERT▶ Be aware that the sustained-release forms (Metadate SR, Ritalin SR) may be given once the daily dose is titrated; the regular tablets and the titrated 8-hour dosage correspond to sustained-release size.

PO
• Do not give drug in afternoon or evening because the drug can cause insomnia.
• Do not crush or break sustained-release capsules.
• Crush tablets as needed.
• Give dose 30 to 45 minutes before meals.
• Open Metadate CD and sprinkle on applesauce, if desired.

Intervention and Evaluation
• Perform a complete blood count (CBC) to assess white blood cell (WBC) count, differential, and platelet count routinely during therapy.

• Discontinue or reduce methylphenidate dosage if a paradoxical return of attention deficit occurs.

Patient Teaching
• Warn the patient to avoid tasks that require mental alertness or motor skills until his or her response to the drug is established.
• Suggest to the patient that taking sips of tepid water and chewing sugarless gum may relieve dry mouth.
• Warn the patient to notify the physician if he or she experiences any increase in seizures, fever, nervousness, palpitations, skin rash, or vomiting.
• Instruct the patient to take the last dose of methylphenidate in the early morning to avoid insomnia.
• Urge the patient to avoid consuming caffeine during methylphenidate therapy.
• Caution the patient against abruptly discontinuing the drug after prolonged use.

modafinil
mode-ah-**feen**-awl
(Alertec, Provigil)

CATEGORY AND SCHEDULE
Pregnancy Risk Category: C

MECHANISM OF ACTION
An alpha$_1$-agonist that binds to dopamine reuptake carrier site, increasing alpha activity, decreasing delta, theta, and beta activity. *Therapeutic Effect:* Reduces the number of sleep episodes and total daytime sleep.

PHARMACOKINETICS
Well absorbed. Protein binding: 60%. Widely distributed. Metabolized in lever. Excreted in the kid-

ney. Unknown if removed by hemo-dialysis. **Half-life:** 8–10 hrs.

AVAILABILITY
Tablets: 100 mg, 200 mg.

INDICATIONS AND DOSAGES
▸ **Narcolepsy, sleep disorders**
PO
Adults, Elderly. 200–400 mg/day.

UNLABELED USES
Depression

CONTRAINDICATIONS
None known

INTERACTIONS
Drug
Central nervous system (CNS) stimulants: May increase CNS stimulation.
Cyclosporine, oral contraceptives, theophylline: May decrease concentrations of cyclosporine, oral contraceptives, theophylline.
Diazepam, phenytoin, propranolol, tricyclic antidepressants, warfarin: May increase concentrations of diazepam, phenytoin, propranolol, tricyclic antidepressants, warfarin.
Herbal
None known.
Food
None known.

DIAGNOSTIC TEST EFFECTS
None known.

SIDE EFFECTS
Frequent
Anxiety, headache, insomnia, nausea, nervousness
Occasional
Anorexia, diarrhea, dizziness, dry mouth or skin, muscle stiffness, increased thirst, rhinitis, tingling of skin, tremor, headache, vomiting

SERIOUS REACTIONS
• Agitation, excitation, increased blood pressure (B/P), and insomnia may occur.

NURSING CONSIDERATIONS
Baseline Assessment
• Obtain the patient's baseline characteristics of narcolepsy or other sleep disorders, including environmental situations, lengths of time of sleep episodes, and pattern.
• Ask the patient about sudden loss of muscle tone or cataplexy precipitated by strong emotional responses.
• Assess the frequency and severity of the patient's sleep episodes prior to drug therapy.
Lifespan Considerations
• Be aware that it is unknown if modafinil is excreted in breast milk. Use caution if giving modafinil to pregnant women.
• Be aware that the safety and efficacy of this drug have not been established in children younger than 16 years of age.
• In the elderly, the age-related liver or renal impairment may require decreased dosage.
Precautions
• Use cautiously in patients with a history of clinically significant mitral valve prolapse or seizures, left ventricular hypertrophy, and liver impairment.
Administration and Handling
• Give modafinil without regard to meals.
Intervention and Evaluation
• Monitor restlessness during sleep, length of insomnia episodes during the night, and sleep pattern.
• Assess the patient for anxiety and dizziness. Institute safety precautions.
• Suggest to the patient that taking sips of tepid water and chewing sugarless gum may relieve dry mouth.

Patient Teaching
• Warn the patient to avoid tasks that require mental alertness or motor skills until his or her response to the drug is established.
• Instruct the patient not to increase the drug dose without first checking with the physician.
• Tell the patient to use alternatives to oral contraceptives during therapy, and 1 month after discontinuing modafinil.

pemoline
pem-oh-leen
(Cylert)

CATEGORY AND SCHEDULE
Pregnancy Risk Category: B
Controlled substance: Schedule IV

MECHANISM OF ACTION
A central nervous system (CNS) stimulant that blocks reuptake of dopaminergic neurons at cerebral cortex and subcortical structures. *Therapeutic Effect:* Reduces motor restlessness, increases mental alertness, provides mood elevation, reduces sense of fatigue.

AVAILABILITY
Tablets: 18.75 mg, 37.5 mg, 75 mg.
Tablets (chewable): 37.5 mg.

INDICATIONS AND DOSAGES
▶ **Attention deficit disorder**
PO
Children 6 yrs and older. Initially, 37.5 mg/day given as single dose in morning. May increase by 18.75 mg at weekly intervals until therapeutic response is achieved. Range: 56.25–75 mg/day. Maximum: 112.5 mg/day.

CONTRAINDICATIONS
Family history of Tourette's disorder, impaired liver function, patients with motor tics

INTERACTIONS
Drug
CNS-stimulating medications: May increase CNS stimulation.
Herbal
None known.
Food
None known.

DIAGNOSTIC TEST EFFECTS
May increase LDH concentrations, SGOT (AST), and SGPT (ALT) levels.

SIDE EFFECTS
Frequent
Anorexia, insomnia
Occasional
Nausea, abdominal discomfort, diarrhea, headache, dizziness, drowsiness

SERIOUS REACTIONS
• Dyskinetic movements of tongue, lips, face, and extremities, visual disturbances, and rash have occurred.
• Large doses may produce extreme nervousness and tachycardia.
• Hepatic effects, such as hepatitis and jaundice, appear to be reversible when drug is discontinued.
• Prolonged administration to children with attention deficit disorder may produce a temporary suppression of weight and height patterns.

NURSING CONSIDERATIONS

Baseline Assessment
• Perform blood serum hepatic enzyme tests before beginning pemoline therapy and periodically during therapy.

• Obtain baseline height and weight, and plan to weigh the patient regularly to monitor for growth retardation.

Precautions

• Use cautiously in patients with history of drug abuse, hypertension, psychosis, renal impairment, and seizures.

Patient Teaching

• Urge the patient to avoid alcohol and caffeine during pemoline therapy.

• Tell the patient that pemoline may cause dizziness and impair his or her ability to perform tasks requiring mental alertness or motor skills.

• Explain to the patient that pemoline may be habit-forming. Caution the patient against abruptly discontinuing the medication.

• Warn the patient to notify the physician if he or she experiences dark urine, gastrointestinal complaints, loss of appetite, or yellow skin.

codeine phosphate, codeine sulfate

fentanyl

hydromorphone hydrochloride

meperidine hydrochloride

methadone hydrochloride

morphine sulfate

oxycodone

propoxyphene hydrochloride, propoxyphene napsylate

Uses: Narcotic analgesics are used to relieve moderate to severe pain related to surgery, myocardial infarction, burns, cancer, and other conditions. These agents may be used as an adjunct to anesthesia, either as preoperative medication or as an intraoperative supplement to anesthesia. They're also used for obstetric analgesia. Codeine may be prescribed for its antitussive effects. Opium tinctures can be used to control severe diarrhea. Although methadone can relieve severe pain, it's used primarily as part of heroin detoxification.

Action: All narcotic analgesics bind to opioid receptors and have actions similar to morphine, which is why they're also referred to as *opioid* analgesics. (See illustration, *Mechanism of Action: Narcotic Analgesics,* page 802.) These agents produce major effects on the central nervous system (causing analgesia, drowsiness, mood changes, mental clouding, analgesia without loss of consciousness, nausea, and vomiting) and the gastrointestinal tract (reducing hydrochloric acid secretion; biliary, pancreatic, and intestinal secretions; and propulsive peristalsis). They also depress respirations and cause such cardiovascular effects as peripheral vasodilation, decreased peripheral resistance, and inhibited baroreceptors reflexes.

COMBINATION PRODUCTS

CAPITAL WITH CODEINE: acetaminophen (a non-narcotic analgesic)/ codeine 120 mg/12 mg per 5 ml.

DARVOCET-N: propoxyphene/ acetaminophen (a non-narcotic analgesic) 50 mg/325 mg; 100 mg/650 mg.

DARVOCET A 500: propoxyphene/ acetaminophen (a non-narcotic analgesic) 100 mg/500 mg.

PERCOCET: oxycodone/ acetaminophen (a non-narcotic analgesic) 2.5 mg/325 mg; 5 mg/ 325 mg; 5 mg/500 mg; 7.5 mg/ 325 mg; 7.5 mg/500 mg; 10 mg/ 325 mg; 10 mg/650 mg.

PERCODAN: oxycodone/aspirin (a non-narcotic analgesic) 2.25 mg/325 mg; 4.5 mg/325 mg.

PHENERGAN WITH CODEINE: codeine/ promethazine (an antihistamine) 10 mg/6.25 mg

PHENERGAN VC WITH CODEINE: codeine/promethazine (an antihistamine)/phenylephrine (a vasopressor) 10 mg/6.25 mg/5 mg.

ROBITUSSIN AC: codeine/guaifenesin (an antitussive) 10 mg/100 mg.

ROXICET: oxycodone/acetaminophen

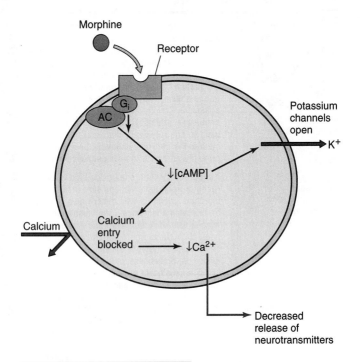

Mechanism of Action: Narcotic Analgesics

Narcotic analgesics bind to three types of opioid receptors: mu, kappa, and delta receptors. They produce analgesia primarily by activating mu receptors. However, they also engage with and activate kappa and delta receptors, producing other effects, such as sedation and vasomotor stimulation.

When morphine or another narcotic analgesic binds to opioid receptors, activation occurs. The receptors send signals to the enzyme adenyl cyclase (AC) to slow activity by way of G proteins (G_i). Decreased adenyl cyclase activity causes less cyclic adenosine monophosphate (cAMP) to be produced. A secondary messenger substance, cAMP, is important for regulating cell membrane channels. A reduced cAMP level allows fewer potassium ions to leave the cell and blocks calcium ions from entering the cell. This ion imbalance—especially the reduced intracellular calcium level—ultimately decreases the release of neurotransmitters from the cell, thereby blocking or reducing pain impulse transmission.

(a non-narcotic analgesic) 5 mg/
500 mg.
TYLENOL WITH CODEINE: acetaminophen (a non-narcotic analgesic)/
codeine 120 mg/12 mg per 5 ml;

300 mg/15 mg; 300 mg/30 mg;
300 mg/60 mg.
TYLOX: oxycodone/acetaminophen
(a non-narcotic analgesic) 5 mg/
500 mg.

codeine phosphate
koe-deen
(Actacode[AUS], Codeine,
Codeine Linctus[AUS])
codeine sulfate
(Contin[CAN])
Do not confuse with Lodine.

CATEGORY AND SCHEDULE
Pregnancy Risk Category: C, D
if used for prolonged periods,
high dosages at term
Controlled substance: Schedule II
(analgesic), Schedule III (fixed-
combination form)

MECHANISM OF ACTION
An opioid agonist that binds at
opiate receptor sites in central
nervous system (CNS). Has direct
action in the medulla. *Therapeutic
Effect:* Inhibits ascending pain
pathways, altering perception of and
response to pain, causes cough
suppression.

AVAILABILITY
Tablets: 15 mg, 30 mg, 60 mg.
Soluble Tablets: 15 mg, 30 mg,
60 mg.
Injection: 30 mg, 60 mg.

INDICATIONS AND DOSAGES
▸ **Analgesia**
PO/Subcutaneous/IM
Adults, Elderly. 30 mg q4–6h.
Range: 15–60 mg.
Children. 0.5–1 mg/kg q4–6h.
Maximum: 60 mg/dose.
▸ **Antitussive**
PO
*Adults, Elderly, Children 12 yrs and
older.* 10–20 mg q4–6h.
Children 6–11 yrs. 5–10 mg
q4–6h.
Children 2–5 yrs. 2.5–5 mg q4–6h.

▸ **Dosage in renal impairment**

Creatinine Clearance	Dosage
10–50 ml/min	75% dose
less than 10 ml/min	50% dose

UNLABELED USES
Treatment of diarrhea

CONTRAINDICATIONS
None known

INTERACTIONS
Drug
*Alcohol, central nervous system
(CNS) depressants:* May increase
CNS or respiratory depression, and
hypotension.
MAOIs: May produce severe, fatal
reaction unless dosage reduced by
one quarter.
Herbal
None known.
Food
None known.

DIAGNOSTIC TEST EFFECTS
May increase serum amylase and
lipase levels.

SIDE EFFECTS
Frequent
Constipation, drowsiness, nausea,
vomiting
Occasional
Paradoxical excitement, confusion,
pounding heartbeat, facial flushing,
decreased urination, blurred vision,
dizziness, dry mouth, headache, hypotension, decreased appetite, redness, burning, pain at injection site
Rare
Hallucinations, depression, stomach
pain, insomnia

SERIOUS REACTIONS
• Too frequent use may result in
paralytic ileus.

• Overdosage results in cold or clammy skin, confusion, convulsions, decreased blood pressure (B/P), restlessness, pinpoint pupils, bradycardia, respiratory depression, decreased level of consciousness (LOC), and severe weakness.
• Tolerance to analgesic effect and physical dependence may occur with repeated use.

NURSING CONSIDERATIONS

Baseline Assessment
• Assess the duration, location, onset, and type of pain.
• Keep in mind that the effect of medication is reduced if full pain response recurs before next dose.
• Assess the frequency, severity, and type of cough, and sputum production.
Precautions
• Use extremely cautiously in patients with acute alcoholism, anoxia, central nervous system (CNS) depression, hypercapnia, respiratory depression, respiratory dysfunction, seizures, shock, and untreated myxedema.
• Use cautiously in patients with acute abdominal conditions, Addison's disease, chronic obstructive pulmonary disease (COPD), hypothyroidism, impaired liver function, increased intracranial pressure, prostatic hypertrophy, and urethral stricture.
Administration and Handling
◄ALERT► Be aware that ambulatory patients and those not in severe pain may experience dizziness, hypotension, nausea, and vomiting more frequently than patients in the supine position or with severe pain.
◄ALERT► Expect to reduce the initial dosage in those with hypothyroidism, concurrent CNS depressants, Addison's disease, renal

insufficiency, elderly, and debilitated.
Intervention and Evaluation
• Assess the patient's daily pattern of daily bowel activity and stool consistency.
• Increase the patient's fluid intake and environmental humidity to help improve viscosity of lung secretions.
• Encourage deep breathing and coughing exercises.
• Assess the patient for clinical improvement. Record the onset of relief of cough or pain.
Patient Teaching
• Instruct the patient to change positions slowly to avoid orthostatic hypotension.
• Warn the patient to avoid tasks that require mental alertness or motor skills until his or her response to the drug is established.
• Explain to the patient that drug dependence or tolerance may occur with prolonged use of high dosages.
• Urge the patient to avoid alcohol during codeine therapy.
• Tell the patient to report the onset of pain because the effect of drug is reduced if full pain response recurs before next dose.

fentanyl
fen-tah-nil
(Actiq, Duragesic, Sublimaze)
Do not confuse with alfentanil.

CATEGORY AND SCHEDULE
Pregnancy Risk Category: C, D if used for prolonged periods or at high dosages at term
Controlled substance: Schedule II

MECHANISM OF ACTION
An opioid, narcotic agonist that binds at opiate receptor sites within

the central nervous system (CNS), reducing stimuli from sensory nerve endings. *Therapeutic Effect:* Increases pain threshold, alters pain reception, inhibits ascending pain pathways.

PHARMACOKINETICS

Route	Onset	Peak	Duration
IM	7–15 min	20–30 min	1–2 hrs
IV	1–2 min	3–5 min	0.5–1 hr
Trans-dermal	6–8 hrs	24 hrs	72 hrs
Trans-mucosal	5–15 min	20–30 min	1–2 hrs

Well absorbed after topical, IM administration. Transmucosal absorbed through mucosal tissue of mouth, GI tract. Protein binding: 80%–85%. Metabolized in liver. Primarily eliminated via biliary system. **Half-life:** IV: 2–4 hrs. Transdermal: 17 hrs. Transmucosal: 6.6 hrs.

AVAILABILITY

Injection: 50 mcg/ml.
Transdermal Patch: 25 mcg/hr, 50 mcg/hr, 75 mcg/hr, 100 mcg/hr.
Lozenges: 200 mcg, 400 mcg, 600 mcg, 800 mcg, 1,200 mcg, 1,600 mcg.

INDICATIONS AND DOSAGES
▸ **Sedation (minor procedures or analgesia)**
IM/IV
Adults, Elderly, Children older than 12 yrs. 0.5–1 mcg/kg/dose; may repeat after 30–60 min.
Children 1–12 yrs. 1–2 mcg/kg/dose.
Children younger than 1 yr. 1–4 mcg/kg/dose.

▸ **Preoperative sedation, adjunct regional anesthesia, postoperative pain**
IM/IV
Adults, Elderly, Children older than 12 yrs. 50–100 mcg/dose.
▸ **Adjunct to general anesthesia**
IV
Adults, Elderly, Children older than 12 yrs. 2–50 mcg/kg.
Transdermal
Adults, Elderly, Children older than 12 yrs. Initially, 25 mcg/hr system. May increase after 3 days.
Transmucosal
Adults, Children. 200–400 mcg for breakthrough cancer pain.
Epidural
Adults, Elderly. Bolus of 100 mcg, then continuous infusion rate of 4–12 ml/hr of a 10 mcg/ml concentration.
▸ **Continuous analgesia**
IV
Adults, Elderly, Children 1–12 yrs. Bolus of 1–2 mcg/kg, then 1 mcg/kg/hr. Range: 1–5 mcg/kg/hr.
Children younger than 1 yr. Bolus of 1–2 mcg/kg, then 0.5–1 mcg/kg/hr.
▸ **Dosage in renal impairment**

Creatinine Clearance	Dosage
10–50 ml/min	75% of dose
less than 10 ml/min	50% of dose

CONTRAINDICATIONS
Increased intracranial pressure, severe liver or renal impairment, severe respiratory depression

INTERACTIONS
Drug
Benzodiazepines: May increase the risk of hypotension and respiratory depression.
Buprenorphine: May decrease the effects of fentanyl.

Central nervous system (CNS) depressants: May increase respiratory depression and hypotension.

Herbal
None known.

Food
None known.

DIAGNOSTIC TEST EFFECTS
May increase serum amylase levels and plasma lipase concentrations.

IV INCOMPATIBILITIES
Phenytoin (Dilantin)

IV COMPATIBILITIES
Atropine, bupivacaine (Marcaine, Sensorcaine), clonidine (Duraclon), diltiazem (Cardizem), diphenhydramine (Benadryl), dobutamine (Dobutrex), dopamine (Intropin), droperidol (Inapsine), heparin, hydromorphone (Dilaudid), ketorolac (Toradol), lorazepam (Ativan), metoclopramide (Reglan), midazolam (Versed), milrinone (Primacor), morphine, nitroglycerin, norepinephrine (Levophed), ondansetron (Zofran), potassium chloride, propofol (Diprivan)

SIDE EFFECTS
Frequent
Transdermal (10%–3%): Headache, itching skin, nausea, vomiting, sweating, difficulty breathing, confusion, dizziness, drowsiness, diarrhea, constipation, decreased appetite
IV: Postoperative drowsiness, nausea, vomiting
Occasional
Transdermal (3%–1%): Chest pain, irregular heartbeat, redness, itching, swelling of skin, fainting, agitation, tingling or burning of skin
IV: Postoperative confusion, blurred vision, chills, orthostatic hypotension, constipation, difficulty urinating

SERIOUS REACTIONS
• Overdosage or too rapid IV administration results in severe respiratory depression, skeletal and thoracic muscle rigidity resulting in apnea, laryngospasm, bronchospasm, cold and clammy skin, cyanosis, and coma.
• Tolerance to the drug's analgesic effect may occur with repeated use.

NURSING CONSIDERATIONS
Baseline Assessment
• Make sure resuscitative equipment and an opiate antagonist (naloxone 0.5 mcg/kg) is readily available before administering the drug.
• Establish the patient's baseline blood pressure (B/P) and respiration rate.
• Assess the duration, intensity, location, and type of pain the patient is experiencing.

Lifespan Considerations
• Be aware that fentanyl readily crosses the placenta and that it is unknown if fentanyl is distributed in breast milk. Know that fentanyl may prolong labor if administered in the latent phase of first stage of labor, or before the cervix has dilated 4 to 5 cm.
• Be aware that respiratory depression may occur in the neonate if the mother received opiates during labor.
• Be aware that the safety and efficacy of the fentanyl patch have not been established in children younger than 12 years.
• Be aware that the transdermal form of fentanyl is not recommended in children younger than 12 years or children younger than

18 years and weighing less than 50 kg.
• Be aware that neonates and the elderly are more susceptible to the respiratory depressant effects of fentanyl.
• In the elderly, age-related renal impairment may require dosage adjustment.

Precautions

• Use cautiously in patients with bradycardia, head injuries, impaired consciousness, and liver, renal, or respiratory disease.
• Use cautiously in patients who use MAOIs within 14 days of fentanyl administration.

Administration and Handling

◀ALERT▶ Keep in mind that fentanyl may be combined with a local anesthetic, such as bupivacaine.

IV

• Store parenteral form at room temperature.
• For initial anesthesia induction dosage, give small amount, via tuberculin syringe, as prescribed.
• Give by slow IV push, over 1 to 2 minutes.
• Too rapid of an IV infusion increases the risk that the patient will experience severe adverse reactions, such as anaphylaxis, marked by bronchospasm, cardiac arrest, laryngospasm, peripheral circulatory collapse, and skeletal and thoracic muscle rigidity resulting in apnea.
• An opiate antagonist, such as naloxone, should be readily available during fentanyl administration.

Transdermal

• Apply to nonhairy area of intact skin of upper torso of the patient.
• Use a flat, nonirritated site.
• Firmly press the patch onto the patient's skin evenly for 10 to 20 seconds, ensuring adhesion is in full contact with skin, and edges are completely sealed.

• Use only water to cleanse the patient's patch site before application because soap and oils may irritate skin.
• Rotate sites of application.
• Carefully fold used patches so that they adhere to themselves; discard in toilet.

Transmucosal

• Patient should suck lozenge vigorously.

Intervention and Evaluation

• Assist the patient with ambulation.
• Encourage the patient to cough, turn, and deep breathe every 2 hours.
• Monitor the patient's blood pressure (B/P), heart rate, oxygen saturation, and respiratory rate.
• Assess the patient for relief of pain.

Patient Teaching

• Urge the patient to avoid alcohol and not to take any other medications during fentanyl therapy without first notifying the physician.
• Warn the patient to avoid tasks requiring mental alertness or motor skills until his or her response to the drug is established.
• Teach the patient the proper application of the transdermal fentanyl patch.
• Tell the patient to use fentanyl as directed to avoid overdosage. Explain to the patient that there is a potential for physical dependence on the drug with its prolonged use.
• Instruct the patient to discontinue fentanyl slowly after long-term use.

hydromorphone hydrochloride
high-dro-**more**-phone
(Dilaudid, Dilaudid HP,
Hydromorph Contin[CAN])

CATEGORY AND SCHEDULE
Pregnancy Risk Category B, D if
used for prolonged periods or at
high dosages at term
Controlled Substance: Schedule II

MECHANISM OF ACTION
An opioid agonist that binds
at opiate receptor sites in the central nervous system (CNS). *Therapeutic Effect:* Reduces intensity
of pain stimuli incoming from
sensory nerve endings, altering
pain perception and emotional
response to pain; suppresses
cough reflex.

PHARMACOKINETICS

Route	Onset	Peak	Duration
PO	30 min	90–120 min	4 hrs
Subcuta-neous	15 min	30–90 min	4 hrs
IM	15 min	30–60 min	4–5 hrs
IV	10–15 min	15–30 min	2–3 hrs
Rectal	15–30 min	N/A	N/A

Well absorbed from the gastrointestinal (GI) tract, after IM administration. Widely distributed. Metabolized in liver. Excreted in urine.
Half-life: 1–3 hrs.

AVAILABILITY
Tablets: 2 mg, 3 mg, 4 mg, 8 mg.
Liquid: 5 mg/5 ml.

Injection: 1 mg/ml, 2 mg/ml,
4 mg/ml, 10 mg/ml.
Suppository: 3 mg.

INDICATIONS AND DOSAGES
▸ **Analgesic**
IV
*Adults, Elderly, Children weighing
more than 50 kg.* 0.2-0.6 mg q2-3h.
PO
*Adults, Elderly, Children weighing
50 kg and more.* 2-4 mg q3-4h.
Range: 2-8 mg/dose.
*Children older than 6 mos, weigh-
ing less than 50 kg.* 0.03-0.08
mg/kg/dose q3-4h
Rectal
Adults, Elderly. 3 mg q4-8h.
▸ **Antitussive**
PO
*Adults, Elderly, Children older than
12 yrs.* 1 mg q3–4h.
Children 6-12 yrs. 0.5 mg q3–4h.
▸ **Patient controlled analgesia (PCA)**
IV
Adults, Elderly. 0.05-0.5 mg at
5-15 min lockout. 4 hr Maximum:
4-6 mg.
Epidural
Adults, Elderly. bolus of 1-1.5 mg.
rate of 0.04-0.4 mg/hr. Demand
dose of 0.15 mg at 30 min lockout.

CONTRAINDICATIONS
None known

INTERACTIONS
Drug
Alcohol, CNS depressants: May
increase CNS or respiratory depres-
sion, hypotension.
MAOIs: May produce severe, fatal
reaction; plan to reduce dose to one
quarter usual dose.
Herbal
None known.
Food
None known.

DIAGNOSTIC TEST EFFECTS

May increase serum amylase levels and plasma lipase concentrations.

IV INCOMPATIBILITIES

Amphotericin B complex (Abelcet, AmBisome, Amphotec), cefazolin (Ancef, Kefzol), diazepam (Valium), phenobarbital, phenytoin (Dilantin)

IV COMPATIBILITIES

Diltiazem (Cardizem), diphenhydramine (Benadryl), dobutamine (Dobutrex), dopamine (Intropin), fentanyl (Sublimaze), furosemide (Lasix), heparin, lorazepam (Ativan), magnesium sulfate, metoclopramide (Reglan), midazolam (Versed), milrinone (Primacor), morphine, propofol (Diprivan)

SIDE EFFECTS

Frequent
Drowsiness, dizziness, hypotension, decreased appetite
Occasional
Confusion, diaphoresis, facial flushing, urinary retention, constipation, dry mouth, nausea, vomiting, headache, pain at injection site
Rare
Allergic reaction, depression

SERIOUS REACTIONS

• Overdosage results in respiratory depression, skeletal muscle flaccidity, cold or clammy skin, cyanosis, extreme somnolence progressing to seizures, stupor, and coma.
• Tolerance to analgesic effect and physical dependence may occur with repeated use.
• Prolonged duration of action and cumulative effect may occur in patients with impaired liver or renal function.

NURSING CONSIDERATIONS

Baseline Assessment
• Obtain the patient's vital signs before administering hydromorphone.
• Withhold the medication, and notify the physician if the adult patient's respirations are 12/minute or less, or 20/minute or less in children.
• Assess the duration, location, onset, and type of pain.
• Know that the effect of hydromorphone is reduced if the patient experiences full pain before the next dose.
• Assess the frequency, severity, and type of cough the patient experiences.
Lifespan Considerations
• Be aware that hydromorphone readily crosses the placenta and it is unknown if hydromorphone is distributed in breast milk.
• Be aware that hydromorphone use may prolong labor if administered in the latent phase of the first stage of labor or before cervical dilation of 4 to 5 cm has occurred.
• Be aware that respiratory depression may occur in neonate if mother receives opiates during labor. Regular use of opiates during pregnancy may produce withdrawal symptoms in the neonate, including diarrhea, excessive crying, fever, hyperactive reflexes, irritability, seizures, sneezing, tremors, vomiting, and yawning.
• Be aware that pediatric patients younger than 2 years of age may be more susceptible to respiratory depression.
• Be aware that elderly patients may be more susceptible to respiratory depression and the drug may cause paradoxical excitement.
• In the elderly, age-related prostatic hypertrophy or obstruction and renal impairment may increase the risk of urinary retention, and dosage adjustment is recommended.

Precautions
• Use extremely cautiously in patients with acute alcoholism, anoxia, CNS depression, hypercapnia, respiratory depression or dysfunction, seizures, shock, and untreated myxedema.
• Use cautiously in patients with acute abdominal conditions, Addison's disease, chronic obstructive pulmonary disease (COPD), hypothyroidism, impaired liver function, increased intracranial pressure, prostatic hypertrophy, and urethral stricture.

Administration and Handling
◀ALERT▶ Keep in mind that hydromorphone's side effects depend on the dosage amount and route of administration, but occur infrequently with oral antitussives.
• Know that patients who are ambulatory or not in severe pain may experience dizziness, hypotension, nausea, and vomiting more frequently than those in supine position or having severe pain.

PO
• Give hydromorphone without regard to meals.
• Crush tablets, as needed.

Subcutaneous/IM
• Use short 30-gauge needle for subcutaneous injection.
• Administer slowly, rotating injection sites.
• Know that patients with circulatory impairment experience higher risk of overdosage because of delayed absorption of repeated subcutaneous or IM injections.

IV
◀ALERT▶ Be aware that a high concentration injection (10 mg/ml) should be used only in patients currently receiving high doses of another opiate agonist for severe, chronic pain caused by cancer or tolerance to opiate agonists.

• Store at room temperature; protect from light.
• Slight yellow discoloration of parenteral form does not indicate loss of potency.
• May give undiluted as IV push.
• May further dilute with 5 ml sterile water for injection or 0.9% NaCl.
• Administer IV push very slowly, over 2 to 5 minutes.
• Be aware that rapid IV administration increases risk of severe anaphylactic reaction, marked by apnea, cardiac arrest, and circulatory collapse.

Rectal
• Refrigerate suppositories.
• Moisten suppository with cold water before inserting well up into rectum.

Intervention and Evaluation
• Monitor and assess the patient's vital signs.
• Assess the patient for cough and pain relief.
• Auscultate the patient's lungs for adventitious breath sounds.
• Increase the patient's fluid intake and environmental humidity to decrease the viscosity of patient lung secretions.
• Assess the patient's pattern of daily bowel activity and stool consistency, especially with long-term use.
• Initiate deep breathing and coughing exercises, particularly in patients with impaired pulmonary function.
• Assess the patient for clinical improvement and record the onset of relief of cough or pain.

Patient Teaching
• Urge the patient to avoid alcohol during hydromorphone therapy.
• Warn the patient to avoid tasks that require mental alertness and motor skills until his or her response to the drug is established.

• Explain to the patient that drug dependence and tolerance may occur with prolonged use at high dosages.
• Instruct the patient to change positions slowly to avoid orthostatic hypotension.
• Tell the patient to alert you to pain at its onset because the effect of hydromorphone is reduced if the patient experiences full pain before the next dose.

meperidine hydrochloride

meh-**pear**-ih-deen
(Demerol, Pethidine Injection[AUS])

CATEGORY AND SCHEDULE

Pregnancy Risk Category: B, D if used for prolonged periods or at high dosages at term
Controlled Substance: Schedule II

MECHANISM OF ACTION

A narcotic agonist that binds with opioid receptors within the central nervous system (CNS). *Therapeutic Effect:* Alters processes, affecting pain perception, emotional response to pain.

PHARMACOKINETICS

Route	Onset	Peak	Duration
PO	15 min	60 min	2–4 hrs
Subcuta-neous	10–15 min	30–50 min	2–4 hrs
IM	10–15 min	30–50 min	2–4 hrs
IV	less than 5 min	5–7 min	2–3 hrs

Variably absorbed from the gastro-intestinal (GI) tract, well absorbed after IM administration. Protein binding: 60%–80%. Widely distributed. Metabolized in liver to active metabolite. Primarily excreted in urine. Not removed by hemodialysis. **Half-life:** 2.4–4 hrs (half-life is increased in elderly). Metabolite: 8–16 hrs.

AVAILABILITY

Tablets: 50 mg, 100 mg.
Syrup: 50 mg/5 ml.
Injection: 25 mg/ml, 50 mg/ml, 75 mg/ml, 100 mg/ml.

INDICATIONS AND DOSAGES
▸ **Pain**
PO/IM/Subcutaneous
Adults, Elderly. 50–150 mg q3–4h.
Children. 1.1–1.5 mg/kg q3–4h.
Do not exceed single pediatric dose 100 mg.
▸ **Patient controlled analgesia (PCA)**
IV
Adults. Loading dose: 50–100 mg. Intermittent bolus: 5–30 mg. Lock-out interval: 10–20 min. Continuous infusion: 5–40 mg/hr. 4-hr limit: 200–300 mg.
▸ **Dosage in renal impairment**

Creatinine Clearance	% Normal Dose
10–50 ml/min	75
less than 10 ml/min	50

CONTRAINDICATIONS

Delivery of premature infant, diarrhea due to poisoning, those receiving MAOIs in past 14 days

INTERACTIONS
Drug
Alcohol, CNS depressants: May increase CNS or respiratory depression and hypotension.
MAOIs: May produce severe, fatal reaction; plan to reduce dose to one quarter the usual dose.

Herbal
Valerian: May increase CNS depression.
Food
None known.

DIAGNOSTIC TEST EFFECTS

May increase serum amylase and lipase levels. Therapeutic serum level is 100–550 ng/ml; toxic serum level is greater than 1,000 ng/ml.

IV INCOMPATIBILITIES

Allopurinol (Aloprim), amphotericin B complex (Abelcet, AmBisome, Amphotec), cefepime (Maxipime), cefoperazone (Cefobid), doxorubicin liposome (Doxil), furosemide (Lasix), idarubicin (Idamycin), nafcillin (Nafcil)

IV COMPATIBILITIES

Bumetanide (Bumex), diltiazem (Cardizem), dobutamine (Dobutrex), dopamine (Intropin), heparin, insulin, lidocaine, magnesium, oxytocin (Pitocin), potassium

SIDE EFFECTS

Frequent
Sedation, decreased blood pressure (B/P), diaphoresis, flushed face, dizziness, nausea, vomiting, constipation
Occasional
Confusion, irregular heartbeat, tremors, decreased urination, abdominal pain, dry mouth, headache, irritation at injection site, euphoria, dysphoria
Rare
Allergic reaction, marked by rash and itching, insomnia

SERIOUS REACTIONS

• Overdosage results in respiratory depression, skeletal muscle flaccidity, cold or clammy skin, cyanosis, extreme somnolence progressing to convulsions, stupor, and coma. The overdosage antidote is 0.4 mg naloxone (Narcan).
• Tolerance to the drug's analgesic effect and physical dependence may occur with repeated use.

NURSING CONSIDERATIONS

Baseline Assessment
• Place patient in a recumbent position before giving parenteral meperidine.
• Assess the duration, location, onset, and type pain the patient is experiencing.
• Obtain the patient's vital signs before giving meperidine.
• Withhold the medication and notify the physician if the adult patient's respirations are 12/minute or less, or 20/minute or less in children.
• Know that the effects of meperidine are reduced if the patient experiences full pain before the next dose of the drug.
Lifespan Considerations
• Be aware that meperidine crosses the placenta and is distributed in breast milk.
• Be aware that respiratory depression may occur in the neonate if the mother received opiates during labor. Regular use of opiates during pregnancy may produce withdrawal symptoms in neonate, such as diarrhea, excessive crying, fever, hyperactive reflexes, irritability, seizures, sneezing, tremors, vomiting, and yawning.
• Be aware that children may experience paradoxical excitement.
• Know that children younger than 2 years of age and the elderly are more susceptible to the respiratory depressant effects of meperidine.
• In the elderly, age-related renal

impairment may increase the risk of urinary retention.

Precautions

• Use cautiously in patients with acute abdominal conditions, cor pulmonale, history of seizures, increased intracranial pressure, liver or renal impairment, respiratory abnormalities, and supraventricular tachycardia.

• Use cautiously in elderly or debilitated patients.

Administration and Handling

◀ALERT▶ Be aware that meperidine's side effects are dependent on dosage amount and route of administration.

• Know that patients that are ambulatory and not in severe pain may experience dizziness, nausea, and vomiting more frequently than those in supine position or having severe pain.

◀ALERT▶ Keep in mind that the IM route is preferred over the subcutaneous route because the subcutaneous injection can produce induration, local irritation, and pain.

PO

• Give meperidine without regard to meals.

• Dilute syrup in glass of water to prevent an anesthetic effect on mucous membranes.

Subcutaneous/IM

• Inject slowly.

• Know that patients with circulatory impairment experience a higher risk of overdosage because of delayed absorption of repeated injection.

IV

◀ALERT▶ Give by slow IV push or infusion.

• Store at room temperature.

• May give undiluted or may dilute in D_5W, lactated Ringer's, a dextrose-saline combination, such as 2.5%, 5%, or 10% dextrose with 0.45% or 0.9% NaCl, Ringer's, lactated

Ringer's, or molar sodium lactate diluent for IV injection or infusion.

• Administer IV push very slowly, over 2 to 3 minutes.

• Be aware that rapid IV administration increases risk of severe anaphylactic reaction, marked by apnea, cardiac arrest, and circulatory collapse.

Intervention and Evaluation

• Monitor the patient's vital signs 15 to 30 minutes after subcutaneous/IM dose, 5 to 10 minutes after IV dose. Monitor for decreased blood pressure (B/P), as well as a change in quality and rate of pulse.

• Monitor the patient's pain level and sedation.

• Assess the patient's daily pattern of bowel activity and stool consistency.

• Evaluate the patient for adequate voiding.

• Initiate deep breathing and coughing exercises, particularly in patients with impaired pulmonary function. Therapeutic serum level is 100 to 550 ng/ml; toxic serum level is greater than 1,000 ng/ml.

Patient Teaching

• Instruct the patient to take meperidine before the pain fully returns, within prescribed intervals.

• Explain to the patient that discomfort may occur with injection.

• Instruct the patient to change positions slowly to avoid orthostatic hypotension.

• Urge the patient to increase his or her fluid intake and consumption of fiber, bulking agents to prevent constipation.

• Tell the patient that dependence and tolerance of the drug may occur with prolonged use of high doses.

• Urge the patient to avoid alcohol and other CNS depressants while taking meperidine.

• Warn the patient to avoid tasks that require mental alertness or motor skills until his or her response to the drug is established.

methadone hydrochloride
meth-ah-doan
(Dolophine, Metadol[CAN], Methadose, Physeptone[AUS])

CATEGORY AND SCHEDULE
Pregnancy Risk Category: B, D if used for prolonged periods or at high dosages at term
Controlled Substance: Schedule II

MECHANISM OF ACTION
A narcotic agonist that binds with opioid receptors within the central nervous system (CNS). *Therapeutic Effect:* Alters processes affecting analgesia, emotional response to acute withdrawal syndrome.

PHARMACOKINETICS

Route	Onset	Peak	Duration
PO	30–60 min	0.5–1 hr	6–8 hrs
Subcutaneous	10–15 min	1–2 hrs	4–6 hrs
IM	10–15 min	1–2 hrs	4–6 hrs

Well absorbed after IM injection. Protein binding: 80%–85%. Metabolized in liver. Primarily excreted in urine. Not removed by hemodialysis. **Half-life:** 15–25 hrs.

AVAILABILITY
Tablets: 5 mg, 10 mg.
Tablets (dispersible): 40 mg.
Oral Solution: 5 mg/5 ml, 10 mg/5 ml.
Oral Concentrate: 10 mg/ml.
Injection: 10 mg/ml.

INDICATIONS AND DOSAGES
▶ **Analgesia**
PO/IM/IV/Subcutaneous
Adults. 2.5–10 mg q3–8h as needed up to 5–20 mg q6–8h.
Elderly. 2.5 mg q8–12h.
Children. Initially, 0.1 mg/kg/dose q4h for 2–3 doses, then q6–12h. Maximum: 10 mg/dose.
▶ **Detoxification**
PO
Adults, Elderly. 15–40 mg/day.
▶ **Maintenance of opiate dependence**
PO
Adults, Elderly. 20–120 mg/day.

CONTRAINDICATIONS
Delivery of premature infant, during labor, diarrhea due to poisoning, hypersensitivity to narcotics

INTERACTIONS
Drug
Alcohol, CNS depressants: May increase CNS or respiratory depression and hypotension.
MAOIs: May produce severe, fatal reaction; plan to reduce to one quarter usual dose.
Herbal
Valerian: May increase CNS depression.
Food
None known.

DIAGNOSTIC TEST EFFECTS
May increase serum amylase and lipase levels.

SIDE EFFECTS
Frequent
Sedation, decreased blood pressure [B/P], diaphoresis, flushed face, constipation, dizziness, nausea, vomiting
Occasional
Confusion, decreased urination, pounding heartbeat, stomach

cramps, visual changes, dry mouth, headache, decreased appetite, nervousness, inability to sleep
Rare
Allergic reaction, such as rash or itching

SERIOUS REACTIONS

• Overdosage results in respiratory depression, skeletal muscle flaccidity, cold or clammy skin, cyanosis, extreme somnolence progressing to convulsions, stupor, and coma. The antidote for overdosage is 0.4 mg naloxone.
• Tolerance to the drug's analgesic effect and physical dependence may occur with repeated use.

NURSING CONSIDERATIONS

Baseline Assessment

• Place the patient in the recumbent position before giving parenteral methadone.
• Obtain the patient's vital signs before giving medication.
• Withhold the medication, and notify the physician if the adult patient's respirations are 12/minute or less, or 20/minute or less in children.

Lifespan Considerations

• Be aware that methadone crosses the placenta and is distributed in breast milk.
• Be aware that respiratory depression may occur in the neonate if the mother received opiates during labor. Know that regular use of opiates during pregnancy may produce withdrawal symptoms in neonate, such as diarrhea, excessive crying, fever, hyperactive reflexes, irritability, seizures, sneezing, tremors, vomiting, and yawning.
• Be aware that children may experience paradoxical excitement.
• Be aware that children younger

than 2 years and the elderly are more susceptible to the respiratory depressant effects of methadone.
• In the elderly, age-related renal impairment may increase the risk of urine retention.

Precautions

• Use extremely cautiously in patients with acute abdominal conditions, cor pulmonale, history of seizures, impaired liver or renal function, increased intracranial pressure, respiratory abnormalities, and supraventricular tachycardia.
• Use cautiously in debilitated and elderly patients.

Administration and Handling

PO
• Give methadone without regard to meals.
• Dilute syrup in glass of water to prevent anesthetic effect on mucous membranes.
Subcutaneous/IM
◀ALERT▶ Be aware that the IM route is preferred over subcutaneous route because the subcutaneous route can produce induration, local irritation, and pain.
• Do not use if solution appears cloudy or contains a precipitate.
• Inject slowly.
• Know that patients with circulatory impairment experience higher risk of overdosage because of delayed absorption of repeated subcutaneous or IM injections.

Intervention and Evaluation

• Monitor the patient's vital signs 15 to 30 minutes after subcutaneous/IM dose, 5 to 10 minutes after IV dose.
• Know that oral methadone is one-half as potent as parenteral methadone.
• Assess the patient for adequate voiding.

• Assess the patient for clinical improvement and record the onset of relief of pain.
• Provide support to the patient in a detoxification program. Monitor the patient for withdrawal symptoms.

Patient Teaching
• Urge the patient to avoid alcohol.
• Caution the patient against abruptly discontinuing the drug after prolonged use.
• Explain to the patient that methadone may cause drowsiness and dry mouth.
• Warn the patient that methadone may impair his or her ability to perform activities requiring mental alertness and motor skills.

morphine sulfate

(Anamorph[AUS], Astramorph, Avinza, Duramorph, Infumorph, Kadian, Kapanol[AUS], M-Eslon, Morphine Mixtures[AUS], MS Contin, MSIR, MS Mono[AUS], Oramorph SR, RMS, Roxanol, Statex[CAN])
Do not confuse with hydromorphone or Roxicet.

CATEGORY AND SCHEDULE
Pregnancy Risk Category: C, D if used for prolonged periods or at high dosages at term
Controlled Substance: Schedule II

MECHANISM OF ACTION
A narcotic agonist that binds with opioid receptors within the central nervous system (CNS). *Therapeutic Effect:* Alters processes affecting pain perception, emotional response to pain; produces generalized CNS depression.

PHARMACOKINETICS

Route	Onset	Peak	Duration
Tablets	N/A	1 hr	3–5 hrs
Oral Solution	N/A	1 hr	3–5 hrs
Epidural	N/A	1 hr	12–20 hrs
ER Tabs	N/A	3–4 hrs	8–12 hrs
Rectal	N/A	0.5–1 hr	3–7 hrs
Subcutaneous	N/A	1.1–5 hrs	3–5 hrs
IM	5–30 min	0.5–1 hr	3–5 hrs
IV	Rapid	0.3 hr	3–5 hrs

Variably absorbed from the gastrointestinal (GI) tract. Readily absorbed after subcutaneous, IM administration. Protein binding: 20%–35%. Widely distributed. Metabolized in liver. Primarily excreted in urine. Removed by hemodialysis. **Half-life:** 2–3 hrs.

AVAILABILITY
Capsules (sustained release): 20 mg (Kadian), 30 mg (Kadian), 50 mg (Kadian), 60 mg (Kadian), 100 mg (Kadian).
Capsules (extended-release): 30 mg (Avinza), 60 mg (Avinza), 90 mg (Avinza), 120 mg (Avinza).
Solution for Injection: 0.5 mg/ml, 1 mg/ml, 2 mg/ml, 4 mg/ml, 5 mg/ml, 8 mg/ml, 10 mg/ml, 15 mg/ml, 25 mg/ml, 50 mg/ml.
Solution for Injection (preservative-free): 0.5 mg/ml, 1 mg/ml, 10 mg/ml, 25 mg/ml, 50 mg/ml.
Epidural and Intrathecal via Infusion Device: 10 mg/ml (Infumorph), 25 mg/ml (Infumorph).
Epidural, Intrathecal, IV Infusion: 0.5 mg/ml (Astramorph, Duramorph), 1 mg/ml (Astramorph, Duramorph), 4 mg/ml (Astramorph, Duramorph).
IV Infusion (via patient-controlled

analgesia [PCA]): 1 mg/ml,
5 mg/ml.
Oral Solution: 10 mg/5 ml (Roxanol), 20 mg/5 ml (Roxanol),
20 mg/ml (Roxanol), 100 mg/5 mg
(Roxanol).
Suppository (RMS): 5 mg, 10 mg,
20 mg, 30 mg.
Tablets: 15 mg/30 mg (MSIR).
Tablets (extended-release): 15 mg
(MS Contin, Oramorph SR),
30 mg (MS Contin, Oramorph SR),
60 mg (MS Contin, Oramorph SR),
100 mg (MS Contin, Oramorph
SR), 200 mg (MS Contin,
Oramorph SR).

INDICATIONS AND DOSAGES
▸ **Pain**
PO
Adults, Elderly (prompt-release).
10–30 mg q4h as needed.
Adults, Elderly (sustained-release).
0.2–0.5 mg/kg/dose q4–6h.
Children (sustained-release). 15–30
mg q8–12h.
Children. 0.3–0.6 mg/kg/dose q12h.
IV/IM/Subcutaneous
Adults, Elderly. 2.5–20 mg/dose
q2–6h.
Children. 0.1–0.2 mg/kg/dose   ·
q2–4h. Maximum: 15 mg/dose.
IV continuous infusion
Adults, Elderly. 0.8–10 mg/hr.
Range: Up to 80 mg/hr.
Children. 0.025–2.6 mg/kg/hr.
Epidural
Adults, Elderly. Initially, 5 mg. May
give 1–2 mg in 1 hr if no relief.
Maximum: 10 mg/24 hrs.
Intrathecal
Adults, Elderly. One-tenth of the
epidural dose: 0.2–1 mg/dose.
▸ **PCA**
IV
Adults, Elderly. Loading dose: 5–10
mg. Intermittent bolus: 0.5–3 mg.
Lockout interval: 5–12 min. Contin-

uous infusion: 1–10 mg/hr. 4-hr
limit: 20–30 mg.

CONTRAINDICATIONS
Severe respiratory depression, acute
or severe asthma, severe liver or
renal impairment, GI obstruction.

INTERACTIONS
Drug
*Alcohol, central nervous system
(CNS) depressants:* May increase
CNS or respiratory depression and
hypotension.
MAOIs: May produce severe, fatal
reaction; plan to reduce dose to one
quarter of usual dose.
Herbal
None known.
Food
None known.

DIAGNOSTIC TEST EFFECTS
May increase serum amylase and
lipase levels.

IV INCOMPATIBILITIES
Amphotericin B complex (Abelcet,
AmBisome, Amphotec), cefepime
(Maxipime), doxorubicin liposome
(Doxil), thiopental

IV COMPATIBILITIES
Amiodarone (Cordarone), bumetanide (Bumex), bupivacaine
(Marcaine, Sensorcaine), diltiazem
(Cardizem), dobutamine (Dobutrex),
dopamine (Intropin), heparin, lidocaine, lorazepam (Ativan), magnesium, midazolam (Versed), milrinone (Primacor), nitroglycerin,
potassium, propofol (Diprivan)

SIDE EFFECTS
Frequent
Sedation, decreased blood pressure
(B/P), diaphoresis, flushed face,
constipation, dizziness, drowsiness,
nausea, vomiting

Occasional
Allergic reaction, such as rash and itching, difficulty breathing, confusion, pounding heartbeat, tremors, decreased urination, stomach cramps, vision changes, dry mouth, headache, decreased appetite, pain/burning at injection site
Rare
Paralytic ileus

SERIOUS REACTIONS

• Overdosage results in respiratory depression, skeletal muscle flaccidity, cold or clammy skin, cyanosis, extreme somnolence progressing to convulsions, stupor, and coma.
• Tolerance to analgesic effect and physical dependence may occur with repeated use.
• Prolonged duration of action and cumulative effect may occur in those with impaired liver and renal function.

NURSING CONSIDERATIONS

Baseline Assessment
• Place the patient in a recumbent position before giving parenteral morphine.
• Assess the duration, location, onset, and type of pain the patient is experiencing.
• Obtain the patient's vital signs before giving morphine.
• Withhold the medication and notify the physician if the adult patient's respirations are 12/minute or less, or 20/minute or less in children.
• Be aware that the effect of the medication is reduced if the patient experiences full pain before next dose.

Lifespan Considerations
• Be aware that morphine crosses the placenta and is distributed in breast milk.

• Be aware that morphine may prolong labor if administered in latent phase of first stage of labor or before cervical dilation of 4 to 5 cm has occurred. Respiratory depression may occur in neonate if mother received opiates during labor.
• Be aware that regular use of opiates during pregnancy may produce withdrawal symptoms in neonate, such as diarrhea, excessive crying, fever, hyperactive reflexes, irritability, seizures, sneezing, tremors, vomiting, and yawning.
• Be aware that children and the elderly may experience paradoxical excitement.
• Be aware that children younger than 2 years of age and the elderly are more susceptible to respiratory depressant effects.
• In the elderly, age-related renal impairment may increase the risk of urine retention.

Precautions
• Use extremely cautiously in patients with chronic obstructive pulmonary disease (COPD), cor pulmonale, head injury, hypoxia, hypercapnia, increased intracranial pressure, preexisting respiratory depression, and severe hypotension.
• Use cautiously in patients with Addison's disease, alcoholism, biliary tract disease, CNS depression, hypothyroidism, pancreatitis, prostatic hypertrophy, seizure disorders, toxic psychosis, and urethral stricture.
• Use cautiously in debilitated patients.

Administration and Handling
◀ALERT▶ Expect to reduce the drug dosage in the debilitated and elderly and those on concurrent CNS depressants. Titrate to desired effect, as prescribed.
◀ALERT▶ Be aware that meperidine's side effects are dependent on

dosage amount and route of administration.

• Know that patients that are ambulatory and not in severe pain may experience dizziness, nausea, and vomiting more frequently than those in supine position or having severe pain.

PO

• Mix liquid form with fruit juice to improve taste.

• Do not crush, open, or break extended-release capsule.

• May mix Kadian with applesauce immediately prior to administration.

Subcutaneous/IM

• Give injection slowly, rotating injection sites.

• Know that patients with circulatory impairment experience a higher risk of overdosage because of delayed absorption of repeated injections.

IV

• Store at room temperature.

• May give undiluted as IV push.

• For IV push, may dilute 2.5 to 15 mg morphine in 4 to 5 ml sterile water for injection.

• For continuous IV infusion, dilute to concentration of 0.1 to 1 mg/ml in D_5W and give through controlled infusion device.

• Always administer very slowly. Be aware that rapid IV administration increases risk of severe anaphylactic reaction, marked by apnea, cardiac arrest, and circulatory collapse.

Rectal

• If suppository is too soft, chill for 30 minutes in refrigerator or run cold water over foil wrapper.

• Moisten suppository with cold water before inserting well into rectum.

Intervention and Evaluation

• Monitor the patient's vital signs 5 to 10 minutes after IV administration, and 15 to 30 minutes after subcutaneous or IM injection.

• Be alert for decreased patient respirations or blood pressure (B/P).

• Evaluate the patient for difficulty voiding.

• Assess the patient's daily pattern of bowel activity and stool consistency.

• Initiate deep breathing and coughing exercises, particularly in patients with impaired pulmonary function.

• Assess the patient for clinical improvement and record the onset of pain relief.

• Consult with the physician if the patient's pain relief is not adequate.

Patient Teaching

• Tell the patient that discomfort may occur with injection.

• Instruct the patient to change positions slowly to avoid orthostatic hypotension.

• Warn the patient to avoid tasks that require mental alertness or motor skills until his or her response to the drug is established.

• Urge the patient to avoid alcohol and CNS depressants during morphine therapy.

• Explain to the patient that dependence and tolerance may occur with prolonged use of high morphine doses.

oxycodone

ox-ih-koe-doan
(Endone[AUS], Intensol, OxyContin, OxyFast, OxyIR, Perolone, Roxicodone, Supeudol[CAN])
Do not confuse with oxybutynin.

CATEGORY AND SCHEDULE

Pregnancy Risk Category: B, D if used for prolonged periods or at high dosages at term
Controlled Substance: Schedule II

MECHANISM OF ACTION

An opioid analgesic that binds with opioid receptors within the central nervous system (CNS). *Therapeutic Effect:* Alters processes affecting pain perception, emotional response to pain.

PHARMACOKINETICS

Route	Onset	Peak	Duration
Immediate-release	N/A	N/A	4–5 hrs
Controlled-release	N/A	N/A	12 hrs

Moderately absorbed from the gastrointestinal (GI) tract. Protein binding: 38%–45%. Widely distributed. Metabolized in liver. Excreted in urine. Unknown if removed by hemodialysis. **Half-life:** 2–3 hrs (controlled-release: 3.2 hrs).

AVAILABILITY

Capsules (immediate-release): 5 mg (OxyIR).
Oral Concentrate: 20 mg/ml (Oxy-Fast, Roxicodone, Intensol).
Oral Solution: 5 mg/ml (Roxicodone).
Tablets (immediate-release): 5 mg (Percolone, Roxicodone), 15 mg (Percolone, Roxicodone), 30 mg (Percolone, Roxicodone).
Tablets (controlled-release): 10 mg (Oxycontin), 20 mg (Oxycontin), 40 mg (Oxycontin), 80 mg (Oxycontin), 160 mg (Oxycontin).

INDICATIONS AND DOSAGES

▸ **Analgesia**
PO
Adults, Elderly (controlled-release). Initially, 10 mg q12h. May increase q1–2 days by 25%–50%. Usual: 40 mg/day. Cancer pain:100 mg/day.
Adults, Elderly (immediate-release).

Initially, 5 mg q6h as needed. May increase up to 30 mg q4h. Usual: 10–30 mg q4h as needed.
Children. 0.05–0.15 mg/kg/dose q4–6h.

CONTRAINDICATIONS

None known

INTERACTIONS

Drug
Alcohol, CNS depressants: May increase CNS or respiratory depression and hypotension.
MAOIs: May produce severe, fatal reaction; expect to reduce dose to one quarter usual dose.
Herbal
None known.
Food
None known.

DIAGNOSTIC TEST EFFECTS

May increase serum amylase and lipase levels.

SIDE EFFECTS

Frequent
Drowsiness, dizziness, hypotension, anorexia
Occasional
Confusion, diaphoresis, facial flushing, urinary retention, constipation, dry mouth, nausea, vomiting, headache
Rare
Allergic reaction, depression, paradoxical CNS hyperactivity or nervousness in children, excitement and restlessness in elderly and debilitated patients

SERIOUS REACTIONS

• Overdose results in respiratory depression, skeletal muscle flaccidity, cold or clammy skin, cyanosis, extreme somnolence progressing to convulsions, stupor, and coma.
• Liver toxicity may occur with

overdosage of acetaminophen component.
• Tolerance to analgesic effect and physical dependence may occur with repeated use.

NURSING CONSIDERATIONS

Baseline Assessment
• Assess the duration, location, onset, and type of pain the patient is experiencing.
• Know that the effect of oxycodone is reduced if the patient experiences full pain before next dose.
• Obtain the patient's vital signs before giving the medication.
• Withhold the medication and notify the physician if the adult patient's respirations are 12/minute or less, or 20/minute or less in children.

Lifespan Considerations
• Be aware that oxycodone readily crosses the placenta and is distributed in breast milk.
• Be aware that respiratory depression may occur in neonate if mother received opiates during labor.
• Be aware that regular use of opiates during pregnancy may produce withdrawal symptoms in neonate, including irritability, diarrhea, excessive crying, fever, hyperactive reflexes, irritability, seizures, sneezing, tremors, vomiting, and yawning.
• Be aware that children may experience paradoxical excitement.
• Be aware that children younger than 2 years of age and the elderly are more susceptible to the respiratory depressant effects of oxycodone.
• In the elderly, age-related renal impairment may increase the risk of urine retention.

Precautions
• Use extremely cautiously in patients with acute alcoholism, anoxia, CNS depression, hypercapnia, respiratory depression or dysfunction, seizures, shock, and untreated myxedema.
• Use cautiously in patients with acute abdominal conditions, Addison's disease, chronic obstructive pulmonary disease (COPD), hypothyroidism, impaired liver function, increased intracranial pressure, prostatic hypertrophy, and urethral stricture.

Administration and Handling
◀ALERT▶ Be aware that oxycodone's effects are dependent on the dosage amount.
• Know that ambulatory patients and patients not in severe pain may experience dizziness, hypotension, nausea, and vomiting more frequently than those in supine position or having severe pain.

PO
• Give oxycodone without regard to meals.
• Crush immediate-release tablets as needed.
• Have the patient swallow controlled-release tablets whole; do not crush, break, chew.

Intervention and Evaluation
• Palpate the patient's bladder for urine retention.
• Monitor the patient's pattern of daily bowel activity and stool consistency.
• Initiate deep breathing and coughing exercises, particularly in patients with impaired pulmonary function.
• Monitor the patient's blood pressure (B/P), mental status, respiratory rate, and pain relief.

Patient Teaching
• Tell the patient that oxycodone may cause drowsiness and dry mouth.

• Warn the patient to avoid performing tasks that require mental alertness or motor skills.
• Urge the patient to avoid alcohol while taking oxycodone.
• Caution the patient that oxycodone may be habit-forming.
• Instruct the patient not to break, chew, or crush controlled-release tablets.
• Instruct the patient to take meperidine before the pain fully returns, within prescribed intervals.

propoxyphene hydrochloride
pro-**pox**-ih-feen
(Darvon)

propoxyphene napsylate
(Darvon-N[CAN])

CATEGORY AND SCHEDULE
Pregnancy Risk Category: C (D if used for prolonged periods)
Controlled Substance: Schedule IV

MECHANISM OF ACTION
An opioid agonist that binds with opioid receptors within the central nervous system (CNS). *Therapeutic Effect:* Alters processes affecting pain perception, emotional response to pain.

PHARMACOKINETICS

Route	Onset	Peak	Duration
PO	15–60 min	N/A	4–6 hrs

Well absorbed from the gastrointestinal (GI) tract. Protein binding: High. Widely distributed. Metabolized in liver. Primarily excreted in urine. Not removed by hemodialysis. **Half-life:** 6–12 hrs; metabolite: 30–36 hrs.

AVAILABILITY
Capsules (Hydrochloride): 65 mg.
Tablets (Napsylate): 100 mg.

INDICATIONS AND DOSAGES
▶ **Relief of mild to moderate pain**
PO (propoxyphene hydrochloride)
Adults, Elderly. 65 mg q4h, as needed. Maximum: 390 mg/day.
PO (propoxyphene napsylate)
Adults, Elderly. 100 mg q4h, as needed. Maximum: 600 mg/day.

CONTRAINDICATIONS
None known

INTERACTIONS
Drug
Alcohol, CNS depressants: May increase CNS or respiratory depression and risk of hypotension.
Buprenorphine: Effects may be decreased with buprenorphine.
Carbamazepine: May increase the blood concentration and risk of toxicity of carbamazepine.
MAOIs: May produce severe, fatal reaction; plan to reduce to one quarter usual dose.
Herbal
None known.
Food
None known.

DIAGNOSTIC TEST EFFECTS
May increase serum alkaline phosphatase, amylase, bilirubin, LDH, lipase, SGOT (AST), and SGPT (ALT) levels. Therapeutic blood serum level is 100–400 ng/ml; toxic blood serum level is greater than 500 ng/ml.

SIDE EFFECTS
Frequent
Dizziness, drowsiness, dry mouth,

euphoria, hypotension, nausea, vomiting, unusual tiredness

Occasional

Histamine reaction, including decreased blood pressure (B/P), increased sweating, flushing, and wheezing, trembling, decreased urination, altered vision, constipation, headache

Rare

Confusion, increased B/P, depression, stomach cramps, anorexia

SERIOUS REACTIONS

• Overdosage results in respiratory depression, skeletal muscle flaccidity, cold or clammy skin, cyanosis, extreme somnolence progressing to convulsions, stupor, and coma.

• Liver toxicity may occur with overdosage of acetaminophen component of fixed-combination.

• Tolerance to propoxyphene's analgesic effect and physical dependence may occur with repeated use.

NURSING CONSIDERATIONS

Baseline Assessment

• Obtain the patient's vital signs before giving the medication.

• Withhold the medication and notify the physician if the adult patient's respirations are 12/minute or less, or 20/minute or less in children.

• Assess the duration, location, onset, and type of pain the patient is experiencing.

• Know that the effect of the medication is reduced if the patient experiences full pain before next dose.

• Expect to obtain baseline blood serum chemistry tests to assess liver function.

Lifespan Considerations

• Be aware that propoxyphene crosses the placenta and a minimal amount of the drug is distributed in breast milk.

• Be aware that respiratory depression may occur in the neonate if the mother received opiates during labor.

• Be aware that regular use of opiates during pregnancy may produce withdrawal symptoms in neonate, including diarrhea, excessive crying, fever, hyperactive reflexes, irritability, seizures, sneezing, tremors, vomiting, and yawning.

• Be aware that the pediatric dosage of this drug has not been established.

• The elderly may be more susceptible to propoxyphene's CNS effects and constipation.

• Avoid use in the elderly, if possible.

Precautions

• Use cautiously in patients with liver or renal impairment and substitution for opiates in narcotic-dependent patients.

Administration and Handling

◀ALERT▶ Be alert that propoxyphene's side effects are dependent on the dosage amount.

• Know that ambulatory patients and patients not in moderate pain may experience dizziness, hypotension, nausea, and vomiting more frequently than patients in the supine position or having moderate pain.

◀ALERT▶ Expect to reduce the drug's initial dosage in patients with Addison's disease, hypothyroidism, and renal insufficiency, in debilitated or elderly patients, and in patients concurrently taking CNS depressants.

PO

• Give propoxyphene without regard to meals.

• Empty capsules and mix with food as needed.

• Shake oral suspension well.
• Do not crush or break film-coated tablets.

Intervention and Evaluation

• Palpate the patient's bladder for urine retention.
• Monitor the patients' pattern of daily bowel activity and stool consistency.
• Initiate deep breathing and coughing exercises, particularly in patients with impaired pulmonary function.
• Assess the patient for clinical improvement and record the onset of relief of pain, and contact the physician if the patient's pain is not adequately relieved.

• Know the therapeutic serum level of propoxyphene is 100 to 400 ng/ml, and the toxic serum level of propoxyphene is over 500 ng/ml.

Patient Teaching

• Urge the patient to avoid alcohol during propoxyphene therapy.
• Caution the patient that propoxyphene may be habit-forming.
• Warn the patient that propoxyphene may impair his or her ability to perform tasks requiring mental alertness or motor skills.
• Caution the patient not to abruptly discontinue the drug.
• Instruct the patient to take meperidine before the pain fully returns, within prescribed intervals.

naloxone hydrochloride
naltrexone hydrochloride

Uses: Narcotic antagonists are primarily used to reverse the respiratory depression caused by narcotic overdosage. Naloxone is the drug of choice for reversal of respiratory depression. In patients with severe respiratory depression, treatment requires additional measures, including oxygen administration and mechanical ventilation.

Action: By displacing narcotics (opioid agonists) at receptor sites in the central nervous system, narcotic antagonists prevent and reverse their effects on mu receptors. For example, they increase respiration and reverse sedative effects.

COMBINATION PRODUCTS
SUBOXONE: naloxone/buprenorphine (a non-narcotic analgesic) 0.5 mg/2 mg; 2 mg/8 mg.

naloxone hydrochloride
nay-**lox**-own
(Narcan)
Do not confuse with Norcuron.

CATEGORY AND SCHEDULE
Pregnancy Risk Category: B

MECHANISM OF ACTION
A narcotic antagonist that displaces opiates at opiate-occupied receptor sites in the central nervous system (CNS). *Therapeutic Effect:* Blocks narcotic effects. Reverses opiate-induced sleep or sedation. Increases respiratory rate, returns depressed blood pressure (B/P) to normal rate.

PHARMACOKINETICS

Route	Onset	Peak	Duration
Subcuta-neous	2–5 min	N/A	20–60 min
IM	2–5 min	N/A	20–60 min
IV	1–2 min	N/A	20–60 min

Well absorbed after subcutaneous, IM administration. Metabolized in liver. Primarily excreted in urine. **Half-life:** 60–100 min.

AVAILABILITY
Injection: 0.02 mg/ml, 0.4 mg/ml, 1 mg/ml.

INDICATIONS AND DOSAGES
▸ **Opioid toxicity**
Subcutaneous/IM/IV
Adults, Elderly. 0.4–2 mg q2–3min as needed. May repeat q20–60 min. *Children 5 yrs and older or weighing 20 kg and more.* 2 mg/dose; if no response may repeat q2–3min. May need to repeat q20–60 min. *Children younger than 5 yrs or weighing less than 20 kg.* 0.1 mg/kg, repeat q2–3min. May need to repeat q20–60min.

▸ **Postanesthesia narcotic reversal**
IV
Children. 0.01 mg/kg, may repeat
q2–3min.
▸ **Neonatal opioid-induced depression**
IV
Neonates. 0.01 mg/kg. May repeat
q2–3min as needed. May need to
repeat q1–2h.

CONTRAINDICATIONS
Respiratory depression due to non-opiate drugs

INTERACTIONS
Drug
*Butorphanol, nalbuphine, opioid
agonist analgesics, pentazocine:*
Reverses the analgesic and side
effects and may precipitate withdrawal symptoms of butorphanol,
nalbuphine, opioid agonist analgesics, and pentazocine.
Herbal
None known.
Food
None known.

DIAGNOSTIC TEST EFFECTS
None known.

IV INCOMPATIBILITIES
Amphotericin B complex (Abelcet,
AmBisome, Amphotec)

IV COMPATIBILITIES
Heparin, ondansetron (Zofran),
propofol (Diprivan)

SIDE EFFECTS
None known, little or no pharmacologic effect in absence of narcotics

SERIOUS REACTIONS
• Too rapid reversal of narcotic
depression may result in nausea,
vomiting, tremulousness, sweating,
increased blood pressure (B/P), and
tachycardia.
• Excessive dosage in postoperative
patients may produce significant
reversal of analgesia, excitement,
and tremulousness.
• Hypotension or hypertension,
ventricular tachycardia and fibrillation, and pulmonary edema may
occur in patients with cardiovascular disease.

NURSING CONSIDERATIONS
Baseline Assessment
• Maintain the patient's airway.
• Obtain the body weight of pediatric patients to calculate expected
drug dosage.
Lifespan Considerations
• Be aware that it is unknown if
naloxone crosses the placenta or is
distributed in breast milk.
• There are no age-related precautions noted in children or the
elderly.
Precautions
• Use cautiously in patients with
chronic cardiac or pulmonary
disease and coronary artery
disease.
• Use cautiously in postoperative
patients—to avoid potential cardiovascular complications—and patients suspected of being opioid
dependent.
Administration and Handling
◀ALERT▶ The American Academy of
Pediatrics recommends initial dose
of 0.1 mg/kg for infants and children 5 years of age and younger
and weighing less than 20 kg. For
children older than 5 yrs or weighing more than 20 kg the recommended initial dose is 2 mg.
IM
• Give IM injection in upper, outer
quadrant of buttock.

IV
• Store parenteral form at room temperature.
• Use mixture within 24 hours; discard unused solution.
• Protect from light. Stable in D_5W or 0.9% NaCl at 4 mcg/ml for 24 hours.
• May dilute 1 mg/ml with 50 ml Sterile Water for Injection to provide a concentration of 0.02 mg/ml.
• For continuous IV infusion, dilute each 2 mg of naloxone with 500 ml of D_5W 0.9% NaCl, producing solution containing 0.004 mg/ml.
• May administer undiluted.
• Give each 0.4 mg as IV push over 15 seconds.
• Use the 0.4 mg/ml and 1 mg/ml for injection for adults, the 0.02 mg/ml concentration for neonates.

Intervention and Evaluation
• Monitor the patient's vital signs, especially the depth, rate, and rhythm of respirations, during and frequently after administration.
• Carefully observe the patient after satisfactory response because the duration of opiate may exceed duration of naloxone, resulting in recurrence of respiratory depression.
• Assess the patient for increased pain with reversal of the opiate.

Patient Teaching
• Instruct the patient to let you know if he or she experiences pain or feelings of increased sedation.
• Review potential source of opiate overdose; whether or not it was caused by taking too much of a drug, or if the drug overdose was intentional.

naltrexone hydrochloride
nal-**trex**-own
(Revia)

CATEGORY AND SCHEDULE
Pregnancy Risk Category: C

MECHANISM OF ACTION
A narcotic antagonist that binds to opioid receptors. *Therapeutic Effect:* Blocks physical effects of opioid analgesics. Acts to decrease craving, drinking days, relapse rate in alcoholism.

AVAILABILITY
Tablets: 50 mg.

INDICATIONS AND DOSAGES
▸ **Naloxone challenge test**
IV
Adults, Elderly. Draw 2 amps naloxone, 2 ml (0.8 mg) into syringe. Inject 0.5 ml (0.2 mg); while needle is still in vein, observe for 30 sec for withdrawal signs/symptoms. If no evidence of withdrawal, inject remaining 1.5 ml (0.6 mg); observe for additional 20 min for withdrawal signs or symptoms.
Subcutaneous
Adults, Elderly. Give 2 ml (0.8 mg); observe for 45 min for withdrawal signs or symptoms.
▸ **Opioid free state**
PO
Adults, Elderly. Initially, 25 mg. Observe patient for 1 hour. If no withdrawal signs appear, give another 25 mg. May be given as 100 mg every other day or 150 mg every 3 days.
▸ **Adjunct in treatment of alcohol dependence**
PO
Adults, Elderly. 50 mg once a day.

UNLABELED USES
Treatment of eating disorders, post-concussional syndrome unresponsive to other treatments

CONTRAINDICATIONS
Acute hepatitis, acute opioid withdrawal, failed naloxone challenge, history of sensitivity to naltrexone, liver failure, opioid dependent, opioid withdrawal, positive urine screen for opioids

INTERACTIONS
Drug
Opioid containing products, including antidiarrheals, cold and cough preparations, and opioid analgesics: Benefits of opioid containing drugs are negated.
Thioridazine: Concurrent use with this drug may produce lethargy and somnolence.
Herbal
None known.
Food
None known.

DIAGNOSTIC TEST EFFECTS
May increase SGOT (AST) and SGPT (ALT) levels.

SIDE EFFECTS
Frequent
Alcoholism (10%–7%): Nausea, headache, depression
Narcotic addiction (10%–5%): Insomnia, anxiety, nervousness, headache, low energy, abdominal cramps, nausea, vomiting, joint or muscle pain
Occasional
Alcoholism (4%–2%): Dizziness, nervousness, fatigue, insomnia, vomiting, anxiety, suicidal ideation
Narcotic addiction (5%–2%): Irritability, increased energy, dizziness, anorexia, diarrhea or constipation, rash, chills, increased thirst

SERIOUS REACTIONS
• Signs and symptoms of opioid withdrawal include stuffy or runny nose, tearing, yawning, sweating, tremor, vomiting, piloerection, feeling of temperature change, joint, bone or muscle pain, abdominal cramps, and feeling of skin crawling.
• May cause hepatocellular injury if given in large doses.
• Accidental naltrexone overdose produces withdrawal symptoms within 5 minutes of ingestion, lasts up to 48 hours. Symptoms present as confusion, visual hallucinations, somnolence, and significant vomiting and diarrhea.

NURSING CONSIDERATIONS
Baseline Assessment
• Perform a naloxone challenge test on the patient if there is any question of opioid dependence.
• Begin treatment with naltrexone after the patient is opioid free for 7 to 10 days.
• Establish the patient's medication history, especially for opioid use, and determine the patient's other medical conditions, including hepatitis or other liver disease.
• Plan to perform baseline lab tests, including creatinine clearance, serum bilirubin, SGOT (AST), and SGPT (ALT) levels.
Precautions
• Use cautiously in patients with active liver disease.
Administration and Handling
PO
• Give with antacids, after meals, or with food to avoid adverse gastrointestinal (GI) effects.
Intervention and Evaluation
• Monitor the patient closely for evidence of liver toxicity. Assess the results of liver function studies.

• Monitor the patient's creatinine clearance, serum bilirubin, SGOT (AST), and SGPT (ALT) levels.

Patient Teaching

• Tell the patient that if he or she self administers heroin or other opiates, these drugs will have no effect during naltrexone therapy. Stress that any attempt to overcome naltrexone's prolonged 24 to 72 hour blockade of opioid effects by taking large amount of opioids is very dangerous and may result in coma, serious injury, or fatal overdose.

• Warn the patient to notify the physician if he or she experiences abdominal pain that lasts longer than 3 days, dark-colored urine, white bowel movements, or yellow of the whites of the eyes.

• Instruct the patient to take the oral form with antacids, after meals, or with food to avoid adverse gastrointestinal (GI) effects.

• Help the patient obtain a referral to an alcohol or drug rehab center.

43 Non-Narcotic Analgesics

acetaminophen
aspirin
  (acetylsalicylic
  acid, ASA)
buprenorphine
  hydrochloride
butorphanol tartrate
diflunisal
nalbuphine
  hydrochloride
salsalate
tramadol
  hydrochloride

Uses: Non-narcotic analgesics are used to relieve mild to moderate pain. Acetaminophen and salicylates, such as aspirin, also have anti-inflammatory and antipyretic effects. By virtue of its action on platelet function, aspirin is also used to prevent and treat diseases associated with hypercoagulability and to reduce the risk of stroke and myocardial infarction.

Actions: Different non-narcotic analgesics act in distinct ways. *Agonist-antagonists,* such as nalbuphine, primarily act as antagonists at mu receptors and as agonists at kappa receptors. Although these agents have less abuse potential and cause less respiratory depression than narcotic analgesics, they generally produce weaker analgesic effects. (See illustration, *Mechanism of Action: Agonist-Antagonists,* page 831.) *Acetaminophen* may act by inhibiting prostaglandin synthesis in the central nervous system (CNS). *Salicylates,* such as aspirin, inhibit cyclooxygenase, thereby inhibiting prostaglandin synthesis in the CNS and periphery.

COMBINATION PRODUCTS

AGGRENOX: aspirin/dipyridamole (an antiplatelet agent) 25 mg/ 200 mg.

ANEXSIA: acetaminophen/ hydrocodone (a narcotic analgesic) 500 mg/6 mg; 650 mg/7.5 mg; 660 mg/10 mg.

CAPITAL WITH CODEINE: acetaminophen/codeine (a narcotic analgesic) 120 mg/12 mg per 5 ml.

DARVOCET A 500: acetaminophen/ propoxyphene (a narcotic analgesic) 500 mg/100 mg.

DARVOCET-N: acetaminophen/ propoxyphene (a narcotic analgesic) 325 mg/50 mg; 650 mg/100 mg.

FIORICET: acetaminophen/caffeine (a CNS stimulant)/butabarbital (a sedative-hypnotic) 325 mg/ 40 mg/50 mg.

FIORINAL: aspirin/butabarbital (a sedative-hypnotic)/caffeine (a CNS stimulant) 325 mg/50 mg/40 mg.

LORTAB: acetaminophen/ hydrocodone (a narcotic analgesic) 500 mg/2.5 mg; 500 mg/5 mg; 500 mg/7.5 mg.

LORTAB/ASA: aspirin/hydrocodone (a narcotic analgesic) 325 mg/5 mg.

LORTAB ELIXIR: acetaminophen/ hydrocodone (a narcotic analgesic) 167 mg/2.5 mg per 5 ml.

NORCO: acetaminophen/hydrocodone (a narcotic analgesic) 325 mg/ 10 mg.

PERCOCET: acetaminophen/ oxycodone (a narcotic analgesic) 325 mg/5 mg.

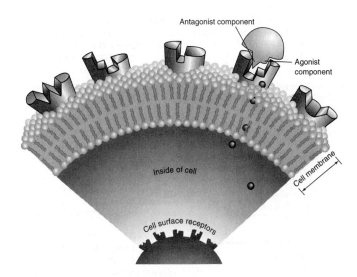

Mechanism of Action: Agonist-Antagonists

Cell membranes have different types of opioid receptors, such as mu, kappa, and delta receptors. Opioid agonist-antagonists, such as butorphanol and nalbuphine, work by stimulating one type of receptor, while simultaneously blocking another type. As agonists, they work primarily by activating kappa receptors to produce analgesia and such other effects as central nervous system and respiratory depression, decreased gastrointestinal motility, and euphoria. As antagonists, they compete with opioids at mu receptors, helping to reverse or block some of the other effects of agonists.

PERCODAN: aspirin/oxycodone (a narcotic analgesic) 325 mg/2.25 mg; 325 mg/4.5 mg.

PRAVIGARD: aspirin/pravastatin (an antihyperlipidemic) 81 mg/20 mg; 325 mg/20 mg; 81 mg/40 mg; 325 mg/40 mg; 81 mg/80 mg; 325 mg/80 mg.

ROXICET: acetaminophen/oxycodone (a narcotic analgesic) 325 mg/5 mg.

SUBOXONE: buprenorphine/naloxone (a narcotic antagonist) 2 mg/ 0.5 mg; 8 mg/2 mg.

TYLENOL WITH CODEINE: acetaminophen/codeine (a narcotic analgesic) 120 mg/12 mg per 5 ml;

300 mg/15 mg; 300 mg/30 mg; 300 mg/60 mg.

TYLOX: acetaminophen/oxycodone (a narcotic analgesic) 500 mg/5 mg.

ULTRACET: acetaminophen/tramadol (a non-narcotic analgesic) 325 mg/ 37.5 mg.

VICODIN: acetaminophen/ hydrocodone (a narcotic analgesic) 500 mg/5 mg.

VICODIN ES: acetaminophen/ hydrocodone (a narcotic analgesic) 750 mg/7.5 mg.

VICODIN HP: acetaminophen/ hydrocodone (a narcotic analgesic) 660 mg/10 mg.

ZYDONE: acetaminophen/ hydrocodone (a narcotic analgesic) 400 mg/5 mg; 400 mg/7.5 mg; 400 mg/10 mg.

acetaminophen
ah-see-tah-**min**-oh-fen
(Abenol[CAN], Apo-Acetaminophen[CAN], Atasol[CAN], Dymadon[AUS], Feverall, Panadol[AUS], Panamax[AUS], Paralgin [AUS], Setamol[AUS], Tempra, Tylenol)
Do not confuse with Fiorinal, Hycodan, Indocin, Percodan, or Tuinal.

CATEGORY AND SCHEDULE
Pregnancy Risk Category: B
OTC

MECHANISM OF ACTION
A central analgesic whose exact mechanism is unknown, but appears to inhibit prostaglandin synthesis in the central nervous system (CNS) and, to a lesser extent, block pain impulses through peripheral action. Acetaminophen acts centrally on hypothalamic heat-regulating center, producing peripheral vasodilation (heat loss, skin erythema, sweating). *Therapeutic Effect:* Results in antipyresis. Produces analgesic effect.

PHARMACOKINETICS

Route	Onset	Peak	Duration
PO	15–30 mins	1–1.5 hrs	4–6 hrs

Rapidly, completely absorbed from gastrointestinal (GI) tract; rectal absorption variable. Protein binding: 20%–50%. Widely distributed to most body tissues. Metabolized in liver; excreted in urine. Removed by hemodialysis. **Half-life:** 1–4 hrs (half-life is increased in those with liver disease, elderly, neonates; decreased in children).

AVAILABILITY
Capsules: 80 mg, 160 mg, 325 mg, 500 mg.
Drops: 100 mg/ml.
Elixir: 100 mg/ml, 130 mg/5 ml, 160 mg/5 ml, 500 mg/5 ml.
Liquid: 32 mg/ml, 100 mg/ml, 160 mg/5 ml.
Suppository: 80 mg, 120 mg, 325 mg, 650 mg.
Suspension: 100 mg/ml, 160 mg/ 5 ml.
Syrup: 160 mg/5 ml.
Tablets: 80 mg, 160 mg, 325 mg, 500 mg, 650 mg.
Tablets (chewable): 80 mg, 160 mg.
Tablets (controlled release): 650 mg.

INDICATIONS AND DOSAGES
▸ **Analgesia and antipyresis**
PO
Adults, Elderly. 325–650 mg q4–6h or 1 g 3–4 times/day. Maximum: 4 g/day.
Children. 10–15 mg/kg/dose q4-6h as needed. Maximum: 5 doses/ 24 hrs.
Neonates. 10–15 mg/kg/dose q6-8h as needed.
Rectal
Adults. 650 mg q4–6h. Maximum: 6 doses/24 hrs.
Children. 10–20 mg/kg/dose q4-6h as needed.
Neonates. 10–15 mg/kg/dose q6-8h as needed.
▸ **Dosage in renal impairment**

Creatinine Clearance	Frequency
10–50 ml/min	q6h
less than 10 ml/min	q8h

CONTRAINDICATIONS
Active alcoholism, liver disease, or viral hepatitis, all of which increase the risk of hepatotoxicity

INTERACTIONS
Drug
Alcohol (chronic use), hepatotoxic medications (e.g., phenytoin), liver enzyme inducers (e.g., cimetidine): May increase risk of hepatotoxicity with prolonged high dose or single toxic dose.
Warfarin: May increase the risk of bleeding with regular use.
Herbal
None known.
Food
None known.

DIAGNOSTIC TEST EFFECTS
May increase serum bilirubin, prothrombin time (may indicate hepatotoxicity), SGOT (AST), and SGPT (ALT). Therapeutic serum level: 10–30 mcg/ml; toxic serum level: greater than 200 mcg/ml.

SIDE EFFECTS
Rare
Hypersensitivity reaction

SERIOUS REACTIONS
• Acetaminophen toxicity is the primary serious reaction.
• Early signs and symptoms of acetaminophen toxicity include anorexia, nausea, diaphoresis, and generalized weakness within the first 12 to 24 hrs.
• Later signs of acetaminophen toxicity include vomiting, right upper quadrant tenderness, and elevated liver function tests within 48 to 72 hrs after ingestion.
• The antidote to acetaminophen toxicity is acetylcysteine.

NURSING CONSIDERATIONS
Baseline Assessment
• Assess onset, type, location, and duration of pain before acetaminophen is given for analgesia. The effect of the medication is reduced if full pain response recurs before the next dose.
• Expect to obtain the patient's vital signs before giving any of acetaminophen's fixed combinations. If respirations are 12 per minute or lower (20 per minute or lower in children), withhold the medication and contact the physician.
Lifespan Considerations
• Acetaminophen crosses the placenta and is distributed in breast milk.
• Acetaminophen is routinely used in all stages of pregnancy and appears safe for short-term use.
• There are no age-related precautions noted in children or the elderly.
◀ALERT▶ Children may receive repeat doses 4 to 5 times a day to a maximum of 5 doses in 24 hours.
Precautions
• Use cautiously in patients with G6PD deficiency, phenylketonuria, sensitivity to acetaminophen, or severe impaired renal function.
Administration and Handling
PO
• Give without regard to meals.
• Tablets may be crushed.
Rectal
• Moisten suppository with cold water before inserting well up into the rectum.
Intervention and Evaluation
• Assess for clinical improvement and relief of pain or fever.
• Monitor serum levels. A therapeutic serum level is 10 to 30 mcg/ml and a toxic serum level is greater than 200 mcg/ml.

Patient Teaching
• Caution the patient to consult with the physician before using acetaminophen in children under 2 years of age; oral use for more than 5 days in children, more than 10 days in adults, or fever lasting more than 3 days. Monitor patient for severe or recurrent pain or high, continuous fever, which may indicate a serious illness.

aspirin (acetylsalicylic acid, ASA)

ass-purr-in

(Ascriptin, Aspro[AUS], Bayer, Bex[AUS], Bufferin, Disprin[AUS], Ecotrin, Entrophen[CAN], Halfprin, Novasen[CAN], Solprin[AUS], Spren[AUS])

CATEGORY AND SCHEDULE

Pregnancy Risk Category: C (D if full dose used in third trimester of pregnancy)
OTC

MECHANISM OF ACTION

A nonsteroidal salicylate that inhibits prostaglandin synthesis, acts on the hypothalamus heat-regulating center, and blocks prostaglandin synthetase action. *Therapeutic Effect:* Reduces inflammatory response and intensity of pain stimulus reaching sensory nerve endings. Decreases elevated body temperature. Inhibits platelet aggregation.

PHARMACOKINETICS

Route	Onset	Peak	Duration
PO	1 hr	2–4 hrs	24 hrs

Rapidly, completely absorbed from gastrointestinal (GI) tract; enteric-coated absorption delayed; rectal absorption delayed, incomplete. Protein binding: High. Widely distributed. Rapidly hydrolyzed to salicylate. **Half-life** (aspirin): 15–20 min; salicylate half-life is 2–3 hrs at low dose; greater than 20 hrs at high dose.

AVAILABILITY

Tablets: 81 mg, 325 mg, 500 mg, 650 mg.
Tablets (chewable): 81 mg.
Tablets (enteric-coated): 81 mg, 162 mg, 325 mg, 500 mg, 650 mg, 975 mg.
Tablets (controlled-release): 650 mg, 800 mg, 975 mg.
Suppository: 60 mg, 120 mg, 200 mg, 300 mg, 600 mg.

INDICATIONS AND DOSAGES
▶ **Analgesic, antipyretic**
PO/Rectal
Adults, Elderly. 325–1000 mg q4-6h.
Children. 10–15 mg/kg/dose q4-6h.
Maximum: 4 g/day.
▶ **Antiinflammatory**
PO
Adults, Elderly. Initially, 2.4–3.6 g/day in divided doses, then 3.6–5.4 g/day.
Children. 60–90 mg/kg/day in divided doses, then 80–100 mg/kg/day.
▶ **Suspected myocardial infarction (MI)**
PO
Adults, Elderly. Initially, 162 mg as soon as the MI is suspected, then daily for 30 days post-MI.
▶ **MI prophylaxis**
PO
Adults, Elderly. 75–325 mg/day.
▶ **Stroke prevention following transischemic attack (TIA)**
PO
Adults, Elderly. 50–325 mg/day.

▸ **Kawasaki disease**
PO
Children. 80–100 mg/kg/day in
divided doses.

UNLABELED USES
Prophylaxis against thromboembolism, treatment of Kawasaki disease

CONTRAINDICATIONS
Allergy to tartrazine dye, bleeding disorders, chickenpox or flu in children and teenagers, GI bleeding or ulceration, history of hypersensitivity to aspirin or NSAIDs, impaired liver function

INTERACTIONS
Drug
Alcohol, NSAIDs: May increase the risk of adverse GI effects, including ulceration.
Antacids, urinary alkalinizers: Increase the excretion of aspirin.
Anticoagulants, heparin, thrombolytics: Increase the risk of bleeding.
Insulin, oral hypoglycemics: Large doses of aspirin may increase the effect of insulin or oral hypoglycemics.
Methotrexate, zidovudine: May increase the risk of toxicity of these drugs.
Ototoxic medications, vancomycin: May increase the risk of ototoxicity of aspirin.
Platelet aggregation inhibitors, valproic acid: May increase the risk of bleeding.
Probenecid, sulfinpyrazone: May decrease the effect of these drugs.
Herbal
None known.
Food
None known.

DIAGNOSTIC TEST EFFECTS
May alter serum alkaline phosphatase, SGOT (AST), SGPT (ALT),
and serum uric acid levels. May prolong bleeding time, and prothrombin time (PT). May decrease blood levels of cholesterol, serum potassium, and T_3 and T_4 levels.

SIDE EFFECTS
Occasional
GI distress, including abdominal distention, cramping, heartburn, and mild nausea; allergic reaction, including bronchospasm, pruritus, and urticaria

SERIOUS REACTIONS
• High doses of aspirin may produce GI bleeding and gastric mucosal lesions.
• High doses of aspirin may produce low-grade toxicity characterized by ringing in ears, generalized pruritus (may be severe), headache, dizziness, flushing, tachycardia, hyperventilation, sweating, and thirst.
• Toxic aspirin levels may be reached quickly in dehydrated, febrile children. Marked toxicity is manifested as hyperthermia, restlessness, abnormal breathing patterns, convulsions, respiratory failure, and coma.

NURSING CONSIDERATIONS
Baseline Assessment
• Do not give aspirin to children or teenagers who have the chickenpox or flu as this increases the risk of developing Reye's syndrome.
• Do not use aspirin that smells of vinegar because this odor indicates chemical breakdown in the medication.
• Assess the duration, location, and type of inflammation or pain.
• Inspect the appearance of affected joints for deformities, immobility, and skin condition.

• The therapeutic serum aspirin level for antiarthritic effect is 20 to 30 mg/dl. Aspirin toxicity occurs if levels are over 30 mg/dl.

Lifespan Considerations
• Be aware that aspirin readily crosses the placenta and is distributed in breast milk.
• Be aware that aspirin may decrease fetal birth weight, increase the incidence of hemorrhage, neonatal mortality, and stillbirths, and prolong gestation and labor.
• Be aware that aspirin use should be avoided during the last trimester of pregnancy because the drug may adversely affect the fetal cardiovascular system causing premature closure of ductus arteriosus.
• Use caution in giving aspirin to children with acute febrile illness because this increases the risk of developing Reye's syndrome.
• Be aware that lower aspirin dosages are recommended in the elderly because this age group may be more susceptible to aspirin toxicity.

Precautions
• Use cautiously in patients with chronic renal insufficiency or Vitamin K deficiency.
• Use cautiously in those patients diagnosed with the "aspirin triad" of asthma, nasal polyps, and rhinitis.

Administration and Handling
PO
• Do not crush or break enteric-coated or sustained-release forms.
• May give with water, milk, or meals if GI distress occurs.
Rectal
• Refrigerate suppositories.
• If the suppository is too soft, chill it for 30 minutes in the refrigerator or run cold water over the foil wrapper.
• Moisten the suppository with cold water before inserting well into the rectum.

Intervention and Evaluation
• Monitor the patient's urine pH levels for signs of sudden acidification, indicated by a pH of 6.5 to 5.5. Sudden acidification may cause the serum salicylate level to greatly increase, leading to toxicity.
• Assess the patient's skin for evidence of bruising.
• If aspirin is given as an antipyretic, assess the patient's temperature directly before and 1 hour after giving the medication.
• Evaluate the patient for a therapeutic response to the drug manifested as improved grip strength, increased joint mobility, reduced joint tenderness, and relief of pain, stiffness, or swelling.

Patient Teaching
• Instruct the patient not to crush or chew sustained-release or enteric-coated aspirin.
• Caution the patient to report ringing in the ears or persistent GI pain to the physician.
• Advise the patient that the therapeutic anti-inflammatory effect of aspirin should be noticed within 1 to 3 weeks.

buprenorphine hydrochloride
byew-**pren**-or-phen
(Buprenex, Subutex, Temgesic[CAN])

CATEGORY AND SCHEDULE
Pregnancy Risk Category: C
Controlled Substance: Schedule V (opioid agonist), Schedule III (tablet)

MECHANISM OF ACTION
An opioid agonist that binds with opioid receptors within the central nervous system (CNS). *Therapeutic*

Effect: Alters pain perception, emotional response to pain.

AVAILABILITY
Injection: 0.3 mg/ml.
Tablets (sublingual): 2 mg, 8 mg.

INDICATIONS AND DOSAGES
▸ **Analgesic**
IM/IV
Adults, Children older than 12 yrs.
0.3 mg q6-8h as needed. May repeat once in 30–60 min. Range: 0.15–0.6 mg q4-8h as needed.
Children 2–12 yrs. 2–6 mcg/kg q4-6h as needed.
Elderly. 0.15 mg q6h as needed.
▸ **Opioid dependence**
Sublingual
Adults, Elderly, Children older than 16 yrs. Initially, 12–16 mg/day. Begin at least 4 hrs after last use of heroin or short acting opioid. Maintenance: 16 mg/day. Range: 4–24 mg/day. Patients should be switched to buprenorphine and naloxone combination.

CONTRAINDICATIONS
None significant

INTERACTIONS
Drug
CNS depressants, MAOIs: May increase CNS or respiratory depression and hypotension.
Other opioid analgesics: May decrease the effects of other opioid analgesics.
Herbal
Kava kava, St. John's wort, valerian: May increase CNS depression.
Food
None significant.

DIAGNOSTIC TEST EFFECTS
May increase serum amylase and lipase.

SIDE EFFECTS
Frequent
Injection (greater than 10%): Sedation
Tablet: Headache, pain, insomnia, anxiety, depression, nausea, abdominal pain, constipation, back pain, weakness, rhinitis, withdrawal syndrome, infection, sweating
Occasional
Injection: Hypotension, respiratory depression, dizziness, headache, vomiting, nausea, vertigo

SERIOUS REACTIONS
• Overdosage results in cold, clammy skin, weakness, confusion, severe respiratory depression, cyanosis, pinpoint pupils, extreme somnolence progressing to convulsions, stupor, and coma.

NURSING CONSIDERATIONS
Baseline Assessment
• Assess the duration, location, onset, and type of pain.
• Know that the effect of buprenorphine is reduced if full pain recurs before next dose.
Precautions
• Use cautiously in patients with impaired liver function and in patients with possible neurologic injury.
Administration and Handling
IV
• Administer slowly, over at least 2 minutes.
PO
• Place tablet under the patient's tongue until dissolved. If 2 or more tablets are needed, may place all under the tongue at the same time.
Intervention and Evaluation
• Monitor the patient for change in blood pressure (B/P), rate and quality of pulse, and respiration.
• Have the patient initiate deep

breathing and coughing exercises, particularly in patients with impaired pulmonary function.
• Assess the patient for clinical improvement and record the onset of pain relief.
Patient Teaching
• Instruct the patient to change positions slowly to avoid dizziness.
• Warn the patient to avoid tasks requiring mental alertness or motor skills until his or her response to the drug is established.

---

butorphanol tartrate
byew-**tore**-phen-awl
(Stadol, Stadol NS)
Do not confuse with Haldol.

CATEGORY AND SCHEDULE
Pregnancy Risk Category: C, D if used for prolonged time, high dose at term
Controlled Substance: Schedule IV

MECHANISM OF ACTION
An opioid that binds to opiate receptor sites in the central nervous system (CNS). Reduces intensity of pain stimuli incoming from sensory nerve endings. *Therapeutic Effect:* Alters pain perception and emotional response to pain.

PHARMACOKINETICS

Route	Onset	Peak	Duration
IM	10–30 min	30–60 min	3–4 hrs
IV	less than 1 min	30 min	2–4 hrs
Nasal	15 min	1–2 hrs	4–5 hrs

Rapidly absorbed from IM injection. Protein binding: 80%. Extensively metabolized in liver. Primar-

ily excreted in urine. **Half-life:** 2.5–4 hrs.

AVAILABILITY
Injection: 1 mg/ml, 2 mg/ml.
Nasal Spray: 10 mg/ml.

INDICATIONS AND DOSAGES
▸ **Analgesia**
IM
Adults. 1–4 mg q3–4h as needed.
Elderly. 1 mg q4–6h as needed.
IV
Adults. 0.5–2 mg q3–4h as needed.
Elderly. 1 mg q4–6h as needed.
Nasal
Adults. 1 mg or 1 spray in one nostril. May repeat in 60–90 min. May repeat 2-dose sequence q3–4h as needed. Alternatively, 2 mg or 1 spray each nostril if patient remains recumbent, may repeat in 3–4 hrs.

CONTRAINDICATIONS
CNS disease that affects respirations, physical dependence on other opioid analgesics, preexisting respiratory depression, pulmonary disease

INTERACTIONS
Drug
Alcohol, CNS depressants: May increase CNS or respiratory depression and hypotension.
Buprenorphine: Effects may be decreased with buprenorphine.
MAOIs: May produce severe, fatal reaction unless dose is reduced by one-fourth.
Herbal
None known.
Food
None known.

DIAGNOSTIC TEST EFFECTS
None known.

IV INCOMPATIBILITIES
Amphotericin B complex (Abelcet, AmBisome, Amphotec)

IV COMPATIBILITIES
Atropine, diphenhydramine (Benadryl), droperidol (Inapsine), hydroxyzine (Vistaril), morphine, promethazine (Phenergan), propofol (Diprivan)

SIDE EFFECTS
Frequent
Parenteral: Drowsiness (43%), dizziness (19%)
Nasal: Nasal congestion (13%), insomnia (11%)
Occasional
Parenteral (3%–9%): Confusion, sweating/clammy skin, lethargy, headache, nausea, vomiting, dry mouth
Nasal (3%–9%): Vasodilation, constipation, unpleasant taste, dyspnea, epistaxis, nasal irritation, upper respiratory infection, tinnitus
Rare
Parenteral: Hypotension, pruritus, blurred vision, sensation of heat, CNS stimulation, insomnia
Nasal: Hypertension, tremor, ear pain, paresthesia, depression, sinusitis

SERIOUS REACTIONS
• Abrupt withdrawal after prolonged use may produce symptoms of narcotic withdrawal, such as abdominal cramping, rhinorrhea, lacrimation, anxiety, increased temperature, and piloerection or goose bumps.
• Overdosage results in severe respiratory depression, skeletal muscle flaccidity, cyanosis, extreme somnolence progressing to convulsions, stupor, and coma.
• Tolerance to analgesic effect and physical dependence may occur with chronic use.

NURSING CONSIDERATIONS
Baseline Assessment
• Obtain the patient's vital signs before giving medication.
• Withhold the medication and notify the physician if the adult patient's respirations are 12/minute or less, or 20/minute or less in children.
• Assess duration, location, onset, and type of pain the patient is experiencing.
• Know that the effect of the medication is reduced if the patient experiences full pain before the next dose.
• Protect the patient from falls.
• During labor, assess fetal heart tones, and the patient's uterine contractions.
Lifespan Considerations
• Be aware that butorphanol readily crosses the placenta and is distributed in breast milk. Breast-feeding is not recommended in this patient population.
• Be aware that the safety and efficacy of butorphanol have not been established in children younger than 18 years of age.
• Be aware that the elderly may be more sensitive to effects. Adjust drug dose and interval in the elderly.
Precautions
• Use cautiously in patients who are debilitated or elderly.
• Use cautiously in patients with head injury, hypertension, impaired liver or renal function, myocardial infarction, and prior to biliary tract surgery, because the drug produces spasm of sphincter of Oddi.

Administration and Handling
◀ **ALERT** ▶ May be given by IM or IV push.

Intranasal

• Instruct patient to blow nose to clear nasal passages as much as possible.

• Tilt the patient's head slightly forward and insert spray tip into nostril, pointing toward nasal passages, away from nasal septum.

• Spray into nostril while holding other nostril closed and instruct patient to concurrently inspire through nose to permit medication as high into nasal passages as possible.

IV

• Store at room temperature.

• May give undiluted.

• Administer over 3 to 5 minutes.

Intervention and Evaluation

• Monitor the patient for a change in blood pressure (B/P), pulse rate and quality, and respirations.

• Initiate deep breathing and coughing exercises, particularly in patients with impaired pulmonary function.

• Help the patient change position every 2 to 4 hours.

• Assess the patient for clinical improvement and record the onset of relief of pain.

Patient Teaching

• Instruct the patient to change positions slowly to avoid dizziness.

• Warn the patient to avoid tasks that require mental alertness or motor skills until his or her response to the drug is established.

• Teach the patient the proper use of nasal spray.

• Urge the patient to avoid alcohol or CNS depressants during butorphanol therapy.

• Instruct the patient to alert you to the onset of pain, and not to wait until the pain is unbearable. Butorphanol is more effective when given at the onset of pain.

---

diflunisal
dye-**flew**-neh-sol
(Apo-Diflunisal[CAN], Dolobid, Novo-Diflunisal[CAN])
Do not confuse with Slo-bid.

CATEGORY AND SCHEDULE
Pregnancy Risk Category: C, D if used in third trimester or near delivery

---

MECHANISM OF ACTION
A nonsteroidal anti-inflammatory that inhibits prostaglandin synthesis, reducing inflammatory response and intensity of pain stimulus reaching sensory nerve endings. *Therapeutic Effect:* Produces analgesic and anti-inflammatory effect.

PHARMACOKINETICS

Route	Onset	Peak	Duration
PO	1 hr	2–3 hrs	8–12 hrs

Completely absorbed from the gastrointestinal (GI) tract. Widely distributed. Protein binding: greater than 99%. Metabolized in liver. Primarily excreted in urine. Not removed by hemodialysis. **Half-life:** 8–12 hrs.

AVAILABILITY
Tablets: 250 mg, 500 mg.

INDICATIONS AND DOSAGES
▸ **Mild to moderate pain**
PO
Adults, Elderly. Initially, 0.5–1 g, then 250–500 mg q8–12h. Maximum: 1.5 g/day.

▸ **Rheumatoid arthritis, osteoarthritis**
PO
Adults, Elderly. 0.5–1 g/day in 2 divided doses. Maximum: 1.5 g/day.

UNLABELED USES
Treatment of psoriatic arthritis, vascular headache

CONTRAINDICATIONS
Active GI bleeding, factor VII or factor IX deficiencies, hypersensitivity to aspirin or NSAIDs

INTERACTIONS
Drug
Antihypertensives, diuretics: May decrease the effects of antihypertensives and diuretics.
Aspirin, salicylates: May increase the risk of GI bleeding and side effects.
Bone marrow depressants: May increase the risk of hematologic reactions.
Heparin, oral anticoagulants, thrombolytics: May increase the effects of heparin, oral anticoagulants, and thrombolytics.
Lithium: May increase the blood concentration and risk of toxicity of lithium.
Methotrexate: May increase the risk of toxicity of methotrexate.
Probenecid: May increase diflunisal blood concentration.
Herbal
Ginkgo biloba: May increase the risk of bleeding.
Food
None known.

DIAGNOSTIC TEST EFFECTS
May increase serum transaminase levels. May decrease serum uric acid levels.

SIDE EFFECTS
Side effects appear less frequently with short-term treatment.
Occasional (9%–3%)
Nausea, dyspepsia (heartburn, indigestion, epigastric pain), diarrhea, headache, rash
Rare (3%–1%)
Vomiting, constipation, flatulence, dizziness, somnolence, insomnia, fatigue, tinnitus

SERIOUS REACTIONS
• Overdosage may produce drowsiness, vomiting, nausea, diarrhea, hyperventilation, tachycardia, diaphoresis, stupor, and coma.
• Peptic ulcer, GI bleeding, gastritis, and severe hepatic reaction, including cholestasis, jaundice occur rarely.
• Nephrotoxicity, including dysuria, hematuria, proteinuria, and nephrotic syndrome, and severe hypersensitivity reaction, marked by bronchospasm and facial edema, occur rarely.

NURSING CONSIDERATIONS
Baseline Assessment
• Assess the patient for the duration, location, onset, and type of inflammation or pain the patient is experiencing.
• Inspect the appearance of the patient's affected joints for deformities, immobility, and skin condition.
• Plan to obtain baseline lab tests, including aPT, aPTT, renal and liver function studies, and complete blood count (CBC).
Lifespan Considerations
• Be aware that diflunisal crosses the placenta and is distributed in breast milk. Avoid diflunisal use during the last trimester of pregnancy as the drug may adversely affect the fetal cardiovascular sys-

tem, causing premature closure of ductus arteriosus.
• Be aware that the safety and efficacy of this drug have not been established in children.
• In the elderly GI bleeding or ulceration is more likely to cause serious adverse effects.
• In the elderly, age-related renal impairment may increase risk of liver or renal toxicity; a decreased drug dosage is recommended.

Precautions
• Use cautiously in patients with edema, elevated liver function tests, erosive gastritis, impaired renal or liver function, peptic ulcer disease, platelet and bleeding disorders, and vitamin K deficiency.

Administration and Handling
PO
• May give diflunisal with meals, milk, or water.
• Do not crush or break film-coated tablets.

Intervention and Evaluation
• Monitor the patient for dyspepsia and nausea.
• Assess the patient's skin for evidence of rash.
• Assess the patient's pattern of daily bowel activity and stool consistency.
• Evaluate the patient for therapeutic response, improved grip strength, increased joint mobility, reduced joint tenderness, and relief of pain, stiffness, and swelling.

Patient Teaching
• Instruct the patient to swallow tablets whole; do not chew or crush.
• Teach the patient that if he or she experiences GI upset occurs, that he or she may take diflunisal with food or milk.
• Warn the patient to notify the

physician if he or she experiences GI distress, headache, or rash.
• Tell the patient to inform the physician if she suspects pregnancy, or plans to become pregnant.

nalbuphine hydrochloride
nail-**byew**-phin
(Nubain)
Do not confuse with Navane.

CATEGORY AND SCHEDULE
Pregnancy Risk Category: B, D if used for prolonged periods or at high dosages at term

MECHANISM OF ACTION
A narcotic agonist and antagonist that binds with opioid receptors within the central nervous system (CNS). May displace opioid agonists and competitively inhibit their action; may precipitate withdrawal symptoms. *Therapeutic Effect:* Alters pain perception, emotional response to pain.

PHARMACOKINETICS

Route	Onset	Peak	Duration
Subcuta-neous	less than 15 min	N/A	3–6 hrs
IM	less than 15 min	60 min	3–6 hrs
IV	2–3 min	30 min	3–6 hrs

Well absorbed after subcutaneous, IM administration. Protein binding: 50%. Metabolized in liver. Primarily eliminated in feces via biliary secretion. **Half-life:** 3.5–5 hrs.

AVAILABILITY
Injection: 10 mg/ml, 20 mg/ml.

INDICATIONS AND DOSAGES
▶ **Analgesia**
Subcutaneous/IM/IV
Adults, Elderly. 10 mg q3–6h as
needed. Do not exceed maximum
single dose of 20 mg, maximum
daily dose of 160 mg. In patients
chronically receiving narcotic analgesics of similar duration of action,
give 25% of usual dosage.
Children. 0.1–0.15 mg/kg q3–6h as
needed.
▶ **Supplement to anesthesia**
IV
Adults, Elderly. Induction:
0.3–3 mg/kg over 10–15 min.
Maintenance: 0.25–0.5 mg/kg as
needed.

CONTRAINDICATIONS
Respirations less than 12/min

INTERACTIONS
Drug
Alcohol, CNS depressants: May
increase CNS or respiratory depres-
sion and hypotension.
Buprenorphine: Effects may be
decreased with this drug.
MAOIs: May produce severe
reaction; plan to reduce dose to one
quarter usual dose.
Herbal
None known.
Food
None known.

DIAGNOSTIC TEST EFFECTS
May increase serum amylase and
lipase levels.

IV INCOMPATIBILITIES
Amphotericin B complex (Abelcet,
AmBisome, Amphotec), cefepime
(Maxipime), docetaxel (Doxil),
methotrexate, nafcillin (Nafcil),
piperacillin/tazobactam (Zosyn),
sargramostim (Leukine, Prokine),
sodium bicarbonate

IV COMPATIBILITIES
Diphenhydramine (Benadryl), droperidol (Inapsine), glycopyrrolate
(Robinul), hydroxyzine (Vistaril),
ketorolac (Toradol), lidocaine,
midazolam (Versed), propofol
(Diprivan)

SIDE EFFECTS
Frequent (35%)
Sedation
Occasional (9%–3%)
Sweaty or clammy feeling, nausea,
vomiting, dizziness, vertigo, dry
mouth, headache
Rare (1% or less)
Restlessness, crying, euphoria,
hostility, confusion, numbness,
tingling, flushing, paradoxical reac-
tion

SERIOUS REACTIONS
• Abrupt withdrawal after prolonged
use may produce symptoms of
narcotic withdrawal, marked by
abdominal cramping, rhinorrhea,
lacrimation, anxiety, increased
temperature, and piloerection or
goose bumps.
• Overdose results in severe respiratory depression, skeletal muscle
flaccidity, cyanosis, extreme somnolence progressing to convulsions,
stupor, and coma.
• Tolerance to analgesic effect and
physical dependence may occur
with chronic use.

NURSING CONSIDERATIONS
Baseline Assessment
• Obtain the patient's vital signs
before giving nalbuphine.
• Withhold the medication and
notify the physician if the adult
patient's respirations are 12/minute
or less, or 20/minute or less in
children.

• Assess the duration, location, onset, and type of pain the patient is experiencing.
• Know that the effect of the medication is reduced if the patient experiences full pain before the next dose.
• Know that nalbuphine has a low abuse potential.

Lifespan Considerations
• Be aware that nalbuphine readily crosses the placenta and is distributed in breast milk. Breast-feeding is not recommended in this patient population.
• Be aware that children may experience paradoxical excitement.
• Be aware that children younger than 2 years of age and the elderly are more susceptible to respiratory depression.
• In the elderly, age-related impaired renal function may increase risk of urinary retention.

Precautions
• Use cautiously in patients with head trauma, increased intracranial pressure, liver or renal impairment, recent biliary tract surgery, recent myocardial infarction (MI), and respiratory depression.
• Use cautiously in pregnant patients and patients suspected to be opioid dependent.

Administration and Handling
◀ALERT▶ Keep in mind that nalbuphine dosage is based on the patient's concurrent use of other medications, physical condition, and severity of pain.

IM
• Rotate IM injection sites.

IV
• Store at room temperature.
• May give undiluted.
• For IV push, administer each 10 mg over 3 to 5 minutes.

Intervention and Evaluation
• Monitor the patient for change in blood pressure (B/P), pulse rate or quality, and respirations.
• Assess the patient's pattern of daily bowel activity and stool consistency.
• Initiate deep breathing and coughing exercises, particularly in patients with impaired pulmonary function.
• Assess the patient for clinical improvement and record the onset of relief of pain.
• Consult the physician if the patient's pain relief is not adequate.

Patient Teaching
• Urge the patient to avoid alcohol during nalbuphine therapy.
• Warn the patient that nalbuphine use may cause drowsiness, and impair his or her ability to perform activities requiring mental alertness or motor skills.
• Tell the patient that nalbuphine may cause dry mouth.
• Caution the patient that nalbuphine may be habit-forming.
• Tell the patient to alert you to the onset of pain because the effect of the medication is reduced if the patient experiences full pain before the next dose.

salsalate
sal-sah-late
(Disalcid, Mono-Gesic)

CATEGORY AND SCHEDULE
Pregnancy Risk Category: C

MECHANISM OF ACTION
A nonsteroidal anti-inflammatory that inhibits prostaglandin synthesis. Reduces inflammatory response, intensity of pain stimulus reaching

sensory nerve endings. *Therapeutic Effect:* Produces analgesic, anti-inflammatory response.

AVAILABILITY
Capsules: 500 mg.
Tablets: 500 mg, 750 mg.

INDICATIONS AND DOSAGES
▶ **Rheumatoid arthritis, osteo-arthritis**
PO
Adults, Elderly. Initially, 3 g/day in 2–3 divided doses. Maintenance: 2–4 g/day.

CONTRAINDICATIONS
Bleeding disorders, hypersensitivity to salicylates, NSAIDs

INTERACTIONS
Drug
Alcohol, NSAIDs: May increase the risk of gastrointestinal (GI) effects, such as ulceration.
Antacids, urinary alkalinizers: Increase the excretion of salsalate.
Anticoagulants, heparin, thrombolytics: Increase the risk of bleeding.
Insulin, oral hypoglycemics: Large dose may increase the effects of insulin and oral hypoglycemics.
Methotrexate, zidovudine: May increase the toxicity of methotrexate and zidovudine.
Ototoxic medications, vancomycin: May increase the risk of ototoxicity.
Platelet aggregation inhibitors, valproic acid: May increase the risk of bleeding.
Probenecid, sulfinpyrazone: May decrease the effects of probenecid and sulfinpyrazone.
Herbal
Ginkgo biloba: May increase the risk of bleeding.
Food
None known.

DIAGNOSTIC TEST EFFECTS
May alter serum alkaline phosphatase, SGOT (AST), SGPT (ALT), and uric acid levels. May prolong bleeding time and prothrombin time. May decrease serum cholesterol, potassium, T_3, and T_4 levels.

SIDE EFFECTS
Occasional
Nausea, dyspepsia, including heartburn, indigestion, and epigastric pain

SERIOUS REACTIONS
• Tinnitus may be the first sign that serum salicylic acid concentration is reaching or exceeding upper therapeutic range.
• Salsalate use may also produce vertigo, headache, confusion, drowsiness, diaphoresis, hyperventilation, vomiting, and diarrhea.
• Severe overdosage may result in electrolyte imbalance, hyperthermia, dehydration, and blood pH imbalance.
• There is a low incidence of GI bleeding and peptic ulcer occurrence.

NURSING CONSIDERATIONS
Baseline Assessment
• Do not give salsalate to children or teenagers who have chickenpox or the flu because this increases the risk of Reye's syndrome development.
• Assess duration, location, onset, and type of inflammation or pain the patient is experiencing.
• Inspect the appearance of the patient's affected joints for deformities, immobility, and skin condition.
• Expect to obtain baseline liver function and coagulation studies.

Precautions
• Use cautiously in patients with asthma, bleeding disorders, gastritis, history of gastric irritation, liver or renal impairment, peptic ulcer disease, and platelet disorders.

Intervention and Evaluation
• Assess the patient for evidence of dyspepsia and nausea.
• Evaluate the patient for therapeutic response, improved grip strength, increased joint mobility, reduced joint tenderness, and relief of pain, stiffness, or swelling.

Patient Teaching
• Urge the patient to avoid alcohol and using aspirin-containing products during salsalate therapy.
• Instruct the patient to take the drug with food, and to use antacids to relieve stomach upset.
• Warn the patient to notify the physician if he or she experiences persistent GI pain or ringing in the ears.

---

tramadol hydrochloride
tray-mah-doal
(Tramal[AUS], Tramal SR[AUS], Ultram)
Do not confuse with Toradol or Ultane.

CATEGORY AND SCHEDULE
Pregnancy Risk Category: C

MECHANISM OF ACTION
An analgesic that binds to mu-opiate receptors, and inhibits reuptake of norepinephrine and serotonin. *Therapeutic Effect:* Reduces intensity of pain stimuli incoming from sensory nerve endings, altering pain perception and emotional response to pain.

PHARMACOKINETICS

Route	Onset	Peak	Duration
PO	less than 1 hr	2–3 hrs	4–6 hrs

Rapidly, almost completely absorbed after PO administration. Protein binding: 20%. Extensively metabolized in liver to active metabolite (reduced in patients with advanced cirrhosis). Primarily excreted in urine. Minimally removed by hemodialysis. **Half-life:** 6–7 hrs.

AVAILABILITY
Tablets: 50 mg.

INDICATIONS AND DOSAGES
▸ **Moderate to moderately severe pain**
PO
Adults, Elderly. 50–100 mg q4–6h. Maximum younger than 75 yrs: 400 mg/day. Maximum older than 75 yrs: 300 mg/day.
▸ **Renal function impairment, with creatinine clearance of less than 30 ml/min**
PO
Adults, Elderly. Increase dosing interval to 12 hrs. Maximum daily dose: 200 mg.
▸ **Liver function impairment**
PO
Adults, Elderly. 50 mg q12h.

CONTRAINDICATIONS
Acute intoxication with alcohol, centrally acting analgesics, hypnotics, opioids, or psychotropic drugs

INTERACTIONS
Drug
Alcohol, central nervous system (CNS) depressants: May increase CNS effects or respiratory depression and hypotension.

Carbamazepine: Increases tramadol's metabolism, decreases tramadol blood concentration.
MAOIs: Increase tramadol blood concentration.
Herbal
None known.
Food
None known.

DIAGNOSTIC TEST EFFECTS
May increase serum creatinine and liver enzymes. May decrease blood Hgb. May cause proteinuria.

SIDE EFFECTS
Frequent (25%–15%)
Dizziness or vertigo, nausea, constipation, headache, somnolence
Occasional (10%–5%)
Vomiting, pruritus, CNS stimulation, (such as nervousness, anxiety, agitation, tremor, euphoria, mood swings, and hallucinations) asthenia, diaphoresis, dyspepsia, dry mouth, diarrhea
Rare (less than 5%)
Malaise, vasodilation, anorexia, flatulence, rash, visual disturbance, urinary retention/frequency, menopausal symptoms

SERIOUS REACTIONS
• Overdosage results in respiratory depression and seizures.
• Prolonged duration of action and cumulative effect may occur in those with impaired liver or renal function.

NURSING CONSIDERATIONS
Baseline Assessment
• Assess the duration, location, onset, and type of pain the patient is experiencing.
• Know that the effect of the medication is reduced if the patient experiences full pain before the next dose.
• Determine the patient's medication history, especially for carbamazepine, CNS depressant medications, and MAOIs. Review the patient's past medical history, especially for epilepsy and seizures.
• Assess the patient's liver and renal function lab values, as well as a complete blood count.
Lifespan Considerations
• Be aware that tramadol crosses the placenta and is distributed in breast milk.
• Be aware that the safety and efficacy of tramadol have not been established in children.
• In the elderly, age-related renal impairment may require dosage adjustment.
Precautions
• Use extremely cautiously in patients with acute alcoholism, advanced liver cirrhosis, anoxia, CNS depression, epilepsy, respiratory depression, and shock.
• Use cautiously in patients with acute abdominal conditions, impaired liver or renal function, increased intracranial pressure, opioid dependency, and sensitivity to opioids.
Administration and Handling
◀ALERT▶ Be aware that dialysis patients can receive their regular dose on day of dialysis.
PO
• Give tramadol without regard to meals.
Intervention and Evaluation
• Monitor the patient's blood pressure (B/P) and pulse.
• Assist the patient with ambulation if he or she experiences dizziness or vertigo.
• Offer the patient cola and dry crackers to relieve nausea, sips of tepid water to help relieve dry mouth.

• Assess the patient's daily pattern of bowel activity and stool consistency.

• Palpate the patient's bladder for urine retention.

• Monitor pattern of daily bowel activity, stool consistency.

• Assess the patient for clinical improvement and record the onset of relief of pain.

Patient Teaching

• Caution the patient that tramadol use may cause dependence.

• Urge the patient to avoid alcohol and over-the-counter (OTC) medications such as analgesics and sedatives during tramadol therapy.

• Tell the patient that tramadol may cause blurred vision, dizziness, and drowsiness. Warn the patient to avoid tasks requiring mental alertness or motor skills until his or her reaction to the drug is established.

• Warn the patient to notify the physician if he or she experiences chest pain, difficulty breathing, excessive sedation, muscle weakness, palpitation, seizures, severe constipation, or tremors.

44 Nonsteroidal Anti-inflammatory Drugs (NSAIDs)

celecoxib
diclofenac
etodolac
fenoprofen calcium
flurbiprofen
ibuprofen
indomethacin
ketoprofen
ketorolac
  tromethamine
meloxicam
nabumetone
naproxen, naproxen
  sodium
oxaprozin
piroxicam
rofecoxib
sulindac
valdecoxib

Uses: NSAIDs relieve the pain and inflammation of musculoskeletal disorders, such as rheumatoid arthritis, osteoarthritis, and ankylosing spondylitis. They're also used to provide analgesia for mild to moderate pain and to reduce fever. However, many of these agents aren't suited for long-term therapy because of toxicity.

Action: The NSAIDs' exact mechanism of action in relieving inflammation, pain, and fever is unknown. They may work by inhibiting cyclooxygenase, the enzyme responsible for prostaglandin synthesis. Also, these agents may inhibit other mediators of inflammation, such as leukotrienes. In addition, they may have a direct action on the heat-regulating center of the hypothalamus, which may contribute to their antipyretic effects.

COMBINATION PRODUCTS
ARTHROTEC: diclofenac/misoprostol (an antisecretory gastric protectant) 50 mg/200 mcg; 75 mg/200 mcg.
CHILDREN'S ADVIL COLD: ibuprofen/pseudoephedrine (a nasal decongestant) 100 mg/15 mg per 5 ml.
VICOPROFEN: ibuprofen/hydrocodone (a narcotic analgesic) 200 mg/7.5 mg.

celecoxib
sell-eh-**cox**-ib
(Celebrex, DisperDose, Panixine)
Do not confuse with Cerebyx or Celexa.

CATEGORY AND SCHEDULE
Pregnancy Risk Category: C
(D if used in third trimester or near delivery)

MECHANISM OF ACTION
A nonsteroidal anti-inflammatory that inhibits cyclo-oxygenase-2, the enzyme responsible for producing prostaglandins that cause pain and inflammation. *Therapeutic Effect:* Produces anti-inflammatory effects.

PHARMACOKINETICS

Widely distributed. Protein binding: 97%. Metabolized in the liver. Primarily eliminated in feces. **Half-life:** 11.2 hrs.

AVAILABILITY

Capsules: 100 mg, 200 mg, 400 mg.

INDICATIONS AND DOSAGES

▸ **Osteoarthritis**

PO

Adults, Elderly. 200 mg/day as single dose or 100 mg twice a day.

▸ **Rheumatoid arthritis**

PO

Adults, Elderly. 100–200 mg twice a day.

▸ **Familial adenomatous polyposis (FAP)**

PO

Adults, Elderly. 400 mg twice a daily (give with food).

CONTRAINDICATIONS

Hypersensitivity to aspirin, NSAIDs, sulfonamides

INTERACTIONS

Drug

Fluconazole, lithium: Significant interactions may occur with fluconazole and lithium.

Warfarin: May increase the risk of bleeding with warfarin.

Herbal

None known.

Food

None known.

DIAGNOSTIC TEST EFFECTS

May increase liver function test results.

SIDE EFFECTS

Frequent (greater than 5%)

Diarrhea, dyspepsia, headache, upper respiratory tract infection

Occasional (5%–1%)

Abdominal pain, flatulence, nausea, back pain, peripheral edema, dizziness, rash

SERIOUS REACTIONS

• None known.

NURSING CONSIDERATIONS

Baseline Assessment

• Assess the duration, location, onset, and type of inflammation or pain the patient is experiencing.

• Inspect the appearance of the patient's affected joints for deformity, immobility, and skin condition.

Lifespan Considerations

• Be aware that it is unknown if celecoxib crosses the placenta or is distributed in breast milk.

• Be aware that celecoxib use should be avoided during the third trimester of pregnancy as it may adversely affect the fetal cardiovascular system causing premature closure of ductus arteriosus.

• Be aware that the safety and efficacy of celecoxib have not been established in children younger than 18 years of age.

• There are no age-related precautions noted in the elderly.

Precautions

• Use cautiously in patients who are older than 60 years of age, consume alcohol, have a past history of peptic ulcer disease, receive anticoagulant or steroid therapy, and smoke.

Administration and Handling

PO

• May give celecoxib without regard to food.

• Do not crush or break capsules.

Intervention and Evaluation

• Evaluate the patient for therapeutic response, decreased stiffness, swelling, and tenderness, improved grip strength, increased joint mobility, and pain relief.

Patient Teaching

• Teach the patient to take celecoxib with food if he or she experiences gastrointestinal (GI) upset.

• Warn the patient to avoid alcohol and aspirin during celecoxib therapy. These substances increase the risk of GI bleeding.

diclofenac
dye-**klo**-feh-nak
(Cataflam, Diclohexal[AUS], Diclotek[CAN], Fenac[AUS], Novo-Difenac[CAN], Solaraze, Voltaren, Voltaren Emulgel[AUS], Voltaren Rapid[AUS], Voltaren XR)
Do not confuse with Diflucan, Duphalac, or Verelan.

CATEGORY AND SCHEDULE
Pregnancy Risk Category: B, D if used in third trimester or near delivery (oral); C (ophthalmic); B (topical)

MECHANISM OF ACTION
A nonsteroidal anti-inflammatory that inhibits prostaglandin synthesis and the intensity of pain stimulus reaching sensory nerve endings. Constricts iris sphincter. *Therapeutic Effect:* Produces analgesic and anti-inflammatory effect. Prevents miosis during cataract surgery.

PHARMACOKINETICS

Route	Onset	Peak	Duration
PO	30 min	2–3 hrs	Up to 8 hrs

Completely absorbed from the gastrointestinal (GI) tract; penetrates cornea after ophthalmic administration (may be systemically absorbed). Widely distributed. Protein binding: greater than 99%. Metabolized in liver. Primarily excreted in urine. Minimally removed by hemodialysis. **Half-life:** 1.2–2 hrs.

AVAILABILITY
Gel: 3%.
Tablets: 50 mg (Cataflam).
Tablets (delayed-release): 25 mg, 50 mg, 75 mg.
Tablets (extended-release): 100 mg.
Ophthalmic Solution: 0.1%.

INDICATIONS AND DOSAGES
▸ **Osteoarthritis**
PO
Adults, Elderly. 100–150 mg/day in 2–3 divided doses. Extended-release: 100 mg/day as single dose.
▸ **Rheumatoid arthritis**
PO
Adults, Elderly. 150–200 mg/day in 2–4 divided doses. Extended-release: 100 mg/day. Maximum: 200 mg.
▸ **Ankylosing spondylitis**
PO
Adults, Elderly. 100–125 mg/day in 4–5 divided doses.
▸ **Analgesic, primary dysmenorrhea**
PO
Adults. 150 mg/day in 3 divided doses.
▸ **Usual pediatric dosage**
Children. 2–3 mg/kg/day in divided doses 2–4 times/day.
Ophthalmic
Adults, Elderly. Apply 1 drop to eye 4 times/day commencing 24 hrs after cataract surgery. Continue for 2 wks after surgery.
▸ **Actinic keratoses**
Topical
Adults, Adolescents. Apply 2 times/day to lesion for 60–90 days.
▸ **Photophobia**
Ophthalmic
Adults, Elderly. 1 drop to affected

eye 1 hr preoperative, within 15 min postoperative, then 4 times/day for 3 days.

UNLABELED USES
Ophthalmic: Reduces occurrence and severity of cystoid macular edema post cataract surgery
PO: Treatment of vascular headaches

CONTRAINDICATIONS
Hypersensitivity to aspirin, diclofenac, and NSAIDs, porphyria

INTERACTIONS
Drug
Acetylcholine, carbachol: Ophthalmic diclofenac may decrease the effects of acetylcholine and carbachol.
Antihypertensives, diuretics: May decrease the effects of antihypertensives and diuretics.
Aspirin, salicylates: May increase the risk of GI bleeding and side effects.
Bone marrow depressants: May increase the risk of hematologic reactions.
Epinephrine, other antiglaucoma medications: May decrease the antiglaucoma effect of these drugs.
Heparin, oral anticoagulants, thrombolytics: May increase the effects of heparin, oral anticoagulants and thrombolytics.
Lithium: May increase the blood concentration and risk of toxicity of lithium.
Methotrexate: May increase the risk of toxicity of methotrexate.
Probenecid: May increase diclofenac blood concentration.
Herbal
Ginkgo biloba: May increase the risk of bleeding.
Food
None known.

DIAGNOSTIC TEST EFFECTS
May increase BUN, LDH, serum potassium levels, urine protein, and serum alkaline phosphatase, creatinine, and transaminase. May decrease serum uric acid levels.

SIDE EFFECTS
Frequent (9%–4%)
PO: Headache, abdominal cramping, constipation, diarrhea, nausea, dyspepsia
Ophthalmic: Burning, stinging on instillation, ocular discomfort
Occasional (3%–1%)
PO: Flatulence, dizziness, epigastric pain
Ophthalmic: Itching, tearing
Rare (less than 1%)
PO: Rash, peripheral edema or fluid retention, visual disturbances, vomiting, drowsiness

SERIOUS REACTIONS
• Overdosage may result in acute renal failure.
• In patients treated chronically, peptic ulcer disease, GI bleeding, gastritis, severe hepatic reaction, marked by jaundice, nephrotoxicity, characterized by hematuria, dysuria, or proteinuria, and severe hypersensitivity reaction, manifested by bronchospasm or facial edema, occur rarely.

NURSING CONSIDERATIONS
Baseline Assessment
• Assess the duration, location, onset, and type of inflammation or pain the patient is experiencing.
• Inspect the appearance of the patient's affected joints for deformity, immobility, and skin condition.
• Plan to obtain baseline BUN, LDH, serum potassium levels, urine protein, and serum alkaline phos-

phatase, creatinine, and transaminase, as well as serum uric acid levels.

Lifespan Considerations
• Be aware that diclofenac crosses the placenta and it is unknown if the drug is distributed in breast milk.
• Be aware that diclofenac use should be avoided during the last trimester of pregnancy as the drug may adversely affect the fetal cardiovascular system causing premature closure of ductus arteriosus.
• Be aware that the safety and efficacy of diclofenac have not been established in children.
• Be aware that GI bleeding or ulceration is more likely to cause serious adverse effects in elderly patients.
• In the elderly, age-related renal impairment may increase the risk of liver or renal toxicity and a reduced dosage is recommended.

Precautions
• Use cautiously in patients with congestive heart failure (CHF), history of GI disease, hypertension, and impaired liver or renal function.
• Avoid applying diclofenac topical gel to children, eyes, exfoliative dermatitis, infants, infections, neonates, and open skin wounds.

Administration and Handling
PO
• Do not crush or break enteric-coated form.
• May give with food, milk, or antacids if the patient experiences GI distress.
Ophthalmic
• Place a gloved finger on the patient's lower eyelid and pull it out until a pocket is formed between the eye and lower lid.
• Hold the dropper above the pocket and place the prescribed number of drops in the pocket.

• Gently close the patient's eye, and apply digital pressure to the lacrimal sac for 1 to 2 minutes to minimize drainage into the nose and throat and reduce the risk of systemic effects.
• Remove excess solution with tissue.

Intervention and Evaluation
• Monitor the patient for dyspepsia and headache.
• Assess the patient's pattern of daily bowel activity and stool consistency.
• Evaluate the patient for therapeutic response, improved grip strength, increased joint mobility, reduced joint tenderness, and relief of pain, stiffness, and swelling.

Patient Teaching
• Instruct the patient to swallow diclofenac tablet whole and not to crush or chew tablets.
• Warn the patient to avoid alcohol and aspirin during diclofenac therapy as these substances increase the risk of GI bleeding.
• Instruct the patient to take diclofenac with food or milk if he or she experiences GI upset.
• Warn the patient to notify the physician if he or she experiences black stools, changes in vision, itching, persistent headache, skin rash, or weight gain.
• Instruct the patient not to use hydrogel soft contact lenses during ophthalmic diclofenac therapy.
• Warn the patient to notify the physician if he or she experiences a rash during diclofenac topical therapy.
• Instruct female patients to notify the physician if she suspects pregnancy or plans to become pregnant.

etodolac
eh-**toe**-doe-lack
(Apo-Etodolac[CAN], Lodine,
Lodine XL, Ultradol[CAN])
**Do not confuse with codeine or
iodine.**

CATEGORY AND SCHEDULE
Pregnancy Risk Category: C, D
if used in third trimester or near
delivery

MECHANISM OF ACTION
A nonsteroidal anti-inflammatory
drug that produces analgesic and
anti-inflammatory effect by inhibiting prostaglandin synthesis. *Therapeutic Effect:* Reduces inflammatory
response and intensity of pain stimulus reaching sensory nerve endings.

PHARMACOKINETICS

Route	Onset	Peak	Duration
PO (analgesic)	30 min	N/A	4–12 hrs

Completely absorbed from the
gastrointestinal (GI) tract. Widely
distributed. Protein binding: greater
than 99%. Metabolized in liver.
Primarily excreted in urine. Not
removed by hemodialysis. **Half-life:**
6–7 hrs.

AVAILABILITY
Capsules: 200 mg, 300 mg.
Tablets: 400 mg, 500 mg.
Tablets (extended-release): 400 mg,
500 mg, 600 mg.

INDICATIONS AND DOSAGES
▶ **Osteoarthritis**
PO
Adults, Elderly. Initially, 800–
1,200 mg/day in 2–4 divided doses.
Maintenance: 600–1,200 mg/day.

▶ **Rheumatoid arthritis**
PO
Adults, Elderly. Initially, 300 mg
2–3 times/day or 400–500 mg
2 times/day. Maintenance:
600–1,200 mg/day.
▶ **Analgesia**
PO
Adults, Elderly. 200–400 mg q6–8h
as needed. Maximum: 1,200 mg/
day.

UNLABELED USES
Treatment of acute gouty arthritis,
vascular headache

CONTRAINDICATIONS
Active peptic ulcer disease, chronic
inflammation of GI tract, GI bleeding disorders, GI ulceration, history
of hypersensitivity to aspirin or
NSAIDs

INTERACTIONS
Drug
Antihypertensives, diuretics: May
decrease the effects of antihypertensives and diuretics.
Aspirin, salicylates: May increase
the risk of GI bleeding and side
effects.
Bone marrow depressants: May
increase the risk of hematologic
reactions.
*Heparin, oral anticoagulants,
thrombolytics:* May increase the
effects of heparin, oral anticoagulants, and thrombolytics.
Lithium: May increase the blood
concentration and risk of toxicity of
lithium.
Methotrexate: May increase the risk
of toxicity with methotrexate.
Probenecid: May increase etodolac
blood concentration.
Herbal
Feverfew, ginkgo biloba: May
increase the risk of bleeding.

Food
None known.

DIAGNOSTIC TEST EFFECTS
May increase bleeding time, liver function tests, and serum creatinine levels. May decrease serum uric acid levels.

SIDE EFFECTS
Occasional (9%–4%)
Dizziness, headache, abdominal pain or cramps, bloated feeling, diarrhea, nausea, indigestion
Rare (3%–1%)
Constipation, rash, itching, visual changes, ringing in ears

SERIOUS REACTIONS
• Overdosage may result in acute renal failure.
• In those treated chronically, peptic ulcer disease, GI bleeding, gastritis, severe hepatic reactions, such as jaundice, nephrotoxicity, marked by hematuria, dysuria, proteinuria, and severe hypersensitivity reaction, including bronchospasm, and facial edema occur rarely.

NURSING CONSIDERATIONS
Baseline Assessment
• Assess the duration, location, onset, and type of inflammation or pain the patient is experiencing.
• Inspect the appearance of the patient's affected joints for deformity, immobility, and skin condition.
Lifespan Considerations
• Be aware that it is unknown if etodolac crosses the placenta or is distributed in breast milk.
• Be aware that etodolac use should be avoided during the last trimester of pregnancy as the drug may adversely affect the fetal cardiovas-

cular system causing premature closure of ductus arteriosus.
• Be aware that the safety and efficacy of the drug have not been established in children.
• Be aware that GI bleeding and ulceration is more likely to cause serious adverse effects in elderly patients.
• In the elderly, age-related renal impairment may increase risk of liver or renal toxicity and a decreased dosage is recommended.
Precautions
• Use cautiously in patients with a history of GI tract disease, impaired liver or renal function, and predisposition to fluid retention.
Administration and Handling
◀ALERT▶ Expect to reduce etodolac dosage in the elderly. Know that the maximum dose for patients weighing less than 60 kg is 20 mg/kg.
PO
• Do not crush, open, or break capsules, extended-release capsules.
• May give with antacids, food, or milk if the patient experiences GI distress.
Intervention and Evaluation
• Monitor the patient's complete blood count (CBC) and serum chemistry lab values to access liver and renal function.
• Evaluate the patient for bleeding and bruising.
• Assess the patient for therapeutic response, improved grip strength, increased joint mobility, reduced joint tenderness, and relief of pain, stiffness, and swelling.
Patient Teaching
• Instruct the patient to swallow etodolac capsules whole and not to open, chew, or crush capsules.
• Warn the patient to avoid alcohol and aspirin during etodolac therapy. These substances increase the risk of GI bleeding.

• Warn the patient to notify the physician if he or she experiences edema, GI distress, headache, rash, signs of bleeding or visual disturbances.

• Teach the patient to take etodolac with antacids, food, or milk if he or she experiences GI distress.

• Warn the patient to use caution performing tasks that require mental alertness or motor skills until his or her response to the drug is established.

• Tell the patient to notify the physician if she suspects pregnancy or if she plans to become pregnant.

---

fenoprofen calcium
fen-oh-pro-fen
(Nalfon)
Do not confuse with Naldecon.

CATEGORY AND SCHEDULE
Pregnancy Risk Category: B, D if used in third trimester or near delivery

MECHANISM OF ACTION
A nonsteroidal anti-inflammatory drug that produces analgesic and anti-inflammatory effect by inhibiting prostaglandin synthesis. *Therapeutic Effect:* Reduces inflammatory response and intensity of pain stimulus reaching sensory nerve endings.

AVAILABILITY
Capsules: 200 mg, 300 mg.
Tablets: 600 mg.

INDICATIONS AND DOSAGES
▸ **Mild to moderate pain**
PO
Adults, Elderly. 200 mg q4–6h as needed.

▸ **Rheumatoid arthritis, osteoarthritis**
PO
Adults, Elderly. 300–600 mg 3–4 times/day.

UNLABELED USES
Treatment of ankylosing spondylitis, psoriatic arthritis, vascular headaches

CONTRAINDICATIONS
Active peptic ulcer disease, chronic inflammation of GI tract, GI bleeding disorders, GI ulceration, history of hypersensitivity to aspirin and NSAIDs, history of significantly impaired renal function

INTERACTIONS
Drug
Antihypertensives, diuretics: May decrease the effects of antihypertensives and diuretics.
Aspirin, salicylates: May increase the risk of GI bleeding and side effects.
Bone marrow depressants: May increase the risk of hematologic reactions.
Heparin, oral anticoagulants, thrombolytics: May increase the effects of heparin, oral anticoagulants, and thrombolytics.
Lithium: May increase the blood concentration and risk of toxicity of lithium.
Methotrexate: May increase the risk of toxicity of methotrexate.
Probenecid: May increase fenoprofen blood concentrations.
Herbal
None known.
Food
None known.

DIAGNOSTIC TEST EFFECTS
May increase bleeding time, blood glucose levels, BUN, LDH, serum

protein, alkaline phosphatase, creatinine, and transaminase levels.

SIDE EFFECTS
Frequent (9%–3%)
Headache, somnolence or drowsiness, dyspepsia (heartburn, indigestion, epigastric pain), nausea, vomiting, constipation
Occasional (2%–1%)
Dizziness, pruritus, nervousness, asthenia (loss of strength), diarrhea, abdominal cramps, flatulence, tinnitus, blurred vision, peripheral edema and fluid retention

SERIOUS REACTIONS
• Overdosage may result in acute hypotension and tachycardia.
• Peptic ulcer disease, GI bleeding, nephrotoxicity, dysuria, cystitis, hematuria, proteinuria, nephrotic syndrome, gastritis, severe hepatic reaction, such as cholestasis or jaundice, and severe hypersensitivity reaction, marked by bronchospasm and facial edema, occur rarely.

NURSING CONSIDERATIONS
Baseline Assessment
• Assess the duration, location, onset, and type of inflammation or pain the patient is experiencing.
• Inspect the appearance of the patient's affected joints for deformity, immobility, and skin condition.
• Plan to check baseline bleeding time, blood glucose levels, BUN, LDH, serum protein, alkaline phosphatase, creatinine, and transaminase levels.
Precautions
• Use cautiously in patients with a history of GI tract diseases, impaired liver or renal function, and a predisposition to fluid retention.

Administration and Handling
◀ALERT▶ Do not exceed fenoprofen dose of 3.2 g/day, as prescribed.
Intervention and Evaluation
• Assist the patient with ambulation if he or she experiences dizziness, drowsiness, or somnolence.
• Monitor the patient for dyspepsia.
• Assess the patient's pattern of daily bowel activity and stool consistency.
• Examine the area behind the patient's medial malleolus for fluid.
• Evaluate the patient for therapeutic response, improved grip strength, increased joint mobility, and relief of pain, stiffness, and swelling.
Patient Teaching
• Instruct the patient to swallow fenoprofen capsules whole and not to chew or crush capsules.
• Warn the patient to avoid tasks that require mental alertness or motor skills until his or her response to the drug is established.
• Teach the patient that if he or she experiences GI upset, to take fenoprofen with food or milk.
• Warn the patient to avoid alcohol and aspirin during fenoprofen therapy as these substances increase the risk of GI bleeding.

flurbiprofen
fleur-bih-pro-fen
(Ansaid, Froben[CAN], Ocufen, Strepfen[AUS])

CATEGORY AND SCHEDULE
Pregnancy Risk Category: B; D if used in third trimester or near delivery; C for Ophthalmic solution

MECHANISM OF ACTION
A phenylalkanoic acid that produces analgesic and anti-inflammatory

effect by inhibiting prostaglandin synthesis. Relaxes iris sphincter. *Therapeutic Effect:* Reduces inflammatory response and the intensity of pain stimulus reaching sensory nerve endings. Prevents, reduces miosis.

PHARMACOKINETICS
Well absorbed from the gastrointestinal (GI) tract, penetrates cornea after ophthalmic administration, which may be systemically absorbed. Widely distributed. Protein binding: 99%. Metabolized in liver. Primarily excreted in urine. **Half-life:** 3–4 hrs.

AVAILABILITY
Tablets: 50 mg, 100 mg.
Ophthalmic Solution: 0.03%.

INDICATIONS AND DOSAGES
▸ **Rheumatoid arthritis, osteoarthritis**
PO
Adults, Elderly. 200–300 mg/day in 2–4 divided doses. Do not give more than 100 mg/dose or 300 mg/day.
▸ **Dysmenorrhea**
PO
Adults. 50 mg 4 times/day
Ophthalmic
Adults, Elderly, Children. 1 drop q30min starting 2 hrs before surgery for total of 4 doses.

CONTRAINDICATIONS
Active peptic ulcer, chronic inflammation of GI tract, GI bleeding disorders, GI ulceration, history of hypersensitivity to aspirin or NSAIDs

INTERACTIONS
Drug
Acetylcholine, carbachol: Ophthalmic flurbiprofen may decrease the effects of acetylcholine and carbachol.
Antihypertensives, diuretics: May decrease the effects of antihypertensives and diuretics.
Aspirin, salicylates: May increase the risk of GI bleeding and side effects.
Bone marrow depressants: May increase the risk of hematologic reactions.
Epinephrine, other antiglaucoma medications: May decrease antiglaucoma effect.
Heparin, oral anticoagulants, thrombolytics: May increase the effects of heparin, oral anticoagulants, and thrombolytics.
Lithium: May increase the blood concentration and risk of toxicity of lithium.
Methotrexate: May increase the risk of toxicity of methotrexate.
Probenecid: May increase flurbiprofen blood concentration.
Herbal
Feverfew: May have decreased effect.
Ginkgo biloba: May increase the risk of bleeding.
Food
None known.

DIAGNOSTIC TEST EFFECTS
May increase bleeding time, serum LDH, serum alkaline phosphatase, and serum transaminase levels.

SIDE EFFECTS
Occasional
PO (9%–3%): Headache, abdominal pain, diarrhea, indigestion, nausea, fluid retention
Ophthalmic: Burning, stinging on instillation, keratitis, elevated intraocular pressure
Rare (less than 3%)
Blurred vision, flushed skin, dizziness, drowsiness, nervousness,

insomnia, unusual weakness, constipation, decreased appetite, vomiting, confusion

SERIOUS REACTIONS
• Overdosage may result in acute renal failure.
• In patients treated chronically, peptic ulcer, GI bleeding, gastritis, severe hepatic reaction, marked by jaundice, nephrotoxicity, hematuria, dysuria, proteinuria, severe hypersensitivity reaction, characterized by bronchospasm and facial edema, and cardiac arrhythmias occur rarely.

NURSING CONSIDERATIONS

Baseline Assessment
• Assess the duration, location, onset, and type of inflammation or pain the patient is experiencing.
• Inspect the appearance of the patient's affected joints for deformity, immobility, and skin condition.

Lifespan Considerations
• Be aware that flurbiprofen crosses the placenta and it is unknown whether the drug is distributed in breast milk.
• Be aware that flurbiprofen use should be avoided during the last trimester of pregnancy as the drug may adversely affect the fetal cardiovascular system causing premature closure of ductus arteriosus.
• Be aware that the safety and efficacy of flurbiprofen have not been established in children.
• Be aware that GI bleeding or ulceration is more likely to cause serious adverse effects in elderly patients.
• In the elderly, age-related renal impairment may increase the risk of liver or renal toxicity and a decreased dosage is recommended.

Precautions
• Use cautiously in patients with history of GI tract disease, impaired liver or renal function, predisposition to fluid retention, soft contact lens wearers, and surgical patients with bleeding tendencies.

Administration and Handling
PO
• Do not crush or break enteric-coated form.
• May give with antacids, food, or milk if the patient experiences GI distress.
Ophthalmic
• Place a gloved finger on the patient's lower eyelid, and pull it out until a pocket is formed between the eye and lower lid.
• Hold the dropper above the pocket, and place the prescribed number of drops into the pocket.
• Close the patient's eye gently and apply digital pressure to the lacrimal sac for 1 to 2 minutes to minimize drainage into the nose and throat, reducing the risk of systemic effects.
• Remove excess solution with tissue.

Intervention and Evaluation
• Monitor the patient for dizziness, dyspepsia, and headache.
• Assess the patient's pattern of daily bowel activity and stool consistency.
• For patients taking oral flurbiprofen, monitor the patient's BUN, complete blood count (CBC), serum alkaline phosphatase, bilirubin, creatinine, SGOT (AST), and SGPT (ALT) levels. Check stools for occult blood.
• Perform periodic eye exams in patients on ophthalmic flurbiprofen therapy.
• Evaluate the patient for therapeutic response, improved grip strength, increased joint mobility, and relief of pain, stiffness, and swelling.

Patient Teaching
• Instruct the patient to swallow flurbiprofen tablets whole and not to chew or crush tablets.
• Warn the patient to avoid alcohol and aspirin during flurbiprofen therapy. These substances increase the risk of GI bleeding.
• Teach the patient to take flurbiprofen with food or milk if he or she experiences GI upset.
• Warn the patient to notify the physician if he or she experiences edema, GI distress, headache, rash, or visual disturbances.
• Tell patients taking ophthalmic flurbiprofen that his or her eye may momentarily sting during drug instillation.
• Instruct the patient to notify the physician if she suspects pregnancy or plans to become pregnant.

ibuprofen
eye-byew-**pro**-fen
(Act-3[AUS], Advil, Apo-Ibuprofen, Brufen[AUS], Codral Period Pain [AUS], Motrin, Novoprofen[CAN], Nuprin, Nurofen[AUS], Rafen[AUS])

CATEGORY AND SCHEDULE
Pregnancy Risk Category: B, D if used in third trimester or near delivery
OTC (Tablets: 200 mg, Oral Suspension: 100 mg/5 ml)

MECHANISM OF ACTION
A nonsteroidal anti-inflammatory that inhibits prostaglandin synthesis. Produces vasodilation in hypothalamus. *Therapeutic Effect:* Produces analgesic and anti-inflammatory effect, decreases elevated body temperature.

PHARMACOKINETICS

Route	Onset	Peak	Duration
PO (analgesic)	0.5 hr	N/A	4–6 hrs
PO (antirheumatic)	2 days	1–2 wks	N/A

Rapidly absorbed from the gastrointestinal (GI) tract. Protein binding: greater than 90%. Metabolized in liver. Primarily excreted in urine. Not removed by hemodialysis.
Half-life: 2–4 hrs.

AVAILABILITY
Capsules: 200 mg.
Tablets: 20 mg, 100 mg, 200 mg (OTC), 300 mg, 400 mg, 600 mg, 800 mg.
Tablets (chewable): 50 mg, 100 mg.
Oral Suspension: 100 mg/5 ml (OTC).
Oral Drops: 40 mg/ml.

INDICATIONS AND DOSAGES
▶ **Acute and chronic rheumatoid arthritis, osteoarthritis**
PO
Adults, Elderly. 400–800 mg 3–4 times/day. Maximum: 3.2 g.
▶ **Mild to moderate pain, primary dysmenorrhea**
PO
Adults, Elderly. 200–400 mg q4–6h as needed. Maximum: 1.6 g.
▶ **Fever, minor aches, pain**
PO
Adults, Elderly. 200–400 mg q4–6h. Maximum: 1.6 g/day.
Children. 5–10 mg/kg/dose q6–8h. Maximum: 40 mg/kg/day. OTC: 7.5 mg/kg/dose q6–8h. Maximum: 30 mg/kg/day.
▶ **Juvenile arthritis**
PO
Children. 30–70 mg/kg/24h in 3–4 divided doses. Maximum in

children weighing less than 20 kg: 400 mg/day. Maximum in children weighing 20–30 kg: 600 mg/day. Maximum in children weighing greater than 30–40 kg: 800 mg/day.

UNLABELED USES
Treatment of psoriatic arthritis, vascular headaches

CONTRAINDICATIONS
Active peptic ulcer, chronic inflammation of GI tract, GI bleeding disorders, GI ulceration, history of hypersensitivity to aspirin or NSAIDs

INTERACTIONS
Drug
Antihypertensives, diuretics: May decrease the effects of antihypertensives and diuretics.
Aspirin, salicylates: May increase the risk of GI bleeding and side effects.
Bone marrow depressants: May increase the risk of hematologic reactions.
Heparin, oral anticoagulants, thrombolytics: May increase the effects of heparin, oral anticoagulants, and thrombolytics.
Lithium: May increase the blood concentration and risk of toxicity of lithium.
Methotrexate: May increase the risk of toxicity of methotrexate.
Probenecid: May increase ibuprofen blood concentration.
Herbal
Feverfew: May decrease the effects of feverfew
Ginkgo biloba: May increase the risk of bleeding.
Food
None known.

DIAGNOSTIC TEST EFFECTS
May prolong bleeding time. May alter blood glucose levels. May increase BUN, liver function test results, and serum creatinine and potassium levels. May decrease blood Hgb and Hct.

SIDE EFFECTS
Occasional (9%–3%)
Nausea with or without vomiting, dyspepsia, including heartburn, indigestion, and epigastric pain, dizziness, rash
Rare (less than 3%)
Diarrhea or constipation, flatulence, abdominal cramping or pain, itching

SERIOUS REACTIONS
• Acute overdosage may result in metabolic acidosis.
• Peptic ulcer disease, GI bleeding, gastritis, and severe hepatic reaction (cholestasis, jaundice) occur rarely.
• Nephrotoxicity, including dysuria, hematuria, proteinuria, and nephrotic syndrome and severe hypersensitivity reaction, particularly those with systemic lupus erythematosus, other collagen diseases occur rarely.

NURSING CONSIDERATIONS
Baseline Assessment
• Assess the duration, location, onset, and type of inflammation or pain the patient is experiencing.
• Inspect the appearance of the patient's affected joints for deformity, immobility, and skin condition.
Lifespan Considerations
• Be aware that it is unknown if ibuprofen crosses the placenta or is distributed in breast milk.
• Be aware that ibuprofen use should be avoided during the third trimester of pregnancy as this drug may adversely affect the fetal cardiovascular system causing premature closure of ductus arteriosus.

• Be aware that the safety and efficacy of this drug have not been established in children younger than 6 months of age.
• Be aware that GI bleeding or ulceration is more likely to cause serious adverse effects in elderly patients.
• In the elderly, age-related renal impairment may increase the risk of liver or renal toxicity and a reduced dosage is recommended.

Precautions
• Use cautiously in patients with congestive heart failure (CHF), concurrent anticoagulant use, dehydration, GI disease, such as GI bleeding or ulcers, hypertension, and impaired liver or renal function.

Administration and Handling
PO
• Do not crush or break enteric-coated form.
• Give ibuprofen with antacids, food, or milk if the patient experiences GI distress.

Intervention and Evaluation
• Monitor the patient for dyspepsia and nausea.
• Monitor the patient's complete blood count (CBC), platelet count, serum alkaline phosphatase, bilirubin, creatinine, SGOT (AST), and SGPT (ALT) levels.
• Assess the patient's pattern of daily bowel activity and stool consistency.
• Examine the patient's skin for rash.
• Evaluate the patient for therapeutic response, improved grip strength, increased joint mobility, reduced joint tenderness, and relief of pain, stiffness, and swelling.
• Monitor the patient's body temperature for fever.

Patient Teaching
• Warn the patient to avoid alcohol and aspirin during ibuprofen ther-

apy. These substances increase the risk of GI bleeding.
• Instruct the patient to take ibuprofen with antacids, food, or milk if the patient experiences GI upset.
• Teach the patient not to chew or crush enteric-coated ibuprofen tablets.
• Tell the patient that ibuprofen use may cause dizziness.

indomethacin
in-doe-**meth**-ah-sin
(Apo-Indomethacin[CAN],
Arthrexin[AUS], Indocid[CAN],
Indocin, Indocin-SR,
Novomethacin[CAN])

CATEGORY AND SCHEDULE
Pregnancy Risk Category: B
(D if used after 34 wks'
gestation, close to delivery, or
longer than 48 hrs)

MECHANISM OF ACTION
A nonsteroidal anti-inflammatory that produces analgesic and anti-inflammatory effect by inhibiting prostaglandin synthesis. *Therapeutic Effect:* Reduces inflammatory response and intensity of pain stimulus reaching sensory nerve endings. Patent ductus in neonates: Inhibits prostaglandin synthesis, increases sensitivity of premature ductus to dilating effects of prostaglandins. *Therapeutic Effect:* Causes closure of patent ductus arteriosus.

AVAILABILITY
Capsules: 25 mg, 50 mg.
Capsules (sustained-release): 75 mg.
Oral Suspension: 25 mg/5 ml.
Suppository: 50 mg.
Powder for Injection: 1 mg.

INDICATIONS AND DOSAGES
▶ **Moderate to severe rheumatoid arthritis, osteoarthritis, ankylosing spondylitis**
PO
Adults, Elderly. Initially, 25 mg 2–3 times/day. Increase by 25–50 mg/wk up to 150–200 mg/day.
Children. 1–2 mg/kg/day.
Maximum: 150–200 mg/day.
PO (extended-release)
Adults, Elderly. Initially, 75 mg/day up to 75 mg 2 times/day.
▶ **Acute gouty arthritis**
PO
Adults, Elderly. Initially, 100 mg, then 50 mg 3 times/day.
▶ **Acute painful shoulder**
PO
Adults, Elderly. 75–150 mg/day in 3–4 divided doses.
Rectal
Adults, Elderly. 50 mg 4 times/day.
Children. Initially, 1.5–2.5 mg/kg/day, up to 4 mg/kg/day. Do not exceed 150–200 mg/day.
▶ **Patent ductus arteriosus**
IV
Neonates. Initially, 0.2 mg/kg.
Neonates older than 7 days.
0.25 mg/kg for 2nd and 3rd doses.
Neonates 2–7 days. 0.2 mg/kg for 2nd and 3rd doses.
Neonates less than 48 hrs.
0.1 mg/kg for 2nd and 3rd doses.

UNLABELED USES
Treatment of fever due to malignancy, pericarditis, psoriatic arthritis, rheumatic complications associated with Paget's disease of bone, vascular headache

CONTRAINDICATIONS
Active GI bleeding and ulcers, hypersensitivity to aspirin, indomethacin, other NSAIDs, impaired renal function, thrombocytopenia

INTERACTIONS
Drug
Aminoglycosides: May increase the blood concentration of these drugs in neonates.
Antihypertensives, diuretics: May decrease the effects of antihypertensives and diuretics.
Aspirin, salicylates: May increase the risk of GI bleeding and side effects.
Bone marrow depressants: May increase the risk of hematologic reactions.
Heparin, oral anticoagulants, thrombolytics: May increase the effects of heparin, oral anticoagulants, and thrombolytics.
Lithium: May increase the blood concentration and risk of toxicity of lithium.
Methotrexate: May increase the toxicity of methotrexate.
Probenecid: May increase indomethacin blood concentration.
Triamterene: Do not give concurrently with this drug as this may potentiate acute renal failure.
Herbal
Feverfew: The effect on this herb may be decreased.
Ginkgo biloba: May increase the risk of bleeding.
Food
None known.

DIAGNOSTIC TEST EFFECTS
May prolong bleeding time. May alter blood glucose levels. May increase BUN, liver function test results, and serum creatinine and potassium levels. May decrease sodium levels and platelet count.

IV INCOMPATIBILITIES
Amino acid injection, calcium gluconate, cimetidine (Tagamet), dobutamine (Dobutrex), dopamine

(Intropin), gentamicin (Garamycin), tobramycin (Nebcin)

IV COMPATIBILITIES
Insulin, potassium

SIDE EFFECTS
Frequent (11%–3%)
Headache, nausea, vomiting, dyspepsia, as well as heartburn, indigestion, and epigastric pain, dizziness
Occasional (less than 3%)
Depression, tinnitus, diaphoresis, drowsiness, constipation, diarrhea
Patent ductus arteriosus: bleeding disturbances
Rare
Increased blood pressure (B/P), confusion, hives, itching, rash, blurred vision

SERIOUS REACTIONS
• Paralytic ileus and ulceration of esophagus, stomach, duodenum, or small intestine may occur.
• In those with impaired renal function, hyperkalemia along with worsening of impairment may occur.
• May aggravate depression or psychiatric disturbances, epilepsy, and parkinsonism.
• Nephrotoxicity, including dysuria, hematuria, proteinuria, and nephrotic syndrome, occurs rarely.
• In patent ductus arteriosus, acidosis, apnea, bradycardia, and alkalosis occur rarely.

NURSING CONSIDERATIONS

Baseline Assessment
• Know that indomethacin use may mask signs of infection.
• Assess the duration, location, onset, and type of fever, inflammation, or pain the patient is experiencing.

• Inspect the appearance of the patient's affected joints for deformity, immobility, and skin condition.
• Expect to obtain baseline laboratory values, especially a complete blood count (CBC) and blood chemistry, including aPT, APTT, and liver and renal function studies.
• In neonates with patent ductus arteriosus, assess baseline heart sounds. For murmurs, note the location, intensity, quality, and timing.

Precautions
• Use cautiously inpatients with cardiac dysfunction, concurrent anticoagulant therapy, epilepsy, hypertension, and liver or renal impairment.

Administration and Handling
PO
• Give indomethacin after meals or with antacids or food.
• Do not crush sustained-release capsules.
Rectal
• If suppository is too soft, chill for 30 minutes in refrigerator, or run cold water over foil wrapper.
• Moisten suppository with cold water before inserting into rectum.
IV
◀ALERT▶ IV injection is the preferred route for neonatal patients with patent ductus arteriosus. May give dose PO by NG tube or rectally.
◀ALERT▶ May give up to 3 doses at 12- to 24-hour intervals.
• IV solutions made without preservatives should be used immediately.
• Use IV immediately after reconstitution. IV solution normally appears clear; discard if cloudy or if precipitate forms.
• Discard unused portion.
• To 1-mg vial, add 1 to 2 ml preservative-free sterile water for

injection, or 0.9% NaCl to provide concentration of 1 mg or 0.5 mg/ml, respectively.
• Do not further dilute.
• Administer over 5 to 10 seconds.
• Restrict the patient's fluid intake, as ordered.

Intervention and Evaluation
• Monitor the patient for dyspepsia and nausea.
• Assist the patient with ambulation if he or she experiences dizziness.
• Evaluate the patient for therapeutic response, improved grip strength, increased joint mobility, reduced joint tenderness, and relief of pain, stiffness, and swelling.
• Monitor the patient's BUN, and serum alkaline phosphatase, bilirubin, creatinine, potassium, SGOT (AST), and SGPT (ALT) levels.
• Monitor the blood pressure (B/P), EKG, heart rate and, platelet count, serum sodium and blood glucose levels, and urine output in neonatal patients. Assess heart sounds for the presence of a murmur, or changes in the intensity.

Patient Teaching
• Warn the patient to avoid alcohol and aspirin during indomethacin therapy. These substances increase the risk of GI bleeding.
• Instruct the patient to swallow capsules whole and not to chew, open, or crush capsules.
• Teach the patient to take indomethacin with food or milk if he or she experiences GI upset.
• Warn the patient to avoid tasks that require mental alertness or motor skills until his or her response to the drug is established.

ketoprofen
key-toe-**pro**-fen
(Actron, Apo-Keto[CAN], Novo-Keto-EC, Orudis, Orudis KT[CAN], Orudis SR[AUS], Oruvail, Oruvail SR[AUS], Rhodis[CAN])

CATEGORY AND SCHEDULE
Pregnancy Risk Category: B, D if used in third trimester or near delivery
OTC (tablets)

MECHANISM OF ACTION
A nonsteroidal anti-inflammatory that produces analgesic and anti-inflammatory effect by inhibiting prostaglandin synthesis. *Therapeutic Effect:* Reduces inflammatory response and intensity of pain stimulus reaching sensory nerve endings.

AVAILABILITY
Tablets: 12.5 mg (OTC).
Capsules: 50 mg, 75 mg.
Capsules (extended-release): 100 mg, 150 mg, 200 mg.

INDICATIONS AND DOSAGES
▸ **Acute and chronic rheumatoid arthritis, osteoarthritis**
PO
Adults. Initially, 75 mg 3 times/day or 50 mg 4 times/day.
Elderly. Initially, 25–50 mg 3–4 times/day. Maintenance: 150–300 mg/day in 3–4 divided doses. Extended-release: 100–200 mg/day as single dose.
▸ **Mild to moderate pain, dysmenorrhea**
PO
Adults, Elderly. 25–50 mg q6–8h. Maximum: 300 mg/day.

UNLABELED USES

Treatment of acute gouty arthritis, ankylosing spondylitis, psoriatic arthritis, vascular headache

CONTRAINDICATIONS

Active peptic ulcer disease, chronic inflammation of the gastrointestinal (GI) tract, GI bleeding disorders, GI ulceration, history of hypersensitivity to aspirin or NSAIDs

INTERACTIONS
Drug

Antihypertensives, diuretics: May decrease the effects of antihypertensives and diuretics.
Aspirin, salicylates: May increase the risk of GI bleeding and side effects.
Bone marrow depressants: May increase the risk of hematologic reactions.
Heparin, oral anticoagulants, thrombolytics: May increase the effects of heparin, oral anticoagulants, and thrombolytics.
Lithium: May increase the blood concentration and risk of toxicity of lithium.
Methotrexate: May increase the risk of toxicity of methotrexate.
Probenecid: May increase ketoprofen blood concentration.
Herbal
Feverfew: The effects of this herb may be decreased.
Ginkgo biloba: May increase the risk of bleeding.
Food
None known.

DIAGNOSTIC TEST EFFECTS

May prolong bleeding time. May increase LDH, liver function tests, and serum alkaline phosphatase levels. May decrease blood Hgb and Hct, and serum sodium levels.

SIDE EFFECTS

Frequent (11%)
Dyspepsia, including heartburn, indigestion, epigastric pain
Occasional (less than 3%)
Nausea, diarrhea or constipation, flatulence, abdominal cramping, headache
Rare (less than 2%)
Anorexia, vomiting, visual disturbances, fluid retention

SERIOUS REACTIONS

• Peptic ulcer, GI bleeding, gastritis, and severe hepatic reaction, such as cholestasis and jaundice, occur rarely.
• Nephrotoxicity, including dysuria, hematuria, proteinuria, and nephrotic syndrome and severe hypersensitivity reaction, marked by bronchospasm, and angioedema occur rarely.

NURSING CONSIDERATIONS
Baseline Assessment
• Assess the duration, location, onset, and type of inflammation or pain the patient is experiencing.
• Inspect the appearance of the patient's affected joints for deformity, immobility, and skin condition.
• Plan to obtain baseline lab tests, especially a complete blood count (CBC) and blood chemistry, including aPT, APTT, and renal and liver function studies.
Precautions
• Use cautiously in patients with a history of GI tract disease, impaired liver or renal function, and a predisposition to fluid retention.
Administration and Handling
◀ALERT▶ Do not exceed ketoprofen dose of 300 mg/day. Oruvail is not recommended as initial therapy in patients who are small, older than 75 years, or with renal impairment.

PO
• May give ketoprofen with food, full glass (8 oz) of water, or milk to minimize the potential GI distress.
• Do not break, open, or chew extended-release capsules.
Intervention and Evaluation
• Monitor the patient for dyspepsia and nausea.
• Evaluate the patient for therapeutic response, improved grip strength, increased mobility and range of motion, and pain relief.
• Monitor the patient's liver and renal function test results and mental function.
Patient Teaching
• Warn the patient to avoid alcohol and aspirin during ketoprofen therapy. These substances increase the risk of GI bleeding.
• Instruct the patient to swallow capsules whole and not to chew or crush capsules.
• Teach the patient to take the drug with food or milk if he or she experiences GI upset.
• Tell the patient to inform the physician if she suspects pregnancy or plans to become pregnant.

ketorolac tromethamine

key-**tore**-oh-lack
(Acular, Acular PF, Toradol)
Do not confuse with Acthar.

CATEGORY AND SCHEDULE
Pregnancy Risk Category: C, D if used in third trimester

MECHANISM OF ACTION

A nonsteroidal anti-inflammatory that inhibits prostaglandin synthesis, reduces prostaglandin levels in aqueous humor. *Therapeutic Effect:* Reduces intensity of pain stimulus reaching sensory nerve endings, reduces intraocular inflammation.

PHARMACOKINETICS

Route	Onset	Peak	Duration
PO	30–60 min	1.5–4 hrs	4–6 hrs
IV/IM	30 min	1–2 hrs	4–6 hrs

Readily absorbed from the gastrointestinal (GI) tract, after IM administration. Protein binding: greater than 99%. Partially metabolized primarily in kidneys. Primarily excreted in urine. Not removed by hemodialysis. **Half-life:** 3.8–6.3 hrs, half-life is increased with impaired renal function, in elderly.

AVAILABILITY
Tablets: 10 mg.
Injection: 15 mg/ml, 30 mg/ml.
Ophthalmic Solution: 0.4%, 0.5%.

INDICATIONS AND DOSAGES
▶ **Analgesic for short term relief of mild to moderate pain (multiple dosing)**
PO
Adults, Elderly. 10 mg q4–6h. Maximum: 40 mg/24 hrs.
IV/IM
Adults younger than 65 yrs. 30 mg q6h. Maximum: 120 mg/24 hrs.
Adults 65 yrs and older, with renal impairment, weighing less than 50 kg. 15 mg q6h. Maximum: 60 mg/24 hrs.
Children 2–16 yrs. 0.5 mg/kg q6h.
▶ **Analgesic (single dose)**
IM
Adults younger than 65 yrs. 60 mg.
Adults 65 yrs and older, with renal impairment, weighing less than 50 kg. 30 mg.
Children 2–16 yrs. 0.4–1 mg/kg.

IV
Adults younger than 65 yrs. 30 mg.
Adults 65 yrs and older, with renal impairment, weighing more than 50 kg. 15 mg.
Children. 0.4–1 mg/kg.
Ophthalmic
Adults, Elderly. 1 drop 4 times/day.

UNLABELED USES
Ophthalmic: Prophylaxis or treatment of ocular inflammation

CONTRAINDICATIONS
Active peptic ulcer disease, chronic inflammation of GI tract, GI bleeding disorders, GI ulceration, history of hypersensitivity to aspirin or NSAIDs

INTERACTIONS
Drug
Antihypertensives, diuretics: May decrease the effects of antihypertensives.
Aspirin, salicylates: May increase the risk of GI bleeding and side effects.
Bone marrow depressants: May increase the risk of hematologic reactions.
Heparin, oral anticoagulants, thrombolytics: May increase the effects of heparin, oral anticoagulants, and thrombolytics.
Lithium: May increase the blood concentration and risk of toxicity of lithium.
Methotrexate: May increase the risk of toxicity of methotrexate.
Probenecid: May increase ketorolac blood concentration.
Herbal
Feverfew: The effects of this herb may be decreased.
Ginkgo biloba: May increase the risk of bleeding.
Food
None known.

DIAGNOSTIC TEST EFFECTS
May prolong bleeding time. May increase liver function tests.

IV INCOMPATIBILITIES
Promethazine (Phenergan)

IV COMPATIBILITIES
Fentanyl (Sublimaze), hydromorphone (Dilaudid), morphine, nalbuphine (Nubain)

SIDE EFFECTS
Frequent (17%–12%)
Headache, nausea, abdominal cramping/pain, dyspepsia (heartburn, indigestion, epigastric pain)
Occasional (9%–3%)
Diarrhea
Ophthalmic: Transient stinging and burning
Rare (3%–1%)
Constipation, vomiting, flatulence, stomatitis
Ophthalmic: Ocular irritation, allergic reactions, superficial ocular infection, keratitis

SERIOUS REACTIONS
• GI bleeding and peptic ulcer occur infrequently.
• Nephrotoxicity, including glomerular nephritis, interstitial nephritis, and nephrotic syndrome may occur in patients with preexisting impaired renal function.
• Acute hypersensitivity reaction, such as fever, chills, and joint pain, occurs rarely.

NURSING CONSIDERATIONS

Baseline Assessment
• Assess the duration, location, onset, and type of pain the patient is experiencing.
Lifespan Considerations
• Be aware that it is unknown if ketorolac is excreted in breast milk.

• Be aware that ketorolac use should be avoided during the third trimester of pregnancy as the drug may adversely affect the fetal cardiovascular system causing premature closure of ductus arteriosus.

• Be aware that the safety and efficacy of ketorolac have not been established in children, but doses of 0.5 mg/kg have been used.

• Be aware that GI bleeding or ulceration is more likely to cause serious adverse effects in the elderly.

• In the elderly, age-related renal impairment may increase risk of liver or renal toxicity and a decreased dosage is recommended.

Precautions

• Use cautiously in patients with a history of GI tract disease, impaired liver or renal function, and predisposition to fluid retention.

Administration and Handling

◀ALERT▶ Be aware that the combined duration of IM, IV and PO administration should not exceed 5 days. May give as single dose, routine, or as-needed schedule, as prescribed.

PO

• Give ketorolac with antacids, food, or milk if the patient experiences GI distress.

IM

• Give injection deeply and slowly into large muscle mass.

IV

• Give undiluted as IV push over at least 15 seconds.

Ophthalmic

• Place a gloved finger on the patient's lower eyelid and pull it out until pocket is formed between the eye and lower lid.

• Hold the dropper above the pocket and place the prescribed number of drops in the pocket.

• Close the patient's eye gently and apply digital pressure to lacrimal sac for 1 to 2 minutes to minimize drainage into the nose and throat, reducing the risk of systemic effects.

• Remove excess solution with tissue.

Intervention and Evaluation

• Monitor the patient's liver and renal function, BUN, serum alkaline phosphatase, bilirubin, creatinine, SGOT (AST), SGPT (ALT) levels to assess complete blood count (CBC) and urine output.

• Evaluate the patient for therapeutic response, improved grip strength, increased joint mobility, reduced joint tenderness, and relief of pain, stiffness, and swelling.

• Be alert to signs of bleeding, which may also occur with ophthalmic route due to systemic absorption.

Patient Teaching

• Warn the patient to avoid alcohol and aspirin during ketorolac therapy with oral or ophthalmic ketorolac which increase the tendency to bleed.

• Instruct the patient to take ketorolac with food or milk if he or she experiences GI upset.

• Warn the patient to avoid tasks that require mental alertness or motor skills until his or her response to the drug is established.

• Advise patients receiving ophthalmic ketorolac that transient burning and stinging may occur upon instillation.

• Instruct patients receiving ophthalmic ketorolac not to administer the drug while wearing soft contact lenses.

• Tell the patient to inform the physician if she suspects pregnancy or plans to become pregnant.

meloxicam
meh-**locks**-ih-cam
(Mobic)

CATEGORY AND SCHEDULE
Pregnancy Risk Category: C, D
if used in third trimester or near
term

MECHANISM OF ACTION
A nonsteroidal anti-inflammatory
that produces analgesic and anti-
inflammatory effect by inhibiting
prostaglandin synthesis. *Therapeutic
Effect:* Reduces inflammatory response and intensity of pain stimulus reaching sensory nerve endings.

PHARMACOKINETICS

Route	Onset	Peak	Duration
PO anal- gesic	30 min	4–5 hrs	N/A

Well absorbed after PO administration. Protein binding: 99%. Metabolized in liver. Eliminated via the
kidney and feces. Not removed by
hemodialysis. **Half-life:** 15–20 hrs.

AVAILABILITY
Tablets: 7.5 mg, 15 mg.

INDICATIONS AND DOSAGES
▶ **Osteoarthritis**
PO
Adults. Initially, 7.5 mg/day.
Maximum: 15 mg/day.

CONTRAINDICATIONS
Aspirin-induced nasal polyps associated with bronchospasm

INTERACTIONS
Drug
None known.

Herbal
Ginkgo biloba: May increase the
risk of bleeding.
Food
None known.

DIAGNOSTIC TEST EFFECTS
May increase serum creatinine, SGOT
(AST), and SGPT (ALT) levels.

SIDE EFFECTS
Frequent (9%–7%)
Dyspepsia, including heartburn,
indigestion, and epigastric pain,
headache, diarrhea, nausea
Occasional (4%–3%)
Dizziness, insomnia, rash, pruritus,
flatulence, constipation, vomiting
Rare (less than 2%)
Somnolence and drowsiness, urti-
caria, photosensitivity

SERIOUS REACTIONS
• In patients treated chronically, peptic ulcer disease, GI bleeding, gastritis, severe hepatic reaction, characterized by jaundice, nephrotoxicity,
including hematuria, dysuria, and
proteinuria, and severe hypersensitivity reaction, marked by bronchospasm and angioedema, occur rarely.

NURSING CONSIDERATIONS
Baseline Assessment
• Assess the duration, location,
onset, and type of inflammation or
pain the patient is experiencing.
• Inspect the appearance of the
patient's affected joints for deformity, immobility, and skin condition.
Lifespan Considerations
• Be aware that meloxicam is excreted in breast milk.
• Be aware that the safety and
efficacy of meloxicam have not
been established in children.
• In the elderly, age-related renal

impairment may require dosage adjustment.
• Be aware that the elderly are more susceptible to GI toxicity and a lower dosage of the drug is recommended for this patient population.
Precautions
• Use cautiously in patients with asthma, congestive heart failure (CHF), dehydration, hemostatic disease, history of GI disease, such as ulcers, hypertension, and impaired liver or renal function.
• Use cautiously in patients who concurrently use anticoagulants.
Administration and Handling
PO
• Give meloxicam without regard to meals.
Intervention and Evaluation
• Monitor the patient's complete blood count (CBC) and chemistry lab values, especially BUN, serum alkaline phosphatase, bilirubin, creatinine, SGOT (AST), and SGPT (ALT) levels.
• Evaluate the patient for therapeutic response, improved grip strength, increased joint mobility, reduced joint tenderness, and relief of pain, stiffness, and swelling.
Patient Teaching
• Instruct the patient to take meloxicam with food or milk to reduce GI upset.
• Warn the patient to notify the physician if he or she experiences chest pain, difficulty breathing, palpitations, persistent cramping or pain in the stomach, rash, ringing in ears, severe nausea or vomiting, swelling of the extremities, and unusual bleeding or bruising.
• Tell the patient to inform the physician if she suspects pregnancy or plans to become pregnant.
• Warn the patient to avoid tasks that require mental alertness or motor skills until his or her response to the drug is established.

nabumetone
nah-**byew**-meh-tone
(Relafen)

CATEGORY AND SCHEDULE
Pregnancy Risk Category: C, D if used in third trimester or near delivery

MECHANISM OF ACTION
A nonsteroidal anti-inflammatory that produces analgesic and anti-inflammatory effect by inhibiting prostaglandin synthesis. *Therapeutic Effect:* Reduces inflammatory response and intensity of pain stimulus reaching sensory nerve endings.

PHARMACOKINETICS
Readily absorbed from the gastrointestinal (GI) tract. Protein binding: greater than 99%. Widely distributed. Metabolized in liver to active metabolite. Primarily excreted in urine. Not removed by hemodialysis. **Half-life:** 22–30 hrs.

AVAILABILITY
Tablets: 500 mg, 750 mg.

INDICATIONS AND DOSAGES
▶ **Acute and chronic treatment of rheumatoid arthritis and osteoarthritis**
PO
Adults, Elderly. Initially, 1,000 mg as single dose or in 2 divided doses. May increase up to 2,000 mg/day as single or in 2 divided doses.

CONTRAINDICATIONS
Active peptic ulcer disease, chronic inflammation of GI tract, GI bleeding disorders, GI ulceration, history of hypersensitivity to aspirin or NSAIDs, history of significantly impaired renal function

INTERACTIONS
Drug
Antihypertensives, diuretics: May decrease the effects of antihypertensives and diuretics.

Aspirin, salicylates: May increase the risk of GI bleeding and side effects.

Bone marrow depressants: May increase the risk of hematologic reactions.

Heparin, oral anticoagulants, thrombolytics: May increase the effects of heparin, oral anticoagulants, and thrombolytics.

Lithium: May increase the blood concentration and risk of toxicity of lithium.

Methotrexate: May increase the risk of toxicity of methotrexate.

Probenecid: May increase nabumetone blood concentration.

Herbal
Feverfew: The effects of feverfew may be decreased.

Ginkgo biloba: May increase the risk of bleeding.

Food
None known.

DIAGNOSTIC TEST EFFECTS
May increase BUN, serum LDH concentration, serum alkaline phosphatase, serum creatinine, potassium, and transaminase levels, and urine protein levels. May decrease serum uric acid levels.

SIDE EFFECTS
Frequent (14%–12%)
Diarrhea, abdominal cramping and pain, dyspepsia, including heartburn, indigestion, and epigastric pain
Occasional (9%–4%)
Nausea, constipation, flatulence, dizziness, headache
Rare (3%–1%)
Vomiting, stomatitis

SERIOUS REACTIONS
• Overdose may result in acute hypotension and tachycardia.
• Peptic ulcer, GI bleeding, nephrotoxicity, including dysuria, cystitis, hematuria, proteinuria, or nephrotic syndrome, gastritis, severe hepatic reaction, such as cholestasis and jaundice, and severe hypersensitivity reaction, including bronchospasm or facial edema, occur rarely.

NURSING CONSIDERATIONS
Baseline Assessment
• Assess the duration, location, onset, and type of inflammation or pain the patient is experiencing.
• Inspect the appearance of the patient's affected joints for deformity, immobility, and skin condition.
• Plan to obtain baseline lab tests, such as blood chemistry, renal and liver function studies, and complete blood count.
Lifespan Considerations
• Be aware that nabumetone is distributed in low concentration in breast milk.
• Be aware that nabumetone use should be avoided during the last trimester of pregnancy as this drug may adversely affect the fetal cardiovascular system causing premature closing of ductus arteriosus.
• Be aware that the safety and efficacy of this drug have not been established in children.
• In the elderly, age-related renal impairment may increase the risk of liver or renal toxicity and a reduced drug dosage is recommended.
• Be aware that the elderly are more likely to have serious adverse effects with GI bleeding and ulceration.

Precautions
• Use cautiously in patients with congestive heart failure (CHF), decreased liver or renal function, and hypertension.
• Use cautiously in patients on concurrent anticoagulant therapy.

Administration and Handling
PO
• Give nabumetone with antacids, food, or milk if the patient experiences GI distress.
• Do not crush tablets; instead have patient swallow whole.

Intervention and Evaluation
• Assist the patient with ambulation if he or she experiences dizziness, drowsiness, or somnolence.
• Monitor the patient for dyspepsia.
• Assess the patient's pattern of daily bowel activity and stool consistency.
• Evaluate the patient for therapeutic response, improved grip strength, increased joint mobility, reduced joint tenderness, and relief of pain, stiffness, and swelling.

Patient Teaching
• Advise the patient that nabumetone may cause serious GI bleeding with or without pain.
• Warn the patient to avoid aspirin during nabumetone therapy.
• Instruct the patient to take nabumetone with food if he or she experiences GI upset.
• Advise the patient that nabumetone may cause confusion or dizziness. Warn the patient to use caution when performing tasks requiring mental alertness or motor skills.
• Tell the patient to inform the physician if she suspects pregnancy or plans to become pregnant.

naproxen
nah-**prox**-en
(Crysanal[AUS], EC-Naprosyn, Inza[AUS], Naprelan, Naprosyn, Naxem[CAN])

naproxen sodium
(Aleve, Anaprox, Apo-Napro[CAN], Naprogesic[AUS], Novonaprox[CAN])

CATEGORY AND SCHEDULE
Pregnancy Risk Category: B (D if used in third trimester or near delivery)
OTC (gelcaps, 200 mg tablets)

MECHANISM OF ACTION
A nonsteroidal anti-inflammatory that produces analgesic and anti-inflammatory effect by inhibiting prostaglandin synthesis. *Therapeutic Effect:* Reduces inflammatory response and intensity of pain stimulus reaching sensory nerve endings.

PHARMACOKINETICS

Route	Onset	Peak	Duration
PO (analgesic)	less than 1 hr	N/A	7 hrs or less
PO (antirheumatic)	14 days or less	2–4 wks	N/A

Completely absorbed from the gastrointestinal (GI) tract. Protein binding: 99%. Metabolized in liver. Primarily excreted in urine. Not removed by hemodialysis. **Half-life:** 13 hrs.

AVAILABILITY
Gelcaps: 220 mg (OTC).
Tablets: 200 mg (OTC), 250 mg, 375 mg, 500 mg.

Tablets (delayed-release): 375 mg, 500 mg.
Oral Suspension: 125 mg/5 ml.

INDICATIONS AND DOSAGES
▸ **Rheumatoid arthritis, osteoarthritis, ankylosing spondylitis**
PO
Adults, Elderly. 250–500 mg (275–550 mg) 2 times/day or 250 mg (275 mg) in morning and 500 mg (550 mg) in evening. Naprelan: 750–1,000 mg daily as single dose.
▸ **Juvenile rheumatoid arthritis (naproxen only)**
PO
Children. 10–15 mg/kg/day in 2 divided doses. Maximum: 1,000 mg/day.
▸ **Acute gouty arthritis**
PO
Adults, Elderly. Initially, 750 (825) mg, then 250 (275) mg q8h until attack subsides. Naprelan: Initially, 1,000–1,500 mg, then 1,000 mg/day as single dose until attack subsides.
▸ **Mild to moderate pain, dysmenorrhea, bursitis, tendinitis**
PO
Adults, Elderly. Initially, 500 (550) mg, then 250 (275) mg q6–8h as needed. Total daily dose not to exceed 1.25 (1.375) g. Naprelan: 1,000 mg/day as single dose.

UNLABELED USES
Treatment of vascular headaches

CONTRAINDICATIONS
Hypersensitivity to aspirin, naproxen, or other NSAIDs

INTERACTIONS
Drug
Antihypertensives, diuretics: May decrease the effects of antihypertensives and diuretics.
Aspirin, salicylates: May increase the risk of GI bleeding and side effects.
Bone marrow depressants: May increase risk of hematologic reactions.
Heparin, oral anticoagulants, thrombolytics: May increase the effects of heparin, oral anticoagulants, and thrombolytics.
Lithium: May increase the blood concentration and risk of toxicity of lithium.
Methotrexate: May increase the risk of toxicity of methotrexate.
Probenecid: May increase naproxen blood concentration.
Herbal
Feverfew: May decrease the effects of feverfew.
Ginkgo biloba: May increase the risk of bleeding.
Food
None known.

DIAGNOSTIC TEST EFFECTS
May prolong bleeding time, alter blood glucose levels. May increase liver function tests. May decrease serum sodium and uric acid levels.

SIDE EFFECTS
Frequent (9%–4%)
Nausea, constipation, abdominal cramps/pain, heartburn, dizziness, headache, drowsiness
Occasional (3%–1%)
Stomatitis, diarrhea, indigestion
Rare (less than 1%)
Vomiting, confusion

SERIOUS REACTIONS
• Peptic ulcer disease, GI bleeding, gastritis, and severe hepatic reaction, such as cholestasis and jaundice, occur rarely.
• Nephrotoxicity, including dysuria, hematuria, proteinuria, and nephrotic syndrome, and severe hypersensitivity reaction, marked by

---

fever, chills, and bronchospasm, occur rarely.

NURSING CONSIDERATIONS

Baseline Assessment
• Assess the duration, location, onset, and type of inflammation or pain that the patient is experiencing.
• Inspect the appearance of the patient's affected joints for deformity, immobility, and skin condition.

Lifespan Considerations
• Be aware that naproxen crosses the placenta and is distributed in breast milk.
• Be aware that naproxen use should be avoided during the third trimester of pregnancy as this drug may adversely affect the fetal cardiovascular system causing premature closing of ductus arteriosus.
• Be aware that the safety and efficacy of naproxen have not been established in children younger than 2 years of age.
• Be aware that children older than 2 years of age are at an increased risk of developing skin rash during naproxen therapy.
• In the elderly, age-related renal impairment may increase the risk of liver and renal toxicity and a reduced drug dosage is recommended.
• Be aware that the elderly are more likely to have serious adverse effects with GI bleeding and ulceration.

Precautions
• Use cautiously in patients with cardiac disease, GI disease, and impaired liver or renal function.
• Use cautiously in patients concurrently on anticoagulant therapy.

Administration and Handling
◀ALERT▶ Be aware that each 275- or 550-mg tablet of naproxen so-

dium equals 250 or 500 mg naproxen, respectively.
PO
• Have patient swallow enteric-coated form whole; scored tablets may be broken or crushed.
• May give naproxen with food, milk, or antacids if the patient experiences GI distress.

Intervention and Evaluation
• Assist the patient with ambulation if he or she experiences dizziness.
• Monitor the patient's complete blood count (CBC), particularly BUN, including Hgb, Hct, platelet count, and serum alkaline phosphatase, bilirubin, creatinine, SGOT (AST), and SGPT (ALT) levels to assess liver and renal function.
• Assess the patient's pattern of daily bowel activity and stool consistency.
• Evaluate the patient for therapeutic response, improved grip strength, increased joint mobility, reduced joint tenderness, and relief of pain, stiffness, and swelling.

Patient Teaching
• Instruct the patient to take naproxen with food or milk if he or she experiences GI upset.
• Caution the patient to avoid alcohol and aspirin during naproxen therapy. These substances increase the risk of GI bleeding.
• Warn the patient to notify the physician if he or she experiences black stools, persistent headache, rash, visual disturbances, and weight gain.
• Warn the patient to avoid tasks that require mental alertness or motor skills until his or her response to the drug is established.
• Tell the patient to inform the physician if she suspects pregnancy or plans to become pregnant.

oxaprozin
ox-ah-**pro**-zin
(Daypro)
Do not confuse with oxazepam.

CATEGORY AND SCHEDULE
Pregnancy Risk Category: C, D
if used in third trimester or near
delivery

MECHANISM OF ACTION
A nonsteroidal anti-inflammatory
that produces analgesic and anti-
inflammatory effect by inhibiting
prostaglandin synthesis. *Therapeutic
Effect:* Reduces inflammatory
response and intensity of pain
stimulus reaching sensory nerve
endings.

PHARMACOKINETICS
Well absorbed from the gastrointestinal (GI) tract. Protein binding:
greater than 99%. Widely distributed. Metabolized in liver. Primarily excreted in urine; partially
eliminated in feces. Not removed
by hemodialysis. **Half-life:**
42–50 hrs.

AVAILABILITY
Tablets: 600 mg.

INDICATIONS AND DOSAGES
▸ **Osteoarthritis**
PO
Adults, Elderly. 1,200 mg once a
day; 600 mg in patients with low
body weight, mild disease.
Maximum: 1,800 mg/day.
▸ **Rheumatoid arthritis**
PO
Adults, Elderly. 1,200 mg once a
day. Range: 600–1,800 mg/day.

▸ **Juvenile rheumatoid arthritis**

Weight	Dose/Day
22–31 kg	600 mg
32–54 kg	900 mg
greater than 54 kg	1200 mg

▸ **Dosage in renal impairment**
PO
Adults, Elderly. 600 mg/day. May
increase up to 1200 mg/day.

CONTRAINDICATIONS
Active peptic ulcer disease, chronic
inflammation of GI tract, GI bleeding disorders, GI ulceration, history
of hypersensitivity to aspirin or
NSAIDs

INTERACTIONS
Drug
Antihypertensives, diuretics: May
decrease the effects of antihypertensives and diuretics.
Aspirin, salicylates: May increase
the risk of GI bleeding and side
effects.
Bone marrow depressants: May
increase risk of hematologic reactions.
*Heparin, oral anticoagulants,
thrombolytics:* May increase the
effects of heparin, oral anticoagulants, and thrombolytics.
Lithium: May increase the blood
concentration and risk of toxicity of
lithium.
Methotrexate: May increase the risk
of toxicity of methotrexate.
Probenecid: May increase oxaprozin blood concentration.
Herbal
Feverfew: May decrease the effects
of feverfew.
Ginkgo biloba: May increase the
risk of bleeding.
Food
None known.

DIAGNOSTIC TEST EFFECTS

May increase BUN, serum creatinine, SGOT (AST), and SGPT (ALT) levels.

SIDE EFFECTS

Occasional (9%–3%)
Nausea, diarrhea, constipation, dyspepsia, including heartburn, indigestion, and epigastric pain
Rare (less than 3%)
Vomiting, abdominal cramping or pain, flatulence, anorexia, confusion, ringing in ears, insomnia, drowsiness

SERIOUS REACTIONS

• GI bleeding and coma may occur.
• Hypertension, acute renal failure, and respiratory depression occur rarely.

NURSING CONSIDERATIONS

Baseline Assessment

• Assess the duration, location, onset, and type of inflammation or pain that the patient is experiencing.
Lifespan Considerations
• Be aware that it is unknown if oxaprozin is excreted in breast milk.
• Be aware that oxaprozin use should be avoided during the third trimester of pregnancy as this drug may adversely affect the fetal cardiovascular system causing premature closing of ductus arteriosus.
• Be aware that the safety and efficacy of oxaprozin have not been established in children.
• In the elderly, age-related renal impairment may increase risk of liver or renal toxicity and a decreased dosage is recommended.
• Be aware that GI bleeding or ulceration is more likely to cause serious adverse effects in the elderly.

Precautions

• Use cautiously in patients with a history of GI tract disease, impaired liver or renal function, and a predisposition to fluid retention.
Administration and Handling
PO
• May give oxaprozin with antacids, food, or milk if the patient experiences GI distress.
Intervention and Evaluation
• Assess the patient for bleeding, bruising, edema, mental confusion and weight gain.
• Monitor the patient's BUN, serum alkaline phosphatase, bilirubin, creatinine, SGOT (AST), and SGPT (ALT) levels to assess liver and renal function.
• Evaluate the patient for therapeutic response, improved grip strength, increased joint mobility, reduced joint tenderness, and relief of pain, stiffness, and swelling.
Patient Teaching
• Tell the patient to use caution performing tasks that require mental alertness or motor skills as this drug causes drowsiness.
• Instruct the patient to take oxaprozin with food or milk if he or she experiences GI upset.
• Caution the patient to avoid alcohol and aspirin during oxaprozin therapy. These substances increase the risk of GI bleeding.
• Warn the patient to notify the physician if he or she experiences persistent GI effects, especially black, tarry stools.
• Tell the patient to inform the physician if she suspects pregnancy or plans to become pregnant.

piroxicam

purr-**ox**-i-kam
(Apo-Piroxicam[CAN], Candyl-
D[AUS], Feldene, Fexicam[CAN],
Mobilis[AUS], Novopirocam[CAN],
Pirohexal-D[AUS], Rosig[AUS],
Rosig-D[AUS])

CATEGORY AND SCHEDULE

Pregnancy Risk Category: C
(D if used in third trimester)

MECHANISM OF ACTION

A nonsteroidal anti-inflammatory
that produces analgesic and anti-
inflammatory effect by inhibiting
prostaglandin synthesis. *Therapeutic
Effect:* Reduces inflammatory response and intensity of pain stimulus reaching sensory nerve endings.

AVAILABILITY

Capsules: 10 mg, 20 mg.

INDICATIONS AND DOSAGES

▸ **Acute or chronic rheumatoid
arthritis, osteoarthritis**
PO
Adults, Elderly. Initially, 10–20 mg/
day as single/divided doses. Some
patients may require up to
30–40 mg/day.
Children. 0.2–0.3 mg/kg/day.
Maximum: 15 mg/day.

UNLABELED USES

Treatment of acute gouty arthritis,
ankylosing spondylitis, dysmenorrhea

CONTRAINDICATIONS

Active peptic ulcer disease, chronic
inflammation of the gastrointestinal
(GI) tract, GI bleeding disorders, GI
ulceration, history of hypersensitivity to aspirin or NSAIDs

INTERACTIONS
Drug

Antihypertensives, diuretics: May
decrease the effects of antihypertensives and diuretics.
Aspirin, salicylates: May increase
the risk of GI bleeding and side
effects.
Bone marrow depressants: May
increase risk of hematologic reactions.
*Heparin, oral anticoagulants,
thrombolytics:* May increase the
effects of heparin, oral anticoagulants, and thrombolytics.
Lithium: May increase the blood
concentration and risk of toxicity of
lithium.
Methotrexate: May increase the risk
of toxicity of methotrexate.
Probenecid: May increase piroxicam blood concentration.
Herbal
Feverfew: May decrease the effects
of feverfew.
Ginkgo biloba: May increase the
risk of bleeding.
St. John's wort: May increase the
risk of phototoxicity.
Food
None known.

DIAGNOSTIC TEST EFFECTS

May increase serum transaminase
activity. May decrease serum uric
acid levels.

SIDE EFFECTS

Frequent (9%–4%)
Dyspepsia, nausea, dizziness
Occasional (3%–1%)
Diarrhea, constipation, abdominal
cramping/pain, flatulence, stomatitis
Rare (less than 1%)
Increased blood pressure (B/P),
hives, painful or difficult urination,
ecchymosis, blurred vision, insom-
nia

SERIOUS REACTIONS
• Peptic ulcer disease, GI bleeding, gastritis, and severe hepatic reaction, such as cholestasis and jaundice, occur rarely.
• Nephrotoxicity, including dysuria, hematuria, proteinuria, and nephrotic syndrome, and severe hypersensitivity reaction, marked by fever, chills, and bronchospasm, occur rarely.
• Hematologic toxicity, characterized by anemia, leukopenia, eosinophilia, and thrombocytopenia, may occur rarely with long-term treatment.

NURSING CONSIDERATIONS
Baseline Assessment
• Assess the duration, location, onset, and type of inflammation or pain that the patient is experiencing.
• Inspect the appearance of the patient's affected joints for deformity, immobility, and skin condition.
• Expect to obtain baseline complete blood count (CBC) and serum chemistry tests, especially BUN, serum alkaline phosphatase, bilirubin, creatinine, SGOT (AST), and SGPT (ALT) levels to assess liver and renal function.
Precautions
• Use cautiously in patients with GI disease, hypertension, and impaired cardiac or liver function.
• Use cautiously in patients concurrently on anticoagulant therapy.
Administration and Handling
PO
• Do not crush or break capsule form.
• May give piroxicam with antacids, food, or milk if the patient experiences GI distress.
Intervention and Evaluation
• Monitor the patient for GI distress and nausea.
• Monitor the patient's complete blood count (CBC) and liver and renal function test results.

• Assess the patient's pattern of daily bowel activity and stool consistency.
• Evaluate the patient for therapeutic response, improved grip strength, increased joint mobility, reduced joint tenderness, and relief of pain, stiffness, and swelling.
Patient Teaching
• Warn the patient to avoid tasks that require mental alertness or motor skills until his or her response to the drug is established.
• Instruct the patient to take piroxicam with antacids, food, or milk if he or she experiences GI upset.
• Caution the patient to avoid alcohol and aspirin during piroxicam therapy. These substances increase the risk of GI bleeding.
• Tell the patient to inform the physician if she suspects pregnancy or plans to become pregnant.

rofecoxib
row-feh-**cox**-ib
(Vioxx)
Do not confuse with Zyvox.

CATEGORY AND SCHEDULE
Pregnancy Risk Category: C, D if used in third trimester or near delivery

MECHANISM OF ACTION
A nonsteroidal anti-inflammatory that produces analgesic and anti-inflammatory effect by inhibiting prostaglandin synthesis. *Therapeutic Effect:* Reduces inflammatory response and intensity of pain stimulus reaching sensory nerve endings.

PHARMACOKINETICS
Rapid, complete absorption from the gastrointestinal (GI) tract. Pro-

tein binding: 87%. Primarily metabolized in liver. Primarily eliminated in urine with a lesser amount excreted in feces. Not removed by hemodialysis. **Half-life:** 17 hrs.

AVAILABILITY
Tablets: 12.5 mg, 25 mg, 50 mg.
Suspension: 12.5 mg/5 ml, 25 mg/5 ml.

INDICATIONS AND DOSAGES
▸ **Osteoarthritis**
PO
Adults. Initially, 12.5 mg/day. May increase dosage to 25 mg/day. Maximum is 25 mg/day.
▸ **Rheumatoid arthritis**
PO
Adults, Elderly. 25 mg/day.
▸ **Acute pain, dysmenorrhea**
PO
Adults. Initially, 50 mg/day.

CONTRAINDICATIONS
Hypersensitivity to aspirin and NSAIDs

INTERACTIONS
Drug
Anticoagulants: May increase the effects of anticoagulants.
Aspirin: May increase the risk of GI bleeding and side effects.
Herbal
Feverfew: May decrease the effects of this herb.
Ginkgo biloba: May increase the risk of bleeding.
Food
None known.

DIAGNOSTIC TEST EFFECTS
May prolong bleeding time. May increase LDH, liver function tests, and serum alkaline phosphatase. May decrease blood Hgb, Hct, and serum sodium levels.

SIDE EFFECTS
Frequent (6%–5%)
Nausea (with or without vomiting), diarrhea, abdominal distress
Occasional (3%)
Dyspepsia, including heartburn, indigestion, epigastric pain
Rare (less than 2%)
Constipation, flatulence

SERIOUS REACTIONS
• None known.

NURSING CONSIDERATIONS
Baseline Assessment
• Assess the duration, location, onset, and type of inflammation or pain that the patient is experiencing.
• Inspect the appearance of the patient's affected joints for deformity, immobility, and skin condition.
• Plan to obtain a baseline aPT, APTT, BUN, serum alkaline phosphatase, bilirubin, creatinine, LDH concentration, SGOT (AST) and SGPT (ALT) levels to assess renal and liver function as well as serum sodium levels and a complete blood count (CBC), particularly Hct and Hgb levels.
Lifespan Considerations
• Be aware that it is unknown if rofecoxib is distributed in breast milk.
• Be aware that rofecoxib use should be avoided during the third trimester of pregnancy as this drug may adversely affect the fetal cardiovascular system causing premature closing of ductus arteriosus.
• Be aware that the safety and efficacy of rofecoxib have not been established in children.
• Be aware that the elderly are more likely to have serious adverse effects with GI bleeding and ulceration.

• In the elderly, age-related renal impairment may increase the risk of liver and renal toxicity and a reduced drug dosage is recommended.
Precautions
• Use cautiously in patients with a history of GI tract disease, impaired liver or renal function, and a predisposition to fluid retention.
Administration and Handling
PO
• Give rofecoxib without regard to meals.
Intervention and Evaluation
• Monitor the patient for dyspepsia and nausea.
• Assess the patient's pattern of daily bowel activity and stool consistency.
• Evaluate the patient for therapeutic response, improved grip strength, increased joint mobility, reduced joint tenderness, and relief of pain, stiffness, and swelling.
• Monitor the patient's blood pressure (B/P).
Patient Teaching
• Instruct the patient to take rofecoxib with antacids, food, or milk if he or she experiences GI upset.
• Caution the patient to avoid alcohol and aspirin during rofecoxib therapy. These substances increase the risk of GI bleeding.
• Warn the patient to notify the physician if he or she experiences persistent GI upset.
• Tell the patient to inform the physician if she suspects she's pregnant or plans to become pregnant.

sulindac
suel-**in**-dak
(Aclin[AUS], Apo-Sulin[CAN], Clinoril, Novo Sundac[CAN])
Do not confuse with Clozaril.

CATEGORY AND SCHEDULE
Pregnancy Risk Category: B
(D if used in third trimester or near delivery)

MECHANISM OF ACTION
A nonsteroidal anti-inflammatory that produces analgesic and anti-inflammatory effect by inhibiting prostaglandin synthesis. *Therapeutic Effect:* Reduces inflammatory response and intensity of pain stimulus reaching sensory nerve endings.

PHARMACOKINETICS

Route	Onset	Peak	Duration
PO (Anti-rheumatic)	7 days	2–3 wks	N/A

Well absorbed from the gastrointestinal (GI) tract. Metabolized in liver to active metabolite. Primarily excreted in urine. Not removed by hemodialysis. **Half-life:** 7.8 hrs; metabolite: 16.4 hrs.

AVAILABILITY
Tablets: 150 mg, 200 mg.

INDICATIONS AND DOSAGES
▸ **Rheumatoid arthritis, osteoarthritis, ankylosing spondylitis**
PO
Adults, Elderly. Initially, 150 mg 2 times/day, up to 400 mg/day.
▸ **Acute painful shoulder, gouty arthritis, bursitis, tendinitis**
PO
Adults, Elderly. 200 mg 2 times/day.

CONTRAINDICATIONS

Active peptic ulcer disease, chronic inflammation of GI tract, concurrent anticoagulant use, GI bleeding disorders, GI ulceration, history of hypersensitivity to aspirin or NSAIDs

INTERACTIONS

Drug

Antacids: May decrease sulindac blood concentration.

Antihypertensives, diuretics: May decrease the effects of antihypertensives and diuretics.

Aspirin, salicylates: May increase the risk of GI bleeding and side effects.

Bone marrow depressants: May increase risk of hematologic reactions.

Heparin, oral anticoagulants, thrombolytics: May increase the effects of heparin, oral anticoagulants, and thrombolytics.

Lithium: May increase the blood concentration and risk of toxicity of lithium.

Methotrexate: May increase the risk of toxicity of methotrexate.

Probenecid: May increase sulindac blood concentration.

Herbal

Feverfew: May decrease the effects of feverfew.

Ginkgo biloba: May increase the risk of bleeding.

Food

None known.

DIAGNOSTIC TEST EFFECTS

May increase liver function test results and serum alkaline phosphatase levels.

SIDE EFFECTS

Frequent (9%–4%)
Diarrhea or constipation, indigestion, nausea, maculopapular rash, dermatitis, dizziness, headache

Occasional (3%–1%)
Anorexia, GI cramps, flatulence

SERIOUS REACTIONS

• GI bleeding and peptic ulcer disease occur infrequently.

• Nephrotoxicity, including glomerular nephritis, interstitial nephritis, and nephrotic syndrome, may occur in those with preexisting impaired renal function.

• Acute hypersensitivity reaction, marked by fever, chills, and joint pain, occurs rarely.

NURSING CONSIDERATIONS

Baseline Assessment

• Assess the duration, location, onset, and type of inflammation or pain that the patient is experiencing.

• Inspect the appearance of the patient's affected joints for deformity, immobility, and skin condition.

• Expect to obtain baseline complete blood count (CBC), particularly platelet count, and baseline blood chemistry values, especially BUN, serum alkaline phosphatase, bilirubin, creatinine, SGOT (AST), SGPT (ALT) levels to assess liver and renal function.

Lifespan Considerations

• Be aware that it is unknown if sulindac is excreted in breast milk.

• Be aware that sulindac use should be avoided during the third trimester of pregnancy as this drug may adversely affect the fetal cardiovascular system causing premature closing of ductus arteriosus.

• Be aware that the safety and efficacy of naproxen have not been established in children.

• In the elderly, age-related renal impairment may increase the risk of liver and renal toxicity and a reduced drug dosage is recommended.

• Be aware that the elderly are more likely to have serious adverse effects with GI bleeding and ulceration.

Precautions
• Use cautiously in patients with history of GI tract disease, impaired liver or renal function, and a predisposition to fluid retention.

Administration and Handling
PO
• Give sulindac with antacids, food, or milk if the patient experiences GI distress.

Intervention and Evaluation
• Assist the patient with ambulation if he or she experiences dizziness.
• Monitor the patient's complete blood count (CBC), especially platelet count, and liver and renal function test results.
• Assess the patient's pattern of daily bowel activity and stool consistency.
• Evaluate the patient for therapeutic response, improved grip strength, increased joint mobility, reduced joint tenderness, and relief of pain, stiffness, and swelling.
• Assess the patient's skin for evidence of rash.

Patient Teaching
• Advise the patient that the therapeutic antiarthritic effect will be noted 1 to 3 weeks after sulindac therapy begins.
• Caution the patient to avoid alcohol and aspirin during naproxen therapy. These substances increase the risk of GI bleeding.
• Instruct the patient to take sulindac with food or milk if he or she experiences GI upset.
• Tell the patient to inform the physician if she suspects pregnancy or plans to become pregnant.

valdecoxib
val-deh-**cox**-ib
(Bextra)

CATEGORY AND SCHEDULE
Pregnancy Risk Category: B, D if used in third trimester or near delivery

MECHANISM OF ACTION
A nonsteroidal anti-inflammatory drug that inhibits cyclo-oxygenase-2, the enzyme responsible for producing prostaglandins that cause pain and inflammation. *Therapeutic Effect:* Reduces inflammatory response and intensity of pain stimulus reaching sensory nerve endings.

PHARMACOKINETICS
Rapidly and almost completely absorbed. Widely distributed. Extensively metabolized in the liver. Primarily eliminated in urine. **Half-life:** 8–11 hrs.

AVAILABILITY
Tablets: 10 mg, 20 mg.

INDICATIONS AND DOSAGES
▶ **Osteoarthritis, rheumatoid arthritis**
PO
Adults, Elderly. 10 mg once a day.
▶ **Primary dysmenorrhea**
PO
Adults, Elderly. 20 mg twice a day.

CONTRAINDICATIONS
Hypersensitivity to aspirin or NSAIDs, severe liver impairment, severe renal disease

INTERACTIONS
Drug
Anticoagulants: May increase the effects of anticoagulants.

Aspirin: May increase the risk of GI bleeding and side effects.

Dextromethorphan: May increase the plasma levels of dextromethorphan.

Fluconazole, ketoconazole: May increase valdecoxib plasma concentration.

Herbal
None known.

Food
None known.

DIAGNOSTIC TEST EFFECTS
May increase BUN, liver function levels, and serum creatinine.

SIDE EFFECTS
Frequent (8%–4%)
Headache
Occasional (3%–2%)
Dizziness
Rare (less than 2%)
Dyspepsia, marked by heartburn, epigastric pain, and indigestion, nausea, diarrhea, sinusitis, and peripheral edema

SERIOUS REACTIONS
• None known.

NURSING CONSIDERATIONS

Baseline Assessment
• Assess the duration, location, onset, and type of inflammation or pain that the patient is experiencing.
• Inspect the appearance of the patient's affected joints for deformity, immobility, and skin condition.

Lifespan Considerations
• Be aware that valdecoxib is excreted in breast milk.
• Be aware that valdecoxib use should be avoided during the third trimester of pregnancy as this drug may adversely affect the fetal cardiovascular system causing premature closing of ductus arteriosus.
• Be aware that the safety and

efficacy of valdecoxib have not been established in children younger than 18 years of age.
• In the elderly, there is an increased possibility of adverse reactions to NSAIDs.

Precautions
• Use cautiously in patients with moderate liver impairment.
• Use cautiously in patients who are older than 65 years of age, consume alcohol, receive anticoagulant therapy or steroids, and smoke.

Administration and Handling
• Do not crush or break film-coated tablets.
• May be given with or without food.

Intervention and Evaluation
• Assist the patient with ambulation if he or she experiences dizziness.
• Monitor the patient's BUN, serum creatinine, and hepatic enzyme test results.
• Assess the patient's pattern of daily bowel activity and stool consistency.
• Evaluate the patient for therapeutic response, improved grip strength, increased joint mobility, reduced joint tenderness, and relief of pain, stiffness, and swelling.
• Monitor the patient for headache.
• Assess the patient for relief of abdominal cramping due to dysmenorrhea.

Patient Teaching
• Instruct the patient to take valdecoxib with food or milk if he or she experiences GI upset.
• Caution the patient to avoid alcohol and aspirin during valdecoxib therapy. These substances increase the risk of GI bleeding.
• Tell the patient to inform the physician if she suspects she's pregnant or plans to become pregnant.

chloral hydrate
dexmedetomidine
  hydrochloride
flurazepam
  hydrochloride
temazepam
triazolam
zaleplon
zolpidem tartrate

Uses: Sedative-hypnotics are used to treat insomnia, which includes difficulty falling asleep initially, frequent awakening, and awakening too early. Benzodiazepines, such as flurazepam and triazolam, are the most widely used agents. As sedative-hypnotics, they have largely replaced barbiturates because they offer greater safety and a lower risk of drug dependence. Nonbenzodiazepines, including zaleplon and zolpidem, have a rapid onset and short duration of action and are used to treat short-term insomnia.

Action: Sedatives decrease motor activity, moderate excitement, and have calming effects. Hypnotics produce drowsiness and enhance the onset and maintenance of sleep, resembling natural sleep. *Benzodiazepines* potentiate gamma-aminobutyric acid (GABA), which inhibits impulse transmission in the reticular formation in the brain. They increase the total sleep time by decreasing sleep latency (time before the onset of sleep), the number of awakenings, and the time spent in the awake stage of sleep (light sleep). *Nonbenzodiazepines* bind selectively to a subunit of GABA to enhance its action.

chloral hydrate
klor-al **high**-drate
(Aquachloral Supprettes, PMS-Chloral Hydrate[CAN], Somnote)

CATEGORY AND SCHEDULE
Pregnancy Risk Category: C

MECHANISM OF ACTION
A nonbarbiturate chloral derivative that produces central nervous system (CNS) depression. *Therapeutic Effect:* Induces quiet, deep sleep, with only slight decrease in respiration and blood pressure (B/P).

AVAILABILITY
Capsules: 500 mg.
Syrup: 500 mg/5 ml.
Suppository: 324 mg, 500 mg, 648 mg.

INDICATIONS AND DOSAGES
▸ **Premedication for dental or medical procedures**
PO/Rectal
Adults. 0.5–1 g.
Children. 75 mg/kg up to 1 g total.
▸ **Premedication for EEG**
PO/Rectal
Adults. 0.5–1.5 g.
Children. 25–50 mg/kg/dose.

CONTRAINDICATIONS

Marked hepatic, presence of gastritis, renal impairment, severe cardiac disease

INTERACTIONS
Drug

Alcohol, CNS depressants: May increase the effects of chloral hydrate.
IV furosemide: This drug, given within 24 hrs following chloral hydrate, may alter B/P and cause diaphoresis.
Warfarin: May increase the effect of warfarin.
Herbal
None known.
Food
None known.

DIAGNOSTIC TEST EFFECTS

None known.

SIDE EFFECTS

Occasional
Gastric irritation, including nausea, vomiting, flatulence, and diarrhea, rash, sleepwalking
Rare
Headache, paradoxical CNS hyperactivity or nervousness in children, excitement or restlessness in elderly, particularly noted when given in presence of pain

SERIOUS REACTIONS

• Overdosage may produce somnolence, confusion, slurred speech, severe incoordination, respiratory depression, and coma.
• Tolerance and psychological dependence may occur by second week of therapy.

NURSING CONSIDERATIONS

Baseline Assessment
• Assess the patient's B/P, pulse, and respirations immediately before beginning chloral hydrate administration.
• Raise the patient's bed rails and provide call bell.
• Provide the patient with an environment conducive to sleep. For example, offer a back rub, quiet environment, and low lighting.
• Expect to obtain baseline chemistry lab values to assess renal and liver function.
Precautions
• Use cautiously in patients with clinical depression and a history of drug abuse.
Intervention and Evaluation
• Monitor the patient's mental status and vital signs.
• Dilute the drug dose in water to decrease gastric irritation.
• Assess the patient's sleep pattern, including time it takes to fall asleep and nocturnal awakenings.
• Assess pediatric and elderly patients for paradoxical reaction, such as excitability.
• Evaluate the patient for therapeutic response to insomnia, a decrease in number of nocturnal awakenings and an increase in length of sleep.
Patient Teaching
• Instruct the patient to take chloral hydrate capsule with a full glass of fruit juice or water.
• Teach the patient to swallow capsules whole and not to chew them.
• Tell the patient not to drive if he or she is taking chloral hydrate before a procedure.
• Caution the patient against abruptly withdrawing the medication after long-term use.
• Tell the patient that dependence and tolerance may occur with prolonged use.

dexmedetomidine hydrochloride

decks-meh-deh-**tome**-ih-deen
(Precedex)
Do not confuse with Peridex or Percocet.

CATEGORY AND SCHEDULE
Pregnancy Risk Category: C

MECHANISM OF ACTION
A selective alpha$_2$-adrenergic agonist. *Therapeutic Effect:* Produces analgesic, hypnotic, sedative effects.

AVAILABILITY
Injection: 100 mcg/ml.

INDICATIONS AND DOSAGES
▸ **Sedation before, during, and after intubation and mechanical ventilation while in ICU**
IV infusion
Adults. Loading dose of 1 mcg/kg over 10 min followed by maintenance dose of 0.2–0.7 mcg/kg/hr.
Elderly. May decrease dosage. No guidelines available.

CONTRAINDICATIONS
None known

INTERACTIONS
Drug
Anesthetics, hypnotics, opioids, sedatives: Concurrent administration with these drugs may enhance the effects of dexmedetomidine.
Herbal
None known.
Food
None known.

DIAGNOSTIC TEST EFFECTS
May increase serum potassium levels, serum alkaline phosphatase, SGOT (AST), and SGPT (ALT) levels.

IV INCOMPATIBILITIES
Do not mix with any other medications

SIDE EFFECTS
Frequent
Hypotension (30%), nausea (11%)
Occasional (3%–2%)
Pain, fever, oliguria, thirst

SERIOUS REACTIONS
• Bradycardia, atrial fibrillation, hypoxia, anemia, pain, and pleural effusion may occur if IV is infused too rapidly.

NURSING CONSIDERATIONS
Baseline Assessment
• Obtain baseline vital signs, including BP and heart rate.
• Expect to perform a baseline EKG to help rule out underlying cardiac disease.
Precautions
• Use cautiously in patients with advanced heart block, hypovolemia, impaired liver or renal function, and congestive heart failure (CHF).
• Expect to obtain baseline hepatic function enzyme tests as well as serum electrolytes.
• Make sure that the patient is closely monitored before administering drug. Place patient on a continuous cardiac monitor and pulse oximeter to assess for arrhythmias and hypoxemia.
Administration and Handling
◂ALERT▸ Dilute with 48 ml 0.9% NaCl before use. Do not infuse longer than 24 hours.
IV
• Store at room temperature.

• Dilute 2 ml of dexmedetomidine with 48 ml of 0.9 NaCl.
• Give as maintenance infusion, as prescribed.

Intervention and Evaluation
• Monitor the patient's EKG for atrial fibrillation, blood pressure for hypotension, level of sedation, and pulse for bradycardia.
• Assess the patient's respiratory rate and rhythm.

Patient Teaching
• Explain to the patient that he or she is receiving a drug to provide relaxation and sedation before, during, and after insertion of the endotracheal tube, and during mechanical ventilation.
• Provide comfort measures, such as mouth care and repositioning while patient is sedated. Tell the patient that his hands and arms will be restrained during mechanical ventilation.

---

flurazepam hydrochloride
flur-**ah**-zah-pam
(Apo-Flurazepam[CAN], Dalmane)
Do not confuse with Dialume.

CATEGORY AND SCHEDULE
Pregnancy Risk Category: X
Controlled substance: Schedule IV

MECHANISM OF ACTION
A benzodiazepine that enhances action of inhibitory neurotransmitter gamma-aminobutyric acid (GABA). *Therapeutic Effect:* Produces hypnotic effect due to central nervous system (CNS) depression.

PHARMACOKINETICS

Route	Onset	Peak	Duration
PO	15–20 min	3–6 hrs	7–8 hrs

Well absorbed from the gastrointestinal (GI) tract. Protein binding: 97%. Crosses blood-brain barrier. Widely distributed. Metabolized in liver to active metabolite. Primarily excreted in urine. Not removed by hemodialysis. **Half-life:** 2.3 hrs; metabolite: 40–114 hrs.

AVAILABILITY
Capsules: 15 mg, 30 mg.

INDICATIONS AND DOSAGES
▸ **Insomnia**
PO
Adults. 15–30 mg at bedtime.
Elderly, debilitated, liver disease, low serum albumin, Children older than 15 yrs. 15 mg at bedtime.

CONTRAINDICATIONS
Acute alcohol intoxication, acute narrow-angle glaucoma

INTERACTIONS
Drug
Alcohol, CNS depressants: May increase CNS depressant effect.
Herbal
Kava kava, valerian: May increase CNS depression.
Food
None known.

DIAGNOSTIC TEST EFFECTS
None known.

SIDE EFFECTS
Frequent
Drowsiness, dizziness, ataxia, sedation
Morning drowsiness may occur initially.

Occasional
GI disturbances, nervousness, blurred vision, dry mouth, headache, confusion, skin rash, irritability, slurred speech
Rare
Paradoxical CNS excitement or restlessness, particularly noted in elderly or debilitated

SERIOUS REACTIONS

• Abrupt or too rapid withdrawal after long-term use may result in pronounced restlessness and irritability, insomnia, hand tremors, abdominal or muscle cramps, sweating, vomiting, and seizures.
• Overdosage results in somnolence, confusion, diminished reflexes, and coma.

NURSING CONSIDERATIONS

Baseline Assessment
• Assess the patient's B/P, pulse, and respirations immediately before beginning flurazepam administration.
• Raise the patient's bed rails and place the call bell within reach.
• Provide the patient with an environment conducive to sleep. For example, offer a back rub, quiet environment, and low lighting.

Lifespan Considerations
• Be aware that flurazepam crosses the placenta and may be distributed in breast milk.
• Be aware that chronic flurazepam ingestion during pregnancy may produce withdrawal symptoms and CNS depression in neonates.
• Be aware that the safety and efficacy of flurazepam have not been established in children younger than 15 years of age.
• Use small initial doses with gradual dose increases to avoid ataxia or excessive sedation in the elderly.

Precautions
• Use cautiously in patients with impaired liver or renal function.

Administration and Handling
PO
• Give flurazepam without regard to meals.
• If desired, empty capsules and mix with food.

Intervention and Evaluation
• Assess patients for paradoxical reaction, such as excitability, particularly during early therapy.
• Evaluate the patient for therapeutic response to insomnia, a decrease in number of nocturnal awakenings and an increase in length of sleep.

Patient Teaching
• Tell the patient that smoking reduces the drug's effectiveness.
• Caution the patient against abruptly withdrawing the medication after long-term use.
• Explain to the patient that he or she may have disturbed sleep 1 to 2 nights after discontinuing the drug.
• Instruct the patient to notify the physician if she becomes pregnant or plans to become pregnant. Explain to the patient that flurazepam is pregnancy risk category X and the drug cannot be taken due to its risk factor.
• Urge the patient to avoid alcohol and other CNS depressants during flurazepam therapy.
• Advise the patient that flurazepam may be habit-forming.

temazepam
tem-**az**-eh-pam
(Apo-Temazepam[CAN], Novo-
Temazepam[CAN], PMS-
Temazepam[CAN], Restoril)
**Do not confuse with Vistaril or
Zestril.**

CATEGORY AND SCHEDULE
Pregnancy Risk Category: X
Controlled substance: Schedule IV

MECHANISM OF ACTION
A benzodiazepine that enhances
action of inhibitory neurotransmitter
gamma-aminobutyric acid (GABA).
Therapeutic Effect: Produces hypnotic effect due to central nervous
system (CNS) depression.

PHARMACOKINETICS
Well absorbed from the gastrointestinal (GI) tract. Protein binding:
96%. Widely distributed. Crosses
blood-brain barrier. Metabolized in
liver. Primarily excreted in urine.
Not removed by hemodialysis.
Half-life: 4–18 hrs.

AVAILABILITY
Capsules: 7.5 mg, 15 mg, 30 mg.

INDICATIONS AND DOSAGES
▸ **Insomnia**
PO
Adults, Children older than 18 yrs.
15–30 mg at bedtime.
Elderly, debilitated. 7.5–15 mg at
bedtime.

CONTRAINDICATIONS
CNS depression, narrow-angle
glaucoma, severe uncontrolled pain,
sleep apnea

INTERACTIONS
Drug
Alcohol, CNS depressants: May
increase CNS depressant effect.
Herbal
Kava kava, valerian: May increase
CNS effects.
Food
None known.

DIAGNOSTIC TEST EFFECTS
None known.

SIDE EFFECTS
Frequent
Drowsiness, sedation, rebound
insomnia that may occur for
1–2 nights after drug is discontin-
ued, dizziness, confusion, euphoria
Occasional
Weakness, anorexia, diarrhea
Rare
Paradoxical CNS excitement, rest-
lessness, particularly noted in el-
derly or debilitated

SERIOUS REACTIONS
• Abrupt or too rapid withdrawal may
result in pronounced restlessness, irritability, insomnia, hand tremors, abdominal or muscle cramps, diaphoresis, vomiting, and seizures.
• Overdosage results in somnolence,
confusion, diminished reflexes,
respiratory depression, and coma.

NURSING CONSIDERATIONS
Baseline Assessment
• Determine if the patient is preg-
nant before beginning temazepam
therapy.
• Assess the patient's blood pressure
(B/P), pulse, and respirations before
temazepam administration.
• Provide the patient with an en-
vironment conducive to sleep.
For example, offer a back rub,

low lighting, and a quiet environment.
• Assess the patient's baseline sleep pattern, including time to fall asleep and nocturnal awakenings.

Lifespan Considerations
• Be aware that temazepam crosses the placenta and may be distributed in breast milk.
• Be aware that chronic temazepam ingestion during pregnancy may produce withdrawal symptoms and CNS depression in neonates.
• Be aware that temazepam use is not recommended in children younger than 18 years of age.
• Plan to use small initial doses with gradual dosage increases to avoid ataxia or excessive sedation in the elderly.

Precautions
• Use cautiously in patients with drug dependence potential and mental impairment.

Administration and Handling
PO
• Give temazepam without regard to meals.
• Capsules may be emptied and mixed with food.

Intervention and Evaluation
• Assess elderly or debilitated patients for paradoxical reaction, particularly during early drug therapy.
• Monitor the patient's cardiovascular, mental, and respiratory statuses.
• Evaluate the patient for therapeutic response, a decrease in the number of nocturnal awakenings and an increase in the length of sleep.

Patient Teaching
• Urge the patient to avoid alcohol and other CNS depressants.
• Advise the patient that temazepam may cause daytime drowsiness.

• Warn the patient to avoid activities requiring mental alertness or motor skills until his or her response to the drug is established.
• Instruct the patient to take temazepam about 30 minutes before bedtime.
• Caution the patient to notify the physician if she becomes pregnant or plans to become pregnant during temazepam therapy.

---

triazolam
try-**aye**-zoe-lam
(Apo-Triazo[CAN], Halcion)
Do not confuse with Haldol or Healon.

CATEGORY AND SCHEDULE
Pregnancy Risk Category: X
Controlled substance: Schedule IV

MECHANISM OF ACTION
A benzodiazepine that enhances action of inhibitory neurotransmitter gamma-aminobutyric acid (GABA). *Therapeutic Effect:* Produces hypnotic effect due to central nervous system (CNS) depression.

AVAILABILITY
Tablets: 0.125 mg, 0.25 mg.

INDICATIONS AND DOSAGES
▶ **Hypnotic**
PO
Adults, Children older than 18 yrs.
0.125–0.5 mg at bedtime.
Elderly. 0.0625–0.125 mg at bedtime.

CONTRAINDICATIONS
CNS depression, narrow-angle glaucoma, pregnancy or lactation, severe uncontrolled pain, sleep apnea

INTERACTIONS
Drug
Alcohol, CNS depressants: May increase CNS depressant effect.
Herbal
Kava kava, valerian: May increase CNS depression.
Food
Grapefruit or grapefruit juice: May alter the absorption of triazolam.

DIAGNOSTIC TEST EFFECTS
None known.

SIDE EFFECTS
Frequent
Drowsiness, sedation, dry mouth, headache, dizziness, nervousness, lightheadedness, incoordination, nausea
Occasional
Euphoria, tachycardia, abdominal cramps, visual disturbances
Rare
Paradoxical CNS excitement, restlessness, particularly noted in elderly, debilitated

SERIOUS REACTIONS
• Abrupt or too rapid withdrawal may result in pronounced restlessness, irritability, insomnia, hand tremors, abdominal or muscle cramps, diaphoresis, vomiting, and seizures.
• Overdosage results in somnolence, confusion, diminished reflexes, respiratory depression, and coma.

NURSING CONSIDERATIONS

Baseline Assessment
• Determine if the patient is pregnant before beginning triazolam therapy.
• Assess the patient's vital signs immediately before triazolam administration.

• Raise the patient's bed rails and provide a call bell.
• Provide the patient with an environment conducive to sleep. For example, offer a back rub, quiet environment, and low lighting.
Precautions
• Use cautiously in patients with a potential for drug abuse.
Administration and Handling
PO
• Give triazolam without regard to meals.
• Crush tablets as needed.
• Keep in mind that grapefruit juice may alter absorption.
Intervention and Evaluation
• Assess the patient's sleep pattern.
• Assess elderly or debilitated patients for paradoxical reaction, particularly during early drug therapy.
• Monitor the patient's cardiovascular, mental, and respiratory status and liver function with prolonged triazolam use.
• Evaluate the patient for therapeutic response, a decrease in the number of nocturnal awakenings and an increase in the length of sleep.
Patient Teaching
• Urge the patient to avoid alcohol and other CNS depressants.
• Inform the patient that triazolam may cause drowsiness.
• Warn the patient to avoid activities requiring mental alertness or motor skills until his or her response to the drug is established.
• Caution the patient to notify the physician if she becomes pregnant, or plans to become pregnant during triazolam therapy.
• Tell the patient that triazolam may cause dry mouth and physical or psychological dependence.
• Explain to the patient that smoking reduces the drug's effectiveness.

• Inform the patient that rebound insomnia may occur when this drug is discontinued after short-term therapy. Explain further to the patient that he or she may experience disturbed sleep patterns for 1 to 2 nights after discontinuing triazolam.

• Urge the patient to avoid consuming grapefruit or grapefruit juice during triazolam therapy. Explain to the patient that these foods decrease the absorption of triazolam.

zaleplon
zale-eh-plon
(Sonata, Stamoc[CAN])

CATEGORY AND SCHEDULE
Pregnancy Risk Category: C

MECHANISM OF ACTION
A nonbenzodiazepine that enhances action of inhibitory neurotransmitter gamma-aminobutyric acid (GABA). *Therapeutic Effect:* Produces hypnotic effect.

AVAILABILITY
Capsules: 5 mg, 10 mg.

INDICATIONS AND DOSAGES
▸ **Hypnotic**
PO
Adults. 10 mg at bedtime. Range: 5–20 mg.
Elderly. 5 mg at bedtime.

CONTRAINDICATIONS
Severe liver impairment

INTERACTIONS
Drug
Alcohol, central nervous system (CNS) depressants: May increase CNS depressant effect.

Cimetidine: Increases the effect of zaleplon.
Rifampin: Reduces zaleplon blood concentration.
Herbal
None known.
Food
High-fat, heavy meals: Delays sleep onset time by approximately 2 hrs.

DIAGNOSTIC TEST EFFECTS
None known.

SIDE EFFECTS
Expected
Drowsiness, sedation, mild rebound insomnia on first night after drug is discontinued
Frequent (28%–7%)
Nausea, headache, myalgia, dizziness
Occasional (5%–3%)
Abdominal pain, asthenia or a loss of strength and energy, dyspepsia, eye pain, paresthesia
Rare (2%)
Tremors, amnesia, hyperacusis or an acute sense of hearing, fever, dysmenorrhea

SERIOUS REACTIONS
• May produce abnormal thinking or behavior changes.
• Taking medication while ambulating may result in memory impairment, hallucination, impaired coordination, dizziness, and lightheadedness.
• Overdosage results in somnolence, confusion, diminished reflexes, and coma.

NURSING CONSIDERATIONS
Baseline Assessment
• Raise the patient's bed rails and provide a call light immediately after drug administration.
• Provide the patient with an envi-

ronment conducive to sleep. For example, offer a back rub, quiet environment, and low lighting.

Precautions
• Use cautiously in patients with hypersensitivity to aspirin (allergic-type reaction) and mild to moderate liver function impairment, and patients experiencing signs or symptoms of depression.

Administration and Handling
PO
• Keep in mind that giving this drug with or immediately after a high-fat meal results in slower absorption.
• Capsules may be emptied and mixed with food.

Intervention and Evaluation
• Assess the patient's sleep pattern, including amount of time it takes to fall asleep and nocturnal awakenings.

Patient Teaching
• Urge the patient to avoid alcohol and other CNS depressants.
• Warn the patient to avoid activities requiring mental alertness or motor skills until his or her response to the drug is established.
• Tell the patient that rebound insomnia may occur when this drug is discontinued after short-term therapy.
• Instruct the patient to take zaleplon right before bedtime or when in bed and not falling asleep.
• Warn the patient not to exceed the prescribed drug dosage.
• Teach the patient not to take zaleplon with or immediately after a high-fat or heavy meal.

zolpidem tartrate
zole-pih-dem
(Ambien, Stilnox[AUS])
Do not confuse with Amen.

CATEGORY AND SCHEDULE
Pregnancy Risk Category: B
Controlled substance: Schedule IV

MECHANISM OF ACTION
A nonbenzodiazepine that enhances action of gamma-aminobutyric acid (GABA), an inhibitory neurotransmitter in the central nervous system (CNS). *Therapeutic Effect:* Produces hypnotic effect, induces sleep with fewer nightly awakenings, improves sleep quality.

PHARMACOKINETICS

Route	Onset	Peak	Duration
PO	30 min	N/A	6–8h

Rapidly absorbed from the gastrointestinal (GI) tract. Protein binding: 92%. Metabolized in liver; excreted in urine. Not removed by hemodialysis. **Half-life:** 1.4–4.5 hrs, half-life is increased with impaired liver function.

AVAILABILITY
Tablets: 5 mg, 10 mg.
Oral Disintegrating Tablets: 5 mg, 10 mg.

INDICATIONS AND DOSAGES
▸ **Hypnotic**
PO
Adults. 10 mg at bedtime.
Elderly, debilitated. 5 mg at bedtime.

CONTRAINDICATIONS
None known

INTERACTIONS
Drug
CNS depressants: Potentiate the effects when used with these drugs.
Herbal
None known.
Food
None known.

DIAGNOSTIC TEST EFFECTS
None known.

SIDE EFFECTS
Occasional (7%)
Headache
Rare (less than 2%)
Dizziness, nausea, diarrhea, muscle pain

SERIOUS REACTIONS
• Overdosage may produce severe ataxia, marked clumsiness and unsteadiness, bradycardia, diplopia, altered vision, severe drowsiness, nausea, vomiting, difficulty breathing, and unconsciousness.
• Abrupt withdrawal of drug after long-term use may produce weakness, facial flushing, diaphoresis, vomiting, and tremor.
• Tolerance or dependence may occur with prolonged use of high dosages.

NURSING CONSIDERATIONS
Baseline Assessment
• Assess the patient's blood pressure (B/P), pulse, and respirations immediately before zolpidem administration.
• Raise the patient's bed rails and provide a call light.
• Provide the patient with an environment conducive to sleep. For example, offer a back rub, quiet environment, and low lighting.

Lifespan Considerations
• Be aware that it is unknown if zolpidem crosses the placenta or is distributed in breast milk.
• Be aware that the safety and efficacy of zolpidem have not been established in children.
• Be aware that the elderly are more likely to experience falls or confusion and decreased initial drug doses are recommended.
• In the elderly, age-related liver impairment may require dosage adjustment.
Precautions
• Use cautiously in patients with depression, a history of drug dependence, and impaired liver function.
Administration and Handling
PO
• For faster sleep onset, do not give with or immediately after a meal.
Intervention and Evaluation
• Assess the patient's sleep pattern, including amount of time it takes to fall asleep and nocturnal awakenings.
• Evaluate the patient for therapeutic response, a decrease in the number of nocturnal awakenings and an increase in the length of sleep.
Patient Teaching
• Urge the patient to avoid alcohol during zolpidem therapy.
• Warn the patient to avoid activities requiring mental alertness or motor skills until his or her response to the drug is established.
• Caution the patient against abruptly withdrawing the medication after long-term use.
• Tell the patient that dependence on or tolerance to the drug may occur with prolonged use of high dosages.

baclofen
carisoprodol
cyclobenzaprine
  hydrochloride
dantrolene sodium
tizanidine

Uses: As adjuncts to rest and physical therapy, *central-acting skeletal muscle relaxants*, such as carisoprodol, relieve discomfort in acute, painful musculoskeletal disorders, such as local spasms from muscle injury. *Baclofen and dantrolene* are used to treat spasticity characterized by heightened muscle tone, spasm, and loss of dexterity caused by multiple sclerosis, cerebral palsy, spinal cord lesions, or stroke.

Action: *Central-acting skeletal muscle relaxants* work by a mechanism that's not fully understood. They may act at various levels of the central nervous system to depress polysynaptic reflexes, and their sedative effect may be responsible for their ability to relax muscles. *Baclofen* may mimic the actions of gamma-aminobutyric acid on spinal neurons; it doesn't directly affect skeletal muscles. *Dantrolene* acts directly on skeletal muscles, relieving spasticity.

baclofen
back-low-fin
(Apo-Baclofen[CAN], Baclo[AUS], Clofen[AUS], Kemstro, Liotec[CAN])
Do not confuse with Bactroban, Beclovent, or lisinopril.

CATEGORY AND SCHEDULE
Pregnancy Risk Category: C

MECHANISM OF ACTION
A skeletal muscle relaxant that inhibits transmission of reflexes at the spinal cord level. *Therapeutic Effect:* Relieves muscle spasticity.

PHARMACOKINETICS
Well absorbed from the gastrointestinal (GI) tract. Protein binding: 30%. Partially metabolized in liver. Primarily excreted in urine. **Half-life:** 2.5–4 hrs. Intrathecal: 1.5 hrs.

AVAILABILITY
Tablets: 10 mg, 20 mg.
Ampules: 500 mcg/ml.
Oral disintegrating tablet: 10 mg.

INDICATIONS AND DOSAGES
▸ **Musculoskeletal spasm**
PO
Adults. Initially, 5 mg 3 times a day. May increase by 15 mg/day at 3-day intervals. Range: 40–80 mg/day. Total dose not to exceed 80 mg/day.
Elderly. Initially, 5 mg 2–3 times a day. May gradually increase dosage.
Children 2–7 yrs. Initially 10–15 mg/day in divided dose q8h. May increase at 3-day intervals by 5–15 mg/day. Maximum: 40 mg/day.
Children 8 yrs and older. Maximum: 60 mg/day.
Intrathecal
Adults, Elderly, Children older than 12 yrs. Usual dose 300–800 mcg/day.

Children 12 yrs or younger. Usual dose 100–300 mcg/day.

UNLABELED USES
Treatment of trigeminal neuralgia

CONTRAINDICATIONS
Cerebral palsy, Parkinson's disease, skeletal muscle spasm due to rheumatic disorders, stroke

INTERACTIONS
Drug
CNS depressants, including alcohol: Potentiate effects when used with other CNS depressants, including alcohol.
Herbal
None known.
Food
None known.

DIAGNOSTIC TEST EFFECTS
May increase serum alkaline phosphatase, blood glucose, SGOT (AST), and SGPT (ALT) levels.

SIDE EFFECTS
Frequent (greater than 10%)
Transient drowsiness, weakness, dizziness, lightheadedness, nausea, vomiting
Occasional (10%–2%)
Headache, paresthesia of hands and feet, constipation, anorexia, hypotension, confusion, nasal congestion
Rare (less than 1%)
Paradoxical CNS excitement and restlessness, slurred speech, tremor, dry mouth, diarrhea, nocturia, impotence

SERIOUS REACTIONS
• Abrupt baclofen withdrawal may produce hallucinations and seizures.
• Baclofen overdosage results in blurred vision, convulsions, myosis, mydriasis, severe muscle weakness, strabismus, respiratory depression, and vomiting.

NURSING CONSIDERATIONS
Baseline Assessment
• Record the duration, location, onset, and type of muscular spasm.
• Evaluate the patient for signs and symptoms of immobility, stiffness, or swelling.
Lifespan Considerations
• Be aware that it is unknown if baclofen crosses the placenta or is distributed in breast milk.
• Be aware that the safety and efficacy of baclofen have not been established in children younger than 12 years.
• In the elderly, there is an increased risk of central nervous system (CNS) toxicity, manifested as confusion, hallucinations, mental depression, and sedation.
• In the elderly, age-related renal impairment may require a decreased dosage.
Precautions
• Use cautiously in patients with a history of stroke, diabetes mellitus, epilepsy, impaired renal function, and preexisting psychiatric disorders.
Administration and Handling
PO
• Give without regard to meals.
• Tablets may be crushed.
Intervention and Evaluation
• Assess the patient for paradoxical reaction.
• Assist the patient with ambulation at all times.
• Expect to obtain blood counts and liver and renal function tests periodically for those on long-term therapy.
• Evaluate the patient for a therapeutic response, such as decreased intensity of skeletal muscle pain.
• Assess the patient for signs and symptoms of developing infection.

Patient Teaching
• Explain to the patient that the side effect of drowsiness usually diminishes with continued therapy.
• Warn the patient to avoid tasks that require mental alertness or motor skills until his or her response to baclofen is established.
• Caution the patient against abruptly discontinuing baclofen after long-term therapy.
• Urge the patient to avoid alcohol and CNS depressants.

carisoprodol
kar-is-oh-**pro**-dole
(Soma)

CATEGORY AND SCHEDULE
Pregnancy Risk Category: C

MECHANISM OF ACTION
A central depressant whose exact mechanism is unknown. Many effects due to its central depressant actions. *Therapeutic Effect:* Relieves pain or muscle spasms.

AVAILABILITY
Tablets: 350 mg.

INDICATIONS AND DOSAGES
▸ **Muscle relaxant**
PO
Adults, Elderly. 350 mg 4 times/day.

CONTRAINDICATIONS
Acute intermittent porphyria, sensitivity to meprobamate

INTERACTIONS
Drug
Alcohol, central nervous system (CNS) depressants: May increase CNS depression.

Herbal
None known.
Food
None known.

DIAGNOSTIC TEST EFFECTS
None known.

SIDE EFFECTS
Frequent (greater than 10%)
Drowsiness
Occasional (10%–1%)
Tachycardia, flushing of face, dizziness, headache, lightheadedness, dermatitis, nausea, vomiting, stomach cramps, dyspnea

SERIOUS REACTIONS
• Overdose may cause CNS depression, coma, shock, and respiratory depression.

NURSING CONSIDERATIONS
Baseline Assessment
• Assess the patient's use of other medications, especially other CNS depressants.
• Expect to obtain baseline lab values, reflecting liver and renal function.
Precautions
• Use cautiously in patients with liver or renal impairment.
Administration and Handling
PO
• May give carisoprodol without regard to meals.
• Give last dose at bedtime.
Intervention and Evaluation
• Assess the patient for relief of pain and muscle spasm.
• Institute safety measures.
• Assist the patient with ambulation.
Patient Teaching
• Tell the patient that this drug may cause dizziness or drowsiness.
• Warn the patient to avoid alcohol

and other CNS depressants during carisoprodol therapy.

cyclobenzaprine hydrochloride
cy-klow-**benz**-ah-preen
(Flexeril, Flexitec[CAN], Novo-Cycloprine[CAN])
Do not confuse with cyclo-serine, cyproheptadine, or Floxin.

CATEGORY AND SCHEDULE
Pregnancy Risk Category: B

MECHANISM OF ACTION
A centrally acting skeletal muscle relaxant that reduces tonic somatic motor activity influencing motor neurons. *Therapeutic Effect:* Relieves local skeletal muscle spasm.

PHARMACOKINETICS

Route	Onset	Peak	Duration
PO	1 hr	3–4 hrs	12–24 hrs

Well (but slowly) absorbed from the gastrointestinal (GI) tract. Protein binding: 93%. Metabolized in GI tract, liver. Primarily excreted in urine. **Half-life:** 1–3 days.

AVAILABILITY
Tablets: 5 mg, 10 mg.

INDICATIONS AND DOSAGES
▶ **Acute, painful musculoskeletal conditions**
PO
Adults, Elderly. 10 mg 3 times/day. Range: 20–40 mg/day in 2–4 divided doses. Maximum: 60 mg/day.

UNLABELED USES
Treatment of fibromyalgia

CONTRAINDICATIONS
Acute recovery phase of myocardial infarction (MI), arrhythmias, congestive heart failure (CHF), concurrent use of MAOIs or within 14 days after their discontinuation, heart blocks or conduction disturbances, hyperthyroidism

INTERACTIONS
Drug
Central nervous system (CNS) depression-producing medications, tricyclic antidepressants: May increase CNS depression.
MAOIs: May increase the risk of hypertensive crisis and severe seizures.
Herbal
None known.
Food
None known.

DIAGNOSTIC TEST EFFECTS
None known.

SIDE EFFECTS
Frequent
Drowsiness (39%), dry mouth (27%), dizziness (11%)
Rare (3%–1%)
Fatigue, tiredness, asthenia, blurred vision, headache, nervousness, confusion, nausea, constipation, dyspepsia, unpleasant taste

SERIOUS REACTIONS
• Overdosage may result in visual hallucinations, hyperactive reflexes, muscle rigidity, vomiting, and hyperpyrexia.

NURSING CONSIDERATIONS
Baseline Assessment
• Record the duration, location, onset, and type of muscular spasm.
• Examine the patient for immobility, stiffness, and swelling.

Lifespan Considerations
• Be aware that it is unknown if cyclobenzaprine crosses the placenta or is distributed in breast milk.
• Be aware that the safety and efficacy of cyclobenzaprine have not been established in children.
• The elderly have an increased sensitivity to the drug's anticholinergic effects, such as confusion and urine retention.

Precautions
• Use cautiously in patients with angle-closure glaucoma, history of urine retention, impaired liver or renal function, and increased intraocular pressure.

Administration and Handling
◀ALERT▶ Do not use cyclobenzaprine longer than 2 to 3 weeks.
PO
• Give cyclobenzaprine without regard to food.

Intervention and Evaluation
• Assist the patient with ambulation at all times.
• Evaluate the patient for therapeutic response, decreased intensity of skeletal muscle pain, stiffness, and tenderness and improved mobility.

Patient Teaching
• Tell the patient that drowsiness usually diminishes with continued therapy.
• Warn the patient to avoid tasks that require mental alertness or motor skills until his or her response to the drug is established.
• Urge the patient to avoid alcohol or other depressants while taking cyclobenzaprine.
• Instruct the patient to avoid sudden changes in posture to help avoid hypotensive effects.
• Suggest to the patient sips of tepid water and sugarless gum may relieve dry mouth.

dantrolene sodium
dan-trow-lean
(Dantrium)
Do not confuse with Daraprim.

CATEGORY AND SCHEDULE
Pregnancy Risk Category: C

MECHANISM OF ACTION
A skeletal muscle relaxant that reduces muscle contraction by interfering with release of calcium ion. Reduces calcium ion concentration. *Therapeutic Effect:* Dissociates excitation-contraction coupling. Interferes with catabolic process associated with malignant hyperthermic crisis.

PHARMACOKINETICS
Poorly absorbed from the gastrointestinal (GI) tract. Protein binding: High. Metabolized in liver. Primarily excreted in urine. **Half-life:** IV: 4–8 hrs; PO: 8.7 hrs.

AVAILABILITY
Capsules: 25 mg, 50 mg, 100 mg.
Powder for Injection: 20-mg vial.

INDICATIONS AND DOSAGES
▶ **Spasticity**
PO
Adults, Elderly. Initially, 25 mg/day. Increase to 25 mg 2–4 times/day, then by 25-mg increments up to 100 mg 2–4 times/day.
Children. Initially, 0.5 mg/kg 2 times/day. Increase to 0.5 mg/kg 3–4 times/day, then increase by 0.5 mg/kg/day up to 3 mg/kg 2–4 times/day. Maximum: 400 mg/day.
▶ **Prevention of malignant hyperthermia crisis**
PO
Adults, Elderly, Children. 4–8 mg/

kg/day in 3–4 divided doses
1–2 days before surgery; give last
dose 3–4 hrs before surgery.
IV infusion
Adults, Elderly, Children. 2.5 mg/kg
about 1.25 hrs before surgery.
▸ **Management of malignant hyper-thermia crisis**
IV
Adults, Elderly, Children. Initially a
minimum of 1 mg/kg rapid IV; may
repeat up to total cumulative dose
of 10 mg/kg. May follow with
4–8 mg/kg/day PO in 4 divided
doses up to 3 days after crisis.

UNLABELED USES
Relief of exercise-induced pain in
patients with muscular dystrophy,
treatment of flexor spasms and
neuroleptic malignant syndrome

CONTRAINDICATIONS
Active liver disease

INTERACTIONS
Drug
*Central nervous system (CNS)
depressants:* May increase CNS
depression with short-term use.
Liver toxic medications: May increase the risk of liver toxicity with
chronic use.
Herbal
None known.
Food
None known.

DIAGNOSTIC TEST EFFECTS
May alter liver function tests.

IV INCOMPATIBILITIES
None known.

SIDE EFFECTS
Frequent
Drowsiness, dizziness, weakness,
general malaise, diarrhea, which
may be severe

Occasional
Confusion, headache, insomnia,
constipation, urinary frequency
Rare
Paradoxical CNS excitement or
restlessness, paresthesia, tinnitus,
slurred speech, tremor, blurred
vision, dry mouth, diarrhea, nocturia, impotence

SERIOUS REACTIONS
• There is a risk of liver toxicity,
most notably in females, those older
than 35 years of age, and those
taking other medications concurrently.
• Overt hepatitis noted most frequently between 3rd and 12th
month of therapy.
• Overdosage results in vomiting,
muscular hypotonia, muscle twitching, respiratory depression, and
seizures.

NURSING CONSIDERATIONS

Baseline Assessment
• Plan to obtain the patient's baseline liver function tests, including
serum alkaline phosphatase, SGOT
(AST), SGPT (ALT), and total
bilirubin levels.
• Record the duration, location,
onset, and type of muscular spasm
the patient is experiencing.
• Examine the patient for immobility, stiffness, and swelling.
Lifespan Considerations
• Be aware that dantrolene readily
crosses the placenta and should not
be used in breast-feeding mothers.
• There are no age-related precautions noted in children older than
5 years of age.
• There is no information available
on dantrolene use in the elderly.
Precautions
• Use cautiously in patients with a
history of previous liver disease and

impaired cardiac or pulmonary function.

Administration and Handling
◀ALERT▶ Begin with low-dose therapy, as prescribed, then increase gradually at 4- to 7-day intervals to reduces incidence of side effects.

PO
* Give dantrolene without regard to meals.

IV
* Store at room temperature.
* Use within 6 hours after reconstitution.
* Solution normally appears clear, colorless.
* Discard if cloudy or precipitate is present.
* Reconstitute 20-mg vial with 60 ml sterile water for injection to provide a concentration of 0.33 mg/ml.
* For IV infusion, administer over 1 hour.
* Diligently monitor for extravasation because of high pH of IV preparation. May produce severe complications.

Intervention and Evaluation
* Assist the patient with ambulation.
* Perform periodic blood counts and liver and renal function tests, as ordered, in patients on long-term therapy.
* Evaluate the patient for therapeutic response, decreased intensity of skeletal muscle pain or spasm.

Patient Teaching
* Explain to the patient that drowsiness usually diminishes with continued therapy.
* Caution the patient to avoid tasks that require mental alertness or motor skills until his or her response to the drug is established.
* Urge the patient to avoid alcohol or other depressants while taking dantrolene.

* Warn the patient to notify the physician if he or she experiences bloody or tarry stools, continued weakness, diarrhea, fatigue, itching, nausea, or skin rash.

tizanidine
tih-**zan**-ih-deen
(Zanaflex)

CATEGORY AND SCHEDULE
Pregnancy Risk Category: C

MECHANISM OF ACTION
A skeletal muscle relaxant that increases presynaptic inhibition of spinal motor neurons mediated by alpha$_2$-adrenergic agonists, reducing facilitation to postsynaptic motor neurons. *Therapeutic Effect:* Reduces muscle spasticity.

PHARMACOKINETICS

Route	Onset	Peak	Duration
PO	N/A	1–2 hrs	3–6 hrs

Metabolized in liver. **Half-life**: 4–8 hrs.

AVAILABILITY
Tablets: 2 mg, 4 mg.

INDICATIONS AND DOSAGES
▸ **Muscle spasticity**
PO
Adults, Elderly. Initially 2–4 mg, gradually increased in 2- to 4-mg increments and repeated q6–8h. Maximum: 3 doses/day or 36 mg total in 24 hrs.

UNLABELED USES
Spasticity associated with multiple sclerosis and spinal cord injury

CONTRAINDICATIONS
None known

INTERACTIONS
Drug
Alcohol, central nervous system (CNS) depressants: May increase CNS depressant effects.
Antihypertensives: May increase tizanidine's hypotensive potential.
Oral contraceptives: May reduce tizanidine clearance.
Phenytoin: May increase serum levels and risk of toxicity of phenytoin.
Herbal
None known.
Food
None known.

DIAGNOSTIC TEST EFFECTS
May increase serum alkaline phosphatase, SGOT (AST), and SGPT (ALT) levels.

SIDE EFFECTS
Frequent (49%–41%)
Dry mouth, somnolence, asthenia or loss of strength, weakness
Occasional (16%–4%)
Dizziness, urinary tract infection, constipation
Rare (3%)
Nervousness, amblyopia or dimness of vision, pharyngitis, rhinitis, vomiting, urinary frequency

SERIOUS REACTIONS
• Hypotension with a reduction in either diastolic or systolic blood pressure (B/P) and may be associated with bradycardia, orthostatic hypotension, and rarely, syncope. As dosage increases, risk of hypotension increases and is noted within 1 hour after dosing.

NURSING CONSIDERATIONS
Baseline Assessment
• Record the duration, location, onset, and type of muscular spasm the patient is experiencing.
• Examine the patient for immobility, stiffness, and swelling.
• Plan to obtain the patient's baseline liver function tests, that is serum alkaline phosphatase and total bilirubin.
Lifespan Considerations
• Be aware that the safety and efficacy of tizanidine have not been established in children.
• In the elderly, age-related renal impairment may warrant caution.
Precautions
• Use cautiously in patients with cardiac disease, hypotension, and liver or renal disease.
Intervention and Evaluation
• Assist the patient with ambulation at all times.
• Evaluate the patient for therapeutic response, decreased intensity of skeletal muscle pain, stiffness, and tenderness and improved mobility.
• Perform periodic liver and renal function tests for patients on long-term therapy, as ordered.
• Instruct the patient at increased risk of orthostatic hypotension to rise slowly from lying to sitting and from sitting to standing position.
Patient Teaching
• Warn the patient to avoid tasks that require mental alertness or motor skills until his or her response to the drug is established.
• Instruct the patient to avoid sudden changes in posture to help avoid hypotensive effects.
• Explain to the patient that tizanidine may cause hypotension, impaired coordination, and sedation.

47 Miscellaneous CNS Agents

alosetron
botulinum toxin
  type A
botulinum toxin
  type B
flumazenil
fluvoxamine maleate
nicotine
riluzole

Uses: Miscellaneous central nervous system (CNS) agents have a wide variety of uses. *Alosetron* is prescribed to treat severe diarrhea, especially in women with irritable bowel syndrome who don't respond to conventional therapy. Both types of *botulinum toxin* are used to block the neuromuscular effects of cervical dystonia; in addition, type A can reduce brow furrow lines. *Flumazenil* is used as an antidote for benzodiazepine overdosage. *Fluvoxamine* is used to treat obsessive-compulsive disorder. *Nicotine* is helpful as a smoking deterrent. *Riluzole* is ordered to treat amyotrophic lateral sclerosis.

Action: Most of these miscellaneous agents act on receptors in the CNS. *Alosetron* is a 5-HT$_3$ receptor antagonist that affects enteric neurons in the GI tract. Both types of *botulinum toxin* inhibit acetylcholine release to produce neuromuscular blocking effects. *Flumazenil* antagonizes the effect of benzodiazepines on gamma-aminobutyric acid receptors in the CNS. *Fluvoxamine* selectively inhibits serotonin reuptake by neurons in the CNS. *Nicotine* produces autonomic effects by binding with acetylcholine receptors, which causes stimulation followed by and depression of the peripheral and central nervous systems. *Riluzole* inhibits presynaptic glutamate release in the CNS and interferes postsynaptically with the effects of excitatory amino acids.

alosetron
al-**ohs**-eh-tron
(Lotronex)

CATEGORY AND SCHEDULE
Pregnancy Risk Category: B

MECHANISM OF ACTION
A 5-HT$_3$ receptor antagonist
that mediates abdominal pain,

bloating, nausea, peristalsis, secretory reflexes, and vomiting. *Therapeutic Effect:* Alleviates exaggerated
motor responses including diarrhea,
reduces gastric pain.

PHARMACOKINETICS
Rapidly absorbed after PO administration. Extensively metabolized in
liver. Primarily excreted in urine,
with a lesser amount in feces.
Half-life: 1.5 hrs.

AVAILABILITY
Tablets: 1 mg.

INDICATIONS AND DOSAGES
▸ **Irritable bowel syndrome**
PO
Adults (women older than 18 yrs).
1 mg 2 times/day. Maximum: 2 mg/
day.

UNLABELED USES
Carcinoid diarrhea and treatment
of irritable bowel syndrome
in men

CONTRAINDICATIONS
Breast-feeding, constipation, gastrointestinal (GI) bleeding, GI obstruction, GI perforation, history of
colitis, history of ischemic colitis or
Crohn's disease, history of or active
diverticulitis, thrombophlebitis,
ulcerative colitis

INTERACTIONS
Drug
*Hydralazine, isoniazid,
procainamide:* May alter the effects
of these drugs.
Herbal
St. John's wort: May increase alosetron blood concentration.
Food
Concurrent use of food: May decrease the absorption of alosetron or
delay the peak alosetron blood
concentration.

DIAGNOSTIC TEST EFFECTS
May increase serum alkaline phos-
phatase, serum bilirubin, SGPT
(ALT), SGOT (AST).

SIDE EFFECTS
Frequent (28%)
Constipation
Occasional (10%–2%)
Nausea, GI or abdominal discomfort
or pain, dyspepsia, flatulence, in-
creased blood pressure (B/P), clini-
cal depression
Rare
Sedation, abnormal dreams, anxiety

SERIOUS REACTIONS
• Acute ischemic colitis and serious
complications of constipation have
resulted in the need for blood transfusions and surgery.

NURSING CONSIDERATIONS
Baseline Assessment
• Determine the patient's history of
abdominal distress, abdominal pain
or discomfort, bloating, blood in
stools, and diarrhea.
• Check the patient's baseline hydration status including assessing
mucous membranes for dryness,
skin turgor, and urinary status.
Lifespan Considerations
◀ALERT▶ Be aware that the safety

and efficacy of alosetron have not been established in men.

* Be aware that it is unknown if alosetron is excreted in breast milk.
* Be aware that the safety and efficacy of alosetron have not been established in children.
* There are no age-related precautions noted in the elderly.

Precautions
* Use cautiously in patients with liver function impairment.

Administration and Handling
PO
* May give without regard to food.

Intervention and Evaluation
* Encourage the patient to maintain adequate fluid intake.
* Assess the patient's bowel sounds for peristalsis.
* Monitor the patient's daily pattern of bowel activity and stool consistency.
* Assess the patient for a decrease in signs and symptoms.

Patient Teaching
* Advise the patient that the therapeutic response may not be reached for 1 to 4 weeks.
* Explain to the patient that urgency and diarrhea may be reduced within 1 week of treatment. Inform the patient that constipation can become persistent and may require interruption of treatment or medication management.
* Warn the patient to notify the physician or nurse if bloody diarrhea, severe constipation, or a sudden worsening of stomach pain occurs.

botulinum toxin type A
botch-you-lin-em toxin
(Botox, Dysport[AUS])

CATEGORY AND SCHEDULE
Pregnancy Risk Category: C

MECHANISM OF ACTION
A neurotoxin that blocks neuromuscular conduction by binding to receptor sites on motor nerve endings, entering the nerve terminals, inhibiting the release of acetylcholine, and producing denervation of the muscle. *Therapeutic Effect:* Results in reduced muscle activity.

AVAILABILITY
Injection: 100 units.

INDICATIONS AND DOSAGES
▸ **Cervical dystonia, treatment of strabismus and blepharospasm associated with dystonia in patients with known history of tolerating toxin**
IM
Adults, Elderly. Mean dose is 236 units with range of 198–300 units divided among the affected muscles, based on patient's head and neck position, localization of pain, muscle hypertrophy, patient response, adverse event history.
▸ **Cervical dystonia, treatment of strabismus and blepharospasm associated with dystonia in patients without prior use**
IM
Adults, Elderly. Administer at lower dosage than for patients with known history of tolerance.

UNLABELED USES
Treatment of dynamic muscle contracture in pediatric cerebral palsy

patients, focal task-specific dystonia, head and neck tremor unresponsive to drug therapy, hemifacial spasms, laryngeal dystonia, oromandibular dystonia, spasmoditic torticollis, writer's cramp

CONTRAINDICATIONS

Presence of infection at proposed injection sites

INTERACTIONS

Drug

Aminoglycoside antibiotics, other drugs that interfere with neuromuscular transmission, such as curare-like compounds: May potentiate the effects of botulinum toxin A.

Herbal

None known.

Food

None known.

DIAGNOSTIC TEST EFFECTS

None known.

SIDE EFFECTS

◀ALERT▶ Side effects usually occur within first week following injection.
Frequent (15%–11%)
Localized pain, tenderness, bruising at injection site, localized weakness of injected muscle, upper respiratory tract infection, neck pain, headache
Occasional (10%–2%)
Increased cough, flu syndrome, back pain, rhinitis, dizziness, hypertonia, soreness at injection site, asthenia, dry mouth, nausea, drowsiness
Rare
Stiffness, numbness, double vision, ptosis or drooping of upper eyelid

SERIOUS REACTIONS

• Dysphagia, mild to moderate in severity, occurs in approximately 20% of patients.
• Cardiac arrhythmias and severe dysphagia manifested as aspiration,

dyspnea, and pneumonia occur rarely.
• Overdosage produces systemic weakness and muscle paralysis.

NURSING CONSIDERATIONS

Baseline Assessment

• Assess the duration, location, onset, and type of dystonia the patient is experiencing.
• Examine the proposed injection site for signs of infection, such as erythema or swelling.

Precautions

• Use cautiously in patients with neuromuscular junctional disorders, such as amyotrophic lateral sclerosis, Lambert-Eaton syndrome, motor neuropathy, and myasthenia gravis, as these patients may experience significant systemic effects, including respiratory compromise, and severe dysphagia.

Administration and Handling

◀ALERT▶ Plan to have a physician inject the drug into the affected muscle.
• Expect to administer the drug at the lowest effective dosage, and at the longest effective dosing interval to avoid the potential formation of neutralizing antibodies.

IM

• Store in the freezer.
• Administer within 4 hours after removal from freezer and reconstitution.
• May store reconstituted solution in refrigerator for up to 4 hours.
• Normally appears as a clear, colorless solution. Discard if particulate matter is present.
• Dilute drug with 0.9% NaCl.
• To create a concentration in units/0.1 ml, draw up and add 1 ml diluent to provide 10 units, 2 ml to provide 5 units, 4 ml to provide 2.5 units, or 8 ml to provide 1.25 units.

- Slowly and gently inject diluent into the vial, avoid bubbles and rotate vial gently to mix. If a vacuum doesn't pull the diluent into the vial, discard it.
- Assist the physician in injecting drug solution into affected muscle using 25-, 27-, or 30-gauge needle for superficial muscles, and a 22-gauge needle for deeper muscles.

Intervention and Evaluation
- Know that clinical improvement begins within first 2 weeks after injection and that the maximum patient benefit appears at approximately 6 weeks after injection.
- Assess for signs of dysphagia and aspiration pneumonia, including fever, sputum production, and adventitious breath sounds.

Patient Teaching
- Tell the patient to resume normal activity slowly and carefully.
- Warn the patient to seek medical attention immediately if respiratory, speech, or swallowing difficulties appear.

botulinum toxin type B
botch-you-lin-em toxin
(Dysport[AUS], Myobloc)

CATEGORY AND SCHEDULE
Pregnancy Risk Category: C

MECHANISM OF ACTION
A neurotoxin that inhibits acetylcholine release at the neuromuscular junction by binding, internalization, and translocation of the toxin where it acts as an endoprotease, an enzyme. *Therapeutic Effect:* Splits polypeptides essential for neurotransmitter release.

AVAILABILITY
Injection: 2,500 units, 5,000 units, 10,000 units.

INDICATIONS AND DOSAGES
▸ **Cervical dystonia, to reduce severity of abnormal head position and neck pain in patients with history of tolerating toxin**
IM
Adults, Elderly. 2,500–5,000 units divided among the affected muscles.
▸ **Cervical dystonia, to reduce severity of abnormal head position and neck pain in patients without prior use**
IM
Adults, Elderly. Administer at lower dosage than for patients with known history of tolerance.

CONTRAINDICATIONS
None known

INTERACTIONS
Drug
Aminoglycoside antibiotics, other drugs that interfere with neuromuscular transmission, such as curare-like compounds: May potentiate the effects of botulinum toxin B.
Herbal
None known.
Food
None known.

DIAGNOSTIC TEST EFFECTS
None known.

SIDE EFFECTS
Frequent (19%–12%)
Infection, neck pain, headache, injection site pain, dry mouth
Occasional (10%–4%)
Flu syndrome, generalized pain, increased cough, back pain, myasthenia
Rare
Dizziness, nausea, rhinitis, headache, vomiting, edema, allergic reaction

SERIOUS REACTIONS
• Dysphagia, mild to moderate in severity, occurs in approximately 10% of patients.
• Cardiac arrhythmias and severe dysphagia manifested as aspiration, dyspnea, and pneumonia occur rarely.
• Overdosage produces systemic weakness and muscle paralysis.

NURSING CONSIDERATIONS
Baseline Assessment
• Assess the duration, location, onset, and type of dystonia the patient is experiencing.
• Examine the proposed injection site for signs of infection, such as erythema or swelling.
Precautions
• Use cautiously in patients with neuromuscular junctional disorders, such as amyotrophic lateral sclerosis, Lambert-Eaton syndrome, motor neuropathy, and myasthenia gravis, as these patients may experience significant systemic effects, including respiratory compromise, and severe dysphagia.
Administration and Handling
◀ALERT▶ Plan to have a physician inject the drug into the affected muscle.
◀ALERT▶ Side effects usually occur within first week after injection.
IM
• May be refrigerated for up to 21 months. Do not freeze.
• Administer within 4 hours after removal from freezer and reconstitution.
• May store reconstituted solution in refrigerator for up to 4 hours.
• Solution normally appears clear, colorless. Discard if particulate matter is present.
• Dilute drug with 0.9% NaCl.
• Slowly, gently inject diluent into the vial; avoid bubbles, rotate vial gently to mix. If a vacuum doesn't pull the diluent into the vial, discard it.
• Assist the physician in injecting drug solution into affected muscle using 25-, 27-, or 30-gauge needle for superficial muscles, and a 22-gauge needle for deeper muscles.
Intervention and Evaluation
• Know that the duration of effect lasts between 12 to 16 weeks at doses of 5,000 units or 10,000 units.
• Assess for signs of dysphagia and aspiration pneumonia, including fever, sputum production, and adventitious breath sounds.
Patient Teaching
• Tell the patient to resume normal activity slowly and carefully.
• Warn the patient to seek medical attention immediately if respiratory, speech, or swallowing difficulties appear.

flumazenil
flew-**maz**-ah-nil
(Anexate[CAN], Romazicon)

CATEGORY AND SCHEDULE
Pregnancy Risk Category: C

MECHANISM OF ACTION
An antidote that antagonizes the effect of benzodiazepines on the gamma-aminobutyric acid (GABA) receptor complex in the central nervous system (CNS). *Therapeutic Effect:* Reverses sedative effect of benzodiazepines.

PHARMACOKINETICS

Route	Onset	Peak	Duration
IV	1–2 min	6–10 min	less than 1 hr

Duration, degree of benzodiazepine reversal related to dosage, plasma concentration. Protein binding: 50%. Metabolized by liver; excreted in urine.

AVAILABILITY
Injection: 0.1 mg/ml.

INDICATIONS AND DOSAGES
▶ **Reversal of conscious sedation, in general anesthesia**
IV
Adults, Elderly. Initially, 0.2 mg (2 ml) over 15 sec; may repeat 0.2-mg dose in 45 sec; then at 60-sec intervals. Maximum: 1 mg (10 ml total dose).
Children, Neonates. Initially, 0.01 mg/kg (maximum: 0.2 mg) May repeat after 45 sec and then every min. Maximum cumulative dose: 0.05 mg/kg or 1 mg.
▶ **Benzodiazepine overdose**
IV
Adults, Elderly. Initially, 0.2 mg (2 ml) over 30 sec; may repeat after 30 sec with 0.3 mg (3 ml) over 30 sec if desired level of consciousness (LOC) not achieved. Further doses of 0.5 mg (5 ml) over 30 sec may be administered at 60-sec intervals. Maximum: 3 mg (30 ml) total dose.
Children, Neonates. Initially, 0.01 mg/kg (maximum: 0.2 mg) May repeat in 45 seconds, then at 60-sec intervals. Maximum cumulative dose: 1 mg.

CONTRAINDICATIONS
Anticholinergic signs, arrhythmias, cardiovascular collapse, history of hypersensitivity to benzodiazepines, those showing signs of serious cyclic antidepressant overdose manifested by motor abnormalities, those who have been given a benzodiazepine for control of a potentially life-threatening condition, such as control of intracranial pressure and status epilepticus

INTERACTIONS
Drug
Toxic effects, such as seizures and arrhythmias, of drugs taken in overdose, especially tricyclic antidepressants, may emerge with reversal of sedative effect of benzodiazepines.
Herbal
None known.
Food
None known.

DIAGNOSTIC TEST EFFECTS
None known.

IV INCOMPATIBILITIES
No information available via Y-site administration.

IV COMPATIBILITIES
Aminophylline, cimetidine (Tagamet), dobutamine (Dobutrex), dopamine (Intropin), famotidine (Pepcid), heparin, lidocaine, procainamide (Pronestyl), ranitidine (Zantac)

SIDE EFFECTS
Frequent (11%–4%)
Agitation, anxiety, dry mouth, dyspnea, insomnia, palpitations, tremors, headache, blurred vision, dizziness, ataxia, nausea, vomiting, pain at injection site, diaphoresis
Occasional (3%–1%)
Fatigue, flushing, auditory disturbances, thrombophlebitis, skin rash
Rare (less than 1%)
Hives, itching, hallucinations

SERIOUS REACTIONS
• Toxic effects, such as seizures and arrhythmias, of other drugs taken in overdose, especially tricyclic antidepressants, may emerge with reversal of sedative effect of benzodiazepines.

• May provoke panic attack in those with history of panic disorder.

NURSING CONSIDERATIONS

Baseline Assessment
• Obtain arterial blood gasses (ABGs) before and at 30-minute intervals during IV flumazenil administration.
• Prepare to intervene in reestablishing the patient's airway and assisting ventilation because the drug may not fully reverse ventilatory insufficiency induced by benzodiazepines.
• Know that the effects of flumazenil may wear off before the effects of benzodiazepines wear off.

Lifespan Considerations
• Be aware that it is unknown if flumazenil crosses the placenta or is distributed in breast milk. Flumazenil use is not recommended during labor and delivery.
• There are no age-related precautions noted in children.
• In the elderly, benzodiazepine-induced sedation tends to be deeper and more prolonged, requiring careful monitoring.

Precautions
• Use cautiously in patients with alcoholism, drug dependence, head injury, and impaired liver function.

Administration and Handling
• Compatible with D_5W, lactated Ringer's, 0.9% NaCl.
◀ALERT▶ If resedation occurs, repeat dose at 20-min intervals. Maximum: 1 mg, given as 0.2 mg/minute, at any one time, 3 mg in any 1 hour.
IV
• Store parenteral form at room temperature.
• Discard after 24 hours once medication is drawn into syringe, is mixed with any solutions, or if particulate or discoloration is noted.

• Rinse spilled medication from skin with cool water.
• Give over 15 seconds, as prescribed, for reversal of conscious sedation or general anesthesia.
• Give over 30 seconds, as prescribed, for benzodiazepine overdose.
• Administer through freely running IV infusion into large vein because local injection produces pain and inflammation at injection site.

Intervention and Evaluation
• Properly manage the patient's airway, assisted breathing, maintain circulatory access and support, perform internal decontamination by lavage and charcoal, and provide adequate clinical evaluation.
• Monitor the patient for reversal of the benzodiazepine effect.
• Assess the patient for possible hypoventilation, resedation, and respiratory depression.
• Assess the patient closely for return of unconsciousness or narcosis for at least 1 hour after patient is fully alert.

Patient Teaching
• Warn the patient to avoid tasks requiring mental alertness or motor skills until at least 24 hours following discharge.
• Instruct the patient to avoid taking nonprescription drugs until at least 18 to 24 hours after discharge.

fluvoxamine maleate
flew-**vox**-ah-meen
(Faverin[AUS], Luvox)

CATEGORY AND SCHEDULE
Pregnancy Risk Category: C

MECHANISM OF ACTION

An antidepressant, antiobsessional agent that selectively inhibits serotonin neuronal uptake in central nervous system (CNS). *Therapeutic Effect:* Produces antidepressant, antiobsessive effects.

AVAILABILITY

Tablets: 25 mg, 50 mg, 100 mg.

INDICATIONS AND DOSAGES

▶ **Obsessive compulsive disorder (OCD)**

PO

Adults. 50 mg at bedtime; increase by 50 mg q4–7 days. Doses greater than 100 mg/day in 2 divided doses. Maximum: 300 mg/day.

Children 8–17 yrs. 25 mg at bedtime; increase by 25 mg q4–7 days. Doses greater than 50 mg/day in 2 divided doses. Maximum: 200 mg/day.

UNLABELED USES

Treatment of depression

CONTRAINDICATIONS

Within 14 days of MAOI ingestion

INTERACTIONS

Drug

Benzodiazepines, carbamazepine, clozapine, theophylline: May increase the blood concentration and risk of toxicity of benzodiazepines, carbamazepine, clozapine, and theophylline.

Lithium, tryptophan: May enhance serotonergic effects.

MAOIs: May produce serious reactions, including hyperthermia, rigidity, and myoclonus.

Tricyclic antidepressants: May increase fluvoxamine blood concentration.

Warfarin: May increase the effects of warfarin.

Herbal

St. John's wort: May have an additive effect.

Food

None known.

DIAGNOSTIC TEST EFFECTS

None known.

SIDE EFFECTS

Frequent

Nausea (40%), headache, somnolence, insomnia (21%–22%)

Occasional (14%–8%)

Nervousness, dizziness, diarrhea or loose stools, dry mouth, asthenia or loss of strength, weakness, dyspepsia, constipation, abnormal ejaculation

Rare (6%–3%)

Anorexia, anxiety, tremor, vomiting, flatulence, urinary frequency, sexual dysfunction, taste change

SERIOUS REACTIONS

• Overdosage may produce seizures, nausea, vomiting, excessive agitation, and extreme restlessness.

NURSING CONSIDERATIONS

Baseline Assessment

• Plan to perform baseline blood serum chemistry tests to assess liver function.

Precautions

• Use cautiously in elderly patients and patients with impaired liver or renal function.

Administration and Handling

◀ALERT▶ Expect to use lower or less frequent dosing in the elderly and in patients with impaired liver function.

Intervention and Evaluation

• Closely supervise suicidal-risk patients during early therapy. As depression lessens, the patient's

energy level improves, which increases the suicide potential.
• Assess the patient's appearance, behavior, level of interest, mood, and speech pattern.
• Assist the patient with ambulation, if he or she experiences dizziness and somnolence.
• Assess the patient's daily pattern of bowel activity and stool consistency.

Patient Teaching
• Tell the patient that the maximum therapeutic response may require 4 weeks or more to appear.
• Suggest to the patient that taking sips of tepid water and chewing sugarless gum may relieve dry mouth.
• Caution the patient not to abruptly discontinue the medication.
• Warn the patient to avoid tasks that require mental alertness or motor skills until his or her response to the drug is established.

nicotine
nick-oh-teen
(Habitrol Patch, Nicabate[AUS], Nicabate CQ Clear [AUS], Nicoderm CQ Patch, Nicorette DS Gum, Nicorette Inhaler[AUS], Nicorette Plus[CAN], Nicorette Gum, Nicotrol NS, Nicotinell [AUS], Nicotrol Patch)
Do not confuse with Nitroderm.

CATEGORY AND SCHEDULE
Pregnancy Risk Category: C (chewing gum), D (transdermal nicotine)
OTC (Nicoderm transdermal patch, Nicotrol transdermal patch 15 mg/day, chewing gum)

MECHANISM OF ACTION
A cholinergic-receptor agonist that produces autonomic effects by binding to acetylcholine receptors. Produces both stimulating and depressant effects on peripheral and central nervous systems; respiratory stimulant. *Therapeutic Effect:* Low amounts increase heart rate, blood pressure (B/P); high dosages may decrease B/P; may increase motor activity of the gastrointestinal (GI) smooth muscle. Nicotine produces psychological and physical dependence.

PHARMACOKINETICS
Absorption is slow after transdermal administration. Protein binding: 5%. Metabolized in the liver. Excreted primarily in urine. **Half-life:** 4 hrs.

AVAILABILITY
Transdermal patch: 5 mg/day (Nicotrol), 7 mg/day (Nicoderm, OTC), 10 mg/day (Nicotrol), 14 mg/day (Nicoderm, OTC), 15 mg/day (Nicotrol, OTC), 21 mg/day (Nicoderm, OTC).
Chewing gum: 2-mg squares (Nicorette, OTC), 4-mg squares (Nicorette, OTC).
Nasal Spray.
Inhaler (Nicotrol).
Lozenges: 2 mg (Commit), 4 mg (Commit).

INDICATIONS AND DOSAGES
▸ **Smoking deterrent**
PO (lozenge)
Adults, Elderly. 2 mg. Do not use more than 1 lozenge at a time. Maximum: 5/6 hrs, 20/day.
Adults, Elderly who smoke first cigarette within 30 min of waking. 4 mg. Do not use more than 1 lozenge at a time. Maximum: 5 lozenges/6 hrs, 20 lozenges/day.
Week 1–6: one q1–2h
Week 7–9: one q2–4h
Week 10–12: one q4–8h
PO (chewing gum)

Adults, Elderly. Usually,
10–12 pieces/day. Maximum:
30 pieces/day.
Transdermal
*Adults, Elderly who smoke 10 ciga-
rettes or more per day.*
Step One: 21 mg/day for 4–6 wks
Step Two: 14 mg/day for 2 wks.
Step·Three: 7 mg/day for 2 wks.
*Adults, Elderly who smoke less than
10 cigarettes per day.*
Step One: 14 mg/day for 6 wks
Step Two: 7 mg/day for 2 wks
*Initial starting dose for patients
weighing less than 100 lbs, history
of cardiovascular disease.* 14 mg/
day for 4–6 wks, then 7 mg/day for
2–4wks.
Decrease dose in patients taking
more than 600 mg cimetidine
(Tagamet) a day.
Transdermal (Nicotrol)
Adults, Elderly. One patch a day for
6 wks.
Nasal spray
Adults, Elderly. (1 dose = 2 sprays
= 1 mg) 1–2 doses/hr up to
40 doses/day. No more than 5 doses
(10 sprays) per hour.
Inhaler
Adults, Elderly. Puff on nicotine
cartridge mouthpiece for about
20 min as needed.

CONTRAINDICATIONS
During immediate post-myocardial
infarction (MI) period, life-
threatening arrhythmias, severe or
worsening angina

INTERACTIONS
Drug
*Beta-adrenergic blockers, bron-
chodilators, such as theophylline,
insulin, propoxyphene:* Smoking
cessation may increase the effects
of beta-adrenergic blockers, bronchodilators, such as theophylline,
insulin, propoxyphene.

Herbal
None known.
Food
None known.

DIAGNOSTIC TEST EFFECTS
None known.

SIDE EFFECTS
Frequent
Hiccups, nausea
Gum: Mouth or throat soreness,
nausea, hiccups
Transdermal: Erythema, pruritus,
burning at application site
Occasional
Eructation, gastrointestinal (GI)
upset, dry mouth, insomnia, sweat-
ing, irritability
Gum: Hiccups, hoarseness
Inhaler: Mouth or throat irritation,
cough
Rare
Dizziness, muscle or joint pain

SERIOUS REACTIONS
• Overdose produces palpitations,
tachyarrhythmias, convulsions,
depression, confusion, profuse
diaphoresis, hypotension, rapid or
weak pulse, and difficulty breathing.
Lethal dose for adults is 40–60 mg.
Death results from respiratory
paralysis.

NURSING CONSIDERATIONS
Baseline Assessment
• Screen and evaluate patients with
Buerger's disease, coronary heart
disease, including angina pectoris,
and history of MI, Prinzmetal's
variant angina, and serious cardiac
arrhythmias.
• Plan to perform a baseline EKG.
Lifespan Considerations
• Be aware that nicotine passes
freely into breast milk and that the
use of cigarettes or nicotine gum is

associated with a decrease in fetal breathing movements.
• Be aware that nicotine use in children is not recommended.
• In the elderly, age-related decrease in cardiac function may require cautious use.

Precautions
• Use cautiously in patients with eczematous dermatitis, esophagitis, hyperthyroidism, insulin-dependent diabetes mellitus, oral or pharyngeal inflammation, peptic ulcer disease—because it delays healing of ulcers, pheochromocytoma, and severe renal impairment.

Administration and Handling
◄ALERT► Expect to individualize dose, and administer when patient plans to stop smoking.

Transdermal
• Apply promptly upon removal from protective pouch. This wrapping prevents evaporation and loss of nicotine. Use only intact pouch. Do not cut patch.
• Apply only once daily to hairless, clean, dry skin on upper body or outer arm.
• Replace daily at different sites; do not use same site within 7 days; do not use same patch more than 24 hours.
• Wash hands with water alone after applying patch because soap may increase nicotine absorption.
• Discard used patch by folding patch in half with sticky side together, placing in pouch of new patch, and throwing away in such a way as to prevent child or pet accessibility.

Gum
• Do not swallow.
• Chew 1 piece when urge to smoke is present.
• Chew slowly and intermittently for 30 minutes.
• Chew until distinctive, peppery

nicotine taste or slight tingling in mouth is perceived. When tingling is almost gone, after approximately 1 minute, repeat chewing procedure to allow constant slow buccal absorption.
• At too rapid chewing may cause excessive release of nicotine, resulting in adverse effects similar to oversmoking, such as nausea and throat irritation.

Inhaler
• Insert cartridge into mouthpiece.
• Vigorously puff for 20 minutes.

Intervention and Evaluation
• Monitor the patient's application site for burning, erythema, or pruritus if transdermal system is used.
• Obtain baseline vital signs, including blood pressure (B/P) and pulse.
• Assess smoking habits in relation to sleep patterns.

Patient Teaching
• Instruct the patient with the proper application of the nicotine transdermal system. Teach the patient not to cut patches.
• Instruct the patient to chew nicotine gum slowly to avoid jaw ache, nausea, and throat irritation, and to maximize therapeutic benefit.
• Warn the patient to notify the physician if he or she experiences itching or persistent rash during treatment with the transdermal patch.
• Urge the patient not to smoke while wearing nicotine transdermal patches.
• Instruct the patient how to properly dispose used patches.

riluzole
ril-you-zoal
(Rilutek)

CATEGORY AND SCHEDULE
Pregnancy Risk Category: C

MECHANISM OF ACTION

An amyotrophic lateral sclerosis (ALS) agent that inhibits effect on glutamate release, inactivating voltage dependent sodium channels. Interferes with intracellular events that follow transmitter binding at amino acid receptors. *Therapeutic Effect:* Extends survival of ALS patients.

AVAILABILITY

Tablets: 50 mg.

INDICATIONS AND DOSAGES
▸ **ALS**
PO
Adults, Elderly. 50 mg q12h.

CONTRAINDICATIONS

None significant

INTERACTIONS
Drug
Alcohol: May increase central nervous system (CNS) depression.
Amitriptyline, quinolones, theophylline: May increase the effects and risk of toxicity of riluzole.
Omeprazole, rifampin: May decrease the effects of riluzole.
Herbal
None known.
Food
Caffeine: May increase the effects and risk of toxicity of riluzole.
High fat meals: May decrease the absorption and the effects of riluzole.

DIAGNOSTIC TEST EFFECTS

May increase liver function tests.

SIDE EFFECTS

Frequent (greater than 10%)
Nausea, weakness, reduced respiratory function

Occasional (10%–1%)
Edema, tachycardia, headache, dizziness, somnolence, depression, vertigo, tremor, pruritus, alopecia, abdominal pain, diarrhea, anorexia, dyspepsia, vomiting, stomatitis, increased cough

SERIOUS REACTIONS

• None known.

NURSING CONSIDERATIONS
Baseline Assessment
• Assess the patient's baseline blood serum chemisty tests to assess liver function.
Precautions
• Use cautiously in patients with a history or abnormal liver function and impaired renal function.
Administration and Handling
PO
• Remember that the drug is best taken at least 1 hour before or 2 hours after a meal.
Intervention and Evaluation
• Monitor the patient's serum hepatic function enzyme tests.
• Discontinue the drug if alanine aminotransferase (ALT) exceeds 10 times the upper normal limit.
Patient Teaching
• Instruct the patient to take riluzole at least 1 hour before or 2 hours after a meal. Teach the patient to take riluzole at the same times each day.
• Urge the patient to avoid excess alcohol ingestion.
• Tell the patient that riluzole may cause dizziness, somnolence, or vertigo.
• Warn the patient to avoid tasks requiring mental alertness or motor skills until his or her response to the medication is established.
• Caution the patient to notify the physician if he or she experiences any febrile illness.

48 Anticholinergics and Antispasmodics

atropine sulfate
dicyclomine
  hydrochloride
glycopyrrolate
hyoscyamine
scopolamine

Uses: Anticholinergic and antispasmodic agents are used to treat a wide variety of gastrointestinal (GI) conditions that involve bowel irritability and increased tone (spasticity) or motility of the GI tract.

Action: Also known as parasympatholytics, antimuscarinics, and muscarinic blockers, anticholinergics and antispasmodics competitively block the actions of acetylcholine at muscarinic receptors. Through this action, they reduce GI tone and motility and suppress gastric acid secretion.

COMBINATION PRODUCTS

LOMOTIL: atropine sulfate/ diphenoxylate hydrochloride (an antidiarrheal) 0.025 mg/ 2.5 mg.

atropine sulfate
See antiarrhythmic agents

dicyclomine hydrochloride
dye-**sigh**-clo-meen
(Bentyl, Bentylol[CAN], Formulex[CAN], Lomine[CAN],Merbentyl[AUS])
Do not confuse with Aventyl, Benadryl, doxycycline, or dyclonine.

CATEGORY AND SCHEDULE
Pregnancy Risk Category: B

MECHANISM OF ACTION
A gastrointestinal (GI) antispasmodic and anticholinergic agent that directly acts as a relaxant on smooth muscle. *Therapeutic Effect:* Reduces tone, motility of GI tract.

PHARMACOKINETICS

Route	Onset	Peak	Duration
PO	1–2 hrs	N/A	4 hrs

Readily absorbed from GI tract. Widely distributed. Metabolized in liver. **Half-life:** 9–10 hrs.

AVAILABILITY
Capsules: 10 mg.
Tablets: 20 mg.
Syrup: 10 mg/5 ml.
Injection: 10 mg/ml.

INDICATIONS AND DOSAGES
▸ **Functional disturbances of GI motility**
PO
Adults. 10–20 mg 3–4 times/day up to 40 mg 4 times/day.
Children older than 2 yrs. 10 mg 3–4 times/day.
Children 6 mos–2 yrs. 5 mg 3–4 times/day.
Elderly. 10–20 mg 4 times/day. May increase up to 160 mg/day.
IM
Adults. 20 mg q4–6h.

CONTRAINDICATIONS

Bladder neck obstruction due to prostatic hypertrophy, cardiospasm, intestinal atony, myasthenia gravis in those not treated with neostigmine, narrow-angle glaucoma, obstructive disease of GI tract, paralytic ileus, severe ulcerative colitis, tachycardia secondary to cardiac insufficiency or thyrotoxicosis, toxic megacolon, unstable cardiovascular status in acute hemorrhage

INTERACTIONS
Drug

Antacids, antidiarrheals: May decrease the absorption of dicyclomine.
Anticholinergics: May increase the effects of dicyclomine.
Ketoconazole: May decrease the absorption of ketoconazole.
Potassium chloride: May increase the severity of GI lesions with wax matrix formulation of potassium chloride.
Herbal
None known.
Food
None known.

DIAGNOSTIC TEST EFFECTS

None known.

SIDE EFFECTS

Frequent
Dry mouth—sometimes severe, constipation, decreased sweating ability
Occasional
Blurred vision, intolerance to light, urinary hesitancy, drowsiness—with high dosage, agitation, excitement, or drowsiness noted in elderly—even with low dosages
IM: transient lightheadedness, irritation at injection site

Rare
Confusion, hypersensitivity reaction, increased intraocular pressure, nausea, vomiting, unusual tiredness

SERIOUS REACTIONS

• Overdosage may produce temporary paralysis of ciliary muscle, pupillary dilation, tachycardia, palpitation, hot, dry, or flushed skin, absence of bowel sounds, hyperthermia, increased respiratory rate, EKG abnormalities, nausea, vomiting, rash over face or upper trunk, CNS stimulation, and psychosis, marked by agitation, restlessness, rambling speech, visual hallucination, paranoid behavior, and delusions, followed by depression.

NURSING CONSIDERATIONS

Baseline Assessment
• Instruct the patient to void before giving the medication to reduce the risk of urinary retention.
Lifespan Considerations
• Be aware that it is unknown if dicyclomine crosses the placenta or is distributed in breast milk.
• Be aware that infants and young children are more susceptible to the drug's toxic effects.
• Be aware that dicyclomine use in the elderly may cause agitation, confusion, drowsiness, or excitement.
Precautions
• Use extreme caution in patients with autonomic neuropathy, diarrhea, known or suspected GI infections, and mild to moderate ulcerative colitis.
• Use cautiously in patients with chronic obstructive pulmonary disease (COPD), congestive heart failure (CHF), coronary artery disease, esophageal reflux or hiatal hernia associated with reflux esoph-

agitis, gastric ulcer, hyperthyroid-ism, hypertension, liver or renal disease, and tachyarrhythmias.
• Use cautiously in infant and elderly patients.

Administration and Handling
• Store capsules, tablets, syrup, parenteral form at room tempera-ture.

PO
• Dilute oral solution with equal volume of water just before admin-istration.
• May give dicyclomine without regard to meals because food may slightly decrease absorption.

IM
• Injection normally appears color-less.
• Do not administer IV or subcuta-neously.
• Inject IM deep in large muscle mass.
• Do not give for longer than 2 days, as prescribed.

Intervention and Evaluation
• Assess the patient's daily pattern of bowel activity and stool consis-tency.
• Evaluate the patient for urinary retention.
• Monitor changes in the patient's blood pressure (B/P) and body temperature.
• Be alert for fever because it in-creases the risk of hyperthermia.
• Assess the patient's bowel sounds for peristalsis, and mucous mem-branes and skin turgor to evaluate hydration status.
• Encourage adequate fluid intake.

Patient Teaching
• Tell the patient not to become overheated during exercise in hot weather because this may cause heat stroke.
• Urge the patient to avoid hot baths and saunas.
• Warn the patient to avoid tasks

that require mental alertness or motor skills until his or her re-sponse to the drug is established.
• Instruct the patient not to take antacids or antidiarrheals within 1 hour of taking this medication as these drugs decrease dicyclomine's effectiveness.

glycopyrrolate
gly-ko-**pie**-roll-ate
(Robinul, Robinul Forte, Robinul Injection [AUS])

CATEGORY AND SCHEDULE
Pregnancy Risk Category: B

MECHANISM OF ACTION
A quaternary anticholinergic that inhibits action of acetylcholine at postganglionic parasympathetic sites in smooth muscle, secretory glands, and central nervous system (CNS). *Therapeutic Effect:* Reduces saliva-tion and excessive secretions of respiratory tract; reduces gastric secretions, acidity.

AVAILABILITY
Injection: 0.2 mg/ml.

INDICATIONS AND DOSAGES
▸ **Preoperative**
IM
Adults, Elderly. 4.4 mcg/kg 30–60 min before procedure.
Children 2 yrs and older. 4.4 mcg/kg.
Children younger than 2 yrs. 4.4–8.8 mcg/kg.
▸ **Block effects of anticholinester-ase agents**
IV
Adults, Elderly. 0.2 mg for each 1 mg neostigmine or 5 mg pyri-dostigmine.

CONTRAINDICATIONS

Acute hemorrhage, myasthenia gravis, narrow-angle glaucoma, obstructive uropathy, paralytic ileus, tachycardia, ulcerative colitis

INTERACTIONS
Drug

Antacids, antidiarrheals: May decrease the absorption of glycopyrrolate.
Anticholinergics: May increase the effects of glycopyrrolate.
Ketoconazole: May decrease the absorption of ketoconazole.
Potassium chloride: May increase the severity of GI lesions with potassium chloride.
Herbal
None known.
Food
None known.

DIAGNOSTIC TEST EFFECTS

May decrease serum uric acid levels.

IV INCOMPATIBILITIES

None known.

IV COMPATIBILITIES

Diphenhydramine (Benadryl), droperidol (Inapsine), hydromorphone (Dilaudid), hydroxyzine (Vistaril), lidocaine, midazolam (Versed), morphine, promethazine (Phenergan)

SIDE EFFECTS
Frequent
Dry mouth, decreased sweating, constipation
Occasional
Blurred vision, bloated feeling, urinary hesitancy, drowsiness, with high dosage, headache, intolerance to light, loss of taste, nervousness, flushing, insomnia, impotence, mental confusion or excitement, particularly in elderly, children
Parenteral form: temporary light-headedness, local irritation
Rare
Dizziness, faintness

SERIOUS REACTIONS

• Overdosage may produce temporary paralysis of ciliary muscle, pupillary dilation, tachycardia, palpitation, hot, dry, or flushed skin, absence of bowel sounds, hyperthermia, increased respiratory rate, EKG abnormalities, nausea, vomiting, rash over face or upper trunk, CNS stimulation, and psychosis, marked by agitation, restlessness, rambling speech, visual hallucination, paranoid behavior, and delusions, followed by depression.

NURSING CONSIDERATIONS

Baseline Assessment

• Instruct the patient to void before giving the medication to reduce the risk of urinary retention.
• Perform a careful health history that screens for the presence of myasthenia gravis, narrow-angle glaucoma, obstructive uropathy, tachyarrhythmias, and ulcerative colitis.
Precautions
• Use cautiously in patients with congestive heart failure (CHF), diarrhea, fever, gastrointestinal (GI) infections, hyperthyroidism, liver or renal disease, and reflux esophagitis.
Intervention and Evaluation
• Assess the patient's daily pattern of bowel activity and stool consistency.
• Palpate the patient's bladder for signs of urine retention, and monitor his or her urine output.
• Monitor the patient's blood pres-

sure (B/P), body temperature, and heart rate.
• Assess the patient's bowel sounds for peristalsis and mucous membranes and skin turgor to evaluate hydration status.
• Encourage adequate fluid intake.
• Be alert for fever because of an increased risk of hyperthermia.

Patient Teaching
• Inform the patient that glycopyrrolate use may cause dry mouth.
• Instruct the patient to take glycopyrrolate 30 minutes before meals. Explain that food decreases the absorption of glycopyrrolate.
• Instruct the patient not to become overheated during exercise in hot weather as this may result in heat stroke.
• Urge the patient to avoid hot baths and saunas.
• Warn the patient to avoid tasks that require mental alertness or motor skills until his or her response to the drug is established.
• Instruct the patient not to take antacids or antidiarrheals within 1 hour of taking this medication as these drugs decrease glycopyrrolate's effectiveness.

hyoscyamine
high-oh-**sigh**-ah-meen
(Anaspaz, Buscopan[CAN], Cystospaz, Levsin, Levsinex, Nulev)
Do not confuse with Anaprox.

CATEGORY AND SCHEDULE
Pregnancy Risk Category: C

MECHANISM OF ACTION
A gastrointestinal (GI) antispasmodic and anticholinergic agent that inhibits the action of acetylcholine at post-ganglionic (muscarinic) receptor sites. *Therapeutic Effect:* Decreases secretions (bronchial, salivary, sweat glands, gastric juices) and reduces motility of GI and urinary tract.

AVAILABILITY
Tablets: 0.125 mg, 0.15 mg.
Tablets (sublingual): 0.125 mg.
Capsules (time-release): 0.375 mg.
Drops and Oral Solution: 0.125 mg/ml
Elixir: 0.125 mg/5 ml.
Injection: 0.5 mg/ml.

INDICATIONS AND DOSAGES
▸ **GI tract disorders**
IM/Subcutaneous
Adults, Elderly, Children older than 12 yrs. 0.25–0.5 mg q4h for 1–4 doses.
PO/Sublingual
Adults, Elderly, Children older than 12 yrs. 0.125–0.25 mg q4h.
Maximum: 1.5 or 0.375–0.75 mg q12h, time-release capsule.
Children 2-12 yrs. 0.0625–0.125 mg q4h as needed. Maximum: 0.75 mg/ day.
Children younger than 2 yrs. Drops dose q4h, using drop formulation.
▸ **Hypermotility of lower urinary tract**
PO/sublingual
Adults, Elderly. 0.15–0.3 mg 4 times/day or 0.375 mg q12h, time-release capsule.
▸ **Duodenography**
IV
Adults, Elderly. 0.25–0.5 mg 10 min before procedure.
▸ **Preoperative**
IM
Adults, Elderly. 0.5 mg (0.005 mg/ kg) 30–60 min before induction of

anesthesia or administration of preoperative medications.

CONTRAINDICATIONS

GI or genitourinary (GU) obstruction, myasthenia gravis, narrow-angle glaucoma, paralytic ileus, severe ulcerative colitis

INTERACTIONS
Drug

Antacids, antidiarrheals: May decrease the absorption of hyoscyamine.
Anticholinergics: May increase the effects of hyoscyamine.
Ketoconazole: May decrease the absorption of this drug.
Potassium chloride: May increase the severity of GI lesions with this drug.
Herbal
None known.
Food
None known.

DIAGNOSTIC TEST EFFECTS

None known.

SIDE EFFECTS

Frequent
Dry mouth (sometimes severe), decreased sweating, constipation
Occasional
Blurred vision, bloated feeling, urinary hesitancy, drowsiness—with high dosage, headache, intolerance to light, loss of taste, nervousness, flushing, insomnia, impotence, mental confusion or excitement, particularly in elderly, children
Parenteral form: temporary light-headedness, local irritation
Rare
Dizziness, faintness

SERIOUS REACTIONS

• Overdosage may produce temporary paralysis of ciliary muscle, pupillary dilation, tachycardia, palpitations, hot, dry, or flushed skin, absence of bowel sounds, hyperthermia, increased respiratory rate, EKG abnormalities, nausea, vomiting, rash over face or upper trunk, CNS stimulation, and psychosis, marked by agitation, restlessness, rambling speech, visual hallucinations, paranoid behavior, and delusions, followed by depression.

NURSING CONSIDERATIONS

Baseline Assessment
• Instruct the patient to void before giving the medication to reduce the risk of urine retention.
Precautions
• Use cautiously in patients with cardiac arrhythmias, chronic lung disease, congestive heart failure (CHF), hyperthyroidism, neuropathy, and prostatic hypertrophy.
Administration and Handling
PO
• Give hyoscyamine without regard to meals.
• Crush or chew tablets.
• Extended-release capsule should be swallowed whole.
Parenteral
• May give undiluted.
Intervention and Evaluation
• Assess the patient's daily pattern of bowel activity and stool consistency.
• Palpate the patient's bladder for signs of urine retention, and monitor his or her urine output.
• Monitor changes in the patient's blood pressure (B/P) and body temperature.
• Be alert for fever because of an increased risk of hyperthermia.
• Assess the patient's bowel sounds for peristalsis and mucous membranes and skin turgor to evaluate hydration status.

• Encourage adequate fluid intake.

Patient Teaching

• Advise the patient that hyoscyamine may cause dry mouth. Urge the patient to maintain good oral hygiene habits as the lack of saliva may increase risk of cavities.

• Warn the patient to notify the physician if he or she experiences constipation, difficulty urinating, eye pain, or rash.

• Urge the patient to avoid hot baths and saunas.

• Caution the patient to avoid tasks that require mental alertness or motor skills until his or her response to the drug is established.

scopolamine

See antiemetics

bismuth subsalicylate
diphenoxylate
   hydrochloride with
   atropine sulfate
loperamide
   hydrochloride
nitazoxanide

Uses: Antidiarrheals are used to treat acute diarrhea and chronic diarrhea of inflammatory bowel disease. The goal of antidiarrheal therapy is to determine and treat the underlying cause of diarrhea, replenish fluids and electrolytes, relieve gastrointestinal (GI) cramping, and reduce the passage of unformed stools. Some antidiarrheals are also used to reduce fluid from ileostomies.

Action: Systemic and local antidiarrheals act in different ways. *Systemic agents,* such as diphenoxylate, act at receptors in enteric smooth muscles, disrupting peristaltic movements, decreasing GI motility, and decreasing the transit time of intestinal contents. *Local agents,* such as bismuth subsalicylate, adsorb toxic substances and fluids to large surface areas of particles in the preparation. Some of these agents coat and protect irritated intestinal walls. They may also have local anti-inflammatory action. Nitazoxanide interferes with an enzyme-dependent reaction that's essential for anaerobic metabolism in *Cryptosporidium parvum* and *Giardia lamblia,* two organisms responsible for diarrhea.

COMBINATION PRODUCTS

HELIDAC: bismuth/metronidazole (an anti-infective)/tetracycline (an anti-infective) 262 mg/250 mg/ 500 mg.
IMODIUM ADVANCED: loperamide/ simethicone (an antiflatulent) 2 mg/ 125 mg.
LOMOTIL: diphenoxylate/atropine (an anticholinergic and antispasmodic) 2.5 mg/0.025 mg.

bismuth subsalicylate
bis-muth sub-sal-ih-sah-late
(Bismed[CAN], Pepto-Bismol)

CATEGORY AND SCHEDULE
Pregnancy Risk Category: C
OTC

MECHANISM OF ACTION
An antinauseant and antiulcer agent that absorbs water, toxins in large intestine, forms a protective coat in intestinal mucosa. Also possesses antisecretory and antimicrobial effects. *Therapeutic Effect:* Prevents

diarrhea. Helps treat *H. pylori*-associated peptic ulcer disease.

AVAILABILITY
Tablets: 262 mg.
Tablets (chewable): 262 mg, 300 mg.
Suspension: 262 mg/5 ml, 525 mg/5 ml.

INDICATIONS AND DOSAGES
▶ **Diarrhea, gastric distress**
PO
Adults, Elderly. 2 tablets (30 ml) q30–60min up to 8 doses/24 hrs.
Children 9–12 yrs. 1 tablet or 15 ml q30–60min up to 8 doses/24 hrs.
Children 6–8 yrs. Two-thirds of a tablet or 10 ml q30–60min up to 8 doses/24 hrs.
Children 3–5 yrs. One-third of a tablet or 5 ml q30–60min up to 8 doses/24 hrs.
▶ ***H. pylori*–associated duodenal ulcer, gastritis**
PO
Adults, Elderly. 525 mg 4 times/day, with 500 mg amoxicillin and 500 mg metronidazole, 3 times/day after meals, for 7–14 days.

UNLABELED USES
Prevents traveler's diarrhea

CONTRAINDICATIONS
Bleeding ulcers, gout, hemophilia, hemorrhagic states, renal function impairment

INTERACTIONS
Drug
Anticoagulants, heparin, thrombolytics: May increase the risk of bleeding.
Insulin, oral hypoglycemics: Large dose may increase the effects of insulin and oral hypoglycemics.
Other salicylates: May increase the risk of toxicity.

Tetracyclines: May decrease the absorption of tetracyclines.
Herbal
None known.
Food
None known.

DIAGNOSTIC TEST EFFECTS
May alter serum alkaline phosphatase, SGOT (AST), SGPT (ALT), and uric acid levels. May decrease serum potassium levels. May prolong prothrombin time.

SIDE EFFECTS
Frequent
Grayish black stools
Rare
Constipation

SERIOUS REACTIONS
• Debilitated patients and infants may develop impaction.

NURSING CONSIDERATIONS
Baseline Assessment
• Prior to administration, assess the patient's abdomen for signs of tenderness, rigidity, and the presence of bowel sounds.
• Determine when the patient last had a bowel movement, and find out the amount and consistency.
Precautions
• Use cautiously in diabetic and elderly patients.
Intervention and Evaluation
• Encourage the patient to drink and maintain adequate fluid intake.
• Assess the patient's bowel sounds for peristaltic activity.
• Assess the patient's daily pattern of bowel activity and stool consistency.
Patient Teaching
• Explain to the patient that his or her stool may appear black or gray.

- Instruct the patient to chew tablets thoroughly before swallowing.
- Warn the patient to avoid this drug if he or she is taking aspirin or other salicylates, due to an increased risk for toxicity.
- Instruct the patient to ask the physician about taking bismuth if he or she takes anticoagulants because this drug combination can dangerously prolong the bleeding time.

diphenoxylate hydrochloride with atropine sulfate

dye-pen-ox-e-late
(Lofenoxal[aus], Lomotil, Lonox)
Do not confuse with Lamictal, Lanoxin, Loprox, or Lovenox.

CATEGORY AND SCHEDULE
Pregnancy Risk Category: C

MECHANISM OF ACTION
A meperidine derivative that acts locally, centrally, to reduces intestinal motility.

PHARMACOKINETICS
Well absorbed from the gastrointestinal (GI) tract. Metabolized in liver to active metabolite. Primarily eliminated in feces. **Half-life:** 2.5 hrs; metabolite: 12–24 hrs.

AVAILABILITY
Tablets: 2.5 mg.
Liquid: 2.5 mg/5 ml.

INDICATIONS AND DOSAGES
▸ **Antidiarrheal**
PO
Adults, Elderly. Initially, 15–20 mg/ day in 3–4 divided doses, then 5–15 mg/day in 2–3 divided doses.

Children 9–12 yrs. 2 mg 5 times/ day.
Children 6–8 yrs. 2 mg 4 times/day.
Children 2–5 yrs. 2 mg 3 times/day.

CONTRAINDICATIONS
Children younger than 2 yrs, dehydration, jaundice, narrow-angle glaucoma, severe liver disease

INTERACTIONS
Drug
Alcohol, central nervous system (CNS) depressants: May increase the effects of diphenoxylate hydrochloride with atropine sulfate.
Anticholinergics: May increase the effects of atropine.
MAOIs: May precipitate hypertensive crisis.
Herbal
None known.
Food
None known.

DIAGNOSTIC TEST EFFECTS
May increase serum amylase levels.

SIDE EFFECTS
Frequent
Drowsiness, lightheadedness, dizziness, nausea
Occasional
Headache, dry mouth
Rare
Flushing, tachycardia, urinary retention, constipation, paradoxical reaction, marked by restlessness and agitation, blurred vision

SERIOUS REACTIONS
- Dehydration may predispose to toxicity.
- Paralytic ileus, toxic megacolon, marked by constipation, decreased appetite, and stomach pain with nausea or vomiting, occur rarely.
- Severe anticholinergic reaction, manifested by severe lethargy,

hypotonic reflexes, and hyperthermia, may result in severe respiratory depression and coma.

NURSING CONSIDERATIONS

Baseline Assessment
* Check the patient's baseline hydration status. Assess the mucous membranes, skin turgor, and urinary output.
* Perform a baseline abdominal assessment, checking for abdominal tenderness, distension, and guarding, as well as the presence and activity of bowel sounds.

Lifespan Considerations
* Be aware that it is unknown if the drug crosses the placenta or is distributed in breast milk.
* Be aware that this drug is not recommended for use in children because of increased susceptibility to toxicity that can cause respiratory depression.
* Be aware that the elderly are more susceptible to anticholinergic effects, confusion, and respiratory depression.

Precautions
* Use cautiously in patients with acute ulcerative colitis, cirrhosis, liver or renal disease, and renal impairment.

Administration and Handling
PO
* Give without regard to meals. If gastrointestinal (GI) irritation occurs, give with food or meals.
* Administer the liquid form to children 2 to 12 years of age using a graduated dropper for accurate measurement.

Intervention and Evaluation
* Encourage the patient to maintain adequate fluid intake.
* Assess the patient's bowel sounds for peristalsis.

* Assess the patient's daily pattern of bowel activity and stool consistency and record time of evacuation.
* Evaluate the patient for abdominal disturbances.
* Discontinue the medication if the patient experiences abdominal distention.

Patient Teaching
* Warn the patient to avoid tasks that require mental alertness or motor skills until his or her response to the drug is established.
* Urge the patient to avoid alcohol and barbiturates during drug therapy.
* Tell the patient to notify the physician if he or she experiences abdominal distention, fever, palpitations, or persistent diarrhea.

loperamide hydrochloride
low-**pear**-ah-myd
(Apo-Loperamide[CAN], Gastro-Stop[AUS], Imodium A-D, Loperacap[CAN], Novo-Loperamide[CAN])
Do not confuse with Ionamin.

CATEGORY AND SCHEDULE
Pregnancy Risk Category: B
OTC tablets, liquid

MECHANISM OF ACTION
An antidiarrheal that directly affects the intestinal wall muscles. *Therapeutic Effect:* Slows intestinal motility, prolongs transit time of intestinal contents by reducing fecal volume, diminishing loss of fluid and electrolytes, and increasing viscosity and bulk of stool.

PHARMACOKINETICS

Poorly absorbed from the gastrointestinal (GI) tract. Protein binding: 97%. Metabolized in liver. Eliminated in feces, excreted in urine. Not removed by hemodialysis.
Half-life: 9.1–14.4 hrs.

AVAILABILITY

Tablets: 2 mg (OTC).
Capsules: 2 mg.
Liquid: 1 mg/5 ml (OTC).

INDICATIONS AND DOSAGES

▸ **Acute diarrhea (capsules)**
PO
Adults, Elderly. Initially, 4 mg, then 2 mg after each unformed stool. Maximum: 16 mg/day.
Children 9–12 yrs, weighing more than 30 kg. Initially, 2 mg 3 times/day for 24 hrs.
Children 6–8 yrs, weighing 20–30 kg. Initially, 2 mg 2 times/day for 24 hrs.
Children 2–5 yrs, weighing 13–20 kg. Initially, 1 mg 3 times/day for 24 hrs. Maintenance: 1 mg/10 kg only after loose stool.
▸ **Chronic diarrhea**
PO
Adults, Elderly. Initially, 4 mg, then 2 mg after each unformed stool until diarrhea is controlled.
Children. 0.08–0.24 mg/kg/day in 2–3 divided doses. Maximum: 2 mg/dose.
▸ **Traveler's diarrhea**
PO
Adults, Elderly. Initially, 4 mg, then 2 mg after each loose bowel movement (LBM). Maximum: 8 mg/day for 2 days.
Children 9–11 yrs. Initially, 2 mg, then 1 mg after each LBM. Maximum: 6 mg/day for 2 days.
Children 6–8 yrs. Initially, 1 mg, then 1 mg after each LBM. Maximum: 4 mg/day for 2 days.

CONTRAINDICATIONS

Acute ulcerative colitis—may produce toxic megacolon, diarrhea associated with pseudomembranous enterocolitis due to broad-spectrum antibiotics or with organisms that invade intestinal mucosa, such as *Escherichia coli*, shigella, and salmonella, patients who must avoid constipation

INTERACTIONS
Drug
Opioid (narcotic) analgesics: May increase the risk of constipation.
Herbal
None known.
Food
None known.

DIAGNOSTIC TEST EFFECTS

None known.

SIDE EFFECTS
Rare
Dry mouth, drowsiness, abdominal discomfort, allergic reaction, such as rash and itching

SERIOUS REACTIONS

• Toxicity results in constipation, GI irritation, including nausea and vomiting, and central nervous system (CNS) depression. Activated charcoal is the treatment for toxicity.

NURSING CONSIDERATIONS

Baseline Assessment
• Do not administer to the patient in the presence of bloody diarrhea or temperature greater than 101°F.
• Ask the patient if he or she has a history of ulcerative colitis.
• Expect to obtain stool specimens for culture and sensitivity and ova and parasites, if infectious diarrhea is suspected.

Lifespan Considerations
• Be aware that it is unknown if loperamide crosses the placenta or is distributed in breast milk.
• Be aware that loperamide use is not recommended in children younger than 6 years of age, infants under 3 months of age are more susceptible to CNS effects.
• Keep in mind that loperamide use in the elderly may mask dehydration and electrolyte depletion.

Precautions
• Use cautiously in patients with fluid and electrolyte depletion and liver impairment.

Intervention and Evaluation
• Encourage the patient to maintain adequate fluid intake.
• Assess the patient's bowel sounds for peristalsis.
• Assess the patient's daily pattern of bowel activity and stool consistency.
• Withhold the drug and notify the physician promptly in the event the patient experiences abdominal distention, pain, or fever.

Patient Teaching
• Caution the patient not to exceed the prescribed dose.
• Tell the patient that loperamide may cause dry mouth.
• Urge the patient to avoid alcohol during loperamide therapy.
• Instruct the patient to avoid tasks that require mental alertness or motor skills until his or her response to the drug is established.
• Warn the patient to notify the physician if he or she experiences abdominal distention and pain, diarrhea that does not stop within 3 days, or fever.

nitazoxanide
nye-tay-**zocks**-ah-nide
(Alinia)

CATEGORY AND SCHEDULE
Pregnancy Risk Category: B

MECHANISM OF ACTION
An antiparasitic that interferes with the body's reaction to pyruvate ferredoxin oxidoreductase, an enzyme essential for anaerobic energy metabolism. *Therapeutic Effect:* Produces antiprotozoal activity, reducing or terminating diarrheal episodes.

PHARMACOKINETICS
Rapidly hydrolyzed to an active metabolite. Protein binding: 99%. Excreted in the urine, bile, and feces. **Half-life:** 2–4 hrs.

AVAILABILITY
Powder for Oral Suspension: 100 mg/5 ml.

INDICATIONS AND DOSAGES
▶ **Diarrhea**
PO
Children 5–11 yrs. 200 mg (10 ml) q12h for 3 days.
Children 1–4 yrs. 100 mg (5 ml) q12h for 3 days.

CONTRAINDICATIONS
History of sensitivity to aspirin and salicylates

INTERACTIONS
Drug
None known.
Herbal
None known.
Food
None known.

DIAGNOSTIC TEST EFFECTS

May increase serum creatinine and SGPT (ALT) levels.

SIDE EFFECTS

Occasional (8%)
Abdominal pain
Rare (2%–1%)
Diarrhea, vomiting, headache

SERIOUS REACTIONS

• None known.

NURSING CONSIDERATIONS

Baseline Assessment
• Establish the patient's baseline blood glucose and electrolyte levels, blood pressure (B/P), and weight.
• Assess the patient for dehydration.
Lifespan Considerations
• Be aware that it is unknown if nitazoxanide is distributed in breast milk.
• Be aware that the safety and efficacy of nitazoxanide have not been established in children older than 11 years of age.
• Be aware that nitazoxanide is not indicated for use in the elderly.
Precautions
• Use cautiously in patients with biliary or liver disease, gastrointestinal (GI) disorders, and renal impairment.
Administration and Handling
PO
• Store unreconstituted powder at room temperature.

• Reconstitute oral suspension with 48 ml water to provide a concentration of 100 mg/5 ml.
• Shake vigorously to suspend powder.
• Reconstituted solution is stable for 7 days at room temperature.
• Give with food.
Intervention and Evaluation
• Evaluate the diabetic patient's blood glucose levels.
• Assess the patient's electrolyte levels for abnormalities that may have been caused by diarrhea.
• Weigh the patient each day.
• Encourage the patient to maintain adequate fluid intake.
• Assess the patient's bowel sounds for peristalsis.
• Assess the patient's daily pattern of bowel activity and stool consistency.

Patient Teaching
• Tell older children with diabetes mellitus and their parents that the oral suspension of nitazoxanide contains 1.48 grams of sucrose per 5 ml.
• Explain to the patient that nitazoxanide therapy should significantly improve his or her symptoms.
• Instruct the patient and his or her parents to make sure the drug is taken with food.

cimetidine
famotidine
nizatidine
ranitidine, ranitidine bismuth citrate

GASTROINTESTINAL AGENTS

Uses: Histamine (H₂) antagonists are used for short-term treatment of duodenal ulcer and active benign gastric ulcer and for maintenance therapy of duodenal ulcer. They're also used to treat pathologic hypersecretory conditions, such as Zollinger-Ellison syndrome, and gastroesophageal reflux disease (GERD). In addition, these agents are used to prevent upper gastrointestinal bleeding in critically ill patients.

Action: H₂ antagonists inhibit gastric acid secretion by interfering with histamine at H₂ receptors in parietal cells. (See illustration, *Sites of Action: Drugs Used to Treat GERD*, page 932.) They also inhibit acid secretion, which is regulated by the hormone gastrin, whether the secretion is basal (fasting), nocturnal, or stimulated by food or fundic distention. H₂ antagonists decrease the volume and H₂ concentration of gastric juices.

COMBINATION PRODUCTS

PEPCID COMPLETE: famotidine/calcium chloride (an antacid)/magnesium hydroxide (an antacid) 10 mg/800 mg/165 mg.

cimetidine
sih-**met**-ih-deen
(Apo-Cimetidine[CAN], Cimehexal[AUS], Magicul[AUS], Novocimetine[CAN], Peptol[CAN], Sigmetadine[AUS], Tagamet, Tagamet HB)
Do not confuse with simethicone.

CATEGORY AND SCHEDULE
Pregnancy Risk Category: B
OTC Tablets: 100 mg

MECHANISM OF ACTION
An antiulcer and gastric acid secretion inhibitor that inhibits histamine action at H₂ receptor sites of parietal cells. *Therapeutic Effect*: Inhibits gastric acid secretion during fasting, at night, or when stimulated by food, caffeine, or insulin.

PHARMACOKINETICS
Well absorbed from the gastrointestinal (GI) tract. Protein binding: 15%–20%. Widely distributed. Metabolized in liver. Primarily excreted in urine. Not removed by hemodialysis. **Half-life:** 2 hrs, half-life is increased with impaired renal function.

AVAILABILITY
Tablets: 100 mg (OTC), 200 mg, 300 mg, 400 mg, 800 mg.
Oral Liquid: 300 mg/5 ml.
Injection: 300 mg/2 ml.
Suspension: 200 mg/5 ml.

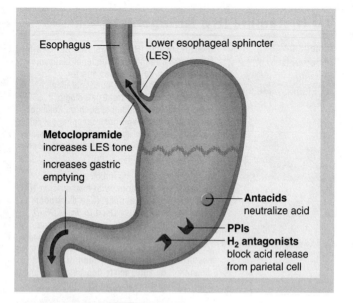

Sites of Action: Drugs Used to Treat GERD

Gastroesophageal reflux disease (GERD) occurs when acidic stomach contents regurgitate into the esophagus, causing heartburn. The disorder may result from a weakness or incompetence of the lower esophageal sphincter (LES). Because the malfunctioning LES makes the reflux leave the esophagus and re-enter the stomach slowly, the esophageal mucosa is exposed to the acid for a long time. Because the enzymatic action of parietal cells in the stomach makes the reflux highly acidic, GERD causes irritation and possible erosion of the esophageal mucosa.

Treatment of GERD can employ drugs from several classes: histamine (H_2) antagonists, proton pump inhibitors (PPIs), the miscellaneous gastrointestinal (GI) agent metoclopramide, and antacids. H_2 antagonists, such as cimetidine, act in parietal cells of the stomach. Normally, H_2-receptor stimulation results in gastric acid secretion. By blocking these receptors, H_2 antagonists decrease the amount and acidity of gastric secretion, including secretion that occurs with fasting, food consumption at night, and stomach distension.

PPIs, such as esomeprazole, also suppress gastric acid secretion. However, they do it by inhibiting the hydrogen-potassium-adenosine triphosphatase (H^+/K^+ ATPase) enzyme system, which is located on the surface of parietal cells and controls their gastric acid secretion. PPIs block acid secretion that results from fasting or stomach distension caused by food ingestion.

Metoclopramide increases the tone and motility of the upper GI tract. It works by stimulating the release of acetylcholine from GI nerve endings, which improves LES tone and leads to decreased reflux. The drug also stimulates gastric emptying, which reduces gastric contents.

Antacids, such as aluminum hydroxide, act primarily in the stomach by chemically combining with the hydrogen ions (H^+) in gastric acid and raising the pH of gastric contents. They don't prevent reflux. However, they make the reflux less acidic, so it causes less damage to the esophageal mucosa.

INDICATIONS AND DOSAGES

▸ **Active ulcer**

IM/IV

Adults, Elderly. 300 mg q6h
or 150 mg as single dose followed by 37.5 mg/hr continuous
infusion.

PO

Adults, Elderly. 300 mg 4 times/day
or 400 mg 2 times/day or 800 mg at
bedtime.

▸ **Prophylaxis duodenal ulcer**

PO

Adults, Elderly. 400–800 mg at
bedtime.

▸ **Gastric hypersecretory
conditions**

IM/IV/PO

Adults, Elderly. 300–600 mg q6h.
Maximum: 2,400 mg/day.

Children. 20–40 mg/kg/day in
divided doses q6h.

Infants. 10–20 mg/kg/day in divided doses q6–12h.

Neonates. 5–10 mg/kg/day in divided doses q8–12h.

▸ **Gastrointestinal reflux disease
(GERD)**

PO

Adults, Elderly. 800 mg 2 times/
day or 400 mg 4 times/day for
12 wks.

▸ **Over-the-counter (OTC) use**

PO

Adults, Elderly. 100 mg up to
30 min before meals. Maximum:
2 doses/day.

▸ **Prevention of upper GI
bleeding**

IV infusion

Adults, Elderly. 50 mg/hr.

▸ **Dosage in renal impairment**

Based on 300-mg dose in
adults.

Creatinine Clearance	Dosage Interval
greater than 40 ml/min	q6h
20–40 ml/min	q8h or decrease dose by 25%
less than 20 ml/min	q12h or decrease dose by 50%

Give after hemodialysis and q12h
between dialysis period

UNLABELED USES

Prophylaxis of aspiration pneumonia, treatment of acute urticaria,
chronic warts, upper GI bleeding

CONTRAINDICATIONS

None known

INTERACTIONS

Drug

Antacids: May decrease the absorption of cimetidine, so do not give
within 30 minutes–1 hr.

*Calcium channel blockers, cyclo-
sporine, lidocaine, metoprolol,
metronidazole, oral anticoagulants,
oral hypoglycemics, phenytoin,
propranolol, theophylline, tricyclic
antidepressants:* May decrease the
metabolism and increase the blood
concentrations of calcium channel
blockers, cyclosporine, lidocaine,
metoprolol, metronidazole, oral
anticoagulants, oral hypoglycemics,
phenytoin, propranolol, theophylline, and tricyclic antidepressants.

Ketoconazole: May decrease the
absorption of ketoconazole, so give
at least 2 hrs after.

Herbal

None known.

Food

None known.

DIAGNOSTIC TEST EFFECTS

Interferes with skin tests using
allergen extracts. May increase

prolactin, serum creatinine, and transaminase levels. May decrease parathyroid hormone concentration.

IV INCOMPATIBILITIES
Allopurinol (Aloprim), amphotericin B complex (AmBisome, Amphotec, Abelcet), cefepime (Maxipime)

IV COMPATIBILITIES
Aminophylline, diltiazem (Cardizem), furosemide (Lasix), heparin, hydromorphone (Dilaudid), insulin (regular), lidocaine, lorazepam (Ativan), midazolam (Versed), morphine, potassium chloride, propofol (Diprivan)

SIDE EFFECTS
Occasional (4%–2%)
Headache
Elderly, severely ill, impaired renal function: Confusion, agitation, psychosis, depression, anxiety, disorientation, hallucinations—effects reverse 3–4 days after discontinuance
Rare (less than 2%)
Diarrhea, dizziness, drowsiness, headache, nausea, vomiting, gynecomastia, rash, impotence

SERIOUS REACTIONS
• Rapid IV may produce cardiac arrhythmias and hypotension.

NURSING CONSIDERATIONS
Baseline Assessment
• Do not administer antacids concurrently. Separate administration of drugs by 1 hour.
Lifespan Considerations
• Be aware that cimetidine crosses the placenta and is distributed in breast milk.
• Be aware that in infants cimetidine use may suppress gastric acidity, inhibit drug metabolism,

and produce central nervous system (CNS) stimulation.
• Be aware that in children long-term use may induce cerebral toxicity and affect hormonal system.
• The elderly are more likely to experience confusion, especially in patients with impaired renal function.
Precautions
• Use cautiously in elderly patients and patients with impaired liver and renal function.
Administration and Handling
PO
• Give cimetidine without regard to meals. Best given with meals and at bedtime.
• Do not administer within 1 hour of antacids.
IM
• Administer undiluted.
• Inject deep into large muscle mass, such as the gluteus maximus muscle.
IV
• Store at room temperature.
• Reconstituted IV is stable for 48 hours at room temperature.
• Dilute each 300 mg (2 ml) with 18 ml 0.9% NaCl, 0.45% NaCl, 0.2% NaCl, D_5W, $D_{10}W$, Ringer's solution, or lactated Ringer's to a total volume of 20 ml.
• For IV push, administer over not less than 2 minutes to prevent arrhythmias and hypotension.
• For intermittent IV (piggyback) administration, infuse over 15 to 20 minutes.
• For IV infusion, dilute with 100 to 1,000 ml 0.9% NaCl, D_5W, or other compatible solution, and infuse over 24 hours.
Intervention and Evaluation
• Monitor the patient's blood pressure (B/P) for hypotension during IV infusion.
• Assess the patient for GI bleeding

manifested as blood in stool and hematemesis.
• Check the mental status in elderly and severely ill patients and patients with impaired renal function.

Patient Teaching
• Warn the patient that IM administration may produce transient discomfort at injection site.
• Instruct the patient not to take antacids within 1 hour of PO cimetidine administration.
• Warn the patient to avoid tasks that require mental alertness or motor skills until his or her response to the drug is established.
• Urge the patient to avoid smoking.
• Caution the patient to notify the physician if he or she experiences any blood in emesis or stool, or dark, tarry stool.

famotidine
fah-mow-**tih**-deen
(Mylanta AR, Novo-Famotidine[CAN] Pepcid, Pepcid AC, Pepcidine[AUS], Pepcid RPD, Ulcidine[CAN])

CATEGORY AND SCHEDULE
Pregnancy Risk Category: B
OTC Tablet, 10 mg

MECHANISM OF ACTION
An antiulcer and gastric acid secretion inhibitor that inhibits histamine action at H$_2$ receptors of parietal cells. *Therapeutic Effect:* Inhibits gastric acid secretion when fasting, at night, or when stimulated by food, caffeine, or insulin.

PHARMACOKINETICS

Route	Onset	Peak	Duration
PO	1 hr	1–4 hrs	10–12 hrs
IV	1 hr	0.5–3 hrs	10–12 hrs

Rapidly, incompletely absorbed from the gastrointestinal (GI) tract. Protein binding: 15%–20%. Partially metabolized in liver. Primarily excreted in urine. Not removed by hemodialysis. **Half-life:** 2.5–3.5 hrs (half-life is increased with impaired renal function).

AVAILABILITY
Tablets: 10 mg (OTC), 20 mg, 40 mg.
Tablet (chewable): 10 mg.
Powder for oral suspension: 40 mg/5 ml.
Injection: 10 mg/ml, 20 mg/50 ml NaCl infusion.

INDICATIONS AND DOSAGES
▶ **Acute therapy—duodenal ulcer**
PO
Adults, Elderly. 40 mg at bedtime or 20 mg q12h. Maintenance: 20 mg at bedtime.
Children 1–16 yrs. 0.5 mg/kg/day. Maximum: 40 mg.
▶ **Acute therapy—benign gastric ulcer**
PO
Adults, Elderly. 40 mg at bedtime.
▶ **Gastroesophageal reflux disease (GERD)**
PO
Adults, Elderly. 20 mg 2 times/day up to 6 wks; 20–40 mg 2 times/day up to 12 wks in patients with esophagitis, including erosions and ulcerations.
Children 1–16 yrs. 1 mg/kg/day in 2 divided doses. Maximum: 80 mg/day.

▸ **Pathologic hypersecretory conditions**
PO
Adults, Elderly. Initially, 20 mg q6h up to 160 mg q6h.
▸ **Acid indigestion, heartburn, sour stomach**
PO
Adults, Elderly. 10 mg 15–60 min before eating. Maximum: 2 tablets/day.
▸ **Usual Parenteral Dosage**
IV
Adults, Elderly. 20 mg q12h.
Children. 0.25 mg/kg q12h.
Maximum: 40 mg/day.
▸ **Dosage in renal impairment**

Creatinine Clearance	Dosing Frequency
10–50 ml/min	q24h
less than 10 ml/min	q36–48h

UNLABELED USES
Autism, prophylaxis for aspiration pneumonitis

CONTRAINDICATIONS
None known

INTERACTIONS
Drug
Antacids: May decrease the absorption of famotidine; do not give within 30 minutes to 1 hr.
Ketoconazole: May decrease the absorption of ketoconazole, give at least 2 hrs after.
Herbal
None known.
Food
None known.

DIAGNOSTIC TEST EFFECTS
Interferes with skin tests using allergen extracts. May increase liver enzymes.

IV INCOMPATIBILITIES
Amphotericin B complex (Abelcet, Amphotec, AmBisome), cefepime (Maxipime), furosemide (Lasix), piperacillin/tazobactam (Zosyn)

IV COMPATIBILITIES
Calcium gluconate, dobutamine (Dobutrex), dopamine (Intropin), heparin, hydromorphone (Dilaudid), insulin (regular), lidocaine, lorazepam (Ativan), magnesium sulfate, midazolam (Versed), morphine, nitroglycerin, norepinephrine (Levophed), potassium chloride, potassium phosphate, propofol (Diprivan)

SIDE EFFECTS
Occasional (5%)
Headache
Rare (2% or less)
Constipation, diarrhea, dizziness

SERIOUS REACTIONS
• None known.

NURSING CONSIDERATIONS
Baseline Assessment
• Do not administer antacids concurrently. Separate administration of drugs by 30 minutes to 1 hour.
Lifespan Considerations
• Be aware that it is unknown if famotidine crosses the placenta or is distributed in breast milk.
• There are no age-related precautions noted in children.
• Be aware that the elderly are more likely to experience confusion, especially patients with impaired liver or renal function.
Precautions
• Use cautiously in patients with impaired liver or renal function.

Administration and Handling
PO
• Store tablets, suspension at room temperature.
• After reconstitution, oral suspension is stable for 30 days at room temperature.
• Give famotidine without regard to meals. Keep in mind that it's best given after meals or at bedtime.
• Shake suspension well before use.
• Pepcid RPD dissolves under tongue; does not require water for dosing.
IV
• Refrigerate unreconstituted vials.
• IV solution normally appears clear, colorless.
• After dilution, IV solution is stable for 48 hours at room temperature.
• For IV push, dilute 20 mg with 5 to 10 ml 0.9% NaCl, D_5W, $D_{10}W$, lactated Ringer's, or 5% sodium bicarbonate.
• For intermittent IV piggyback infusion, dilute with 50 to 100 ml D_5W, or 0.9% NaCl.
• IV push given over at least 2 minutes.
• Infuse piggyback over 15 to 30 minutes.

Intervention and Evaluation
• Monitor the patient's daily pattern of bowel activity and stool consistency.
• Assess the patient for constipation, diarrhea, and headache.

Patient Teaching
• Tell the patient that he or she may take famotidine without regard to meals or antacids.
• Warn the patient to notify the physician if he or she experiences headache.
• Urge the patient to avoid consuming excessive amounts of aspirin and coffee.
• Instruct the patient to contact the physician if he or she experiences persistent acid indigestion, heartburn, or sour stomach despite the medication.

nizatidine
nye-**zah**-tih-deen
(Axid, Axid AR, Tazac[AUS])

CATEGORY AND SCHEDULE
Pregnancy Risk Category: B
OTC (Capsules, 75 mg)

MECHANISM OF ACTION
An antiulcer and gastric acid secretion inhibitor that inhibits histamine action at H_2 receptors of parietal cells. *Therapeutic Effect:* Inhibits basal and nocturnal gastric acid secretion.

PHARMACOKINETICS
Rapidly, well absorbed from the gastrointestinal (GI) tract. Protein binding: 35%. Metabolized in liver. Primarily excreted in urine. Not removed by hemodialysis. **Half-life:** 1–2 hrs, half-life is increased with impaired renal function.

AVAILABILITY
Capsules: 75 mg (OTC), 150 mg, 300 mg.

INDICATIONS AND DOSAGES
▶ **Active duodenal ulcer**
PO
Adults, Elderly. 300 mg at bedtime or 150 mg 2 times/day.
▶ **Maintenance of healed ulcer**
PO
Adults, Elderly. 150 mg at bedtime.
▶ **Gastroesophageal reflux disease (GERD)**
PO
Adults, Elderly. 150 mg 2 times/day.

▸ **Active benign gastric ulcer**
PO
Adults, Elderly. 150 mg 2 times/day
or 300 mg at bedtime.
▸ **Dyspepsia, OTC**
PO
Adults, Elderly. 75 mg 30–60 min
before meals; no more than 2 tab-
lets/day.
▸ **Dosage in renal impairment**

Creatinine Clearance	Active Ulcer	Maintenance Therapy
20–50 ml/min	150 mg at bedtime	150 mg every other day
less than 20 ml/min	150 mg every other day	150 mg q3 days

UNLABELED USES
To decrease weight gain in patients
taking Zyprexa, treatment of gastric
hypersecretory conditions, multiple
endocrine adenoma, Zollinger-
Ellison syndrome

CONTRAINDICATIONS
None known

INTERACTIONS
Drug
Antacids: May decrease the absorp-
tion of nizatidine, do not give
within 1 hr.
Ketoconazole: May decrease the
absorption of ketoconazole, give at
least 2 hrs after.
Herbal
None known.
Food
None known.

DIAGNOSTIC TEST EFFECTS
Interferes with skin tests using
allergen extracts. May increase
serum alkaline phosphatase, SGOT
(AST), and SGPT (ALT) levels.

SIDE EFFECTS
Occasional (2%)
Somnolence, fatigue
Rare (less than 1%)
Sweating, rash

SERIOUS REACTIONS
• Asymptomatic ventricular tachycardia, hyperuricemia, not associated with gout, and nephrolithiasis
occur rarely.

NURSING CONSIDERATIONS
Baseline Assessment
• Expect to obtain baseline blood
chemistry lab tests, including BUN,
serum alkaline phosphatase, bilirubin, creatinine, SGOT (AST), and
SGPT (ALT) levels to assess liver
and renal function.
Lifespan Considerations
• Be aware that it is unknown if
nizatidine crosses the placenta or is
distributed in breast milk.
• Be aware that the safety and
efficacy of nizatidine have not been
established in children younger than
16 years of age.
• There are no age-related precautions noted in the elderly.
Precautions
• Use cautiously in patients with
liver or renal impairment.
Administration and Handling
PO
• Give nizatidine without regard to
meals. Best given after meals or at
bedtime.
• Do not administer within 1 hour of
magnesium-or aluminum-containing
antacids because it can decrease the
absorption of nizatidine.
• Give right before eating for heartburn prevention.

Intervention and Evaluation
• Assess the patient for abdominal pain and GI bleeding. Observe the patient for overt blood in emesis or stool and tarry stools.
• Monitor the patient's blood tests for elevated serum alkaline phosphatase, bilirubin, SGOT (AST), and SGPT (ALT) levels.

Patient Teaching
• Warn the patient to avoid tasks that require mental alertness or motor skills until his or her response to the drug is established.
• Urge the patient to avoid alcohol, aspirin, and smoking during nizatidine therapy.
• Instruct the patient to notify the physician if he or she experiences acid indigestion, gastric distress, or heartburn after 2 weeks of continuous use of nizatidine.

---

ranitidine
rah-**nih**-tih-deen
(Apo-Ranitidine[CAN], Novo-Ranidine[CAN], Zantac, Zantac-75, Zantac EFFERdose)
Do not confuse with Xanax, Ziac, or Zyrtec.

ranitidine bismuth citrate
(Tritec)

CATEGORY AND SCHEDULE
Pregnancy Risk Category: B
OTC (Tablets, 75 mg)

MECHANISM OF ACTION
An antiulcer agent that inhibits histamine action at H$_2$ receptors of gastric parietal cells. *Therapeutic Effect:* Inhibits gastric acid secretion when fasting, at night, or when stimulated by food, caffeine, or insulin. Reduces volume, hydrogen ion concentration of gastric juice.

PHARMACOKINETICS
Rapidly absorbed from the gastrointestinal (GI) tract. Protein binding: 15%. Widely distributed. Metabolized in liver. Primarily excreted in urine. Not removed by hemodialysis. **Half-life:** PO: 2.5 hrs; IV: 2–2.5 hrs (half-life is increased with impaired renal function).

AVAILABILITY
Tablets: 75 mg (OTC), 150 mg, 300 mg, 400 mg (bismuth citrate).
Tablets (effervescent): 150 mg.
Capsules: 150 mg, 300 mg.
Syrup: 15 mg/ml.
Granules (effervescent): 150 mg.
Injection (vial): 25 mg/ml.
Injection (infusion premix): 0.5 mg/ml, 50 ml infusion.

INDICATIONS AND DOSAGES
▸ **Duodenal, gastric ulcers, gastroesophageal reflux disease (GERD)**
PO
Adults, Elderly. 150 mg 2 times/day or 300 mg at qhs. Maintenance: 150 mg at bedtime.
Children. 2–4 mg/kg/day in divided doses 2 times/day. Maximum: 300 mg/day.
▸ **Erosive esophagitis**
PO
Adults, Elderly. 150 mg 4 times/day. Maintenance: 150 mg 2 times/day or 300 mg at bedtime.
Children. 4–10 mg/kg/day in 2 divided doses. Maximum: 600 mg/day.
▸ **Hypersecretory conditions**
PO
Adults, Elderly. 150 mg 2 times/day. May increase up to 6 g/day.
▸ **Usual parenteral dosage**
IV/IM
Adults, Elderly. 50 mg/dose q6-8h. Maximum: 400 mg/day.

Children. 2–4 mg/kg/day in divided doses q6-8h. Maximum: 200 mg/day.

▸ **Usual neonatal dosage**
IV
Neonates. Initially, 1.5 mg/kg/dose, then 1.5–2 mg/kg/day in divided doses q12h.
PO
Neonates. 2 mg/kg/day in divided doses q12h.

▸ **Dosage in renal impairment creatinine clearance less than 50 ml/min**
PO
• 150 mg q24h.
IM/IV
• 50 mg q18–24h.

UNLABELED USES
Prophylaxis of aspiration pneumonia

CONTRAINDICATIONS
History of acute porphyria

INTERACTIONS
Drug
Antacids: May decrease the absorption of ranitidine, therefore do not give within 1 hr.
Ketoconazole: May decrease the absorption of ketoconazole, therefore give at least 2 hrs after.
Herbal
None known.
Food
None known.

DIAGNOSTIC TEST EFFECTS
Interferes with skin tests using allergen extracts. May increase liver function enzymes, gamma-glutamyl transpeptidase, and serum creatinine levels.

IV INCOMPATIBILITIES
Amphotericin B complex (Abelcet, AmBisome, Amphotec)

IV COMPATIBILITIES
Diltiazem (Cardizem), dobutamine (Dobutrex), dopamine (Intropin), heparin, hydromorphone (Dilaudid), insulin, lidocaine, lorazepam (Ativan), morphine, norepinephrine (Levophed), potassium chloride, propofol (Diprivan)

SIDE EFFECTS
Occasional (2%)
Diarrhea
Rare (1%)
Constipation, headache (may be severe)

SERIOUS REACTIONS
• Reversible hepatitis and blood dyscrasias occur rarely.

NURSING CONSIDERATIONS
Baseline Assessment
• Expect to obtain baseline blood chemistry tests including BUN, serum alkaline phosphatase, bilirubin, creatinine, SGOT (AST), and SGPT (ALT) levels to assess liver and renal function.
Lifespan Considerations
• Be aware that it is unknown if ranitidine crosses the placenta or is distributed in breast milk.
• There are no age-related precautions noted in children.
• Be aware that the elderly are more likely to experience confusion, especially in patients with liver or renal impairment.
Precautions
• Use cautiously in elderly patients and patients with impaired liver and renal function.
Administration and Handling
PO
• Give ranitidine without regard to meals. Best given after meals or at bedtime.
• Do not administer within 1 hour

of magnesium- or aluminum-containing antacids because they decrease ranitidine absorption by 33%.

IM

• May be given undiluted.
• Give deep IM into large muscle mass, such as the gluteus maximus.

IV

• IV solutions normally appear clear, colorless to yellow, slight darkening does not affect potency.
• IV infusion (piggyback) is stable for 48 hours at room temperature. Discard if discolored or precipitate forms.
• For IV push, dilute each 50 mg with 20 ml 0.9% NaCl or D_5W.
• For intermittent IV infusion (piggyback), dilute each 50 mg with 50 ml 0.9% NaCl or D_5W.
• For IV infusion, dilute with 250 to 1,000 ml 0.9% NaCl or D_5W.
• Administer IV push over minimum of 5 minutes to prevent arrhythmias and hypotension.

• Infuse IV piggyback over 15 to 20 minutes.
• Infuse IV infusion over 24 hours.

Intervention and Evaluation

• Monitor the patient's serum alkaline phosphatase, bilirubin, SGOT (AST), and SGPT (ALT) levels.
• Assess the elderly patient's mental status.

Patient Teaching

• Tell the patient that smoking decreases the effectiveness of ranitidine.
• Instruct the patient not to take ranitidine within 1 hour of magnesium- or aluminum-containing antacids.
• Warn the patient that transient burning or itching may occur with IV administration.
• Instruct the patient to notify the physician if he or she experiences headache during ranitidine therapy.
• Urge the patient to avoid alcohol and aspirin during ranitidine therapy.

bisacodyl
cascara sagrada
docusate, docusate
   sodium
lactulose
magnesium citrate,
   magnesium
   hydroxide
methylcellulose
polycarbophil
polyethylene glycol-
   electrolyte solution
   (PEG-ES)
psyllium
senna

Uses: Laxatives are used for short-term treatment of constipation and for colon evacuation before rectal or bowel examinations. They're also used to prevent straining, such as after anorectal surgery or myocardial infarction; to prevent fecal impaction; and to reduce painful elimination, such as in patients with recent episiotomy, hemorrhoids, or anorectal lesions. In addition, these agents are helpful in modifying ileostomy effluent and in removing ingested poisons.

Action: Laxatives ease or stimulate defecation by three basic mechanisms. They attract and retain fluid in the colonic contents through their hydrophilic or osmotic properties. They act directly or indirectly on the mucosa to decrease water and sodium absorption. Or they increase intestinal motility and decrease water and sodium absorption. (See illustration, *Mechanisms of Action: Laxatives,* page 944.)
—*Bulk-forming laxatives,* such as psyllium and polycarbophil, act primarily in the small and large intestines. They retain water in stool and may bind with water and ions in the colonic lumen to soften feces and increase stool bulk. They may also increase colonic bacteria growth, which increases fecal mass. Typically, they produce soft stool in 1 to 3 days.
—*Osmotic laxatives,* including lactulose, act in the colon like saline laxatives. Their osmotic action may be enhanced in the distal ileum and colon by bacterial metabolism to lactate and other organic acids. This decreases the pH and increases the osmotic pressure, which in turn increases the stool water content and softens the stool. They produce soft stool in 1 to 3 days.
—*Stimulant laxatives,* such as bisacodyl and senna, act in the colon. They enhance water and electrolyte accumulation in the colonic lumen, which enhances intestinal motility, and may also act directly on the intestinal mucosa. Most of them produce semifluid stool in 6 to 12 hours. However, bisacodyl suppositories act in 15 to 60 minutes.

—*Surfactant laxatives,* such as docusate, act in the small and large intestines. By their surfactant action, they hydrate and soften stool, helping fat and water penetrate it. They produce soft stool in 1 to 3 days.

COMBINATION PRODUCTS

FERRO-SEQUELS: docusate/ferrous fumarate (a hematinic) 100 mg/150 mg.

GELUSIL: magnesium hydroxide/aluminum hydroxide (an antacid)/simethicone (an antiflatulent) 200 mg/200 mg/25 mg.

GENTLAX-S: senna/docusate (a laxative) 8.6 mg/50 mg.

HALEY'S M-O: magnesium/mineral oil (a lubricant laxative) 300 mg/1.25 ml.

PEPCID COMPLETE: magnesium hydroxide/famotidine (a histamine [H$_2$] antagonist)/calcium chloride (an antacid) 165 mg/10 mg/800 mg.

SENOKOT-S: senna/docusate (a laxative) 8.6 mg/50 mg.

bisacodyl

bise-ah-**co**-dahl
(Apo-Bisacodyl[CAN], Bisalax[AUS], Dulcolax)

CATEGORY AND SCHEDULE

Pregnancy Risk Category: C
OTC

MECHANISM OF ACTION

A gastrointestinal (GI) stimulant that has a direct effect on colonic smooth musculature by stimulating the intramural nerve plexi. *Therapeutic Effect:* Promotes fluid and ion accumulation in colon to increase peristalsis, promote a laxative effect.

PHARMACOKINETICS

Route	Onset	Peak	Duration
PO	6–12 hrs	N/A	N/A
Rectal	15–60 min	N/A	N/A

Minimal absorption following PO, rectal administration. Absorbed drug excreted in urine; remainder eliminated in feces.

AVAILABILITY

Tablets (enteric-coated): 5 mg.
Suppository: 10 mg.

INDICATIONS AND DOSAGES

▶ **Laxative**
PO
Adults. 5–15 mg as needed.
Children 3–12 yrs. 5–10 mg or 0.3 mg/kg at bedtime or after breakfast.
Elderly. Initially, 5 mg/day.
Rectal
Adults, Children 12 yrs and older. 10 mg to induce bowel movement.
Children 2–11 yrs. 5–10 mg as a single dose.
Children younger than 2 yrs. 5 mg.
Elderly. 5–10 mg/day.

CONTRAINDICATIONS

Abdominal pain, appendicitis, intestinal obstruction, nausea, undiagnosed rectal bleeding, vomiting

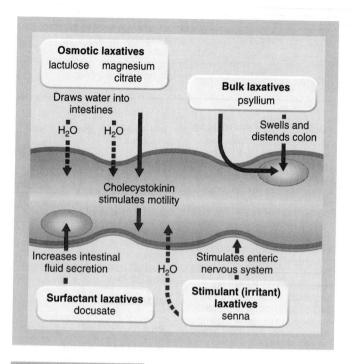

Laxatives ease or stimulate defecation. Typically, they're classified by their mechanism of action as bulk-forming, osmotic, stimulant, or surfactant laxatives.

Bulk-forming laxatives, such as psyllium, act in the small and large bowel. Because ingredients in these laxatives are undigestible, they remain within the stool and increase the fecal mass by drawing in water. These agents also enhance bacterial growth in the colon, further adding to the fecal mass.

Osmotic laxatives, such as lactulose, draw water into the intestinal lumen, causing the fecal mass to soften and swell. This osmotic action may be enhanced by the metabolism of colonic bacteria to lactate and other organic acids. These acids decrease colonic pH and increase colonic motility.

Stimulant (or irritant) laxatives, such as senna, act on the intestinal wall to increase water and electrolytes in the intestinal lumen. In addition, they directly irritate the colon, increasing motility.

Surfactant laxatives (or fecal softeners), such as docusate, reduce the surface tension of the stool, allowing water to enter it. These laxatives may also help to increase water and electrolyte excretion into the intestinal lumen, softening and increasing the fecal mass.

INTERACTIONS
Drug
Antacids, cimetidine, famotidine, ranitidine: May cause rapid dissolution of bisacodyl, producing abdominal cramping, and vomiting.
PO medications: May decrease transit time of concurrently administered PO medications, decreasing absorption of bisacodyl.
Herbal
None known.
Food
Milk: May cause rapid dissolution of bisacodyl.

DIAGNOSTIC TEST EFFECTS
None known

SIDE EFFECTS
Frequent
Some degree of abdominal discomfort, nausea, mild cramps, faintness
Occasional
Rectal administration may produce burning of rectal mucosa, mild proctitis

SERIOUS REACTIONS
• Long-term use may result in laxative dependence, chronic constipation, and loss of normal bowel function.
• Chronic use or overdosage may result in electrolyte or metabolic disturbances, such as hypokalemia, hypocalcemia, metabolic acidosis, or alkalosis, as well as persistent diarrhea, malabsorption, and weight loss. Electrolyte and metabolic disturbance may produce vomiting and muscle weakness.

NURSING CONSIDERATIONS

Baseline Assessment
• Prior to administration, assess the patient's abdomen for signs of tenderness, rigidity, and the presence of bowel sounds.
• Try to determine when the patient last had a bowel movement, and find out the amount and consistency.
Lifespan Considerations
• Be aware that it is unknown if bisacodyl crosses the placenta or is distributed in breast milk.
• Avoid bisacodyl use in children younger than 6 years of age as this patient population is usually unable to describe symptoms or more severe side effects.
• Be aware that the repeated use of bisacodyl in the elderly may cause orthostatic hypotension and weakness due to electrolyte loss.
Precautions
• Know that excessive use may lead to fluid and electrolyte imbalance.
Administration and Handling
PO
• Give bisacodyl on an empty stomach for faster action.
• Offer 6 to 8 glasses of water a day to aid in stool softening.
• Administer tablets whole; do not chew or crush.
• Avoid giving within 1 hour of antacids, milk, or other oral medications.
Rectal
• If suppository is too soft, chill for 30 minutes in refrigerator or run cold water over foil wrapper.
• Moisten suppository with cold water before inserting well into rectum.
Intervention and Evaluation
• Encourage the patient to maintain adequate fluid intake.
• Assess the patient's bowel sounds for peristalsis.
• Assess the patient's daily pattern of daily bowel activity and stool

consistency and record time of evacuation.
• Assess the patient for abdominal disturbances.
• Monitor the serum electrolytes in patients exposed to excessive, frequent, or prolonged use of bisacodyl.

Patient Teaching
• Tell the patient to institute measures to promote defecation such as increasing his or her fluid intake, exercising, and eating a high-fiber diet.
• Instruct the patient not to take antacids, milk, or other medications within 1 hour of taking bisacodyl as these substances may decrease the effectiveness of bisacodyl.
• Warn the patient to notify the physician if he or she experiences unrelieved constipation, dizziness, muscle cramps or pain, rectal bleeding, and weakness.

cascara sagrada
cass-**care**-ah sah-**graud**-ah
(Cascara Sagrada)

CATEGORY AND SCHEDULE
Pregnancy Risk Category: C

MECHANISM OF ACTION
A gastrointestinal (GI) stimulant that increases peristalsis by direct effect on colonic smooth musculature, by stimulating intramural nerve plexi. *Therapeutic Effect:* Promotes fluid and ion accumulation in colon to promote a laxative effect.

AVAILABILITY
Tablets: 325 mg.
Liquid: (18% alcohol).

INDICATIONS AND DOSAGES
▸ **Laxative**
PO
Adults, Elderly. 1 tablet or 5 ml at bedtime.
Children 2-11 yrs. 2.5 ml, 1–3 ml as a single dose.
Infants. 1.25 ml, 0.5–2 ml as a single dose.

CONTRAINDICATIONS
Abdominal pain, appendicitis, intestinal obstruction, nausea, vomiting

INTERACTIONS
Drug
PO medications: May decrease transit time of concurrently administered oral medication, decreasing the absorption of cascara sagrada.
Herbal
None known.
Food
None known.

DIAGNOSTIC TEST EFFECTS
May increase blood glucose levels. May decrease serum calcium and potassium levels.

SIDE EFFECTS
Frequent
Pink-red, red-violet, red-brown, or yellow-brown discoloration of urine
Occasional
Some degree of abdominal discomfort, nausea, mild cramps, faintness

SERIOUS REACTIONS
• Long-term use may result in laxative dependence, chronic constipation, and loss of normal bowel function.
• Chronic use or overdosage may result in electrolyte disturbances,

such as hypokalemia, hypocalcemia, metabolic acidosis or alkalosis, persistent diarrhea, malabsorption, and weight loss. Electrolyte disturbance may produce vomiting and muscle weakness.

NURSING CONSIDERATIONS

Baseline Assessment
• Prior to administration, assess the patient's abdomen for signs of tenderness, rigidity, and the presence of bowel sounds.
• Try to determine when the patient last had a bowel movement, and find out the amount and consistency.

Intervention and Evaluation
• Encourage the patient to maintain adequate fluid intake.
• Assess the patient's bowel sounds for peristalsis.
• Assess the patient's daily pattern of daily bowel activity and stool consistency and record time of evacuation.
• Assess the patient for abdominal disturbances.
• Monitor the serum electrolytes in patients exposed to excessive, frequent, or prolonged use of cascara sagrada.

Patient Teaching
• Explain to the patient that his or her urine may temporarily turn pink-red, red-violet, red-brown, or yellow-brown.
• Tell the patient to institute measures to promote defecation such as increasing his or her fluid intake, exercising, and eating a high-fiber diet.
• Instruct the patient not to take other oral medications within 1 hour of taking cascara sagrada as these substances may decrease the effectiveness of cascara sagrada because of increased peristalsis.

• Warn the patient not to use cascara sagrada if he or she experiences abdominal pain, nausea, or vomiting longer than 1 week.
• Tell the patient that the liquid form contains alcohol.

docusate
dock-cue-sate
(Coloxyl[AUS], Pro-Cal-Sof, Surfak)

docusate sodium
(Colace, Diocto, Selax[CAN], SoFlax[CAN], Surfak)

CATEGORY AND SCHEDULE
Pregnancy Risk Category: C
OTC

MECHANISM OF ACTION
A bulk-producing laxative that decreases surface film tension by mixing liquid and bowel docusate contents. *Therapeutic Effect:* Increases infiltration of liquid to form a softer stool.

PHARMACOKINETICS
Minimal absorption from the gastrointestinal (GI) tract. Acts in small and large intestines. Results occur 1–2 days after first dose, may take 3–5 days.

AVAILABILITY
Capsules: 50 mg (sodium), 100 mg (sodium), 240 mg (calcium), 250 mg (sodium).
Tablets: 100 mg (sodium).
Syrup: 50 mg/15 ml (sodium), 60 mg/15 ml (sodium).
Liquid: 150 mg/15 ml (sodium).
Solution: 50 mg/ml (sodium).
Elixir: 60 mg/15 ml (sodium).

INDICATIONS AND DOSAGES
▶ **Stool softener**
PO
Adults, Elderly, Children older than 12 yrs. 50–500 mg/day in 1–4 divided doses.
Children 6–12 yrs. 40–150 mg/day in 1–4 divided doses.
Children 3–5 yrs. 20–60 mg/day in 1–4 divided doses.
Children younger than 3 yrs. 10–40 mg in 1–4 divided doses.

CONTRAINDICATIONS
Acute abdominal pain, concomitant use of mineral oil, intestinal obstruction, nausea, vomiting

INTERACTIONS
Drug
Danthron, mineral oil: May increase the absorption of danthron or mineral oil.
Herbal
None known.
Food
None known.

DIAGNOSTIC TEST EFFECTS
None known.

SIDE EFFECTS
Occasional
Mild GI cramping, throat irritation with liquid preparation
Rare
Rash

SERIOUS REACTIONS
• None known.

NURSING CONSIDERATIONS

Baseline Assessment
• Prior to administration, assess the patient's abdomen for signs of tenderness, rigidity, and the presence of bowel sounds.
• Try to determine when the patient last had a bowel movement, and find out the amount and consistency.

Lifespan Considerations
• Be aware that it is unknown if docusate is distributed in breast milk.
• Be aware that docusate use is not recommended in children younger than 6 years of age.
• There are no age-related precautions noted in the elderly.

Administration and Handling
• Drink 6 to 8 glasses of water a day to aid in stool softening.
• Give each dose with full glass of water or fruit juice.
• Administer docusate liquid with infant formula, fruit juice, or milk to mask the bitter taste.

Intervention and Evaluation
• Encourage the patient to maintain adequate fluid intake.
• Assess the patient's bowel sounds for peristalsis.
• Assess the patient's daily pattern of daily bowel activity and stool consistency and record time of evacuation.
• Assess the patient for abdominal disturbances.

Patient Teaching
• Advise the patient to institute measures to promote defecation such as increasing his or her fluid intake, exercising, and eating a high-fiber diet.
• Warn the patient to notify the physician if he or she experiences unrelieved constipation, dizziness, muscle cramps or pain, rectal bleeding, and weakness.

lactulose
lack-tyoo-lows
(Acilac[CAN], Actilax[AUS],
Constulose, Duphalac[CAN],
Enulose, Generlac, Genlac[AUS],
Kristalose, Laxilose[CAN])
Do not confuse with lactose.

CATEGORY AND SCHEDULE
Pregnancy Risk Category: B

MECHANISM OF ACTION
A lactose derivative that retains
ammonia in colon and decreases
serum ammonia concentration,
producing osmotic effect. *Therapeutic Effect:* Promotes increased
peristalsis, bowel evacuation, expelling ammonia from colon.

PHARMACOKINETICS

Route	Onset	Peak	Duration
PO	24–48 hrs	N/A	N/A
Rectal	30–60 min	N/A	N/A

Poorly absorbed from the gastrointestinal (GI) tract. Acts in colon.
Primarily excreted in feces.

AVAILABILITY
Syrup: 10 g/15 ml.
Packets: 10 g, 20 g.

INDICATIONS AND DOSAGES
▶ **Constipation**
PO
Adults, Elderly. 15–30 ml/day up to
60 ml/day.
Children. 7.5 ml/day after breakfast.
▶ **Portal-systemic encephalopathy**
PO
Adults, Elderly. Initially, 30–45 ml
every hr. Then, 30–45 ml 3–4
times/day. Adjust dose q1–2 days to
produce 2–3 soft stools/day.

Children. 40–90 ml/day in divided
doses.
Infants. 2.5–10 ml/day in divided
doses.
Rectal (as retention enema)
Adults, Elderly, 300 ml with 700 ml
water or saline; retain 30–60 min;
repeat q4–6h. If evacuation occurs
too promptly, repeat immediately.

CONTRAINDICATIONS
Abdominal pain, appendicitis,
nausea, patients on a galactose-free
diet, vomiting

INTERACTIONS
Drug
PO medication: May decrease
transit time of concurrently adminis-
tered oral medication, decreasing
absorption.
Herbal
None known.
Food
None known.

DIAGNOSTIC TEST EFFECTS
May decrease serum potassium
levels.

SIDE EFFECTS
Occasional
Cramping, flatulence, increased
thirst, abdominal discomfort
Rare
Nausea, vomiting

SERIOUS REACTIONS
• Diarrhea indicates overdosage.
• Long-term use may result in
laxative dependence, chronic constipation, and loss of normal bowel
function.

NURSING CONSIDERATIONS
Baseline Assessment
• Prior to administration, assess the
patient's abdomen for signs of

tenderness, rigidity, and the presence of bowel sounds.
• Try to determine when the patient last had a bowel movement, and find out the amount and consistency.
• Plan to obtain baseline serum ammonia levels.
• Assess the patient's baseline mental status, and look for signs of high ammonia levels, such as asterixis.

Lifespan Considerations
• Be aware that it is unknown if lactulose crosses the placenta or is distributed in breast milk.
• Be aware that lactulose use should be avoided in children younger than 6 years of age as this patient population is usually unable to describe symptoms.
• There are no age-related precautions noted in the elderly.

Precautions
• Use cautiously in patients with diabetes mellitus.

Administration and Handling
PO
• Store solution at room temperature.
• Solution normally appears pale yellow to yellow in color, and viscous in consistency. Cloudy, darkened solution does not indicate potency loss.
• Drink juice, milk, or water with each dose to aid in stool softening and increase palatability.
Rectal
• Lubricate anus with petroleum jelly before enema insertion.
• Insert carefully, to prevent damage to the rectal wall, with nozzle toward navel.
• Squeeze container until entire dose expelled.
• Retain liquid until definite lower abdominal cramping is felt.

Intervention and Evaluation
• Encourage the patient to maintain adequate fluid intake.
• Assess the patient's bowel sounds for peristalsis.
• Assess the patient's daily pattern of daily bowel activity and stool consistency and record time of evacuation.
• Assess the patient for abdominal disturbances.
• Monitor the serum electrolytes in patients exposed to excessive, frequent, or prolonged use of lactulose.
• Obtain periodic serum ammonia levels, looking for a reduction.
• Assess the patient's mental status, and monitor for signs of reduced ammonia levels, such as lessening of asterixis.

Patient Teaching
• Instruct the patient to retain the liquid until cramping felt.
• Tell the patient that evacuation occurs in 24 to 48 hours of the initial drug dose.
• Instruct the patient to institute measures to promote defecation such as increasing his or her fluid intake, exercising, and eating a high-fiber diet.

magnesium
magnesium chloride
(Citro-Mag[CAN], Phillips'
Magnesia Tablets[CAN], Slow-
Mag)

magnesium citrate
(Citrate of Magnesia, Citroma)

magnesium hydroxide
(MOM)

magnesium oxide
(Mag-Ox 400, Maox 420)

magnesium protein complex
(Mg-PLUS)

magnesium sulfate
(Epsom salt, magnesium sulfate
injection)

**Do not confuse with manganese
sulfate.**

CATEGORY AND SCHEDULE
Pregnancy Risk Category: B

MECHANISM OF ACTION
An antacid, anticonvulsant, electrolyte, and laxative. Antacid: Acts in
stomach to neutralize gastric acid.
Therapeutic Effect: Increases pH.
Laxative: Osmotic effect primarily
in small intestine. Draws water into
intestinal lumen. *Therapeutic Effect:*
Produces distention; promotes peristalsis, bowel evacuation. Systemic
dietary supplement, replacement:
Found primarily in intracellular
fluids. Essential for enzyme activity,
nerve conduction, and muscle contraction. Anticonvulsant: Blocks
neuromuscular transmission, amount
of acetylcholine released at motor
end plate. *Therapeutic Effect:* Produces seizure control.

PHARMACOKINETICS
Antacid, Laxative: Minimal absorption through intestine. Absorbed
dose primarily excreted in urine.
Systemic: Widely distributed. Primarily excreted in urine.

AVAILABILITY
Magnesium chloride
Tablets (delayed release): 64 mg
(Slow-Mag).
Magnesium citrate
Solution: 300 ml.
Magnesium hydroxide
Liquid: 400 mg/5 ml, 800 mg/5 ml.
Chewable Tablets: 311 mg.
Magnesium oxide
Tablets: 400 mg (Mag-Ox)
Magnesium sulfate
Premix Solution: 10 mg/ml, 20 mg/
ml, 40 mg/ml, 80 mg/ml.
Injection Solution: 125 mg/ml,
500 mg/ml.

INDICATIONS AND DOSAGES
▶ **Hypomagnesemia (magnesium
sulfate)**
IM/IV
Adults, Elderly. 1 g q6h for 4 doses.
Children. 25–50 mg/kg/dose q4–6h
for 3–4 doses.
PO
Adults, Elderly. 3 g q6h for 4 doses.
Children. 10–20 mg/kg (elemental
magnesium)/dose 4 times/day.
▶ **Hypertension, seizures (magne-
sium sulfate)**
IM/IV
Adults, Elderly. 1 g q6h for 4 doses
as needed.
Children. 20–100 mg/kg/dose
q4–6h as needed.
▶ **Torsades de pointes (magnesium
sulfate)**
IV
Adults, Elderly. 1–2 g over 60–90
seconds followed by 1–2 g/hr diluted
in 100 ml of 0.9% NaCl or D_5W.
Children, Neonates. 25–50 mg/kg/
dose. Maximum: 2 g.

▶ **Laxative (magnesium citrate)**
PO
Adults, Elderly, Children older than 12 yrs. 150–300 ml.
Children 6–12 yrs. 100–150 ml.
Children younger than 6 yrs. 2–4 ml/kg.

▶ **Laxative (magnesium hydroxide)**
PO
Adults, Elderly, Children 12 yrs and older. 30–60 ml/day.
Children 6–11 yrs. 15–30 ml/day.
Children 2–5 yrs. 5–15 ml/day.
Children younger than 2 yrs. 0.5 ml/kg/dose.

▶ **Antacid (magnesium hydroxide)**
PO
Adults, Elderly. 622–1,244 mg/dose (tablet), 2.5–7.5 ml/dose (liquid concentrate), 5–15 ml/dose (liquid).
Children. 2.5–5 ml/dose (liquid).

CONTRAINDICATIONS

Antacids: Appendicitis or symptoms of appendicitis, ileostomy, intestinal obstruction, severe renal impairment
Laxative: Appendicitis, colostomy, congestive heart failure (CHF), hypersensitivity, ileostomy, intestinal obstruction, undiagnosed rectal bleeding
Systemic: Heart block, myocardial damage, renal failure

INTERACTIONS
Drug

Antacids
Ketoconazole, tetracyclines: May decrease the absorption of ketoconazole and tetracyclines.
Methenamine: May decrease the effects of methenamine.
Antacids, laxatives
Digoxin, oral anticoagulants, phenothiazines: May decrease the effects of digoxin, oral anticoagulants, and phenothiazines.
Tetracyclines: May form nonabsorbable complex with tetracyclines.
Systemic (dietary supplement, replacement)
Calcium: May neutralize the effects of magnesium.
Central nervous system (CNS) depression-producing medications: May increase CNS depression.
Digoxin: May cause changes in cardiac conduction or heart block with digoxin.
Herbal
None known.
Food
None known.

DIAGNOSTIC TEST EFFECTS

Antacid: May increase gastrin, pH.
Laxative: May decrease serum potassium.
Systemic (dietary supplement, replacement): None known.

IV INCOMPATIBILITIES

Amphotericin B complex (Abelcet, AmBisome, Amphotec), cefepime (Maxipime)

IV COMPATIBILITIES

Amikacin (Amikin), cefazolin (Ancef), cefepime (Maxipime), ciprofloxacin (Cipro), dobutamine (Dobutrex), enalapril (Vasotec), gentamicin, heparin, hydromorphone (Dilaudid), insulin, milrinone (Primacor), morphine, piperacillin/tazobactam (Zosyn), potassium chloride, propofol (Diprivan), tobramycin (Nebcin), vancomycin (Vancocin)

SIDE EFFECTS

Frequent
Antacid: Chalky taste, diarrhea, laxative effect
Occasional
Antacid: Nausea, vomiting, stomach cramps
Antacid, laxative: Prolonged use or large dose with renal impairment

may cause increased magnesium levels, marked by dizziness, irregular heartbeat, mental changes, tiredness, and weakness
Laxative: Cramping, diarrhea, increased thirst, gas
Systemic (dietary supplement, replacement): Reduced respiratory rate, decreased reflexes, flushing, hypotension, decreased heart rate

SERIOUS REACTIONS
• Magnesium as an antacid or laxative has no known serious reactions.
• Systemic use of magnesium may produce prolonged PR interval and widening of QRS intervals.
• May cause loss of deep tendon reflexes, heart block, respiratory paralysis, and cardiac arrest. The antidote is 10 to 20 ml 10% calcium gluconate (5 to 10 mEq of calcium).

NURSING CONSIDERATIONS
Baseline Assessment
• Determine if the patient is sensitive to magnesium.
• Assess for the presence of gastrointestinal (GI) pain. Note its pattern, duration, quality, intensity, location, and areas of radiation, as well as factors that relieve or worsen the pain.
• Assess the amount, color, and consistency of the stool of the patient taking magnesium as a laxative.
• Assess the daily pattern of bowel activity and evaluate the bowel sounds for peristalsis of the patient taking magnesium as a laxative.
• Assess the patient for history of recent abdominal surgery, nausea, vomiting, and weight loss.
• Assess the BUN and serum creatinine and magnesium levels of the patient taking magnesium for systemic use.

Lifespan Considerations
• Be aware that it is unknown if antacid forms of magnesium are distributed in breast milk.
• Be aware that parenteral magnesium readily crosses the placenta and is distributed in breast milk for 24 hours after magnesium therapy is discontinued.
• Be aware that continuous IV infusion increases the risk of magnesium toxicity in the neonate.
• Be aware that IV administration of magnesium should not be used 2 hours preceding delivery.
• There are no age-related precautions noted in children.
• Be aware that the elderly are at an increased risk of developing magnesium deficiency, such as decreased absorption, medications, and poor diet.

Precautions
• Use cautiously in children younger than 6 years of age. The safety of magnesium use in this patient population is unknown.
• When magnesium is given as an antacid, use cautiously in patients with chronic diarrhea, colostomy, diverticulitis, ulcerative colitis, and undiagnosed gastrointestinal (GI) or rectal bleeding.
• When magnesium is given as a laxative, use cautiously in patients with diabetes mellitus or patients on a low-salt diet because some magnesium supplements contain sugar or sodium.
• When magnesium is given for systemic use, use cautiously in patients with severe renal impairment.

Administration and Handling
PO (Antacid)
◄ALERT► Keep in mind that antacids may be given up to 4 times/day.
• Shake suspension well before use.
• Make sure that chewable tablets

are chewed thoroughly before swallowing, and followed by full glass of water.

PO (Laxative)

• Drink full glass of liquid (8 oz) with each dose to prevent dehydration.

• Follow dose with citrus carbonated beverage or fruit juice to improve flavor.

• Refrigerate citrate of magnesia to retain potency, palatability.

IM

• For adults, elderly, use 250 mg/ml (25%) or 500 mg/ml (50%) magnesium sulfate concentration, as prescribed.

• For infants, children, do not exceed 200 mg/ml (20%) as prescribed.

IV

• Store at room temperature.

• Must dilute to avoid exceeding 20 mg/ml concentration.

• For IV infusion, do not exceed magnesium sulfate concentration of 200 mg/ml (20%).

• Do not exceed IV infusion rate of 150 mg/min.

Intervention and Evaluation

• Assess the patient taking magnesium antacid for relief of gastric distress.

• Monitor the renal function, especially if dosing is long-term or frequent, of the patient taking magnesium antacid.

• Monitor the patient taking magnesium laxative for constipation or diarrhea.

• Ensure the patient taking magnesium laxative maintains adequate fluid intake.

• Monitor the BUN, electrocardiogram (EKG), and serum creatinine and magnesium levels in patients taking systemic magnesium.

• Test the knee jerk and patellar reflexes before giving repeat parenteral doses of systemic magnesium because these reflexes are used as indication of central nervous system (CNS) depression. Know that a suppressed reflex may be sign of impending respiratory arrest. Make sure that patellar reflexes are present, with a respiratory rate greater than 16 a minute, before giving each parenteral dose.

• Provide seizure precautions to the patient taking systemic magnesium.

Patient Teaching

• Instruct the patient to take magnesium antacids at least 2 hours apart from other medications.

• Tell the patient not to take magnesium antacids longer than 2 weeks, unless directed by the physician.

• Instruct the peptic ulcer disease patient to take magnesium antacids 1 and 3 hours after meals and at bedtime for 4 to 6 weeks. Teach the patient to chew tablets thoroughly followed with glass of water or to shake suspensions well.

• Warn the patient that repeat dosing or large doses of magnesium antacids may have a laxative effect.

• Instruct patient taking magnesium laxatives to drink a full glass (8 oz) of liquid to aid stool softening.

• Tell the patient taking magnesium laxatives that these drugs are for short-term use only.

• Warn the patient taking magnesium laxatives not to use the drug if he or she experiences abdominal pain, nausea, or vomiting.

• Warn the patient taking systemic magnesium to notify the physician if he or she experiences any signs of hypermagnesemia, including confusion, cramping, dizziness, irregular heartbeat, lightheadedness, or unusual tiredness or weakness.

methylcellulose

meth-ill-**cell**-you-los
(Citrucel, Cologel)
Do not confuse with Citracal.

CATEGORY AND SCHEDULE

Pregnancy Risk Category: C
OTC

MECHANISM OF ACTION

A bulk-forming laxative that dissolves and expands in water. *Therapeutic Effect:* Provides increased bulk, moisture content in stool, increasing peristalsis, bowel motility.

PHARMACOKINETICS

Route	Onset	Peak	Duration
PO	12–24 hrs	N/A	N/A

Full effect may not be evident for 2–3 days. Acts in small and large intestines.

AVAILABILITY

Powder.

INDICATIONS AND DOSAGES

▸ **Laxative**
PO
Adults, Elderly. 1 tbsp (15 ml) in 8 oz water 1–3 times/day.
Children 6–12 yrs. 1 tsp (5 ml) in 4 oz water 3–4 times/day.

CONTRAINDICATIONS

Abdominal pain, dysphagia, nausea, partial bowel obstruction, symptoms of appendicitis, vomiting

INTERACTIONS

Drug
Digoxin, oral anticoagulants, salicylates: May decrease the effects of digoxin, oral anticoagulants, and salicylates by decreasing absorption.
Potassium-sparing diuretics, potassium supplements: May interfere with the effects of potassium-sparing diuretics and potassium supplements.
Herbal
None known.
Food
None known.

DIAGNOSTIC TEST EFFECTS

May increase blood glucose levels. May decrease serum potassium levels.

SIDE EFFECTS

Rare
Some degree of abdominal discomfort, nausea, mild cramps, griping, faintness

SERIOUS REACTIONS

• Esophageal or bowel obstruction may occur if administered with insufficient liquid, less than 250 ml or 1 full glass.

NURSING CONSIDERATIONS

Baseline Assessment
• Prior to administration, assess the patient's abdomen for signs of tenderness, rigidity, and the presence of bowel sounds.
• Try to determine when the patient last had a bowel movement, and find out the amount and consistency.
Lifespan Considerations
• This drug may be used safely in pregnancy.
• Be aware that the safety and efficacy of methylcellulose have not been established in children younger than 6 years of age. Methylcellulose use is not recommended in this age group.

• There are no age-related precautions noted in the elderly.

Administration and Handling

PO

• Instruct the patient to drink 6 to 8 glasses of water a day to aid in stool softening.

• Not to be swallowed in dry form; mix with at least 1 full glass (8 oz) of liquid.

Intervention and Evaluation

• Encourage the patient to maintain adequate fluid intake.

• Assess the patient's bowel sounds for peristalsis.

• Assess the patient's daily pattern of daily bowel activity and stool consistency and record time of evacuation.

• Monitor the serum electrolytes in patients exposed to excessive, frequent, or prolonged use of methylcellulose.

Patient Teaching

• Tell the patient to institute measures to promote defecation such as increasing his or her fluid intake, exercising, and eating a high-fiber diet.

• Instruct the patient to take each dose with a full glass of water.

• Warn the patient that inadequate fluid intake may cause choking or swelling in throat.

---

polycarbophil

polly-**car**-bow-fill
(Fibercon, Replens[CAN])

CATEGORY AND SCHEDULE

Pregnancy Risk Category: C
OTC

MECHANISM OF ACTION

A bulk-forming laxative and antidiarrheal. Laxative: Retains water in intestine, opposes dehydrating forces of the bowel. *Therapeutic Effect:* Promotes well-formed stools. Antidiarrheal: Absorbs fecal-free water, restores normal moisture level, provides bulk. *Therapeutic Effect:* Forms gel, produces formed stool.

PHARMACOKINETICS

Route	Onset	Peak	Duration
PO	12–72 hrs	N/A	N/A

Acts in small and large intestines.

AVAILABILITY

Tablets: 500 mg, 625 mg.
Tablets (chewable): 500 mg.

INDICATIONS AND DOSAGES

▶ **Laxative, antidiarrheal**

PO

Adults, Elderly, Children older than 12 yrs. 1 g 1–4 times/day, or as needed. Maximum: 4 g/24 hrs.
Children 6–12 yrs. 500 mg 1–4 times/day, or as needed. Maximum: 2 g/24 hrs.
Children younger than 6 yrs. Consult product labeling.

CONTRAINDICATIONS

Abdominal pain, dysphagia, nausea, partial bowel obstruction, symptoms of appendicitis, vomiting

INTERACTIONS

Drug

Digoxin, oral anticoagulants, salicylates, tetracyclines: May decrease the effects of digoxin, salicylates, and tetracyclines.
Potassium-sparing diuretics, potassium supplements: May interfere with the effects of potassium-sparing diuretics and potassium supplements.

Herbal
None known.
Food
None known.

DIAGNOSTIC TEST EFFECTS

May increase blood glucose levels.
May decrease serum potassium
levels.

SIDE EFFECTS

Rare
Some degree of abdominal discomfort, nausea, mild cramps, griping,
faintness

SERIOUS REACTIONS

• Esophageal or bowel obstruction
may occur if administered with less
than 250 ml or 1 full glass.

NURSING CONSIDERATIONS

Baseline Assessment
• Prior to administration, assess the
patient's abdomen for signs of
tenderness, rigidity, and the presence of bowel sounds.
• Try to determine when the patient
last had a bowel movement, and
find out the amount and consistency.
Lifespan Considerations
• This drug may be used safely in
pregnancy.
• Be aware that polycarbophil use is
not recommended in children younger than 6 years of age.
• There are no age-related precautions noted in the elderly.
Administration and Handling
◀ALERT▶ For severe diarrhea,
give every half hour up to maximum daily dosage; for laxative,
give with 8 oz liquid, as
prescribed.
Intervention and Evaluation
• Encourage the patient to maintain
adequate fluid intake.

• Assess the patient's bowel sounds
for peristalsis.
• Assess the patient's daily pattern
of daily bowel activity and stool
consistency and record time of
evacuation.
• Monitor the serum electrolytes in
patients exposed to excessive,
frequent, or prolonged use of polycarbophil.
Patient Teaching
• Tell the patient to institute measures to promote defecation such as
increasing his or her fluid intake,
exercising, and eating a high-fiber
diet.
• Instruct the patient to drink 6 to
8 glasses of water a day when using
polycarbophil as a laxative to aid in
stool softening.

---

polyethylene glycol-electrolyte solution (PEG-ES)

poly-eth-ah-leen
(CoLyte, GoLYTELY, Klean-Prep[CAN], MiraLax, NuLytely,
Peglyte[CAN], Pro-Lax[CAN])

CATEGORY AND SCHEDULE

Pregnancy Risk Category: C

MECHANISM OF ACTION

A laxative that has an osmotic
effect. *Therapeutic Effect:* Induces
diarrhea, cleanses bowel without
depleting electrolytes.

PHARMACOKINETICS

Indication	Onset	Peak	Duration
Bowel cleansing	1–2 hrs	N/A	N/A
Constipation	2–4 days	N/A	N/A

AVAILABILITY
Powder for Oral Solution.
Oral Solution.

INDICATIONS AND DOSAGES
▶ **Bowel evacuant**
PO
Adults, Elderly. 4 liters before gastrointestinal (GI) examination: 240 ml (8 oz) q10min until 4 liters consumed or rectal effluent clear. NG tube: 20–30 ml/min until 4 liters given.
Children. 25–40 ml/kg/hr until rectal effluent clear.
▶ **Constipation**
PO
Adults. (Miralax): 17 g or 1 heaping tbsp a day.

CONTRAINDICATIONS
Bowel perforation, gastric retention, GI obstruction, toxic colitis, toxic ileus, megacolon

INTERACTIONS
Drug
PO medications: May decrease the absorption of oral medications if given within 1 hour because they may be flushed from GI tract.
Herbal
None known.
Food
None known.

DIAGNOSTIC TEST EFFECTS
None known.

SIDE EFFECTS
Frequent (50%)
Some degree of abdominal fullness, nausea, bloating
Occasional (10%–1%)
Abdominal cramping, vomiting, anal irritation
Rare (less than 1%)
Urticaria, rhinorrhea, dermatitis

SERIOUS REACTIONS
• None known.

NURSING CONSIDERATIONS
Baseline Assessment
• Do not give oral medication within 1 hour of the initiation of polyethylene therapy or the oral medication may not adequately be absorbed before GI cleansing.
Lifespan Considerations
• Be aware that it is unknown if polyethylene crosses the placenta or is distributed in breast milk.
• There are no age-related precautions noted in children or the elderly.
Precautions
• Use cautiously in patients with ulcerative colitis.
Administration and Handling
PO
• Refrigerate reconstituted solutions; use within 48 hours.
• May use tap water to prepare solution. Shake vigorously several minutes to ensure complete dissolution of powder.
• Give nothing by mouth 3 hours or more before ingestion of solution. Give clear liquids only after administration.
• May give via NG tube.
• Rapid drinking preferred. Chilled solution is more palatable.
Intervention and Evaluation
• Assess the patient's bowel sounds for peristalsis.
• Assess the patient's daily pattern of daily bowel activity and stool consistency and record time of evacuation.
• Assess the patient for abdominal disturbances.
• Monitor the patient's blood glucose, BUN, serum electrolytes, and urine osmolality.

Patient Teaching
• Tell the patient chill solution to make more palatable, encourage fast ingestion.
• Instruct the patient to fast 3 hours prior to taking drug, and to only ingest clear liquids afterward, as prescribed.
• Warn the patient to notify the physician if he or she experiences severe abdominal pain or bloating.

psyllium
sill-ee-um
(Fiberall, Hydrocil, Konsyl, Metamucil, Perdiem, Prodiem Plain[CAN])

CATEGORY AND SCHEDULE
Pregnancy Risk Category: B
OTC

MECHANISM OF ACTION
A bulk-forming laxative in powder or wafer form that dissolves and swells in water, and provides increased bulk and moisture content in stool. *Therapeutic Effect:* Increased bulk promotes peristalsis, bowel motility.

PHARMACOKINETICS

Route	Onset	Peak	Duration
PO	12–24 hrs	2–3 days	N/A

Acts in small and large intestines.

AVAILABILITY
Powder.
Wafer.

INDICATIONS AND DOSAGES
▸ Laxative
PO
Adults, Elderly. 1–2 rounded tea-spoons, packet, or wafer in water 1–4 times/day.
Children 6–11 yrs. One half–1 tea-spoon in water 1–3 times/day.

CONTRAINDICATIONS
Fecal impaction, GI obstruction

INTERACTIONS
Drug
Digoxin, oral anticoagulants, salicylates: May decrease the effects of digoxin, oral anticoagulants, and salicylates by decreasing absorption.
Potassium-sparing diuretics, potassium supplements: May interfere with the effects of potassium-sparing diuretics and potassium supplements.
Herbal
None known.
Food
None known.

DIAGNOSTIC TEST EFFECTS
May increase blood glucose levels. May decrease serum potassium levels.

SIDE EFFECTS
Rare
Some degree of abdominal discomfort, nausea, mild cramps, griping, faintness

SERIOUS REACTIONS
• Esophageal or bowel obstruction may occur if administered with insufficient liquid, less than 250 ml or 1 full glass.

NURSING CONSIDERATIONS

Baseline Assessment
• Prior to administration, assess the patient's abdomen for signs of tenderness, rigidity, and the presence of bowel sounds.

• Try to determine when the patient last had a bowel movement, and find out the amount and consistency.

Lifespan Considerations

• This drug may be used safely in pregnancy.

• Be aware that the safety and efficacy of psyllium has not been established in children younger than 6 years of age.

• There are no age-related precautions noted in the elderly.

Precautions

• Use cautiously in patients with esophageal strictures, intestinal adhesions, stenosis, and ulcers.

Administration and Handling

PO

• Drink 6 to 8 glasses of water a day to aid in stool softening.

• Do not swallow in dry form; mix with at least 1 full glass (8 oz) of liquid.

Intervention and Evaluation

• Encourage the patient to maintain adequate fluid intake.

• Assess the patient's bowel sounds for peristalsis.

• Assess the patient's daily pattern of daily bowel activity and stool consistency and record time of evacuation.

• Assess the patient for abdominal disturbances.

• Monitor the serum electrolytes in patients exposed to excessive, frequent, or prolonged use of psyllium.

Patient Teaching

• Tell the patient to institute measures to promote defecation such as increasing his or her fluid intake, exercising, and eating a high-fiber diet.

• Instruct the patient to take each dose with a full glass of water.

• Warn the patient that inadequate fluid intake may cause choking or swelling in throat.

senna
sen-ah
(Senokot, Senolax)

CATEGORY AND SCHEDULE
Pregnancy Risk Category: C
OTC

MECHANISM OF ACTION
A gastrointestinal (GI) stimulant that has a direct effect on intestinal smooth musculature by stimulating the intramural nerve plexi. *Therapeutic Effect:* Increases peristalsis, promotes laxative effect.

PHARMACOKINETICS

Route	Onset	Peak	Duration
PO	6–12 hrs	N/A	N/A
Rectal	0.5–2 hrs	N/A	N/A

Minimal absorption after PO administration. Hydrolyzed to active form by enzymes of colonic flora. Absorbed drug metabolized in liver; eliminated in feces via biliary system.

AVAILABILITY
Granules: 15 mg/3 g.
Liquid: 25 mg/15 ml, 33.3 mg/ml.
Syrup: 8.8 mg/5 ml.
Tablets: 8.6 mg.
Tablets (chewable): 10 mg, 15 mg.

INDICATIONS AND DOSAGES
▸ **Constipation**
PO (tablets)
Adults, Elderly, Children older than 12 yrs. 2 tablets at bedtime up to 4 tablets 2 times/day.

Children 6–12 yrs. 1 tablet at bedtime up to 2 tablets 2 times/day.
Children 2–younger than 6 yrs. one half (1/2) tablet at bedtime up to 1 tablet 2 times/day.
PO (syrup)
Adults, Elderly, Children older than 12 yrs. 10–15 ml at bedtime up to 15 ml 2 times/day.
Children 6–12 yrs. 5–7.5 ml at bedtime up to 7.5 ml 2 times/day.
Children 2–younger than 6 yrs. 2.5–3.75 ml at bedtime up to 3.75 ml 2 times/day.
PO (granules)
Adults, Elderly, Children older than 12 yrs. 1 teaspoon at bedtime up to 2 teaspoons 2 times/day.
Children 6–12 yrs. one half (1/2) teaspoon at bedtime up to 1 teaspoon 2 times/day.
Children 2–younger than 6 yrs. one quarter (1/4) teaspoon at bedtime up to one half (1/2) teaspoon 2 times/day.

CONTRAINDICATIONS
Abdominal pain, appendicitis, intestinal obstruction, nausea, vomiting

INTERACTIONS
Drug
PO medications: May decrease transit time of concurrently administered oral medication, decreasing absorption of senna.
Herbal
None known.
Food
None known.

DIAGNOSTIC TEST EFFECTS
May increase blood glucose levels. May decrease serum potassium levels.

SIDE EFFECTS
Frequent
Pink-red, red-violet, red-brown, or yellow-brown discoloration of urine
Occasional
Some degree of abdominal discomfort, nausea, mild cramps, griping, faintness

SERIOUS REACTIONS
• Long-term use may result in laxative dependence, chronic constipation, and loss of normal bowel function.
• Chronic use or overdosage may result in electrolyte disturbances, such as hypokalemia, hypocalcemia, and metabolic acidosis or alkalosis, persistent diarrhea, malabsorption, and weight loss. Electrolyte disturbance may produce vomiting, muscle weakness.

NURSING CONSIDERATIONS
Baseline Assessment
• Prior to administration, assess the patient's abdomen for signs of tenderness, rigidity, and the presence of bowel sounds.
• Try to determine when the patient last had a bowel movement, and find out the amount and consistency.
Lifespan Considerations
• Be aware that it is unknown if senna is distributed in breast milk.
• Be aware that the safety and efficacy of senna has not been established in children younger than 6 years of age.
• There are no age-related precautions noted in the elderly, but monitor this patient population for signs of dehydration and electrolyte loss.
Precautions
• Use cautiously for extended periods greater than 1 week.
Administration and Handling
PO
• Give senna on an empty stomach for faster results.

• Offer the patient at least 6 to
8 glasses of water a day to aid in
stool softening.
• Avoid giving within 1 hour of
other oral medication because it
decreases drug absorption.

Intervention and Evaluation
• Encourage the patient to maintain
adequate fluid intake.
• Assess the patient's bowel sounds
for peristalsis.
• Assess the patient's daily pattern
of daily bowel activity and stool
consistency and record time of
evacuation.
• Assess the patient for gastrointestinal (GI) disturbances.
• Monitor the serum electrolytes in
patients exposed to excessive,
frequent, or prolonged use of senna.

Patient Teaching
• Explain to the patient that his or
her urine may turn pink-red, red-
violet, red-brown, or yellow-brown.
• Instruct the patient to institute
measures to promote defecation
such as increasing his or her fluid
intake, exercising, and eating a
high-fiber diet.
• Instruct the patient not to take
other oral medications within 1 hour
of taking senna as these substances
may decrease the effectiveness of
senna.
• Tell the patient that senna's laxative effect generally occurs in 6 to
12 hours but may take 24 hours to
appear, and the senna's suppository
produces evacuation in 30 minutes
to 2 hours.

esomeprazole
lansoprazole
omeprazole
pantoprazole
rabeprazole sodium

Uses: Proton pump inhibitors are used to treat various gastric disorders, including gastric and duodenal ulcers, gastroesophageal reflux disease (GERD), and pathologic hypersecretory conditions.

Action: Proton pump inhibitors suppress gastric acid secretion by specifically inhibiting the hydrogen-potassium-adenosine triphosphatase (H^+/K^+ ATPase) enzyme system found at the secretory surface of gastric parietal cells. This enzyme system is considered the acid pump of the gastric mucosa. (See illustration, *Sites of Action: Drugs Used to Treat GERD,* page 932.) Proton pump inhibitors don't have anticholinergic or histamine-receptor antagonistic properties.

---

esomeprazole
es-oh-**mep**-rah-zole
(Nexium)

CATEGORY AND SCHEDULE
Pregnancy Risk Category: B

MECHANISM OF ACTION
A proton pump inhibitor that is converted to active metabolites that irreversibly bind to and inhibit H^+, K^+, ATPase, an enzyme on surface of gastric parietal cells. Inhibits hydrogen ion transport into gastric lumen. *Therapeutic Effect:* Increases gastric pH, reducing gastric acid production.

PHARMACOKINETICS
Well absorbed after PO administration. Protein binding: 97%. Extensively metabolized by the liver. Primarily excreted in urine. **Half-life:** 1–1.5 hrs.

AVAILABILITY
Capsules (delayed-release): 20 mg, 40 mg.

INDICATIONS AND DOSAGES
▸ **Erosive esophagitis**
PO
Adults, Elderly. 20–40 mg once daily for 4–8 wks.
▸ **Maintenance healing of erosive esophagitis**
PO
Adults, Elderly. 20 mg/day.
▸ **Gastroesophageal reflux disease (GERD)**
PO
Adults, Elderly. 20 mg once a day for 4 wks.
▸ *H. Pylori* **duodenal ulcer**
PO
Adults, Elderly. Esomeprazole: 40 mg once a day, with amoxicillin 1,000 mg and clarithromycin 500 mg twice a day for 10 days.

CONTRAINDICATIONS
None known

INTERACTIONS
Drug
Digoxin, iron, ketoconazole: May decrease the concentration of digoxin, iron, and ketoconazole.
Herbal
None known.
Food
None known.

DIAGNOSTIC TEST EFFECTS
None known.

SIDE EFFECTS
Frequent (7%)
Headache
Occasional (3%–2%)
Diarrhea, abdominal pain, nausea
Rare (less than 2%)
Dizziness, asthenia or loss of strength, vomiting, constipation, rash, cough

SERIOUS REACTIONS
• None known.

NURSING CONSIDERATIONS
Baseline Assessment
• Before giving drug, determine if the patient can swallow capsules whole.
Lifespan Considerations
• Be aware that it is unknown if esomeprazole crosses the placenta or is distributed in breast milk.
• Be aware that the safety and efficacy of esomeprazole have not been established in children.
• There are no age-related precautions noted in the elderly.
Administration and Handling
PO
• Give 1 hour or more before eating.
• Do not crush or open capsule. Instruct the patient to swallow the capsule whole. For those with

difficulty swallowing capsules, open capsule and mix pellets with 1 tablespoon of applesauce. Instruct the patient to swallow the spoonful without chewing.
Intervention and Evaluation
• Evaluate the patient for therapeutic response (i.e., relief of gastrointestinal [GI] symptoms).
• Assess the patient for diarrhea, discomfort, or nausea.
Patient Teaching
• Warn the patient to notify the physician if he or she experiences headache during esomeprazole therapy.
• Instruct the patient to take esomeprazole 1 hour or more before eating.
• Teach patients with difficulty swallowing to open the esomeprazole capsule, mix the pellets with 1 tablespoon of applesauce, and swallow the spoonful without chewing.

lansoprazole
lan-sew-**prah**-zoll
(Prevacid, Zoton[AUS])
Do not confuse with Pepcid, Pravachol, or Prevpac.

CATEGORY AND SCHEDULE
Pregnancy Risk Category: B

MECHANISM OF ACTION
A proton pump inhibitor that selectively inhibits parietal cell membrane enzyme system H^+, K^+, ATPase or proton pump. *Therapeutic Effect:* Suppresses gastric acid secretion.

PHARMACOKINETICS

Dosage	Onset	Peak	Duration
15 mg	2–3 hrs	N/A	24 hrs
30 mg	1–2 hrs	N/A	longer than 24 hrs

Once leaving stomach, rapid and complete absorption (food may decrease absorption). Protein binding: 97%. Distributed primarily to gastric parietal cells, converted to two active metabolites. Extensively metabolized in liver. Eliminated from body in bile and urine. Not removed by hemodialysis. **Half-life:** 1.5 hrs (half-life is increased in elderly, those with liver impairment).

AVAILABILITY
Capsules (extended-release): 15 mg, 30 mg.
Granules for Oral Suspension: 15 mg/pack; 30 mg/pack.

INDICATIONS AND DOSAGES
▸ **Duodenal ulcer**
PO
Adults, Elderly. 15 mg/day, before eating, preferably in the morning, for up to 4 wks.
▸ **Erosive esophagitis**
PO
Adults, Elderly. 30 mg/day, before eating, for up to 8 wks. If healing does not occur within 8 wks (5%–10%), may give for additional 8 wks. Maintenance: 15 mg/day.
▸ **Gastric ulcer**
PO
Adults. 30 mg/day for up to 8 wks.
▸ **Healed duodenal ulcer, gastroesophageal reflux disease (GERD)**
PO
Adults. 15 mg/day.
▸ **Usual pediatric dosage**
Children 3 mos–14 yrs, weighing less than 10 kg. 7.5 mg.

Children 3 mos–14 yrs, weighing 10–20 kg. 15 mg.
Children 3 mos–14 yrs, weighing more than 20 kg. 30 mg.
▸ **H. pylori**
PO
Adults. 30 mg 2 times/day for 10 days (with amoxicillin, clarithromycin).
▸ **Pathologic hypersecretory conditions (including Zollinger-Ellison syndrome)**
PO
Adults, Elderly. 60 mg/day. Individualize dosage according to patient needs and for as long as clinically indicated. May increase to more than 120 mg/day in divided doses.

CONTRAINDICATIONS
None known

INTERACTIONS
Drug
Ampicillin, digoxin, iron salts, ketoconazole: May interfere with the absorption of ampicillin, digoxin, iron salts, and ketoconazole.
Sucralfate: May delay the absorption of lansoprazole; give lansoprazole 30 min before sucralfate.
Herbal
None known.
Food
None known.

DIAGNOSTIC TEST EFFECTS
May increase LDH concentrations, serum alkaline phosphatase, bilirubin, cholesterol, creatinine, SGOT (AST), SGPT (ALT), triglycerides, and uric acid levels. May produce abnormal albumin/globulin ratio, electrolyte balance, and platelet, red blood cell (RBC), and white blood cell (WBC) counts. May increase blood Hgb and Hct.

SIDE EFFECTS
Occasional (3%–2%)
Diarrhea, abdominal pain, rash, pruritus, altered appetite
Rare (1%)
Nausea, headache

SERIOUS REACTIONS
• Bilirubinemia, eosinophilia, and hyperlipemia occur rarely.

Baseline Assessment
• Obtain the patient's baseline lab values, including complete blood count (CBC) and blood chemistry.
• Assess the patient's medication history, especially for the use of sucralfate.

Lifespan Considerations
• Be aware that it is unknown if lansoprazole is distributed in breast milk.
• Be aware that the safety and efficacy of lansoprazole have not been established in children.
• There are no age-related precautions noted in the elderly, but doses larger than 30 mg are not recommended in this patient population.

Precautions
• Use cautiously in patients with impaired liver function.

Administration and Handling
PO
• Give lansoprazole while fasting or before meals because food diminishes absorption.
• Instruct the patient not to chew or crush delayed-release capsules.
• If the patient has difficulty swallowing capsules, open capsules and sprinkle granules on 1 tablespoon of applesauce. Instruct the patient to swallow immediately.

Intervention and Evaluation
• Monitor the patient's ongoing laboratory results.
• Assess the patient for therapeutic response, such as relief of gastrointestinal (GI) symptoms.
• Assess the patient for abdominal pain, diarrhea, and nausea.

Patient Teaching
• Instruct the patient not to chew or crush delayed-release capsules.
• Teach patients who have difficulty swallowing capsules to open lansoprazole capsules, sprinkle the granules on 1 tablespoon of applesauce, and swallow immediately.
• Instruct patient to take lansoprazole 30 min before sucralfate.

omeprazole
oh-**mep**-rah-zole
(Losec[CAN], Maxor[AUS], Prilosec, Prilosec DR)
Do not confuse with prilocaine, Prinivil, or Prozac.

CATEGORY AND SCHEDULE
Pregnancy Risk Category: C

MECHANISM OF ACTION
A benzimidazole that is converted to active metabolites that irreversibly bind to and inhibit H^+/K^+ ATPase, an enzyme on surface of gastric parietal cells. Inhibits hydrogen ion transport into gastric lumen. *Therapeutic Effect:* Increases gastric pH, reduces gastric acid production.

PHARMACOKINETICS

Route	Onset	Peak	Duration
PO	1 hr	2 hrs	72 hrs

Rapidly absorbed from the gastrointestinal (GI) tract. Protein binding: 99%. Primarily distributed into gastric parietal cells. Metabolized extensively in liver. Primarily excreted in urine. Unknown if removed by hemodialysis. **Half-life:** 0.5–1 hr (increased in patients with decreased liver function).

AVAILABILITY
Capsules (delayed-release): 10 mg, 20 mg, 40 mg.

INDICATIONS AND DOSAGES
▸ **Erosive esophagitis, poorly responsive gastroesophageal reflux disease (GERD), active duodenal ulcer, prevention and treatment of NSAID-induced ulcers**
PO
Adults, Elderly. 20 mg/day.
▸ **Maintenance healing of erosive esophagitis**
PO
Adults, Elderly. 20 mg/day.
▸ **Pathologic hypersecretory conditions**
PO
Adults, Elderly. Initially, 60 mg/day up to 120 mg, 3 times/day.
▸ **H. Pylori duodenal ulcer**
PO
Adults, Elderly. 20 mg 2 times/day for 10 days.
▸ **Active benign gastric ulcer**
PO
Adults, Elderly. 40 mg/day for 4–8 wks.
▸ **Usual pediatric dosage**
Children older than 2 yrs, weighing less than 20 kg. 10 mg/day.
Children older than 2 yrs, weighing 20 kg and more. 20 mg/day.

UNLABELED USES
Prevention and treatment of NSAID-induced ulcers, treatment of active benign gastric ulcers, H. pylori–associated duodenal ulcer, with amoxicillin and clarithromycin

CONTRAINDICATIONS
None known

INTERACTIONS
Drug
Diazepam, oral anticoagulants, phenytoin: May increase the blood concentration of diazepam, oral anticoagulants, and phenytoin.
Herbal
None known.
Food
None known.

DIAGNOSTIC TEST EFFECTS
May increase serum alkaline phosphatase, SGOT (AST), and SGPT (ALT) levels.

SIDE EFFECTS
Frequent (7%)
Headache
Occasional (3%–2%)
Diarrhea, abdominal pain, nausea
Rare (less than 2%)
Dizziness, asthenia or loss of strength, vomiting, constipation, upper respiratory infection, back pain, rash, cough

SERIOUS REACTIONS
• None known.

NURSING CONSIDERATIONS
Baseline Assessment
• Expect to obtain baseline serum chemistry lab values, particularly serum alkaline phosphatase, SGOT (AST), and SGPT (ALT) levels to assess liver function.
Lifespan Considerations
• Be aware that it is unknown if omeprazole crosses the placenta or is distributed in breast milk.
• Be aware that the safety and efficacy of omeprazole have not been established in children.
• There are no age-related precautions noted in the elderly.

Administration and Handling
PO
* Give omeprazole before meals.
* Do not crush or open capsules; capsules should be swallowed whole.

Intervention and Evaluation
* Evaluate the patient for therapeutic response, relief of gastrointestinal (GI) symptoms.
* Assess the patient for diarrhea, discomfort, and nausea.

Patient Teaching
* Warn the patient to notify the physician if he or she experiences headache during omeprazole therapy.
* Instruct the patient to swallow omeprazole capsules whole and not to open or crush them.
* Teach the patient to take omeprazole capsules prior to eating.

pantoprazole
pan-tow-**pray**-zoll
(Protonix, Pantoloc, Somac[AUS])
Do not confuse with Lotronex.

CATEGORY AND SCHEDULE
Pregnancy Risk Category: B

MECHANISM OF ACTION
A benzimidazole that is converted to active metabolites that irreversibly bind to and inhibit H^+/K^+ ATPase, an enzyme on surface of gastric parietal cells. Inhibits hydrogen ion transport into gastric lumen. *Therapeutic Effect:* Increases gastric pH, reduces gastric acid production.

PHARMACOKINETICS

Route	Onset	Peak	Duration
PO	N/A	N/A	24 hrs

Rapidly absorbed from the gastrointestinal (GI) tract. Protein binding: greater than 98%. Primarily distributed into gastric parietal cells. Metabolized extensively in liver. Primarily excreted in urine. Not removed by hemodialysis. **Half-life:** 1 hr.

AVAILABILITY
Powder for Injection: 40 mg.
Tablets (delayed-release): 20 mg, 40 mg.

INDICATIONS AND DOSAGES
▶ **Erosive esophagitis**
PO
Adults, Elderly. 40 mg/day for up to 8 wks. If not healed after 8 wks, may continue an additional 8 wks.
IV infusion
Adults, Elderly. 40 mg/day for 7–10 days.
▶ **Hypersecretory conditions**
IV
Adults, Elderly. 80 mg 2 times/day. May increase up to 80 mg q8h.
PO
Adults, Elderly. Initially, 40 mg 2 times/day. May increase up to 240 mg/day.

CONTRAINDICATIONS
None known

INTERACTIONS
Drug
None known.
Herbal
None known.
Food
None known.

DIAGNOSTIC TEST EFFECTS
May increase serum creatinine, cholesterol, and uric acid levels.

IV INCOMPATIBILITIES

Do not mix with other medications. Flush IV with D_5W, 0.9% NaCl, or lactated Ringer's before and after administration.

SIDE EFFECTS

Rare (less than 2%)
Diarrhea, headache, dizziness, pruritus, skin rash

SERIOUS REACTIONS

• None known.

NURSING CONSIDERATIONS

Baseline Assessment
• Obtain the patient's baseline serum chemistry lab values, including serum creatinine and cholesterol.

Lifespan Considerations
• Be aware that it is unknown if pantoprazole crosses the placenta or is distributed in breast milk.
• Be aware that the safety and efficacy of pantoprazole have not been established in children.
• There are no age-related precautions noted in the elderly.

Precautions
• Use cautiously in patients with a history of chronic or current liver disease.

Administration and Handling
PO
• Give pantoprazole without regard to meals.
• Do not crush or split tablet; tablet should be swallowed whole.
IV
• Refrigerate vials and protect from light.
• Do not freeze reconstituted vials.
• Once diluted, keep in mind that the drug is stable for 12 hours at room temperature.
• Mix 40-mg vial with 10 ml 0.9% NaCl injection.

• Further dilute with 100 ml D_5W, 0.9% NaCl, or lactated Ringer's to concentration of 0.4 mg/ml.
• Infuse over 15 minutes using in-line filter provided.
• Position filter below the Y-site that is closest to the patient.

Intervention and Evaluation
• Evaluate the patient for therapeutic response, relief of GI symptoms.
• Assess the patient for GI discomfort and nausea.

Patient Teaching
• Warn the patient to notify the physician if he or she experiences headache during pantoprazole therapy.
• Instruct the patient to swallow pantoprazole tablets whole, not to open, chew, or crush them.
• Teach the patient to take pantoprazole tablets before eating.

rabeprazole sodium

rah-**bep**-rah-zole
(Aciphex, Pariet[AUS])
Do not confuse with Accupril or Aricept.

CATEGORY AND SCHEDULE

Pregnancy Risk Category: B

MECHANISM OF ACTION

A proton pump inhibitor that converts to active metabolites that irreversibly binds to and inhibits H^+/K^+ ATPase, an enzyme on surface of gastric parietal cells. Actively secretes hydrogen ions for potassium ions, resulting in an accumulation of H^+ in gastric lumen. *Therapeutic Effect:* Increases gastric pH, reducing gastric acid production.

PHARMACOKINETICS

Rapidly absorbed from the gastro-intestinal (GI) tract after passing through stomach relatively intact. Protein binding: 96%. Metabolized extensively in liver. Primarily excreted in urine. Unknown if removed by hemodialysis. **Half-life:** 1–2 hrs, half-life is increased with impaired liver function.

AVAILABILITY

Tablets (delayed-release):
20 mg.

INDICATIONS AND DOSAGES

▸ **Gastroesophageal reflux disease (GERD)**
PO
Adults, Elderly. 20 mg/day for 4–8 wks. Maintenance: 20 mg/day.
▸ **Duodenal ulcer**
PO
Adults, Elderly. 20 mg/day after morning meal for 4 wks.
▸ **Pathologic hypersecretory conditions**
PO
Adults, Elderly. Initially, 60 mg once a day. May increase up to 60 mg 2 times/day.
▸ **H. pylori**
PO
Adults, Elderly. 20 mg 2 times a day for 7 days (given in combination with amoxicillin 1000 mg and clarithromycin 500 mg)

CONTRAINDICATIONS

None known

INTERACTIONS

Drug
Digoxin: May increase the plasma concentration of digoxin.
Ketoconazole: May decrease the blood concentration of ketoconazole.

Herbal
None known.
Food
None known.

DIAGNOSTIC TEST EFFECTS

May increase serum alkaline phosphatase, SGOT (AST), and SGPT (ALT) levels.

SIDE EFFECTS

Rare (2% or less)
Headache, nausea, dizziness, rash, diarrhea, malaise

SERIOUS REACTIONS

• Hyperglycemia, hypokalemia, hyponatremia, and hyperlipemia occur rarely.

NURSING CONSIDERATIONS

Baseline Assessment
• Obtain the patient's baseline lab values, especially blood chemistries and liver function tests.
Lifespan Considerations
• Be aware that it is unknown if rabeprazole crosses the placenta or is distributed in breast milk.
• Be aware that the safety and efficacy of rabeprazole have not been established in children.
• There are no age-related precautions noted in the elderly.
Precautions
• Use cautiously in patients with impaired liver function.
Administration and Handling
PO
• Give rabeprazole before meals.
• Do not crush, chew, or split tablet; swallow whole.
Intervention and Evaluation
• Monitor the patient's ongoing laboratory results.
• Evaluate the patient for therapeutic response, relief of GI symptoms.

• Assess the patient for diarrhea, GI discomfort, headache, nausea, and skin rash.
• Observe the patient for dizziness and utilize appropriate safety precautions.

Patient Teaching
• Instruct the patient to swallow rabeprazole tablets whole, not to chew, crush, or split them.
• Tell the patient to notify the physician if he or she experiences headache during rabeprazole therapy.

53 Miscellaneous Gastrointestinal Agents

balsalazide
infliximab
mesalamine
 (5-aminosalicylic
 acid, 5-ASA)
metoclopramide
olsalazine sodium
orlistat
pancreatin
pancrelipase
simethicone
sucralfate
sulfasalazine
tegaserod
ursodiol

Uses: Because miscellaneous gastrointestinal (GI) agents come from different classes, their uses vary greatly. *Balsalazide* is used to treat ulcerative colitis. *Infliximab* may be used alone to treat Crohn's disease or with other drugs to treat rheumatoid arthritis. As GI anti-inflammatory agents, *mesalamine, olsalazine, and sulfasalazine* are prescribed to manage ulcerative colitis; other indications include proctosigmoiditis and proctitis (mesalamine) and inflammatory bowel disease and rheumatoid arthritis (sulfasalazine). *Orlistat* is used to manage obesity as an adjunct to calorie reduction. *Metoclopramide* is used to stimulate gastric emptying and intestinal transit, which is helpful in facilitating small bowel intubation and in relieving symptoms of gastroparesis, reflux esophagitis, and gastroesophageal reflux disease (GERD). *Pancreatin and pancrelipase* are used to replace or supplement pancreatic enzymes in chronic pancreatitis and other disorders; they can also treat steatorrhea caused by certain conditions. The antiflatulent *simethicone* is used to treat flatulence, gastric bloating, postoperative gas pain, and other conditions that may cause gas retention. *Sucralfate* is used to treat and prevent duodenal ulcers. *Tegaserod* may be used in short-term treatment of irritable bowel syndrome that features constipation. *Ursodiol* is used primarily to treat gallstone disease and prevent gallstone development.

Action: Miscellaneous GI agents act in different ways. *Balsalazide* diminishes colon inflammation by changing intestinal microflora, altering prostaglandin production, and inhibiting the function of mast cells, neutrophils, and macrophages. *Infliximab* binds to and inhibits tumor necrosis factor, producing GI anti-inflammatory effects. Among the other GI anti-inflammatory drugs, *mesalamine* acts locally to inhibit the production of arachidonic acid metabolites; *olsalazine* is converted to mesalamine by

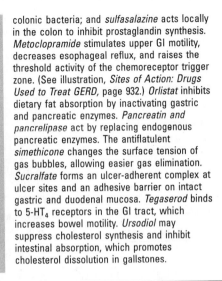

colonic bacteria; and *sulfasalazine* acts locally in the colon to inhibit prostaglandin synthesis. *Metoclopramide* stimulates upper GI motility, decreases esophageal reflux, and raises the threshold activity of the chemoreceptor trigger zone. (See illustration, *Sites of Action: Drugs Used to Treat GERD,* page 932.) *Orlistat* inhibits dietary fat absorption by inactivating gastric and pancreatic enzymes. *Pancreatin and pancrelipase* act by replacing endogenous pancreatic enzymes. The antiflatulent *simethicone* changes the surface tension of gas bubbles, allowing easier gas elimination. *Sucralfate* forms an ulcer-adherent complex at ulcer sites and an adhesive barrier on intact gastric and duodenal mucosa. *Tegaserod* binds to 5-HT$_4$ receptors in the GI tract, which increases bowel motility. *Ursodiol* may suppress cholesterol synthesis and inhibit intestinal absorption, which promotes cholesterol dissolution in gallstones.

COMBINATION PRODUCTS

EXTRA STRENGTH MAALOX: simethicone/magnesium hydroxide (an antacid)/aluminum hydroxide (an antacid) 20 mg/200 mg/200 mg; 40 mg/400 mg/400 mg.

GELUSIL: simethicone/aluminum hydroxide (an antacid)/magnesium hydroxide (an antacid) 25 mg/ 200 mg/200 mg.

IMODIUM ADVANCED: simethicone/ loperamide (an antidiarrheal) 125 mg/2 mg.

MAALOX PLUS: simethicone/aluminum hydroxide (an antacid)/magnesium hydroxide (an antacid) 25 mg/ 200 mg/200 mg.

MYLANTA: simethicone/magnesium hydroxide (an antacid)/aluminum hydroxide (an antacid) 20 mg/ 200 mg/200 mg; 40 mg/400 mg/ 400 mg.

SILAIN-GEL: simethicone/magnesium

hydroxide (an antacid)/aluminum hydroxide (an antacid).

balsalazide
ball-**sall**-ah-zide
(Colazal)

CATEGORY AND SCHEDULE
Pregnancy Risk Category: B

MECHANISM OF ACTION
A 5-aminosalicylic acid derivative that changes intestinal microflora, altering prostaglandin production, inhibiting function of natural killer cells, mast cells, neutrophils, macrophages. *Therapeutic Effect:* Diminishes inflammatory effect in colon.

AVAILABILITY
Capsules: 750 mg.

INDICATIONS AND DOSAGES
▶ **Ulcerative colitis**
PO
Adults, Elderly. Three 750 mg capsules 3 times/day for duration of 8 weeks.

CONTRAINDICATIONS
Hypersensitivity to salicylates

SIDE EFFECTS
Frequent (8%–6%)
Headache, abdominal pain, nausea, diarrhea
Occasional (4%–2%)
Vomiting, arthralgia, rhinitis, insomnia, fatigue, flatulence, coughing, dyspepsia

SERIOUS REACTIONS
• Liver toxicity occurs rarely.

NURSING CONSIDERATIONS
Baseline Assessment
• Assess the patient's serum chemistry lab values including BUN, serum alkaline phosphatase, bilirubin, creatinine, SGOT (AST), and SGPT (ALT) levels to assess liver and renal function.
Precautions
• Use cautiously in patients with liver or renal impairment.
Intervention and Evaluation
• Monitor the patient's bowel sounds for peristalsis.
• Assess the patient's daily pattern of bowel activity and stool consistency.
• Evaluate the patient for abdominal discomfort.
• Monitor the patient's blood serum chemistry for liver function test abnormalities.
Patient Teaching
• Instruct the patient to take balsalazide as directed.
• Teach the patient not to chew or open balsalazide capsules.

• Warn the patient to notify the physician if he or she experiences abdominal pain, severe headache or chest pain, or unresolved diarrhea.

infliximab
in-**flicks**-ih-mab
(Remicade)
Do not confuse with Reminyl.

CATEGORY AND SCHEDULE
Pregnancy Risk Category: C

MECHANISM OF ACTION
A monoclonal antibody that binds to tumor necrosis factor (TNF), inhibits functional activity of TNF. *Therapeutic Effect:* Reduces infiltration of inflammatory cells, decreases inflamed areas of the intestine.

PHARMACOKINETICS

Diagnosis	Onset	Peak	Duration
Crohn's	1–2 wks	N/A	8–48 wks
Rheumatoid arthritis (RA)	3–7 days	N/A	6–12 wks

Absorbed into the gastrointestinal (GI) tissue; primarily distributed in the vascular compartment. **Half-life:** 9.5 days.

AVAILABILITY
Powder for Injection: 100 mg.

INDICATIONS AND DOSAGES
▶ **Moderate to severe Crohn's disease**
IV infusion
Adults, Elderly. 5 mg/kg as a single IV infusion.

▶ **Fistulizing Crohn's disease**
IV infusion
Adults, Elderly. Initially, 5 mg/kg followed with additional 5 mg/kg doses at 2 and 6 wks after the first infusion.
▶ **RA**
IV infusion
Adults, Elderly. 3 mg/kg; follow with additional doses at 2 and 6 wks after the first infusion: Then q8wks thereafter.

UNLABELED USES
Ankylosing spondylitis, sciatica

CONTRAINDICATIONS
Sensitivity to infliximab, murine proteins, sepsis, serious active infection

INTERACTIONS
Drug
Immunosuppressants: May reduce frequency of infusion reactions and antibodies to infliximab.
Live vaccines: May decrease immune response.
Herbal
None known.
Food
None known.

DIAGNOSTIC TEST EFFECTS
None known.

IV INCOMPATIBILITIES
Do not infuse infliximab concurrently in the same IV line with other agents.

SIDE EFFECTS
Frequent (22%–10%)
Headache, nausea, fatigue, fever
Occasional (9%–5%)
Fever or chills during infusion, pharyngitis, vomiting, pain, dizziness, bronchitis, rash, rhinitis, coughing, pruritus, sinusitis, myalgia, back pain

Rare (4%–1%)
Hypotension or hypertension, paresthesia, anxiety, depression, insomnia, diarrhea, urinary tract infection

SERIOUS REACTIONS
• There is a potential for hypersensitivity reaction and lupus-like syndrome.

NURSING CONSIDERATIONS
Baseline Assessment
• Assess the patient's daily pattern of bowel activity and stool consistency.
• Establish the patient's baseline hydration status by examining the mucous membranes for dryness, skin turgor, and urinary status.
Lifespan Considerations
• Be aware that it is unknown if infliximab is distributed in breast milk.
• Be aware that the safety and efficacy of infliximab have not been established in children.
• Use infliximab cautiously in the elderly due to a higher rate of infection.
Precautions
• Use cautiously in patients with a history of recurrent infections.
Administration and Handling
IV
• Refrigerate vials.
• Reconstitute each vial with 10 ml Sterile Water for Injection, using 21-gauge or smaller needle. Direct the stream of sterile water to the glass wall of the vial.
• Swirl the vial gently to dissolve the contents. Do not shake.
• Allow the solution to stand for 5 minutes.
• Because infliximab is a protein, the solution may develop a few translucent particles; do not use if particles are opaque or foreign particles are present.

• Know that the solution normally appears colorless to light yellow and opalescent; do not use if discolored.
• Withdraw and waste a volume of 0.9% NaCl from a 250-ml bag to equal the volume of reconstituted solution to be injected into the 250-ml bag, which is approximately 10 ml. Total dose to be infused should equal 250 ml.
• Slowly add the reconstituted infliximab solution to the 250-ml infusion bag. Gently mix. Infusion concentration should range between 0.4 and 4 mg/ml.
• Begin infusion within 3 hours after reconstitution.
• Administer IV infusion over more than 2 hours, using set with a low-protein-binding filter.

Intervention and Evaluation
• Monitor the patient's blood pressure (B/P), erythrocyte sedimentation rate (ESR), and urinalysis.
• Monitor the patient for signs of infection.
• Evaluate the abdominal pain, C-reactive protein, and stool frequency in patients with Crohn's disease.
• Evaluate the rheumatoid arthritis patient for C-reactive protein and a decrease in pain, stiffness, and swollen joints.

Patient Teaching
• Tell the patient to expect follow-up tests, such as erythrocyte sedimentation rate (ESR), C-reactive protein levels, and urinalysis.
• Tell the patient to report signs of infection, such as fever.
• Instruct the rheumatoid arthritis patient to report an increase in pain, stiffness, and swelling of joints.
• Tell the Crohn's disease patient to report changes in stool pattern, color or consistency.

mesalamine (5-aminosalicylic acid, 5-ASA)
mess-al-ah-meen
(Asacol, Fiv-ASA, Mesasal[CAN], Pentasa, Rowasa, Salofalk[CAN])
Do not confuse with Os-Cal.

CATEGORY AND SCHEDULE
Pregnancy Risk Category: B

MECHANISM OF ACTION
A salicylic acid derivative that produces local inhibitory effect on arachidonic acid metabolite production, which is increased in patients with chronic inflammatory bowel disease. *Therapeutic Effect:* Blocks prostaglandin production, diminishes inflammation in colon.

PHARMACOKINETICS
Poorly absorbed from colon. Moderately absorbed from the gastrointestinal (GI) tract. Metabolized in liver to active metabolite. Unabsorbed portion eliminated in feces; absorbed portion excreted in urine. Unknown if removed by hemodialysis. **Half-life:** 0.5–1.5 hrs; metabolite: 5–10 hrs.

AVAILABILITY
Tablets (delayed-release): 400 mg.
Capsules (controlled-release): 250 mg.
Suppository: 500 mg.
Rectal Suspension: 4 g/60 ml.

INDICATIONS AND DOSAGES
▸ **Ulcerative colitis, proctosigmoiditis, proctitis**
PO (Asacol)
Adults, Elderly. 800 mg 3 times/day for 6 wks.
Children. 50 mg/kg/day q8–12h.
PO (Pentasa)

Adults, Elderly. 1 g 4 times/day for
8 wks.
Children. 50 mg/kg/day q6–12h.
Rectal (retention enema)
Adults, Elderly. 60 ml (4 g) at
bedtime; retain overnight, about
8 hrs, for 3–6 wks.
Rectal (suppository)
Adults, Elderly. 1 suppository
(500 mg) 2 times/day, retain
1–3 hrs for 3–6 wks.
▸ **Maintenance of remission, ulcera-
tive colitis**
PO (Asacol)
Adults, Elderly. 1.6 g/day in divided
doses.
PO (Pentasa)
Adults, Elderly. 1 g 4 times/day

CONTRAINDICATIONS
None known

INTERACTIONS
Drug
None known.
Herbal
None known.
Food
None known.

DIAGNOSTIC TEST EFFECTS
May increase BUN, serum alkaline
phosphatase, creatinine, SGOT
(AST), and SGPT (ALT) levels.

SIDE EFFECTS
Generally well tolerated, with only
mild and transient effects.
Frequent (greater than 6%)
PO: Abdominal cramps or pain,
diarrhea, dizziness, headache, nau-
sea, vomiting, rhinitis, unusual
tiredness
Rectal: Abdominal or stomach
cramps, flatulence, headache, nausea
Occasional (6%–2%)
PO: Hair loss, decreased appetite,
back or joint pain, flatulence, acne
Rectal: Hair loss

Rare (less than 2%)
Rectal: Anal irritation

SERIOUS REACTIONS
• Sulfite sensitivity in susceptible
patients noted as cramping, headache, diarrhea, fever, rash, hives,
itching, and wheezing. Discontinue
drug immediately.
• Hepatitis, pancreatitis, and pericarditis occur rarely with oral dosage.

NURSING CONSIDERATIONS
Baseline Assessment
• Expect to obtain baseline BUN,
serum alkaline phosphatase, creatinine, SGOT (AST), and SGPT
(ALT) levels.
• Ask the patient if he or she has an
allergy to sulfa-based products,
before administering drug.
Lifespan Considerations
• Be aware that it is unknown if
mesalamine crosses the placenta or
is distributed in breast milk.
• Be aware that the safety and
efficacy of mesalamine have not
been established in children.
• In the elderly, age-related renal
impairment may require cautious
use.
Precautions
• Use cautiously in patients with
preexisting renal disease and sul-
fasalazine sensitivity.
Administration and Handling
◀ALERT▶ Store rectal suspension,
suppository, and oral forms at room
temperature.
PO
• Have patient swallow whole; do
not break outer coating of tablet.
• Give mesalamine without regard
to food.
Rectal
• Shake bottle well.
• Instruct patient to lie on left side
with lower leg extended, upper leg

flexed forward, or to assume the knee-chest position.
• Insert applicator tip into rectum, pointing toward umbilicus.
• Squeeze bottle steadily until contents are emptied. Tell the patient to try to retain the enema for as long as tolerable, preferably for a minimum of 8 hours.

Intervention and Evaluation
• Encourage the patient to maintain adequate fluid intake.
• Assess the patient's bowel sounds for peristalsis.
• Assess the patient's daily pattern of bowel activity and stool consistency and record time of evacuation.
• Evaluate the patient for abdominal disturbances.
• Assess the patient's skin for rash and urticaria.
• Discontinue the medication if cramping, diarrhea, fever, or rash occurs.

Patient Teaching
• Warn the patient to avoid tasks that require mental alertness or motor skills until his or her response to the drug is established.
• Tell the patient that mesalamine use may discolor his or her urine yellow-brown.
• Explain to the patient that mesalamine suppositories stain fabrics.

metoclopramide
See antiemetics

olsalazine sodium
ol-**sal**-ah-zeen
(Dipentum)

CATEGORY AND SCHEDULE
Pregnancy Risk Category: C

MECHANISM OF ACTION
A salicylic acid derivative that is converted in colon by bacterial action to mesalamine. Blocks prostaglandin production in bowel mucosa. *Therapeutic Effect:* Reduces colonic inflammation in inflammatory bowel disease.

AVAILABILITY
Capsules: 250 mg.

INDICATIONS AND DOSAGES
▸ **Maintenance of controlled ulcerative colitis**
PO
Adults, Elderly. 1 g/day in 2 divided doses, preferably q12h.

UNLABELED USES
Treatment of inflammatory bowel disease

CONTRAINDICATIONS
History of hypersensitivity to salicylates

INTERACTIONS
Drug
None known.
Herbal
None known.
Food
None known.

DIAGNOSTIC TEST EFFECTS
May increase SGOT (AST) and SGPT (ALT) levels.

SIDE EFFECTS
Frequent (10%–5%)
Headache, diarrhea, abdominal pain or cramps, nausea
Occasional (5%–1%)
Depression, fatigue, dyspepsia, upper respiratory infection, decreased appetite, rash, itching, arthralgia

Rare (less than 1%)
Dizziness, vomiting, stomatitis

SERIOUS REACTIONS
• Sulfite sensitivity in susceptible patients noted as cramping, headache, diarrhea, fever, rash, hives, itching, and wheezing may occur. Discontinue drug immediately.
• Excessive diarrhea associated with extreme fatigue is noted rarely.

NURSING CONSIDERATIONS
Baseline Assessment
• Expect to obtain baseline serum alkaline phosphatase, SGOT (AST), and SGPT (ALT) levels.
• Ask the patient if he or she has an allergy to sulfa-based products, before administering drug.
Precautions
• Use cautiously in patients with preexisting renal disease.
Administration and Handling
PO
• Give olsalazine with food in evenly divided doses.
Intervention and Evaluation
• Assess the patient's bowel sounds for peristalsis.
• Assess the patient's daily bowel activity and stool consistency and record time of evacuation.
• Evaluate the patient for abdominal disturbances.
• Assess the patient's skin for hives and rash.
• Discontinue the medication if the patient experiences cramping, diarrhea, fever, and rash.
Patient Teaching
• Warn the patient to notify physician if he or she experiences persistent or increasing cramping, diarrhea, fever, pruritus, and rash.
• Encourage the patient to maintain adequate fluid intake.

orlistat
ore-leh-stat
(Xenical)

CATEGORY AND SCHEDULE
Pregnancy Risk Category: B

MECHANISM OF ACTION
A gastric and pancreatic lipase inhibitor that inhibits absorption of dietary fats by inactivating gastric and pancreatic enzymes. *Therapeutic Effect:* Results in a caloric deficit that may have a positive effect on weight control.

PHARMACOKINETICS
Minimal absorption after administration. Protein binding: greater than 99%. Primarily eliminated unchanged in feces. Unknown if removed by hemodialysis. **Half-life:** 1–2 hrs.

AVAILABILITY
Capsules: 120 mg.

INDICATIONS AND DOSAGES
▸ **Weight reduction**
PO
Adults, Elderly. 120 mg 3 times/day.

CONTRAINDICATIONS
Cholestasis, chronic malabsorption syndrome

INTERACTIONS
Drug
Pravastatin: May increase the blood concentration and risk of rhabdomyolysis.
Herbal
None known.
Food
None known.

DIAGNOSTIC TEST EFFECTS
Decreases blood glucose and total cholesterol levels, and serum LDL concentrations. Decreases absorption and levels of vitamins A and E.

SIDE EFFECTS
Frequent (30%–20%)
Headache, abdominal discomfort, flatulence, fecal urgency, fatty or oily stool
Occasional (14%–5%)
Back pain, menstrual irregularity, nausea, fatigue, diarrhea, dizziness
Rare (less than 4%)
Anxiety, rash, myalgia, dry skin, vomiting

SERIOUS REACTIONS
• None known.

NURSING CONSIDERATIONS
Baseline assessment
• Expect to obtain baseline lab studies, such as blood glucose levels and a lipid profile.
• Obtain an accurate assessment of height and weight to help determine weight loss goals.
• Plan to consult a registered dietician to review the patient's current diet, and to make dietary recommendations.
Lifespan Considerations
• Be aware that it is unknown if orlistat is excreted in breast milk. Orlistat use is not recommended during pregnancy or in breast-feeding women.
• Be aware that the safety and efficacy of orlistat have not been established in children.
• There are no age-related precautions noted in the elderly.
Administration and Handling
◀ALERT▶ Know that the side effects tend to be mild and transient in nature, gradually diminishing during treatment.
PO
• Give orlistat without regard to food.
Intervention and Evaluation
• Monitor the patient's blood glucose and cholesterol levels, and serum LDL concentrations.
• Monitor the patient for changes in coagulation parameters.
Patient Teaching
• Instruct the patient to maintain a nutritionally balanced, reduced-calorie diet. Teach the patient to distribute his or her daily intake of carbohydrates, fat, and protein over three main meals.
• Tell the patient that some of the unpleasant side effects, such as flatulence and urgency, should diminish with time.

pancreatin
pan-kree-**ah**-tin
(Ku-Zyme, Pancreatin)
pancrelipase
pan-kree-**lie**-pace
(Cotazym, Cotazym-S Forte[AUS], Creon, Pancrease[CAN], Pancrease MT, Ultrase, Viokase)

CATEGORY AND SCHEDULE
Pregnancy Risk Category: C

MECHANISM OF ACTION
A digestive enzyme that replaces endogenous pancreatic enzymes. *Therapeutic Effect:* Assists in digestion of protein, starch, fats.

AVAILABILITY
Tablets.
Capsules.

INDICATIONS AND DOSAGES
▸ **Pancreatic enzyme replacement or supplement when enzymes are absent or deficient, such as with chronic pancreatitis, cystic fibrosis, or ductal obstruction from cancer of the pancreas or common bile duct, reduces malabsorption, treatment of steatorrhea associated with bowel resection or postgastrectomy syndrome**
PO
Adults, Elderly. 1–3 capsules or tablets before or with meals, snacks. May increase up to 8 tablets/dose.
Children. 1–2 tablets with meals, snacks.

CONTRAINDICATIONS
Acute pancreatitis, exacerbation of chronic pancreatitis, hypersensitivity to pork protein

INTERACTIONS
Drug
Antacids: May decrease the effects of pancreatin and pancrelipase.
Iron supplements: May decrease the absorption of iron supplements.
Herbal
None known.
Food
None known.

DIAGNOSTIC TEST EFFECTS
May increase serum uric acid levels.

SIDE EFFECTS
Rare
Allergic reaction, mouth irritation, shortness of breath, wheezing

SERIOUS REACTIONS
• Excessive dosage may produce nausea, cramping, and diarrhea.
• Hyperuricosuria and hyperuricemia have been reported with extremely high dosages.

NURSING CONSIDERATIONS
Baseline Assessment
• Know that spilling Viokase powder on the hands may irritate skin.
• Know that inhaling powder may irritate mucous membranes and produce bronchospasm.
Lifespan Considerations
• Be aware that it is unknown if pancreatin or pancrelipase cross the placenta or are distributed in breast milk.
• Be aware that information is not available on pancreatin or pancrelipase use in children.
• There are no age-related precautions noted in the elderly.
Precautions
• Use pancreatin and pancrelipase cautiously because inhalation of the drug's powder form may precipitate an asthma attack.
Administration and Handling
PO
• Give pancreatin or pancrelipase before or with meals, snacks.
• Crush tablets as needed. Do not crush enteric-coated form.
Intervention and Evaluation
• Evaluate the patient for therapeutic relief from gastrointestinal (GI) symptoms.
• Advise the patient not to change brands of the drug without first consulting the physician.
Patient Teaching
• Instruct the patient not to chew capsules or tablet to minimize irritation to mouth, lips, and tongue. May open capsule and spread over applesauce, mashed fruit, or rice cereal.
• Warn the patient not to spill Viokase powder on the hands because it may irritate skin.
• Instruct the patient to avoid inhaling powder because it may irritate

mucous membranes and produce bronchospasm.

simethicone
sye-**meth**-ih-cone
(Alka-Seltzer Gas Relief, Gas-X, Genasym, Maalox AntiGas, Mylanta Gas, Ovol[CAN], Phazyme)

CATEGORY AND SCHEDULE
Pregnancy Risk Category: C
OTC

MECHANISM OF ACTION
An antiflatulent that changes surface tension of gas bubbles, allowing easier elimination of gas. *Therapeutic Effect:* Disperses, prevents formation of gas pockets in the gastrointestinal (GI) tract.

PHARMACOKINETICS
Does not appear to be absorbed from GI tract. Excreted unchanged in feces.

AVAILABILITY
Softgel: 125 mg, 180 mg.
Oral Suspension Drops: 40 mg/0.6 ml.
Tablets (chewable): 80 mg, 125 mg.

INDICATIONS AND DOSAGES
▸ **Antiflatulent**
PO
Adults, Elderly, Children older than 12 yrs. 40–250 mg after meals and at bedtime. Maximum: 500 mg/day.
Children 2–12 yrs. 40 mg 4 times/day.
Children younger than 2 yrs. 20 mg 4 times/day.

UNLABELED USES
Adjunct to bowel radiography, gastroscopy

CONTRAINDICATIONS
None known

INTERACTIONS
Drug
None known.
Herbal
None known.
Food
None known.

DIAGNOSTIC TEST EFFECTS
None known.

SIDE EFFECTS
None known.

SERIOUS REACTIONS
• None known.

NURSING CONSIDERATIONS
Baseline Assessment
• Prior to administration, assess the patient's abdomen for signs of tenderness, rigidity, and the presence of bowel sounds.
• Determine when the patient last had a bowel movement, and find out the amount and consistency.
Lifespan Considerations
• Be aware that it is unknown if simethicone crosses the placenta or is distributed in breast milk.
• This drug may be used safely in children and the elderly.
Administration and Handling
PO
• Give simethicone after meals and at bedtime as needed. Chew tablets thoroughly before swallowing.
• Shake suspension well before using.

Intervention and Evaluation
• Evaluate the patient for therapeutic response, relief of abdominal bloating and flatulence.

Patient Teaching
• Urge the patient to avoid carbonated beverages during simethicone therapy.
• Instruct the patient to chew tablets thoroughly before swallowing.

sucralfate
sue-**kral**-fate
(Carafate, Novo-Sucralate[CAN], Sulcrate[CAN], Ulcyte[AUS])
Do not confuse with Cafergot.

CATEGORY AND SCHEDULE
Pregnancy Risk Category: B

MECHANISM OF ACTION
An antiulcer agent that forms an ulcer-adherent complex with proteinaceous exudate, such as albumin, at ulcer site. Also forms a viscous, adhesive barrier on surface of intact mucosa of stomach or duodenum. *Therapeutic Effect:* Protects damaged mucosa from further destruction by absorbing gastric acid, pepsin, bile salts.

PHARMACOKINETICS
Minimally absorbed from the gastrointestinal (GI) tract. Eliminated in feces with small amount excreted in urine. Not removed by hemodialysis.

AVAILABILITY
Tablets: 1 g.
Oral Suspension: 500 mg/ 5 ml.

INDICATIONS AND DOSAGES
▶ **Duodenal ulcers, active**
PO
Adults, Elderly. 1 g 4 times/day (before meals and at bedtime) for up to 8 wks.
▶ **Duodenal ulcers, maintenance**
PO
Adults, Elderly. 1 g 2 times/day.

UNLABELED USES
Prevention and treatment of stress-related mucosal damage, especially in acutely ill patients, treatment of gastric ulcer, rheumatoid arthritis—relieves GI symptoms associated with NSAIDs, treatment of gastroesophageal reflux disease (GERD)

CONTRAINDICATIONS
None known

INTERACTIONS
Drug
Antacids: May interfere with binding; do not give within 30 minutes of sucralfate.
Digoxin, phenytoin, quinolones, such as ciprofloxacin, theophylline: May decrease the absorption of digoxin, phenytoin, quinolones, and theophylline; do not give within 2–3 hrs of sucralfate.
Herbal
None known.
Food
None known.

DIAGNOSTIC TEST EFFECTS
None known.

SIDE EFFECTS
Frequent (2%)
Constipation
Occasional (less than 2%)
Dry mouth, backache, diarrhea, dizziness, drowsiness, nausea,

indigestion, skin rash, hives, itching, stomach discomfort

SERIOUS REACTIONS
• None known.

NURSING CONSIDERATIONS

Baseline Assessment
• Prior to administration, assess the patient's abdomen for signs of tenderness, rigidity, and the presence of bowel sounds.
• Determine when the patient last had a bowel movement, and find out the amount and consistency.

Lifespan Considerations
• Be aware that it is unknown if sucralfate crosses the placenta or is distributed in breast milk.
• Be aware that the safety and efficacy of sucralfate have not been established in children.
• There are no age-related precautions noted in the elderly.

Administration and Handling
◀ALERT▶ Know that 1 g equals 10 ml suspension.
PO
• Administer 1 hour before meals and at bedtime.
• Tablets may be crushed or dissolved in water.
• Avoid antacids 30 minutes before or after giving sucralfate.

Intervention and Evaluation
• Assess the patient's daily pattern of bowel activity and stool consistency.

Patient Teaching
• Instruct the patient to take sucralfate on an empty stomach. Teach the patient that antacids may be given as an adjunct to other drugs, but should not be taken for 30 minutes before or after sucralfate because the formation of sucralfate gel is activated by stomach acid.

• Suggest sips of tepid water or sour hard candy to the patient to relieve dry mouth.

sulfasalazine
See miscellaneous anti-infectives

tegaserod
te-**gas**-err-odd
(Zelnorm)

CATEGORY AND SCHEDULE
Pregnancy Risk Category: B

MECHANISM OF ACTION
An anti-irritable bowel syndrome (IBS) agent that binds to 5-HT$_4$ receptors in the gastrointestinal (GI) tract. *Therapeutic Effect:* Triggers a peristaltic reflex in the gut, increasing bowel motility.

PHARMACOKINETICS
Rapidly absorbed. Widely distributed. Protein binding: 98%. Metabolized by hydrolysis in the stomach and oxidation and conjugation of the primary metabolite. Primarily excreted in feces. **Half-life:** 11 hrs.

AVAILABILITY
Tablets: 2 mg, 6 mg.

INDICATIONS AND DOSAGES
▸ **Irritable bowel syndrome (IBS)**
PO
Adults, Elderly women. 6 mg 2 times/day for 4–6 wks.

CONTRAINDICATIONS
Abdominal adhesions, diarrhea, history of bowel obstruction, moderate to severe liver impairment, severe renal impairment, suspected

sphincter of Oddi dysfunction, symptomatic gallbladder disease

INTERACTIONS
Drug
None known.
Herbal
None known.
Food
None known.

DIAGNOSTIC TEST EFFECTS
None known.

SIDE EFFECTS
Frequency (greater than 5%)
Headache, abdominal pain, diarrhea, nausea, flatulence
Occasional (5%–2%)
Dizziness, migraine, back pain, leg pain

SERIOUS REACTIONS
• None known.

NURSING CONSIDERATIONS
Baseline Assessment
• Assess the patient for diarrhea; avoid tegaserod use in these patients.
Lifespan Considerations
• Be aware that it is unknown if tegaserod is distributed in breast milk.
• Be aware that the safety and efficacy of tegaserod have not been established in children.
• There are no age-related precautions noted in the elderly.
Administration and Handling
PO
• Give tegaserod before meals.
• Crush tablets as needed.
Intervention and Evaluation
• Evaluate the patient for an improvement in symptoms, relief from abdominal discomfort, bloating, cramping, and urgency.

Patient Teaching
• Instruct the patient to take tegaserod before meals.
• Warn the patient to notify the physician if he or she experiences new or worsening episodes of abdominal pain.

ursodiol
er-**sew**-dee-ol
(Actigall, Urso)

CATEGORY AND SCHEDULE
Pregnancy Risk Category: B

MECHANISM OF ACTION
A gallstone solubilizing agent that suppresses hepatic synthesis, secretion of cholesterol and inhibits intestinal absorption of cholesterol.
Therapeutic Effect: Changes the bile of patients with gallstones from precipitating—or capable of forming crystals—to cholesterol solubilizing—or capable of being dissolved.

AVAILABILITY
Capsules: 300 mg.
Tablets: 250 mg.

INDICATIONS AND DOSAGES
▸ **Dissolution of radiolucent, non-calcified gallstones when cholescyctectomy is an unacceptable method of treatment, treatment of biliary cirrhosis**
PO
Adults, Elderly. 8–10 mg/kg/day in 2–3 divided doses. Treatment may require months of therapy. Obtain ultrasound image of gallbladder at 6-mo intervals for first year. If dissolved, continue therapy and repeat ultrasound within 1–3 mos.
▸ **Prevention of gallstones**
PO
Adults, Elderly. 300 mg 2 times/day.

UNLABELED USES

Treatment of alcoholic cirrhosis, biliary atresia, chronic hepatitis, gallstone formation, prophylaxis of liver transplant rejection, sclerosing cholangitis

CONTRAINDICATIONS

Allergy to bile acids, calcified cholesterol stones, chronic liver disease, radiolucent bile pigment stones, radiopaque stones

INTERACTIONS

Drug

Aluminum-containing antacids, cholestyramine: May decrease the absorption and effects of ursodiol.
Estrogens, oral contraceptives: May decrease the effects of ursodiol.

Herbal

None known.

Food

None known.

DIAGNOSTIC TEST EFFECTS

May alter liver functions tests.

SIDE EFFECTS

Occasional
Diarrhea

SERIOUS REACTIONS

• None significant.

NURSING CONSIDERATIONS

Baseline Assessment
• Obtain the patient's blood serum chemistry values including BUN, serum alkaline phosphatase, bilirubin, creatinine, SGOT (AST), and SGPT (ALT) levels to assess hepatic function before beginning ursodiol therapy, and after 1 and 3 months of therapy, and every 6 months thereafter.

Intervention and Evaluation
• Monitor the patient's liver function tests.
• Assess the patient for abdominal pain, especially right upper quadrant pain, nausea, and vomiting.

Patient Teaching
• Explain to the patient that treatment requires months of ursodiol therapy.
• Instruct the patient to avoid taking antacids within hours of taking ursodiol.

54 Anticoagulants

argatroban
bivalirudin
dalteparin sodium
desirudin
enoxaparin sodium
fondaparinux sodium
heparin sodium
lepirudin
tinzaparin sodium
warfarin sodium

Uses: Subclasses of anticoagulants have somewhat different indications. *Heparin* is used to treat pulmonary embolism, evolving stroke, and massive deep vein thrombosis (DVT). It's also used as an adjunct to thrombolytics to treat acute myocardial infarction (MI) and in low doses to prevent postoperative venous thrombosis. *Low-molecular-weight (LMW) heparins* are used to prevent DVT after hip or knee replacement surgery and to treat DVT, ischemic stroke, pulmonary embolism, and non Q-wave MI. *Thrombin inhibitors* are prescribed for preventing and treating thrombosis in heparin-induced thrombocytopenia (HIT) and for preventing HIT during percutaneous coronary procedures. *Warfarin* is used to prevent venous thrombosis and associated pulmonary embolism.

Action: Each anticoagulant subclass acts by a different mechanism. *Heparin* combines with antithrombin III, accelerating the anticoagulant cascade that prevents thrombosis formation. (See illustration, *Mechanisms and Sites of Action: Hematologic Agents,* page 988.) It inhibits the action of thrombin and factor Xa. By preventing the conversion of fibrinogen to fibrin, heparin prevents the formation of fibrin clots. *LMW heparins,* such as dalteparin and enoxaparin, are composed of shorter molecules than those in standard heparin. These agents preferentially inactivate factor Xa. *Thrombin inhibitors,* such as argatroban and bivalirudin, reversibly inhibit thrombin by binding to its receptor sites. *Warfarin* suppresses coagulation by acting as a vitamin-K antagonist. It does this by blocking the synthesis of vitamin K-dependent factors (factors VII, IX, X, and prothrombin).

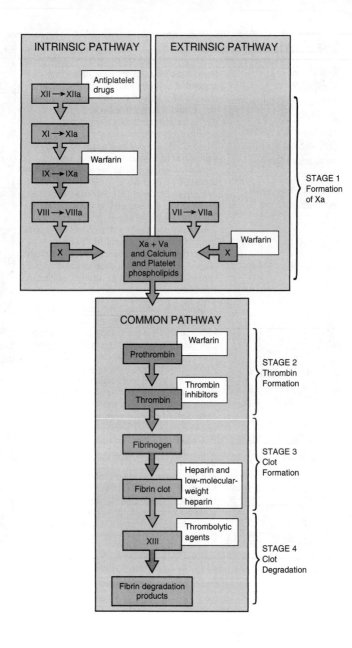

Mechanisms and Sites of Action: Hematologic Agents

Hemostasis causes the formation of a fibrin-platelet meshwork (clot) to stop bleeding. It results from activation of the coagulation cascade, which consists of intrinsic, extrinsic, and common pathways. Drugs that affect hemostasis include anticoagulants and antiplatelets (which prevent clot formation) and thrombolytics (which dissolve already-formed clots).

Different anticoagulants act at various points in the cascade. For example, heparin enhances antithrombin III in the plasma to inactivate factor Xa. As a result, prothrombin can't be converted to thrombin, which prevents fibrinogen from forming fibrin, a major clot component. Low-molecular-weight heparins, such as dalteparin, also inactivate factor Xa and thrombin by enhancing antithrombin III, ultimately preventing fibrinogen from forming fibrin. Thrombin inhibitors, such as argatroban, reversibly inhibit thrombin by binding to its receptor sites. This action prevents the conversion of fibrinogen to a fibrin clot. Warfarin depletes vitamin K-dependent factors X, IX, VII, and prothrombin. Consequently new clots can't form, and pre-existing clots can't extend.

Antiplatelet drugs inhibit platelet aggregation—and clotting—in different ways. Platelet aggregation and adhesion starts at the beginning of the clotting cascade that ultimately results in inactivated factor X. Aspirin inhibits cyclooxygenase and blocks the production of thromboxane A_2, a substance that causes vasoconstriction and platelet aggregation. Ticlopidine alters platelet membranes, preventing them from interacting. Dipyridamole stimulates prostacyclin release, which blocks thromboxane A_2 formation. Adenosine diphosphate (ADP) receptor antagonists, such as clopidogrel, block ADP receptors on platelets, inhibiting their aggregation. GP IIb/IIIa receptor inhibitors, such as abciximab, prevent fibrinogen from binding to GP IIb/IIIa receptors on platelets, rapidly inhibiting platelet aggregation.

Thrombolytic agents, such as streptokinase, break down clots that have already formed. They trigger the conversion of plasminogen to plasmin, an enzyme that dissolves fibrin clots into fibrin degradation products.

argatroban
our-ga-**trow**-ban
(Acova)

CATEGORY AND SCHEDULE
Pregnancy Risk Category: B

MECHANISM OF ACTION
A direct thrombin inhibitor that reversibly binds to thrombin active sites. Inhibits thrombin catalyzed or induced reactions, including fibrin formation, activation of coagulant factors V, VIII, and XIII; protein C; and platelet aggregation. *Therapeutic Effect:* Produces anticoagulation.

PHARMACOKINETICS
Following IV administration, distributed primarily in extracellular fluid. Protein binding: 54%. Metabolized in the liver. Primarily excreted in the feces, presumably through biliary secretion. **Half-life:** 39–51 min.

AVAILABILITY
Injection: 100 mg/ml.

INDICATIONS AND DOSAGES
▶ **Prevent and treat heparin-induced thrombocytopenia (HIT)**
IV infusion
Adults, Elderly. Initially, 2 mcg/kg/min administered as a continuous infusion. After initial infusion, dose may be adjusted until steady state aPTT is 1.5–3 times initial baseline value not to exceed 100 sec.

▸ **Dosage in hepatic impairment**
Adults, Elderly. Initially, 0.5 mcg/kg/min.

CONTRAINDICATIONS
Overt major bleeding

INTERACTIONS
Drug
Antiplatelet agents, thrombolytics, other anticoagulants: May increase the risk of bleeding.
Herbal
None known.
Food
None known.

DIAGNOSTIC TEST EFFECTS
Increased active partial thromboplastin time (aPTT), international normalized ratio (INR), and prothrombin time (PT)

IV INCOMPATIBILITIES
Do not mix with any other medications or solutions.

SIDE EFFECTS
Frequent (8%–3%)
Dyspnea, hypotension, fever, diarrhea, nausea, pain, vomiting, infection, cough

SERIOUS REACTIONS
• Ventricular tachycardia and atrial fibrillation occur occasionally.
• Major bleeding and sepsis occur rarely.

NURSING CONSIDERATIONS

Baseline Assessment
• Evaluate the patient's complete blood count (CBC).
• Check the patient's PT and aPTT levels.
• Expect to obtain the patient's blood pressure (B/P) before beginning therapy.

• Minimize any procedures that involve puncturing the skin. Avoid numerous blood draws, catheter insertions, and drug injection sites.
Lifespan Considerations
• Be aware that it is unknown if argatroban is excreted in breast milk.
• Be aware that the safety and efficacy of argatroban have not been established in children less than 18 years of age.
• There are no age-related precautions noted in the elderly.
Precautions
• Use cautiously in patients with congenital or acquired bleeding disorders, liver function impairment, severe hypertension, or ulcerations.
• Use cautiously in patients immediately following administration of spinal anesthesia, lumbar puncture, and major surgery.
Administration and Handling
IV
• Discard the solution if it appears cloudy or has an insoluble precipitate.
• Following reconstitution, the solution is stable for 24 hours at room temperature, 48 hours if refrigerated.
• Avoid exposing the solution to direct sunlight.
• Dilute the solution 100-fold prior to infusion in 0.9% NaCl, D_5W, or lactated Ringer's to provide a final concentration of 1 mg/ml.
• Mix the solution by repeated inversion of the diluent bag for 1 minute.
• Following reconstitution, the solution may briefly appear hazy from the formation of microprecipitates. These rapidly dissolve when the solution is mixed.
• The rate of administration is based on body weight at 2 mcg/kg/min (e.g., 50-kg patient infuse at 6 ml/hr).

Intervention and Evaluation
• Assess the patient for any signs of bleeding, such as bleeding at a surgical site, bleeding from the gums, bleeding from injection sites, blood in the stool, bruising, hematuria, and petechiae.
• Handle the patient carefully and as infrequently as possible to prevent bleeding. Do not obtain B/P in the lower extremities, because a deep vein thrombi may be present.
• Monitor the patient's ACT, aPTT, PT, and platelet count.
• Observe the patient for any complaints of abdominal or back pain, a decrease in B/P, an increase in pulse rate, and severe headache, which indicates evidence of hemorrhage.
• Monitor the patient for an increase in menstrual flow.
• Test the patient's urine output for hematuria.
• Monitor the patient for any occurring hematomas.
• Gently remove the patient's dressings and tape.

Patient Teaching
• Instruct the patient to use an electric razor and soft toothbrush to prevent bleeding.
• Warn the patient to report any sign of black or red stool, coffee-ground vomitus, red or dark urine, or red-speckled mucus from cough.

---

bivalirudin
bye-**vail**-ih-rhu-din
(Angiomax)

CATEGORY AND SCHEDULE
Pregnancy Risk Category: B

MECHANISM OF ACTION
An anticoagulant that specifically and reversibly inhibits thrombin by binding to its receptor sites. *Therapeutic Effect*: Decreases acute ischemic complications in patients with unstable angina pectoris.

PHARMACOKINETICS

Route	Onset	Peak	Duration
IV	Immediate	N/A	1 hr

Primarily eliminated by kidneys. **Half-life:** 25 min, half-life is increased with moderate to severe renal dysfunction; 25% is removed by hemodialysis.

AVAILABILITY
Injection, lyophilized: 250 mg.

INDICATIONS AND DOSAGES
▶ **Anticoagulant for unstable angina patients undergoing percutaneous transluminal coronary angioplasty (PTCA)**
IV
Adults, Elderly. 1 mg/kg given as IV bolus followed by a 4-hr IV infusion at rate of 2.5 mg/kg/hr. After initial 4-hr infusion is completed, give additional IV infusion at rate of 0.2 mg/kg/hr for 20 hrs or less, if necessary.
▶ **Dosage in renal impairment**

GRF	Dosage Reduced by
30–59 ml/min	20%
10–29 ml/min	60%
Dialysis	90%

CONTRAINDICATIONS
Active major bleeding

INTERACTIONS
Drug
Platelet aggregation inhibitors other than aspirin, thrombolytics,

warfarin: May increase the risk of bleeding complications.
Herbal
Ginkgo biloba: May increase the risk of bleeding.
Food
None known.

DIAGNOSTIC TEST EFFECTS

Prolongs activated partial thromboplastin time (aPTT) and prothrombin time (PT).

IV INCOMPATIBILITIES

Do not mix with any other medication.

SIDE EFFECTS

Frequent (42%)
Back pain
Occasional (15%–12%)
Nausea, headache, hypotension, generalized pain
Rare (8%–4%)
Injection site pain, insomnia, hypertension, anxiety, vomiting, pelvic or abdominal pain, bradycardia, nervousness, dyspepsia, fever, urinary retention

SERIOUS REACTIONS

• A hemorrhagic event occurs rarely and is characterized by fall in blood pressure (B/P) or Hct.

NURSING CONSIDERATIONS

Baseline Assessment
• Assess the patient's bleeding time, BUN, complete blood count (CBC), and serum creatinine to assess renal function.
• Establish the patient's baseline B/P.
Lifespan Considerations
• Be aware that it is unknown if bivalirudin is distributed in breast milk or crosses the placenta.
• Be aware that the safety and

efficacy of bivalirudin have not been established in children.
• In the elderly, age-related renal function impairment may require dosage adjustment.
Precautions
• Use cautiously in patients with conditions associated with increased risk of bleeding, including bacterial endocarditis, cerebrovascular accident (CVA), hemorrhagic diathesis, intracerebral surgery, recent major bleeding, recent major surgery, stroke, severe hypertension, severe liver or renal function impairment, and stroke.
Administration and Handling
◄ALERT► Intended for use with aspirin, 300–325 mg daily.
◄ALERT► Treatment should be initiated just prior to angioplasty.
IV
• Store unreconstituted vials at room temperature.
• Reconstituted solution may only be refrigerated for 24 hours or less.
• Diluted drug with a concentration of 0.5 to 5 mg/ml is stable at room temperature for 24 hours or less.
• To each 250-mg vial add 5 ml Sterile Water for Injection.
• Gently swirl until all material is dissolved.
• Further dilute each vial in 50 ml D_5W or 0.9% NaCl to yield final concentration of 5 mg/ml: 1 vial in 50 ml, 2 vials in 100 ml, 5 vials in 250 ml.
• If low-rate infusion is used after the initial infusion, reconstitute the 250-mg vial with added 5 ml Sterile Water for Injection.
• Gently swirl until all material is dissolved.
• Further dilute each vial in 500 ml D_5W or 0.9% NaCl to yield final concentration of 0.5 mg/ml.
• Produces a clear, colorless

solution; do not use if cloudy or contains a precipitate.
• Expect to adjust IV infusion based on aPTT or patient's body weight.

Intervention and Evaluation
• Monitor the patient's aPTT, BUN, Hct, serum creatinine, and stool or urine cultures for occult blood.
• Assess the patient for a decrease in blood pressure (B/P) and an increase in pulse rate.
• Determine the patient's discharge during menses and monitor for any increase.
• Assess the patient's urine for hematuria.

Patient Teaching
• Warn female patients that their menstrual flow may be heavier than usual.
• Instruct the patient to report signs of bleeding in the urine or stool.
• Urge the patient to report any pain or discomfort, especially chest pain, after treatment.
• Instruct the patient to remain on bed rest and to keep leg used during PTCA immobile, as ordered. Let the patient know to report bleeding from femoral vein site.

---

dalteparin sodium
dawl-teh-pear-in
(Fragmin)

CATEGORY AND SCHEDULE
Pregnancy Risk Category: B

MECHANISM OF ACTION
An antithrombin that in presence of low-molecular-weight heparin inhibits factor Xa and thrombin. Only slightly influences platelet aggregation, prothrombin time (PT), activated partial thromboplastin time (APTT). *Therapeutic Effect:* Produces anticoagulation.

PHARMACOKINETICS

Route	Onset	Peak	Duration
Subcutaneous	N/A	4 hrs	N/A

Protein binding: less than 10%.
Half-life: 3–5 hrs.

AVAILABILITY
Syringe: 2,500 units, 5,000 units, 7,500 units, 10,000 units, 25,000 units/ml.
Vial: 95,000 units (10,000 units/ml).

INDICATIONS AND DOSAGES
▸ **Low- to moderate-risk abdominal surgery**
Subcutaneous
Adults, Elderly. 2,500 units 1–2 hrs before surgery, then daily for 5–10 days.
▸ **High-risk abdominal surgery**
Subcutaneous
Adults, Elderly. 5,000 units 1–2 hrs before surgery, then daily for 5–10 days.
▸ **Total hip surgery**
Subcutaneous
Adults, Elderly. 2,500 units 1–2 hrs before surgery, then 2,500 units 6 hrs after surgery, then 5,000 units/day for 7–10 days.
▸ **Treatment unstable angina, non–Q-wave myocardial infarction (MI)**
Subcutaneous
Adults, Elderly. 120 units/kg q12h (Maximum: 10,000 units/dose) with concurrent aspirin until clinically stable.

CONTRAINDICATIONS
Active major bleeding, concurrent heparin therapy, hypersensitivity to dalteparin, heparin, or pork prod-

ucts, thrombocytopenia associated with positive in vitro test for anti-platelet antibody

INTERACTIONS
Drug
Anticoagulants, platelet inhibitors: May increase risk of bleeding.
Herbal
None known.
Food
None known.

DIAGNOSTIC TEST EFFECTS
Reversible increases in LDH concentrations, serum alkaline phosphatase, SGOT (AST), and SGPT (ALT) levels.

SIDE EFFECTS
Occasional (7%–3%)
Hematoma at injection site
Rare (less than 1%)
Hypersensitivity reaction (chills, fever, pruritus, urticaria, asthma, rhinitis, lacrimation, headache); mild, local skin irritation

SERIOUS REACTIONS
• Accidental overdosage may lead to bleeding complications ranging from local ecchymoses to major hemorrhage.
• Thrombocytopenia occurs rarely.

NURSING CONSIDERATIONS
Baseline Assessment
• Assess the patient's complete blood count (CBC).
• Establish the patient's baseline blood pressure (B/P).
Lifespan Considerations
• Be aware that this drug should be used with caution in pregnant women, particularly during the last trimester of pregnancy and immediately postpartum. Dalteparin use

increases the risk of maternal hemorrhage.
• Be aware that it is unknown if dalteparin is distributed in breast milk.
• Be aware that the safety and efficacy of dalteparin have not been established in children.
• There are no age-related precautions noted in the elderly.
Precautions
• Use cautiously in patients with bacterial endocarditis, conditions with increased risk of hemorrhage, history of heparin-induced thrombocytopenia or recent GI ulceration and hemorrhage, hypertensive or diabetic retinopathy, impaired liver or renal function, and uncontrolled arterial hypertension.
Administration and Handling
Subcutaneous
• Store at room temperature.
• Instruct the patient to sit or lie down before administering by deep subcutaneous injection.
• Inject in U-shaped area around the navel, upper outer side of thigh, or upper outer quadrangle of buttock.
• Use a fine needle (25 to 26 gauge) to minimize tissue trauma.
• Introduce entire length of needle (one half inch) into skin fold held between thumb and forefinger, holding needle during injection at a 45° to 90° angle.
• Do not rub injection site after administration to avoid bruising.
• Alternate the administration site with each injection.
Intervention and Evaluation
• Periodically monitor the patient's complete blood count (CBC) and stool for occult blood; no need for daily monitoring in patients with normal presurgical coagulation parameters.
• Assess the patient for any sign of bleeding, including bleeding at

surgical or injection sites, bleeding from gums, hematuria, blood in stool, bruising, hematuria, and petechiae.

Patient Teaching

• Explain to the patient that the usual length of dalteparin therapy is 5 to 10 days.

• Warn the patient to notify the physician of any signs of bleeding, breathing difficulty, bruising, dizziness, fever, itching, lightheadedness, rash, and swelling.

• Explain to the patient that he or she should not take any medications, including over-the-counter (OTC) drugs, without consulting the physician.

• Instruct the patient to rotate injection sites daily.

• Teach the patient the proper injection technique.

• Instruct the patient to perform an ice massage at the injection site shortly before injection to prevent excessive bruising.

desirudin
deh-**sear**-ew-din
(Iprivask)

CATEGORY AND SCHEDULE
Pregnancy Risk Category: C

MECHANISM OF ACTION
An anticoagulant that binds specifically and directly to thrombin, inhibiting free circulating and clot-bound thrombin. *Therapeutic Effect:* Prolongs the clotting time of human plasma.

PHARMACOKINETICS
Complete absorption. Distributed in extracellular space. Metabolized and eliminated by the kidney. **Half-life:** 2–3 hrs.

AVAILABILITY
Powder for Injection: 15 mg vial with diluent (diluent includes 0.6 ml mannitol (3%) in Water for Injection).

INDICATIONS AND DOSAGES
▸ **Prophylaxis of deep vein thrombosis (DVT) in patients undergoing hip replacement surgery**
Subcutaneous
Adults, Elderly. Initially, 15 mg q12h. Give initial dose 5–15 min prior to surgery, but following induction of regional block anesthesia, if used. May administer up to 12 days postoperative.

▸ **Moderate renal function impairment (31–60 ml/min or higher)**
Subcutaneous
Adults, Elderly. 5 mg q12h.
▸ **Severe renal function impairment (less than 31 ml/min)**
Subcutaneous
Adults, Elderly. 1.7 mg q12h.

CONTRAINDICATIONS
Hypersensitivity to natural or recombinant hirudins (anticoagulation factors), patients with active bleeding or irreversible coagulation disorders

INTERACTIONS
Drug
Anticoagulants, Dextran 40, systemic glucocorticoids, thrombolytics: Increase the risk of bleeding and should be discontinued prior to initiation of desirudin therapy.
Herbal
None known.
Food
None known.

DIAGNOSTIC TEST EFFECTS

May increase activated partial thromboplastin time (aPTT). May decrease blood hemoglobin, hematocrit (Hct) concentrations.

SIDE EFFECTS

Frequent (6%)
Hematoma
Occasional (4%–2%)
Injection site mass, wound secretion, nausea, hypersensitivity reaction

SERIOUS REACTIONS

• Serious or major hemorrhage and anaphylactic reaction occur rarely.

NURSING CONSIDERATIONS

Baseline Assessment
• Discontinue any medication that may enhance the risk of hemorrhage before beginning desirudin therapy.
• Establish the patient's baseline aPTT, BUN, and serum creatinine to assess liver and renal function.
• Avoid overinflating the cuff when monitoring the patient's blood pressure (B/P).
• Remove adhesive tape from any pressure dressing very carefully and slowly.

Lifespan Considerations
• Be aware that desirudin may be teratogenic and it is unknown if the drug is distributed in breast milk.
• Be aware that the safety and efficacy of desirudin have not been established in children.
• In the elderly, age-related renal impairment may require dosage adjustment.

Precautions
• Use cautiously in patients with epidural or spinal anesthesia, increased risk of hemorrhage, including bacterial endocarditis, hemo-philia, history of GI bleeding or pulmonary bleeding within the past 3 months, history of hemorrhagic stroke, intracranial or intraocular bleeding, organ biopsy, puncture of a non-compressible vessel within the last month, recent major surgery, and severe uncontrolled hypertension), and renal function impairment.

Administration and Handling
Subcutaneous
• Store vials at room temperature.
• Reconstitute each vial with 0.5 ml provided diluent. Gently agitate or rotate. Use reconstituted solution immediately but is stable for up to 24 hours if stored at room temperature. Discard unused portion.
• Using a 26- or 27-gauge needle approx. one half inch in length, withdraw reconstituted solution and inject by deep subcutaneous injection, alternating sites between left and right anterolateral and left and right posterolateral abdominal wall. Introduce entire length of needle into skin fold held between thumb and forefinger, holding skin fold during injection.

Intervention and Evaluation
• Monitor the aPTT and serum creatinine daily in patients with an increased risk of bleeding or renal impairment. Expect to reduce dosage if peak aPTT exceeds 2 times control.
• Assess the patient for abdominal or back pain, a decrease in B/P and Hct, an increase in pulse rate, and severe headache because these signs may be evidence of hemorrhage.
• Determine the patient's discharge during menses and monitor for an increase.
• Assess the patient's gums for erythema and gingival bleeding, skin for bruises, and urine for hematuria.

• Examine the patient for excessive bleeding from minor cuts and scratches.

Patient Teaching
• Tell the patient to use an electric razor and soft toothbrush to prevent bleeding during desirudin therapy.
• Explain to the patient that he or she should not take any medications, including over-the-counter (OTC) drugs, especially aspirin, without consulting the physician.
• Warn the patient to notify the physician if he or she experiences black or red stool, coffee-ground vomitus, dark or red urine, or red-speckled mucus from cough.
• Tell female patients that their menstrual flow may be heavier than usual.

---

enoxaparin sodium
en-**ox**-ah-pear-in
(Klexane[CAN], Lovenox)
Do not confuse with Lotronex.

CATEGORY AND SCHEDULE
Pregnancy Risk Category: B

MECHANISM OF ACTION
A low-molecular-weight heparin that potentiates the action of antithrombin III and inactivates coagulation factor Xa. *Therapeutic Effect:* Produces anticoagulation. Does not significantly influence bleeding time, prothrombin time (PT), activated partial thromboplastin time (APTT).

PHARMACOKINETICS

Route	Onset	Peak	Duration
Subcuta-neous	N/A	3–5 hrs	12 hrs

Well absorbed after subcutaneous administration. Eliminated primarily in urine. Not removed by hemodialysis. **Half-life:** 4.5 hrs.

AVAILABILITY
Injection: 30 mg/0.3 ml, 40 mg/0.4 ml, 60 mg/0.6 ml, 80 mg/0.8 ml, 100 mg/1 ml, 120 mg/0.8 ml, 150 mg/1 ml, prefilled syringes.

INDICATIONS AND DOSAGES
▶ **Prevention of deep vein thrombosis (DVT) (hip, knee surgery)**
Subcutaneous
Adults, Elderly. 30 mg twice a day, generally for 7–10 days.
▶ **Prevention of DVT abdominal surgery**
Subcutaneous
Adults, Elderly. 40 mg a day for 7–10 days.
▶ **Prevention of long-term DVT, nonsurgical acute illness**
Subcutaneous
Adults, Elderly. 40 mg once a day for 3 wks.
▶ **Angina, myocardial infarction (MI)**
Subcutaneous
Adults, Elderly. 1 mg/kg q12h (treatment).
▶ **Acute DVT**
Subcutaneous
Adults, Elderly. 1 mg/kg q12h or 1.5 mg/kg once daily.
▶ **Usual dosage for children**
Subcutaneous
Children. 0.5 mg/kg q12h (prophylaxis); 1 mg/kg q12h (treatment).
▶ **Dosage in renal impairment**
Clearance decreased when creatinine clearance is less than 30 ml/min. Monitor, adjust dosage.

UNLABELED USES
Prevents DVT following general surgical procedures

CONTRAINDICATIONS

Active major bleeding, concurrent heparin therapy, hypersensitivity to heparin or pork products, thrombocytopenia associated with positive in vitro test for antiplatelet antibody

INTERACTIONS

Drug

Anticoagulants, platelet inhibitors: May increase bleeding.

Herbal

None known.

Food

None known.

DIAGNOSTIC TEST EFFECTS

Reversible increases in LDH concentrations, serum alkaline phosphatase, SGOT (AST), and SGPT (ALT) levels.

SIDE EFFECTS

Occasional (4%–1%)
Injection site hematoma, nausea, peripheral edema

SERIOUS REACTIONS

• Accidental overdosage may lead to bleeding complications ranging from local ecchymoses to major hemorrhage. Antidote: Protamine sulfate (1% solution) should be equal to the dose of enoxaparin injected. One mg protamine sulfate neutralizes 1 mg enoxaparin. A second dose of 0.5 mg/mg protamine sulfate may be given if APTT tested 2–4 hrs after the first injection remains prolonged.

NURSING CONSIDERATIONS

Baseline Assessment

• Assess the patient's complete blood count (CBC).
• Examine the patient's list of allergies, especially to heparin or pork products.

Lifespan Considerations

• Be aware that enoxaparin should be used with caution in pregnant women, particularly during the last trimester of pregnancy and immediately postpartum. Enoxaparin use increases the risk of maternal hemorrhage.
• Be aware that it is unknown if enoxaparin is excreted in breast milk.
• Be aware that the safety and efficacy of enoxaparin have not been established in children.
• Be aware that the elderly may be more susceptible to bleeding.

Precautions

• Use cautiously in elderly patients and patients with conditions with increased risk of hemorrhage, history of recent GI ulceration and hemorrhage, history of heparin-induced thrombocytopenia, impaired renal function, and uncontrolled arterial hypertension.

Administration and Handling

◀ALERT▶ Do not mix with other injections or infusions. Do not give IM.

◀ALERT▶ Give initial dose as soon as possible after surgery but not more than 24 hours after surgery.

Subcutaneous

• Parenteral form normally appears clear and colorless to pale yellow.
• Store at room temperature.
• Instruct the patient to lie down before administering by deep subcutaneous injection.
• Inject between left and right anterolateral and left and right posterolateral abdominal wall.
• Introduce entire length of needle (one half inch) into skin fold held between thumb and forefinger, holding skin fold during injection.

Intervention and Evaluation
• Periodically monitor the patient's complete blood count (CBC) and stool for occult blood; there is no need for daily monitoring in patients with normal presurgical coagulation parameters.
• Assess the patient for any sign of bleeding, including bleeding at injection or surgical sites, bleeding from gums, blood in stool, bruising, hematuria, and petechiae.

Patient Teaching
• Tell the patient that the usual length of therapy is 7 to 10 days.
• Instruct the patient to let you know if he or she experiences bleeding from surgical site, chest pain, or dyspnea.
• Tell the patient to use an electric razor and soft toothbrush to prevent bleeding during enoxaparin therapy.
• Explain to the patient that he or she should not take any medications, including over-the-counter (OTC) drugs, especially aspirin, without consulting the physician.
• Warn the patient to notify the you if he or she experiences black or red stool, coffee-ground vomitus, dark or red urine, or red-speckled mucus from cough.
• Tell female patients that their menstrual flow may be heavier than usual.

---

fondaparinux sodium
fond-dah-**pear**-in-ux
(Arixtra)

CATEGORY AND SCHEDULE
Pregnancy Risk Category: B

MECHANISM OF ACTION
A factor Xa inhibitor and pentasaccharide that selectively binds to antithrombin, and increases its affinity for and inhibiting factor Xa, stopping the blood coagulation cascade. *Therapeutic Effect:* Indirectly prevents formation of thrombin and subsequently the fibrin clot.

PHARMACOKINETICS
Well absorbed after subcutaneous administration. Undergoes minimal, if any, metabolism. Highly bound to antithrombin III. Distributed mainly in blood and to a minor extent in extravascular fluid. Excreted unchanged in urine. Removed by hemodialysis. **Half-life:** 17–21 hrs (half-life is prolonged in patients with impaired renal function).

AVAILABILITY
Prefilled Syringe: 2.5 mg.

INDICATIONS AND DOSAGES
▸ **Prevention of venous thromboembolism**
Subcutaneous
Adults. 2.5 mg once a day for 5–9 days after surgery. Initial dose should be given 6–8 hrs after surgery. Dosage should be adjusted in elderly, those with renal impairment.

CONTRAINDICATIONS
Active major bleeding, bacterial endocarditis, severe renal impairment with creatinine clearance less than 30 mL/min, thrombocytopenia associated with antiplatelet antibody formation in the presence of fondaparinux, body weight less than 50 kg

INTERACTIONS
Drug
Anticoagulants, platelet inhibitors:
May increase bleeding.
Herbal
None known.
Food
None known.

DIAGNOSTIC TEST EFFECTS
Reversible increases in serum
creatinine levels, SGOT (AST),
and SGPT (ALT) levels. May
decrease Hgb, Hct, and platelet
count.

SIDE EFFECTS
Occasional (14%)
Fever
Rare (4%–1%)
Injection site hematoma, nausea,
peripheral edema

SERIOUS REACTIONS
• Accidental overdosage may lead
to bleeding complications ranging
from local ecchymoses to major
hemorrhage.
• Thrombocytopenia occurs
rarely.

NURSING CONSIDERATIONS
Baseline Assessment
• Assess the patient's baseline
BUN, creatinine, and complete
blood count (CBC).
Lifespan Considerations
• Be aware that fondaparinux
should be used with caution in
pregnant women, particularly during
the last trimester of pregnancy and
immediately postpartum because
fondaparinux increases the risk of
maternal hemorrhage.
• Be aware that it is unknown if
fondaparinux is excreted in breast
milk.
• Be aware that the safety and

efficacy of fondaparinux have not
been established in children.
• In the elderly, age-related decreased renal function may increase
risk of bleeding.
Precautions
• Use cautiously in elderly patients
and patients with conditions with
increased risk of hemorrhage, such
as concurrent use of antiplatelet
agents, gastrointestinal (GI) ulceration, hemophilia, history of cerebrovascular accident (CVA), and severe
uncontrolled hypertension, history
of heparin-induced thrombocytopenia, impaired renal function, indwelling epidural catheter use, and
neuraxial anesthesia.
Administration and Handling
Subcutaneous
• Keep in mind that the parenteral
form normally appears clear and
colorless. Discard if discoloration or
particulate matter is noted.
• Store at room temperature.
• Do not expel the air bubble from
the prefilled syringe before injection
to avoid expelling drug.
• Pinch a fold of patient skin at the
injection site between thumb and
forefinger. Introduce the entire
length of subcutaneous needle
into skin fold during injection.
Inject into fatty tissue between the
left and right anterolateral or the
left and right posterolateral abdominal wall.
• Rotate injection sites.
Intervention and Evaluation
• Periodically monitor the patient's
complete blood count (CBC) and
stool for occult blood, as ordered.
Know that there is no need for daily
monitoring in patients with normal
presurgical coagulation parameters.
• Assess the patient for any sign of
bleeding, including bleeding at
injection or surgical sites, bleeding

from gums, blood in stool, bruising, hematuria, and petechiae.
• Monitor the patient's blood pressure (B/P). Hypotension may indicate bleeding.

Patient Teaching
• Tell the patient that the usual length of therapy is 5 to 9 days.
• Explain to the patient that he or she should not take any medications, including over-the-counter (OTC) drugs, especially aspirin and NSAIDs, without consulting the physician.
• Warn the patient to notify the physician if he or she experiences severe or sudden headache, swelling in the feet or hands, unusual back pain, or unusual bleeding, bruising, or weakness.
• Instruct the patient to let you know if he or she experiences bleeding from surgical site, chest pain, or dyspnea.
• Tell the patient to use an electric razor and soft toothbrush to prevent bleeding during fondaparinux therapy.
• Warn the patient to notify the physician if he or she experiences black or red stool, coffee-ground vomitus, dark or red urine, or red-speckled mucus from cough.
• Tell female patients that their menstrual flow may be heavier than usual.

heparin sodium
hep-ah-rin
(Hepalean[CAN], Heparin injection B.P.[AUS], Heparin Leo, Uniparin[AUS])
Do not confuse with Hespan.

CATEGORY AND SCHEDULE
Pregnancy Risk Category: C

MECHANISM OF ACTION
A blood modifier that interferes with blood coagulation by blocking conversion of prothrombin to thrombin and fibrinogen to fibrin. *Therapeutic Effect:* Prevents further extension of existing thrombi or new clot formation. No effect on existing clots.

PHARMACOKINETICS
Well absorbed following subcutaneous administration. Protein binding: Very high. Metabolized in liver, removed from circulation via uptake by reticuloendothelial system. Primarily excreted in urine. Not removed by hemodialysis. **Half-life:** 1–6 hrs.

AVAILABILITY
Injection: 10 units/ml, 100 units/ml, 1,000 units/ml, 2,500 units/ml, 5,000 units/ml, 7,500 units/ml, 10,000 units/ml, 20,000 units/ml, 40,000 units/ml, 25,000 units/ 500 ml infusion.

INDICATIONS AND DOSAGES
▸ **Line flushing**
IV
Adults, Elderly, Children. 100 units q6–8h.
Infants weighing less than 10 kg. 10 units q6–8h.
▸ **Prophylaxis of venous thrombosis, pulmonary embolism, peripheral arterial embolism, atrial fibrillation with embolism**
Subcutaneous
Adult, Elderly. 5,000 units q8–12h.
▸ **Treatment of venous thrombosis, pulmonary embolism, peripheral arterial embolism, atrial fibrillation with embolism**
Intermittent IV
Adults, Elderly. Initially, 10,000 units, then 50–70 units/kg (5,000–10,000 units) q4–6h.

Children older than 1 yr. Initially, 50–100 units/kg, then 50–100 units q4h.
IV infusion
Adults, Elderly. Loading dose: 80 units/kg, then 18 units/kg/hr with adjustments according to activated partial thromboplastin time (aPTT). Range: 10–30 units/kg/hr.
Children older than 1 yr. Loading dose: 75 units/kg, then 20 units/kg/hr with adjustments according to aPTT.
Children younger than 1 yr. Loading dose: 75 units/kg, then 28 units/kg/hr.

CONTRAINDICATIONS
Intracranial hemorrhage, severe hypotension, severe thrombocytopenia, subacute bacterial endocarditis, uncontrolled bleeding

INTERACTIONS
Drug
Anticoagulants, platelet aggregation inhibitors, thrombolytics: May increase the risk of bleeding.
Antithyroid medications, cefoperazone, cefotetan, valproic acid: May cause hypoprothrombinemia.
Probenecid: May increase the effects of heparin.
Herbal
Feverfew, ginkgo biloba: May have additive effect.
Food
None known.

DIAGNOSTIC TEST EFFECTS
May increase free fatty acid, SGOT (AST), and SGPT (ALT) levels. May decrease serum cholesterol and triglyceride levels.

IV INCOMPATIBILITIES
Amiodarone (Cordarone), amphotericin B complex (Abelcet, AmBisome, Amphotec), ciprofloxacin (Cipro), dacarbazine (DTIC), diazepam (Valium), dobutamine (Dobutrex), doxorubicin (Adriamycin), droperidol (Inapsine), filgrastim (Neupogen), gentamicin (Garamycin), haloperidol (Haldol), idarubicin (Idamycin), labetalol (Trandate), nicardipine (Cardene), phenytoin (Dilantin), quinidine, tobramycin (Nebcin), vancomycin (Vancocin)

IV COMPATIBILITIES
Aminophylline, ampicillin/sulbactam (Unasyn), aztreonam (Azactam), calcium gluconate, cefazolin (Ancef), ceftazidime (Fortaz), ceftriaxone (Rocephin), digoxin (Lanoxin), diltiazem (Cardizem), dopamine (Intropin), enalapril (Vasotec), famotidine (Pepcid), fentanyl (Sublimaze), furosemide (Lasix), hydromorphone (Dilaudid), insulin, lidocaine, lorazepam (Ativan), magnesium sulfate, methylprednisolone (Solu-Medrol), midazolam (Versed), milrinone (Primacor), morphine, nitroglycerin, norepinephrine (Levophed), oxytocin (Pitocin), piperacillin/tazobactam (Zosyn), procainamide (Pronestyl), propofol (Diprivan)

SIDE EFFECTS
Occasional
Itching, burning, particularly on soles of feet—caused by vasospastic reaction
Rare
Pain, cyanosis of extremity 6–10 days after initial therapy, lasts 4–6 hrs; hypersensitivity reaction, including chills, fever, pruritus, urticaria, asthma, rhinitis, lacrimation, and headache

SERIOUS REACTIONS
• Bleeding complications ranging from local ecchymoses to major

hemorrhage occur more frequently in high-dose therapy, intermittent IV infusion, and in women older than 60 yrs.

• Antidote: Protamine sulfate 1–1.5 mg for every 100 units heparin subcutaneous if overdosage occurred before 30 min, 0.5–0.75 mg for every 100 units heparin subcutaneous if overdosage occurred within 30–60 min, 0.25–0.375 mg for every 100 units heparin subcutaneous if 2 hrs have elapsed since overdosage, 25–50 mg if heparin given by IV infusion.

NURSING CONSIDERATIONS

Baseline Assessment

• Cross-check heparin dose with another nurse before administering to the patient. Determine the patient's aPTT before administering heparin, and 24 hours following heparin therapy, then 24 to 48 hours for the first week of heparin therapy or until the maintenance dose is established.

• Monitor the patient's aPTT 1 to 2 times weekly for 3 to 4 weeks. In long-term therapy, monitor the patient's aPTT 1 to 2 times a month.

Lifespan Considerations

• Be aware that heparin should be used with caution in pregnant women, particularly during the last trimester of pregnancy and immediately postpartum because heparin increases the risk of maternal hemorrhage.

• Be aware that it is heparin does not cross the placenta and is not distributed in breast milk.

• There are no age-related precautions noted in children.

• Be aware that the benzyl alcohol preservative may cause gasping syndrome in infants.

• Be aware that the elderly are more susceptible to hemorrhage.

• In the elderly, age-related decreased renal function may increase the risk of bleeding.

Precautions

• Use cautiously in patients with IM injections, menstruation, peptic ulcer disease, recent invasive or surgical procedures, and severe liver or renal disease.

Administration and Handling

◀ALERT▶ Do not give by IM injection because it may cause pain, hematoma, ulceration, and erythema.

Subcutaneous

◀ALERT▶ Keep in mind that the subcutaneous route is used for low-dose therapy.

• After withdrawing heparin from the vial, change the needle before injection to prevent leakage along the needle track.

• Inject heparin dose above the iliac crest or in abdominal fat layer. Do not inject within 2 inches of umbilicus, or any scar tissue.

• Withdraw the needle rapidly and apply prolonged pressure at injection site without massaging. Rotate injection sites.

IV

◀ALERT▶ Be aware that continuous IV therapy is preferred because intermittent IV therapy produces a higher incidence of bleeding abnormalities.

• Store at room temperature.

• Dilute IV infusion in isotonic sterile saline, D_5W, or lactated Ringer's.

• Invert IV bag at least 6 times to ensure mixing, and to prevent pooling of the medication.

• Use constant-rate IV infusion pump.

Intervention and Evaluation

• Monitor the patient's aPTT dili-

gently. The therapeutic heparin dosage causes an aPTT of 1.5–2.5 times normal.
• Assess the patient's Hct, platelet count, SGOT (AST) and SGPT (ALT) levels, and stool and urine cultures for occult blood, regardless of route of administration.
• Determine the patient's discharge during menses and monitor for an increase.
• Assess the patient's gums for erythema and gingival bleeding, skin for bruises or petechiae, and urine for hematuria.
• Examine the patient for excessive bleeding from minor cuts and scratches.
• Evaluate the patient for abdominal or back pain, a decrease in blood pressure (B/P), an increase in pulse rate, and severe headache, which may be evidence of hemorrhage.
• Check the patient's peripheral pulses for loss of peripheral circulation.
• Avoid giving IM injections of other medications to the patient due to potential for hematomas.
• When converting to Coumadin therapy, monitor the patient's prothrombin time (PT) results, as ordered. Keep in mind that the PT will be 10% to 20% higher while heparin is given concurrently.

Patient Teaching
• Tell the patient to use an electric razor and soft toothbrush to prevent bleeding during heparin therapy.
• Explain to the patient that he or she should not take any medications, including over-the-counter (OTC) drugs, without consulting the physician.
• Warn the patient to notify the physician if he or she experiences black or red stool, coffee-ground vomitus, dark or red urine, or red-speckled mucus from cough.

• Suggest to the patient to carry or wear identification that notes he or she is on anticoagulant therapy.
• Stress to the patient that he or she should inform his or her dentist and other physicians of heparin therapy.

lepirudin
leh-**pier**-ruh-din
(Refludan)

CATEGORY AND SCHEDULE
Pregnancy Risk Category: B

MECHANISM OF ACTION
An anticoagulant that inhibits thrombogenic action of thrombin—independent of antithrombin II and not inhibited by platelet factor 4. *Therapeutic Effect.* Produces Increase in activated partial thromboplastin time (APTT).

PHARMACOKINETICS
Distributed primarily in extracellular fluid. Primarily eliminated by kidneys. **Half-life:** 1.3 hrs, half-life is increased with impaired renal function. Removed by hemodialysis.

AVAILABILITY
Powder for Injection: 50 mg.

INDICATIONS AND DOSAGES
▶ **Anticoagulant in patients with heparin-induced thrombocytopenia and associated thromboembolic disease to prevent further thromboembolic complications**
IV/IV infusion
Adults, Elderly. 0.2–0.4 mg/kg, IV slowly over 15–20 sec, followed by IV infusion of 0.1–0.15 mg/kg/hr for 2–10 days or longer.
▶ **Dosage in renal impairment**
Initial dose decreased to 0.2 mg/kg

with infusion rate adjusted based on creatinine clearance.

Creatinine Clearance (ml/min)	% of standard infusion rate	Infusion rate (mg/kg/hr)
45–60	50	0.075
30–44	30	0.045
15–29	15	0.0225

CONTRAINDICATIONS
None known

INTERACTIONS
Drug
Platelet aggregation inhibitors, thrombolytics, warfarin: May increase the risk of bleeding complications.
Herbal
Ginkgo biloba: May increase the risk of bleeding.
Food
None known.

DIAGNOSTIC TEST EFFECTS
Increases APTT and thrombin time.

IV INCOMPATIBILITIES
Do not mix with any other medication.

SIDE EFFECTS
Frequent (14%–5%)
Bleeding from puncture sites or wounds, hematuria, fever, gastrointestinal (GI) and rectal bleeding
Occasional (3%–1%)
Epistaxis, allergic reaction, such as rash and pruritus, vaginal bleeding

SERIOUS REACTIONS
• Overdosage is characterized by excessively high APTT values.
• Intracranial bleeding occurs rarely.
• Abnormal liver function occurs in 6% of patients.

NURSING CONSIDERATIONS
Baseline Assessment
• Assess the patient's complete blood count (CBC), including platelet count, as well as aPTT and thrombin time.
• Determine the patient's initial blood pressure (B/P).
• Assess the patient's baseline serum chemistry lab values including BUN, serum alkaline phosphatase, creatinine, SGOT (AST), and SGPT (ALT) levels to assess liver and renal function.
Lifespan Considerations
• Be aware that it is unknown if lepirudin is distributed in breast milk or crosses the placenta.
• Be aware that the safety and efficacy of lepirudin have not been established in children.
• In the elderly, age-related renal function impairment may require dosage adjustment.
Precautions
• Use cautiously in patients with conditions associated with increased risk of bleeding, such as bacterial endocarditis, cerebrovascular accident (CVA), hemorrhagic diathesis, intracerebral surgery, recent major bleeding, recent major surgery, severe hypertension, severe liver or renal function impairment, and stroke.
Administration and Handling
◀ALERT▶ Give initial dose as soon as possible after surgery but not more than 24 hours after surgery.
◀ALERT▶ Dosage adjusted according to aPTT ratio with target range of 1.5 to 2.5 normal.
◀ALERT▶ Know that for patients weighing more than 110 kg, the maximum initial dose is 44 mg, with maximum rate of 16.5 mg/hr.
IV
• Store unreconstituted vials at room temperature.

• Know that the reconstituted solution should be used immediately, but the IV infusion is stable for up to 24 hours at room temperature.
• Add 1 ml sterile water for injection or 0.9% NaCl to 50-mg vial and shake gently.
• Be aware that reconstitution normally produces a clear, colorless solution; do not use if cloudy.
• For IV push, further dilute by transferring to syringe and adding sufficient sterile water for injection, 0.9% NaCl, or D_5W to produce concentration of 5 mg/ml.
• For IV infusion, add contents of 2 vials (100 mg) to 250 ml or 500 ml 0.9% NaCl or D_5W, providing a concentration of 0.4 or 0.2 mg/ml, respectively.
• Give IV push given over 15 to 20 seconds.
• Expect to adjust IV infusion based on aPTT or patient's body weight.

Intervention and Evaluation
• Monitor the patient's aPTT diligently.
• Assess the patient for abdominal or back pain, a decrease in B/P, an increase in pulse rate, and severe headache that may be evidence of hemorrhage.
• Determine the patient's discharge during menses and monitor for an increase.
• Assess the patient's gums for erythema and gingival bleeding, skin for bruises or petechiae, and urine for hematuria.
• Examine the patient for excessive bleeding from minor cuts and scratches.
• Assess the patient's BUN, Hct, platelet count, renal function studies, serum creatinine SGOT (AST) and SGPT (ALT) levels, and stool and urine cultures for occult blood.
• Check the patient's peripheral pulses for signs of diminished peripheral circulation.

Patient Teaching
• Warn the patient to notify the physician if he or she experiences bleeding, breathing difficulty, bruising, dizziness, fever, itching, lightheadedness, rash, or swelling.
• Instruct the patient to let you know if he or she experiences bleeding from surgical site, chest pain, or dyspnea.
• Tell the patient to use an electric razor and soft toothbrush to prevent bleeding during lepirudin therapy.
• Explain to the patient that he or she should not take any medications, including over-the-counter (OTC) drugs, especially aspirin, without consulting the physician.
• Warn the patient to notify the physician if he or she experiences black or red stool, coffee-ground vomitus, dark or red urine, or red-speckled mucus from cough.
• Tell female patients that their menstrual flow may be heavier than usual.

tinzaparin sodium
tin-zah-**pare**-inn
(Innohep)

CATEGORY AND SCHEDULE
Pregnancy Risk Category: B

MECHANISM OF ACTION
A low-molecular-weight heparin that inhibits factor Xa. Tinzaparin causes less inactivation of thrombin, inhibition of platelets, and bleeding than standard heparin. Does not significantly influence bleeding time, prothrombin time (PT), activated partial thromboplastin time (APTT). *Therapeutic Effect:* Produces anticoagulation.

PHARMACOKINETICS
Well absorbed after subcutaneous administration. Primarily eliminated in urine. **Half-life**: 3–4 hrs.

AVAILABILITY
Injection: 20,000 anti-Xa international units/ml.

INDICATIONS AND DOSAGES
▶ **Deep vein thrombosis (DVT)**
Subcutaneous
Adults, Elderly. 175 anti-Xa international units/kg given once a day. Continue at least 6 days and until patient is sufficiently anticoagulated with warfarin international normalizing ratio (INR) of 2 or higher for 2 consecutive days.

CONTRAINDICATIONS
Active major bleeding, concurrent heparin therapy, hypersensitivity to heparin or pork products, thrombocytopenia associated with positive in vitro test for antiplatelet antibody

INTERACTIONS
Drug
Anticoagulants, platelet inhibitors: May increase the risk of bleeding.
Herbal
Ginkgo biloba: May increase the risk of bleeding.
Food
None known.

DIAGNOSTIC TEST EFFECTS
Reversible increases in LDH concentrations, serum alkaline phosphatase, SGOT (AST), and SGPT (ALT) levels.

SIDE EFFECTS
Frequent (16%)
Injection site reaction, such as inflammation, oozing, nodules, and skin necrosis

Rare (less than 2%)
Nausea, asthenia or unusual tiredness or weakness, constipation, epistaxis or nosebleed

SERIOUS REACTIONS
• Accidental overdosage may lead to bleeding complications ranging from local ecchymoses to major hemorrhage. Antidote: Dose of protamine sulfate (1% solution) should be equal to the dose of tinzaparin injected. One mg protamine sulfate neutralizes 100 units of tinzaparin. A second dose of 0.5 mg/mg protamine sulfate may be given if APTT tested 2–4 hrs after the first infusion remains prolonged.

NURSING CONSIDERATIONS
Baseline Assessment
• Assess the patient's PT/INR and complete blood count (CBC), including platelet count.
• Determine the patient's initial blood pressure (B/P).
Lifespan Considerations
• Be aware that tinzaparin should be used with caution in pregnant women, particularly during the last trimester of pregnancy and immediately postpartum. Tinzaparin use increases the risk of maternal hemorrhage.
• Be aware that it is unknown if tinzaparin is excreted in breast milk.
• Be aware that the safety and efficacy of tinzaparin have not been established in children.
• Be aware that the elderly may be more susceptible to bleeding.
Precautions
• Use cautiously in elderly patients and patients with conditions with increased risk of hemorrhage, history of recent GI ulceration and hemorrhage, history of heparin-

induced thrombocytopenia, impaired renal function, and uncontrolled arterial hypertension.

Administration and Handling

◀ALERT▶ Do not mix with other injections or infusions. Do not give IM.

Subcutaneous

• Remember that the parenteral form normally appears clear and colorless to pale yellow.

• Store at room temperature.

• Instruct patient to lie down before administering by deep subcutaneous injection.

• Introduce entire length of half inch needle into skin fold held between thumb and forefinger, holding patient skin fold during injection.

• Inject between left and right anterolateral and left and right posterolateral abdominal wall.

Intervention and Evaluation

• Periodically monitor the patient's complete blood count (CBC), including platelet count, as ordered.

• Assess the patient for any sign of bleeding, including bleeding at injection or surgical sites, bleeding from gums, blood in stool, bruising, hematuria, and petechiae.

Patient Teaching

• Instruct the patient to only administer tinzaparin subcutaneously.

• Tell the patient that he or she may have a tendency to bleed easily. Suggest that he or she use an electric razor and a soft tissue to prevent bleeding.

• Warn the patient to notify the physician if he or she experiences chest pain, injection site reaction, such as inflammation, nodules, or oozing, numbness, pain, swelling or tingling of joints, or unusual bleeding or bruising.

warfarin sodium

war-fair-in

(Coumadin, Marevan[AUS], Warfilone[CAN])

Do not confuse with Kemadrin.

CATEGORY AND SCHEDULE

Pregnancy Risk Category: D

MECHANISM OF ACTION

A coumarin derivative that interferes with hepatic synthesis of vitamin K–dependent clotting factors, resulting in depletion of coagulation factors II, VII, IX, X. *Therapeutic Effect:* Prevents further extension of formed existing clot; prevents new clot formation or secondary thromboembolic complications.

PHARMACOKINETICS

Route	Onset	Peak	Duration
PO	1.5–3 days	5–7 days	N/A

Well absorbed from the gastrointestinal (GI) tract. Metabolized in liver. Primarily excreted in urine. Not removed by hemodialysis. **Half-life:** 1.5–2.5 days.

AVAILABILITY

Tablets: 1 mg, 2 mg, 2.5 mg, 3 mg, 4 mg, 5 mg, 6 mg, 7.5 mg, 10 mg. *Injection:* 5-mg vials.

INDICATIONS AND DOSAGES

▸ **Anticoagulant**

PO

Adults, Elderly. Initially, 5–15 mg/ day for 2–5 days, then adjust based on international normalized ratio (INR). Maintenance: 2–10 mg/day. *Children.* Initially, 0.1–0.2 mg/kg

(maximum 10 mg). Maintenance:
0.05–0.34 mg/kg/day.
▸ **Usual elderly dosage**
PO/IV
• *Elderly.* 2–5 mg/day (maintenance).

UNLABELED USES
Prophylaxis against the recurrent cerebral embolism, myocardial reinfarction, treatment adjunct in transient ischemic attacks

CONTRAINDICATIONS
Neurosurgical procedures, open wounds, pregnancy, severe hypertension, severe liver or renal damage, uncontrolled bleeding, ulcers

INTERACTIONS
Drug
Acetaminophen, allopurinol, amiodarone, anabolic steroids, androgens, aspirin, cefamandole, cefoperazone, chloral hydrate, chloramphenicol, cimetidine, clofibrate, danazol, dextrothyroxine, diflunisal, disulfiram, erythromycin, fenoprofen, gemfibrozil, indomethacin, methimazole, metronidazole, oral hypoglycemics, phenytoin, plicamycin, propylthiouracil (PTU), quinidine, salicylates, sulfinpyrazone, sulfonamides, sulindac: Warfarin increases the effects of aforementioned drugs.
Barbiturates, carbamazepine, cholestyramine, colestipol, estramustine, estrogens, griseofulvin, primidone, rifampin, vitamin K: Warfarin decreases the effects of aforementioned drugs.
Herbal
Feverfew, garlic, ginkgo biloba, ginseng: May increase the risk of bleeding.
Food
None known.

DIAGNOSTIC TEST EFFECTS
None known.

SIDE EFFECTS
Occasional
GI distress, such as nausea, anorexia, abdominal cramps, and diarrhea
Rare
Hypersensitivity reaction, including dermatitis and urticaria, especially in those sensitive to aspirin

SERIOUS REACTIONS
• Bleeding complications ranging from local ecchymoses to major hemorrhage may occur. Drug should be discontinued immediately and vitamin K or phytonadione administered. Mild hemorrhage: 2.5–10 mg PO/IM/IV. Severe hemorrhage: 10–15 mg IV and repeated q4h, as necessary.
• Hepatotoxicity, blood dyscrasias, necrosis, vasculitis, and local thrombosis occur rarely.

NURSING CONSIDERATIONS
Baseline Assessment
• Cross-check warfarin dose with another nurse before administering the drug to the patient.
• Determine the patient's international normalizing ratio (INR) before administration and daily after therapy initiation. When stabilized, follow with INR determination every 4 to 6 weeks.
Lifespan Considerations
• Be aware that warfarin use is contraindicated in pregnancy because it will cause fetal and neonatal hemorrhage, and intrauterine death.
• Be aware that warfarin crosses the placenta and is distributed in breast milk.
• Be aware that children are more

susceptible to the effects of warfarin.

- In the elderly there is an increased risk of hemorrhage and a lower drug dosage is recommended.

Precautions

- Use cautiously in patients at risk for hemorrhage and patients with active tuberculosis, diabetes, gangrene, heparin-induced thrombocytopenia, and necrosis.

Administration and Handling

◀ALERT▶ Remember that the dosage is highly individualized, based on prothrombin time (aPT), INR.

PO

- Crush scored tablets as needed.
- Give warfarin without regard to food. If gastrointestinal (GI) upset occurs, give with food.

Intervention and Evaluation

- Monitor the patient's INR reports diligently.
- Assess the patient's Hct, platelet count, SGOT (AST) and SGPT (ALT) levels, and stool and urine cultures for occult blood, regardless of route of administration.
- Evaluate the patient for abdominal or back pain, a decrease in blood pressure (B/P), an increase in pulse rate, and severe headache because it may be a sign of hemorrhage.
- Determine the patient's discharge during menses and monitor for an increase.
- Assess the patient's area of thromboembolus for color and temperature.
- Check the patient's peripheral pulses.

- Assess the patient's gums for erythema and gingival bleeding, skin for bruises and petechiae, and urine for hematuria.
- Examine the patient for excessive bleeding from minor cuts or scratches.

Patient Teaching

- Instruct the patient to take warfarin exactly as prescribed.
- Caution the patient against taking or discontinuing any other medication except on the advice of the physician.
- Urge the patient to avoid alcohol, drastic dietary changes, and salicylates.
- Teach the patient not to change from one brand of the drug to another.
- Instruct the patient to consult the physician before having dental work or surgery.
- Explain to the patient that his or her urine may become red-orange.
- Tell the patient to use an electric razor and soft toothbrush to prevent bleeding during warfarin therapy.
- Explain to the patient that he or she should not take any medications, including over-the-counter (OTC) drugs, without consulting the physician.
- Warn the patient to notify the physician if he or she experiences black stool, bleeding, brown, dark, or red urine, coffee-ground vomitus, or red-speckled mucus from cough.

factor VIII
(antihemophilic
factor, AHF)
factor IX complex

Uses: Antihemophilic agents are used to prevent or treat bleeding episodes in patients with hemophilia A, in which factor VIII activity is deficient, or hemophilia B (also called Christmas disease), in which factor IX complex activity is deficient.

Action: Antihemophilic agents promote hemostasis by activating the intrinsic or extrinsic pathway of the coagulation cascade. Factor VIII prevents bleeding by replacing this clotting factor, which is needed to transform prothrombin into thrombin. Factor IX complex raises the plasma level of factor IX, restoring hemostasis in patients with factor IX deficiency.

antihemophilic factor (factor VIII, AHF)

(Alphanate, Hyate, Bioclate, Humate-P, Kogenate, Monoclate-P)

CATEGORY AND SCHEDULE
Pregnancy Risk Category: C

MECHANISM OF ACTION
An antihemophilic agent that assists in conversion of prothrombin to thrombin, essential for blood coagulation, Replaces missing clotting factor. *Therapeutic Effect:* Produces hemostasis, corrects or prevents bleeding episodes.

AVAILABILITY
Injection: Actual number of anti-hemolytic factor (AHF) units listed on each vial.

INDICATIONS AND DOSAGES
▸ **Prevention and treatment of bleeding in patients with hemo-**
philia A factor XIII deficiency, hypofibrinogenemia, von Willebrand disease
Dosage is highly individualized, based on patient weight, severity of bleeding, coagulation studies.

UNLABELED USES
Treatment of disseminated intravascular coagulation (DIC)

CONTRAINDICATIONS
None known

INTERACTIONS
Drug
None known.
Herbal
None known.
Food
None known.

DIAGNOSTIC TEST EFFECTS
None known.

IV INCOMPATIBILITIES
Do not mix with other IV solutions or medications.

SIDE EFFECTS

Occasional

Allergic reaction, including fever, chills, urticaria, wheezing, slight hypotension, nausea, and a feeling of chest tightness, stinging at injection site, dizziness, dry mouth, headache, unpleasant taste

SERIOUS REACTIONS

• There is a risk of transmitting viral hepatitis.

• Possibility of intravascular hemolysis occurring if large or frequent doses used with blood group A, B, or AB.

NURSING CONSIDERATIONS

Baseline Assessment

• Avoid overinflation of cuff when monitoring the patient's B/P. Take blood pressure manually, avoiding automatic blood pressure cuffs.

• Remove adhesive tape from any pressure dressing on the patient very carefully and slowly.

Precautions

• Use cautiously in patients with liver disease and in patients with blood type A, B, or AB. If large doses are given to patients with these blood types, expect to monitor the blood hematocrit and direct Coomb's test to check for hemolytic anemia. If hemolytic anemia occurs, expect to give transfusions with Type O blood.

Administration and Handling

IV

• Refer to individual vials for specific storage requirements.

• Warm concentrate and diluent to room temperature.

• Gently agitate or rotate to dissolve. Do not shake vigorously. Complete dissolution may take 5 to 10 minutes.

• Filter before administration.

• Administer IV at rate of approximately 2 ml/min. Can give up to 10 ml/min.

Intervention and Evaluation

• Monitor the patient's IV site for oozing.

• Assess the patient for allergic reactions.

• Assess the patient's urine for hematuria.

• Monitor the patient's vital signs.

• Assess the patient for complaints of abdominal or back pain or severe headache, a decrease in B/P, and an increase in pulse rate.

• Determine if the patient has an increase in the amount of discharge during menses.

• Assess the patient's skin for bruises and petechiae.

• Examine the patient for excessive bleeding from minor cuts or scratches.

• Assess the patient's gums for erythema and gingival bleeding.

• Evaluate the patient for therapeutic reduction of swelling and restricted joint movement and relief of pain.

Patient Teaching

• Tell the patient to use an electric razor and soft toothbrush to prevent bleeding.

• Warn the patient to notify the physician if he or she experiences any sign of black or red stool, coffee-ground emesis, dark or red urine, or red-speckled mucus from cough.

factor IX complex
Benefix, Propex T, Konyne

CATEGORY AND SCHEDULE
Pregnancy Risk Category: C

MECHANISM OF ACTION

A blood modifier that raises plasma levels of factor IX, restores hemostasis in patients with factor IX deficiency. *Therapeutic Effect:* Increases blood clotting factors II, VII, IX, and X.

AVAILABILITY

Injection: Number of units indicated on each vial.

INDICATIONS AND DOSAGES

▸ **Reversal of anticoagulant effect of coumarin anticoagulants, treatment of bleeding caused by hemophilia B, treatment of bleeding in patients with hemophilia A who have factor VIII inhibitors**

Amount of factor IX required is individualized. Dosage depends on degree of deficiency, level of each factor desired, weight of patient, and severity of bleeding.

CONTRAINDICATIONS

Sensitivity to mouse protein

INTERACTIONS

Drug

Aminocaproic acid: May increase the risk of thrombosis.

Herbal

None known.

Food

None known.

DIAGNOSTIC TEST EFFECTS

None known.

IV INCOMPATIBILITIES

Do not mix with any other medications.

SIDE EFFECTS

Rare

Mild hypersensitivity reaction, marked by, fever, chills, change in blood pressure (B/P) and pulse rate, rash, and urticaria

SERIOUS REACTIONS

- High risk of venous thrombosis during postoperative period.
- Acute hypersensitivity reaction or anaphylactic reaction may occur.
- Risk of transmitting viral hepatitis and other viral diseases.

NURSING CONSIDERATIONS

Baseline Assessment

- Assess the results of the patient's coagulation studies and the extent of existing bleeding, joint pain, overt bleeding or bruising, and swelling.

Precautions

- Use cautiously in patients with liver impairment, recent surgery, and sensitivity to factor IX.

Administration and Handling

IV

- Store in refrigerator.
- Know that reconstituted solution is stable for 12 hours at room temperature.
- Begin administration within 3 hours of reconstitution.
- Do not refrigerate reconstituted solution.
- Before reconstitution, warm diluent to room temperature.
- Gently agitate vial until powder is completely dissolved to prevent the removal of active components during administration through filter.
- Administer by slow IV push or IV infusion.
- Filter before administration.
- Infuse slowly, not to exceed 3 ml/min. Too rapid an IV infusion may produce a change in B/P and pulse rate, headache, flushing, and tingling sensation.

Intervention and Evaluation

- Monitor the patient's intake and output and vital signs.

• Assess the patient for hypersensitivity reaction.

• Monitor the results of the patient's coagulation studies closely.

• Avoid IM or subcutaneous injections.

• Monitor the patient's IV site for oozing every 5 to 15 minutes for 1 to 2 hours after administration.

• Report any evidence of hematuria or change in the patient's vital signs immediately.

Patient Teaching

• Tell the patient to use an electric razor and soft toothbrush to prevent bleeding.

• Warn the patient to notify the physician if he or she experiences any sign of black or red stool, coffee-ground emesis, dark or red urine, and red-speckled mucus from cough.

• Caution the patient against using over-the-counter medications without physician approval.

• Instruct the patient to carry identification that indicates his or her condition or disease.

abciximab
anagrelide
aspirin
cilostazol
clopidogrel
dipyridamole
eptifibatide
ticlopidine
  hydrochloride
tirofiban
treprostinil sodium

Uses: Most antiplatelet agents are used to prevent myocardial infarction (MI) or stroke, repeat MI, and stroke in patients with transient ischemic attacks (TIAs). Cilostazol is prescribed to reduce symptoms of intermittent claudication. The glycoprotein (GP) IIb/IIIa receptor inhibitors are used to prevent ischemic events in patients with acute coronary syndrome and those undergoing percutaneous coronary intervention.

Action: The three major groups of antiplatelet drugs inhibit platelet aggregation by different mechanisms. *Aspirin* irreversibly inhibits cyclooxygenase, thereby blocking the synthesis of thromboxane A_2. *Adenosine diphosphate (ADP) receptor antagonists,* such as clopidogrel, irreversibly block ADP receptors. *GP IIb/IIIa receptor inhibitors,* such as abciximab and tirofiban, reversibly block GP IIb/IIIa receptors. (See illustration, *Mechanisms and Sites of Action: Hematologic Agents,* page 988.)

COMBINATION PRODUCTS
AGGRENOX: dipyridamole/aspirin (an antiplatelet agent) 200 mg/25 mg.

abciximab
ab-**six**-ih-mab
(c7E3 Fab, ReoPro)

CATEGORY AND SCHEDULE
Pregnancy Risk Category: C

MECHANISM OF ACTION
A glycoprotein IIb/IIIa receptor inhibitor that produces rapid inhibition of platelet aggregation by preventing the binding of fibrinogen to GP IIb/IIIa receptor sites on platelets. *Therapeutic Effect:* Prevents closure of treated coronary arteries. Prevents acute cardiac ischemic complications.

PHARMACOKINETICS
Rapidly cleared from plasma with an initial-phase half-life of less than 10 min and a second-phase half-life of 30 min. Platelet function generally returns within 48 hrs.

AVAILABILITY
Injection: 2 mg/ml (5-ml vials).

INDICATIONS AND DOSAGES
▸ **Percutaneous coronary intervention (PCI)**
IV bolus
Adults. 0.25 mg/kg given 10–60 min before angioplasty or atherectomy, then 12-hr IV infusion

of 0.125 mcg/kg/min. Maximum:
10 mcg/min.
▸ **PCI (unstable angina)**
IV bolus
Adults. 0.25 mg/kg, followed
by 18- to 24-hr infusion of
10 mcg/min, end 1 hr after procedure.

CONTRAINDICATIONS

Active internal bleeding, arteriovenous malformation or aneurysm,
cerebrovascular accident (CVA)
with residual neurologic defect,
history of CVA (within the past
2 yrs) or oral anticoagulants within
the past 7 days unless prothrombin
time is less than 1.2 × control,
history of vasculitis, intracranial
neoplasm, prior IV dextran use
before or during PTCA, recent
surgery or trauma (within the past
6 wks), recent (within the past
6 wks) gastrointestinal (GI) or
genitourinary (GU) bleeding,
thrombocytopenia (less than
100,000 cells/mcl), or severe uncontrolled hypertension

INTERACTIONS
Drug

Anticoagulants, including heparin:
May increase risk of hemorrhage.
*Platelet aggregation inhibitors (e.g.,
aspirin, dextran, thrombolytic
agents):* May increase risk of
bleeding.
Herbal
None known.
Food
None known.

DIAGNOSTIC TEST EFFECTS

Increases activated clotting time
(ACT), activated partial thromboplastin time (aPTT), and prothrombin time (PT). Decreases platelet
count.

IV INCOMPATIBILITIES

Administer in separate line; no
other medication should be added to
infusion solution.

SIDE EFFECTS
Frequent
Nausea (16%), hypotension (12%)
Occasional (9%)
Vomiting
Rare (3%)
Bradycardia, abnormal thinking,
dizziness, pain, peripheral edema,
urinary tract infection

SERIOUS REACTIONS

• Major bleeding complications may
occur. If complications occur, stop
the infusion immediately.
• Hypersensitivity reaction may
occur.
• Atrial fibrillation or flutter, pulmonary edema, and complete atrioventricular (AV) block occur occasionally.

NURSING CONSIDERATIONS
Baseline Assessment

• Expect to discontinue heparin
4 hours before the arterial sheath is
removed.
• Maintain patient on bed rest for
6 to 8 hours after the sheath is
removed or the drug is discontinued, whichever is later.
• Check aPTT platelet count, and
PT before abciximab infusion to
assess for preexisting blood abnormalities, 2 to 4 hours after treatment, and at 24 hours or before
discharge, whichever is first.
• Check insertion site, distal pulse
of the affected limb while the femoral artery sheath is in place, and
then routinely for 6 hours after the
femoral artery sheath is removed.
• Minimize the need for invasive
procedures, such as blood draws,

catheters, intubations, and numerous injections.

Lifespan Considerations

• Be aware that it is unknown if abciximab is distributed in breast milk.

• Be aware that the safety and efficacy have not been established in children and that there is an increased risk of bleeding in the elderly.

Precautions

• Use cautiously in patients who weigh less than 75 kg, those over age 65, those with a history of GI disease, and those receiving aspirin, heparin, or thrombolytics. Also use abciximab cautiously in patients who've had a PTCA performed within 12 hours of the onset of signs and symptoms of acute myocardial infarction (MI), who've had a prolonged PTCA (greater than 70 minutes), or who've had a failed PTCA, because they are at increased risk for bleeding.

Administration and Handling

IV

• Store vials in refrigerator.

• Solution normally appears clear and colorless.

• Do not shake.

• Discard any unused portion left in the vial or any preparation that contains opaque particles.

• For bolus injection and continuous infusion, use a sterile, nonpyrogenic, low protein-binding 0.2- or 0.22-micron filter. The continuous infusion may be filtered either during drug preparation or at the time of administration.

• The bolus dose may be given undiluted.

• Withdraw the desired dose and further dilute it in 250 ml of 0.9% NaCl or D_5W (e.g., 10 mg in 250 ml equals a concentration of 40 mcg/ml).

• Give in separate IV line; do not add any other medication to infusion.

• While femoral artery sheath is in position, maintain patient on complete bed rest with head of bed elevated at 30 degrees.

• Maintain affected limb in straight position.

• After the sheath is removed, apply femoral pressure for 30 minutes, either manually or mechanically, then apply a pressure dressing.

Intervention and Evaluation

• Stop abciximab and heparin infusion if any serious bleeding occurs that is uncontrolled by pressure.

• Assess skin for bruises and petechiae. Also, assess for GI, GU, and retroperitoneal bleeding and for bleeding at all puncture sites.

• Avoid the use of IM injections, venipunctures, and the use of indwelling urinary catheters, and nasogastric tubes.

• Handle patient carefully and as infrequently as possible to prevent bleeding.

• Do not obtain blood pressure (B/P) in lower extremities because the patient may have deep vein thrombi.

• Assess for signs and symptoms of hemorrhage, including a decrease in B/P, increase in pulse rate, complaint of abdominal or back pain, or severe headache. Also, monitor laboratory test results, including ACT, aPTT, platelet count, and PT.

• Monitor the patient for an increase in menstrual flow.

• Assess urine for hematuria.

• Monitor for any new or expanding hematomas.

• Gently remove dressings and tape.

Patient Teaching

• Instruct the patient to take precautions to prevent bleeding, such as

the use of an electric razor and soft toothbrush.
• Warn the patient to report any signs of bleeding, including black or red stool, coffee-ground emesis, red or dark urine, or red-speckled mucus from cough.

anagrelide
an-ah-**gree**-lide
(Agrylin)

CATEGORY AND SCHEDULE
Pregnancy Risk Category: C

MECHANISM OF ACTION
A hematologic agent that reduces platelet production and prevents platelet shape changes caused by platelet aggregating agents. *Therapeutic Effect:* Inhibits platelet aggregation.

PHARMACOKINETICS
After PO administration, peak plasma concentration occurs within 1 hr. Extensively metabolized. Primarily excreted in urine. **Half-life:** About 3 days.

AVAILABILITY
Capsules: 0.5 mg, 1 mg.

INDICATIONS AND DOSAGES
▸ **Thrombocythemia**
PO
Adults, Elderly. Initially, 0.5 mg 4 times/day or 1 mg 2 times/day. Adjust to lowest effective dosage, increasing by up to 0.5 mg/day in any 1 wk. Maximum: 10 mg/day or 2.5 mg/dose.

CONTRAINDICATIONS
None known

INTERACTIONS
Drug
None known.
Herbal
None known.
Food
None known.

DIAGNOSTIC TEST EFFECTS
May increase liver enzymes (rare).

SIDE EFFECTS
Frequent (5% or more)
Headache, palpitations, diarrhea, abdominal pain, nausea, flatulence, bloating, asthenia (loss of strength and energy), pain, dizziness
Occasional (less than 5%)
Tachycardia, chest pain, vomiting, paresthesia, peripheral edema, anorexia, dyspepsia, rash
Rare
Confusion, insomnia

SERIOUS REACTIONS
• Angina, heart failure, and arrhythmias occur rarely.

NURSING CONSIDERATIONS
Baseline Assessment
• Expect to obtain Hgb, Hct, platelet count, and white blood cell count (WBC) levels prior to treatment, every 2 days during the first week of treatment, and weekly thereafter until therapeutic range is achieved.
• Determine if the patient is breastfeeding, planning to become pregnant, or pregnant because anagrelide may cause fetal harm.
Lifespan Considerations
• Be aware that it is unknown if anagrelide crosses the placenta or is distributed in breast milk.
• Anagrelide may cause fetal harm.
• Be aware that the safety and efficacy of anagrelide have not been

established in children younger than 16 years.
• Use anagrelide cautiously in the elderly, who have age-related cardiac disease and decreased renal and liver function.

Precautions
• Use cautiously in patients with cardiac disease, or liver or renal impairment.

Administration and Handling
PO
• May give without regard to food.

Intervention and Evaluation
• Expect to monitor BUN, serum creatinine levels, hepatic enzyme test results, and those patients with suspected heart disease.
• Assess the patient's skin for bruises or petechiae, and inspect catheter and needle insertion sites for bleeding. Also assess patient for signs and symptoms of gastrointestinal bleeding.

Patient Teaching
• Inform the patient that his or her platelet count should respond within 7 to 14 days of beginning therapy.
◀ALERT▶ Warn the patient that anagrelide use is not recommended in pregnant women. Strongly urge the patient to use contraceptives while taking anagrelide.

---

cilostazol
sill-oh-**stay**-zole
(Pletal)
Do not confuse with Plendil.

CATEGORY AND SCHEDULE
Pregnancy Risk Category: C

MECHANISM OF ACTION
A phosphodiesterase III inhibitor that inhibits platelet aggregation,

dilation of vascular beds with greatest dilation in femoral beds. *Therapeutic Effect:* Improves walking distance in patients with intermittent claudication.

PHARMACOKINETICS
Moderately absorbed from the gastrointestinal (GI) tract. Protein binding: 95%–98%. Extensively metabolized in the liver. Excreted primarily in the urine and, to a lesser extent, in the feces. Not removed by hemodialysis. **Half-life:** 11–13 hrs. Therapeutic effect noted in 2–4 wks but may take as long as 12 wks before beneficial effect is experienced.

AVAILABILITY
Tablets: 50 mg, 100 mg.

INDICATIONS AND DOSAGES
▶ **Intermittent claudication**
PO
Adults, Elderly. 100 mg 2 times/day at least 30 min before or 2 hrs after meals.

CONTRAINDICATIONS
Congestive heart failure (CHF) of any severity

INTERACTIONS
Drug
None known.
Herbal
None known.
Food
Grapefruit juice: May increase blood concentration and risk of toxicity of cilostazol.

DIAGNOSTIC TEST EFFECTS
May decrease Hgb and Hct. May increase BUN and serum creatinine levels.

SIDE EFFECTS
Frequent (34%–10%)
Headache, diarrhea, palpitations, dizziness, pharyngitis
Occasional (7%–3%)
Nausea, rhinitis, back pain, peripheral edema, dyspepsia, abdominal pain, tachycardia, cough, flatulence, myalgia
Rare (2%–1%)
Leg cramps, paresthesia, rash, vomiting

SERIOUS REACTIONS
• Overdosage is noted by severe headache, diarrhea, hypotension, and cardiac arrhythmias.

NURSING CONSIDERATIONS

Baseline Assessment
• Assess the patient's Hgb, Hct, and platelet count before and periodically during cilostazol treatment.
Lifespan Considerations
• Be aware that it is unknown if cilostazol crosses the placenta or is distributed in breast milk.
• Be aware that the safety and efficacy of cilostazol have not been established in children.
• There are no age-related precautions noted in the elderly.
Administration and Handling
PO
• Give cilostazol at least 30 minutes before or 2 hours after meals.
• Do not take with grapefruit juice.
Patient Teaching
• Instruct the patient to take cilostazol dose on an empty stomach at least 30 minutes before or 2 hours after meals.
• Teach the patient to avoid taking cilostazol with grapefruit juice as this food may increase the drug's blood concentration and risk of toxicity.

clopidogrel
klow-**pih**-duh-grel
(Iscover[AUS], Plavix)

CATEGORY AND SCHEDULE
Pregnancy Risk Category: B

MECHANISM OF ACTION
A thienopyridine derivative that inhibits binding of the enzyme adenosine phosphate (ADP) to its platelet receptor and subsequent ADP-mediated activation of a glycoprotein complex. *Therapeutic Effect:* Inhibits platelet aggregation.

PHARMACOKINETICS

Route	Onset	Peak	Duration
PO	1 hr	2 hrs	N/A

Rapidly absorbed. Protein binding: 98%. Extensively metabolized by the liver. Eliminated equally in the urine and feces. **Half-life:** 8 hrs.

AVAILABILITY
Tablets: 75 mg.

INDICATIONS AND DOSAGES
▶ **Inhibition of platelet aggregation**
PO
Adults, Elderly. 75 mg once a day.

CONTRAINDICATIONS
Active bleeding, coagulation disorders, severe liver disease

INTERACTIONS
Drug
Fluvastatin, other NSAIDs, phenytoin, tamoxifen, tolbutamide, torsemide, warfarin: May interfere with metabolism of fluvastatin, other NSAIDs, phenytoin, tamoxi-

fen, tolbutamide, torsemide, and warfarin.
Herbal
Ginger, ginkgo: May increase the risk of bleeding.
Food
None known.

DIAGNOSTIC TEST EFFECTS
Prolongs bleeding time.

SIDE EFFECTS
Frequent (15%)
Skin disorders
Occasional (8%–6%)
Upper respiratory tract infection, chest pain, flu-like symptoms, headache, dizziness, arthralgia
Rare (5%–3%)
Fatigue, edema, hypertension, abdominal pain, dyspepsia, diarrhea, nausea, epistaxis, dyspnea, rhinitis

SERIOUS REACTIONS
• None known.

NURSING CONSIDERATIONS
Baseline Assessment
• Perform platelet counts prior to clopidogrel therapy, every 2 days during the first week of treatment and weekly thereafter until therapeutic maintenance dose is reached.
• Know that abrupt discontinuation of drug therapy produces an elevation of platelet count within 5 days.
Lifespan Considerations
• Be aware that it is unknown if clopidogrel crosses the placenta or is distributed in breast milk.
• Be aware that the safety and efficacy of clopidogrel have not been established in children.
• There are no age-related precautions noted in the elderly.
Precautions
• Use cautiously in patients sched-uled for surgery and patients with hematologic disorders, history of bleeding, hypertension, and liver or renal impairment.
Administration and Handling
PO
• Give clopidogrel without regard to food.
• Do not crush coated tablets.
Intervention and Evaluation
• Monitor the patient's platelet count for evidence of thrombocytopenia.
• Assess the patient's BUN, Hgb, serum bilirubin, creatinine, SGOT (AST) and SGPT (ALT) levels, and white blood cell (WBC) count.
• Evaluate the patient for signs and symptoms of liver insufficiency during clopidogrel therapy.
Patient Teaching
• Inform the patient that it may take longer to stop bleeding during drug therapy.
• Warn the patient to notify the physician if he or she experiences any unusual bleeding.
• Tell the patient to notify his or her dentist, and other physicians, of clopidogrel therapy before surgery is scheduled or new drugs are prescribed.

dipyridamole
die-pie-**rid**-ah-mole
(Apo-Dipyridamole[CAN], Novodipiradol[CAN], Persantin[AUS], Persantin 100[AUS], Persantin SR[AUS], Persantine)
Do not confuse with Aggrastat, disopyramide, or Periactin.

CATEGORY AND SCHEDULE
Pregnancy Risk Category: C

MECHANISM OF ACTION
A blood modifier and platelet aggregation inhibitor that inhibits the activity of adenosine deaminase and phosphodiesterase, enzymes causing accumulation of adenosine and cyclic adenosine monophosphate (cAMP). *Therapeutic Effect:* Inhibits platelet aggregation, may cause coronary vasodilation.

PHARMACOKINETICS
Slowly, variably absorbed from the gastrointestinal (GI) tract. Widely distributed. Protein binding: 91%–99%. Metabolized in liver. Primarily eliminated via biliary excretion. **Half-life:** 10–15 hrs.

AVAILABILITY
Tablets: 25 mg, 50 mg, 75 mg.
Injection: 5 mg/ml.

INDICATIONS AND DOSAGES
▶ **Prevention of thromboembolic disorders**
PO
Adults, Elderly. 75–100 mg 4 times/day in combination with other medications.
Children. 3–6 mg/kg/day in 3 divided doses.
▶ **Diagnostic**
IV
Adults, Elderly (based on weight). 0.142 mg/kg/min infused over 4 min; doses greater than 60 mg not needed for any patient.

UNLABELED USES
Prophylaxis of myocardial reinfarction, treatment of transient ischemic attacks (TIAs)

CONTRAINDICATIONS
None known

INTERACTIONS
Drug
Anticoagulants, aspirin, heparin, salicylates, thrombolytics: May increase the risk of bleeding with anticoagulants, aspirin, heparin, salicylates, and thrombolytics.
Herbal
None known.
Food
None known.

DIAGNOSTIC TEST EFFECTS
None known.

IV INCOMPATIBILITIES
No information available via Y-site administration.

SIDE EFFECTS
Frequent (14%)
Dizziness
Occasional (6%–2%)
Abdominal distress, headache, rash
Rare (less than 2%)
Diarrhea, vomiting, flushing, pruritus

SERIOUS REACTIONS
• Overdosage produces peripheral vasodilation, resulting in hypotension.

NURSING CONSIDERATIONS
Baseline Assessment
• Assess the patient for chest pain.
• Obtain the patient's baseline blood pressure (B/P) and pulse.
• When used as an antiplatelet, check the patient's hematologic lab levels.
Lifespan Considerations
• Be aware that dipyridamole is distributed in breast milk.
• Be aware that the safety and efficacy of dipyridamole have not been established in children.
• There are no age-related precautions noted in the elderly.

Precautions
• Use cautiously in patients with hypotension.
Administration and Handling
PO
• Give when patient has an empty stomach with full glass of water.
IV
• Dilute to at least 1:2 ratio with 0.9% NaCl or D₅W for total volume of 20 to 50 ml because undiluted solution may cause irritation.
• Infuse over 4 minutes.
• Inject thallium within 5 minutes after dipyridamole infusion, as prescribed.
Intervention and Evaluation
• Assist the patient with ambulation if he or she experiences dizziness.
• Monitor the patient's heart sounds by auscultation.
• Assess the patient's B/P for hypotension.
• Examine the patient's skin for erythema and rash.
Patient Teaching
• Urge the patient to avoid alcohol during dipyridamole therapy.
• Suggest dry toast and unsalted crackers to the patient to relieve nausea.
• Tell the patient that the therapeutic response may not be achieved before 2 to 3 months of continuous therapy.
• Warn the patient to use caution when getting up suddenly from lying or sitting position.

eptifibatide
ep-tih-**fye**-bah-tide
(Integrilin)

CATEGORY AND SCHEDULE
Pregnancy Risk Category: B

MECHANISM OF ACTION
A glycoprotein IIb and IIIa inhibitor that produces rapid inhibition of platelet aggregation by preventing binding of fibrinogen to receptor sites on platelets. *Therapeutic Effect:* Prevents closure of treated coronary arteries. Prevents acute cardiac ischemic complications.

AVAILABILITY
Injection: 0.75 mg/ml, 2 mg/ml.

INDICATIONS AND DOSAGES
▸ **Adjunct percutaneous coronary intervention (PCI)**
IV bolus/IV infusion
Adults, Elderly. 180 mcg/kg before PCI initiation, then continuous drip of 2 mcg/kg/min and a second 180 mcg/kg bolus 10 min after the first.
▸ **Acute coronary syndrome (ACS)**
IV bolus/IV infusion
Adults, Elderly. 180 mcg/kg bolus then 2 mcg/kg/min until discharge or CABG, up to 72 hrs.

CONTRAINDICATIONS
Active internal bleeding, atrioventricular (AV) malformation or aneurysm, history of cerebrovascular accident (CVA) within 2 years or CVA with residual neurologic defect, history of vasculitis, intracranial neoplasm, oral anticoagulants within less than 7 days unless prothrombin time is less than 1.22 times the control, recent (6 wks or less) gastrointestinal (GI) or genitourinary (GU) bleeding, recent surgery or trauma (6 wks or less), prior IV dextran use before or during percutaneous transluminal coronary angioplasty (PTCA), severe uncontrolled hypertension, thrombocytopenia (less than 100,000 cells/mcl)

INTERACTIONS
Drug
Anticoagulants, heparin: May increase the risk of hemorrhage.
Platelet aggregation inhibitors, such as aspirin, dextran, thrombolytic agents: May increase the risk of bleeding.
Herbal
None known.
Food
None known.

DIAGNOSTIC TEST EFFECTS
Increases activated partial thromboplastin time (aPTT), clotting time (ACT), and prothrombin time (PT). Decreases platelet count.

IV INCOMPATIBILITIES
Administer in separate line; no other medication should be added to infusion solution.

SIDE EFFECTS
Occasional (7%)
Hypotension

SERIOUS REACTIONS
• Minor to major bleeding complications may occur, most commonly at arterial access site for cardiac catheterization.

NURSING CONSIDERATIONS

Baseline Assessment
• Obtain the patient's blood Hgb, Hct, and platelet count before treatment. If platelet count is less than 90,000/mm^3, obtain additional platelet counts routinely to avoid thrombocytopenia development.
Lifespan Considerations
• Be aware that it is unknown if eptifibatide causes fetal harm or can affect reproduction capacity.
• Be aware that it is unknown if eptifibatide is distributed in breast milk.
• Be aware that the safety and efficacy of eptifibatide have not been established in children.
• In the elderly the major bleeding risk is increased.
Precautions
• Use cautiously in patients who weigh less than 75 kg, who are older than 65 years of age, have a history of gastrointestinal (GI) disease, and receive aspirin, heparin, or thrombolytics.
• Use cautiously in patients with PTCA less than 12 hours from the onset of symptoms for acute myocardial infarction (MI), prolonged PTCA that's greater than 70 minutes, and failed PTCA.
Administration and Handling
IV
• Store vials in refrigerator. Solution normally appears clear, colorless. Do not shake. Discard any unused portion left in vial or if preparation contains any opaque particles.
• Withdraw bolus dose from 10-ml vial (2 mg/ml); for IV infusion withdraw from 100-ml vial (0.75/ml). IV push and infusion administration may be given undiluted.
• Give IV push over 1 to 2 minutes.
Intervention and Evaluation
• Diligently monitor the patient for potential bleeding, particularly at other arterial and venous puncture sites.
• Avoid nasogastric (NG) tube and urinary catheter use, if possible.
Patient Teaching
• Instruct the patient to let you know if he or she experiences bleeding from surgical site, chest pain, or dyspnea.
• Tell the patient to use an electric razor and soft toothbrush to prevent bleeding during eptifibatide therapy.
• Explain to the patient that he or

she should not take any medications, including over-the-counter (OTC) drugs, especially aspirin, without consulting the physician.
• Warn the patient to notify the you if he or she experiences black or red stool, coffee-ground emesis, dark or red urine, or red-speckled mucus from cough.
• Tell female patients that their menstrual flow may be heavier than usual.

ticlopidine hydrochloride
tie-**clow**-pih-deen
(Apo-Ticlopidine[CAN], Ticlid, Tilodene[AUS])

CATEGORY AND SCHEDULE
Pregnancy Risk Category: B

MECHANISM OF ACTION
An aggregation inhibitor that inhibits adenosine diphosphate (ADP)-induced platelet-fibrinogen binding, further platelet-platelet interactions. *Therapeutic Effect:* Inhibits platelet aggregation.

AVAILABILITY
Tablets: 250 mg.

INDICATIONS AND DOSAGES
▸ **Prevention of stroke**
PO
Adults, Elderly. 250 mg 2 times/day.

UNLABELED USES
Treatment of intermittent claudication, sickle cell disease, subarachnoid hemorrhage

CONTRAINDICATIONS
Active pathologic bleeding, such as bleeding peptic ulcer and intracra-

nial bleeding, hematopoietic disorders, including neutropenia and thrombocytopenia, presence of hemostatic disorder, severe liver impairment

INTERACTIONS
Drug
Aspirin, heparin, oral anticoagulants, thrombolytics: May increase the risk of bleeding with aspirin, heparin, oral anticoagulants, and thrombolytics.
Herbal
None known.
Food
None known.

DIAGNOSTIC TEST EFFECTS
May increase serum cholesterol levels, serum alkaline phosphatase, bilirubin, triglyceride, SGOT (AST), and SGPT (ALT) levels. May prolong bleeding time. May decrease neutrophil and platelet counts.

SIDE EFFECTS
Frequent (13%–5%)
Diarrhea, nausea, dyspepsia, including heartburn, indigestion, GI discomfort, and bloating
Rare (2%–1%)
Vomiting, flatulence, pruritus, dizziness

SERIOUS REACTIONS
• Neutropenia occurs in approximately 2% of patients.
• Thrombotic thrombocytopenia purpura (TTP), agranulocytosis, hepatitis, cholestatic jaundice, and tinnitus occur rarely.

NURSING CONSIDERATIONS
Baseline Assessment
• Discontinue ticlopidine 10–14 days before surgery if antiplatelet effect is not desired.

• Plan to obtain baseline lab studies, particularly hepatic enzyme tests and complete blood count (CBC).

Precautions

• Use cautiously in patients with an increased risk of bleeding and severe liver or renal disease.

Administration and Handling

PO

• Give ticlopidine with food or just after meals to increase bioavailability and decrease gastrointestinal (GI) discomfort.

Intervention and Evaluation

• Assess the patient's daily pattern of bowel activity and stool consistency.

• Assist the patient with ambulation if he or she experiences dizziness.

• Monitor the patient's heart sounds by auscultation.

• Assess the patient's blood pressure (B/P) for hypotension and skin for erythema and rash.

• Monitor the patient's complete blood count (CBC) and hepatic enzyme tests.

• Observe the patient for signs of bleeding.

Patient Teaching

• Instruct the patient to take ticlopidine with food to decrease GI symptoms.

• Stress to the patient that periodic blood tests are essential to treatment.

• Warn the patient to notify the physician if he or she experiences chills, fever, sore throat, or unusual bleeding.

tirofiban

tie-**row**-fih-ban
(Aggrastat)
Do not confuse with Aggrenox.

CATEGORY AND SCHEDULE

Pregnancy Risk Category: B

MECHANISM OF ACTION

An antiplatelet and antithrombotic agent that binds to platelet receptor glycoprotein IIb and IIIa, preventing binding of fibrinogen. *Therapeutic Effect*: Inhibits platelet aggregation.

PHARMACOKINETICS

Poorly bound to plasma proteins; unbound fraction in plasma: 35%. Limited metabolism. Primarily eliminated in the urine (65%) and, to a lesser amount, in the feces. **Half-life:** 2 hrs. Clearance is significantly decreased in severe renal impairment (creatinine clearance less than 30 ml/min). Removed by hemodialysis.

AVAILABILITY

Injection Premix: 12.5 mg/250 ml, 25 mg/500 ml (50 mcg/ml).
Vial: 250 mcg/ml.

INDICATIONS AND DOSAGES

▸ **Inhibition of platelet aggregation**
IV
Adults, Elderly. Give at initial rate of 0.4 mcg/kg/min for 30 min and then continue at 0.1 mcg/kg/min through procedure and for 12–24 hrs after procedure.
▸ **Severe renal insufficiency** (creatinine clearance less than 30 ml/min) Half the usual rate of infusion.

CONTRAINDICATIONS

Active internal bleeding or a history of bleeding diathesis within previous 30 days, arteriovenous malformation or aneurysm, history of intracranial hemorrhage, history of thrombocytopenia after prior exposure to tirofiban, intracranial neoplasm, major surgical procedure within previous 30 days, severe hypertension, stroke

INTERACTIONS
Drug
Drugs that affect hemostasis, such as aspirin, heparin, NSAIDs, and warfarin: May increase the risk of bleeding
Herbal
None known.
Food
None known.

DIAGNOSTIC TEST EFFECTS
Decreases blood Hct and Hgb and platelet count.

IV INCOMPATIBILITIES
Do not mix with any other medications.

SIDE EFFECTS
Occasional (6%–3%)
Pelvis pain, bradycardia, dizziness, leg pain
Rare (2%–1%)
Edema and swelling, vasovagal reaction, diaphoresis, nausea, fever, headache

SERIOUS REACTIONS
* Overdosage is manifested as primarily minor mucocutaneous bleeding and bleeding at the femoral artery access site.
* Thrombocytopenia occurs rarely.

NURSING CONSIDERATIONS

Baseline Assessment
* Assess the patient's activated partial thromboplastin time (aPTT), blood Hct, Hgb, platelet count, and serum creatinine prior to tirofiban treatment, within 6 hours after the loading dose, and at least daily thereafter during therapy. If the patient's platelet count is less than 90,000/mm^3, obtain additional platelet counts routinely to avoid thrombocytopenia. If the patient

develops thrombocytopenia, discontinue tirofiban therapy and heparin, as prescribed.
Lifespan Considerations
* Be aware that it is unknown if tirofiban is distributed in breast milk.
* Be aware that the safety and efficacy of tirofiban have not been established in children.
* There is an increased risk of bleeding in the elderly. Use tirofiban with caution in this patient population.
Precautions
* Use cautiously in patients with hemorrhagic retinopathy, platelet counts less than 150,000/mm^3, and renal function impairment.
* Use cautiously in patients who concomitantly use drugs affecting hemostasis, such as warfarin.
Administration and Handling
◀ALERT▶ Remember that heparin and tirofiban can be administered through the same IV line.
IV
* Store at room temperature.
* Protect from light.
* Use only clear solution.
* Discard unused solution 24 hours after start of infusion.
* For injection for solution (250 mcg/ml), withdraw and discard 100 ml from a 500-ml bag of 0.9% NaCl or D$_5$W and replace this volume with 100 ml of tirofiban drawn from two 50-ml vials, or withdraw and discard 50 ml from a 250-ml bag and replace with 50 ml of tirofiban drawn from one 50-ml vial to achieve a final concentration of 50 mcg/ml.
* Mix injection for solution (250 mcg/ml) well before administration.
* For injection (50 mcg/ml) premix in 500-ml IntraVia container, tear

off the dust cover to open the Intra-Via container.

• Check the IntraVia container for leaks by squeezing the inner bag firmly; if any leak is found or if the solution is not clear, discard the solution.

• Do not add other drugs or remove injection (50 mcg/ml) premix solution directly from the bag with a syringe. Do not use plastic containers in series connections because it may result in air embolism caused by drawing air from the first container that holds no solution.

• For loading dose, give 0.4 mcg/kg/min for 30 minutes.

• For maintenance infusion, give 0.1 mcg/kg/min.

Intervention and Evaluation

• Monitor the patient's activated partial thromboplastin time (aPTT) 6 hours after the beginning of the heparin infusion.

• Adjust heparin dosage to maintain aPTT at approximately 2 times control.

• Closely monitor the patient for bleeding, particularly at other arterial and venous puncture sites and IM injection sites.

• Avoid nasol gastric (NG) tube and urinary catheter use, if possible.

• Maintain complete bed rest of the patient with head of the bed elevated at 30 degrees.

Patient Teaching

• Inform the patient that it may take longer to stop bleeding during drug therapy.

• Warn the patient to notify the physician if he or she experiences any unusual bleeding.

• Tell the patient to notify his or her dentist, and other physicians, of tirofiban therapy before surgery is scheduled or new drugs are prescribed.

treprostinil sodium
tre-**pros**-tin-il
(Remodulin)

CATEGORY AND SCHEDULE
Pregnancy Risk Category: B

MECHANISM OF ACTION
An antiplatelet that directly vasodilates pulmonary and systemic arterial vascular beds, inhibits platelet aggregation. *Therapeutic Effect:* Reduces symptoms of pulmonary arterial hypertension associated with exercise.

PHARMACOKINETICS
Rapidly, completely absorbed after subcutaneous infusion; 91% bound to plasma protein. Metabolized by the liver. Excreted mainly in the urine with a lesser amount eliminated in the feces. **Half-life:** 2–4 hrs.

AVAILABILITY
Injection: 1 mg/ml, 2.5 mg/ml, 5 mg/ml, 10 mg/ml.

INDICATIONS AND DOSAGES
▶ **Pulmonary arterial hypertension**
Continuous subcutaneous infusion
Adults, Elderly. Initially, 1.25 ng/kg/min. Reduce infusion rate to 0.625 ng/kg/min if initial dose cannot be tolerated. Increase infusion rate in increments of no more than 1.25 ng/kg/min per week for the first 4 wks and then no more than 2.5 ng/kg/min per week for the remaining duration of infusion.
▶ **Liver function impairment**
In mild to moderate hepatic insufficiency, decrease the initial dose to 0.625 ng/kg/min ideal body weight and increase cautiously.

CONTRAINDICATIONS
None known

INTERACTIONS
Drug
Anticoagulants, aspirin, heparin, thrombolytics: May increase the risk of bleeding.
Drugs that alter blood pressure (B/P), including antihypertensive agents, diuretics, vasodilators: Reduction in B/P caused by treprostinil may be exacerbated by other drugs that alter blood pressure.
Herbal
None known.
Food
None known.

DIAGNOSTIC TEST EFFECTS
None known.

SIDE EFFECTS
Frequent
Infusion site pain, erythema, induration, rash
Occasional
Headache, diarrhea, jaw pain, vasodilation, nausea
Rare
Dizziness, hypotension, pruritus, edema

SERIOUS REACTIONS
• Abrupt withdrawal or sudden large reductions in dosage may result in worsening of pulmonary arterial hypertension symptoms.

NURSING CONSIDERATIONS
Baseline Assessment
• Expect to obtain baseline lab tests, including BUN, hepatic enzymes, and serum creatinine.
Lifespan Considerations
• Be aware that it is unknown if treprostinil is distributed in breast milk.

• Be aware that the safety and efficacy of treprostinil have not been established in children.
• In the elderly, age-related decreased cardiac, liver, and renal function may require dosage adjustment.
• In the elderly, concurrent disease or other drug therapy may require treprostinil dosage adjustment.
Precautions
• Use cautiously in elderly patients older than 65 years of age with liver or renal impairment.
Administration and Handling
Subcutaneous
• Store at room temperature.
• Administer without further dilution.
• Do not use a single vial for longer than 14 days after initial use.
• To avoid potential interruptions in drug delivery, provide the patient with immediate access to a backup infusion pump and spare subcutaneous infusion sets.
• Give as a continuous subcutaneous infusion via a subcutaneous catheter, using an infusion pump designed for subcutaneous drug delivery.
• Calculate the infusion rate using following formula: Infusion rate (ml/hr) = Dose (ng/kg/min) multiplied by Weight (kg) multiplied by (0.00006/treprostinil dosage strength concentration [mg/ml]).
Patient Teaching
• Instruct the patient regarding drug administration as a delivery system via a self-inserted subcutaneous catheter using an ambulatory pump.
• Teach the patient how to care for the subcutaneous catheter and troubleshoot infusion pump problems.
• Tell the patient to notify the physician if he or she experiences signs of increased pulmonary artery pressure, such as dyspnea, cough, or chest pain.

57 Hematinics

sodium ferric gluconate complex
ferrous fumarate,
ferrous gluconate,
ferrous sulfate
iron dextran
iron sucrose

Uses: Hematinics (iron supplements) are used to prevent and treat iron deficiency, which may result from improper diet, pregnancy, impaired absorption, or prolonged blood loss.

Action: Hematinics provide supplementary iron to ensure adequate supplies for the formation of hemoglobin, which is needed for erythropoiesis and oxygen transport.

COMBINATION PRODUCTS

FERRO-SEQUELS: ferrous fumarate/docusate (a stool softener) 150 mg/100 mg.

sodium ferric gluconate complex
(Ferrlecit)

CATEGORY AND SCHEDULE
Pregnancy Risk Category: B

MECHANISM OF ACTION

A trace element that repletes total body content of iron. *Therapeutic Effect:* Replaces iron found in Hgb, myoglobin, and specific enzymes; allows oxygen transport via hemoglobin.

AVAILABILITY

Ampoules: 12.5 mg/ml elemental iron.

INDICATIONS AND DOSAGES
▶ **Iron deficiency anemia**
IV infusion
Adults, Elderly. 125 mg in 100 ml 0.9% NaCl infused over 1 hr. Minimum cumulative dose 1 g elemental iron given over 8 sessions at sequential dialysis treatment. May be given during dialysis session itself.

CONTRAINDICATIONS

All anemias not associated with iron deficiency

INTERACTIONS
Drug
None known.
Herbal
None known.
Food
None known.

DIAGNOSTIC TEST EFFECTS
None known.

IV INCOMPATIBILITIES
Do not mix with any other medications.

SIDE EFFECTS
Frequent (greater than 3%)
Flushing, hypotension, hypersensitivity reaction
Occasional (3%–1%)
Injection site reaction, headache, abdominal pain, chills, flu-like syndrome, dizziness, leg cramps, dyspnea, nausea, vomiting, diarrhea, myalgia, pruritus, edema

SERIOUS REACTIONS
• Rarely, potentially fatal hypersensitivity reaction characterized by cardiovascular collapse, cardiac arrest, dyspnea, bronchospasm, angioedema, and urticaria occurs.

• Hypotension associated with flushing, lightheadedness, fatigue, weakness, or severe pain in chest, back, or groin with rapid administration of iron may occur.

NURSING CONSIDERATIONS

Baseline Assessment
• Do not give concurrently with oral iron form. Excessive iron may produce excessive iron storage or hemosiderosis.
• Assess patients with rheumatoid arthritis or iron deficiency anemia for acute exacerbation of joint pain and swelling.

Lifespan Considerations
• Be aware that it is unknown if sodium ferric gluconate complex is distributed in breast milk.
• Be aware that the safety and efficacy of sodium ferric gluconate complex have not been established in children.
• There are no age-related precautions noted in the elderly. Be aware that lower initial dosages of sodium ferric gluconate complex are recommended in the elderly.

Precautions
• Use cautiously in patients with asthma, iron overload, liver impairment, rheumatoid arthritis, and significant allergies.

Administration and Handling
◀ALERT▶ Plan to initially administer a 25-mg test dose that's diluted in 50 ml 0.9% NaCl and given over 60 minutes.
• May give IV undiluted without test dose.
IV
• Store at room temperature.
• Use immediately after dilution.
• Must be diluted.
• Know that the test dose is dilute 25 mg (2 ml) with 50 ml 0.9% NaCl.
• Remember that the standard

recommended dose is diluted 125 mg (10 ml) with 100 ml 0.9% NaCl.
• Infuse both test dose and standard dose over 1 hour.

Intervention and Evaluation
• Monitor the patient's lab tests, especially complete blood count (CBC), serum iron concentrations, and vital signs. Remember that lab test results may not be meaningful for 3 weeks after beginning sodium ferric gluconate complex administration.

Patient Teaching
• Tell the patient that his or her stools may become black with iron therapy. Explain to the patient that this effect is harmless unless accompanied by abdominal cramping or pain, red streaking, and sticky consistency of stool.
• Warn the patient to notify the physician if he or she experiences abdominal cramping or pain, red streaking, and sticky consistency of stool.
• Tell the patient that the drug may be administered during dialysis treatments.

---

ferrous fumarate
fair-us **fume**-ah-rate
(Feostat, Femiron, Palafer[CAN])

ferrous gluconate
fair-us **glue**-kuh-nate
(Apo-Ferrous Gluconate[CAN], Fergon, Ferralet, Simron)

ferrous sulfate
fair-us **sul**-fate
(Apo-Ferrous Sulfate[CAN], Feosol, Fer-In-Sol, Ferro-Gradumet[AUS], Slow-Fe)

CATEGORY AND SCHEDULE
Pregnancy Risk Category: A
OTC

MECHANISM OF ACTION

An enzymatic mineral that acts as an essential component in formation of Hgb, myoglobin, and enzymes. *Therapeutic Effect:* Necessary for effective erythropoiesis and for transport and utilization of oxygen (O_2).

PHARMACOKINETICS

Absorbed in duodenum and upper jejunum; 10% absorbed in those with normal iron stores, increased to 20%–30% in those with inadequate iron stores. Primarily bound to serum transferrin. Excreted in urine, sweat, sloughing of intestinal mucosa and by menses. **Half-life:** 6 hrs.

AVAILABILITY

Ferrous fumarate
Tablets: 63 mg, 195 mg, 200 mg, 324 mg, 350 mg.
Tablets (chewable): 100 mg.
Capsules (controlled-release): 325 mg.
Suspension: 100 mg/5 ml.
Oral Drops: 45 mg/0.6 ml.
Ferrous gluconate
Tablets: 300 mg, 320 mg.
Tablets (sustained release): 320 mg.
Ferrous sulfate
Tablets: 195 mg, 300 mg, 324 mg.
Capsules: 250 mg.
Tablets (timed-release): 325 mg.
Syrup: 90 mg/5 ml.
Elixir: 220 mg/5 ml.
Oral Drops: 125 mg/ml.
Ferrous sulfate (exsiccated)
Tablets: 200 mg.
Tablets (slow-release): 160 mg.
Capsules: 190 mg.
Capsules (timed-release): 159 mg, 250 mg.

INDICATIONS AND DOSAGES

▸ **Iron deficiency**
PO
Adults, Elderly. 2–3 mg/kg/day or 50–100 mg elemental iron 2 times/day up to 100 mg 4 times/day.
Children. 3 mg/kg/day elemental iron in 1–3 divided doses.
▸ **Prophylaxis, iron deficiency**
PO
Adults, Elderly. 60–100 mg elemental iron/day.
Children. 1–2 mg/kg/day elemental iron. Maximum: 15 mg elemental iron/day.

CONTRAINDICATIONS

Hemochromatosis, hemosiderosis, hemolytic anemias, peptic ulcer, regional enteritis, ulcerative colitis

INTERACTIONS

Drug
Antacids, calcium supplements, pancreatin, pancrelipase: May decrease the absorption of ferrous fumarate, ferrous gluconate, and ferrous sulfate.
Etidronate, quinolones, tetracyclines: May decrease the absorption of etidronate, quinolones, and tetracyclines.
Herbal
None known.
Food
Eggs and milk: Inhibit ferrous fumarate absorption.

DIAGNOSTIC TEST EFFECTS

May increase serum bilirubin. May decrease serum calcium levels. May obscure occult blood in stools.

SIDE EFFECTS

Occasional
Mild, transient nausea
Rare
Heartburn, anorexia, constipation, or diarrhea

SERIOUS REACTIONS

• Large doses may aggravate existing gastrointestinal (GI) tract disease, such as peptic ulcer disease, regional enteritis, and ulcerative colitis.

• Severe iron poisoning occurs mostly in children and is manifested as vomiting, severe abdominal pain, diarrhea, dehydration, followed by hyperventilation, pallor or cyanosis, and cardiovascular collapse.

NURSING CONSIDERATIONS

Baseline Assessment

• Use dropper or straw and allow the drug solution to drop on the back of the patient's tongue to prevent mucous membrane and teeth staining with liquid preparation.

• Know that eggs and milk inhibit drug absorption.

Lifespan Considerations

• Be aware that ferrous fumarate, ferrous sulfate, and ferrous gluconate cross the placenta and are distributed in breast milk.

• There are no age-related precautions noted in children and the elderly.

Precautions

• Use cautiously in patients with bronchial asthma and iron hypersensitivity.

Administration and Handling

◄ALERT► Keep in mind that dosage is expressed in terms of elemental iron. Elemental iron content for ferrous fumarate is 33% (99 mg iron/300 mg tablet); ferrous gluconate is 11.6% (35 mg iron/300 mg tablet); ferrous sulfate is 20% (60 mg iron/300 mg tablet).

PO

• Store all forms, including tablets, capsules, suspension, and drops, at room temperature.

• Give between meals with water unless GI discomfort occurs; if so, give with meals.

• To avoid transient staining of mucous membranes and teeth, place liquid on back of tongue with dropper or straw.

• Avoid simultaneous administration of antacids or tetracycline.

• Do not crush sustained-release preparations.

Intervention and Evaluation

• Monitor the patient's blood Hgb, ferritin, reticulocyte count, serum iron, and total iron-binding capacity.

• Assess the patient's daily pattern of bowel activity and stool consistency.

• Evaluate the patient for clinical improvement and record relief of iron deficiency symptoms, fatigue, headache, irritability, pallor, and paresthesia of extremities.

Patient Teaching

• Tell the patient that his or her stools will darken in color.

• Teach the patient to take the drug after meals, or with food if he or she experiences GI discomfort.

• Instruct the patient not to take the drug within 2 hours of antacids as antacids prevent the absorption of this drug.

• Teach the patient not to take the drug with milk or eggs.

iron dextran

iron **dex**-tran

(Dexiron[CAN], Infed, Infufer[CAN])

CATEGORY AND SCHEDULE

Pregnancy Risk Category: C

MECHANISM OF ACTION

A trace element and essential component of formation of Hgb. Necessary for effective erythropoiesis and oxygen (O_2) transport capacity of blood. Serves as cofactor of several essential enzymes. *Therapeutic Effect:* Replenishes hemoglobin and depleted iron stores.

PHARMACOKINETICS

Readily absorbed after IM administration. Major portion of absorption occurs within 72 hrs; remainder within 3–4 wks. Iron is bound to protein to form hemosiderin, ferritin, or transferrin. No physiologic system of elimination. Small amounts lost daily in shedding of skin, hair, and nails and in feces, urine, and perspiration. **Half-life:** 5–20 hrs.

AVAILABILITY

Injection: 50 mg/ml.

INDICATIONS AND DOSAGES

▶ **Iron deficiency anemia (no blood loss)**
IM/IV
Adults, Elderly. Mg iron = 0.66 × weight (kg) × (100 – Hgb [g/dl]/ 14.8

▶ **Replacement secondary to blood loss**
IM/IV
Adults, Elderly. Replacement iron (mg) = blood loss (ml) times Hct.

CONTRAINDICATIONS

All anemias except iron deficiency anemia, including pernicious, aplastic, normocytic, and refractory

INTERACTIONS

Drug
None known.
Herbal
None known.
Food
None known.

DIAGNOSTIC TEST EFFECTS

None known.

IV INCOMPATIBILITIES

No information available via Y-site administration.

SIDE EFFECTS

Frequent
Allergic reaction, such as rash and itching, backache, muscle pain, chills, dizziness, headache, fever, nausea, vomiting, flushed skin, pain or redness at injection site, brown discoloration of skin, metallic taste

SERIOUS REACTIONS

• Anaphylaxis has occurred during the first few minutes after injection, causing death on rare occasions.
• Leukocytosis and lymphadenopathy occur rarely.

NURSING CONSIDERATIONS

Baseline Assessment
• Do not give concurrently with oral iron form because excessive iron may produce excessive iron storage, called hemosiderosis.
• Be alert to patients with rheumatoid arthritis or iron deficiency anemia as acute exacerbation of joint pain and swelling may occur.
• Know that inguinal lymphadenopathy may occur with IM injection.
• Assess the patient for adequate muscle mass before injecting medication.
Lifespan Considerations
• Be aware that iron dextran may cross the placenta in some form and trace amounts of the drug are distributed in breast milk.
• There are no age-related precautions noted in children and the elderly.
Precautions
• Use extremely cautiously in patients with serious liver impairment.

• Use cautiously in patients with bronchial asthma, a history of allergies, and rheumatoid arthritis.

Administration and Handling

◀**ALERT**▶ Know that a test dose is generally given before the full dosage; stay with patient for several minutes after injection due to potential for anaphylactic reaction.

◀**ALERT**▶ Plan to discontinue oral iron form before administering iron dextran. Know that the dosage is expressed in terms of milligrams of elemental iron, degree of anemia, patient weight, and presence of any bleeding. Expect to use periodic hematologic determinations as guide to therapy.

IM

• Draw up medication with one needle; use new needle for injection to minimize skin staining.

• Administer deep IM in upper outer quadrant of buttock only.

• Use Z-tract technique by displacing subcutaneous tissue lateral to injection site before inserting needle to minimize skin staining.

IV

• Store at room temperature.

• May give undiluted or dilute in 0.9% NaCl for infusion.

• Do not exceed IV administration rate of 50 mg/min (1 ml/min). A too rapid IV rate may produce flushing, chest pain, shock, hypotension, tachycardia.

• Keep patient recumbent 30 to 45 minutes after IV administration to avoid postural hypotension.

Intervention and Evaluation

• Monitor the patient's IM site for abscess formation, atrophy, brownish skin color, necrosis, and swelling.

• Evaluate the patient for inflammation, pain, and soreness at or near IM injection site.

• Examine the patient's IV site for phlebitis.

• Monitor the patient's serum ferritin levels.

Patient Teaching

• Tell the patient that he or she may experience pain and brown staining of the skin at the injection site.

• Caution the patient that oral iron should not be taken when receiving iron injections.

• Instruct the patient that his or her stools may become black with iron therapy. Explain that this side effect is harmless unless accompanied by abdominal cramping or pain, red streaking, and sticky consistency of stool.

• Warn the patient to notify the physician if he or she experiences abdominal cramping or pain, back pain, fever, headache, or red streaking or a sticky consistency of stool.

• Suggest gum, hard candy, and maintaining good oral hygiene to prevent or reduce the metallic taste.

iron sucrose
iron **sue**-crose
(Venofer)

CATEGORY AND SCHEDULE
Pregnancy Risk Category: B

MECHANISM OF ACTION
A trace element that is an essential component of formation of Hgb, is necessary for effective erythropoiesis and oxygen transport capacity of blood, and serves as cofactor of several essential enzymes. *Therapeutic Effect:* Replenishes body iron stores in patients on chronic hemodialysis who have iron deficiency anemia and are receiving erythropoietin.

AVAILABILITY
Injection: 20 mg/ml or 100 mg elemental iron in 5-ml single-dose vial.

INDICATIONS AND DOSAGES
▸ **Iron deficiency anemia**
IV
Adults, Elderly. 5 ml iron sucrose, or 100 mg elemental iron, delivered by IV during dialysis; administer 1–3 times/wk to total dose of 1,000 mg in 10 doses. Give no more than 3 times/wk.

UNLABELED USES
Treatment of dystrophic epidermolysis bullosa

CONTRAINDICATIONS
All anemias except iron deficiency anemia, including pernicious, aplastic, normocytic, and refractory anemia, evidence of iron overload

INTERACTIONS
Drug
None known.
Herbal
None known.
Food
None known.

DIAGNOSTIC TEST EFFECTS
Increases blood Hgb, Hct, serum ferritin levels, and serum transferrin saturation.

IV INCOMPATIBILITIES
Do not mix with other medication or add to parenteral nutrition solution for IV infusion.

SIDE EFFECTS
Frequent (36%–23%)
Hypotension, leg cramps, diarrhea

SERIOUS REACTIONS
• A too rapid IV administration may produce severe hypotension, headache, vomiting, nausea, dizziness, paresthesia, abdominal and muscle pain, edema, and cardiovascular collapse.
• Hypersensitivity reaction occurs rarely.

NURSING CONSIDERATIONS
Baseline Assessment
• Plan to obtain baseline lab tests, including blood Hgb, Hct, serum ferritin levels, and serum transferrin saturation.
• Make sure that the patient has patent dialysis access before preparing drug.
Precautions
• Use cautiously in patients with cardiac dysfunction, bronchial asthma, history of allergies, and liver or renal impairment.
Administration and Handling
◂ALERT▸ Administer directly into dialysis line during hemodialysis, as prescribed.
◂ALERT▸ Be aware that the dosage is expressed in terms of milligrams of elemental iron.
IV
• Store at room temperature.
• May give undiluted as slow IV injection or IV infusion. For IV infusion, dilute each vial in maximum of 100 ml 0.9% NaCl immediately before infusion.
• For IV injection, administer into the dialysis line at a rate of 1 ml, or 20 mg iron, undiluted solution per min. Allow 5 minutes per vial, and do not exceed 1 vial per injection.
• For IV infusion, administer into dialysis line at a rate of 100 mg iron over at least 15 minutes be-

cause it reduces the risk of hypotensive episodes.

Intervention and Evaluation
• Initially, monitor the patient's Hct, Hgb, serum ferritin, and serum transferrin levels monthly, then every 2 to 3 months thereafter.
• Obtain reliable patient serum iron values 48 hours after administration.

Patient Teaching
• Tell the patient to expect follow-up blood tests to monitor the results of treatment.
• Explain that iron sucrose is administered during dialysis.
• Ask the patient to report any leg cramps or diarrhea.

darbepoetin alfa
epoetin alfa
filgrastim
oprelvekin
  (interleukin-2, IL-2)
pegfilgrastim
sargramostim
  (granulocyte
  macrophage colony-
  stimulating factor,
  GM-CSF)

Uses: Hematopoietic agents are used to accelerate neutrophil repopulation after cancer chemotherapy, to accelerate bone marrow recovery after autologous bone marrow transplant, and to stimulate erythrocyte production in patients with chronic renal failure.

Action: Hematopoietic agents act by stimulating the proliferation and differentiation of hematopoietic growth factors (naturally occurring hormones) and by enhancing the function of mature forms of neutrophils, monocytes, macrophages, and erythrocytes.

---

darbepoetin alfa
dar-bee-eh-poe-ee-tin alfa
(Aranesp)
Do not confuse with Aricept.

CATEGORY AND SCHEDULE
Pregnancy Risk Category: C

MECHANISM OF ACTION
A glycoprotein that stimulates formation of red blood cells (RBCs) in bone marrow; increases serum half-life of epoetin. *Therapeutic Effect:* Induces erythropoiesis, release of reticulocytes from marrow.

PHARMACOKINETICS
Well absorbed after subcutaneous administration. **Half-life:** 48.5 hrs.

AVAILABILITY
Injection: 25 mcg/ml, 40 mcg/ml, 60 mcg/ml, 100 mcg/ml, 200 mcg/ml, 300 mcg/ml.

INDICATIONS AND DOSAGES
▸ **Anemia in chronic renal failure**
Subcutaneous/IV bolus

Adults, Elderly. Initially, 0.45 mcg/kg once weekly. Adjust dosage to achieve and maintain a target Hgb not to exceed 12 g/dl. Do not increase dose more frequently than once monthly. Limit increases in Hgb by less than 1 g/dl over any 2 week period.
▸ **Anemia associated with chemotherapy**
IV/Subcutaneous
Adults, Elderly. 2.25 mcg/kg/dose once a week.

CONTRAINDICATIONS
History of sensitivity to mammalian cell-derived products or human albumin, uncontrolled hypertension

INTERACTIONS
Drug
None known.
Herbal
None known.
Food
None known.

DIAGNOSTIC TEST EFFECTS
May decrease bleeding time, iron concentration, serum ferritin. May increase BUN, serum phosphorus,

potassium, serum creatinine, serum
uric acid, and sodium levels.

IV INCOMPATIBILITIES
Do not mix with any other medications.

SIDE EFFECTS
Frequent
Myalgia, hypertension/hypotension,
headache, diarrhea
Occasional
Fatigue, edema, vomiting, reaction
at administration site, asthenia,
dizziness

SERIOUS REACTIONS
• Vascular access thrombosis, congestive heart failure (CHF), sepsis,
arrhythmias, and anaphylactic reaction occur rarely.

NURSING CONSIDERATIONS

Baseline Assessment
• Assess the patient's blood pressure
(B/P) before drug administration.
Know that 80% of patients with
chronic renal failure have a history
of hypertension. Expect that B/P
often rises during early therapy
in patients with a history of hypertension.
• Assess the patient's serum iron
and keep in mind that transferrin
saturation should be greater than
20%, and serum ferritin should be
greater than 100 ng/ml, before and
during therapy.
• Consider that all patients will
eventually need supplemental iron
therapy.
• Establish the patient's baseline
complete blood count (CBC), especially note the patient's blood Hct.
Lifespan Considerations
• Be aware that it is unknown if
darbepoetin alfa crosses the placenta
or is distributed in breast milk.

• Be aware that the safety and
efficacy of darbepoetin alfa have
not been established in children.
• In the elderly, age-related renal
impairment may require dosage
adjustment.
Precautions
• Use cautiously in patients with
hemolytic anemia, history of seizures, known porphyria or impairment of erythrocyte formation in
bone marrow or responsible for
liver impairment, sickle cell anemia,
and thalassemia.
Administration and Handling
◀ALERT▶ Avoid excessive agitation
of vial; do not shake because it will
cause foaming.
Subcutaneous
• Use 1 dose per vial; do not reenter vial. Discard unused portion.
May be mixed in a syringe with
bacteriostatic 0.9% NaCl with
benzyl alcohol 0.9% or bacteriostatic saline at a 1:1 ratio; benzyl
alcohol acts as a local anesthetic;
may reduce injection site discomfort.
IV
• Refrigerate vials. Know that
vigorous shaking may denature
medication, rendering it inactive.
• Know that reconstitution is not
necessary.
• May be given as an IV bolus.
Intervention and Evaluation
• Monitor the patient's blood Hct
level diligently. Reduce the drug
dosage if the patient's Hct level
increases more than 4 points in
2 weeks.
• Monitor the patient's BUN, CBC
with differential, Hgb, phosphorus,
potassium, reticulocyte count, serum
creatinine, and serum ferritin.
• Monitor the patient's blood pressure (B/P) aggressively for increase
because 25% of patients taking

medication require antihypertension therapy and dietary restrictions.

Patient Teaching

• Stress to the patient that frequent blood tests are needed to determine correct drug dose.

• Warn the patient to notify the physician if he or she develops a severe headache.

• Caution the patient to avoid hazardous activities, such as driving, during first 90 days of therapy.

epoetin alfa
eh-po-**ee**-tin
(Epogen, Eprex[CAN], Procrit)
Do not confuse with Neupogen.

CATEGORY AND SCHEDULE
Pregnancy Risk Category: C

MECHANISM OF ACTION
A glycoprotein that stimulates division, differentiation of erythroid progenitor cells in bone marrow. *Therapeutic Effect:* Induces erythropoiesis, releases reticulocytes from marrow.

PHARMACOKINETICS
Well absorbed after subcutaneous administration. After administration, an increase in reticulocyte count seen within 10 days, increases in blood Hgb and Hct, and red blood cell (RBC) count within 2–6 wks. **Half-life:** 4–13 hrs.

AVAILABILITY
Injection: 2,000 units/ml, 3000 units/ml, 4,000 units/ml, 10,000 units/ml, 20,000 units/ml, 40,000 units/ml.

INDICATIONS AND DOSAGES
▶ **Chemotherapy patients**
IV/Subcutaneous
Adults, Elderly, Children. 150 units/kg/dose 3 times/wk. Maximum: 1200 units/kg/wk.
▶ **Reduction of allogenic blood transfusions in elective surgery**
Subcutaneous
Adults, Elderly. 300 units/kg/day 10 days before, on day of, and 4 days after surgery.
▶ **Chronic renal failure**
Subcutaneous/IV bolus
Adults, Elderly. Initially, 50–100 units/kg 3 times/wk. Target Hct range: 30%–36%. Dosage adjustments not earlier than 1-mo intervals unless prescribed. Decrease Dose: Hct increasing and approaching 36%: Plan to temporarily hold doses if Hct continues to rise, reinstate lower dose when Hct begins to decrease; Hct increases by more than 4 points in 2 wks: monitor Hct 2 times/wk for 2–6 wks. Increase Dose: Hct does not increase 5–6 points after 8 wks—with adequate iron stores—and Hct below target range. Maintenance: *(Dialysis):* 75 units/kg 3 times/wk. Range: 12.5–525 units/kg. *(Nondialysis):* 75–150 units/kg/wk.
▶ **AZT-treated, HIV-infected patients**
Subcutaneous/IV
Adults. Initially, 100 units/kg 3 times/wk for 8 wks; may increase by 50–100 units/kg 3 times/wk. Evaluate response q4–8wks thereafter; adjust dose by 50–100 units/kg 3 times/wk. If doses larger than 300 units/kg 3 times/wk are not eliciting response, it is unlikely patient will respond. Maintenance: Titrate to maintain desired Hct.

UNLABELED USES
Prevents anemia in patients donating blood before elective surgery or autologous transfusion, treatment of anemia associated with neoplastic diseases.

CONTRAINDICATIONS
History of sensitivity to mammalian cell-derived products or human albumin, uncontrolled hypertension

INTERACTIONS
Drug
Heparin: May need to increase heparin. An increase in RBC volume may enhance blood clotting.
Herbal
None known.
Food
None known.

DIAGNOSTIC TEST EFFECTS
May decrease bleeding time, iron concentration, serum ferritin. May increase BUN, serum phosphorus, potassium, serum creatinine, serum uric acid, and sodium levels.

IV INCOMPATIBILITIES
Do not mix with any other medications.

SIDE EFFECTS
▸ **Cancer patients on chemotherapy**
Frequent (20%–17%)
Fever, diarrhea, nausea, vomiting, edema
Occasional (13%–11%)
Asthenia (loss of strength, energy), shortness of breath, paresthesia
Rare (5%–3%)
Dizziness, trunk pain
▸ **Chronic renal failure patients**
Frequent (24%–11%)
Hypertension, headache, nausea, arthralgia
Occasional (9%–7%)
Fatigue, edema, diarrhea, vomiting,

chest pain, skin reactions at administration site, asthenia or loss of energy and strength, dizziness
▸ **AZT-treated HIV-infected patients**
Frequent (38%–15%)
Fever, fatigue, headache, cough, diarrhea, rash, nausea
Occasional (14%–9%)
Shortness of breath, asthenia or loss of strength, skin reaction at injection site, dizziness

SERIOUS REACTIONS
• Hypertensive encephalopathy, thrombosis, cerebrovascular accident, myocardial infarction (MI), and seizures have occurred rarely.
• Hyperkalemia occurs occasionally in patients with chronic renal failure, usually in those who do not conform to medication compliance, dietary guidelines, and frequency of dialysis.

NURSING CONSIDERATIONS
Baseline Assessment
• Assess the patient's blood pressure (B/P) before giving the drug. Know that 80% of patients with chronic renal failure have a history of hypertension. Expect that B/P often rises during early therapy in patients with history of hypertension.
• Assess the patient's serum iron, keeping in mind that the transferrin saturation should be greater than 20%, and serum ferritin should be greater than 100 ng/ml, before and during therapy.
• Consider that all patients will eventually need supplemental iron therapy.
• Establish the patient's baseline complete blood count (CBC), especially note the patient's blood Hct.
• Monitor the patient aggressively for increased B/P. Know that 25% of patients on medication require

antihypertensive therapy and dietary restrictions.

Lifespan Considerations
• Be aware that it is unknown if epoetin alfa crosses the placenta or is distributed in breast milk.
• Be aware that the safety and efficacy of epoetin alfa have not been established in children younger than 12 years of age.
• There are no age-related precautions noted in the elderly.

Precautions
• Use cautiously in patients with a history of seizures and known porphyria, an impairment of erythrocyte formation in bone marrow.

Administration and Handling
◀ALERT▶ Avoid excessive agitation of vial; do not shake because it can cause foaming.

◀ALERT▶ Be aware that patients receiving AZT with serum erythropoietin levels greater than 500 milliunits are likely not to respond to therapy.

Subcutaneous
• Use 1 dose per vial; do not reenter vial. Discard unused portion. May be mixed in a syringe with Bacteriostatic 0.9% NaCl with benzyl alcohol 0.9% (Bacteriostatic Saline) at a 1:1 ratio. Know that benzyl alcohol acts as a local anesthetic and may reduce injection site discomfort.

IV
• Refrigerate vials. Vigorous shaking may denature medication, rendering it inactive.
• No reconstitution necessary.
• May be given as an IV bolus.

Intervention and Evaluation
• Monitor the patient's blood Hct level diligently. Reduce the drug dosage if the patient's Hct level increases more than 4 points in 2 weeks.

• Assess the patient's complete blood count (CBC) routinely.
• Monitor the patient's body temperature, especially in cancer patients on chemotherapy and zidovudine-treated HIV patients, and BUN, phosphorus, potassium, serum creatinine, and serum uric acid, especially in chronic renal failure patients.

Patient Teaching
• Stress to the patient that frequent blood tests will be needed to determine the correct drug dosage.
• Warn the patient to notify the physician if he or she experiences severe headache.
• Caution the patient to avoid any potentially hazardous activity during first 90 days of therapy as there is an increased risk of seizure development in renal patients during the first 90 days of epoetin alfa therapy.

filgrastim
fill-**grass**-tim
(Neupogen)
Do not confuse with Epogen and Nutramigen.

CATEGORY AND SCHEDULE
Pregnancy Risk Category: C

MECHANISM OF ACTION
A biologic modifier that stimulates production, maturation, and activation of neutrophils. *Therapeutic Effect:* Activates neutrophils to increase their migration and cytotoxicity.

PHARMACOKINETICS
Readily absorbed after subcutaneous administration. Not removed by hemodialysis. **Half-life:** 3.5 hrs.

AVAILABILITY
Injection: 300 mcg/ml, 480 mcg/ 0.8 ml.

INDICATIONS AND DOSAGES
▶ **Myelosuppressive**
Subcutaneous/IV or Subcutaneous infusion
Adults, Elderly. Initially, 5 mcg/ kg/day. May increase by 5 mcg/ kg for each chemotherapy cycle based on duration/severity of absolute neutrophil count (ANC) nadir.
▶ **Bone marrow transplant (BMT)**
IV/Subcutaneous infusion
Adults, Elderly. 5–10 mcg/kg/day. Adjust dose daily during period of neutrophil recovery based on neutrophil response.
▶ **Mobilize progenitor cells**
IV/Subcutaneous
Adults. 10 mcg/kg/day beginning at least 4 days before first leukapheresis and continuing until last leukapheresis.

UNLABELED USES
Treatment of AIDS-related neutropenia; chronic, severe neutropenia; drug-induced neutropenia; myelodysplastic syndrome

CONTRAINDICATIONS
24 hrs before or after cytotoxic chemotherapy, hypersensitivity to *Escherichia coli*–derived proteins, use with other drugs that may result in lowered platelet count

INTERACTIONS
Drug
None known.
Herbal
None known.
Food
None known.

DIAGNOSTIC TEST EFFECTS
May increase LDH concentrations, leukocyte (LAP) scores, and serum alkaline phosphatase and uric acid levels.

IV INCOMPATIBILITIES
Amphotericin (Fungizone), cefepime (Maxipime), cefotaxime (Claforan), cefoxitin (Mefoxin), ceftizoxime (Ceflzox), ceftriaxone (Rocephin), cefuroxime (Zinacef), clindamycin (Cleocin), dactinomycin (Cosmegen), etoposide (VePesid), fluorouracil, furosemide (Lasix), heparin, mannitol, methylprednisolone (Solu-Medrol), mitomycin (Mutamycin), prochlorperazine (Compazine)

IV COMPATIBILITIES
Bumetanide (Bumex), calcium gluconate, hydromorphone (Dilaudid), lorazepam (Ativan), morphine, potassium chloride

SIDE EFFECTS
Frequent
Nausea or vomiting (57%), mild to severe bone pain (22%) occurs more frequently in those receiving high dose via IV form, less frequently in low-dose, subcutaneous form; alopecia (18%), diarrhea (14%), fever (12%), fatigue (11%)
Occasional (9%–5%)
Anorexia, dyspnea, headache, cough, skin rash
Rare (less than 5%)
Psoriasis, hematuria/proteinuria, osteoporosis

SERIOUS REACTIONS
• Chronic administration occasionally produces chronic neutropenia and splenomegaly.
• Thrombocytopenia, myocardial infarction (MI), and arrhythmias occur rarely.

• Adult respiratory distress syndrome may occur in septic patients.

NURSING CONSIDERATIONS

Baseline Assessment
• Obtain a complete blood count (CBC) prior to filgrastim therapy, and twice weekly thereafter.

Lifespan Considerations
• Be aware that it is unknown if filgrastim crosses the placenta or is distributed in breast milk.
• There are no age-related precautions noted in children or the elderly.

Precautions
• Use cautiously in patients with gout, malignancy with myeloid characteristics due to granulocyte colony-stimulating factor (G-CSF) potential to act as a growth factor, preexisting cardiac conditions, and psoriasis.

Administration and Handling
◀ALERT▶ May be given by subcutaneous injection or short IV infusion (15–30 min) or by continuous IV infusion.

◀ALERT▶ Begin at least 24 hours after last dose of chemotherapy; discontinue at least 24 hours before next dose of chemotherapy.

◀ALERT▶ Begin at least 24 hours after last dose of chemotherapy and at least 24 hours after bone marrow infusion.

Subcutaneous
• Store in refrigerator, but remove before use and allow to warm to room temperature.
• Aspirate syringe before injecting drug to avoid intra-arterial administration.

IV
• Refrigerate vials.
• Know that the drug is stable for up to 24 hours at room temperature, provided vial contents are clear and contain no particulate matter. Be aware that the drug remains stable if accidentally exposed to freezing temperature.
• Use single-dose vial, do not reenter vial. Do not shake.
• Dilute with 10 to 50 ml D_5W to concentration of 15 mcg/ml and higher. For concentration from 5 to 15 mcg/ml, add 2 ml of 5% albumin to each 50 ml D_5W to provide a final concentration of 2 mg/ml. Do not dilute to a final concentration of less than 5 mcg/ml.
• For intermittent infusion (piggyback), infuse over 15 to 30 minutes.
• For continuous infusion, give single dose over 4 to 24 hours.
• In all situations, flush IV line with D_5W before and after administration.

Intervention and Evaluation
• In septic patients, be alert to adult respiratory distress syndrome.
• Closely monitor patients with preexisting cardiac conditions.
• Monitor the patient's blood pressure (B/P) because a transient decrease in B/P may occur. Also assess his or her temperature, blood Hct, CBC, hepatic enzyme studies, and serum uric acid levels.

Patient Teaching
• Warn the patient to notify the physician if he or she experiences chest pain, chills, fever, palpitations, or severe bone pain.
• Instruct the patient to avoid situations that might place them at risk for contracting an infectious disease, such as influenza.

oprelvekin (interleukin-2, IL-2)
oh-**prel**-vee-kinn
(Neumega)
Do not confuse with Neupogen.

CATEGORY AND SCHEDULE
Pregnancy Risk Category: C

MECHANISM OF ACTION
A hematopoietic that stimulates production of blood platelets, essential in the blood-clotting process. *Therapeutic Effect:* Results in increased platelet production.

AVAILABILITY
Injection: 5 mg.

INDICATIONS AND DOSAGES
▸ **Prevention of thrombocytopenia**
Subcutaneous
Adults. 50 mcg/kg once a day.
Children. 75–100 mcg/kg once a day. Continue for 14–28 days or until platelet count reaches 50,000 cells/mcl after its nadir.

CONTRAINDICATIONS
None known

INTERACTIONS
Drug
None known.
Herbal
None known.
Food
None known.

DIAGNOSTIC TEST EFFECTS
May decrease blood Hgb and Hct, usually begins 3–5 days of initiation of therapy, reverses about 1 wk after discontinuance of therapy.

SIDE EFFECTS
Frequent
Nausea or vomiting (77%); fluid retention (59%); neutropenic fever (48%); diarrhea (43%); rhinitis (42%); headache (41%); dizziness (38%); fever (36%); insomnia (33%); cough (29%); rash, pharyngitis (25%); tachycardia (20%); vasodilation (19%)

SERIOUS REACTIONS
• Transient atrial fibrillation or flutter occurs in 10% of patients and may be caused by increased plasma volume; drug is not directly arrhythmogenic.
• Arrhythmias usually are brief in duration and convert to normal sinus rhythm spontaneously.
• Papilledema may occur in children.

NURSING CONSIDERATIONS
Baseline Assessment
• Plan to obtain the patient's complete blood count (CBC) prior to chemotherapy and at regular intervals thereafter.
• Expect to obtain a baseline EKG to assess for an underlying arrhythmia.
Precautions
• Use cautiously in patients with congestive heart failure (CHF), history of atrial arrhythmia, history of heart failure, and patients susceptible to developing CHF.
Administration and Handling
◂ALERT▸ Know that dosing should begin 6 to 24 hours following completion of chemotherapy dosing.
Subcutaneous
• Store in refrigerator. Once reconstituted, use within 3 hours.
• Give single injection in abdomen, thigh, hip, or upper arm.
• Add 1 ml sterile water for injec-

tion to provide concentration of 5 mg/ml oprelvekin. Inject along inside surface of vial, and swirl contents gently to avoid excessive agitation.

• Discard unused portion.

Intervention and Evaluation

• Monitor the patient's platelet counts and electrolyte levels.

• Closely monitor the patient's fluid and electrolyte status, particularly in those receiving diuretic therapy.

• Assess the patient for fluid retention evidenced by dyspnea on exertion and peripheral edema, which generally occurs during first week of therapy and continues for duration of treatment.

• Monitor the patient's platelet count periodically to assess therapeutic duration of therapy.

• Continue drug dosing until post-nadir platelet count is greater than 50,000 cells/mcl.

• Stop treatment more than 2 days before starting next round of chemotherapy.

Patient Teaching

• Tell the patient that follow-up blood tests will be performed to assess the results of therapy.

• Instruct the patient to use an electric razor and soft toothbrush to prevent bleeding until platelet count is within normal range.

• Tell the patient to report any palpitations or dyspnea.

---

pegfilgrastim
peg-fill-**grass**-tim
(Neulasta)

CATEGORY AND SCHEDULE
Pregnancy Risk Category: C

MECHANISM OF ACTION

A colony-stimulating factor that regulates production of neutrophils within bone marrow. A glycoprotein, primarily affects neutrophil progenitor proliferation, differentiation, and selected end-cell functional activation. *Therapeutic Effect:* Increases phagocytic ability, antibody-dependent destruction.

PHARMACOKINETICS

Readily absorbed after subcutaneous administration. **Half-life:** 15–80 hrs.

AVAILABILITY

Solution for Injection: 10 mg/ml.

INDICATIONS AND DOSAGES
▸ **Myelosuppression**
Subcutaneous
Adults, Elderly. Give as a single 6-mg injection once per chemotherapy cycle.

CONTRAINDICATIONS

Hypersensitivity to *Escherichia coli*–derived proteins, within 14 days before and 24 hrs after administration of cytotoxic chemotherapy

INTERACTIONS
Drug
Lithium: May potentiate the release of neutrophils.
Herbal
None known.
Food
None known.

DIAGNOSTIC TEST EFFECTS

May increase LDH concentrations, leukocyte (LAP) scores, serum alkaline phosphatase and uric acid levels.

SIDE EFFECTS
Frequent (72%–15%)
Bone pain, nausea, fatigue, alopecia,

diarrhea, vomiting, constipation, anorexia, abdominal pain, arthralgia, generalized weakness, peripheral edema, dizziness, stomatitis, mucositis, neutropenic fever

SERIOUS REACTIONS
• Allergic reactions, such as anaphylaxis, rash, and urticaria, occur rarely.
• Cytopenia resulting from an antibody response to growth factors occurs rarely.
• Splenomegaly occurs rarely; assess for left upper abdominal or shoulder pain.
• Adult respiratory distress syndrome (ARDS) may occur in septic patients.

NURSING CONSIDERATIONS

Baseline Assessment
• Obtain a complete blood count (CBC) and platelet count before initiation of pegfilgrastim therapy and routinely thereafter.

Lifespan Considerations
• Be aware that it is unknown if pegfilgrastim crosses the placenta or is distributed in breast milk.
• Be aware that the safety and efficacy of pegfilgrastim have not been established in children.
• Be aware that pegfilgrastim use should be avoided in infants, children, and adolescents weighing less than 45 kg.
• There are no age-related precautions noted in the elderly.

Precautions
• Use cautiously in patients who concurrently use medications with mycelioid properties and patients with sickle cell disease.

Administration and Handling
◀ALERT▶ Do not administer in the period between 14 days before and 24 hours after administration of cytotoxic chemotherapy, as prescribed.
◀ALERT▶ Do not use pegfilgrastim in infants, children, and adolescents weighing less than 45 kg.
Subcutaneous
• Store in refrigerator, but may warm to room temperature up to a maximum of 48 hours before use. Discard if left at room temperature for longer than 48 hours.
• Protect from light.
• Avoid freezing, but if accidentally frozen, may allow to thaw in refrigerator before administration. Discard if freezing takes place a second time.
• Discard if discoloration or precipitate is present.

Intervention and Evaluation
• Monitor the patient for allergic reactions.
• Examine the patient for peripheral edema, particularly behind medial malleolus, usually the first area to show peripheral edema.
• Assess the patient's mucous membranes for evidence of mucositis, such as red mucous membranes, white patches, and extreme mouth soreness, and stomatitis.
• Evaluate the patient's muscle strength.
• Assess the patient's pattern of daily bowel activity and stool consistency.
• Evaluate septic patients for signs of adult respiratory distress syndrome (ARDS), such as dyspnea.

Patient Teaching
• Tell the patient of pegfilgrastim's possible side effects, as well as the signs and symptoms of allergic reactions.
• Stress to the patient the importance of compliance with pegfilgrastim treatment, including regular monitoring of blood counts.

sargramostim (granulocyte macrophage colony-stimulating factor, GM-CSF)

sar-gra-**moh**-stim
(Leukine)
Do not confuse with Leukeran.

CATEGORY AND SCHEDULE
Pregnancy Risk Category: C

MECHANISM OF ACTION
A colony-stimulating factor that stimulates proliferation and differentiation of hematopoietic cells to activate mature granulocytes and macrophages. *Therapeutic Effect*: Assists bone marrow in making new white blood cells (WBCs); increases their chemotactic, antifungal, antiparasitic activity. Increases cytoneoplastic cells, activates neutrophils to inhibit tumor cell growth.

PHARMACOKINETICS

Effect	Onset	Peak	Duration
Increase WBCs	7–14 days	N/A	1 wk

Detected in serum within 5 min after subcutaneous administration. **Half-life:** IV: 1 hr; Subcutaneous: 3 hrs.

AVAILABILITY
Powder for Injection: 250 mcg, 500 mcg.
Liquid for Injection: 500 mcg/ml.

INDICATIONS AND DOSAGES
▸ **Accelerates myeloid recovery in patients with acute lymphoblastic leukemia, Hodgkin's disease undergoing autologous bone marrow transplantation, non-Hodgkin's lymphoma**
Usual parenteral dosage
IV infusion
Adults, Elderly. 250 mcg/m²/day for 21 days (as a 2-hr infusion). Begin 2–4 hrs after autologous bone marrow infusion and not less than 24 hrs after last dose of chemotherapy or not less than 12 hrs after last radiation treatment. Discontinue if blast cells appear or underlying disease progresses.
▸ **Bone marrow transplantation failure, engraftment delay**
IV infusion
Adults, Elderly. 250 mcg/m²/day for 14 days. Infuse over 2 hrs. May repeat after 7 days of therapy if engraftment has not occurred with 500 mcg/m²/day for 14 days.
▸ **Mobilization or post peripheral blood progenitor cells (PBPC) transplant**
IV/Subcutaneous
Adults. 250 mcg/m²/day.
▸ **Allogeneic transplantation**
IV infusion
Adults. 250 mcg/m²/day for 21 days starting 2–4 hrs after bone marrow infusion and not less than 24 hrs after last chemotherapy dose or 12 hrs after last radiation dose.
▸ **Aplastic anemia**
IV/Subcutaneous
Adults, Elderly. 15–480 mcg/m²/day.
▸ **Cancer chemotherapy recovery**
IV/Subcutaneous
Adults, Elderly. 3–15 mcg/kg/day for 10 days.

UNLABELED USES
Treatment of AIDS-related neutropenia, chronic, severe neutropenia, drug-induced neutropenia; myelodysplastic syndrome

CONTRAINDICATIONS

12 hrs before or after radiation therapy, 24 hrs before or after chemotherapy, excessive leukemic myeloid blasts in bone marrow or peripheral blood (greater than 10%), known hypersensitivity to GM-CSF, yeast-derived products, or any component of the drug

INTERACTIONS
Drug
Lithium, steroids: May increase the effects of sargramostim.
Herbal
None known.
Food
None known.

DIAGNOSTIC TEST EFFECTS

May decrease serum albumin levels. May increase serum bilirubin and creatinine levels, and liver enzymes.

IV INCOMPATIBILITIES

Amphotericin B complex (Abelcet, AmBisome, Amphotec), hydromorphone (Dilaudid), lorazepam (Ativan), morphine

IV COMPATIBILITIES

Calcium gluconate, dopamine (Intropin), heparin, magnesium, potassium chloride

SIDE EFFECTS
Frequent
GI disturbances, including nausea, diarrhea, vomiting, stomatitis, anorexia, and abdominal pain, arthralgia or myalgia, headache, malaise, rash, pruritus
Occasional
Peripheral edema, weight gain, dyspnea, asthenia or loss of strength, fever, leukocytosis, capillary leak syndrome, such as fluid retention, irritation at local injection site, and peripheral edema

Rare
Rapid or irregular heartbeat, thrombophlebitis

SERIOUS REACTIONS
• Pleural or pericardial effusion occurs rarely after infusion.

NURSING CONSIDERATIONS
Baseline Assessment
• Monitor the patient for supraventricular arrhythmias during administration, especially in patients with a history of cardiac arrhythmias.
• Assess the patient closely for dyspnea during and immediately after infusion, particularly in patients with a history of lung disease. Expect to cut the infusion rate by half if dyspnea occurs during infusion. Stop the infusion immediately if dyspnea continues, and notify the physician.
• Stop the dose or reduce it by half, as prescribed, based on the clinical condition of the patient, if his or her neutrophil count exceeds 20,000 cells/mm^3 or platelet count exceeds 500,000/mm^3.
• Know that patient blood counts return to normal or baseline 3 to 7 days after discontinuation of therapy.
Lifespan Considerations
• Be aware that it is unknown if sargramostim crosses the placenta or is distributed in breast milk.
• Be aware that the safety and efficacy of this drug have not been established in children.
• There are no age-related precautions noted in the elderly.
Precautions
• Use cautiously in patients with congestive heart failure (CHF), hypoxia, impaired liver or renal function, preexisting cardiac dis-

ease, preexisting fluid retention, and pulmonary infiltrates.

Administration and Handling

IV

• Refrigerate powder, reconstituted solution, diluted solution for injection. Do not shake. Do not use past expiration date.

• Reconstituted solutions normally are clear, colorless.

• Use within 6 hours; discard unused portions. Use 1 dose/vial; do not reenter vial.

• To 250 mcg/500 mcg vial, add 1 ml preservative-free sterile water for injection.

• Direct sterile water for injection to side of vial, gently swirl contents to avoid foaming; do not shake or vigorously agitate.

• After reconstitution, further dilute with 0.9% NaCl. If final concentration less than 10 mcg/ml, add 1 mg albumin/ml 0.9% NaCl to provide a final albumin concentration of 0.1%.

◀**ALERT**▶ Know that albumin is added before addition of sargramostim to prevent drug adsorption to components of drug delivery system.

• Give each single dose over 2, 4, or 24 hours, as directed by physician.

Intervention and Evaluation

• Monitor the patient's complete blood count (CBC), liver and renal function tests, platelet count, pulmonary function tests, vital signs, and weight.

Patient Teaching

• Tell the patient to expect frequent follow-up blood tests to evaluate the effectiveness of drug therapy.

• Warn the patient to notify the physician if he or she experiences chest pain, chills, fever, palpitations, or dyspnea.

• Instruct the patient to avoid situations that might place them at risk for contracting an infectious disease, such as influenza.

albumin, human	**Uses:** Plasma expanders are used to treat hypovolemia, to expand plasma volume and maintain cardiac output in shock or impending shock, and to treat hypoproteinemia-induced edema or decreased intravascular volume.
dextran, low molecular weight (dextran 40); dextran, high molecular weight (dextran 75)	
hetastarch	**Action:** Plasma expanders stay in the vascular space and restore plasma volume by maintaining the colloidal osmotic pressure.

albumin, human

al-**byew**-min
(Albumex[AUS], Albuminar, Albutein, Buminate, Plasbumin)

CATEGORY AND SCHEDULE

Pregnancy Risk Category: C

MECHANISM OF ACTION

A plasma protein fraction that acts as a blood volume expander. *Therapeutic Effect:* Provides temporary increase in blood volume, reduces hemoconcentration and blood viscosity.

PHARMACOKINETICS

Route	Onset	Peak	Duration
IV	15 min	N/A	N/A

Distributed throughout extracellular fluid. Onset of action: 15 min provided patient is well hydrated.
Half-life: 15–20 days.

AVAILABILITY

Injection: 5%, 25%.

INDICATIONS AND DOSAGES

▸ **Hypovolemia**
IV
Adults, Elderly. Initially, 25 g, may repeat in 15–30 min. Maximum: 250 g within 48 hr.
Children. 0.5–1 g/kg/dose (10–20 ml/kg/dose of 5% albumin) Maximum: 6 g/kg/day.

▸ **Hypoproteinemia**
IV
Adults, Elderly, Children. 0.5–1 g/kg/dose (10–20 ml/kg/dose of 5% albumin) repeat in 1–2 days.

▸ **Burns**
IV
Adults, Elderly, Children. Initially, begin with administration of large volumes of crystalloid infusion to maintain plasma volume. After 24 hrs, an initial dose of 25 g with dosage adjusted to maintain plasma albumin concentration of 2–2.5 g/100 ml.

▸ **Cardiopulmonary bypass**
IV
Adults, Elderly. 5% or 25%: With crystalloid to maintain plasma albumin concentration of 2.5 g/100 ml.

▸ **Acute nephrosis, Nephrotic syndrome**
IV
Adults, Elderly. 25 g of 25% injection, with diuretic once a day for 7–10 days.

▸ **Hemodialysis**
IV
Adults, Elderly: 25%: 100 ml (25 g).

▸ **Hyperbilirubinemia, Erythroblastosis fetalis**
IV
Infants. 1 g/kg 1–2 hrs before transfusion.

CONTRAINDICATIONS
Heart failure, history of allergic reaction to albumin, hypervolemia, normal serum albumin, pulmonary edema, severe anemia

INTERACTIONS
Drug
None known.
Herbal
None known.
Food
None known.

DIAGNOSTIC TEST EFFECTS
May increase serum alkaline phosphatase concentrations.

IV INCOMPATIBILITIES
Midazolam (Versed), vancomycin (Vancocin), verapamil (Isoptin)

IV COMPATIBILITIES
Diltiazem (Cardizem), lorazepam (Ativan)

SIDE EFFECTS
Occasional
Hypotension
Rare
High dose, repeated therapy may result in altered vital signs, chills, fever, increased salivation, nausea, vomiting, urticaria, tachycardia

SERIOUS REACTIONS
• Fluid overload evidenced by signs and symptoms including headache, weakness, blurred vision, behavioral changes, incoordination, and isolated muscle twitching may occur.
• Congestive heart failure (CHF) as evidenced by rapid breathing, rales, wheezing, coughing, increased blood pressure (B/P), and distended neck veins may occur.

NURSING CONSIDERATIONS
Baseline Assessment
• Expect to obtain B/P, pulse, and respirations immediately before administration.
• Ensure adequate hydration before albumin is administered.
Lifespan Considerations
• Be aware that it is unknown if albumin crosses the placenta or is distributed in breast milk.
• There are no age-related precautions noted in children or the elderly.
Precautions
• Use cautiously in patients with liver or renal impairment, hypertension, normal serum albumin concentration, poor heart function, or pulmonary disease.
Administration and Handling
IV
◀ALERT▶ Be aware that the dosage is based on the patient's condition and the duration of administration is based on the patient's response.
• Store at room temperature. Albumin normally appears as a clear, brownish, odorless, and moderate viscous fluid.
• Do not use if solution has been frozen, appears turbid, contains sediment, or is not used within 4 hours of opening the vial.
• Make a 5% solution from 25% solution by adding 1 volume 25% to 4 volumes 0.9% NaCl or D_5W (NaCl preferred). Do not use sterile water for injection because life-threatening acute renal failure and hemolysis can occur.
• Give by IV infusion. The rate is variable and depends on the therapeutic use, the patient's blood volume, and the concentration of solute.

• Give 5% solution at 5 to 10 ml/min; 25%: usually at 2 to 3 ml/min.
• Administer 5% solution undiluted; 25% solution may be administered undiluted or diluted with 0.9% NaCl or D$_5$W. Dilution of with NaCl is preferred.
• May give without regard to patient blood group or Rh factor.

Intervention and Evaluation
• Monitor B/P for hypertension or hypotension.
• Assess the patient frequently for signs and symptoms of fluid overload and pulmonary edema.
• Check the patient's skin for flushing and urticaria.
• Monitor the patient's intake and output and in particular, watch for decreased urine output.
• Assess for therapeutic response as evidenced by an increased B/P and decreased edema.

Patient Teaching
• Advise the patient to immediately report difficulty breathing or skin itching or rash.

---

dextran, low molecular weight (dextran 40)
dex-tran
(Gentran, Rheomacrodex[CAN])
dextran, high molecular weight (dextran 75)
(Macrodex)

CATEGORY AND SCHEDULE
Pregnancy Risk Category: C

MECHANISM OF ACTION
A branched polysaccharide that produces plasma volume expansion due to high colloidal osmotic effect.

Draws interstitial fluid into the intravascular space. May also increase blood flow in microcirculation. *Therapeutic Effect:* Increases central venous pressure, cardiac output, stroke volume, blood pressure (B/P), urine output, capillary perfusion, and pulse pressure. Decreases heart rate, peripheral resistance, and blood viscosity. Corrects hypovolemia.

AVAILABILITY
Injection: 10% dextran 40 in NaCl or D$_5$W, 6% dextran 75 in NaCl or D$_5$W.

INDICATIONS AND DOSAGES
▸ **Volume expansion, shock**
IV
Adults, Elderly. 500–1,000 ml at rate of 20–40 ml/min. Maximum dose: 20 ml/kg first 24 hrs, 10 ml/kg thereafter.
Children. Total dose not to exceed 20 ml/kg on day 1, 10 ml/kg/day thereafter.

CONTRAINDICATIONS
Hypervolemia, renal failure, severe bleeding disorders, severe congestive heart failure (CHF), severe thrombocytopenia

INTERACTIONS
Drug
None known.
Herbal
None known.
Food
None known.

DIAGNOSTIC TEST EFFECTS
Prolongs bleeding time, depresses platelet count. Decreases factors VIII, V, and IX.

IV INCOMPATIBILITIES
Do not add any medications to dextran solution.

SIDE EFFECTS
Occasional
Mild hypersensitivity reaction, including urticaria, nasal congestion, wheezing

SERIOUS REACTIONS
• Severe or fatal anaphylaxis, manifested by marked hypotension, cardiac or respiratory arrest, may occur, noted early during IV infusion, generally in those not previously exposed to IV dextran.

NURSING CONSIDERATIONS
Baseline Assessment
• Expect to obtain baseline laboratory values, such bleeding time, platelet count, and clotting factors.
Precautions
• Use cautiously in patients with chronic liver disease and extreme dehydration.
Administration and Handling
◀ALERT▶ Therapy should not continue longer than 5 days.
IV
• Store at room temperature.
• Use only clear solutions.
• Discard partially used containers.
• Give by IV infusion only.
• Monitor the patient closely during first minutes of infusion for anaphylactic reaction.
• Monitor the patient's vital signs every 5 minutes.
• Monitor the patient's urine flow rates during administration. Discontinue dextran 40 and give an osmotic diuretic, as prescribed, if oliguria or anuria occurs to minimize vascular overloading.
• Monitor the patient's central venous pressure (CVP) when given by rapid infusion. Immediately discontinue the drug and notify the physician if there is a precipitous

rise in CVP caused by overexpansion of blood volume.
• Monitor the patient's blood pressure (B/P) diligently during infusion. Stop the infusion immediately if marked hypotension occurs, a sign of imminent anaphylactic reaction.
• Discontinue drug until blood volume adjusts via diuresis if evidence of blood volume overexpansion occurs.
Intervention and Evaluation
• Monitor the patient's urine output closely. An increase in output generally occurs in oliguric patients after dextran administration. Discontinue dextran until the patient experiences diuresis if there is not an increase in urine output observed after 500 ml dextran is infused.
• Monitor the patient for signs of fluid overload, such as peripheral or pulmonary edema, and impending congestive heart failure [CHF] symptoms.
• Assess the patient's lung sounds for crackles.
• Monitor the patient's CVP to detect overexpansion of blood volume.
• Monitor the patient's vital signs and observe the patient closely for signs of allergic reaction.
• Assess the patient for overt bleeding, especially at the surgical site, as well as bruising and petechiae development, especially following surgery or in patients on anticoagulant therapy.
Patient Teaching:
• Instruct the patient to let you know if he or she experiences bleeding from surgical site, chest pain, or dyspnea.
• Tell the patient to use an electric razor and soft toothbrush to prevent bleeding during dextran therapy.
• Explain to the patient that he or

she should not take any medications, including over-the-counter (OTC) drugs, especially aspirin, without consulting the physician.
• Warn the patient to notify the you if he or she experiences black or red stool, coffee-ground emesis, dark or red urine, or red-speckled mucus from cough.
• Tell female patients that their menstrual flow may be heavier than usual.

hetastarch
het-ah-starch
(Hespan, Hextend)

CATEGORY AND SCHEDULE
Pregnancy Risk Category: C

MECHANISM OF ACTION
A plasma volume expander that exerts osmotic pull on tissue fluids. *Therapeutic Effect:* Reduces hemoconcentration and blood viscosity, increases circulating blood volume.

PHARMACOKINETICS
Smaller molecules, less than 50,000 molecular weight, rapidly excreted by kidneys; larger molecules, greater than 50,000 molecular weight, slowly degraded to smaller sized molecules, then excreted. **Half-life:** 17 days.

AVAILABILITY
Injection: 6 g/100 ml 0.9% NaCl, 500 ml infusion container

INDICATIONS AND DOSAGES
▶ **Plasma volume expansion**
IV
Adults, Elderly. 500–1000 ml/day up to 1,500 ml/day (20 mg/kg) at a rate up to 20 ml/kg/hr in hemor-

rhagic shock, slower rates for burns or septic shock.

▶ **Leukapheresis**
IV
Adults, Elderly. 250–700 ml infused at constant rate, usually 1:8 to venous whole blood.

CONTRAINDICATIONS
Anuria, oliguria, severe bleeding disorders, severe congestive heart failure (CHF)

INTERACTIONS
Drug
None significant.
Herbal
None known.
Food
None known.

DIAGNOSTIC TEST EFFECTS
May prolong bleeding, and clotting times, partial thromboplastin time (PTT), and prothrombin time (PT). May decrease blood hematocrit concentration.

IV INCOMPATIBILITIES
Amikacin (Amikin), ampicillin (Polycillin), cefazolin (Ancef, Kefzol), cefotaxime (Claforan), cefoxitin (Mefoxin), gentamicin (Garamycin), ranitidine (Zantac), tobramycin (Nebcin)

SIDE EFFECTS
Rare
Allergic reaction resulting in vomiting, mild temperature elevation, chills, itching, submaxillary and parotid gland enlargement, peripheral edema of lower extremities, mild flu-like symptoms, headache, muscle aches

SERIOUS REACTIONS
• Fluid overload, marked by headache, weakness, blurred vision,

behavioral changes, incoordination, and isolated muscle twitching and pulmonary edema, manifested by rapid breathing, crackles, wheezing, coughing, increased blood pressure (B/P), and distended neck veins may occur.
• Anaphylactic reaction may be observed as periorbital edema, urticaria, and wheezing.

NURSING CONSIDERATIONS

Baseline Assessment
• Expect to obtain baseline lab tests, including coagulation studies and complete blood count.
• Assess the patient's vitals signs, including the blood pressure, as well as the central venous pressure (CVP).
Precautions
• Use cautiously in patients with congestive heart failure (CHF), liver disease, pulmonary edema, sodium-restricted diets, and thrombocytopenia.
• Use cautiously in the elderly or very young.
Administration and Handling
IV
• Store solutions at room temperature
• Solution normally appears clear, pale yellow to amber. Do not use if discolored a deep turbid brown, or if precipitate forms.
• Administer only by IV infusion.
• Do not add drugs or mix with other IV fluids.
• In acute hemorrhagic shock, administer at rate approaching 1.2 g/kg (20 ml/kg) per hour, as prescribed. Expect to use slower rates for burns or septic shock.
• Monitor the patient's central

venous pressure (CVP) when given by rapid infusion. If there is a precipitous rise in CVP, immediately discontinue the drug, as prescribed, to prevent overexpansion of blood volume.
Intervention and Evaluation
• Monitor the patient for signs of fluid overload, such as peripheral and pulmonary edema and impending CHF symptoms.
• Assess the patient's lung sounds for crackles and wheezing.
• During leukapheresis, monitor the patient's activated partial thromboplastin time (aPTT), complete blood count (CBC), particularly Hct and Hgb, fluid intake and output, leukocyte and platelet counts, and prothrombin time (PT).
• Monitor the patient's CVP to detect overexpansion of blood volume.
• Monitor the patient's urine output closely. An increase in output generally occurs in oliguric patients after administration.
• Assess the patient for itching, periorbital edema, wheezing, and urticaria, signs of an allergic reaction.
• Monitor the patient for anuria, any change in output ratio, and oliguria.
• Monitor the patient for bleeding from surgical or trauma sites.
Patient Teaching
• Tell the patient to use an electric razor and soft toothbrush to prevent bleeding.
• Warn the patient to notify the physician if he or she experiences any sign of black or red stool, coffee-ground vomitus, dark or red urine, or red-speckled mucus from cough.

alteplase, recombinant
reteplase, recombinant
streptokinase
tenecteplase

Uses: Thrombolytic agents are used to treat acute and severe thrombotic diseases, including acute coronary thrombosis, acute myocardial infarction, massive pulmonary emboli, and ischemic stroke.

Action: Thrombolytics act directly or indirectly on the fibrinolytic system to convert plasminogen to plasmin, an enzyme that degrades the fibrin matrix of thrombi, or clots. (See illustration, *Mechanisms and Sites of Action: Hematologic Agents,* page 988.) This action dissolves thrombi that have already formed.

alteplase, recombinant
all-teh-place
(Activase, Actilyse[AUS], Cathflo Activase)

CATEGORY AND SCHEDULE
Pregnancy Risk Category: C

MECHANISM OF ACTION
A tissue plasminogen activator (tPA) that acts as a thrombolytic by binding to the fibrin in a thrombus and converting entrapped plasminogen to plasmin. This process initiates fibrinolysis. *Therapeutic Effect:* Degrades fibrin clots, fibrinogen, and other plasma proteins.

PHARMACOKINETICS
Rapidly metabolized in liver. Primarily excreted in urine. **Half-life:** 35 min.

AVAILABILITY
Powder for Injection: 2 mg, 50 mg, 100 mg.

INDICATIONS AND DOSAGES
▸ **Acute myocardial infarction**
IV infusion
Adults. 100 mg over 90 min (in patients weighing greater than 67 kg): 15-mg bolus given over 1–2 min; then 50 mg over 30 min; then 35 mg over 60 min (in patients weighing 67 kg or less): 15-mg bolus, then 0.75 mg/kg over next 30 min (Maximum: 50 mg), then 0.5 mg/kg over 60 min (Maximum: 35 mg). Three-hour infusion (in patients weighing greater than 67 kg): 60 mg over first hr (6–10 mg as bolus over 1–2 min), 20 mg over second hr, and 20 mg over third hr (in patients weighing 67 kg or less): 1.25 mg/kg given over 3 hrs as 60% of dose over first hr (6%–10% as 1- to 2-min bolus), 20% over second hr, and 20% over third hr.

▸ **Acute pulmonary emboli**
IV infusion
Adults. 100 mg over 2 hrs. Institute or reinstitute heparin near end or immediately after infusion when activated partial thromboplastin time (aPTT) or thrombin time returns to twice normal or less.

▶ **Acute ischemic stroke**
IV infusion
Adults. 0.9 mg/kg over 60 min
(10% total dose as initial IV bolus
over 1 min).
▶ **Central venous catheter clearance**
IV
Adults, Elderly. 2 mg; may repeat in
greater than 120 min.

UNLABELED USES
Coronary thrombolysis, decrease
ischemic events in unstable angina

CONTRAINDICATIONS
Active internal bleeding, atrioventricular (AV) malformation or aneurysm, bleeding diathesis, intracranial
neoplasm, intracranial or intraspinal
surgery or trauma, recent (within
the past 2 mos) cerebrovascular
accident, severe uncontrolled hypertension

INTERACTIONS
Drug
*Anticoagulants, including cefotetan,
heparin, plicamycin, valproic acid:*
May increase risk of hemorrhage.
*Platelet aggregation inhibitors,
including aspirin, NSAIDs,
ticlopidine:* May increase risk of
bleeding.
Herbal
None known.
Food
None known.

DIAGNOSTIC TEST EFFECTS
Decreases plasminogen and fibrinogen levels during infusion, which
decreases clotting time (confirms
the presence of lysis), decreases
Hgb levels and Hct.

IV INCOMPATIBILITIES
Do not add any other medication to
the container of alteplase solution or
administer other medications
through the same IV line.

IV COMPATIBILITIES
Lidocaine, metoprolol (Lopressor),
morphine, nitroglycerin, propranolol
(Inderal)

SIDE EFFECTS
Frequent
Superficial bleeding at puncture
sites, decreased blood pressure
(B/P)
Occasional
Allergic reaction such as rash or
wheezing, bruising

SERIOUS REACTIONS
• Severe internal hemorrhage may
occur.
• Lysis of coronary thrombi may
produce atrial or ventricular arrhythmias or stroke.

NURSING CONSIDERATIONS
Baseline Assessment
• Obtain baseline apical pulse rate
and B/P.
• Record the patient's weight.
• Expect to evaluate the patient's
12-lead echocardiogram (EKG) and
serum CPK, CPK-MB, and electrolytes.
• Assess Hct, platelet count, thrombin time (TT), activated partial
thromboplastin time (aPTT), prothrombin time (PT), and fibrinogen
level before therapy is instituted.
• Expect to obtain a sample of the
patient's blood for blood type,
crossmatch, and hold.
Lifespan Considerations
• Be aware that this drug is used only
when the benefit outweighs the potential risk to a fetus. Also, it is unknown
if alteplase crosses the placenta or is
distributed in breast milk.
• Be aware that the safety and

efficacy have not been established in children.
* In the elderly, there is an increased risk of bleeding with thrombolytic therapy. Patients must be carefully selected and monitored.

Precautions
* Use cautiously in patients who are pregnant or within the first 10 days postpartum. Also, use cautiously in patients with recent (within the past 10 days) major surgery or GI bleeding, organ biopsy, trauma, cerebrovascular disease, or cardiopulmonary resuscitation (CPR); in patients with diabetic retinopathy, endocarditis, left heart thrombus, occluded AV cannula at infected site, severe liver or renal disease, or thrombophlebitis; and in the elderly.

Administration and Handling
IV
* Store vials at room temperature.
* Reconstitute immediately before use with Sterile Water for Injection.
* Reconstitute 100-mg vial with 100 ml Sterile Water for Injection (50-mg vial with 50 ml sterile water) without preservative to provide a concentration of 1 mg/ml. May be further diluted with equal volume D_5W or 0.9% NaCl to provide a concentration of 0.5 mg/ml.
* Avoid excessive agitation; gently swirl or slowly invert vial to reconstitute.
* After reconstitution, solution normally appears colorless to pale yellow.
* Solution is stable for 8 hours after reconstitution. Discard unused portions.
* Give by IV infusion via infusion pump. (See individual dosages.)
* If minor bleeding occurs at puncture sites, apply pressure for 30 seconds; if unrelieved, apply a pressure dressing.

* If uncontrolled hemorrhage occurs, discontinue the infusion immediately. Keep in mind that slowing the rate of infusion may worsen the hemorrhage.
* Avoid undue pressure when the drug is injected into the catheter because the catheter can rupture or expel a clot into circulation.

Intervention and Evaluation
* Perform continuous cardiac monitoring and assess for arrhythmias. Check the patient's B/P, pulse, and respirations every 15 minutes until stable, and then hourly.
* Assess the patient's peripheral pulses and heart and lung sounds.
* Monitor the patient's chest pain relief and notify the physician of any continuation or recurrence of chest pain. Be sure to note the location, type, and intensity of any chest pain.
* Assess for bleeding manifested as overt blood or blood in any body substance.
* Monitor the aPTT per your facility's protocol.
* Maintain the patient's B/P.
* Avoid any trauma that might increase risk of bleeding, such as IM injections or invasive procedures.
* Assess the patient's neurologic status frequently.

Patient Teaching
* Encourage the patient to strictly follow measures to reduce the risk of bleeding, such as using an electric razor and a soft toothbrush.
* Advise the patient to immediately report signs of bleeding, such as oozing from cuts or gums.

reteplase, recombinant

rhet-eh-place
(Rapilysin[AUS], Retavase)
Do not confuse with Restasis.

CATEGORY AND SCHEDULE
Pregnancy Risk Category: C

MECHANISM OF ACTION
A tissue plasminogen activator that activates fibrinolytic system by directly cleaving plasminogen to generate plasmin, an enzyme that degrades the fibrin of the thrombus. *Therapeutic Effect:* Exerts thrombolytic action.

PHARMACOKINETICS
Rapidly cleared from plasma. Eliminated primarily by the liver and kidney. **Half-life:** 13–16 min.

AVAILABILITY
Powder for Injection: 10.8 units (18.8 mg).

INDICATIONS AND DOSAGES
▶ **Acute myocardial infarction (MI)**
IV bolus
Adults, Elderly. 10 units over 2 min, then repeat 10 units 30 min after administration of first bolus injection.

CONTRAINDICATIONS
Active internal bleeding, arteriovenous malformation or aneurysm, bleeding diathesis, history of cerebrovascular accident (CVA), intracranial neoplasm, recent intracranial or intraspinal surgery or trauma, severe uncontrolled hypertension—increases risk of bleeding

INTERACTIONS
Drug
Heparin, platelet aggregation antagonists, such as abciximab, aspirin, dipyridamole, warfarin: Increase the risk of bleeding.
Herbal
Ginkgo biloba: May increase the risk of bleeding.
Food
None known.

DIAGNOSTIC TEST EFFECTS
Fibrinogen and plasminogen levels may decrease.

IV INCOMPATIBILITIES
Do not mix with any other medications.

SIDE EFFECTS
Frequent
Bleeding at superficial sites, such as venous injection sites, catheter insertion sites, venous cutdowns, arterial punctures, and sites of recent surgical procedures

SERIOUS REACTIONS
• Bleeding at internal sites, including intracranial, retroperitoneal, gastrointestinal (GI), genitourinary (GU), or respiratory may occur.
• Lysis or coronary thrombi may produce atrial or ventricular arrhythmias and stroke.

NURSING CONSIDERATION
Baseline Assessment
• Obtain the patient's baseline apical pulse and blood pressure (B/P).
• Evaluate the patient's 12-lead electrocardiogram (EKG), creatine phosphokinase (CPK), CPK-MB, and electrolytes.
• Assess the patient's activated thromboplastin (aPTT), blood Hct,

plasminogen and fibrinogen level, platelet count, prothrombin time (PT), and thrombin (TT) before therapy is instituted.

• Type and hold patient blood.

Lifespan Considerations

• Be aware that it is unknown if reteplase is distributed in breast milk.

• Be aware that the safety and efficacy of reteplase have not been established in children.

• Be aware that the elderly are more susceptible to bleeding. Use reteplase cautiously in this patient population.

Precautions

• Use cautiously in patients with acute pericarditis, bacterial endocarditis, cerebrovascular disease, diabetic retinopathy, hypertension, liver or renal impairment, major surgery, including coronary artery bypass graft, obstetric (OB) delivery, and organ biopsy, mitral stenosis with atrial fibrillation, occluded atrioventricular (AV) cannula at an infected site, ophthalmic hemorrhage, recent GI or GU bleeding, and septic thrombophlebitis.

• Use cautiously in elderly patients of advanced age and in patients receiving oral anticoagulants.

Administration and Handling

◀ALERT ▶ Withhold the second dose if the patient experiences anaphylaxis or bleeding.

IV

• Use within 4 hours of reconstitution.

• Discard any unused portion.

• Reconstitute only with sterile water for injection immediately before use.

• Reconstituted solution contains 1 unit/ml.

• Slight foaming may occur; let stand for a few minutes to allow bubbles to dissipate.

• Give through a dedicated IV line.

• Give as a 10 unit plus 10 unit double bolus, with each IV bolus administered over 2-minute period.

• Give the second bolus 30 minutes after the first bolus injection.

• Do not add other medications to the bolus injection solution.

• Do not give second bolus if serious bleeding occurs after first IV bolus is given.

Intervention and Evaluation

• Carefully monitor all of the patient's needle puncture sites and catheter insertion sites for bleeding.

• Perform continuous cardiac monitoring of the patient for arrhythmias, B/P, pulse, and respiration until the patient is stable.

• Evaluate the patient's lung sounds and peripheral pulses.

• Monitor the patient for chest pain relief. Notify the physician of any continuation or recurrence of patient chest pain. Note intensity, location, and quality.

• Avoid any trauma to the patient that may increase risk of bleeding, such as injections, and shaving.

Patient Teaching

• Tell the patient to use an electric razor and soft toothbrush to prevent bleeding during drug therapy.

• Warn the patient to notify you if he or she experiences black or red stool, coffee-ground vomitus, dark or red urine, red-speckled mucus from cough, or other signs of bleeding.

• Tell the patient to immediately report any chest pain, headache, palpitations, or shortness of breath.

streptokinase
strep-toe-**kine**-ace
(Streptase)

CATEGORY AND SCHEDULE
Pregnancy Risk Category: C

MECHANISM OF ACTION
An enzyme that activates the fibrinolytic system by converting plasminogen to plasmin, an enzyme that degrades fibrin clots. Acts indirectly by forming complex with plasminogen, which converts plasminogen to plasmin. Action occurs within thrombus, on its surface, and in circulating blood. *Therapeutic Effect:* Resultant effect destroys thrombi.

PHARMACOKINETICS
Rapidly cleared from plasma by antibodies, reticuloendothelial system. Route of elimination unknown. Duration of action continues for several hours after discontinuing medication. **Half-life:** 23 min.

AVAILABILITY
Powder for Injection: 250,000 units, 600,000 units, 750,000 units, 1.5 million units.

INDICATIONS AND DOSAGES
▶ **Acute evolving transmural myocardial infarction (MI) (give as soon as possible after symptoms occur)**
IV infusion
Adults, Elderly (1.5 million units diluted to 45 ml). 1.5 million units infused over 60 min.
Intracoronary infusion
Adults, Elderly (250,000 units diluted to 125 ml). Initially, 20,000 units (10 ml) bolus; then, 2,000 units/min for 60 min. Total dose: 140,000 units.
▶ **Pulmonary embolism, deep vein thrombosis, arterial thrombosis and embolism (give within 7 days after onset)**
IV infusion
Adults, Elderly (1.5 million units diluted to 90 ml). Initially, 250,000 units infused over 30 min; then, 100,000 units/hr for 24–72 hrs for arterial thrombosis or embolism, 24–72 hrs for pulmonary embolism, 72 hrs for deep vein thrombosis.
Intracoronary infusion
Adults, Elderly (1.5 million units diluted to 45 ml). Initially, 250,000 units infused over 30 min; then, 100,000 units/hr for maintenance.

CONTRAINDICATIONS
Carcinoma of the brain, cerebrovascular accident (CVA), internal bleeding, intracranial surgery, recent streptococcal infection, internal bleeding, severe hypertension

INTERACTIONS
Drug
Anticoagulants, heparin: May increase the risk of hemorrhage. *Platelet aggregation inhibitors, such as aspirin:* May increase the risk of bleeding.
Herbal
None known.
Food
None known.

DIAGNOSTIC TEST EFFECTS
Decreases plasminogen and fibrinogen level during infusion, decreasing clotting time and confirms presence of lysis

IV INCOMPATIBILITIES
Do not mix with any other medications.

IV COMPATIBILITIES

Dobutamine (Dobutrex), dopamine (Intropin), heparin, lidocaine, nitroglycerin

SIDE EFFECTS

Frequent
Fever, superficial bleeding at puncture sites, decreased blood pressure (B/P)
Occasional
Allergic reaction, including rash and wheezing, bruising

SERIOUS REACTIONS

• Severe internal hemorrhage may occur.
• Lysis of coronary thrombi may produce arrhythmias.

NURSING CONSIDERATIONS

Baseline Assessment

• Assess the patient's activated thromboplastin (aPTT), blood Hct, fibrinogen level, platelet count, prothrombin time (PT), and thrombin time (TT) before beginning streptokinase therapy.
• Discontinue heparin, if heparin is a component of treatment, before giving streptokinase. TT/aPTT should be less than twice normal value before institution of therapy.

Lifespan Considerations

• Be aware that streptokinase should only be used in pregnant women when the benefit outweighs potential risk to fetus.
• Be aware that it is unknown if streptokinase crosses the placenta or is distributed in breast milk.
• Be aware that the safety and efficacy of streptokinase have not been established in children.
• Be aware that the elderly may have an increased risk of intracranial hemorrhage. Use streptokinase cautiously in this patient population.

Precautions

• Use cautiously in patients with gastrointestinal (GI) bleeding, who've had major surgery within 10 days, and with recent trauma.

Administration and Handling

◀ALERT▶ Must be administered within 12 to 14 hours of clot formation (little effect on older, organized clots).

◀ALERT▶ Do not use from 5 days to 6 months of previous streptokinase treatment of streptococcal infection, such as acute glomerulonephritis secondary to streptococcal infection, pharyngitis, and rheumatic fever.

IV
• Store unopened vials at room temperature. Refrigerate reconstituted solution. Use within 24 hours.
• For AV cannula occlusion, dilute 250,000-units vial with 2 ml 0.9% NaCl. Add diluent slowly to side of vial, roll and tilt to avoid foaming. Do not shake vial.
• For AV cannula occlusion, give IV push slowly into each occluded limb of cannula. Then clamp for 2 hours, aspirate contents, and flush with 0.9% NaCl.
• For uses other than cannula occlusion, reconstitute vial with 5 ml D_5W or preferably 0.9% NaCl. Add diluent slowly to side of vial, roll and tilt to avoid foaming. Do not shake vial. May further dilute with 50 to 500 ml in 45-ml increments of D_5W or 0.9% NaCl.
• For IV injection for coronary artery thrombi, give 1.5 million units over 60 minutes.
• For alternative treatment of coronary artery thrombi, give bolus dose over 25 to 30 seconds using coronary catheter. Follow with 2,000 units per minute for 60 minutes.

• For treatment of deep vein thrombosis (DVT), pulmonary arterial embolism, or arterial thrombi, give single dose over 25 to 30 minutes. Follow with maintenance dose of 100,000 or more units every hour for 24 to 72 hours.

• Monitor the patient's blood pressure (B/P) during infusion. Hypotension, which may be severe, occurs in 1% to 10% of patients. Decrease the infusion rate if necessary.

• Discontinue the infusion immediately if the patient experiences uncontrolled hemorrhage. Note that slowing the rate of infusion instead of discontinuing it altogether may produce worsening hemorrhage. Do not use dextran to control hemorrhage.

Intervention and Evaluation

• Evaluate the patient for clinical response and monitor the patient's vital signs per protocol.

• Handle the patient carefully and as infrequently as possible to prevent bleeding and bruising.

• Do not obtain B/P in lower extremities because a deep vein thrombi may be present.

• Monitor the patient's aPTT, fibrinogen level, PT, and TT every 4 hours after therapy begins.

• Examine the patient's stool for occult blood.

• Assess the patient for abdominal or back pain, a decrease in B/P, an increase in pulse rate, and severe headache, which may be evidence of hemorrhage.

• Determine the patient's discharge amount during menses and monitor for an increase.

• Assess the patient's area of thromboembolus for color and temperature.

• Assess the patient's peripheral pulses, skin for bruises and petechiae, and urine for hematuria.

• Examine the patient for excessive bleeding from minor cuts and scratches and any signs of bleeding.

• Monitor the patient's blood Hgb and Hct, B/P, and platelets.

Patient Teaching

• Tell the patient to use an electric razor and soft toothbrush to prevent bleeding during drug therapy.

• Warn the patient to notify you if he or she experiences black or red stool, coffee-ground vomitus, dark or red urine, red-speckled mucus from cough, or other signs of bleeding.

• Tell the patient to immediately report any chest pain, headache, palpitations or shortness of breath.

tenecteplase
ten-**eck**-teh-place
(Metalyse[AUS], TNKase)

CATEGORY AND SCHEDULE
Pregnancy Risk Category: C

MECHANISM OF ACTION
A tissue plasminogen activator (tPA) produced by recombinant DNA, binds to fibrin and converts plasminogen to plasmin. *Therapeutic Effect:* Initiates fibrinolysis by degrading fibrin clots, fibrinogen, other plasma proteins.

PHARMACOKINETICS
Extensively distributed to tissues. Completely eliminated by hepatic metabolism. **Half-life:** 11–20 min.

AVAILABILITY
Powder for Injection: 50 mg.

INDICATIONS AND DOSAGES
▶ **Acute myocardial infarction (AMI)**
IV
Adults. Dosage is based on the weight of the patient. Treatment to be initiated as soon as possible after onset of AMI symptoms.

Weight (kg)	(mg)	(ml)
less than 60	30	6
60 to less than 70	35	7
70 to less than 80	40	8
80 to less than 90	45	9
90 or more	50	10

CONTRAINDICATIONS
Active internal bleeding, history of cerebrovascular accident (CVA), aneurysm, atrioventricular (AV) malformation, intracranial or intraspinal surgery or trauma within 2 mos, intracranial neoplasm, known bleeding diathesis, severe uncontrolled hypertension

INTERACTIONS
Drug
Anticoagulants (e.g., heparin, warfarin), aspirin, dipyridamole, glycoprotein (GP) IIb/IIIa inhibitors: Increase the risk of bleeding.
Herbal
Ginkgo biloba: May increase the risk of bleeding.
Food
None known.

DIAGNOSTIC TEST EFFECTS
Decreases plasminogen and fibrinogen level during infusion, decreasing clotting time—confirms presence of lysis. Decreases blood Hct and Hgb.

IV INCOMPATIBILITIES
Do not mix with any other medications.

SIDE EFFECTS
Frequent
Bleeding (major: 4.7%; minor 21.8%)

SERIOUS REACTIONS
• Bleeding at internal sites, including intracranial, retroperitoneal, gastrointestinal (GI), genitourinary (GU), or respiratory may occur.
• Lysis or coronary thrombi may produce atrial or ventricular dysrhythmias and stroke.

NURSING CONSIDERATIONS
Baseline Assessment
• Obtain the patient's baseline apical pulse and blood pressure (B/P).
• Record the patient's weight.
• Evaluate the patient's 12-lead electrocardiogram (EKG), cardiac enzymes, and electrolytes.
• Assess the patient's activated thromboplastin (aPTT), blood Hct, fibrinogen level, hemoglobin (Hgb), platelet count, and thrombin time (TT) before beginning tenecteplase therapy.
• Type and hold patient blood.
Lifespan Considerations
• Be aware that it is unknown if tenecteplase is distributed in breast milk.
• Be aware that the safety and efficacy of tenecteplase have not been established in children.
• Be aware that the elderly may have an increased risk of intracranial hemorrhage, major bleeding, and stroke. Use tenecteplase cautiously in this patient population.
Precautions
• Use cautiously in patients who previously received tenecteplase and in patients with severe liver impairment.

Administration and Handling

◀ALERT▶ Give as a single IV bolus over 5 seconds. Precipitate may occur when given in an IV line containing dextrose. Flush with saline before and after administration.

IV

• Store at room temperature.
• If possible, use immediately but may refrigerate up to 8 hours after reconstitution.
• Remember that the drug normally appears as colorless to pale yellow solution. Do not use if discolored or contains particulates.
• Discard after 8 hours.
• Add 10 ml sterile water for injection without preservative to vial to provide concentration of 5 mg/ml. Gently swirl until dissolved. Do not shake.
• If foaming occurs, leave vial undisturbed for several minutes.
• Administer as IV push over 5 seconds.

Intervention and Evaluation

• Perform continuous cardiac monitoring of the patient for arrhythmias, blood pressure (B/P), pulse, and respirations every 15 minutes until the patient is stable, then hourly.
• Evaluate the patient's heart and lung sounds and peripheral pulses.
• Monitor the patient for chest pain relief, and notify the physician of any continuation or recurrence. Note the intensity, location, and quality of chest pain.
• Assess the patient for bleeding, including blood in any body substance and overt blood.
• Monitor the patient's PTT per protocol.
• Maintain the patient's B/P and avoid any trauma to the patient that might increase the risk of bleeding, such as injections, shaving.
• Assess the patient's neurologic status with vital signs.

Patient Teaching

• Tell the patient to use an electric razor and soft toothbrush to prevent bleeding during drug therapy.
• Warn the patient to notify you if he or she experiences black or red stool, coffee-ground vomitus, dark or red urine, red-speckled mucus from cough, or other signs of bleeding.
• Tell the patient to immediately report any chest pain, headache, palpitations or shortness of breath.

aminocaproic acid
pentoxifylline
protamine sulfate

Uses: Miscellaneous hematologic agents serve different purposes. *Aminocaproic acid* is used to treat excessive bleeding from hyperfibrinolysis or urinary fibrinolysis. The hemorheologic drug *pentoxifylline* is used to treat the symptoms of intermittent claudication. *Protamine* is used to treat severe heparin overdose and neutralize the effects of heparin given during extracorporeal circulation.

Action: Each miscellaneous agent acts in a different way on the hematologic system. *Aminocaproic acid* inhibits the activation of plasminogen activator substances and blocks antiplasmin activity by inhibiting fibrinolysis. *Pentoxifylline* alters erythrocyte flexibility and inhibits tumor necrosis factor production, neutrophil activation, and platelet aggregation; these actions reduce blood viscosity. *Protamine* complexes with heparin to form a stable salt, which reduces heparin's anticoagulant activity.

aminocaproic acid
ah-meen-oh-kah-**pro**-ick
(Amicar)
Do not confuse with amikacin or Amikin.

CATEGORY AND SCHEDULE
Pregnancy Risk Category: C

MECHANISM OF ACTION
A systemic hemostatic that acts as an antifibrinolytic and antihemorrhagic by inhibiting the activation of plasminogen activator substances. *Therapeutic Effect:* Prevents fibrin clots from forming.

AVAILABILITY
Tablets: 500 mg.
Syrup: 250 mg/ml.
Injection: 250 mg/ml.

INDICATIONS AND DOSAGES
▸ **Acute bleeding**
PO/IV infusion
Adults, Elderly. Initially, 4–5 g over 1 hr, then 1–1.25 g/hr. Continue for 8 hrs or until bleeding is controlled. Maximum: Up to 30 g/24 hrs.
Children. 3 g/m^2 over first hr, then 1 g/m^2/hr. Maximum: 18 g/m^2/24 hrs.
▸ **Dosage in renal impairment**
Decrease dose to 25% of normal.

UNLABELED USES
Prevents reoccurrence of subarachnoid hemorrhage, prevents hemorrhage in hemophiliacs following dental surgery

CONTRAINDICATIONS
Evidence of active intravascular clotting process, disseminated intravascular coagulation without con-

current heparin therapy, hematuria of upper urinary tract origin (unless benefits outweigh risk). Parenteral: Newborns.

INTERACTIONS
Drug
None known.
Herbal
None known.
Food
None known.

DIAGNOSTIC TEST EFFECTS
May elevate serum potassium level.

IV INCOMPATIBILITIES
Sodium lactate. Do not mix with other medications.

SIDE EFFECTS
Occasional
Nausea, diarrhea, cramps, decreased urination, decreased blood pressure (B/P), dizziness, headache, muscle fatigue and weakness, myopathy, bloodshot eyes

SERIOUS REACTIONS
• Too rapid IV administration produces tinnitus, skin rash, arrhythmias, unusual tiredness, and weakness.
• Rarely, a grand mal seizure occurs, generally preceded by weakness, dizziness, and headache.

NURSING CONSIDERATIONS
Precautions
• Use cautiously in patients with hyperfibrinolysis or impaired cardiac, liver, or renal disease.
Administration and Handling
◀ALERT▶ Expect to administer a reduced aminocaproic acid dose if the patient has cardiac, renal, or liver impairment.

IV
• Dilute each 1 g in up to 50 ml 0.9% NaCl, D_5W, Ringer's, or Sterile Water for Injection. Do not use Sterile Water for Injection in patients with subarachnoid hemorrhage.
• Do not give by direct injection. Give only by IV infusion.
• Infuse less than or equal to 5 g over the first hour in 250 ml of solution. Give each succeeding 1 g over 1 hour in 50 to 100 ml solution.
• Monitor the patient for hypotension during infusion.
• Be aware that rapid infusion may produce arrhythmias, including bradycardia.
Intervention and Evaluation
• Assess the patient for severe and continuous muscular pain or weakness, which may indicate myopathy.
• Monitor creatine kinase and SGOT (AST) serum levels frequently to determine if myopathy is present. Myopathy is characterized by an increase in serum creatine kinase and SGOT (AST) levels.
• Monitor the patient's B/P, heart rate and rhythm, and pulse rate. Any abdominal or back pain, decrease in B/P, increase in pulse rate, and severe headache may be evidence of hemorrhage. Assess the quality of the patient's peripheral pulses.
• Check for bruising of the skin, excessive bleeding from minor cuts or scratches, and petechiae.
• Monitor the patient for an increase in menstrual flow.
• Evaluate the patient's gums for erythema and gingival bleeding.
• Examine the patient's urine output for hematuria.
Patient Teaching
• Instruct the patient to report any signs of red or dark urine, black or

red stool, coffee-ground vomit, or red-speckled mucus produced from a cough.

pentoxifylline
pen-tox-ih-**fill**-in
(Pentoxyl, Trental)
Do not confuse with Tegretol.

CATEGORY AND SCHEDULE
Pregnancy Risk Category: C

MECHANISM OF ACTION
A blood viscosity-reducing agent that alters the flexibility of red blood cells (RBCs); inhibits production of tumor necrosis factor, neutrophil activation, platelet aggregation. *Therapeutic Effect:* Reduces blood viscosity, improves blood flow.

PHARMACOKINETICS
Well absorbed after PO administration. Undergoes first-pass metabolism in liver. Primarily excreted in urine. Unknown if removed by hemodialysis. **Half-life:** 24–48 min, metabolite: 60–90 min.

AVAILABILITY
Tablets (controlled-release): 400 mg.

INDICATIONS AND DOSAGES
▸ **Intermittent claudication**
PO
Adults, Elderly. 400 mg 3 times/day. Decrease to 400 mg 2 times/day if gastrointestinal (GI) or central nervous system (CNS) side effects occur. Continue for at least 8 wks.

CONTRAINDICATIONS
History of intolerance to xanthine derivatives, such as caffeine, the-

ophylline, or theobromine, recent cerebral or retinal hemorrhage

INTERACTIONS
Drug
Antihypertensives: May increase the effects of antihypertensives.
Herbal
None known.
Food
None known.

DIAGNOSTIC TEST EFFECTS
None known.

SIDE EFFECTS
Occasional (5%–2%)
Dizziness, nausea, bad taste, dyspepsia, marked by heartburn, epigastric pain, indigestion
Rare (less than 2%)
Rash, pruritus, anorexia, constipation, dry mouth, blurred vision, edema, nasal congestion, anxiety

SERIOUS REACTIONS
• Angina and chest pain occur rarely and may be accompanied by palpitations, tachycardia, arrhythmias.
• Overdosage signs and symptoms, such as flushing, hypotension, nervousness, agitation, hand tremor, fever, and somnolence, are noted 4–5 hrs after ingestion and last 12 hrs.

NURSING CONSIDERATIONS
Baseline Assessment
• Determine if the patient has a sensitivity or allergy to xanthine derivatives, such as caffeine, theophylline, or theobromine.
• Ask the patient about his or her baseline signs and symptoms, such as intermittent claudication, such as aching, cramping, and pain in calf muscles, buttocks, thigh, and feet.

Lifespan Considerations
• Be aware that it is unknown if pentoxifylline crosses the placenta and is distributed in breast milk.
• Be aware that the safety and efficacy of pentoxifylline have not been established in children.
• In the elderly, age-related renal impairment may require cautious use.

Precautions
• Use cautiously in patients with chronic occlusive arterial disease, insulin-treated diabetes, liver or renal impairment, peptic ulcer disease, and recent surgery.

Administration and Handling
PO
• Do not crush or break film-coated tablets.
• Give pentoxifylline with meals to avoid GI upset.

Intervention and Evaluation
• Assist the patient with ambulation if he or she experiences dizziness.
• Assess the patient for hand tremor.
• Monitor the patient for relief of symptoms of intermittent claudication, such as aching, cramping, and pain in calf muscles, buttocks, thigh, and feet. Symptoms generally occur while walking or exercising and not at rest or with weight bearing in absence of walking or exercising.

Patient Teaching
• Tell the patient that pentoxifylline's therapeutic effect is generally noted in 2 to 4 weeks.
• Warn the patient to avoid tasks requiring mental alertness or motor skills until his or her response is established.
• Urge the patient not to smoke and to limit his or her caffeine intake. Explain that smoking causes constriction and occlusion of peripheral blood vessels.

protamine sulfate
pro-tah-meen
(Protamine[CAN], Protamine sulfate)
Do not confuse with ProAmatine, Protopam, or Protropin.

CATEGORY AND SCHEDULE
Pregnancy Risk Category: C

MECHANISM OF ACTION
A protein that complexes with heparin to form a stable salt. *Therapeutic Effect:* Results in reduction of anticoagulant activity of heparin.

AVAILABILITY
Injection: 10 mg/ml.

INDICATIONS AND DOSAGES
▸ **Antidote, treatment of severe heparin overdose**
IV
Adults, Elderly. 1 mg protamine sulfate neutralizes 90–115 units of heparin. Heparin disappears rapidly from circulation, reducing the dosage demand for protamine as time elapses.

UNLABELED USES
Treatment of enoxaparin toxicity

CONTRAINDICATIONS
None known

INTERACTIONS
Drug
None known.
Herbal
None known.
Food
None known.

DIAGNOSTIC TEST EFFECTS
None known.

SIDE EFFECTS
Frequent
Decreased blood pressure (B/P),
dyspnea
Occasional
Hypersensitivity reaction: urticaria,
angioedema; nausea, vomiting,
which generally occurs in those
sensitive to fish, men who have
undergone vasectomy, infertile men,
those on isophane (NPH) insulin, or
previous protamine therapy
Rare
Back pain

SERIOUS REACTIONS
• A too rapid IV administration may
produce acute hypotension, bradycardia, pulmonary hypertension,
dyspnea, transient flushing, and
feeling of warmth.
• Heparin rebound may occur several hours after heparin has been
neutralized by protamine (usually
evident 8–9 hrs after protamine
administration). Heparin rebound
occurs most often after arterial or
cardiac surgery.

NURSING CONSIDERATIONS

Baseline Assessment
• Evaluate the patient's activated
partial thromboplastin time (aPTT),
blood Hct, and prothrombin
time (PT).

• Assess the patient for bleeding.
• Make sure the patient is supine
while administering drug, to prevent
injury from a hypotensive episode
or other complication.
Precautions
• Use cautiously in patients with a
history of allergy to fish and previous protamine therapy, because of a
propensity to hypersensitivity reaction.
• Use cautiously in infertile or
vasectomized men and patients on
isophane (NPH) or insulin therapy.
Administration and Handling
IV
• Store vials at room temperature.
• May give undiluted over 10 minutes. Do not exceed 5 mg/min or
50 mg in any 10-minute period.
Intervention and Evaluation
• Monitor the patient's activated
clotting time (ACT), aPTT, B/P,
cardiac function, and other coagulation tests.
Patient Teaching
• Tell the patient to use an electric
razor and soft toothbrush to prevent
bleeding until coagulation studies
normalize.
• Warn the patient to notify the
physician if he or she experiences
black or red stool, coffee-ground
vomitus, dark or red urine, or red-
speckled mucus from cough.

62 Adrenocortical Steroids

betamethasone
cortisone acetate
dexamethasone
fludrocortisone
hydrocortisone,
  hydrocortisone
  acetate,
  hydrocortisone
  sodium phosphate,
  hydrocortisone
  valerate, sodium
  succinate
methylprednisolone,
  methylprednisolone
  acetate,
  methylprednisolone
  sodium succinate
prednisolone
prednisone
triamcinolone,
  triamcinolone
  acetonide,
  triamcinolone
  diacetate,
  triamcinolone
  hexacetonide

Uses: Adrenocortical steroids are used as replacement therapy in adrenal insufficiency, including Addison's disease. Because these agents have anti-inflammatory and immunosuppressant properties, they're also used to treat the symptoms of multiorgan diseases and conditions, such as rheumatoid arthritis, osteoarthritis, severe psoriasis, ulcerative colitis, lupus erythematosus, anaphylactic shock, and status asthmaticus, and to prevent the rejection of transplanted organs.

Action: Adrenocortical steroids suppress the migration of polymorphonuclear leukocytes and reverse increased capillary permeability by their anti-inflammatory effects. They suppress the immune system by decreasing lymphatic system activity.

COMBINATION PRODUCTS

BLEPHAMIDE: prednisolone/
sulfacetamide (an anti-infective)
0.2%/10%.

CIPRO HC OTIC: hydrocortisone/
ciprofloxacin (an anti-infective)
1%/0.2%.

CIPRODEX OTIC: dexamethasone/
ciprofloxacin (an anti-infective)
0.1%/0.3%.

CORTISPORIN: hydrocortisone/
neomycin (an anti-infective)/
polymyxin (an anti-infective) 5 mg/
10,000 units/5 mg; 10 mg/10,000
units/5 mg.

DEXACIDIN: dexamethasone/neomycin
(an anti-infective)/polymyxin
(an anti-infective): 0.1%/3.5 mg/
10,000 units per g or ml.

LOTRISONE: betamethasone/
clotrimazole (an antifungal)
0.05%/1%.

MAXITROL: dexamethasone/neomycin
(an anti-infective)/polymyxin
(an anti-infective) 0.1%/3.5 mg/
10,000 units per g or ml.

MYCO-II: triamcinolone/nystatin (an
antifungal) 0.1%/100,000 units/g.

MYCOLOG II: triamcinolone/nystatin
(an antifungal) 0.1%/100,000
units/g.

MYCO-TRIACET: triamcinolone/
nystatin (an antifungal) 0.1%/
100,000 units/g.

TOBRADEX: dexamethasone/ tobramycin (an aminoglycoside) 1%/3%.

VASOCIDIN: prednisolone/ sulfacetamide (an anti-infective) 0.25%/10%.

betamethasone

bay-tah-**meth**-a-sone

(Betaderm[CAN], Beta-Val, Betnesol[CAN], Celestone, Diprolene, Diprosone, Luxig Foam)

CATEGORY AND SCHEDULE
Pregnancy Risk Category: C (D if used in first trimester)

MECHANISM OF ACTION
An adrenocorticosteroid that controls the rate of protein synthesis; depresses migration of polymorphonuclear leukocytes and fibroblasts; reduces capillary permeability; prevents or controls inflammation. *Therapeutic Effect:* Decreases tissue response to inflammatory process.

AVAILABILITY
Aerosol: 0.1%.
Cream: 0.1%, 0.05%.
Foam: 0.12%.
Lotion: 0.1%, 0.05%.
Ointment: 0.05%.
Syrup: 0.6 mg/5 ml.

INDICATIONS AND DOSAGES
▶ **Anti-inflammatory, immunosuppressant, corticosteroid replacement therapy**
PO
Adults, Elderly. 0.6–7.2 mg/day.
Children. 0.063–0.25 mg/kg/day in 3–4 divided doses.

CONTRAINDICATIONS
Hypersensitivity to betamethasone, systemic fungal infections

INTERACTIONS
Drug
Amphotericin: May increase hypokalemia.
Digoxin: May increase the toxicity of digoxin secondary to hypokalemia.
Diuretics, insulin, oral hypoglycemics, potassium supplements: May decrease the effects of diuretics, insulin, oral hypoglycemics, and potassium supplements.
Hepatic enzyme inducers: May decrease the effect of betamethasone.
Live virus vaccines: May decrease the patient's antibody response to vaccine, increase vaccine side effects, and potentiate virus replication.
Herbal
None known.
Food
None known.

DIAGNOSTIC TEST EFFECTS
May decrease serum calcium, potassium, and thyroxine levels. May increase blood glucose levels, serum lipids, amylase, and sodium levels.

SIDE EFFECTS
Frequent
Systemic: Increased appetite, abdominal distention, nervousness, insomnia, false sense of well-being
Foam: Burning, stinging, pruritus
Occasional
Systemic: Dizziness, facial flushing, diaphoresis, decreased or blurred vision, mood swings
Topical: Allergic contact dermatitis, purpura or blood-containing blisters, thinning of skin with easy bruising,

telangiectasis or raised dark red spots on skin

SERIOUS REACTIONS
• When taken in excessive quantities, systemic hypercorticism and adrenal suppression may occur.

NURSING CONSIDERATIONS

Baseline Assessment
• Determine if the patient has a hypersensitivity to any corticosteroids and sulfite.
• Obtain the patient's baselines for blood glucose levels, blood pressure (B/P), serum electrolyte levels, height, and weight.
• Evaluate the results of initial tests, such as tuberculosis (TB) skin test, x-rays, and EKG.
• Determine if the patient has diabetes mellitus, and anticipate an increase in his or her antidiabetic drug regimen due to raised blood glucose levels.
• Find out if your patient takes digoxin, and if so plan to draw serum digoxin levels.

Precautions
• Use cautiously in patients at increased risk of peptic ulcer disease and patients with cirrhosis, hypothyroidism, cirrhosis, and nonspecific ulcerative colitis.

Administration and Handling
PO
• Give betamethasone with milk or food because it decreases gastrointestinal (GI) upset.
• Give single doses prior to 9 a.m.; multiple doses should be given at evenly spaced intervals.
Topical
• Gently cleanse area prior to application.
• Use occlusive dressings only as ordered.

• Apply sparingly and rub into area thoroughly.
• When using aerosol, spray area 3 seconds from 15 cm distance; avoid inhalation.

Intervention and Evaluation
• Monitor the patient's blood glucose, B/P, and electrolytes. If your patient takes digoxin, closely follow his or her digoxin levels.
• Apply topical preparation sparingly. Do not use topical betamethasone on broken skin or in areas of infection and do not apply to the face, inguinal areas, or wet skin.

Patient Teaching
• Instruct the patient to take betamethasone with food or milk.
• Teach the patient to take a single daily dose in the morning.
• Caution the patient against abruptly discontinuing the drug.
• Instruct the patient to apply topical preparations in a thin layer.
• Explain that steroids often cause mood swings, ranging from euphoria to depression.

---

cortisone acetate
kore-tih-zone
(Cortate[AUS], Cortone[CAN])
Do not confuse with Cort-Dome.

CATEGORY AND SCHEDULE
Pregnancy Risk Category: C
(D if used in the first trimester)

MECHANISM OF ACTION
An adrenocortical steroid that inhibits the accumulation of inflammatory cells at inflammation sites, phagocytosis, lysosomal enzyme release and synthesis and release of mediators of inflammation. *Thera-*

peutic Effect: Prevents or suppresses cell-mediated immune reactions. Decreases or prevents tissue response to inflammatory process.

AVAILABILITY
Tablets: 25 mg.

INDICATIONS AND DOSAGES
Dosage is dependent on the condition being treated and patient response.
▸ **Anti-inflammatory, immunosuppressive**
PO
Adults, Elderly. 25–300 mg/day in divided doses q12-24h.
Children. 2.5–10 mg/kg/day in divided doses q6-8h.
▸ **Physiologic replacement**
PO
Adults, Elderly. 25–35 mg/day.
Children. 0.5–0.75 mg/kg/day in divided doses q8h.

CONTRAINDICATIONS
Hypersensitivity to any corticosteroid, live virus vaccine, peptic ulcers—except in life-threatening situations, systemic fungal infection

INTERACTIONS
Drug
Amphotericin: May increase hypokalemia.
Digoxin: May increase the toxicity of digoxin caused by hypokalemia.
Diuretics, insulin, oral hypoglycemics, potassium supplements: May decrease the effects of diuretics, insulin, oral hypoglycemics, and potassium supplements.
Hepatic enzyme inducers: May decrease the effects of cortisone.
Live virus vaccines: May decrease the patient's antibody response to vaccine, increase vaccine side effects, and potentiate virus replication.

Herbal
None known.
Food
None known.

DIAGNOSTIC TEST EFFECTS
May decrease serum calcium, potassium, and thyroxine levels. May increase blood glucose levels, serum lipids, amylase, and sodium levels.

SIDE EFFECTS
Frequent
Insomnia, heartburn, nervousness, abdominal distention, increased sweating, acne, mood swings, increased appetite, facial flushing, delayed wound healing, increased susceptibility to infection, diarrhea or constipation
Occasional
Headache, edema, change in skin color, frequent urination
Rare
Tachycardia, allergic reaction, such as rash and hives, psychological changes, hallucinations, depression

SERIOUS REACTIONS
• The serious reactions of long-term therapy are hypocalcemia, hypokalemia, muscle wasting in arms and legs, osteoporosis, spontaneous fractures, amenorrhea, cataracts, glaucoma, peptic ulcer, and congestive heart failure (CHF).
• Abrupt withdrawal following long-term therapy may cause anorexia, nausea, fever, headache, joint pain, rebound inflammation, fatigue, weakness, lethargy, dizziness, and orthostatic hypertension.

NURSING CONSIDERATIONS
Baseline Assessment
• Determine if the patient is hypersensitive to any of the corticosteroids.

• Obtain the patient's baseline values for blood glucose levels, blood pressure (B/P), serum electrolyte levels, height, and weight.
• Determine if the patient has diabetes mellitus, and anticipate an increase in his or her antidiabetic drug regimen because of raised blood glucose levels.
• Find out if your patient takes digoxin, and if so plan to draw serum digoxin levels.

Precautions
• Use cautiously in patients with cirrhosis, CHF, history of tuberculosis—because it may reactivate disease, hypertension, hypothyroidism, nonspecific ulcerative colitis, psychosis, seizure disorders, and thromboembolic disorders.
• Discontinue prolonged therapy slowly.

Intervention and Evaluation
• Be alert to signs of infection caused by reduced immune response, including fever, sore throat, or vague symptoms.
• For those on long-term therapy, monitor for signs and symptoms of hypocalcemia, such as muscle twitching, cramps, positive Chvostek's or Trousseau's signs, or hypokalemia, including weakness and muscle cramps, numbness or tingling, especially in the lower extremities, nausea and vomiting, irritability, and electrocardiogram (EKG) changes.
• Assess the patient's ability to sleep and emotional status.

Patient Teaching
• Instruct the patient not to change the dose or schedule of cortisone.
• Caution the patient against discontinuing the drug. Taper off cortisone under medical supervision.
• Warn the patient to notify the physician if he or she experiences fever, muscle aches, sore throat, and sudden weight gain or swelling.
• Tell the patient to inform his or her dentist and other physicians of cortisone therapy now or within past 12 months.
• Explain that steroids often cause mood swings, ranging from euphoria to depression.

dexamethasone
dex-a-**meth**-a-sone
(Decadron, Dexasone[CAN], Dexmethsone[AUS], Diodex [CAN], Hexadrol [CAN], Maxidex)
Do not confuse with desoximetasone, dextramethophan, or Maxzide.

CATEGORY AND SCHEDULE
Pregnancy Risk Category: C
(D if used in the first trimester)

MECHANISM OF ACTION
A long-acting glucocorticoid that inhibits accumulation of inflammatory cells at inflammation sites, phagocytosis, lysosomal enzyme release and synthesis and release of mediators of inflammation. *Therapeutic Effect:* Prevents and suppresses cell and tissue immune reactions, inflammatory process.

PHARMACOKINETICS
Rapidly, completely absorbed from the gastrointestinal (GI) tract after PO administration. Widely distributed. Protein binding: High. Metabolized in liver. Primarily excreted in urine. Minimally removed by hemodialysis. **Half-life:** 3–4.5 hrs.

AVAILABILITY
Tablets: 0.25 mg, 0.5 mg, 0.75 mg, 1 mg, 1.5 mg, 2 mg, 4 mg, 6 mg.

Elixir: 0.5 mg/5 ml, 1 mg/ml.
Oral Solution: 0.5 mg/5 ml,
0.5 mg/0.5 ml.
Injection: 4 mg/ml.
Inhalant, Intranasal, Ophthalmic:
Solution, suspension, ointment.
Topical: Aerosol, cream.

INDICATIONS AND DOSAGES
▸ **Anti-inflammatory**
PO/IM/IV
Adults, Elderly. 0.75–9 mg/day in
divided doses q6–12h.
Children. 0.08–0.3 mg/kg/day in
divided doses q6–12h.
▸ **Cerebral edema**
IV
Adults, Elderly. Initially, 10 mg,
then 4 mg (IM/IV) q6h.
PO/IM/IV
Children. Loading dose of 1–2 mg/
kg, then 1–1.5 mg/kg/day in di-
vided doses q4–6h.
▸ **Chemotherapy antiemetic**
IV
Adults, Elderly. 8–20 mg once, then
4 mg (PO) q4–6h or 8 mg q8h.
Children. 10 mg/m²/dose
(Maximum: 20 mg), then 5 mg/m²/
dose q6h.
▸ **Physiologic replacement**
PO/IM/IV
Adults, Elderly. 0.03–0.15 mg/kg/
day in divided doses q6–12h.
▸ **Usual ophthalmic dosage, ocular
inflammatory conditions**
Ointment
Adults, Elderly, Children. Thin
coating 3–4 times/day.
Suspension
Adults, Elderly, Children. Initially,
2 drops q1h while awake and q2h at
night for 1 day, then reduce to 3–4
times/day.

CONTRAINDICATIONS
Active untreated infections, fungal,
tuberculosis, or viral diseases of the
eye

INTERACTIONS
Drug
Amphotericin: May increase hypokalemia.
Digoxin: May increase the toxicity
of this drug caused by hypokalemia.
*Diuretics, insulin, oral hypoglyce-
mics, potassium supplements:* May
decrease the effects of diuretics,
insulin, oral hypoglycemics, and
potassium supplements.
Hepatic enzyme inducers: May
decrease the effects of dexamethasone.
Live virus vaccines: May decrease
the patient's antibody response to
vaccine, increase vaccine side
effects, and potentiate virus replication.
Herbal
None known.
Food
None known.

DIAGNOSTIC TEST EFFECTS
May decrease serum calcium, potassium, and thyroxine levels. May
increase blood glucose levels, serum
lipids, amylase, and sodium levels.

IV INCOMPATIBILITIES
Ciprofloxacin (Cipro), daunorubicin
(Cerubidine), idarubicin (Idamycin),
midazolam (Versed)

IV COMPATIBILITIES
Aminophylline, cimetidine (Tagamet), cisplatin (Platinol), cyclophosphamide (Cytoxan), cytarabine
(Cytosar), docetaxel (Taxotere),
doxorubicin (Adriamycin), etoposide (VePesid), granisetron (Kytril),
heparin, hydromorphone (Dilaudid), lorazepam (Ativan), morphine,
ondansetron (Zofran), paclitaxel
(Taxol), potassium chloride, propofol (Diprivan)

SIDE EFFECTS

Frequent

Inhalation: Cough, dry mouth, hoarseness, throat irritation

Intranasal: Burning, mucosal dryness

Ophthalmic: Blurred vision

Systemic: Insomnia, facial swelling or cushingoid appearance, moderate abdominal distention, indigestion, increased appetite, nervousness, facial flushing, diaphoresis

Occasional

Inhalation: Localized fungal infection, such as thrush

Intranasal: Crusting inside nose, nosebleed, sore throat, ulceration of nasal mucosa.

Ophthalmic: Decreased vision, watering of eyes, eye pain, burning, stinging, redness of eyes, nausea, vomiting

Systemic: Dizziness, decreased or blurred vision

Topical: Allergic contact dermatitis, purpura or blood-containing blisters, thinning of skin with easy bruising, telangiectasis or raised dark red spots on skin

Rare

Inhalation: Increased bronchospasm, esophageal candidiasis

Intranasal: Nasal and pharyngeal candidiasis, eye pain

Systemic: General allergic reaction, such as rash and hives, pain, redness, swelling at injection site, psychological changes, false sense of well-being, hallucinations, depression

SERIOUS REACTIONS

• The serious reactions of long-term therapy are muscle wasting, especially in the arms and legs, osteoporosis, spontaneous fractures, amenorrhea, cataracts, glaucoma, peptic ulcer disease, and congestive heart failure (CHF).

• Abrupt withdrawal following long-term therapy may cause severe joint pain, severe headache, anorexia, nausea, fever, rebound inflammation, fatigue, weakness, lethargy, dizziness, and orthostatic hypotension.

• The serious reactions of the ophthalmic form of dexamethasone are glaucoma, ocular hypertension, and cataracts.

NURSING CONSIDERATIONS

Baseline Assessment

• Determine if the patient is hypersensitive to any corticosteroids.

• Obtain the patient's baselines for blood glucose levels, blood pressure (B/P), serum electrolyte levels, height, and weight.

• Evaluate the results of initial tests, such as tuberculosis (TB) skin test, x-rays, and EKG.

• Determine if the patient has diabetes mellitus, and anticipate an increase in his or her antidiabetic drug regimen because of raised blood glucose levels.

• Find out if your patient takes digoxin, and if so plan to draw serum digoxin levels.

Lifespan Considerations

• Be aware that dexamethasone crosses the placenta and is distributed in breast milk.

• Be aware that prolonged treatment with high-dose therapy may decrease the short-term growth rate and cortisol secretion in children.

• Be aware that the elderly are at higher risk for developing hypertension or osteoporosis.

Precautions

• Use cautiously in patients with cirrhosis, CHF, diabetes mellitus, hypertension, hyperthyroidism, ocular herpes simplex, osteoporosis, patients at high thromboembolic

risk, peptic ulcer disease, respiratory tuberculosis, seizure disorders, ulcerative colitis, and untreated systemic infections.
• Use cautiously in patients on long-term therapy as prolonged ophthalmic dexamethasone use may result in cataracts or glaucoma.

Administration and Handling

PO
• Give dexamethasone with milk or food.

IM
• Give deep IM, preferably in the gluteus maximus.

IV
◀ **ALERT** ▶ Dexamethasone sodium phosphate may be given by IV push or IV infusion.
• For IV push, give over 1 to 4 minutes.
• For IV infusion, mix with 0.9% NaCl or D5W and infuse over 15 to 30 minutes.
• For neonate, solution must be preservative free.
• IV solution must be used within 24 hours.

Ophthalmic
• Place a gloved finger on the patient's lower eyelid and pull it out until a pocket is formed between the patient's eye and lower lid.
• Hold the dropper above the pocket and place the correct number of drops—one quarter to half inch ointment—into pocket. Close the patient's eye gently.
• For the ophthalmic solution apply digital pressure to lacrimal sac for 1 to 2 minutes to minimize the drainage to the nose and throat, thereby reducing the risk of systemic effects.
• For the ophthalmic ointment, close the patient's eye for 1 to 2 minutes. Instruct the patient to roll his or her eyeball to increase the contact area of drug to eye.

• Remove excess solution or ointment around the patient's eye with a tissue.
• Use ointment at night to reduce the frequency of solution administration.
• Taper the drug dosage off slowly when discontinuing the drug.

Topical
• Gently cleanse area before application.
• Use occlusive dressings only as ordered.
• Apply sparingly and rub into area thoroughly.

Intervention and Evaluation
• Monitor the patient's intake and output and record his or her daily body weight.
• Evaluate the patient for edema.
• Evaluate the patient's food tolerance. Assess the patient's daily pattern of bowel activity.
• Report any hyperacidity the patient experiences promptly.
• Check the patient's vital signs at least 2 times a day.
• Be alert to signs and symptoms of infection such as fever, sore throat, or vague symptoms.
• Monitor the patient's electrolyte levels.
• Assess the patient's ability to sleep and emotional status.
• Monitor the patient for hypercalcemia, including cramps and muscle twitching, or hypokalemia, such as irritability, numbness or tingling—especially of the lower extremities, muscle cramps and weakness, nausea and vomiting.

Patient Teaching
• Caution the patient against abruptly discontinuing the drug and changing the drug dose or schedule. Explain to the patient that the drug dose must taper off gradually under medical supervision.
• Warn the patient to notify the

physician if he or she experiences fever, muscle aches, sore throat, and sudden weight gain or swelling.

• Explain to the patient that any severe stress, including serious infection, surgery, or trauma, may require an increase in dexamethasone dosage.

• Tell the patient to inform his or her dentist and other physicians of dexamethasone therapy now or within past 12 months.

• Instruct patients taking topical dexamethasone to apply the drug after a batch or shower for best absorption.

• Explain that steroids often cause mood swings, ranging from euphoria to depression.

---

fluidrocortisone
floo-droe-**kor**-tih-sone
(Florinef)
Do not confuse with Fioricet or Florinal.

CATEGORY AND SCHEDULE
Pregnancy Risk Category: C

MECHANISM OF ACTION
A mineralocorticoid that acts at distal tubules. *Therapeutic Effect:* Increases potassium, hydrogen ion excretion, sodium reabsorption, and water retention.

PHARMACOKINETICS
Well absorbed from the gastrointestinal (GI) tract. Protein binding: 42%. Widely distributed. Metabolized in liver, kidney. Primarily excreted in urine. **Half-life:** 3.5 hrs.

AVAILABILITY
Tablets: 0.1 mg.

INDICATIONS AND DOSAGES
▸ **Addison's disease**
PO
Adults, Elderly. 0.05–0.1 mg/day. Range: 0.1 mg 3 times/wk–0.2 mg/day. Administration with cortisone or hydrocortisone preferred.
▸ **Salt-losing adrenogenital syndrome**
PO
Adults, Elderly. 0.1–0.2 mg/day.
▸ **Usual pediatric dosage**
Children. 0.05–0.1 mg/day.

UNLABELED USES
Treatment of acidosis in renal tubular disorders, idiopathic orthostatic hypotension

CONTRAINDICATIONS
Congestive heart failure (CHF), systemic fungal infection

INTERACTIONS
Drug
Digoxin: May increase the risk of toxicity of digoxin caused by hypokalemia.
Hypokalemia-causing medications: May increase the effects of fludrocortisone.
Liver enzyme inducers (e.g., phenytoin): May increase the metabolism of fludrocortisone.
Sodium-containing medications: May increase blood pressure (B/P), incidence of edema, and serum sodium levels.
Herbal
None known.
Food
None known.

DIAGNOSTIC TEST EFFECTS
May increase serum sodium levels. May decrease blood Hct and serum potassium levels.

SIDE EFFECTS
Frequent
Increased appetite, exaggerated sense of well-being, abdominal distention, weight gain, insomnia, mood swings
High-dose, prolonged therapy, too rapid withdrawal: Increased susceptibility to infection, with masked signs and symptoms, delayed wound healing, hypokalemia, hypocalcemia, GI distress, diarrhea or constipation, hypertension
Occasional
Frontal or occipital headache, dizziness, menstrual difficulty or amenorrhea, gastric ulcer development
Rare
Hypersensitivity reaction

SERIOUS REACTIONS
• The serious reactions of long-term therapy are muscle wasting, especially in the arms and legs, osteoporosis, spontaneous fractures, amenorrhea, cataracts, glaucoma, peptic ulcer disease, and CHF.
• Abruptly withdrawing the drug after long-term therapy may cause anorexia, nausea, fever, headache, joint pain, rebound inflammation, fatigue, weakness, lethargy, dizziness, and orthostatic hypotension.

NURSING CONSIDERATIONS
Baseline Assessment
• Obtain the patient's baseline blood glucose levels, B/P, chest x-ray, electrocardiogram (EKG), serum electrolytes, and body weight.
Lifespan Considerations
• Be aware that it is unknown if fludrocortisone crosses the placenta or is distributed in breast milk.
• Be aware that fludrocortisone use in children may cause growth suppression and inhibition of endogenous steroid production.
• Be aware that fludrocortisone use in the elderly studies have not been performed.
Precautions
• Use cautiously in patients with edema, hypertension, and impaired renal function.
Administration and Handling
PO
• Give fludrocortisone with food or milk.
Intervention and Evaluation
• Monitor the patient's blood glucose levels, B/P, serum renin, and electrolyte levels.
• Taper the drug dosage slowly if fludrocortisone is to be discontinued.
Patient Teaching
• Warn the patient not to alter the drug dose or schedule. Also caution the patient not to abruptly discontinue the drug. Explain to the patient that fludrocortisone dosages must taper off gradually.
• Tell the patient to notify the physician if he or she experiences continuing headaches, fever, muscle aches, sore throat, or sudden weight gain or swelling.
• Instruct the patient to maintain careful personal hygiene and to avoid exposure to disease or trauma.
• Explain that severe stress such as serious infection, surgery, or trauma may require the fludrocortisone dosage to be increased.
• Explain that steroids often cause mood swings, ranging from euphoria to depression.

hydrocortisone
high-droe-**core**-tah-sewn
(Colifoam[AUS], Cortef
cream[AUS], Cortic cream[AUS],
Derm-Aid cream[AUS],
Dermaid[AUS], Dermaid soft
cream [AUS], Egocort cream[AUS],
Hycor[AUS], Hycor eye
ointment[AUS], Siquent
Hycor[AUS], Squibb HC[AUS],
WestCort)

CATEGORY AND SCHEDULE
Pregnancy Risk Category: C
(D if used in first trimester)
OTC (Hydrocortisone 0.5% and
1% Cream, Gel, and Ointment)

MECHANISM OF ACTION
An adrenal corticosteroid that inhibits accumulation of inflammatory
cells at inflammation sites, phagocytosis, lysosomal enzyme release and
synthesis or release of mediators of
inflammation. *Therapeutic Effect:*
Prevents or suppresses cell-mediated
immune reactions. Decreases or
prevents tissue response to inflammatory process.

PHARMACOKINETICS

Route	Onset	Peak	Duration
IV	N/A	4–6 hrs	8–12 hrs

Well absorbed after IM administration. Widely distributed. Metabolized in liver. **Half-life:** plasma:
1.5–2 hrs; biologic: 8–12 hrs.

AVAILABILITY
Hydrocortisone
Gel: 0.5%, 1%.
Lotion: 0.25%, 0.5%, 1%, 2%,
2.5%.
Cream: 0.5%, 1%, 2.5%.
Ointment: 0.5%, 1%, 2.5%.

Topical Solution: 1%.
Oral Suspension: 10 mg/5 ml.
Hydrocortisone Sodium Phosphate
Injection: 50 mg/ml.
Hydrocortisone Sodium Succinate
Injection: 100 mg, 250 mg, 500 mg,
1,000 mg.
Hydrocortisone Acetate
Injection: 25 mg/ml, 50 mg/ml.
Suppository: 10 mg, 25 mg, 30 mg.
Cream: 0.5%, 1%.
Ointment: 0.5%, 1%.
Hydrocortisone Valerate
Cream: 0.2%.

INDICATIONS AND DOSAGES
▶ **Acute adrenal insufficiency**
IV
Adults, Elderly. 100 mg IV bolus,
then 300 mg/day in divided doses
q8h.
Children. 1–2 mg/kg IV bolus, then
150–250 mg/day in divided doses
q6–8h.
Infants. 1–2 mg/kg/dose IV bolus,
then 25–150 mg/day in divided
doses q6–8h.
▶ **Anti-inflammatory and immuno-suppression**
IM/IV
Adults, Elderly. 15–240 mg q12h.
Children. 1–5 mg/kg/day in divided
doses q12h.
▶ **Physiologic replacement**
IM
Children. 0.25–0.35 mg/kg/day as a
single daily dose.
PO
Children. 0.5–0.75 mg/kg/day in
divided doses q8h.
▶ **Status asthmaticus**
IV
Adults, Elderly. 100–500 mg q6h.
Children. 2 mg/kg/dose q6h.
▶ **Shock**
IV
*Adults, Elderly, Children 12 yrs and
older.* 100–500 mg q6h.

Children younger than 12 yrs.
50 mg/kg. May repeat in 4 hrs, then
q24h as needed.
▸ **Adjunctive treatment of ulcerative colitis**
Rectal
Adults, Elderly. 100 mg at bedtime
for 21 nights or until clinical and
proctologic remission occurs (may
require 2–3 mos of therapy).
Adults, Elderly (Cortifoam). 1 applicator 1–2 times/day for 2–3 wks,
then every second day thereafter.
Topical
Adults, Elderly. Apply sparingly
2–4 times/day.

CONTRAINDICATIONS
Fungal, tubercular, or viral skin
lesions, serious infections

INTERACTIONS
Drug
Amphotericin: May increase hypokalemia.
Digoxin: May increase the risk of
toxicity of this drug caused by
hypokalemia.
Diuretics, insulin, oral hypoglycemics, potassium supplements: May
decrease the effects of diuretics,
insulin, oral hypoglycemics, and
potassium supplements.
Liver enzyme inducers: May decrease the effects of hydrocortisone.
Live virus vaccines: May decrease
the patient's antibody response to
vaccine, increase vaccine side
effects, and potentiate virus replication.
Herbal
None known.
Food
None known.

DIAGNOSTIC TEST EFFECTS
May decrease serum calcium, potassium, and thyroxine levels. May

increase blood glucose levels, serum
lipids, amylase, and sodium levels.

IV INCOMPATIBILITIES
Ciprofloxacin (Cipro), diazepam
(Valium), idarubicin (Idamycin),
midazolam (Versed), phenytoin
(Dilantin)

IV COMPATIBILITIES
Aminophylline, amphotericin, calcium gluconate, cefepime (Maxipime), digoxin (Lanoxin), diltiazem
(Cardizem), diphenhydramine
(Benadryl), dopamine (Intropin),
insulin, lidocaine, lorazepam (Ativan), magnesium sulfate, morphine,
norepinephrine (Levophed),
procainamide (Pronestyl), potassium
chloride, propofol (Diprivan)

SIDE EFFECTS
Frequent
Insomnia, heartburn, nervousness,
abdominal distention, diaphoresis,
acne, mood swings, increased appetite, facial flushing, delayed wound
healing, increased susceptibility to
infection, diarrhea or constipation
Occasional
Headache, edema, change in skin
color, frequent urination
Topical: Itching, redness, irritation
Rare
Tachycardia, allergic reaction rash
and hives, psychic changes, hallucinations, depression
Topical: Allergic contact dermatitis,
purpura
Systemic: Absorption more likely
with occlusive dressings or extensive application in young children

SERIOUS REACTIONS
• The serious reactions of long-term
therapy are hypocalcemia, hypokalemia, muscle wasting, especially in
arms and legs, osteoporosis, spontaneous fractures, amenorrhea, cata-

racts, glaucoma, peptic ulcer disease, and congestive heart failure (CHF).

• Abruptly withdrawing the drug after long-term therapy may cause anorexia, nausea, fever, headache, sudden severe joint pain, rebound inflammation, fatigue, weakness, lethargy, dizziness, and orthostatic hypotension.

NURSING CONSIDERATIONS

Baseline Assessment

• Determine if the patient has a hypersensitivity to any corticosteroids.

• Obtain the patient's baselines for blood glucose levels, blood pressure (B/P), serum electrolyte levels, height, and weight.

• Evaluate the results of initial tests, such as tuberculosis (TB) skin test, x-rays, and EKG.

• Determine if the patient has diabetes mellitus, and anticipate an increase in his or her antidiabetic drug regimen because of raised blood glucose levels.

• Find out if your patient takes digoxin, and if so plan to draw serum digoxin levels.

Lifespan Considerations

• Be aware that hydrocortisone crosses the placenta and is distributed in breast milk.

• Be aware that chronic hydrocortisone use during the first trimester of pregnancy may produce cleft palate in the neonate.

• Be aware that breast-feeding is contraindicated in this patient population.

• Be aware that prolonged treatment or high dosages may decrease the cortisol secretion and short-term growth rate in children.

• Be aware that the elderly may be more susceptible to developing hypertension or osteoporosis.

Precautions

• Use cautiously in patients with cirrhosis, CHF, diabetes mellitus, hypertension, hyperthyroidism, osteoporosis, peptic ulcer, seizure disorders, thromboembolic tendencies, thrombophlebitis, and ulcerative colitis.

Administration and Handling

IV

• Store at room temperature.

• After reconstitution, use hydrocortisone sodium succinate solution within 72 hours. Use immediately if further diluted with D_5W, 0.9% NaCl, or other compatible diluent.

• Once reconstituted, hydrocortisone sodium succinate solution is stable for 72 hours at room temperature.

• May further dilute hydrocortisone sodium succinate solution with D_5W or 0.9% NaCl. For IV push, dilute to 50 mg/ml; for intermittent infusion, dilute to 1 mg/ml.

• Administer hydrocortisone sodium succinate solution IV push over 3 to 5 minutes. Give intermittent infusion over 20 to 30 minutes.

Topical

• Gently cleanse area before application.

• Use occlusive dressings only as ordered.

• Apply sparingly, and rub into area thoroughly.

Rectal

• Shake homogeneous suspension well.

• Instruct patient to lie on his or her left side with left leg extended and right leg flexed.

• Gently insert applicator tip into rectum, pointed slightly toward umbilicus and slowly instill medication.

Intervention and Evaluation

• Examine the patient for edema.

• Be alert to signs and symptoms of infection such as fever and sore

throat that indicate reduced immune response.
• Assess the patient's daily pattern of bowel activity.
• Monitor the patient's electrolyte levels.
• Observe the patient for evidence of hypocalcemia, such as cramps, muscle twitching, or hypokalemia, such as EKG changes, irritability, nausea and vomiting, numbness or tingling of lower extremities, and weakness.
• Evaluate the patient's ability to sleep and emotional status.

Patient Teaching
• Warn the patient to notify the physician if he or she experiences fever, muscle aches, sore throat, or sudden weight gain or swelling.
• Instruct the patient to consult with the physician before he or she takes aspirin or any other medication during hydrocortisone therapy.
• Urge the patient to avoid alcohol and limit his or her caffeine intake during hydrocortisone therapy.
• Tell the patient to notify his or her dentist and other physicians of his or her use of cortisone therapy now or within past 12 months.
• Caution the patient against overuse of joints injected for symptomatic relief.
• Instruct the patient to apply topical hydrocortisone valerate after a bath or shower for best absorption. Teach the patient not to cover the affected area with any coverings, plastic pants, or tight diapers unless the physician instructs otherwise.
• Warn the patient to avoid getting the medication in contact with his or her eyes.
• Explain that steroids often cause mood swings, ranging from euphoria to depression.

methylprednisolone
meth-ill-pred-**niss**-oh-lone
(Medrol)
methylprednisolone acetate
(Depo-Medrol, Depo-Nisolone[AUS])
methylprednisolone sodium succinate
(A-Methapred, Solu-Medrol)
Do not confuse with Mebaral or medroxyprogesterone.

CATEGORY AND SCHEDULE
Pregnancy Risk Category: C

MECHANISM OF ACTION
An adrenal corticosteroid that suppresses migration of polymorphonuclear leukocytes, reverses increased capillary permeability. *Therapeutic Effect:* Decreases inflammation.

PHARMACOKINETICS

Route	Onset	Peak	Duration
PO	N/A	1–2 hrs	30–36 hrs
IM	N/A	4–8 days	1–4 wks

Well absorbed from the gastrointestinal (GI) tract after IM administration. Widely distributed. Metabolized in liver. Excreted in urine. Removed by hemodialysis. **Half-life:** longer than 3.5 hrs.

AVAILABILITY
Tablets: 2 mg, 4 mg, 8 mg, 16 mg, 24 mg, 32 mg.
Succinate
Powder for Injection: 40 mg, 125 mg, 500 mg, 1 g, 2 g.
Acetate
Injection: 20 mg/ml, 40 mg/ml, 80 mg/ml.

INDICATIONS AND DOSAGES

▶ **Substitution therapy of deficiency states: acute or chronic adrenal insufficiency, adrenal insufficiency secondary to pituitary insufficiency, congenital adrenal hyperplasia, and nonendocrine disorders, such as allergic, collagen, intestinal tract, liver, ocular, renal, and skin diseases, arthritis, bronchial asthma, cerebral edema, malignancies, and rheumatic carditis**

PO
Adults, Elderly. Initially, 4–48 mg/day.

IV (Methylprednisolone Sodium Succinate)
Adults, Elderly. 40–250 mg q4–6h. High dose: 30 mg/kg over at least 30 min. Repeat q4–6h for 48–72 hrs.

IM (Methylprednisolone Acetate)
Adults, Elderly. 10–80 mg/day.

Intra-articular, intralesional
Adults, Elderly. 4–40 mg, up to 80 mg q1–5wks.

CONTRAINDICATIONS

Administration of live virus vaccines, systemic fungal infection

INTERACTIONS

Drug

Amphotericin: May increase hypokalemia.
Digoxin: May increase the risk of toxicity of this drug caused by hypokalemia
Diuretics, insulin, oral hypoglycemics, potassium supplements: May decrease the effects of diuretics, insulin, oral hypoglycemics, and potassium supplements.
Liver enzyme inducers: May decrease the effects of methylprednisolone.
Live virus vaccines: May decrease the patient's antibody response to

vaccine, increase vaccine side effects, and potentiate virus replication.

Herbal

None known.

Food

None known.

DIAGNOSTIC TEST EFFECTS

May decrease serum calcium, potassium, and thyroxine levels. May increase blood glucose levels, serum lipids, amylase, and sodium levels.

IV INCOMPATIBILITIES

Ciprofloxacin (Cipro), diltiazem (Cardizem), docetaxel (Taxotere), etoposide (VePesid), filgrastim (Neupogen), gemcitabine (Gemzar), paclitaxel (Taxol), potassium chloride, propofol (Diprivan), vinorelbine (Navelbine)

IV COMPATIBILITIES

Dopamine (Intropin), heparin, midazolam (Versed), theophylline

SIDE EFFECTS

Frequent
Insomnia, heartburn, nervousness, abdominal distention, diaphoresis, acne, mood swings, increased appetite, facial flushing, GI distress, delayed wound healing, increased susceptibility to infection, diarrhea or constipation
Occasional
Headache, edema, tachycardia, change in skin color, frequent urination, depression
Rare
Psychosis, increased blood coagulability, hallucinations

SERIOUS REACTIONS

• The serious reactions of long-term therapy are hypocalcemia, hypokalemia, muscle wasting, especially in arms and legs, osteoporosis, spontaneous fractures, amenorrhea, cataracts, glaucoma, peptic ulcer disease, and congestive heart failure (CHF).

• Abruptly withdrawing the drug after long-term therapy may cause anorexia, nausea, fever, headache, sudden severe joint pain, rebound inflammation, fatigue, weakness, lethargy, dizziness, and orthostatic hypotension.

NURSING CONSIDERATIONS

Baseline Assessment

• Determine if the patient has a hypersensitivity to any corticosteroids.

• Obtain the patient's baselines for blood glucose levels, blood pressure (B/P), serum electrolyte levels, height, and weight.

• Evaluate the results of initial tests, such as tuberculosis (TB) skin test, x-rays, and EKG.

• Determine if the patient has diabetes mellitus, and anticipate an increase in his or her antidiabetic drug regime because of raised blood glucose levels.

• Find out if your patient takes digoxin, and if so plan to draw serum digoxin levels.

Lifespan Considerations

• Be aware that methylprednisolone crosses the placenta and is distributed in breast milk.

• Be aware that chronic methylprednisolone use in the first trimester of pregnancy may cause cleft palate in the neonate.

• Be aware that breast-feeding is contraindicated in this patient population.

• Be aware that prolonged treatment or high dosages may decrease cortisol secretion and short-term growth rate in children.

• There are no age-related precautions noted in the elderly.

Precautions

• Use cautiously in patients with cirrhosis, CHF, diabetes mellitus, hypertension, hypothyroidism, thromboembolic disorders, and ulcerative colitis.

Administration and Handling

◄ ALERT ► Individualize the drug dose based on the disease, patient, and response.

PO

• Give methylprednisolone with food or milk.

• Give single doses before 9 a.m., give multiple doses at evenly spaced intervals.

IM

• Methylprednisolone acetate should not be further diluted.

• Methylprednisolone sodium succinate should be reconstituted with bacteriostatic water for injection.

• Give deep IM injection in gluteus maximus.

IV

• Store vials at room temperature.

• Follow directions with Mix-o-vial.

• For infusion, add to D_5W, 0.9% NaCl.

• Give IV push over 2 to 3 minutes.

• Give IV piggyback over 10 to 20 minutes.

• Do not give methylprednisolone acetate via IV.

Intervention and Evaluation

• Monitor the patient's intake and output and record the patient's daily weight.

• Assess the patient for edema.

• Evaluate the patient's daily pattern of bowel activity.

• Check the patient's vital signs at east 2 times a day.

• Be alert to signs and symptoms of infection such as fever, sore throat, or vague symptoms.

• Monitor the patient's electrolytes.

• Observe the patient for evidence of hypocalcemia, such as cramps, muscle twitching, or hypokalemia, such as EKG changes, irritability, nausea and vomiting, numbness or tingling of lower extremities, and weakness.

• Assess the patient's ability to sleep and emotional status.

• Check the patient's lab results for blood coagulability and clinical evidence of thromboembolism.

Patient Teaching

• Instruct the patient to take oral methylprednisolone with food or milk.

• Caution the patient against abruptly discontinuing the drug or changing the drug dose or schedule. Explain to the patient that methylprednisolone doses must taper off gradually under medical supervision.

• Warn the patient to notify the physician if he or she experiences fever, muscle aches, sore throat, or sudden weight gain or swelling.

• Tell the patient to maintain good personal hygiene and to avoid exposure to disease or trauma. Explain to the patient that severe stress, such as serious infection, surgery, or trauma may require an increase in methylprednisolone dosage.

• Stress to the patient that follow-up visits and lab tests are a necessary part of treatment and that children must be assessed for growth retardation.

• Tell the patient to inform his or her dentist or other physicians of methylprednisolone therapy now or within past 12 months.

• Explain that steroids often cause mood swings, ranging from euphoria to depression.

prednisolone

pred-**niss**-oh-lone
(AK-Pred, AK-Tate[CAN], Econopred, Inflamase, Minims-Prednisolone[CAN], Novo-Prednisolone[CAN], Pediapred, Pred Mild, Prelone)

CATEGORY AND SCHEDULE

Pregnancy Risk Category: C (D if used in first trimester)

MECHANISM OF ACTION

An adrenal corticosteroid that inhibits accumulation of inflammatory cells at inflammation sites, phagocytosis, lysosomal enzyme release and synthesis, and release of mediators of inflammation. *Therapeutic Effect:* Prevents or suppresses cell-mediated immune reactions. Decreases or prevents tissue response to inflammatory process.

AVAILABILITY

Ophthalmic Suspension: 0.12%, 1%.
Ophthalmic Solution: 0.125%, 1%.
Oral Solution: 5 mg/5 ml, 15 mg/5 ml.
Tablets: 5 mg, 20 mg.

INDICATIONS AND DOSAGES

▸ **Substitution therapy in deficiency states: acute or chronic adrenal insufficiency, congenital adrenal hyperplasia, adrenal insufficiency secondary to pituitary insufficiency and nonendocrine disorders: arthritis; rheumatic carditis; allergic, collagen, intestinal tract, liver, ocular, renal, skin diseases; bronchial asthma; cerebral edema; malignancies**
PO
Adults. 5–60 mg/day.

▸ **Acute asthma**
PO
Children. 1–2 mg/kg/day in divided doses.
▸ **Anti-inflammation or immunosuppression**
PO
Children. 0.1–2 mg/kg/day in divided doses.
Ophthalmic
Adults, Elderly. Solution: 1–2 drops q1h during day; q2h during night; after response, decrease dosage to 1 drop q4h, then 1 drop 3–4 times/day.

CONTRAINDICATIONS
Acute superficial herpes simplex keratitis, systemic fungal infections, varicella

INTERACTIONS
Drug
Amphotericin: May increase hypokalemia.
Digoxin: May increase the risk of toxicity of this drug caused by hypokalemia
Diuretics, insulin, oral hypoglycemics, potassium supplements: May decrease the effects of diuretics, insulin, oral hypoglycemics, and potassium supplements.
Liver enzyme inducers: May decrease the effects of prednisolone.
Live virus vaccines: May decrease the patient's antibody response to vaccine, increase vaccine side effects, and potentiate virus replication.
Herbal
None known.
Food
None known.

DIAGNOSTIC TEST EFFECTS
May decrease serum calcium, potassium, and thyroxine levels. May increase blood glucose levels, serum lipids, amylase, and sodium levels.

SIDE EFFECTS
Frequent
Insomnia, heartburn, nervousness, abdominal distention, increased sweating, acne, mood swings, increased appetite, facial flushing, delayed wound healing, increased susceptibility to infection, diarrhea or constipation
Occasional
Headache, edema, change in skin color, frequent urination
Rare
Tachycardia, allergic reaction, such as rash and hives, psychic changes, hallucinations, depression
Ophthalmic: stinging or burning, posterior subcapsular cataracts

SERIOUS REACTIONS
• The serious effects of long-term therapy are hypocalcemia, hypokalemia, muscle wasting, especially in the arms and legs, osteoporosis, spontaneous fractures, amenorrhea, cataracts, glaucoma, peptic ulcer disease, and congestive heart failure (CHF).
• Abruptly withdrawing the drug after long-term therapy may cause anorexia, nausea, fever, headache, severe or sudden joint pain, rebound inflammation, fatigue, weakness, lethargy, dizziness, and orthostatic hypotension.
• Sudden discontinuance may be fatal.

NURSING CONSIDERATIONS
Baseline Assessment
• Determine if the patient has a hypersensitivity to any corticosteroids.
• Obtain the patient's baselines for blood glucose levels, blood pressure (B/P), serum electrolyte levels, height, and weight.

• Evaluate the results of initial tests, such as tuberculosis (TB) skin test, x-rays, and EKG.
• Determine if the patient has diabetes mellitus, and anticipate an increase in his or her antidiabetic drug regimen because of raised blood glucose levels.
• Find out if your patient takes digoxin, and if so plan to draw serum digoxin levels.
• Remember never to give this patient population a live virus vaccine, such as smallpox.

Precautions
• Use cautiously in patients with cirrhosis, CHF, diabetes mellitus, hypertension, hypothyroidism, myasthenia gravis, ocular herpes simplex, osteoporosis, peptic ulcer disease, thromboembolic disorders, and ulcerative colitis.

Intervention and Evaluation
• Be alert to signs and symptoms of infection such as fever, sore throat, or vague symptoms.
• Assess the patient's mouth daily for signs of candida infection, such as white patches and painful mucous membranes and tongue.

Patient Teaching
• Warn the patient to notify the physician if he or she experiences fever, muscle aches, sore throat, and sudden weight gain, or swelling.
• Urge the patient to avoid alcohol and to limit his or her caffeine intake during prednisolone therapy.
• Caution the patient against abruptly discontinuing the drug without physician's approval.
• Tell the patient to avoid exposure to chickenpox or measles.
• Explain that steroids often cause mood swings, ranging from euphoria to depression.

prednisone
pred-nih-sewn
(Apo-Prednisone[CAN], Deltasone, Meticorten, Panafcort[AUS], Sone[AUS], Winpred[CAN])
Do not confuse with prednisolone, Primidone.

CATEGORY AND SCHEDULE
Pregnancy Risk Category: C, D if used in first trimester

MECHANISM OF ACTION
An adrenal corticosteroid that inhibits accumulation of inflammatory cells at inflammation sites, phagocytosis, lysosomal enzyme release and synthesis, and release of mediators of inflammation. *Therapeutic Effect:* Prevents or suppresses cell-mediated immune reactions. Decreases or prevents tissue response to inflammatory process.

PHARMACOKINETICS
Well absorbed from the gastrointestinal (GI) tract. Protein binding: 70%–90%. Widely distributed. Metabolized in liver and converted to prednisolone. Primarily excreted in urine. Not removed by hemodialysis. **Half-life:** 3.4–3.8 hrs.

AVAILABILITY
Tablets: 1 mg, 2.5 mg, 5 mg, 10 mg, 20 mg, 50 mg.
Oral Solution: 5 mg/5 ml, 5 mg/ml.

INDICATIONS AND DOSAGES
▶ **Substitution therapy in deficiency states: acute or chronic adrenal insufficiency, congenital adrenal hyperplasia, adrenal insufficiency secondary to pituitary insufficiency and nonendocrine disorders: arthritis; rheumatic carditis, allergic, collagen, intestinal tract, liver,**

ocular, renal, skin diseases, bron-
chial asthma, cerebral edema,
malignancies
PO
Adults. 5–60 mg/day.
▸ **Acute asthma**
PO
Children. 1–2 mg/kg/day in divided
doses.
▸ **Anti-inflammation and immuno-
suppression**
PO
Children. 0.05–2 mg/kg/day in
divided doses.

CONTRAINDICATIONS
Acute superficial herpes simplex
keratitis, systemic fungal infections,
varicella

INTERACTIONS
Drug
Amphotericin: May increase hypokalemia.
Digoxin: May increase the risk of
toxicity of this drug caused by
hypokalemia
*Diuretics, insulin, oral hypoglyce-
mics, potassium supplements:* May
decrease the effects of diuretics,
insulin, oral hypoglycemics, and
potassium supplements.
Liver enzyme inducers: May decrease the effects of prednisone.
Live virus vaccines: May decrease
the patient's antibody response to
vaccine, increase vaccine side
effects, and potentiate virus replication.
Herbal
None known.
Food
None known.

DIAGNOSTIC TEST EFFECTS
May decrease serum calcium, potassium, and thyroxine levels. May
increase blood glucose levels, serum
lipids, amylase, and sodium levels.

SIDE EFFECTS
Frequent
Insomnia, heartburn, nervousness,
abdominal distention, increased
sweating, acne, mood swings, increased appetite, facial flushing,
delayed wound healing, increased
susceptibility to infection, diarrhea
or constipation
Occasional
Headache, edema, change in skin
color, frequent urination
Rare
Tachycardia, allergic reaction,
including rash and hives, psychic
changes, hallucinations, depression

SERIOUS REACTIONS
• The serious reactions of long-term
therapy are muscle wasting in the
arms and legs, osteoporosis, spontaneous fractures, amenorrhea, cataracts, glaucoma, peptic ulcer disease, and congestive heart failure
(CHF).
• Abruptly withdrawing the drug
following long-term therapy may
cause anorexia, nausea, fever, headache, sudden or severe joint pain,
rebound inflammation, fatigue,
weakness, lethargy, dizziness, and
orthostatic hypotension.
• Sudden discontinuance of the drug
may be fatal.

NURSING CONSIDERATIONS
Baseline Assessment
• Determine if the patient has a hypersensitivity to any corticosteroids.
• Obtain the patient's baselines for
blood glucose levels, blood pressure
(B/P), serum electrolyte levels,
height, and weight.
• Determine if the patient has diabetes mellitus, and anticipate an increase in his or her antidiabetic
drug regimen because of raised
blood glucose levels.

• Find out if your patient takes digoxin, and if so plan to draw serum digoxin levels.

• Check the results of initial patient tests, such as tuberculosis skin test, x-rays, electrocardiogram (EKG).

• Remember never to give this patient population live virus vaccine, such as smallpox.

Lifespan Considerations

• Be aware that prednisone crosses the placenta and is distributed in breast milk.

• Be aware that chronic prednisone use in the first trimester of pregnancy causes cleft palate in the neonate.

• Be aware that prolonged treatment or high dosages may decrease the cortisol secretion and short-term growth rate of children.

• Be aware that the elderly may be more susceptible to developing hypertension or osteoporosis.

Precautions

• Use cautiously in patients with cirrhosis, congestive heart failure (CHF), hypertension, hyperthyroidism, myasthenia gravis, ocular herpes simplex, osteoporosis, peptic ulcer disease, thromboembolic disorders, and ulcerative colitis.

Administration and Handling

PO

• Give prednisone without regard to meals; give with food if GI upset occurs.

• Give single doses before 9 a.m., give multiple doses at evenly spaced intervals.

Intervention and Evaluation

• Monitor the patient's blood glucose, B/P, electrolytes, and height. In pediatric patients also monitor weight.

• Be alert to signs and symptoms of infection such as fever, sore throat, or vague symptoms.

• Assess the patient's mouth daily

for signs of candida infection, such as white patches and painful mucous membranes and tongue.

Patient Teaching

• Warn the patient to notify the physician if he or she experiences fever, muscle aches, sore throat, or sudden weight gain or swelling.

• Urge the patient to avoid alcohol and limit his or her caffeine intake during prednisone therapy.

• Caution the patient against abruptly discontinuing prednisone without the physician's approval.

• Warn the patient to avoid exposure to chickenpox or measles.

• Explain that steroids often cause mood swings, ranging from euphoria to depression.

triamcinolone
try-am-**sin**-oh-lone
(Aristocort)

triamcinolone acetonide
(Aristocort, Azmacort, Kenalog, Nasacort AQ, Triaderm[CAN])

triamcinolone diacetate
(Amcort, Aristocort Intralesional)

triamcinolone hexacetonide
(Aristospan)

Do not confuse with Triaminicin or Triaminicol.

CATEGORY AND SCHEDULE
Pregnancy Risk Category: C, D if used in first trimester

MECHANISM OF ACTION
An adrenocortical steroid that inhibits accumulation of inflammatory cells at inflammation sites, phagocytosis, lysosomal enzyme release and

synthesis and release of mediators of inflammation. *Therapeutic Effect:* Prevents or suppresses cell-mediated immune reactions. Decreases or prevents tissue response to inflammatory process.

AVAILABILITY
Tablets: 4 mg.
Syrup: 2 mg/5 ml.
Aerosol or respiratory inhalant, nasal spray, ointment: 0.1%.
Cream: 0.025%, 0.1%, 0.5%.
Lotion: 0.025%, 0.1%.
Acetonide
Injection: 10 mg/ml, 40 mg/ml.
Diacetate
Injection: 40 mg/ml.
Hexacetone
Injection: 5 mg/ml, 20 mg/ml.

INDICATIONS AND DOSAGES
▶ **Immunosuppressant, relief of acute inflammation**
PO
Adults, Elderly. 4–60 mg/day.
IM
Adults, Elderly. 40 mg/wk (triamcinolone diacetate)
Intra-articular, intralesional
Adults, Elderly. 5–40 mg.
IM
Adults, Elderly. Initially, 2.5–60 mg/day (triamcinolone acetonide).
Initially, 2.5–40 mg up to 100 mg; 2–20 mg (triamcinolone hexacetonide).
▶ **Control of bronchial asthma**
Inhalation
Adults, Elderly. 2 inhalations 3–4 times/day.
Children 6–12 yrs. 1–2 inhalations 3–4 times/day. Maximum: 12 inhalations/day.
▶ **Rhinitis**
Intranasal
Adults, Children older than 6 yrs. 2 sprays each nostril each day.

▶ **Relief of inflammation or pruritus associated with corticoid responsive dermatoses**
Topical
Adults, Elderly. Sparingly 2–4 times/day. May give 1–2 times/day or intermittent therapy.

CONTRAINDICATIONS
Avoid immunizations, especially smallpox vaccination; hypersensitivity to any corticosteroid or tartrazine, IM injection, oral inhalation not for children younger than 6 yrs, peptic ulcers—except life-threatening situations, systemic fungal infection
Topical: Marked circulation impairment

INTERACTIONS
Drug
Amphotericin: May increase hypokalemia.
Digoxin: May increase the risk of toxicity of this drug caused by hypokalemia.
Diuretics, insulin, oral hypoglycemics, potassium supplements: May decrease the effects of diuretics, insulin, oral hypoglycemics, and potassium supplements.
Liver enzyme inducers: May decrease the effects of triamcinolone.
Live virus vaccines: May decrease the patient's antibody response to vaccine, increase vaccine side effects, and potentiate virus replication.
Herbal
None known.
Food
None known.

DIAGNOSTIC TEST EFFECTS
May decrease serum calcium, potassium, and thyroxine levels. May increase blood glucose levels, serum lipids, amylase, and sodium levels.

SIDE EFFECTS
Frequent
Insomnia, dry mouth, heartburn, nervousness, abdominal distention, diaphoresis, acne, mood swings, increased appetite, facial flushing, delayed wound healing, increased susceptibility to infection, diarrhea or constipation
Occasional
Headache, edema, change in skin color, frequent urination
Rare
Tachycardia, allergic reaction, including rash and hives, mental changes, hallucinations, depression
Topical: Allergic contact dermatitis.

SERIOUS REACTIONS
• The serious reactions of long-term therapy are muscle wasting in the arms or legs, osteoporosis, spontaneous fractures, amenorrhea, cataracts, glaucoma, peptic ulcer disease, and congestive heart failure (CHF).
• Abruptly withdrawing the drug following long-term therapy may cause anorexia, nausea, fever, headache, joint pain, rebound inflammation, fatigue, weakness, lethargy, dizziness, and orthostatic hypotension.
• Anaphylaxis with parenteral administration occurs rarely.
• Sudden discontinuance of the drug may be fatal.
• Blindness has occurred rarely after intralesional injection around face and head.

NURSING CONSIDERATIONS
Baseline Assessment
• Determine if the patient is hypersensitive to any corticosteroids or tartrazine (Kenacort).
• Obtain the patient's baselines for blood glucose levels, blood pressure (B/P), serum electrolyte levels, height, and weight.
• Determine if the patient has diabetes mellitus, and anticipate an increase in his or her antidiabetic drug regimen because of raised blood glucose levels.
• Find out if your patient takes digoxin, and if so plan to draw serum digoxin levels.
• Check the results of initial patient tests, such as tuberculosis skin test, x-rays, electrocardiogram (EKG).
• Remember never to give this patient population live virus vaccine, such as smallpox.
Precautions
• Use cautiously in patients with cirrhosis, CHF, history of tuberculosis—because it may reactivate disease, hypertension, hypothyroidism, nonspecific ulcerative colitis, psychosis, and renal insufficiency.
• Discontinue prolonged therapy slowly.
Administration and Handling
PO
• Give triamcinolone with food or milk.
• Give single doses before 9 a.m., multiple doses at evenly spaced intervals.
IM
• Do not give IV.
• Give deep IM injection in gluteus maximus.
Inhalation
• Shake container well; instruct the patient to exhale as completely as possible.
• Place mouthpiece fully into the patient's mouth and while holding the inhaler upright, have the patient inhale deeply and slowly while pressing the top of the canister. Instruct the patient to hold his or her breath as long as possible before slowly exhaling.

• Wait 1 minute between inhalations when multiple inhalations ordered to allow for deeper bronchial penetration.

• Rinse the patient's mouth with water immediately after inhalation to prevent thrush.

Topical

• Gently cleanse area before application.

• Use occlusive dressings only as ordered.

• Apply sparingly and rub into area thoroughly.

Intervention and Evaluation

• Monitor the patient's blood glucose, B/P, and intake and output. Record the patient's daily weight.

• Assess the patient for edema.

• Check the patient's vital signs at least 2 times a day.

• Be alert to signs and symptoms of infection such as fever, sore throat, or vague symptoms.

• Evaluate the patient for signs and symptoms of hypocalcemia, such as cramps, muscle twitching, positive Chvostek's or Trousseau's signs, or hypokalemia, such as EKG changes, irritability, muscle cramps and weakness, nausea and vomiting, numbness and tingling in the lower extremities.

• Assess the patient's ability to sleep and emotional status.

• Check the mucous membranes for signs of fungal infection in patients taking triamcinolone for oral inhalation.

• Monitor the growth rate in pediatric patients.

• Check patient lab results for blood coagulability and clinical evidence of thromboembolism.

• Assist the patient with ambulation.

Patient Teaching

• Tell the patient taking oral triamcinolone to notify the physician if he or she experiences difficulty breathing, muscle weakness, sudden weight gain, and swelling of the face.

• Instruct the patient taking oral triamcinolone to take the drug with food or after meals.

• Warn the patient to notify the physician if his or her condition worsens.

• Caution the patient against abruptly discontinuing oral triamcinolone without physician approval.

• Explain to the patient that oral triamcinolone may cause dry mouth.

• Urge the patient to avoid alcohol during oral triamcinolone therapy.

• Instruct patients taking inhaled triamcinolone not to take the drug for acute asthma attacks.

• Tell the patient taking inhaled triamcinolone to rinse his or her mouth after drug administration to decrease the risk of mouth soreness.

• Warn the patient taking inhaled triamcinolone to notify the physician if he or she experiences mouth lesions or soreness.

• Warn the patient taking nasal triamcinolone to notify the physician if he or she experiences persistent nasal bleeding, burning, or infection, or unusual cough or spasm.

• Explain that steroids often cause mood swings, ranging from euphoria to depression.

acarbose
glimepiride
glipizide
glyburide
insulin
metformin
  hydrochloride
miglitol
nateglinide
pioglitazone
repaglinide
rosiglitazone maleate

Uses: All antidiabetic agents are used to treat diabetes. *Insulin* is used to manage insulin-dependent diabetes mellitus (type 1) and non-insulin-dependent diabetes mellitus (type 2). It's also used in acute situations, such as ketoacidosis, severe infections, and major surgery in otherwise non-insulin-dependent diabetes mellitus. It's administered to patients receiving parenteral nutrition and is the drug of choice during pregnancy.

Sulfonylureas, such as glimepiride and glyburide, are used to control hyperglycemia in type 2 diabetes mellitus that's not controlled by weight management and diet alone.

Alpha-glucosidase inhibitors, such as acarbose and miglitol, and *biguanides,* such as metformin, are used along with diet to lower the blood glucose level in patients with type 2 diabetes mellitus whose hyperglycemia can't be managed by diet alone.

Meglitinides, such as nateglinide and repaglinide, are used alone or with other antidiabetic agents to control the blood glucose level in patients with type 2 diabetes mellitus whose hyperglycemia can't be managed by diet and exercise.

Thiazolidinediones, such as pioglitazone and rosiglitazone, are used as adjunct therapy in patients with type 2 diabetes who are currently receiving insulin.

Action: Antidiabetic agents act in different ways to control diabetes. *Insulin* is a hormone synthesized and secreted by beta cells in the islets of Langerhans in the pancreas. It controls the storage and use of glucose, amino acids, and fatty acids by activated transport systems and enzymes. It also inhibits the breakdown of glycogen, fat, and protein. Insulin lowers the blood glucose level by inhibiting glycogenolysis and gluconeogenesis in the liver and by stimulating glucose uptake by muscle and adipose tissue. Insulin activity is initiated by binding to cell surface receptors.

Sulfonylureas stimulate insulin release from beta cells and increase insulin sensitivity in

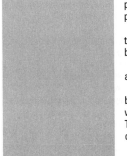

peripheral tissues. Endogenous insulin must be present for these oral drugs to be effective.

Alpha-glucosidase inhibitors work locally in the small intestine, slowing carbohydrate breakdown and glucose absorption.

Biguanides decrease hepatic glucose output and enhance peripheral glucose uptake.

Meglitinides stimulate the release of insulin by depolarizing beta cells in the pancreas, which prompts their calcium channels to open. This action causes an influx of intracellular calcium and stimulates insulin secretion.

Thiazolidinediones decrease insulin resistance.

COMBINATION PRODUCTS

AVANDAMET: metformin/rosiglitazone (an antidiabetic) 500 mg/1 mg; 500 mg/2 mg; 500 mg/4 mg; 1 g/2 mg; 1 g/4 mg.
GLUCOVANCE: glyburide/metformin (an antidiabetic) 1.25 mg/250 mg; 2.5 mg/500 mg; 5 mg/500 mg.
METAGLIP: glipizide/metformin (an antidiabetic) 2.5 mg/250 mg; 2.5 mg/500 mg; 5 mg/500 mg.

acarbose
ah-**car**-bose
(Glucobay[AUS], Prandase[CAN], Precose)
Do not confuse with PreCare.

CATEGORY AND SCHEDULE
Pregnancy Risk Category: B

MECHANISM OF ACTION
An alpha glucosidase inhibitor that delays glucose absorption and digestion of carbohydrates. *Therapeutic Effect:* Results in smaller rise in blood glucose concentration after meals, lowers postprandial hyperglycemia.

AVAILABILITY
Tablets: 25 mg, 50 mg, 100 mg.

INDICATIONS AND DOSAGES
▸ **Diabetes mellitus**
PO
Adults, Elderly. Initially, 25 mg 3 times/day at the start (with first bite) of each main meal. Increase at 4- to 8-wk intervals. Maximum: 60 kg or less, 50 mg 3 times/day; greater than 60 kg, 100 mg 3 times/day.

CONTRAINDICATIONS
Chronic intestinal diseases associated with marked disorders of digestion or absorption, cirrhosis, colonic ulceration, conditions that may deteriorate as a result of increased gas formation in the intestine, diabetic ketoacidosis, hypersensitivity to the drug, inflammatory bowel disease, partial intestinal obstruction or predisposition to intestinal obstruction, and significant renal dysfunction (serum creatinine greater than 2 mg/dl)

INTERACTIONS
Drug
Digestive enzymes, intestinal absorbents (e.g., charcoal): Reduces effect of acarbose. Do not use concurrently.
Herbal
None known.
Food
None known.

DIAGNOSTIC TEST EFFECTS
May increase serum glutamic-oxaloacetic transaminase (SGOT) levels.

SIDE EFFECTS
Frequent
Transient GI disturbances: flatulence (77%), diarrhea (33%), abdominal pain (21%)
Symptoms tend to diminish in frequency and intensity over time.

SERIOUS REACTIONS
• None known.

NURSING CONSIDERATIONS
Baseline Assessment
• Expect to check blood glucose level.
• Discuss lifestyle to determine extent of learning and emotional needs.
Precautions
• Use cautiously in patients with fever or infection or who've had surgery or trauma as these states may cause loss of glycemic control.
Administration and Handling
PO
• Give with the first bite of each main meal.
Intervention and Evaluation
• Monitor blood glucose, food intake, glycosylated hemoglobin, and SGOT (AST) values.
• Assess for signs and symptoms of hypoglycemia as evidenced by anxiety, cool wet skin, diplopia, dizziness, headache, hunger, numbness in mouth, tachycardia, and tremors or hyperglycemia as evidenced by deep rapid breathing, dim vision, fatigue, nausea, polydipsia, polyphagia, polyuria, and vomiting.
• Be alert to conditions that alter glucose requirements, including fever, increased activity or stress, fever, or a surgical procedure.
Patient Teaching
• Advise the patient not to skip or delay meals.
• Stress that the patient check with his or her physician when glucose demands are altered (fever, heavy physical activity, infection, stress, trauma).
• Warn the patient to avoid alcoholic beverages.
• Explain to the patient that exercise, hygiene (including foot care), not smoking, and weight control are essential parts of therapy.

glimepiride
glim-**eh**-purr-eyd
(Amaryl)
Do not confuse with glipizide.

CATEGORY AND SCHEDULE
Pregnancy Risk Category: C

MECHANISM OF ACTION
A second-generation sulfonylurea that promotes release of insulin from beta cells of pancreas, increases insulin sensitivity at peripheral sites. *Therapeutic Effect:* Lowers blood glucose concentration.

PHARMACOKINETICS

Route	Onset	Peak	Duration
PO	N/A	2–3 hrs	24 hrs

Completely absorbed from the gastrointestinal (GI) tract. Protein binding: greater than 99%. Metabolized in liver. Excreted in urine and eliminated in feces. **Half-life:** 5–9.2 hrs.

AVAILABILITY
Tablets: 1 mg, 2 mg, 4 mg.

INDICATIONS AND DOSAGES
▸ **Diabetes mellitus**
PO
Adults, Elderly. Initially, 1–2 mg once a day, with breakfast or first main meal. Maintenance: 1–4 mg once a day. After dose of 2 mg is reached, dosage should be increased in increments of up to 2 mg q1–2wks, based on blood glucose response. Maximum: 8 mg/day.
▸ **Renal function impairment**
PO
Adults. 1 mg once/day.

CONTRAINDICATIONS
Diabetic complications, such as ketosis, acidosis, and diabetic coma, severe liver or renal impairment, sole therapy for type 1 diabetes mellitus, stress situations, including severe infection, trauma, and surgery

INTERACTIONS
Drug
Beta-blockers: May increase the hypoglycemic effect and mask signs of hypoglycemia.
Cimetidine, ciprofloxacin, fluconazole, MAOIs, quinidine, ranitidine, large doses of salicylates: May increase the effects of glimepiride.
Corticosteroids, lithium, thiazide diuretics: May decrease the effects of glimepiride.
Oral anticoagulants: May increase the effects of oral anticoagulants.

Herbal
None known.
Food
None known.

DIAGNOSTIC TEST EFFECTS
May increase BUN, LDH concentrations, serum alkaline phosphatase, creatinine, and SGOT (AST) levels.

SIDE EFFECTS
Frequent
Altered taste sensation, dizziness, drowsiness, weight gain, constipation, diarrhea, heartburn, nausea, vomiting, stomach fullness, headache
Occasional
Increased sensitivity of skin to sunlight, peeling of skin, itching, rash

SERIOUS REACTIONS
• Hypoglycemia may occur due to overdosage, insufficient food intake, especially with increased glucose demands.
• GI hemorrhage, cholestatic hepatic jaundice, leukopenia, thrombocytopenia, pancytopenia, agranulocytosis, aplastic or hemolytic anemia occurs rarely.

NURSING CONSIDERATIONS

Baseline Assessment
• Check the patient's blood glucose levels, as ordered.
• Discuss the patient's lifestyle to determine the extent of his or her emotional and learning needs regarding diabetes mellitus.
Lifespan Considerations
• Be aware that glimepiride use is not recommended during pregnancy.
• Be aware that it is unknown if glimepiride is distributed in breast milk.
• Be aware that the safety and

efficacy of glimepiride have not been established in children.
• Be aware that hypoglycemia may be difficult to recognize in the elderly.
• In the elderly, age-related renal impairment may increase sensitivity to glucose lowering effect.

Precautions
• Use cautiously in patients with adrenal insufficiency, debilitation, impaired renal function, intestinal obstruction, liver disease, malnutrition, pituitary insufficiency, prolonged vomiting, severe diarrhea, and uncontrolled hyperthyroidism.

Administration and Handling
PO
• Give glimepiride with breakfast or first main meal.

Intervention and Evaluation
• Monitor the patient's blood glucose and food intake.
• Assess the patient for signs and symptoms of hypoglycemia, such as anxiety, cool, wet skin, diplopia, dizziness, headache, hunger, numbness in mouth, tachycardia, and tremors, or hyperglycemia, including deep, rapid breathing, dim vision, fatigue, nausea, polydipsia, polyphagia, polyuria, and vomiting.
• Be alert to conditions that alter blood glucose requirements, such as fever, increased activity, stress, or a surgical procedure.

Patient Teaching
• Stress to the patient that the prescribed diet is a principal part of treatment. Warn the patient not to skip or delay meals.
• Make sure the patient is aware of the typical signs and symptoms of hypoglycemia and hyperglycemia.
• Instruct the patient to carry candy, sugar packets, or other sugar supplements for immediate response to hypoglycemia.

• Urge the patient to wear medical alert identification.
• Instruct the patient to notify the physician when his or her glucose demands are altered, such as with fever, heavy physical activity, infection, stress, or trauma.
• Ensure follow-up instruction if the patient or family does not thoroughly understand diabetes management or blood glucose-testing technique.
• Teach the patient to wear sunscreen and protective eyewear to prevent the effects of light sensitivity.

glipizide
glip-ih-zide
(Glucotrol, Glucotrol XL, Melizide[AUS], Minidiab[AUS])
Do not confuse with glimepiride or glyburide.

CATEGORY AND SCHEDULE
Pregnancy Risk Category: C

MECHANISM OF ACTION
A second-generation sulfonylurea that promotes the release of insulin from beta cells of pancreas, increases insulin sensitivity at peripheral sites. *Therapeutic Effect:* Lowers blood glucose concentration.

PHARMACOKINETICS

Route	Onset	Peak	Duration
PO	15–30 min	2–3 hrs	12–24 hrs
Extended-release	2–3 hrs	6–12 hrs	24 hrs

Well absorbed from the gastrointestinal (GI) tract. Protein binding:

99%. Metabolized in liver. Excreted in urine. **Half-life:** 2–4 hrs.

AVAILABILITY
Tablets: 5 mg, 10 mg.
Tablets (extended-release): 2.5 mg, 5 mg, 10 mg.

INDICATIONS AND DOSAGES
▸ **Diabetes mellitus**
PO
Adults. Initially, 5 mg/day or 2.5 mg in the elderly or those with liver disease. Adjust dosage in 2.5- to 5-mg increments at intervals of several days. Maximum single dose: 15 mg. Maximum dose/day: 40 mg. Maintenance (ER Tablet): 20 mg/day.
Elderly. Initially, 2.5–5 mg/day. May increase by 2.5–5 mg/day q1–2wks.

CONTRAINDICATIONS
Diabetic ketoacidosis with or without coma, Type 1 diabetes mellitus

INTERACTIONS
Drug
Beta-blockers: May increase the hypoglycemic effect and mask signs of hypoglycemia.
Cimetidine, ciprofloxacin, fluconazole, MAOIs, quinidine, ranitidine, large doses of salicylates: May increase the effects of glimepiride.
Corticosteroids, lithium, thiazide diuretics: May decrease the effects of glimepiride.
Oral anticoagulants: May increase the effects of oral anticoagulants.
Herbal
None known.
Food
None known.

DIAGNOSTIC TEST EFFECTS
May increase BUN, LDH concentrations, serum alkaline phosphatase, creatinine, and SGOT (AST) levels.

SIDE EFFECTS
Frequent
Altered taste sensation, dizziness, drowsiness, weight gain, constipation, diarrhea, heartburn, nausea, vomiting, stomach fullness, headache
Occasional
Increased sensitivity of skin to sunlight, peeling of skin, itching, rash

SERIOUS REACTIONS
• Hypoglycemia may occur because of overdosage or insufficient food intake, especially with increased glucose demands.
• GI hemorrhage, cholestatic hepatic jaundice, leukopenia, thrombocytopenia, pancytopenia, agranulocytosis, aplastic or hemolytic anemia occurs rarely.

NURSING CONSIDERATIONS
Baseline Assessment
• Check the patient's blood glucose level.
• Discuss the patient's lifestyle to determine the extent of his or her emotional and learning needs.
Lifespan Considerations
• Be aware that insulin is the drug of choice during pregnancy.
• Be aware that glipizide given within 1 month of delivery may produce neonatal hypoglycemia.
• Be aware that glipizide crosses the placenta and is distributed in breast milk.
• Be aware that the safety and efficacy of this drug have not been established in children.
• Be aware that hypoglycemia may be difficult to recognize in the elderly.
• In the elderly, age-related renal impairment may increase sensitivity to glucose-lowering effect.

Precautions
• Use cautiously in patients with adrenal or pituitary insufficiency, hypoglycemic reactions, and impaired liver or renal function.

Administration and Handling
PO
• May give glipizide with food, the response better if taken 15 to 30 minutes before meals.
• Do not crush extended-release tablets.

Intervention and Evaluation
• Monitor the patient's blood glucose and food intake.
• Assess the patient for signs and symptoms of hypoglycemia, such as anxiety, cool, wet skin, diplopia, dizziness, headache, hunger, numbness in mouth, tachycardia, and tremors, or hyperglycemia, including deep, rapid breathing, dim vision, fatigue, nausea, polydipsia, polyphagia, polyuria, and vomiting.
• Be alert to conditions that alter blood glucose requirements, such as fever, increased activity, stress, or a surgical procedure.

Patient Teaching
• Stress to the patient that the prescribed diet is a principal part of treatment. Warn the patient not to skip or delay meals.
• Make sure the patient is aware of the typical signs and symptoms of hypoglycemia and hyperglycemia.
• Instruct the patient to carry candy, sugar packets, or other sugar supplements for immediate response to hypoglycemia.
• Urge the patient to wear medical alert identification.
• Instruct the patient to notify the physician when his or her glucose demands are altered, such as with fever, heavy physical activity, infection, stress, or trauma.
• Ensure follow-up instruction if the patient or family does not thoroughly understand diabetes management or blood glucose-testing technique.
• Teach the patient to wear sunscreen and protective eyewear to prevent the effects of light sensitivity.

glyburide
glye-byoo-ride
(Daonil[CAN], DiaBeta, Euglucon[CAN], Glimel[AUS], Glynase, Micronase, Semi-Daonil[AUS], Semi-Euglucon[AUS])
Do not confuse with Micro-K, Micronor, or Zebeta.

CATEGORY AND SCHEDULE
Pregnancy Risk Category: C

MECHANISM OF ACTION
A second-generation sulfonylurea that promotes release of insulin from beta cells of pancreas, increases insulin sensitivity at peripheral sites. *Therapeutic Effect:* Lowers blood glucose concentration.

PHARMACOKINETICS

Route	Onset	Peak	Duration
PO	0.25–1 hr	1–2 hrs	12–24 hrs

Well absorbed from the gastrointestinal (GI) tract. Protein binding: 99%. Metabolized in liver to weakly active metabolite. Primarily excreted in urine. Not removed by hemodialysis. **Half-life:** 1.4–1.8 hrs.

AVAILABILITY
Tablets: 1.25 mg, 1.5 mg (Glynase), 2.5 mg, 3 mg (Glynase), 5 mg, 6 mg (Glynase).

INDICATIONS AND DOSAGES
▸ **Diabetes mellitus**
PO
Adults. Initially 2.5–5 mg. May increase by 2.5 mg/day at weekly intervals. Maintenance: 1.25–20 mg/day. Maximum: 20 mg/day.
Elderly. Initially, 1.25–2.5 mg/day. May increase by 1.25–2.5 mg/day at 1–3 week intervals.
PO (micronized tablets [Glynase])
Adults, Elderly. Initially 0.75–3 mg/day. May increase by 1.5 mg/day at weekly intervals. Maintenance: 0.75–12 mg/day as single dose or in divided doses.
▸ **Dosage in renal impairment**
Not recommended in patients with creatinine clearance less than 50 ml/min.

CONTRAINDICATIONS
Diabetic ketoacidosis with or without coma, sole therapy for type 1 diabetes mellitus

INTERACTIONS
Drug
Beta-blockers: May increase the hypoglycemic effect and mask signs of hypoglycemia.
Cimetidine, ciprofloxacin, fluconazole, MAOIs, quinidine, ranitidine, large doses of salicylates: May increase the effects of glimepiride.
Corticosteroids, lithium, thiazide diuretics: May decrease the effects of glimepiride.
Oral anticoagulants: May increase the effects of oral anticoagulants.
Herbal
None known.
Food
None known.

DIAGNOSTIC TEST EFFECTS
May increase BUN, LDH concentrations, serum alkaline phosphatase, creatinine, and SGOT (AST) levels.

SIDE EFFECTS
Frequent
Altered taste sensation, dizziness, drowsiness, weight gain, constipation, diarrhea, heartburn, nausea, vomiting, stomach fullness, headache
Occasional
Increased sensitivity of skin to sunlight, peeling of skin, itching, rash

SERIOUS REACTIONS
• Overdosage or insufficient food intake may produce hypoglycemia, especially in patients with increased glucose demands.
• Cholestatic jaundice, leukopenia, thrombocytopenia, pancytopenia, agranulocytosis, aplastic or hemolytic anemia occurs rarely.

NURSING CONSIDERATIONS
Baseline Assessment
• Check the patient's blood glucose level.
• Discuss the patient's lifestyle to determine the extent of his or her emotional and learning needs.
Lifespan Considerations
• Be aware that glyburide crosses the placenta and is distributed in breast milk.
• Be aware that glyburide use within 2 weeks of delivery may produce neonatal hypoglycemia.
• Be aware that the safety and efficacy of glyburide have not been established in children.
• Be aware that hypoglycemia may be difficult to recognize in the elderly.
• In the elderly, age-related renal impairment may increase sensitivity to glucose-lowering effect.
Precautions
• Use cautiously in patients with adrenal or pituitary insufficiency,

hypoglycemic reactions, and impaired liver or renal function.

Intervention and Evaluation

• Monitor the patient's blood glucose and food intake.

• Assess the patient for signs and symptoms of hypoglycemia, such as anxiety, cool, wet skin, diplopia, dizziness, headache, hunger, numbness in mouth, tachycardia, and tremors, or hyperglycemia, including deep, rapid breathing, dim vision, fatigue, nausea, polydipsia, polyphagia, polyuria, and vomiting.

• Be alert to conditions that alter blood glucose requirements, such as fever, increased activity, stress, or a surgical procedure.

Patient Teaching

• Stress to the patient that the prescribed diet is a principal part of treatment. Warn the patient not to skip or delay meals.

• Make sure the patient is aware of the typical signs and symptoms of hypoglycemia and hyperglycemia.

• Instruct the patient to carry candy, sugar packets, or other sugar supplements for immediate response to hypoglycemia.

• Urge the patient to wear medical alert identification.

• Instruct the patient to notify the physician when his or her glucose demands are altered, such as with fever, heavy physical activity, infection, stress, or trauma.

• Ensure follow-up instruction if the patient or family does not thoroughly understand diabetes management or blood glucose-testing technique.

• Teach the patient to wear sunscreen and protective eyewear to prevent the effects of light sensitivity.

insulin
in-sull-in

Rapid acting: Insulin Lispro (Humalog), Insulin Aspart (Novolog, Novorapid[AUS]),
Regular Insulin (Actrapid[AUS], Humulin R, Novolin R, Regular Iletin II,)
Intermediate acting: NPH (Humulin N, Novolin N, Pork), Lente: (Humulin L, Lente Iletin II, Monotard[AUS], Novolin L)
NPH/regular mixture (70%/30%): Humulin 70/30, Novolin 70/30
NPH/regular mixture (50%/50%): Humulin 50/50
NPH/Lispro mixture (75%/25%): Humalog Mix 75/25, Novalog Mix 70/30
Long acting: Insulin Glargine (Lantus)

CATEGORY AND SCHEDULE
Pregnancy Risk Category: B
OTC

MECHANISM OF ACTION
An exogenous insulin that facilitates passage of glucose, potassium, magnesium across cellular membranes of skeletal and cardiac muscle, adipose tissue; controls storage and metabolism of carbohydrates, protein, fats. Promotes conversion of glucose to glycogen in liver.
Therapeutic Effect: Controls glucose levels in diabetic patients.

PHARMACOKINETICS

Drug Form	Onset (hrs)	Peak (hrs)	Duration (hrs)
Lispro		–1	4–5
Insulin aspart	1/6	1–3	3–5
Regular	–1	2–4	5–7
NPH	1–2	6–14	24+
Lente	1–3	6–14	24+
Insulin glargine	N/A	N/A	24

AVAILABILITY

Humalog.
Novolog regular.
NPH, 70/30, 50/50.
Lente: 100 units/ml.

INDICATIONS AND DOSAGES

▸ **Treatment of insulin-dependent type 1 diabetes mellitus, non–insulin-dependent type 2 diabetes mellitus when diet or weight control therapy has failed to maintain satisfactory blood glucose levels or in event of fever, infection, pregnancy, severe endocrine, liver or renal dysfunction, surgery, or trauma, regular insulin used in emergency treatment of ketoacidosis, to promote passage of glucose across cell membrane in hyperalimentation, to facilitate intracellular shift of potassium in hyperkalemia**
Subcutaneous
Adults, Elderly, Children.
0.5–1 units/kg/day.
Adolescents (during growth spurt).
0.8–1.2 units/kg/day.

CONTRAINDICATIONS

Hypersensitivity or insulin resistance may require change of type or species source of insulin

INTERACTIONS
Drug

Alcohol: May increase the effects of insulin.
Beta-adrenergic blockers: May increase the risk of hyperglycemia or hypoglycemia, mask signs of hypoglycemia, and prolong the period of hypoglycemia.
Glucocorticoids, thiazide diuretics: May increase blood glucose.
Herbal
None known.
Food
None known.

DIAGNOSTIC TEST EFFECTS

May decrease serum magnesium, phosphate, and potassium concentrations.

IV INCOMPATIBILITIES

Digoxin (Lanoxin), diltiazem (Cardizem), dopamine (Intropin), nafcillin (Nafcil)

IV COMPATIBILITIES

Amiodarone (Cordarone), ampicillin/sulbactam (Unasyn), cefazolin (Ancef), cimetidine (Tagamet), digoxin (Lanoxin), dobutamine (Dobutrex), famotidine (Pepcid), gentamicin, heparin, magnesium sulfate, metoclopramide (Reglan), midazolam (Versed), milrinone (Primacor), morphine, nitroglycerin, potassium chloride, propofol (Diprivan), vancomycin (Vancocin)

SIDE EFFECTS
Occasional
Local redness, swelling, itching, caused by improper injection technique or allergy to cleansing solution or insulin
Infrequent
Somogyi effect, including rebound hyperglycemia with chronically

excessive insulin doses. Systemic allergic reaction, marked by rash, angioedema, and anaphylaxis, lipodystrophy or depression at injection site due to breakdown of adipose tissue, lipohypertrophy or accumulation of subcutaneous tissue at injection site due to lack of adequate site rotation

Rare
Insulin resistance

SERIOUS REACTIONS

• Severe hypoglycemia caused by hyperinsulinism may occur in overdose of insulin, decrease or delay of food intake, excessive exercise, or those with brittle diabetes.

• Diabetic ketoacidosis may result from stress, illness, omission of insulin dose, or long-term poor insulin control.

NURSING CONSIDERATIONS

Baseline Assessment

• Check the patient's blood glucose level.

• Discuss the patient's lifestyle to determine the extent of his or her emotional and learning needs.

Lifespan Considerations

• Be aware that insulin is the drug of choice for treating diabetes mellitus during pregnancy but close medical supervision is needed. Following delivery, the patient's insulin needs may drop for 24 to 72 hours, then rise to pre-pregnancy levels.

• Be aware that insulin is not secreted in breast milk and that lactation may decrease insulin requirements.

• Be aware that there are no age-related precautions noted in children.

• Be aware that in the elderly decreased vision and shakiness may lead to inaccurate dosage administration.

Administration and Handling

◄ **ALERT** ► Know that insulin dosages are individualized and monitored. Adjust dosage, as prescribed, to achieve premeal and bedtime glucose level of 80 to140 mg/dl in adults, and 100 to 200 mg/dl in children younger than 5 yrs.

Subcutaneous

• Store currently used insulin at room temperature, avoiding extreme temperatures and direct sunlight. Store extra vials in refrigerator.

• Discard unused vials if not used for several weeks. No insulin should have precipitate or discoloration.

• Give subcutaneous only. Regular insulin is the only insulin that may be given IV or IM for ketoacidosis or other specific situations.

• Warm the drug to room temperature—do not give cold insulin.

• Roll the drug vial gently between hands; do not shake. Regular insulin normally appears clear. No insulin should have precipitate or discoloration.

• Administer insulin approximately 30 minutes before a meal. Insulin Lispro may be given up to 15 minutes before meals. Check the patient's blood glucose concentration before administration. Insulin dosages are highly individualized.

• Always draw regular insulin first when insulin is mixed. Mixtures must be administered at once because binding can occur within 5 minutes. Humalog may be mixed with Humulin N and Humulin L.

• Give subcutaneous injections in the abdomen, buttocks, thigh, upper arm, or upper back if there is adequate adipose tissue.

• Maintain a careful record of rotated injection sites.

• For home situations, prefilled syringes are stable for 1 week under refrigeration, including stabilized mixtures, 15 minutes for NPH/Regular and 24 hours for Lente/Regular. Prefilled syringes should be stored in vertical or oblique position to avoid plugging; plunger should be pulled back slightly and the syringe rocked to remix the solution before injection.

IV (Regular)

• Use only if solution is clear.

• May give undiluted.

Intervention and Evaluation

• Monitor the sleeping patient for diaphoresis and restlessness.

• Assess the patient for hypoglycemia, such as anxiety, cool, wet skin, diplopia, dizziness, headache, hunger, numbness in mouth, tachycardia, and tremors, or hyperglycemia, including deep, rapid breathing, dim vision, fatigue, nausea, polydipsia, polyphagia, polyuria, and vomiting.

• Be alert to conditions that alter blood glucose requirements, such as fever, increased activity, stress, or a surgical procedure.

Patient Teaching

• Make sure that the patient adept at drawing up the prescribed dose of insulin, as well as the proper injection technique. Also ensure that he or she can perform self blood glucose testing at the prescribed intervals.

• Stress to the patient that the exercise, hygiene, including foot care, the prescribed diet, and weight control are integral parts of treatment. Warn the patient to avoid smoking and not to skip or delay meals.

• Ensure that the patient knows the signs and symptoms of hypo- and hyperglycemia. Tell the patient to carry candy, sugar packets, or other sugar supplements for immediate response to hypoglycemia.

• Urge the patient to wear medical alert identification.

• Instruct the patient to notify the physician when his or her glucose demands are altered, such as fever, heavy physical activity, infection, stress, and trauma.

• Tell the patient to inform his or her dentist, other physicians, or surgeons of insulin therapy before any treatment is given.

metformin hydrochloride

met-**for**-min

(Diabex[AUS], Diaformin[AUS], Glucohexal[AUS], Glucomet[AUS], Glucophage, Glucophage XL, Glycon[CAN], Novo-Metformin[CAN], Riomet)

CATEGORY AND SCHEDULE

Pregnancy Risk Category: B

MECHANISM OF ACTION

An antihyperglycemic that decreases liver production of glucose, decreases absorption of glucose, improves insulin sensitivity. *Therapeutic Effect:* Provides improvement in glycemic control, stabilizes or decreases body weight, improves lipid profile.

PHARMACOKINETICS

Slowly, incompletely absorbed after PO administration, food delays or decreases extent of absorption. Protein binding: Negligible. Primarily distributed to intestinal mucosa, salivary glands. Primarily excreted unchanged in urine. Removed by hemodialysis. **Half-life:** 3–6 hrs.

AVAILABILITY
Tablets: 500 mg, 850 mg, 1,000 mg.
Tablets (extended-release): 500 mg, 750 mg.
Oral Solution: 100 mg/ml.

INDICATIONS AND DOSAGES
▸ **Diabetes mellitus (500-mg, 1,000-mg tablet)**
PO
Adults, Elderly. Initially, 500 mg twice a day, with morning and evening meals. May increase dosage in 500-mg increments every week, in divided doses. Can be given twice a day up to 2,000 mg/day, for example, 1,000 mg twice a day with morning and evening meals. If 2,500 mg/day dose is required, give 3 times/day with meals. Maximum dose/day: 2,500 mg/day.
Children 10–16 yrs. Initially, 500 mg 2 times/day. May increase by 500 mg/day at weekly intervals. Maximum: 2,000 mg/day.
▸ **Diabetes mellitus (850-mg tablet)**
PO
Adults, Elderly. Initially, 850-mg/day, with morning meal. May increase dosage in 850-mg increments every other week, in divided doses. Maintenance: 850 mg twice a day, with morning and evening meals. Maximum dose/day: 2,550 mg (850 mg 3 times/day).
▸ **Diabetes mellitus (extended-release tablets)**
PO
Adults, Elderly. Initially, 500 mg once a day. May increase by 500 mg/day at weekly intervals. Maximum: 2,000 mg/day once a day.

▸ **Adjunct to insulin therapy**
PO
Adults, Elderly. Initially, 500 mg/day. May increase by 500 mg at 7-day intervals. Maximum: 2,500 mg (2,000 mg for extended release).

UNLABELED USES
Treatment of metabolic complications of AIDS, prediabetes, weight reduction

CONTRAINDICATIONS
Acute myocardial infarction (MI), acute congestive heart failure (CHF), cardiovascular collapse, renal disease or dysfunction, respiratory failure, septicemia

INTERACTIONS
Drug
Alcohol, amiloride, cimetidine, digoxin, furosemide, morphine, nifedipine, procainamide, quinidine, quinine, ranitidine, triamterene, trimethoprim, vancomycin: Increase metformin blood concentration.
Furosemide, hypoglycemia-causing medications: May decrease the dosage of metformin needed.
Iodinated contrast studies: May produce acute renal failure, increases risk of lactic acidosis.
Herbal
None known.
Food
None known.

DIAGNOSTIC TEST EFFECTS
None known.

SIDE EFFECTS
Occasional (greater than 3%)
Gastrointestinal (GI) disturbances are transient and resolve spontaneously during therapy, including diarrhea, nausea, vomiting, abdomi-

nal bloating, flatulence, and anorexia
Rare (3%–1%)
Unpleasant or metallic taste that resolves spontaneously during therapy

SERIOUS REACTIONS
• Lactic acidosis occurs rarely (0.03 cases/1,000 patients) but is a serious, often fatal (50%) complication. Lactic acidosis is characterized by an increase in blood lactate levels (greater than 5 mmol/L), a decrease in blood pH, and electrolyte disturbances. Symptoms include unexplained hyperventilation, myalgia, malaise, and somnolence. May advance to cardiovascular collapse (shock), acute CHF, acute MI, and prerenal azotemia.

NURSING CONSIDERATIONS
Baseline Assessment
• Inform the patient of the potential advantages and risks of metformin therapy and of alternative modes of therapy.
• Assess the patient's blood Hgb and Hct, red blood cell (RBC) count, and serum creatinine levels before beginning metformin therapy and annually thereafter.
Lifespan Considerations
• Be aware that insulin is the drug of choice during pregnancy.
• Be aware that metformin is distributed in breast milk in animals.
• Be aware that the safety and efficacy of metformin have not been established in children.
• In the elderly, age-related renal impairment or peripheral vascular disease may require dosage adjustment or discontinuation.
Precautions
• Use cautiously in patients with conditions that cause hyperglycemia

or hypoglycemia or delay food absorption, such as diarrhea, high fever, malnutrition, gastroparesis, and vomiting.
• Use cautiously in cardiovascular patients, in debilitated, elderly, liver-impaired, or malnourished patients with renal impairment, and in patients concurrently taking drugs that affect renal function.
• Use cautiously in patients with CHF, chronic respiratory difficulty, and uncontrolled hyperthyroidism or hypothyroidism.
• Use cautiously in patients who consume excessive amounts of alcohol.
Administration and Handling
◀ALERT▶ Plan to decrease the insulin dosage if blood glucose levels falls below 120 mg/dl.
◀ALERT▶ Be aware that lactic acidosis, is a rare but potentially severe consequence of metformin therapy. Withhold metformin in patients with conditions that may predispose to lactic acidosis, such as dehydration, hypoperfusion, hypoxemia, and sepsis.
PO
• Do not crush film-coated tablets.
• Give metformin with meals.
Intervention and Evaluation
• Monitor the patient's fasting blood glucose, Hgb A, folic acid, and renal function.
• Assess the patient concurrently taking oral sulfonylureas for signs and symptoms of hypoglycemia, including anxiety, cool, wet skin, diplopia, dizziness, headache, hunger, numbness in mouth, tachycardia, and tremors.
• Be alert to conditions that alter blood glucose requirements, such as fever, increased activity, stress, or a surgical procedure.
Patient Teaching
• Warn the patient to notify the

physician and discontinue metformin therapy, as prescribed, if he or she experiences signs or symptoms of lactic acidosis, such as extreme tiredness, muscle aches, unexplained hyperventilation, and unusual sleepiness.
• Stress to the patient that the prescribed diet is a principal part of treatment. Warn the patient not to skip or delay meals.
• Tell the patient that diabetes mellitus requires lifelong control.
• Urge the patient to avoid consuming alcohol.
• Instruct the patient to notify the physician if he or she experiences diarrhea, easy bleeding or bruising, change in color of stool or urine, headache, nausea, persistent skin rash, and vomiting.

miglitol
mig-lih-toll
(Glyset)

CATEGORY AND SCHEDULE
Pregnancy Risk Category: B

MECHANISM OF ACTION
An alpha-glucosidase inhibitor that delays the digestion of ingested carbohydrates into simple sugars such as glucose. *Therapeutic Effect:* Produces smaller rise in blood glucose concentration after meals.

AVAILABILITY
Tablets: 25 mg, 50 mg, 100 mg.

INDICATIONS AND DOSAGES
▸ **Diabetes mellitus**
PO
Adults, Elderly. Initially, 25 mg 3 times/day with first bite of each main meal. Maintenance: 50 mg

3 times/day. Maximum: 100 mg 3 times/day.

CONTRAINDICATIONS
Colonic ulceration, diabetic ketoacidosis, hypersensitivity to miglitol, inflammatory bowel disease, partial intestinal obstruction

INTERACTIONS
Drug
Digoxin, propranolol, ranitidine: May decrease the blood concentrations and effects of digoxin, propranolol, and ranitidine.
Herbal
None known.
Food
None known.

DIAGNOSTIC TEST EFFECTS
None known.

SIDE EFFECTS
Frequent (40%–10%)
Flatulence, soft stools, diarrhea, abdominal pain
Occasional (5%)
Rash

NURSING CONSIDERATIONS
Baseline Assessment
• Check the patient's blood glucose levels, as ordered.
• Discuss the patient's lifestyle to determine the extent of his or her emotional and learning needs.
• Establish the patient's use of medications, especially digoxin, propranolol, ranitidine.
Precautions
• Use cautiously in patients with renal function impairment.
Intervention and Evaluation
• Monitor the patient's blood glucose and food intake.
• Assess the patient for signs and symptoms of hypoglycemia, such as

anxiety, cool, wet skin, diplopia, dizziness, headache, hunger, numbness in mouth, tachycardia, and tremors, or hyperglycemia, including deep, rapid breathing, dim vision, fatigue, nausea, polydipsia, polyphagia, polyuria, and vomiting.

• Be alert to conditions that alter blood glucose requirements, such as fever, increased activity, stress or a surgical procedure.

Patient Teaching

• Make sure the patient knows to take the drug with the first bite of food with each meal because taking the drug later will greatly alter its effectiveness.

• Stress to the patient that the prescribed diet is a principal part of treatment. Warn the patient not to skip or delay meals.

• Urge the patient to wear medical alert identification.

• Instruct the patient to notify the physician when his or her glucose demands are altered, such as with fever, heavy physical activity, infection, stress, or trauma.

nateglinide
nah-**teg**-glih-nide
(Starlix)

CATEGORY AND SCHEDULE
Pregnancy Risk Category: C

MECHANISM OF ACTION
An antihyperglycemic that stimulates release of insulin from beta cells of the pancreas by depolarizing beta cells, leading to an opening of calcium channels. Resulting calcium influx induces insulin secretion. *Therapeutic Effect*: Lowers glucose concentration.

AVAILABILITY
Tablets: 60 mg, 120 mg.

INDICATIONS AND DOSAGES
▶ **Diabetes mellitus**
PO
Adult, Elderly. 120 mg 3 times/day before meals. Initially, 60 mg may be given.

CONTRAINDICATIONS
Diabetic ketoacidosis, type 1 diabetes mellitus

INTERACTIONS
Drug
Beta-blockers, MAOIs, NSAIDs, salicylates: May increase hypoglycemic effect.
Corticosteroids, thiazide diuretics, thyroid medication, sympathomimetics: May decrease hypoglycemic effect.
Herbal
None known.
Food
Liquid meal: Peak plasma levels may be significantly reduced if administered 10 min before a liquid meal.

DIAGNOSTIC TEST EFFECTS
None known.

SIDE EFFECTS
Frequent (10%)
Upper respiratory tract infection
Occasional (4%–3%)
Back pain, flu symptoms, dizziness, arthropathy, diarrhea
Rare (2% or less)
Bronchitis, cough

SERIOUS REACTIONS
• Hypoglycemia occurs in less than 2% of patients.

NURSING CONSIDERATIONS

Baseline Assessment
• Check the patient's fasting blood glucose level and glycosylated Hgb (HbA$_{1C}$) periodically to determine minimum effective dose.
• Discuss the patient's lifestyle to determine the extent of his or her emotional and learning needs.
• Know that at least 1 week should elapse to assess the patient's response to the drug before new dose adjustment is made.

Precautions
• Use cautiously in patients with liver or renal function impairment.

Administration and Handling
PO
• Ideally, give within 15 minutes of a meal, but may be given immediately before a meal to as long as 30 minutes before a meal.

Intervention and Evaluation
• Monitor the patient's blood glucose and food intake.
• Assess the patient for signs and symptoms of hypoglycemia, such as anxiety, cool, wet skin, diplopia, dizziness, headache, hunger, numbness in mouth, tachycardia, and tremors, or hyperglycemia, including deep, rapid breathing, dim vision, fatigue, nausea, polydipsia, polyphagia, polyuria, and vomiting.
• Be alert to conditions that alter blood glucose requirements, such as fever, increased activity, stress, or a surgical procedure.

Patient Teaching
• Stress to the patient that the prescribed diet is a principal part of treatment. Warn the patient not to skip or delay meals.
• Make sure the patient is aware of the typical signs and symptoms of hypoglycemia and hyperglycemia.
• Instruct the patient to carry candy, sugar packets, or other sugar supplements for immediate response to hypoglycemia.
• Urge the patient to wear medical alert identification.
• Instruct the patient to notify the physician when his or her glucose demands are altered, such as with fever, heavy physical activity, infection, stress, or trauma.
• Ensure follow-up instruction if the patient or family does not thoroughly understand diabetes management or blood glucose-testing technique.

pioglitazone
pie-oh-**glit**-ah-zone
(Actos)

CATEGORY AND SCHEDULE
Pregnancy Risk Category: C

MECHANISM OF ACTION
An antidiabetic that improves target-cell response to insulin without increasing pancreatic insulin secretion. Decreases hepatic glucose output, increases insulin-dependent glucose utilization in skeletal muscle. *Therapeutic Effect:* Lowers blood glucose concentration.

PHARMACOKINETICS
Rapidly absorbed. Highly protein bound (greater than 99%), primarily to albumin. Metabolized in liver. Excreted in urine. Unknown if removed by hemodialysis. **Half-life:** 16–24 hrs.

AVAILABILITY
Tablets: 15 mg, 30 mg, 45 mg.

INDICATIONS AND DOSAGES
▶ **Diabetes mellitus, combination therapy**
PO
Adult, Elderly. Insulin: Initially, 15–30 mg once a day. Initially, continue current insulin dose, then decrease insulin dose by 10% to 25% if hypoglycemia or plasma glucose levels decrease to less than 100 mg/dl. Maximum: 45 mg/day. Sulfonylureas: Initially, 15–30 mg/day. Decrease sulfonylurea if hypoglycemia occurs. Metformin: Initially, 15–30 mg/day. Monotherapy: Monotherapy is not to be used if patient is well controlled with diet and exercise alone. Initially, 15–30 mg/day. May increase dosage in increments up to 45 mg/day.

CONTRAINDICATIONS
Active liver disease, diabetic keto-acidosis, increased serum transaminase levels, including SGPT (ALT) greater than 2.5 times normal serum level, type 1 diabetes mellitus

INTERACTIONS
Drug
Ketoconazole: May significantly inhibit metabolism of pioglitazone. *Oral contraceptives:* May alter the effects of oral contraceptives.
Food
None known.
Herbal
None known.

DIAGNOSTIC TEST EFFECTS
May decrease blood Hgb levels by 2%–4%, serum alkaline phosphatase, bilirubin, and SGOT (ALT) levels. Less than 1% of patients experience SGPT (ALT) values that are 3 times normal level. May increase creatine phosphokinase (CPK) levels.

SIDE EFFECTS
Frequent (13%–9%)
Headache, upper respiratory tract infection
Occasional (6%–5%)
Sinusitis, myalgia (muscle aches), pharyngitis, aggravated diabetes mellitus

SERIOUS REACTIONS
• None known.

NURSING CONSIDERATIONS
Baseline Assessment
• Check the patient's hepatic enzyme levels, as ordered, before beginning pioglitazone therapy and periodically thereafter.
Lifespan Considerations
• Be aware that it is unknown if pioglitazone crosses the placenta or is distributed in breast milk, and that pioglitazone use is not recommended in pregnant or breast-feeding women.
• Be aware that the safety and efficacy of pioglitazone have not been established in children.
• There are no age-related precautions noted in the elderly.
Precautions
• Use cautiously in patients with congestive heart failure (CHF), edema, and liver function impairment.
Administration and Handling
PO
• Give pioglitazone without regard to meals.
Intervention and Evaluation
• Monitor the patient's blood glucose levels, Hgb, and liver function tests, especially SGOT (AST) and SGPT (ALT) levels.
• Assess the patient for signs and symptoms of hypoglycemia, such as anxiety, cool, wet skin, diplopia, dizziness, headache, hunger, numb-

ness in mouth, tachycardia, and tremors, or hyperglycemia, including deep, rapid breathing, dim vision, fatigue, nausea, polydipsia, polyphagia, polyuria, and vomiting.
• Be alert to conditions that alter blood glucose requirements, such as fever, increased activity, stress, or a surgical procedure.

Patient Teaching
• Ensure follow-up instruction if the patient or family does not thoroughly understand diabetes management or blood glucose-testing technique.
• Stress to the patient that the prescribed diet is a principal part of treatment. Warn the patient not to skip or delay meals.
• Make sure the patient is aware of the typical signs and symptoms of hypoglycemia and hyperglycemia.
• Instruct the patient to carry candy, sugar packets, or other sugar supplements for immediate response to hypoglycemia.
• Urge the patient to avoid consuming alcohol.
• Warn the patient to notify the physician if he or she experiences abdominal or chest pain, dark urine or light stool, hypoglycemic reactions, fever, nausea, palpitations, rash, vomiting, or yellowing of the eyes or skin.

repaglinide
reh-**pah**-glih-nide
(Novonorm[AUS], Prandin)

CATEGORY AND SCHEDULE
Pregnancy Risk Category: C

MECHANISM OF ACTION
An antihyperglycemic that stimulates release of insulin from beta cells of the pancreas by depolarizing beta cells, leading to an opening of calcium channels. Resulting calcium influx induces insulin secretion. *Therapeutic Effect:* Lowers glucose concentration.

PHARMACOKINETICS
Rapidly, completely absorbed from the gastrointestinal (GI) tract. Protein binding: 98%. Metabolized in liver to inactive metabolites. Excreted primarily in feces with a lesser amount in urine. Unknown if removed by hemodialysis. **Half-life:** 1 hr.

AVAILABILITY
Tablets: 0.5 mg, 1 mg, 2 mg.

INDICATIONS AND DOSAGES
▸ **Diabetes mellitus**
PO
Adults, Elderly. 0.5–4 mg 2–4 times/day. Maximum: 16 mg/day.

CONTRAINDICATIONS
Diabetic ketoacidosis, type 1 diabetes mellitus

INTERACTIONS
Drug
Beta-blockers, chloramphenicol, gemfibrozil, MAOIs, NSAIDs, probenecid, salicylates, sulfonamides, warfarin: May increase the effects of repaglinide.
Herbal
None known.
Food
Food: Decreases repaglinide plasma concentration.

DIAGNOSTIC TEST EFFECTS
None known.

SIDE EFFECTS
Frequent (10%–6%)
Upper respiratory infection, head-

ache, rhinitis, bronchitis, back pain
Occasional (5%–3%)
Diarrhea, dyspepsia, sinusitis,
nausea, arthralgia, urinary tract
infection
Rare (2%)
Constipation, vomiting, paresthesia,
allergy

SERIOUS REACTIONS
• Hypoglycemia occurs in 16% of
patients.
• Chest pain occurs rarely.

NURSING CONSIDERATIONS

Baseline Assessment
• Check the patient's fasting blood
glucose and glycosylated Hgb
(HbA$_1$C) periodically to determine
the minimum effective dose of
repaglinide.
• Allow at least 1 week to elapse to
assess the patient's response to drug
before new dosage adjustment is
made.
Lifespan Considerations
• Be aware that it is unknown if
repaglinide is distributed in breast
milk.
• Be aware that the safety and
efficacy of repaglinide have not
been established in children.
• There are no age-related precautions noted in the elderly, but hypoglycemia may be more difficult to
recognize in this patient population.
Precautions
• Use cautiously in patients with
liver or renal function impairment.
Administration and Handling
PO
• Ideally, give repaglinide within
15 minutes of a meal but may be
given immediately before a meal to
as long as 30 minutes before a
meal.

Intervention and Evaluation
• Monitor the patient's blood glucose and food intake.
• Assess the patient for signs and
symptoms of hypoglycemia, such as
anxiety, cool, wet skin, diplopia,
dizziness, headache, hunger, numbness in mouth, tachycardia, and
tremors, or hyperglycemia, including deep, rapid breathing, dim
vision, fatigue, nausea, polydipsia,
polyphagia, polyuria, and vomiting.
• Be alert to conditions that alter
blood glucose requirements, such as
fever, increased activity, stress, or a
surgical procedure.
Patient Teaching
• Stress to the patient that the
prescribed diet is a principal part of
treatment. Warn the patient not to
skip or delay meals.
• Make sure the patient is aware of
the typical signs and symptoms of
hypoglycemia and hyperglycemia.
• Urge the patient to wear medical
alert identification.
• Instruct the patient to notify the
physician when his or her glucose
demands are altered, such as with
fever, heavy physical activity, infection, stress, or trauma.
• Explain to the patient that diabetes
mellitus requires lifelong control.
Urge the patient to continue to
adhere to dietary instructions, a
regular exercise program, and regular testing of urine or blood glucose.
• Tell the patient taking combination drug therapy with insulin or
sulfonylurea to always have a
source of glucose available to treat
symptoms of low blood sugar.

rosiglitazone maleate
rose-ih-**glit**-ah-zone
(Avandia)

CATEGORY AND SCHEDULE
Pregnancy Risk Category: C

MECHANISM OF ACTION
An antidiabetic that improves target-cell response to insulin without increasing pancreatic insulin secretion. Decreases hepatic glucose output, increases insulin-dependent glucose utilization in skeletal muscle. *Therapeutic Effect:* Lowers blood glucose concentration.

PHARMACOKINETICS
Rapidly absorbed. Protein binding: greater than 99%. Metabolized in liver. Excreted primarily in urine with a lesser amount in feces. Not removed by hemodialysis. **Half-life:** 3–4 hrs.

AVAILABILITY
Tablets: 2 mg, 4 mg, 8 mg.

INDICATIONS AND DOSAGES
▶ **Diabetes mellitus, combination therapy**
PO
Adults, Elderly. Initially, 4 mg as a single daily dose or in divided doses twice a day. May increase to 8 mg/day after 12 wks of therapy if fasting glucose is not adequately controlled.
▶ **Diabetes mellitus, monotherapy**
Adults, Elderly. Initially, 4 mg as single daily dose or in divided doses twice a day. May increase to 8 mg/day after 12 wks of therapy.

CONTRAINDICATIONS
Active liver disease, diabetic ketoacidosis, increased serum transaminase levels, including SGPT (ALT) greater than 2.5 times the normal serum level, type 1 diabetes mellitus

INTERACTIONS
Drug
None known.
Herbal
None known.
Food
None known.

DIAGNOSTIC TEST EFFECTS
May decrease blood Hct and Hgb, serum alkaline phosphatase, bilirubin, and SGOT (AST) levels. Less than 1% of patients experience SGPT (ALT) values that are 3 times normal level.

SIDE EFFECTS
Frequent (9%)
Upper respiratory tract infection
Occasional (4%–2%)
Headache, edema, back pain, fatigue, sinusitis, diarrhea

SERIOUS REACTIONS
• None known.

NURSING CONSIDERATIONS
Baseline Assessment
• Plan to obtain the patient's hepatic enzyme levels before beginning rosiglitazone therapy and periodically thereafter.
Lifespan Considerations
• Be aware that it is unknown if rosiglitazone crosses the placenta or is distributed in breast milk and that rosiglitazone use is not recommended in pregnant or breast-feeding women.
• Be aware that the safety and efficacy of rosiglitazone have not been established in children.

• There are no age-related precautions noted in the elderly.

Precautions

• Use cautiously in patients with congestive heart failure (CHF), edema, and liver function impairment.

Administration and Handling

PO

• Give rosiglitazone without regard to meals.

Intervention and Evaluation

• Monitor the patient's blood glucose levels, Hgb, and liver function tests, especially SGOT (AST) and SGPT (ALT) levels.

• Assess the patient for signs and symptoms of hypoglycemia, such as anxiety, cool, wet skin, diplopia, dizziness, headache, hunger, numbness in mouth, tachycardia, and tremors, or hyperglycemia, including deep, rapid breathing, dim vision, fatigue, nausea, polydipsia, polyphagia, polyuria, and vomiting.

• Be alert to conditions that alter blood glucose requirements, such as fever, increased activity, stress, or a surgical procedure.

Patient Teaching

• Ensure follow-up instruction if the patient or family does not thoroughly understand diabetes management or blood glucose-testing technique.

• Stress to the patient that the prescribed diet is a principal part of treatment. Warn the patient not to skip or delay meals.

• Make sure the patient is aware of the typical signs and symptoms of hypoglycemia and hyperglycemia.

• Instruct the patient to carry candy, sugar packets, or other sugar supplements for immediate response to hypoglycemia.

• Urge the patient to avoid consuming alcohol.

• Warn the patient to notify the physician if he or she experiences abdominal or chest pain, dark urine or light stool, hypoglycemic reactions, fever, nausea, palpitations, rash, vomiting, and yellowing of the eyes or skin.

• Urge the patient to wear medical alert identification.

• Instruct the patient taking combination drug therapy with insulin or sulfonylurea to always have a source of glucose available to treat symptoms of low blood sugar.

64 Antigout Agents

allopurinol
colchicine
probenecid

Uses: Antigout agents play different roles in the treatment of gout. *Allopurinol and probenecid* are used to reduce hyperuricemia, which helps prevent acute gout attacks. *Colchicine* is used to treat acute gout attacks, reduce the incidence of attacks in chronic gout, and abort an impending gout attack. In addition, probenecid may be given with penicillins or cephalosporins to increase and prolong the plasma antibiotic levels.

Action: Antigout agents act in slightly different ways. *Allopurinol* reduces hyperuricemia by inhibiting uric acid formation. *Colchicine* provides an anti-inflammatory action specific to gout. *Probenecid* reduces hyperuricemia by promoting uric acid excretion. (See illustration, *Mechanism of Action: Antigout Agents,* page 1119.)

allopurinol
al-low-**pure**-ih-nawl
(Aloprim, Allohexal[AUS],Apo-Allopurinol[CAN], Capurate[AUS], Progout[AUS] Purinol[CAN], Zyloprim)

CATEGORY AND SCHEDULE
Pregnancy Risk Category: C

MECHANISM OF ACTION
A xanthine oxidase inhibitor that decreases uric acid production by inhibiting xanthine oxidase, an enzyme. *Therapeutic Effect:* Reduces uric acid concentrations in both serum and urine.

PHARMACOKINETICS

Route	Onset	Peak	Duration
PO/IV	2–3 days	1–3 weeks	1–2 weeks

Well absorbed from GI tract. Widely distributed. Metabolized in liver to active metabolite. Excreted primarily in urine. Removed by hemodialysis. **Half-life:** 1–3 hrs; metabolite: 12–30 hours.

AVAILABILITY
Tablets: 100 mg, 300 mg.
Powder for Injection: 500 mg.

INDICATIONS AND DOSAGES
▶ **Chronic gouty arthritis**
PO
Adults, Children older than 10 yrs.
Initially, 100 mg/day; may increase by 100 mg/day at weekly intervals.
Maximum: 800 mg/day.
Maintenance: 100–200 mg
2–3 times/day or 300 mg/day.
▶ **To prevent uric acid nephropathy during cancer chemotherapy**
PO
Adults: Initially, 600–800 mg/day starting 2–3 days prior to initiation of chemotherapy or radiation therapy.
Children 6–10 yrs. 100 mg 3 times/day or 300 mg once a day.

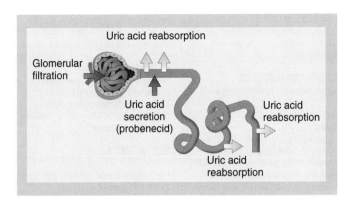

Uric acid reabsorption

Glomerular filtration

Uric acid secretion (probenecid)

Uric acid reabsorption

Uric acid reabsorption

Several drugs are used to manage gout, a disorder of purine metabolism that increases uric acid production or decreases its renal excretion. The result is hyperuricemia (an increased serum uric acid level). When the balance between uric acid formation and excretion is disturbed, uric acid precipitates and forms urate crystals. Then leukocytes and other inflammatory cells move to the area, producing inflammation that can cause gout attacks.

Three drugs are commonly used to manage gout: allopurinol, probenecid, and colchicine. Allopurinol and probenecid help prevent gout attacks by decreasing the uric acid level. Allopurinol interferes with uric acid production by binding to and inhibiting xanthine oxidase, an enzyme that converts adenine and guanine to uric acid. This action leads to decreased uric acid levels in blood and urine. Probenecid competitively inhibits uric acid reabsorption in the proximal tubules of the nephrons, as illustrated here. This action increases uric acid excretion.

Unlike the other antigout agents, colchicine doesn't influence uric acid synthesis or reabsorption. Instead, it acts as an anti-inflammatory agent to treat a gout attack. It does this by inhibiting the action of leukocytes on urate crystals and diminishing inflammation.

Children less than 6 yrs. 50 mg 3 times/day.

IV
Adults. 200–400 mg/m²/day beginning 24–48 hrs prior to initiation of chemotherapy.
Children. 200 mg/m²/day.
Maximum: 600 mg/day.
▸ **Prevention of uric acid calculi**
PO
Adults. 100–200 mg 1–4 times/day or 300 mg once a day.

▸ **Recurrent calcium oxalate calculi**
PO
Adults. 200–300 mg/day.
Elderly. Initially, 100 mg/day, gradually increased to optimal uric acid level.
▸ **Dosage in renal impairment**

Creatinine Clearance	Dosage Adjustment
Greater than 50 ml/min	No change
10–50 ml/min	50%
Less than 10 ml/min	30%

UNLABELED USES
Used in mouthwash following fluorouracil therapy to prevent stomatitis

CONTRAINDICATIONS
Asymptomatic hyperuricemia

INTERACTIONS
Drug
Amoxicillin, ampicillin: May increase incidence of skin rash.
Azathioprine, mercaptopurine: May increase therapeutic effect and toxicity of azathioprine and mercaptopurine.
Oral anticoagulants: May increase anticoagulant effect.
Thiazide diuretics: May decrease the effect of allopurinol.
Herbal
None known.
Food
None known.

DIAGNOSTIC TEST EFFECTS
May increase BUN, serum creatinine levels, serum alkaline phosphatase, SGOT (AST), and SGPT (ALT).

IV INCOMPATIBILITIES
Amikacin (Amikin), carmustine (BiCNU), cefotaxime (Claforan), chlorpromazine (Thorazine), cimetidine (Tagamet), clindamycin (Cleocin), cytarabine (Ara-C), dacarbazine (DTIC), diphenhydramine (Benadryl), doxorubicin (Adriamycin), doxycycline (Vibramycin), droperidol (Inapsine), fludarabine (Fludara), gentamicin (Garamycin), haloperidol (Haldol), hydroxyzine (Vistaril), idarubicin (Idamycin), imipenem-cilastatin (Primaxin), meperidine (Demerol), methylprednisolone (Solu-Medrol), metoclopramide (Reglan), ondansetron (Zofran), prochlorperazine (Compazine), promethazine (Phenergan), streptozocin (Zanosar), tobramycin (Nebcin), vinorelbine (Navelbine)

IV COMPATIBILITIES
Bumetanide (Bumex), calcium gluconate, furosemide (Lasix), heparin, hydromorphone (Dilaudid), lorazepam (Ativan), morphine, potassium chloride

SIDE EFFECTS
Occasional
Oral: Drowsiness, unusual hair loss
IV: Rash, nausea, vomiting
Rare
Diarrhea, headache

SERIOUS REACTIONS
• Pruritic maculopapular rash should be considered a toxic reaction.
• May be accompanied by malaise, fever, chills, joint pain, nausea, and vomiting.
• Severe hypersensitivity may follow appearance of rash.
• Bone marrow depression, liver toxicity, peripheral neuritis or acute renal failure occur rarely.

NURSING CONSIDERATIONS
Baseline Assessment
• Ensure that patient drinks 10 to 12 glasses (eight ounces) of fluid daily while taking this medication.
Lifespan Considerations
• Be aware that it is unknown if drug crosses placenta or is distributed in breast milk.
• There are no age-related precautions noted in children or the elderly.
Precautions
• Use cautiously in patients with congestive heart failure (CHF), diabetes mellitus, hypertension, or impaired renal or liver function.

Administration and Handling
PO
• May give with or immediately after meals or milk.
• Be sure that the patient drinks at least 10 to 12 eight-ounce glasses of water a day.
• Administer dosages greater than 300 mg/day in divided doses.
IV
• Store unreconstituted vials at room temperature.
• May store reconstituted solution at room temperature and give within 10 hours. Do not use if precipitate forms or solution is discolored.
• Reconstitute 500-mg vial with 25 ml sterile water for injection, giving a clear, almost colorless solution (concentration of 20 mg/ml).
• Further dilute with 0.9% NaCl or D_5W (19 ml of added diluent yields 1 mg/ml, 9 ml yields 2 mg/ml, 2.3 ml yields maximum concentration of 6 mg/ml).
• Infuse over 30 to 60 minutes.

Intervention and Evaluation
• Discontinue medication immediately if rash or other evidence of allergic reaction appears.
• Encourage high fluid intake (3,000 ml/day). Monitor the patient's intake and output. The patient's output should be at least 2,000 ml/day.
• Assess the patient's complete blood count (CBC), hepatic enzyme test results, and serum uric acid levels.
• Examine the patient's urine for cloudiness and unusual color and odor.
• Assess the patient for signs and symptoms of a therapeutic response, including reduced joint limitation of motion, redness, swelling, and tenderness.

Patient Teaching
• Inform the patient it may take 1 week or longer of administration of the drug for it to reach full therapeutic effect.
• Encourage the patient to drink 10 to 12 eight-ounce glasses of fluid daily while taking medication.
• Warn the patient to avoid tasks that require mental alertness or motor skills until his or her response to the drug is established.

colchicine
coal-cheh-seen
(Colchicine, Colgout[AUS])

CATEGORY AND SCHEDULE
Pregnancy Risk Category: D

MECHANISM OF ACTION
An alkaloid that decreases leukocyte motility, phagocytosis, lactic acid production. *Therapeutic Effect:* Results in decreased urate crystal deposits, inflammatory process.

PHARMACOKINETICS
Rapidly absorbed from the gastrointestinal (GI) tract. Highest concentration in liver, spleen, kidney. Protein binding: 30%–50%. Reenters intestinal tract by biliary secretion, reabsorbed from intestines. Partially metabolized in liver. Eliminated primarily in feces.

AVAILABILITY
Tablets: 0.5 mg, 0.6 mg.
Injection: 1 mg.

INDICATIONS AND DOSAGES
▸ **Acute gouty arthritis**
PO
Adults, Elderly. 0.5–1.2 mg, then 0.5–0.6 mg q1–2h or 1–1.2 mg q2h,

until pain relieved or nausea, vomiting, or diarrhea occurs. Total dose: 4–8 mg.

IV

Adults, Elderly. Initially, 2 mg, then 0.5 mg q6h until satisfactory response. Maximum: 4 mg/24 hrs or 4 mg/one course of treatment. If pain recurs, may give 1–2 mg/day for several days but no sooner than 7 days after a full course of IV therapy (4 mg).

▶ **Chronic gouty arthritis**

PO

Adults, Elderly. 0.5–0.6 mg once weekly up to once a day, dependent on number of attacks per year.

UNLABELED USES

Reduce frequency of familial Mediterranean fever; treatment of acute calcium pyrophosphate deposition, amyloidosis, biliary cirrhosis, recurrent pericarditis, sarcoid arthritis

CONTRAINDICATIONS

Blood dyscrasias, severe cardiac, gastrointestinal (GI), liver, or renal disorders

INTERACTIONS

Drug

Bone marrow depressants: May increase risk of blood dyscrasias. *NSAIDs:* May increase the risk of bone marrow depression, neutropenia, and thrombocytopenia.

Herbal

None known.

Food

None known.

DIAGNOSTIC TEST EFFECTS

May decrease platelet count. May increase serum alkaline phosphatase and SGOT (AST) levels.

IV INCOMPATIBILITIES

No information available via Y-site administration.

SIDE EFFECTS

Frequent

PO: Nausea, vomiting, abdominal discomfort

Occasional

PO: Anorexia

Rare

Hypersensitivity reaction, including angioedema

Parenteral: Nausea, vomiting, diarrhea, abdominal discomfort, pain or redness at injection site, neuritis in injected arm

SERIOUS REACTIONS

• Bone marrow depression, including aplastic anemia, agranulocytosis, and thrombocytopenia, may occur with long-term therapy.

• Overdose initially causes a burning feeling in the skin or throat, severe diarrhea, and abdominal pain. Then, the patient experiences fever, seizures, delirium, and renal impairment, marked by hematuria and oliguria. The third stage of overdose causes hair loss, leukocytosis, and stomatitis.

NURSING CONSIDERATIONS

Baseline Assessment

• Instruct the patient to drink 8 to 10 glasses (8 oz) of fluid a day while taking medication to help renal excretion of uric acid.

• Prepare to discontinue colchicine if gastrointestinal (GI) symptoms occur.

Lifespan Considerations

• Be aware that it is unknown if colchicine crosses the placenta or is distributed in breast milk.

• Be aware that the safety and efficacy of colchicine have not been established in children.

• Be aware that the elderly may be more susceptible to cumulative toxicity.

• In the elderly, age-related renal impairment may increase risk of myopathy.

Precautions

• Use cautiously in debilitated or elderly patients and in patients with impaired liver function.

Administration and Handling

◀ALERT▶ Those with impaired renal function may exhibit myopathy and neuropathy manifested as generalized weakness.

◀ALERT▶ Subcutaneous or IM administration produces severe local reaction. Use via IV route only.

PO

• Give colchicine without regard to meals.

IV

• Store at room temperature.

• May dilute with 0.9% NaCl or sterile water for injection; do not dilute with D₅W.

• Administer over 2 to 5 minutes.

Intervention and Evaluation

• Discontinue colchicine immediately when the patient experiences GI symptoms.

• Encourage the patient to maintain a high fluid intake (3,000 ml/day).

• Monitor the patient's fluid intake and output; output should be at least 2,000 ml/day.

• Assess the patient's serum uric acid levels.

• Assess the patient for therapeutic response, reduced joint tenderness, limitation of motion, redness, and swelling.

Patient Teaching

• Encourage the patient to limit his intake of high purine food, such as fish and organ meat, and to drink 8 to 10 glasses (8 oz) of fluid daily while taking this medication.

• Warn the patient to notify the

physician if he or she experiences a fever, numbness, skin rash, sore throat, tiredness, unusual bleeding or bruising, and weakness.

• Instruct the patient to discontinue the drug as soon as gout pain is relieved, or at first sign of diarrhea, nausea, or vomiting.

probenecid
pro-**ben**-ah-sid
(Benuryl[CAN], Pro-cid[AUS])
Do not confuse with procainamide.

CATEGORY AND SCHEDULE
Pregnancy Risk Category: C

MECHANISM OF ACTION
An uricosuric that competitively inhibits reabsorption of uric acid at proximal convoluted tubule. Inhibits renal tubular secretion of weak organic acids, such as penicillins. *Therapeutic Effect:* Promotes uric acid excretion, reduces serum uric acid levels, increases plasma levels of penicillins, cephalosporins.

AVAILABILITY
Tablets: 500 mg.

INDICATIONS AND DOSAGES
▶ **Gout**
PO
Adults, Elderly. Initially, 250 mg 2 times/day for 1 wk; then 500 mg 2 times/day. May increase by 500 mg q4wks. Maximum: 2–3 g/day. Maintenance: Dosage that maintains normal uric acid levels.
▶ **Penicillin or cephalosporin therapy**
PO
Adults, Elderly. 2 g/day in divided doses.

Children 2–14 yrs. Initially, 25 mg/kg. Maintenance: 40 mg/kg/day in 4 divided doses.
Children weighing more than 50 kg. Receive adult dosage.
▶ **Gonorrhea**
PO
Adults, Elderly. 1 g 30 min before penicillin, ampicillin, or amoxicillin.

CONTRAINDICATIONS

Blood dyscrasias, children younger than 2 yrs, concurrent high-dose aspirin therapy, severe renal impairment, uric acid kidney stones

INTERACTIONS
Drug

Antineoplastics: May increase the risk of uric acid nephropathy.
Cephalosporins, methotrexate, nitrofurantoin, NSAIDs, penicillins, zidovudine: May increase blood concentrations of cephalosporins, methotrexate, nitrofurantoin, NSAIDs, penicillins, and zidovudine.
Heparin: May increase and prolong the effects of heparin.
Salicylates: May decrease uricosuric effect.
Herbal
None known.
Food
None known.

DIAGNOSTIC TEST EFFECTS

May inhibit renal excretion of PSP (phenolsulfonphthalein), 17-ketosteroids, and BSP (sulfobromophthalein) tests.

SIDE EFFECTS

Frequent (10%–6%)
Headache, anorexia, nausea, vomiting
Occasional (5%–1%)
Lower back or side pain, rash, hives, itching, dizziness, flushed face, frequent urge to urinate, gingivitis

SERIOUS REACTIONS

• Severe hypersensitivity reactions, including anaphylaxis, occur rarely and usually within a few hours after readministration following previous use. If severe hypersensitivity reactions develop, discontinue the drug immediately and contact the physician.
• Pruritic maculopapular rash should be considered a toxic reaction and may be accompanied by malaise, fever, chills, joint pain, nausea, vomiting, leukopenia, and aplastic anemia.

NURSING CONSIDERATIONS
Baseline Assessment
• Do not initiate therapy until acute gouty attack has subsided.
• Determine if the patient is hypersensitive to probenecid or is taking cephalosporin or penicillin antibiotics.
Precautions
• Use cautiously in patients with hematuria, peptic ulcer, and renal colic.
Administration and Handling
◀**ALERT**▶ Do not start taking probenecid until acute gout attack subsides; continue if acute attack occurs during therapy.
◀**ALERT**▶ Do not use in presence of renal impairment.
PO
• Give probenecid with or immediately after meals or milk.
• Instruct the patient to drink at least 6 to 8 glasses (8 oz) of water each day to prevent renal stone development.
Intervention and Evaluation
• Use other agents for gout if the patient experiences an exacer-

bation of gout that recurs after therapy.
• Discontinue the medication immediately if the patient experiences rash or other evidence of an allergic reaction.
• Encourage the patient to maintain a high fluid intake (3,000 ml/day).
• Monitor the patient's intake and urine output, which should be at least 2,000 ml/day.
• Assess the patient's complete blood count (CBC) and serum uric acid levels.
• Evaluate the patient's urine for cloudiness, odor, and unusual color.
• Assess the patient for therapeutic response, reduced joint tenderness, limitation of motion, redness, and swelling.

Patient Teaching
• Tell the patient to drink plenty of fluids to decrease risk of uric acid renal stones.
• Urge the patient to avoid alcohol and large doses of aspirin or other salicylates.
• Tell the patient to avoid eating high-purine foods, such as anchovies, kidneys, liver, meat extracts, sardines, and sweetbreads.
• Explain to the patient that it may take 1 week or more for the full therapeutic effect of the drug to be evident.
• Instruct the patient to drink 6 to 8 glasses (8 oz) of fluid a day during probenecid therapy.

65 Bisphosphonates

alendronate sodium
etidronate disodium
ibandronate sodium
pamidronate disodium
risedronate sodium
tiludronate
zoledronic acid

Uses: Bisphosphonates are used to treat Paget's disease and hypercalcemia. Some of these agents can be used to prevent and treat postmenopausal and other forms of osteoporosis. Pamidronate can also be used to treat breast cancer and osteolytic bone lesions of multiple myeloma.

Action: Bisphosphonates primarily act on bone. Their major effect is inhibition of normal and abnormal bone resorption, which leads to increased bone mineral density and a decreased serum calcium level.

alendronate sodium
ah-**len**-drew-nate
(Fosamax)
Do not confuse with Flomax.

CATEGORY AND SCHEDULE
Pregnancy Risk Category: C

MECHANISM OF ACTION
A bisphosphonate that inhibits normal and abnormal bone resorption, without retarding mineralization. *Therapeutic Effect:* Leads to significant increased bone mineral density, reverses the progression of osteoporosis.

PHARMACOKINETICS
Poorly absorbed after PO administration. Protein binding: 78%. After PO administration, rapidly taken into bone, with uptake greatest at sites of active bone turnover. Excreted in urine. **Terminal half-life:** Greater than 10 yrs (reflects release from skeleton as bone is resorbed).

AVAILABILITY
Tablets: 5 mg, 10 mg, 35 mg, 40 mg, 70 mg.

INDICATIONS AND DOSAGES
▶ **Osteoporosis**
PO
Adults, Elderly. 10 mg/day, in the morning or 70 mg once/wk.
▶ **Paget's disease**
PO
Adults, Elderly. 40 mg/day, in the morning.
▶ **Glucocorticoid-induced osteoporosis**
PO
Adults, Elderly. 5 mg/day (10 mg/day in post-menopausal women not receiving estrogen).
▶ **Prevention of osteoporosis**
PO
Adults, Elderly. 5 mg/day, in the morning or 35 mg once/week.

UNLABELED USES
Treatment of breast cancer

CONTRAINDICATIONS
Gastrointestinal (GI) disease, including dysphagia, frequent heartburn, gastrointestinal reflux disorder (GERD), hiatal hernia, and ulcers, inability to stand or sit upright for at least 30 min, renal function impairment, sensitivity to alendronate

INTERACTIONS
Drug
Aspirin: May increase GI disturbances.
IV ranitidine: May double the bioavailability of alendronate.
Herbal
None known.
Food
Concurrent beverages, dietary supplements, food: May interfere with the absorption of alendronate.

DIAGNOSTIC TEST EFFECTS
Reduces serum calcium and serum phosphate concentrations. Significant decreases in serum alkaline phosphatase levels are noted in those with Paget's disease.

SIDE EFFECTS
Frequent (8%–7%)
Back pain, abdominal pain
Occasional (3%–2%)
Nausea, abdominal distention, constipation, diarrhea, flatulence
Rare (Less than 2%)
Skin rash

SERIOUS REACTIONS
• Hypocalcemia, hypophosphatemia, and significant GI disturbances result from overdosage.
• Esophageal irritation occurs if alendronate is not given with 6–8 oz of plain water or if the patient lies down within 30 min of drug administration.

NURSING CONSIDERATIONS
Baseline Assessment
• Hypocalcemia and vitamin D deficiency must be corrected before therapy.
Lifespan Considerations
• Be aware that alendronate sodium may cause decreased maternal weight gain, delay delivery, and cause incomplete fetal ossification.
• Be aware that it is unknown if alendronate sodium is excreted in breast milk. Do not give to women who are breast-feeding.
• Be aware that safety and efficacy have not been established in children.
• There are no age-related precautions noted in the elderly.
Precautions
• Use cautiously in patients with hypocalcemia or vitamin D deficiency.
Administration and Handling
PO
◀ALERT▶ Give first thing in the morning, at least 30 minutes before the first food, beverage, or medication of the day.
• Give with 6 to 8 ounces of plain water because mineral water, coffee, tea, and juice will decrease the drug's absorption.
• Be sure that the patient does not lie down for at least 30 minutes after receiving the medication and until he or she eats the first food of the day. By drinking plain water and remaining upright, the medication will reach the stomach quickly, which minimizes the risk of esophageal irritation.
Intervention and Evaluation
• Monitor the patient's serum electrolytes, including serum alkaline phosphatase and serum calcium levels.
Patient Teaching
• Instruct the patient that expected benefits occur only when medication is taken with a full glass (6 to 8 ounces) of plain water, first thing in the morning and at least 30 minutes before the first food, beverage, or medication of the day is taken. Explain that any other beverage, including mineral water, orange juice, and coffee, significantly reduces absorption of the medication.

• Advise the patient not to lie down for at least 30 minutes after taking the medication and explain that this helps the drug move quickly to stomach and reduces the risk of esophageal irritation.

• Encourage the patient to consider weight-bearing exercises and modifying behavioral factors, such as smoking cessation and moderate alcohol consumption.

etidronate disodium
eh-**tye**-droe-nate
(Didronel)
Do not confuse with etidocaine or etomidate.

CATEGORY AND SCHEDULE
Pregnancy Risk Category: C (parenteral), B (oral)

MECHANISM OF ACTION
A bisphosphonate that decreases mineral release and matrix in bone and inhibits osteocytic osteolysis. *Therapeutic Effect:* Decreases bone resorption.

AVAILABILITY
Tablets: 200 mg, 400 mg.
Injection: 300 mg amps (50 mg/ml).

INDICATIONS AND DOSAGES
▸ **Paget's disease**
PO
Adults, Elderly. Initially, 5–10 mg/kg/day not to exceed 6 mos or 11–20 mg/kg/day not to exceed 3 mos. Repeat only after drug-free period of at least 90 days.
▸ **Heterotopic ossification caused by spinal cord injury**
PO
Adult, Elderly. 20 mg/kg/day for 2 wks; then 10 mg/kg/day for 10 wks.

▸ **Heterotopic ossification complicating total hip replacement**
PO
Adults, Elderly. 20 mg/kg/day for 1 mo preop; follow with 20 mg/kg/day for 3 mos postop.
▸ **Hypercalcemia associated with malignancy**
IV
Adults, Elderly. 7.5 mg/kg/day for 3 days; retreatment no sooner than 7-day intervals between courses. Follow with oral therapy on day after last infusion. Begin with 20 mg/kg/day for 30 days; may extend up to 90 days.

CONTRAINDICATIONS
Clinically overt osteomalacia

INTERACTIONS
Drug
Antacids with aluminum, calcium, magnesium, mineral supplements: May decrease the absorption of etidronate.
Herbal
None known.
Food
Foods with calcium: May decrease the absorption of etidronate.

DIAGNOSTIC TEST EFFECTS
None known.

IV INCOMPATIBILITIES
Do not mix with other medications.

SIDE EFFECTS
Frequent
Nausea, diarrhea, continuing or more frequent bone pain in those with Paget's disease
Occasional
Bone fractures, especially of the femur
Parenteral: Metallic, altered, or loss of taste

Rare
Hypersensitivity reaction

SERIOUS REACTIONS
• Nephrotoxicity, including hematuria, dysuria, and proteinuria, noted with parenteral route.

NURSING CONSIDERATIONS
Baseline Assessment
• Expect to obtain the patient's baseline lab values, especially electrolyte levels and renal function.
Precautions
• Use cautiously in patients with hyperphosphatemia, impaired renal function, and restricted calcium and vitamin D intake.
Administration and Handling
IV
• Store at room temperature.
• Must dilute with at least 250 ml 0.9% NaCl or D₅W.
• Infuse over at least 2 hours.
Intervention and Evaluation
• Assess the patient for diarrhea.
• Monitor the patient's electrolytes.
• Monitor BUN, and fluid intake and output for the patient with impaired renal function.
• Evaluate pain in patients with Paget's disease.
Patient Teaching
• Tell the patient that it may take up to 3 months for a therapeutic response to be evident.
• Instruct the patient to consume calcium-rich foods, such as dairy products and milk.
• Teach the patient to take oral etidronate on an empty stomach, 2 hours before ingesting antacids, food, and vitamins.

ibandronate sodium
eye-**band**-droh-nate
(Boniva)

CATEGORY AND SCHEDULE
Pregnancy Risk Category: C

MECHANISM OF ACTION
A bisphosphonate that binds to bone hydroxyapatite—part of the mineral matrix of bone—and inhibits osteoclast activity. *Therapeutic Effect:* Reduces rate of bone turnover and bone resorption, resulting in a net gain in bone mass.

PHARMACOKINETICS
Absorbed in the upper gastrointestinal (GI) tract. Extent of absorption impaired by food or beverages (other than plain water). Rapidly binds to bone. The portion not absorbed is eliminated in the urine. Protein binding: 90%. **Half-life:** 10–60 hrs.

AVAILABILITY
Tablets: 2.5 mg

INDICATIONS AND DOSAGES
▶ **Osteoporosis**
PO
Adults, Elderly. 2.5 mg a day.

CONTRAINDICATIONS
Hypersensitivity to other bisphosphonates, including alendronate, etidronate, pamidronate, risedronate, and tiludronate, inability to stand or sit upright for at least 60 min, severe renal impairment with a creatinine clearance less than 30 ml/min, uncorrected hypocalcemia

INTERACTIONS
Drug
Antacids with aluminum, calcium, magnesium, vitamin D: Decrease the absorption of ibandronate.
Herbal
None known.
Food
Beverages other than plain water, concurrent dietary supplements, food: Interfere with the absorption of ibandronate.

DIAGNOSTIC TEST EFFECTS
May decrease serum alkaline phosphatase levels. May increase blood cholesterol levels.

SIDE EFFECTS
Frequent (13%–6%)
Back pain, dyspepsia, including epigastric distress, and heartburn, peripheral discomfort, diarrhea, headache, myalgia
Occasional (4%–3%)
Dizziness, arthralgia, asthenia or lack of strength and energy
Rare (2% or less)
Vomiting, hypersensitivity reaction

SERIOUS REACTIONS
• Upper respiratory infection occurs occasionally.
• Overdosage results in hypocalcemia, hypophosphatemia, and significant GI disturbances

NURSING CONSIDERATIONS
Baseline Assessment
• Plan to correct hypocalcemia and vitamin D deficiencies before beginning ibandronate therapy.
• Expect to obtain the patient's laboratory baselines, especially BUN, electrolytes, and serum creatinine results.

• Prepare the patient for a baseline bone density study.
Lifespan Considerations
• Be aware that ibandronate has the potential for teratogenic effects.
• Be aware that it is unknown if ibandronate is excreted in breast milk. Breast-feeding is not recommended in this patient population.
• Be aware that the safety and efficacy of this drug have not been established in children.
• There are no age-related precautions noted in the elderly.
Precautions
• Use cautiously in patients with gastrointestinal diseases including duodenitis, dysphagia, esophagitis, gastritis, ulcers, and mild to moderate renal impairment.
Administration and Handling
• Give ibandronate 60 minutes before the patient receives his or her first food or beverage of the day, on an empty stomach with 6 to 8 oz of plain—not mineral—water while the patient is standing or sitting in an upright position. The patient cannot lie down for 60 minutes following drug administration. Patient should not chew or suck the tablet due to the potential for oropharyngeal ulceration.
Intervention and Evaluation
• Monitor the patient's serum electrolyte levels, especially calcium and serum alkaline phosphatase levels.
Patient Teaching
• Tell the patient that the drug's expected benefits occur only when the medication is taken with full glass (6–8 oz) of plain water, first thing in the morning and at least 60 minutes before the first beverage, food, or medications of the day. Explain to the patient that any beverage other than plain water,

including coffee, mineral water, and orange juice, significantly reduces the absorption of ibandronate.
• Instruct the patient not to lie down for at least 60 minutes after taking ibandronate to potentiate delivery to the stomach and reduce the risk of esophageal irritation.
• Encourage the patient to consider beginning weight-bearing exercises and modifying behavioral factors, such as reducing alcohol consumption and stopping cigarette smoking.

pamidronate disodium
pam-ih-**drow**-nate
(Aredia)

CATEGORY AND SCHEDULE
Pregnancy Risk Category: D

MECHANISM OF ACTION
A biphosphate that binds to bone, inhibits osteoclast-mediated calcium resorption. *Therapeutic Effect:* Lowers serum calcium concentrations.

PHARMACOKINETICS

Route	Onset	Peak	Duration
IV	24–48 hrs	5–7 days	N/A

After IV administration, rapidly absorbed by bone. Slowly excreted unchanged in urine. Unknown if removed by hemodialysis. Bone half-life: 300 days. Unmetabolized **half-life:** 2.5 hrs.

AVAILABILITY
Powder for Injection: 30 mg, 90 mg.

INDICATIONS AND DOSAGES
▶ **Hypercalcemia**
IV infusion
Adults, Elderly. Moderate corrected serum calcium 12–13.5 mg/dl: 60–90 mg. Severe corrected serum calcium greater than 13.5 mg/dl: 90 mg.
▶ **Paget's disease**
IV infusion
Adults, Elderly. 30 mg/day for 3 days.
▶ **Osteolytic bone lesion**
IV infusion
Adults, Elderly. 90 mg over 2–4 hrs.

CONTRAINDICATIONS
Hypersensitivity to other bisphosphonates, such as etidronate, tiludronate, risedronate, and alendronate

INTERACTIONS
Drug
Calcium-containing medications, vitamin D: May antagonize effects in treatment of hypercalcemia.
Herbal
None known.
Food
None known.

DIAGNOSTIC TEST EFFECTS
May decrease serum phosphate, magnesium, calcium, and potassium levels.

IV INCOMPATIBILITIES
Calcium-containing IV fluids

SIDE EFFECTS
Frequent (greater than 10%)
Temperature elevation (at least 1°C) 24–48 hrs after administration (27%), drug-related redness, swelling, induration, pain at catheter site with 18% of patients receiving 90 mg, anorexia, nausea, fatigue
Occasional (10%–1%)
Constipation, rhinitis

SERIOUS REACTIONS
• Hypophosphatemia, hypokalemia, hypomagnesemia, and hypocalcemia occur more frequently with higher dosage.
• Anemia, hypertension, tachycardia, atrial fibrillation, and somnolence occur more often with 90 mg dosages.
• Gastrointestinal (GI) hemorrhage occurs rarely.

NURSING CONSIDERATIONS

Baseline Assessment
• Establish the patient's baseline electrolyte levels, including BUN, serum calcium and creatinine levels.

Lifespan Considerations
• Be aware that there are no adequate and well-controlled studies in pregnant women and it is unknown if pamidronate causes fetal harm or is excreted in breast milk.
• Be aware that the safety and efficacy of pamidronate have not been established in children.
• Be aware that the elderly may become overhydrated and require careful monitoring of fluid and electrolytes. Dilute the drug in a smaller volume for elderly patients.

Precautions
• Use cautiously in patients with cardiac failure and renal function impairment.

Administration and Handling
IV
• Store parenteral form at room temperature.
• Remember that the reconstituted vial is stable for 24 hours refrigerated, and that the IV solution is stable for 24 hours after dilution.
• Reconstitute each 30-mg vial with 10 ml sterile water for injection to provide concentration of 3 mg/ml.

• Allow the drug to dissolve before withdrawing.
• Further dilute with 1,000 ml sterile 0.45% or 0.9% NaCl or D_5W.
• Remember that adequate hydration is essential in conjunction with pamidronate therapy. Avoid overhydration in patients with the potential for heart failure.
• Administer as IV infusion over 2 to 24 hours for treatment of hypercalcemia; over 2 to 4 hours for other indications.

Intervention and Evaluation
• Monitor the patient's blood Hct and Hgb, magnesium, and serum creatinine.
• Provide the patient with adequate hydration, and take precautions to avoid overhydrating the patient.
• Monitor the patient's fluid intake and output carefully.
• Examine the patient's lungs for crackles and dependent body parts for edema.
• Monitor the patient's blood pressure (B/P), pulse, and temperature.
• Assess the patient's catheter site for pain, redness, and swelling.
• Assess the patient's daily pattern of bowel activity and stool consistency.
• Be alert for potential GI hemorrhage with 90 mg dosage.

Patient Teaching
• Explain to the patient the need for follow-up testing.
• Tell the patient to avoid drugs containing calcium and vitamin D, such as antacids, because they might antagonize the effects of zoledronic acid.

risedronate sodium
rize-droe-nate
(Actonel)

CATEGORY AND SCHEDULE
Pregnancy Risk Category: C

MECHANISM OF ACTION
A bisphosphonate that binds to bone hydroxyapatite and inhibits osteoclasts. *Therapeutic Effect:* Reduces bone turnover, or the number of sites at which bone is remodeled, and bone resorption.

AVAILABILITY
Tablets: 5 mg, 30 mg, 35 mg.

INDICATIONS AND DOSAGES
▶ **Paget's disease**
PO
Adults, Elderly. 30 mg/day for 2 mos. Retreatment may occur after 2-mo post-treatment observation period.
▶ **Osteoporosis (postmenopausal, prevention and treatment)**
PO
Adults, Elderly. 5 mg/day or 35 mg once weekly.
▶ **Osteoporosis (glucocorticoid induced)**
PO
Adults, Elderly. 5 mg/day.

CONTRAINDICATIONS
Hypersensitivity to other bisphosphonates, including etidronate, tiludronate, risedronate, and alendronate, hypocalcemia, inability to stand or sit upright for at least 20 min, renal impairment when serum creatinine clearance greater than 5-mg/dl

INTERACTIONS
Drug
Antacids with aluminum, calcium, magnesium, vitamin D: May decrease the absorption of risedronate.
Herbal
None known.
Food
None known.

DIAGNOSTIC TEST EFFECTS
None known.

SIDE EFFECTS
Frequent (30%)
Arthralgia
Occasional (12%–8%)
Rash, flu-like symptoms, peripheral edema
Rare (5%–3%)
Bone pain, sinusitis, asthenia, (loss of strength, energy), dry eye, tinnitus

SERIOUS REACTIONS
• Hypocalcemia, hypophosphatemia, and significant gastrointestinal (GI) disturbances result from overdosage.

NURSING CONSIDERATIONS
Baseline Assessment
• Correct hypocalcemia and vitamin D deficiency before beginning risedronate therapy.
• Plan to obtain the patient's lab baselines, especially electrolytes and renal function.
Precautions
• Use cautiously in patients with GI diseases including duodenitis, dysphagia, esophagitis, gastritis, and ulcers, and severe renal impairment.
Administration and Handling
PO
• Administer 30 to 60 minutes before consuming drink, food, or other medications orally to avoid interference with absorption.

• Give on empty stomach with full glass of water, but not mineral water.

• Avoid lying down for 30 minutes after swallowing tablet to help drug delivery to the stomach.

Intervention and Evaluation

• Expect to check the patient's electrolytes, especially serum alkaline phosphatase and calcium levels.

• Monitor the BUN, intake and output, and serum creatinine levels in patients with renal impairment, as ordered.

Patient Teaching

• Instruct the patient to take the drug with a full glass (6–8 oz) of plain water, first thing in the morning and at least 30 minutes before first beverage, food, or medication of the day. Explain to the patient that any other beverage, including coffee, mineral water, and orange juice, significantly reduces the absorption of the drug.

• Teach the patient not to lie down for at least 30 minutes after taking risedronate to potentiate delivery to the stomach and reduce the risk of esophageal irritation.

• Explain to the patient that the drug's therapeutic effect depends on his or her adherence to administration instructions.

• Urge the patient to consider performing weight-bearing exercises and modifying his or her behavioral factors, such as avoiding alcohol consumption and cigarette smoking.

tiludronate
tie-**lew**-dro-nate
(Skelid)

CATEGORY AND SCHEDULE
Pregnancy Risk Category: C

MECHANISM OF ACTION
A calcium regulator that inhibits functioning osteoclasts through disruption of cytoskeletal ring structure and inhibition of osteoclastic proton pump. *Therapeutic Effect:* Inhibits bone resorption.

AVAILABILITY
Tablets: 200 mg.

INDICATIONS AND DOSAGES
▸ **Paget's disease**
PO
Adults, Elderly. 400 mg once a day for 3 mos. Must take with 6–8 oz plain water. Do not take within 2 hrs of food intake. Avoid taking aspirin, calcium supplements, mineral supplements, and antacids within 2 hrs of taking tiludronate.

CONTRAINDICATIONS
Gastrointestinal (GI) disease, such as dysphagia and gastric ulcer, impaired renal function.

INTERACTIONS
Drug
Aluminum- or magnesium-containing antacids, calcium, salicylates: May interfere with the absorption of tiludronate.
Herbal
None known.
Food
None known.

DIAGNOSTIC TEST EFFECTS
None known.

SIDE EFFECTS
Frequent (9%–6%)
Nausea, diarrhea, generalized body pain, back pain, headache
Occasional
Rash, dyspepsia, vomiting, rhinitis, sinusitis, dizziness

NURSING CONSIDERATIONS

Baseline Assessment
• Determine if the patient is pregnant and using other medications, especially aluminum, magnesium, calcium, and salicylates.
• Obtain the patient's baseline BUN and serum creatinine to assess renal function.
• Assess the patient for evidence of gastrointestinal (GI) abnormalities.

Precautions
• Use cautiously in patients with hyperparathyroidism, hypocalcemia, and vitamin D deficiency.

Intervention and Evaluation
• Monitor the patient's adjusted serum calcium, serum alkaline phosphatase, osteocalcin, and urinary hydroxyproline to assess the effectiveness of tiludronate.

Patient Teaching
• Instruct the patient take the drug dose with 6 to 8 oz water.
• Warn the patient to avoid taking other medications for 2 hours before or after taking tiludronate.
• Instruct the patient to consult with the physician to determine if he or she needs calcium and vitamin D supplements.

---

zoledronic acid
zole-eh-**dron**-ick
(Zometa)

CATEGORY AND SCHEDULE
Pregnancy Risk Category: C

MECHANISM OF ACTION
A bisphosphonate that inhibits the resorption of mineralized bone and cartilage; inhibits increased osteoclastic activity and skeletal calcium release induced by stimulatory factors released by tumors. *Therapeutic Effect:* Increases urinary calcium and phosphorus excretion; decreases serum calcium and phosphorus levels.

AVAILABILITY
Injection: 4 mg/vial of lyophilized powder.

INDICATIONS AND DOSAGES
▸ **Hypercalcemia**
IV infusion
Adults, Elderly. 4 mg given as an IV infusion over no less than 15 min. Retreatment may be considered, but wait at least 7 days to allow for full response to initial dose.

CONTRAINDICATIONS
Hypersensitivity to other bisphosphonates, including alendronate, etidronate, pamidronate, risedronate, tiludronate

INTERACTIONS
Drug
Calcium-containing medications, vitamin D: May antagonize the effects in treatment of hypercalcemia.
Herbal
None known.
Food
None known.

DIAGNOSTIC TEST EFFECTS
May decrease serum magnesium, calcium, and phosphate levels.

IV INCOMPATIBILITIES
Do not mix with any other medications.

SIDE EFFECTS

Frequent (44%–26%)
Fever, nausea, vomiting, constipation
Occasional (15%–10%)
Hypotension, anxiety, insomnia, flu-like syndrome, such as fever, chills, bone pain, joint pain, and muscle aches, nausea, vomiting, constipation
Rare
Conjunctivitis

SERIOUS REACTIONS

• Renal toxicity may occur if IV infusion is administered in less than 15 minutes.

NURSING CONSIDERATIONS

Baseline Assessment
• Establish the patient's baseline electrolyte levels, including serum calcium, as well as renal function tests.
◀ALERT▶ Make sure the patient is adequately hydrated before administering zoledronic acid.
Precautions
• Use cautiously in patients with a history of aspirin-sensitive asthma, hypoparathyroidism, renal impairment, and risk of hypocalcemia.
Administration and Handling
IV
• Store at room temperature.
• If not used immediately, reconstituted solution should be refrigerated; time from reconstitution to end of administration should not exceed 24 hours.
• Reconstitute 4-mg vial with 5 ml Sterile Water for Injection. Allow drug to dissolve before withdrawing.
• Further dilute with 100 ml 0.9% NaCl or D_5W.
• Adequate hydration is essential in conjunction with zoledronic acid.
• Administer as an IV infusion over not less than 15 minutes to increase the risk of deterioration in renal function.
Intervention and Evaluation
• Monitor the patient's complete blood count (CBC), including blood Hgb, and Hct, serum electrolytes, including, serum calcium, magnesium, and phosphate levels, and renal function tests.
• Assess the patient's vertebral bone mass and document its improvement or stabilization.
• Assess the patient for fever.
• Evaluate the fluid intake and output, especially in patients with impaired renal function.
Patient Teaching
• Explain to the patient the need for follow-up testing.
• Tell the patient to avoid drugs containing calcium and vitamin D, such as antacids, because they might antagonize the effects of zoledronic acid.

conjugated estrogens
estradiol, estradiol cypionate, estradiol transdermal, estradiol valerate
estropipate
medroxyprogesterone acetate
megestrol acetate
progesterone

Uses: Estrogens and progestins are commonly used for contraception and hormone replacement therapy after menopause. They're also used to treat dysfunctional uterine bleeding, female hypogonadism, and prostate and other forms of cancer.

Actions: As ovarian sex hormones, estrogens and progestins provide different actions.

Estrogens, such as estradiol, mainly promote proliferation and growth of specific cells in the body and are responsible for the development of most secondary sex characteristics, such as the breasts and milk-producing apparatus. These agents primarily cause the cellular proliferation and growth of female reproductive organs, including the ovaries, fallopian tubes, uterus, and vagina.

Progestins, such as progesterone, stimulate secretion by the uterine endometrium during the latter half of the female sexual cycle, preparing the uterus for implantation of the fertilized ovum. These hormones decrease the frequency of uterine contractions, which helps prevent expulsion of the implanted ovum. Progesterone also promotes breast development.

Both types of hormones protect women against coronary heart disease and osteoporosis.

COMBINATION PRODUCTS

ACTIVELLA: estradiol/norethindrone (a hormone) 1 mg/0.5 mg.
COMBIPATCH: estradiol/norethindrone (a hormone) 0.05 mg/0.14 mg; 0.05 mg/0.25 mg.
FEMHRT: estradiol/norethindrone (a hormone) 5 mcg/1 mg.
LUNELLE: estradiol/ medroxyprogesterone (a progestin) 5 mg/25 mg per 0.5 ml.
PREMPHASE: conjugated estrogens/ medroxyprogesterone (an androgen): 0.625 mg/5 mg.
PREMPRO: conjugated estrogens/

medroxyprogesterone (an androgen): 0.3 mg/1.5 mg; 0.45 mg/1.5 mg; 0.625 mg/2.5 mg; 0.625 mg/5 mg.

conjugated estrogens
ess-troe-jenz
(Cenestin, C.E.S.[CAN], Congest[CAN], Premarin, Premarin Crème[AUS])

CATEGORY AND SCHEDULE
Pregnancy Risk Category: X

MECHANISM OF ACTION

An estrogen that increases synthesis of DNA, RNA, and various proteins in responsive tissues. Reduces release of gonadotropin-releasing hormone, reducing follicle-stimulating hormone (FSH) and leuteinizing hormone (LH). *Therapeutic Effect:* Promotes vasomotor stability, maintains genitourinary (GU) function, normal growth, development of female sex organs. Prevents accelerated bone loss by inhibiting bone resorption, restoring balance of bone resorption and formation. Inhibits LH, decreases serum concentration of testosterone.

PHARMACOKINETICS

Well absorbed from the gastrointestinal (GI) tract. Widely distributed. Protein binding: 50%–80%. Metabolized in liver. Primarily excreted in urine.

AVAILABILITY

Tablets: 0.3 mg, 0.45 mg, 0.625 mg, 0.9 mg, 1.25 mg, 2.5 mg.
Injection: 25 mg.
Vaginal Cream.

INDICATIONS AND DOSAGES

▸ **Vasomotor symptoms associated with menopause, atrophic vaginitis, kraurosis vulvae**
PO
Adults, Elderly. 0.3–0.625 mg/day cyclically (21 days on; 7 days off or continuously).
Intravaginal
Adults, Elderly. 0.5–2 g/day cyclically.
▸ **Female hypogonadism**
PO
Adults. 0.3–0.625 mg/day in divided doses for 20 days; rest 10 days.

▸ **Female castration, primary ovarian failure**
PO
Adults. Initially, 1.25 mg/day cyclically.
▸ **Osteoporosis**
PO
Adults, Elderly. 0.3–0.625 mg/day, cyclically.
▸ **Breast cancer**
PO
Adults, Elderly. 10 mg 3 times/day for at least 3 mos.
▸ **Prostate cancer**
PO
Adults, Elderly. 1.25–2.5 mg 3 times/day.
▸ **Abnormal uterine bleeding**
IM/IV
Adults. 25 mg, may repeat once in 6–12 hrs.
PO
Adults. 1.25 mg q4h for 24 hrs, then 1.25 mg/day for 7–10 days.

UNLABELED USES

Prevents estrogen deficiency–induced premenopausal osteoporosis Cream: Prevention of nosebleeds

CONTRAINDICATIONS

Breast cancer with some exceptions, liver disease, thrombophlebitis, undiagnosed vaginal bleeding

INTERACTIONS

Drug
Bromocriptine: May interfere with the effects of bromocriptine.
Cyclosporine: May increase the blood concentration and liver and nephrotoxicity of cyclosporine.
Liver toxic medications: May increase the risk of liver toxicity.
Herbal
None known.
Food
None known.

DIAGNOSTIC TEST EFFECTS

May affect metapyrone testing, thyroid function tests. May decrease serum cholesterol levels, and LDH concentrations. May increase blood glucose levels, HDL concentrations, serum calcium, and triglyceride levels.

IV INCOMPATIBILITIES

No information available via Y-site administration.

SIDE EFFECTS

Frequent
Change in vaginal bleeding, such as spotting or breakthrough bleeding, breast pain or tenderness, gynecomastia
Occasional
Headache, increased blood pressure (B/P), intolerance to contact lenses
High-dose therapy: Anorexia, nausea
Rare
Loss of scalp hair, clinical depression

SERIOUS REACTIONS

• Prolonged administration may increase risk of gallbladder, thromboembolic disease, breast, cervical, vaginal, endometrial, and liver carcinoma.

NURSING CONSIDERATIONS

Baseline Assessment

• Determine if the patient is hypersensitive to estrogen, and whether he or she has had previous jaundice or thromboembolic disorders associated with pregnancy or estrogen therapy.

Precautions

• Use cautiously in patients with asthma, cardiac dysfunction, diabetes mellitus, epilepsy, migraine headaches, and renal impairment.

Lifespan Considerations

• Be aware that conjugated estrogen is distributed in breast milk and may be harmful to fetus. Conjugated estrogen should not be used during breast-feeding.
• Be aware that the safety and efficacy of this drug have not been established in children.
• There are no age-related precautions noted in the elderly.

Administration and Handling

PO
• Administer at the same time each day.
• Give conjugated estrogen with food or milk if the patient experiences nausea.

IV
• Refrigerate vials for IV use.
• Remember that the reconstituted solution is stable for 60 days refrigerated.
• Do not use if solution darkens or precipitate forms.
• Reconstitute with the diluent provided—5 ml sterile water for injection containing benzyl alcohol.
• Slowly add diluent, shaking gently. Avoid vigorous shaking.
• Give slowly to prevent flushing reaction.

Intervention and Evaluation

• Assess the patient's blood pressure (B/P) periodically.
• Examine the patient for edema and record the patient's weight.
• Promptly report signs and symptoms of thromboembolic or thrombotic disorders in the patient as evidenced by loss of coordination, numbness or weakness of an extremity, pain in the chest, leg, or groin, shortness of breath, speech or vision disturbance, and sudden severe headache.

Patient Teaching

• Urge the patient to avoid smoking

due to the increased risk of blood clots and myocardial infarction (MI).
• Explain to the patient the importance of diet and exercise when conjugated estrogens are taken to retard osteoporosis.
• Teach the patient how to recognize the signs and symptoms of blood clots, such as tenderness and swelling.
• Warn the patient to notify the physician if he or she experiences abnormal vaginal bleeding, depression, or signs and symptoms of blood clots.
• Teach female patients to perform breast self-exams monthly.
• Instruct the patient to report to the physician any weekly weight gain of more than 5 lbs.
• Instruct the female patient to notify the physician and plan to discontinue the drug if she suspects she is pregnant.

estradiol
ess-tra-**dye**-ole
(Estrace, Estraderm MX[AUS], Sandrena Gel[AUS], Zumenon[AUS])
estradiol cypionate
(Depo Estradiol, Depogen)
estradiol transdermal
(Alora, Climara, Esclim, Estraderm, Vivelle, Vivelle Dot)
estradiol valerate
(Delestrogen, Valogen)
Do not confuse with Testoderm.

CATEGORY AND SCHEDULE
Pregnancy Risk Category: X

MECHANISM OF ACTION
An estrogen that increases synthesis of DNA, RNA, proteins in target tissues; reduces release of gonadotropin-releasing hormone from hypothalamus; reduces follicle-stimulating hormone (FSH) and luteinizing hormone (LH) release from the pituitary. *Therapeutic Effect:* Promotes normal growth, development of female sex organs, maintaining genitourinary (GU) function, vasomotor stability. Prevents accelerated bone loss by inhibiting bone resorption, restoring balance of bone resorption and formation. Inhibits LH, decreases serum concentration of testosterone.

PHARMACOKINETICS
Well absorbed from the gastrointestinal (GI) tract. Widely distributed. Protein binding: 50%–80%. Metabolized in liver. Primarily excreted in urine. **Half-life:** Unknown.

AVAILABILITY
Tablets: 0.5 mg (Estrace), 1 mg (Estrace), 2 mg (Estrace).
Injection: 5 mg/ml (Cypionate), 10 mg/ml (Valerate), 20 mg/ml (Valerate), 40 mg/ml (Valerate).
Transdermal: 0.025 mg, 0.0375 mg, 0.05 mg, 0.075 mg, 0.1 mg.
Vaginal Cream: 100 mcg/g.
Vaginal Ring: 0.05 mg, 0.1 mg, 2 mg.

INDICATIONS AND DOSAGES
▸ **Female hypogonadism**
IM
Adults. 1.5–2 mg/mo (Cypionate), 10–20 mg/mo (Valerate).
PO
Adults. 0.5–2 mg/day cyclically (3 wks on, 1 wk off).
Transdermal
Adults. 0.025–0.05 mg once a week (Climara), 0.05 mg 2 times/wk cyclically in patients with intact uterus, continuous in patients without a uterus (other transdermals).

▸ **Vaginal or vulvae atrophy**
Intravaginal
Adults. Initially, 200–400 mcg/day
(2–4 g of cream) estradiol daily for
1–2 wks; then 100–200 mcg (1–2 g)
daily for 1–2 wks. Maintenance:
After vaginal mucosa restored:
100 mcg 1–3 times/wk for 3 wks,
off 1 wk per cycle.
▸ **Menopausal symptoms**
IM
Adults. 1–5 mg/day cyclically
(3 wks on, 1 wk off) (Cypionate),
10–20 mg q4wks (Valerate).
PO
Adults. 0.5–2 mg/day cyclically or
continuously.
Transdermal
Adults. 25–50 mcg 1–2 times/wk
depending on product used.
▸ **Breast cancer**
PO
Adults. 10 mg 3 times/day for at
least 3 mos.
▸ **Prostate cancer**
PO
Adults. 1–2 mg 3 times/day.
IM
Adults. 30 mg q1–2wks (Valerate).
▸ **Prevention of postmenopausal
osteoporosis**
PO
Adults. 0.5 mg/day, cyclically
(23 days on, 5 days off).
Transdermal
Adults. 25–100 mcg/day (Alora,
Climara, Vivelle).

UNLABELED USES
Treatment of Turner's syndrome

CONTRAINDICATIONS
Abnormal vaginal bleeding, active
arterial thrombosis, blood dyscrasias, estrogen-dependent cancer,
known or suspected breast cancer,
pregnancy, thrombophlebitis or
thromboembolic disorders, thyroid
dysfunction

INTERACTIONS
Drug
Bromocriptine: May interfere with
the effects of bromocriptine.
Cyclosporine: May increase the
blood concentration and risk of
liver toxicity and nephrotoxicity of
cyclosporine.
Liver toxic medications: May increase the risk of liver toxicity.
Herbal
Saw palmetto: Increases the effects
of saw palmetto.
Food
None known.

DIAGNOSTIC TEST EFFECTS
May affect metapyrone testing,
thyroid function tests. May decrease
serum cholesterol levels, LDH
concentrations. May increase blood
glucose levels, HDL concentrations,
serum calcium and triglyceride
levels.

SIDE EFFECTS
Frequent
Anorexia, nausea, swelling of
breasts, peripheral edema, evidenced
by swollen ankles, feet
Transdermal route: Skin irritation,
redness
Occasional
Vomiting, especially with high
dosages, headache that may be
severe, intolerance to contact lenses,
increased blood pressure (B/P),
glucose intolerance, brown spots on
exposed skin
Vaginal route: Local irritation,
vaginal discharge, changes in
vaginal bleeding, including spotting, breakthrough or prolonged
bleeding
Rare
Chorea or involuntary movements,
hirsutism or abnormal hairiness,
loss of scalp hair, depression

SERIOUS REACTIONS
• Prolonged administration increases risk of gallbladder disease, thromboembolic disease, and breast, cervical, vaginal, endometrial, and liver carcinoma.
• Cholestatic jaundice occurs rarely.

NURSING CONSIDERATIONS

Baseline Assessment
• Determine if the patient is hypersensitive to estrogen and whether she has had previous jaundice or thromboembolic disorders associated with pregnancy or estrogen therapy.
• Determine if the patient is pregnant.

Lifespan Considerations
• Be aware that estradiol is distributed in breast milk and may be harmful to offspring. Estradiol should not be used during breastfeeding.
• Be aware that estradiol should be used cautiously in children whose bone growth is not complete as the drug may accelerate epiphyseal closure.
• There are no age-related precautions noted in the elderly.

Precautions
• Use cautiously in pediatric patients whose bone growth is incomplete.
• Use cautiously in patients with diseases exacerbated by fluid retention and liver or renal insufficiency.

Administration and Handling
PO
• Administer estradiol at the same time each day.
IM
• Rotate the vial to disperse drug in solution.
• Give deep IM injection into the gluteus maximus.

Vaginal
• Apply estradiol cream at bedtime for best absorption.
• Insert the end of the filled applicator into the patient's vagina, directed slightly toward sacrum; push plunger down completely.
• Avoid skin contact with cream to prevent skin absorption of the drug.
Transdermal
◀ALERT▶ Transdermal Climara is administered once weekly; others are twice weekly.
• Remove the old patch and select a new site. Consider using the buttocks as an alternative application site.
• Peel off the protective strip on the patch to expose the adhesive surface.
• Apply to clean, dry, intact skin on the trunk of the patient's body in an area with as little hair as possible.
• Press in place for at least 10 seconds. Do not apply the patch to the patient's breasts or waistline.

Intervention and Evaluation
• Monitor the patient's blood glucose levels, B/P, hepatic enzymes, serum calcium levels, and weight.

Patient Teaching
• Urge the patient to limit his or her alcohol and caffeine intake.
• Encourage the patient to stop smoking tobacco.
• Warn the patient to notify the physician if he or she experiences calf or chest pain, mental depression, numbness or weakness of an extremity, severe abdominal pain, shortness of breath, speech or vision disturbance, sudden headache, unusual bleeding, and vomiting.

estropipate
ess-troe-**pie**-pate
(Genoral[AUS], Ogen)

CATEGORY AND SCHEDULE
Pregnancy Risk Category: X

MECHANISM OF ACTION
An estrogen that increases synthesis of DNA, RNA, various proteins in responsive tissues. Reduces release of gonadotropin-releasing hormone, reducing follicle-stimulating hormone (FSH) and luteinizing hormone (LH). *Therapeutic Effect:* Promotes normal growth, development of female sex organs, maintaining genitourinary (GU) function, vasomotor stability. Prevents accelerated bone loss by inhibiting bone resorption, restoring balance of bone resorption and formation.

AVAILABILITY
Tablets: 0.625 mg, 0.75 mg, 1.25 mg, 1.5 mg, 2.5 mg, 3 mg.

INDICATIONS AND DOSAGES
▸ **Vasomotor symptoms, atrophic vaginitis, kraurosis vulvae**
PO
Adults, Elderly. 0.625–5 mg/day cyclically.
▸ **Atrophic vaginitis, kraurosis vulvae**
Intravaginal
Adults, Elderly. 2–4 g/day cyclically.
▸ **Female hypogonadism, castration, primary ovarian failure**
PO
Adults, Elderly. 1.25–7.5 mg/day for 21 days; off 8–10 days. Repeat if bleeding does not occur by end of off cycle.

▸ **Osteoporosis prevention**
PO
Adults, Elderly. 0.625 mg/day (25 days of 31 day cycle/mo).

CONTRAINDICATIONS
Abnormal vaginal bleeding, active arterial thrombosis, blood dyscrasias, estrogen-dependent cancer, known or suspected breast cancer, pregnancy, thrombophlebitis or thromboembolic disorders, thyroid dysfunction

INTERACTIONS
Drug
Bromocriptine: May interfere with the effects of bromocriptine.
Cyclosporine: May increase the blood concentration and risk of liver and nephrotoxicity of cyclosporine.
Liver toxic medications: May increase the risk of liver toxicity.
Herbal
Saw palmetto: Increases the effects of saw palmetto.
Food
None known.

DIAGNOSTIC TEST EFFECTS
May affect metapyrone testing, thyroid function tests. May decrease serum cholesterol levels, LDH concentrations. May increase blood glucose levels, HDL concentrations, serum calcium and triglyceride levels.

SIDE EFFECTS
Frequent
Anorexia, nausea, swelling of breasts, peripheral edema evidenced by swollen ankles, feet
Occasional
Vomiting, especially with high dosages, headache that may be severe, intolerance to contact lenses, increased blood pressure (B/P),

glucose intolerance, brown spots on exposed skin
Vaginal route: Local irritation, vaginal discharge, changes in vaginal bleeding, including spotting, breakthrough or prolonged bleeding
Rare
Chorea or involuntary movements, hirsutism or abnormal hairiness, loss of scalp hair, depression

SERIOUS REACTIONS
• Prolonged administration increases risk of gallbladder disease, thromboembolic disease and breast, cervical, vaginal, endometrial, and liver carcinoma.
• Cholestatic jaundice occurs rarely.

NURSING CONSIDERATIONS
Baseline Assessment
• Determine if the patient is hypersensitive to estrogen and whether she has had previous jaundice or thromboembolic disorders associated with pregnancy or estrogen therapy.
• Determine if the patient is pregnant.
Precautions
• Use cautiously in patients with diseases exacerbated by fluid retention and liver or renal insufficiency.
Intervention and Evaluation
• Promptly report signs and symptoms of thromboembolic or thrombotic disorders including peripheral paresthesia, shortness of breath, speech or vision disturbance, and sudden headache.
Patient Teaching
• Urge the patient to avoid smoking due to the increased risk of blood clots and myocardial infarction (MI).
• Warn the patient to notify the physician if she experiences depres-

sion, or if she experiences abnormal vaginal bleeding.
• Teach the patient to remain recumbent for at least 30 minutes after vaginal application and not to use tampons.
• Instruct the female patient to discontinue the drug and notify the physician if she suspects she is pregnant.

medroxyprogesterone acetate
meh-drocks-ee-pro-**jes**-ter-own
(Depo-Provera, Novo-Medrone[CAN], Provera, Ralovera[AUS])
Do not confuse with Ambien, hydroxyprogesterone, methylprednisolone, or methyltestosterone.

CATEGORY AND SCHEDULE
Pregnancy Risk Category: X

MECHANISM OF ACTION
A hormone that transforms endometrium from proliferative to secretory in an estrogen-primed endometrium; inhibits secretion of pituitary gonadotropins. *Therapeutic Effect:* Prevents follicular maturation and ovulation. Stimulates growth of mammary alveolar tissue; relaxes uterine smooth muscle. Restores hormonal imbalance.

PHARMACOKINETICS
Slow absorption after IM administration. Protein binding: 90%. Metabolized in liver. Primarily excreted in urine. **Half-life:** 30 days.

AVAILABILITY
Tablets: 2.5 mg, 5 mg, 10 mg.
Injection: 150 mg/ml, 400 mg/ml.

INDICATIONS AND DOSAGES
▸ **Endometrial hyperplasia**
PO
Adults. 2–10 mg/day for 14 days.
▸ **Secondary amenorrhea**
PO
Adults. 5–10 mg/day for 5–10 days
to begin at any time during men-
strual cycle or 2.5 mg/day.
▸ **Abnormal uterine bleeding**
PO
Adults. 5–10 mg/day for 5–10 days
to begin on calculated day 16 or
day 21 of menstrual cycle.
▸ **Endometrial, renal carcinoma**
IM
Adults, Elderly. Initially,
400–1,000 mg, repeat at 1-wk
intervals. If improvement occurs,
disease stabilized, begin mainte-
nance with as little as 400 mg/mo.
▸ **Pregnancy prevention**
IM
Adults. 150 mg q3mos.

UNLABELED USES
Hormonal replacement therapy in
estrogen-treated menopausal
women, treatment of endometriosis

CONTRAINDICATIONS
Carcinoma of breast, estrogen-
dependent neoplasm, history of or
active thrombotic disorders, such as
cerebral apoplexy, thrombophlebitis,
or thromboembolic disorders, hypersensitivity to progestins, known or
suspected pregnancy, missed abortion, severe liver dysfunction, undiagnosed abnormal genital bleeding,
undiagnosed vaginal bleeding, use
as pregnancy test

INTERACTIONS
Drug
Bromocriptine: May interfere with
the effects of bromocriptine.
Herbal
None known.

Food
None known.

DIAGNOSTIC TEST EFFECTS
Altered thyroid and liver function
tests, prothrombin time, metapyrone
test

SIDE EFFECTS
Frequent
Transient menstrual abnormalities,
including spotting, change in menstrual flow or cervical secretions,
and amenorrhea, at initiation of
therapy
Occasional
Edema, weight change, breast tenderness, nervousness, insomnia,
fatigue, dizziness
Rare
Alopecia, mental depression, dermatologic changes, headache, fever,
nausea

SERIOUS REACTIONS
• Thrombophlebitis, pulmonary or
cerebral embolism, and retinal
thrombosis occur rarely.

NURSING CONSIDERATIONS
Baseline Assessment
• Determine if the patient is hypersensitive to progestins or pregnant
before beginning medroxyprogesterone therapy.
• Plan to obtain the patient's baseline blood glucose level, blood
pressure (B/P), and weight.
Lifespan Considerations
• Be aware that medroxyprogesterone use should be avoided during
pregnancy, especially in the first
4 months as the drug may cause
congenital heart and limb reduction
defects in the neonate.
• Be aware that medroxyprogesterone is distributed in breast milk.
• Be aware that the safety and

efficacy of this drug have not been established in children.
• There are no age-related precautions noted in the elderly.

Precautions
• Use cautiously in patients with conditions aggravated by fluid retention, including asthma, seizures, migraine, and cardiac or renal dysfunction, diabetes mellitus, and a history of mental depression.

Administration and Handling
PO
• Give medroxyprogesterone without regard to meals.

IM
• Shake vial immediately before administering to ensure complete suspension.
• Inject IM only in upper arm or upper outer aspect of buttock. Rarely, a residual lump, change in skin color, or sterile abscess occurs at injection site.

Intervention and Evaluation
• Monitor the patient's weight daily and report weekly gain of 5 lbs or more.
• Monitor the patient's B/P periodically.
• Assess the patient's skin for rash and urticaria.
• Immediately report pain, redness, swelling, or warmth in the calf, chest pain, migraine headache, numbness of an arm or leg, sudden decrease in vision, and sudden shortness of breath.

Patient Teaching
• Warn the patient to notify the physician if she experiences chest pain, hemoptysis, numbness in the arm or leg, severe headache, severe pain or swelling in the calf, severe pain or tenderness in the abdominal area, sudden loss of vision, or unusually heavy vaginal bleeding.

• Encourage the patient to stop smoking tobacco.

megestrol acetate
See hormones

progesterone
proe-**jess**-ter-one
(Crinone, Gesterol, Gesterolla, Prochieve, Prometrium)

CATEGORY AND SCHEDULE
Pregnancy Risk Category: D

MECHANISM OF ACTION
A natural steroid hormone. *Therapeutic Effect:* Transforms endometrium from proliferative to secretory in an estrogen-primed endometrium, promotes mammary gland development, relaxes uterine smooth muscle.

AVAILABILITY
Injection: 50 mg/ml, 250 mg/ml (Gesterol LA).
Capsules: 100 mg, 200 mg.
Vaginal Gel: 4%, 8%.

INDICATIONS AND DOSAGES
▸ **Amenorrhea**
IM
Adults. 5–10 mg for 6–8 days. Withdrawal bleeding expected in 48–72 hrs if ovarian activity produced proliferative endometrium.
Vaginal
Adults. Apply every other day for 6 doses or less.
PO
Adults. 400 mg daily in evening for 10 days.
▸ **Abnormal uterine bleeding**
IM
Adults. 5–10 mg for 6 days. When

estrogen given concomitantly, begin progesterone after 2 wks of estrogen therapy; discontinue when menstrual flow begins.

▸ **Prevention of endometrial hyperplasia**

PO

Adults. 200 mg in evening for 12 days per 28-day cycle in combination with daily conjugated estrogen.

UNLABELED USES

Treatment of corpus luteum dysfunction

CONTRAINDICATIONS

Breast cancer, cerebral apoplexy or history of these conditions, missed abortion, severe liver dysfunction, thromboembolic disorders, thrombophlebitis, undiagnosed vaginal bleeding, use as a diagnostic test for pregnancy

INTERACTIONS

Drug

Bromocriptine: May interfere with the effects of bromocriptine.

Herbal

None known.

Food

None known.

DIAGNOSTIC TEST EFFECTS

May increase LDL concentrations and serum alkaline phosphatase levels. May decrease glucose tolerance and HDL concentrations. May cause abnormal thyroid, metapyrone, liver, and endocrine function tests.

SIDE EFFECTS

Frequent

Breakthrough bleeding or spotting at beginning of therapy, amenorrhea, change in menstrual flow, breast tenderness

Occasional

Edema, weight gain or loss, rash, pruritus, photosensitivity, skin pigmentation

Rare

Pain or swelling at injection site, acne, mental depression, alopecia, hirsutism

SERIOUS REACTIONS

• Thrombophlebitis, cerebrovascular disorders, retinal thrombosis, and pulmonary embolism occur rarely.

NURSING CONSIDERATIONS

Baseline Assessment

• Determine if the patient is hypersensitive to progestins or pregnant before beginning progesterone therapy.

• Plan to obtain the patient's baseline blood glucose, blood pressure (B/P), and weight.

Precautions

• Use cautiously in patients with conditions aggravated by fluid retention, diabetes mellitus, and a history of mental depression.

Intervention and Evaluation

• Monitor the patient's weight daily and report weekly gain of 5 lbs or more.

• Monitor the patient's B/P periodically.

• Assess the patient's skin for rash and urticaria.

• Immediately report pain, redness, swelling, or warmth in the calf, chest pain, migraine headache, peripheral paresthesia, sudden decrease in vision, and sudden shortness of breath.

• Note progesterone therapy on pathology specimens.

Patient Teaching

• Tell the patient to use sunscreen, and wear protective clothing to protect from sunlight and ultraviolet light until her tolerance is determined.

• Warn the patient to notify the physician of abnormal vaginal bleeding or other symptoms.

• Instruct the female patient to contact the physician, and stop taking the drug, as prescribed, if she suspects she is pregnant.

• Encourage the patient to stop smoking tobacco.

dinoprostone
methylergonovine
mifepristone
oxytocin

Uses: Oxytocic agents are used to induce or augment labor when maternal or fetal need exists. They're also used to control postpartum hemorrhage, cause uterine contractions after cesarean delivery or during other uterine surgery, and to induce therapeutic abortion. In addition, oxytocin is used to promote breast milk ejection.

Action: Oxytocics stimulate the frequency and force of contractions of uterine smooth muscle. They increase the responsiveness of the uterus closer to term. Some agents, such as oxytocin, stimulate the breasts to release milk by causing myoepithelial cells around the mammary glands to contract.

dinoprostone
dye-noe-**pros**-tone
(Cervidil, Prepidil Gel, Prostin E₂)
Do not confuse with bepridil.

CATEGORY AND SCHEDULE
Pregnancy Risk Category: C

MECHANISM OF ACTION
A prostaglandin that directly acts on the myometrium. Direct softening, dilation effect on cervix.
Therapeutic Effect: Stimulates myometrial contractions in gravid uterus.

PHARMACOKINETICS
Undergoes rapid enzymatic deactivation primarily in maternal lungs. Protein binding: 73%. Primarily excreted in urine.

AVAILABILITY
Vaginal Suppository: 20 mg.
Vaginal Gel: 0.5 mg (Prepidil).
Vaginal Inserts: 10 mg (Cervidil).

INDICATIONS AND DOSAGES
▶ **Abortifacient**
Intravaginal
Adults. 20 mg or one suppository high into vagina. May repeat at 3- to 5-hr intervals until abortion occurs. Do not administer more than 2 days.
▶ **Ripening unfavorable cervix**
Intracervical
Adults. Initially, 0.5 mg (2.5 ml) (Prepidil); if no cervical or uterine response, may repeat 0.5-mg dose in 6 hrs. Maximum: 1.5 mg (7.5 ml) for a 24-hr period; 10 mg over 12-hr period (Cervidil). Remove upon onset of active labor or 12 hrs following insertion.

CONTRAINDICATIONS
Active cardiac, liver, pulmonary or renal disease, acute pelvic inflammatory disease, fetal malpresentation, hypersensitivity to dinoprostone or other prostaglandins, significant cephalopelvic disproportion

INTERACTIONS
Drug
Oxytocics: May cause uterine hypertonus, possibly causing uterine rupture or cervical laceration.
Herbal
None known.
Food
None known.

DIAGNOSTIC TEST EFFECTS
None known.

SIDE EFFECTS
Frequent
Vomiting (66%), diarrhea (40%), nausea (33%)
Occasional
Headache (10%), chills or shivering (10%), hives, bradycardia, increased uterine pain accompanying abortion, peripheral vasoconstriction
Rare
Flushing, vulvae edema

SERIOUS REACTIONS
• Excessive dosage may cause uterine hypertonicity with spasm and tetanic contraction, leading to cervical laceration or perforation, and uterine rupture or hemorrhage.

NURSING CONSIDERATIONS

Baseline Assessment
• Offer the patient emotional support.
• Obtain orders for antidiarrheals, antiemetics, meperidine, and other pain medication for abdominal cramps when giving the patient dinoprostone as a suppository.
• Assess the patient for any uterine activity or vaginal bleeding.
• Assess the patient's Bishop score when giving dinoprostone gel.
• Assess the patient's degree of effacement to determine the size of shielded endocervical catheter

when giving the patient dinoprostone gel.
Lifespan Considerations
• Be aware that dinoprostone suppository is teratogenic, therefore the abortion must complete.
• Be aware that sustained uterine hyperstimulation from dinoprostone gel may affect the fetus, such as an abnormal heart rate.
• Remember that dinoprostone is not used in children or the elderly.
Precautions
• Use cautiously in patients with anemia, cardiovascular disease, cervicitis, compromised or scarred uterus, diabetes mellitus, epilepsy, history of asthma, hypertension or hypotension, infected endocervical lesions or acute vaginitis, jaundice, liver disease, renal disease, and uterine fibroids.
Administration and Handling
Suppository
• Keep frozen (less than 4°F); bring to room temperature just before use.
• Administer only in hospital setting with emergency equipment available.
• Warm suppository to room temperature before removing foil wrapper.
• Avoid skin contact due to risk of absorption.
• Insert high in the patient's vagina.
• Keep patient supine for 10 minutes after administration.
Gel
• Refrigerate.
• Use caution in handling, prevent skin contact. Wash hands thoroughly with soap and water following administration.
• Bring to room temperature just before use and avoid forcing the warming process.
• Assemble dosing apparatus as described in manufacturer insert.
• Have patient in the dorsal position

with cervix visualized using a speculum.
• Introduce gel into cervical canal just below level of internal os.
• Have the patient remain in supine position at least 15 to 30 minutes to minimize leakage of the drug from the cervical canal.

Intervention and Evaluation
• Check the duration, frequency, and strength of the contractions in patients receiving dinoprostone suppository.
• Monitor the vital signs of the patient receiving dinoprostone suppository every 15 minutes until stable, then hourly until abortion is complete.
• Check the resting uterine tone of the patient receiving dinoprostone suppository.
• Give medications for relief of gastrointestinal (GI) effects if indicated for abdominal cramps in the patient receiving dinoprostone suppository.
• Monitor the character of cervix, including dilation and effacement, fetal status, including heart rate, and uterine activity, including the onset of uterine contractions, of the patient receiving dinoprostone gel.
• Have the patient receiving dinoprostone gel remain recumbent 12 hours after application with continuous electronic monitoring of fetal heart rate and uterine activity.
• Record the vital signs of the maternal patient receiving dinoprostone gel at least hourly in presence of uterine activity.
• Reassess the Bishop score of the patient receiving dinoprostone gel.

Patient Teaching
• Warn the patient receiving dinoprostone suppository to notify the physician if she experiences chills, fever, foul-smelling or increased vaginal discharge, or uterine cramps or pain.

methylergonovine
meth-ill-er-go-**noe**-veen
(Methergine)

CATEGORY AND SCHEDULE
Pregnancy Risk Category: C

MECHANISM OF ACTION
An ergot alkaloid that stimulates alpha-adrenergic, serotonin receptors, producing arterial vasoconstriction. Causes vasospasm of coronary arteries. Directly stimulates uterine muscle. *Therapeutic Effect:* Increases strength, frequency of contractions, decreases uterine bleeding.

PHARMACOKINETICS

Route	Onset	Peak	Duration
PO	5–10 min	N/A	N/A
IM	2–5 min	N/A	N/A
IV	Immediate	N/A	3 hrs

Rapidly absorbed from the gastrointestinal (GI) tract, after IM administration. Distributed rapidly to plasma, extracellular fluid, tissues. Metabolized in liver, undergoes first-pass effect. Primarily excreted in urine.

AVAILABILITY
Tablets: 0.2 mg.
Injection: 0.2 mg/ml.

INDICATIONS AND DOSAGES
▶ **Prevents and treats postpartum, postabortion hemorrhage due to atony or involution; not for induction or augmentation of labor**
PO
Adults. 0.2 mg 3–4 times/day. Continue for up to 7 days.
IM/IV
Adults. Initially, 0.2 mg. May repeat

no more often than q2–4h for no more than 5 doses total.

UNLABELED USES
Treatment of incomplete abortion

CONTRAINDICATIONS
Hypertension, pregnancy, toxemia, untreated hypocalcemia

INTERACTIONS
Drug
Vasoconstrictors, vasopressors: May increase the effects of methylergonovine.
Herbal
None known.
Food
None known.

DIAGNOSTIC TEST EFFECTS
May decrease prolactin concentration.

IV INCOMPATIBILITIES
No information available for Y-site administration.

IV COMPATIBILITIES
Heparin, potassium

SIDE EFFECTS
Frequent
Nausea, uterine cramping, vomiting
Occasional
Abdominal or stomach pain, diarrhea, dizziness, diaphoresis, tinnitus, bradycardia, chest pain
Rare
Allergic reaction, such as rash and itching, dyspnea, severe or sudden hypertension

SERIOUS REACTIONS
• Severe hypertensive episodes may result in cerebrovascular accident, serious arrhythmias, and seizures. Hypertensive effects are more frequent with patient susceptibility, rapid IV administration, and concurrent use of regional anesthesia or vasoconstrictors.
• Peripheral ischemia may lead to gangrene.

NURSING CONSIDERATIONS
Baseline Assessment
• Determine the patient's baseline blood pressure (B/P), pulse, and serum calcium level.
• Assess the patient's bleeding prior to administration.
Lifespan Considerations
• Be aware that methylergonovine use is contraindicated during pregnancy and that small amounts of the drug are found in breast milk.
• There is no information available on methylergonovine use in children or the elderly.
Precautions
• Use cautiously in patients with coronary artery disease, liver or renal impairment, occlusive peripheral vascular disease, and sepsis.
Administration and Handling
• May give PO, IM, or IV.
• Refrigerate ampoules.
• Initial dose may be given parenterally, followed by oral regimen.
• Use IV in life-threatening emergencies only, as prescribed.
• Dilute to volume of 5 ml with 0.9% NaCl.
• Give over at least 1 minute, carefully monitoring the patient's B/P.
Intervention and Evaluation
• Monitor the patient's bleeding, B/P, pulse, and uterine tone every 15 minutes until stable for 1 to 2 hours.
• Assess the patient's extremities for color, movement, pain, and warmth.
• Report any chest pain the patient experiences promptly.
• Assist the patient with ambulation if she experiences dizziness.

Patient Teaching
• Urge the patient to avoid smoking because of added effects of vaso-constriction.
• Warn the patient to notify the physician if she experiences increased bleeding, cold or pale feet or hands, cramping, or foul-smelling lochia.

mifepristone
my-fih-**priss**-tone
(Mifeprex)
Do not confuse with Mirapex.

CATEGORY AND SCHEDULE
Pregnancy Risk Category: X

MECHANISM OF ACTION
An abortifacient that has antipro-gestational activity resulting from competitive interaction with progesterone; inhibits the activity of endogenous or exogenous pro-gesterone. Also has antiglucocorti-coid and weak antiandrogenic activity. *Therapeutic Effect:* Termi-nates pregnancy.

AVAILABILITY
Tablets: 200 mg.

INDICATIONS AND DOSAGES
▶ **Termination of pregnancy**
PO
Adults. Day 1: 600 mg as single dose. Day 3: 400 mcg misoprostol. Day 14: Post-treatment examination.

UNLABELED USES
Cushing's syndrome, endometriosis, intrauterine fetal death or nonviable early pregnancy, postcoital contra-ception or contragestation, unresect-able meningioma

CONTRAINDICATIONS
Chronic adrenal failure, concurrent long-term steroid or anticoagulant therapy, confirmed or suspected ectopic pregnancy, intrauterine device (IUD) in place, hemorrhagic disorders, inherited porphyries

INTERACTIONS
Drug
Carbamazepine, phenobarbital, phenytoin, rifampin: May increase the metabolism of mifepristone. *Erythromycin, itraconazole, ketoconazole:* May inhibit the metabolism of mifepristone.
Herbal
St. John's wort: May increase the metabolism of mifepristone.
Food
Grapefruit: May inhibit the metabo-lism of mifepristone.

DIAGNOSTIC TEST EFFECTS
May decrease blood Hgb and Hct and red blood cell (RBC) count.

SIDE EFFECTS
Frequent (greater than 10%)
Headache, dizziness, abdominal pain, nausea, vomiting, diarrhea, fatigue
Occasional (10%–3%)
Uterine hemorrhage, back pain, insomnia, vaginitis, dyspepsia, back pain, fever, viral infections, rigors (chills or shaking)
Rare (2%–1%)
Anxiety, syncope, anemia, asthenia, leg pain, sinusitis, leukorrhea

SERIOUS REACTIONS
• None known.

NURSING CONSIDERATIONS

Baseline Assessment
• Determine if the patient is taking anticonvulsants, erythromycin,

itraconazole, ketoconazole, or rifampin as these drugs may inhibit the metabolism of mifepristone.

• Ask the patient if she has an IUD in place, and don't give the drug until its removed.

• Make sure that an ectopic pregnancy has been ruled out.

Precautions

• Use cautiously in female patients older than 35 years of age or who smoke more than 10 cigarettes a day.

• Use cautiously in patients with cardiovascular disease, diabetes, hypertension, liver or renal impairment, and severe anemia.

Administration and Handling

◄ALERT► Be aware that treatment with mifepristone and misoprostol requires three office visits.

Intervention and Evaluation

• Monitor the patient's blood Hgb and Hct levels.

Patient Teaching

• Explain the treatment procedure, its effects, and the need for a follow-up visit to the patient.

• Tell the patient that she may experience uterine cramping and vaginal bleeding.

---

oxytocin
ox-ih-**toe**-sin
(Pitocin, Syntocinon INJ[AUS])
Do not confuse with Pitressin.

CATEGORY AND SCHEDULE
Pregnancy Risk Category: X

MECHANISM OF ACTION
An oxytocic that acts on uterine myofibril activity. Stimulates mammary smooth muscle. *Therapeutic Effect:* Contracts uterine smooth muscle. Enhances milk ejection from breasts.

PHARMACOKINETICS

Route	Onset	Peak	Duration
IM	3–5 min	N/A	2–3 hrs
IV	Immediate	N/A	1 hr
Intranasal	Few minutes	N/A	20 min

Rapidly absorbed through nasal mucous membranes. Protein binding: 30%. Distributed in extracellular fluid. Metabolized in liver, kidney. Primarily excreted in urine. **Half-life:** 1–6 min.

AVAILABILITY
Injection: 10 units/ml.
Nasal Spray: 40 units/ml

INDICATIONS AND DOSAGES
▶ **Induction or stimulation of labor**
IV infusion
Adults. Initially, 0.001–0.002 units/min. May increase by 0.001–0.002 units q15–30min until contraction pattern has been established.
▶ **Incomplete or inevitable abortion**
IV infusion
Adults. 10 units in 500 ml (20 mUnits/ml) D₅W or 0.9% NaCl infused at 20–40 mUnits/min.
▶ **Control of postpartum bleeding**
IV infusion
Adults. 10–40 units (Maximum: 40 units/1,000 ml) infused at rate of 20–40 mUnits/min after delivery of infant.
IM
Adults. 10 units after delivery of placenta.
▶ **Postabortion hemorrhage**
IV infusion
Adults. 10 units infused at rate of 20–100 mUnits/min.

▸ **Promote milk ejection**
Nasal
Adults. 1 spray to one or both
nostrils 2–3 min before nursing or
pumping breasts.

CONTRAINDICATIONS
Adequate uterine activity that fails
to progress, cephalopelvic disproportion, fetal distress without imminent delivery, grand multiparity,
hyperactive or hypertonic uterus,
nasal spray during pregnancy, obstetric emergencies that favor surgical intervention, prematurity, unen-
gaged fetal head, unfavorable fetal
position or presentation, when
vaginal delivery is contraindicated,
such as active genital herpes infection, placenta previa, and cord
presentation

INTERACTIONS
Drug
*Caudal block anesthetics,
vasopressors:* May increase pressor
effects.
Other oxytocics: May cause cervical
lacerations, uterine hypertonus, or
uterine rupture.
Herbal
None known.
Food
None known.

DIAGNOSTIC TEST EFFECTS
None known.

IV INCOMPATIBILITIES
No known incompatibilities via
Y-site administration.

IV COMPATIBILITIES
Heparin, insulin, multivitamins,
potassium chloride

SIDE EFFECTS
Occasional
Tachycardia, premature ventricular

contractions (PVCs), hypotension,
nausea, vomiting
Rare
Nasal: Lacrimation or tearing, nasal
irritation, rhinorrhea, unexpected
uterine bleeding or contractions

SERIOUS REACTIONS
• Hypertonicity with tearing of
uterus, increased bleeding, abruptio
placenta, and cervical and vaginal
lacerations may occur.
• In the fetus, bradycardia, central
nervous system (CNS) or brain
damage, trauma due to rapid pro-
pulsion, low Apgar at 5 minutes,
and retinal hemorrhage occur rarely.
• Prolonged IV infusion of oxytocin
with excessive fluid volume has
caused severe water intoxication
with seizures, coma, and death.

NURSING CONSIDERATIONS
Baseline Assessment
• Assess the patient's baseline blood
pressure (B/P), pulse, and fetal heart
rate.
• Determine the duration, frequency,
and strength of patient contractions.
Lifespan Considerations
• Be aware that oxytocin should be
used as indicated, and is not ex-
pected to present the risk of fetal
abnormalities.
• Be aware that oxytocin is present
in small amounts in breast milk.
Breast-feeding is not recommended
in this patient population.
• Be aware that oxytocin is not used
in children or the elderly.
Precautions
• Induction should be for medical,
not elective reasons.
Administration and Handling
IV
• Store at room temperature.
• Dilute 10 to 40 units (1 to 4 ml)
in 1,000 ml of 0.9% NaCl, lactated

Ringer's, or D$_5$W to provide a concentration of 10 to 40 mUnits/ml solution.

• Give by IV infusion and use an infusion device to carefully control rate of flow as ordered by physician.

Intervention and Evaluation

• Monitor the patient's blood pressure (B/P), contractions, including duration, frequency, strength, fetal heart rate, intrauterine pressure, pulse, respirations, fetal heart rate, and intrauterine pressure every 15 minutes.

• Notify the physician of any patient contractions that last longer than 1 minute, occur more frequently than every 2 minutes, or stop.

• Maintain careful intake and output records for the patient.

• Be alert to potential water intoxication of the patient.

• Check the patient for blood loss.

Patient Teaching

• Explain the labor progress to the patient and family.

• Teach the patient the proper use of the oxytocin nasal spray.

• Explain that the drug will be present in the breast milk, so breast-feeding isn't recommended.

desmopressin
somatrem
somatropin
vasopressin

Uses: Pituitary hormones have various uses. *Antidiuretic hormones,* such as desmopressin and vasopressin, are used to treat diabetes insipidus, postoperative abdominal distention, nocturnal enuresis, hemophilia A, and von Willebrand's disease. *Growth hormones,* such as somatrem and somatropin, are used to treat pediatric growth hormone (GH) deficiency, chronic renal insufficiency, Turner's syndrome, and cachexia or wasting in patients with acquired immunodeficiency syndrome.

Action: The actions of pituitary hormones also vary greatly. *Antidiuretic hormones* act on the collecting ducts of the kidneys to increase their permeability to water, resulting in increased water reabsorption. In higher concentrations, these agents constrict arterioles throughout the body, which increases blood pressure. *Growth hormones* cause growth in almost all body tissues: a childhood deficiency of GH results in dwarfism; an excess results in acromegaly. Metabolic effects of these agents include an increased rate of protein synthesis, mobilization of fatty acids from adipose tissue, and a decreased rate of glucose use.

desmopressin
des-moe-**press**-in
(DDAVP, Minirin[AUS], Octostim [CAN], Stimate)

CATEGORY AND SCHEDULE
Pregnancy Risk Category: B

MECHANISM OF ACTION
A synthetic pituitary hormone that increases reabsorption of water by increasing permeability of collecting ducts of the kidneys. Plasminogen activator. *Therapeutic Effect:* Decreases urinary output. Increases plasma factor VIII (antihemophilic factor).

PHARMACOKINETICS

Route	Onset	Peak	Duration
PO	1 hr	2–7 hrs	6–8 hrs
Intra-nasal	15 min–1 hr	1–5 hrs	5–21 hrs
IV	15–30 min	1.5–3 hrs	N/A

Poorly absorbed after PO/nasal administration. Metabolism: Unknown. **Half-life:** Oral: 1.5–2.5 hrs. Nasal: 3.3–3.5 hrs. IV: 0.4–4 hrs.

AVAILABILITY
Tablets (DDAVP): 0.1 mg, 0.2 mg.
Injection (DDAVP): 4 mcg/ml.

Nasal Solution (DDAVP): 100 mcg/ml.
Nasal Spray: 1.5 mg/ml (150 mcg/spray) (Stimate), 100 mcg/ml (10 mcg/spray) (DDAVP).

INDICATIONS AND DOSAGES
▶ **Primary nocturnal enuresis**
Intranasal
Children 6 yrs and older. Initially, 20 mcg (0.2 ml) at bedtime; use one half dose each nostril. Adjust up to 40 mcg.
PO
Children older than 12 yrs. 0.2–0.6 mg once before bedtime.
▶ **Central cranial diabetes insipidus**
PO
Adults, Elderly, Children 12 yrs and older. Initially, 0.05 mg 2 times/day. Range: 0.1–1.2 mg/day in 2–3 divided doses.
Children younger than 12 yrs. 0.05 mg initially, then 2 times/day. Range: 0.1–0.8 mg daily.
Intranasal
Adults, Elderly, Children older than 12 yrs. 5–40 mcg (0.05–0.4 ml) in 1–3 doses/day.
Children 3 mo–12 yrs. Initially, 5 mcg (0.05 ml)/day. Range: 5–30 mcg (0.05–0.3 ml)/day.
Subcutaneous/IV
Adults, Elderly, Children older than 12 yrs. 2–4 mcg/day in 2 divided doses or of maintenance intranasal dose.
▶ **Hemophilia A, Von Willebrand's Disease (Type I)**
IV infusion
Adults, Elderly, Children weighing 10 kg or more. 0.3 mcg/kg diluted in 50 ml 0.9% NaCl.
Children weighing less than 10 kg. 0.3 mcg/kg diluted in 10 ml 0.9% NaCl.
Intranasal
Adults, Elderly, Children 12 yrs and older weighing more than 50 kg.
300 mcg; use 1 spray each nostril.
Adults, Elderly, Children 12 yrs and older weighing less than 50 kg. 150 mcg as single spray.

CONTRAINDICATIONS
Hemophilia A with factor VIII levels less than 5% or hemophilia B, severe type I, type IIB, or platelet-type von Willebrand disease

INTERACTIONS
Drug
Carbamazepine, chlorpropamide, clofibrate: May increase the effects of desmopressin.
Demeclocycline, lithium, norepinephrine: May decrease effects of desmopressin.
Herbal
None known.
Food
None known.

DIAGNOSTIC TEST EFFECTS
None known.

IV INCOMPATIBILITIES
Information not available.

SIDE EFFECTS
Occasional
IV: Pain, redness, or swelling at injection site, headache, abdominal cramps, vulval pain, flushed skin, mild elevation of blood pressure (B/P), nausea with high dosages
Nasal: Rhinorrhea, nasal congestion, slight elevation of B/P

SERIOUS REACTIONS
• Water intoxication or hyponatremia, marked by headache, drowsiness, confusion, decreased urination, rapid weight gain, seizures, and coma, may occur in overhydration. Children, elderly, and infants are especially at risk.

NURSING CONSIDERATIONS

Baseline Assessment
• Establish the patient's baseline B/P, electrolytes, pulse, urine specific gravity, and weight.
• Plan to check the patient's lab values for factor VIII coagulant concentration for hemophilia A and von Willebrand's disease, and bleeding times.

Lifespan Considerations
• Use cautiously in neonates younger than 3 months as this age group is at an increased risk of fluid balance problems.
• Be aware that careful fluid restrictions are recommended in infants.
• Be aware that the elderly are at increased risk of hyponatremia and water intoxication.

Precautions
• Use cautiously in patients with conditions with fluid or electrolyte imbalance, coronary artery disease, hypertensive cardiovascular disease, and predisposition to thrombus formation.

Administration and Handling
Intranasal
• Refrigerate DDAVP nasal solution and Stimate nasal spray. Nasal solution and Stimate nasal spray are stable for 3 weeks at room temperature if unopened.
• Remember that DDAVP nasal spray is stable at room temperature.
• Draw up a measured quantity of desmopressin with a calibrated catheter (rhinyle). Insert one end in the patient's nose and have the patient blow on the other end to deposit the solution deep in the nasal cavity. For infants, young children, obtunded patients, an air-filled syringe may be attached to the catheter to deposit the solution.

Subcutaneous
• Estimate therapeutic response by adequacy of sleep duration.
• Plan to adjust morning and evening doses separately.
IV
• Refrigerate. Know that the drug is stable for 2 weeks at room temperature.
• For IV infusion, dilute in 10 to 50 ml 0.9% NaCl.
• Prepare to infuse over 15 to 30 minutes.
• For preoperative use, administer 30 minutes before procedure, as prescribed.
• Monitor the patient's blood pressure (B/P) and pulse during IV infusion.
• Remember that the IV dose is one tenth the intranasal dose.

Intervention and Evaluation
• Check the patient's B/P and pulse with IV infusion.
• Monitor for signs of diabetes insipidus, as well as the patient's serum electrolytes, fluid intake, serum osmolality, urine volume, urine specific gravity, and body weight.
• Assess the patient's factor VIII antigen levels, APTT, and factor VIII activity level for hemophilia.

Patient Teaching
• Caution the patient to avoid overhydration.
• Teach the patient the proper technique for intranasal administration.
• Warn the patient to notify the physician if he or she experiences abdominal cramps, headache, heartburn, nausea, or shortness of breath.
• Tell the parent of a child treated for nocturnal enuresis to carefully monitor the child's sleeping pattern.

somatrem

soe-ma-trem
(Protropin)
Do not confuse with Proloprim, Protamine, Protopam, or somatropin.

CATEGORY AND SCHEDULE
Pregnancy Risk Category: C

MECHANISM OF ACTION
A polypeptide hormone that increases the number, size of muscle cells; increases red blood cell (RBC) mass. Affects carbohydrate metabolism by antagonizing action of insulin, increasing the mobilization of fats, and increasing cellular protein synthesis. *Therapeutic Effect:* Stimulates linear growth.

AVAILABILITY
Powder for Injection: 5 mg, 10 mg.

INDICATIONS AND DOSAGES
▸ **Long-term treatment of children who have growth failure due to endogenous growth hormone deficiency**
IM/Subcutaneous
Children. Up to 0.1 mg/kg (0.26 IU/kg) 3 times/wk.

CONTRAINDICATIONS
None known

INTERACTIONS
Drug
Corticosteroids: May inhibit growth response.
Herbal
None known.
Food
None known.

DIAGNOSTIC TEST EFFECTS
May increase serum parathyroid hormone levels, serum alkaline phosphatase, and inorganic phosphorus levels.

SIDE EFFECTS
Frequent (30%)
Persistent antibodies to growth hormone, but generally does not cause failure to respond to somatrem
Occasional
Headache, muscle pain, weakness, mild hyperglycemia, allergic reaction, including rash and itching, pain and swelling at injection site, pain in hip or knee

NURSING CONSIDERATIONS
Baseline Assessment
• Establish the patient's baseline blood glucose levels and thyroid function studies.
Precautions
• Use cautiously in patients with diabetes mellitus, malignancy, and untreated hypothyroidism.
Intervention and Evaluation
• Monitor the patient's blood glucose levels, bone age, growth rate, parathyroid, phosphorus, renal function, serum calcium, and thyroid function studies.
Patient Teaching
• Instruct the patient or caregiver in the correct reconstitution procedure for IM/Subcutaneous administration.
• Teach the patient or caregiver the safe handling and disposal of needles.
• Stress to the patient or caregiver the importance of regular follow-up appointments with physician.

somatropin
soe-mah-**troe**-pin
(Humatrope, Norditropin, Nutropin, Nutropin AQ, Nutropin Depot)
Do not confuse with somatrem or sumatriptan.

CATEGORY AND SCHEDULE
Pregnancy Risk Category: C

MECHANISM OF ACTION
A polypeptide hormone that increases the number, size of muscle cells; increases red blood cell (RBC) mass. Affects carbohydrate metabolism by antagonizing action of insulin, increasing the mobilization of fats, and increasing cellular protein synthesis. *Therapeutic Effect:* Stimulates linear growth.

AVAILABILITY
Injection: 4 mg, 5 mg, 8 mg, 10 mg.
Injection (Depot): 13.5 mg, 18 mg, 22.5 mg.

INDICATIONS AND DOSAGES
▸ **Growth hormone deficiency**
IM/Subcutaneous
Children. Up to 0.06 mg/kg 3 times/wk (Humatrope).
Subcutaneous
Adults. 0.04 mg/kg/wk in 6–7 injections/wk. Maximum: 0.08 mg/kg/wk.
Children. 0.3 mg/kg/wk (Nutropin), 1.5 mg/kg/mo or 0.75 mg/kg 2 times/mo (Nutropin Depot).
▸ **Chronic renal insufficiency**
Subcutaneous
Children. 0.35 mg/kg/wk (Nutropin).
▸ **Turner's syndrome**
Subcutaneous
Children. 0.375 mg/kg/wk divided into 3–7 equal doses/wk.

▸ **AIDS-wasting syndrome**
Subcutaneous
Adults. 4–6 mg at bedtime.

CONTRAINDICATIONS
None known

INTERACTIONS
Drug
Corticosteroids: May inhibit growth response.
Herbal
None known.
Food
None known.

DIAGNOSTIC TEST EFFECTS
May increase serum parathyroid hormone levels, serum alkaline phosphatase and inorganic phosphorus levels.

SIDE EFFECTS
Frequent
Development of persistent antibodies to growth hormone, generally does not cause failure to respond to somatropin; hypercalciuria during first 2–3 mos of therapy
Occasional
Headache, muscle pain, weakness, mild hyperglycemia, allergic reaction, including rash and itching, pain or swelling at injection site, pain in hip or knee

NURSING CONSIDERATIONS
Baseline Assessment
• Establish the patient's baseline blood glucose levels and thyroid function studies.
Precautions
• Use cautiously in patients with diabetes mellitus, malignancy, and untreated hypothyroidism.
Intervention and Evaluation
• Monitor the patient's blood glu-

cose levels, bone age, growth rate, parathyroid, phosphorus, renal function, serum calcium, and thyroid function studies.
• Observe the HIV positive patient for decreased wasting.
Patient Teaching
• Instruct the patient or caregiver in the correct reconstitution procedure and injection technique for IM or subcutaneous administration.
• Teach the patient or caregiver the safe handling and disposal of needles.
• Stress to the patient or caregiver the importance of regular follow-up appointments with physician.

vasopressin
vay-sew-**press**-in
(Pitressin, Pressyn[CAN])

CATEGORY AND SCHEDULE
Pregnancy Risk Category: B

MECHANISM OF ACTION
A posterior pituitary hormone that increases reabsorption of water by the renal tubules. Directly stimulates smooth muscle in the gastrointestinal (GI) tract. *Therapeutic Effect:* Increases water permeability at the distal tubule and collecting duct decreasing urine volume. Causes peristalsis. Causes vasoconstriction.

PHARMACOKINETICS

Route	Onset	Peak	Duration
IM/Subcutaneous	1–2 hrs	N/A	2–8 hrs
IV	N/A	N/A	0.5–1 hr

Distributed throughout extracellular fluid. Metabolized in liver, kidney.

Primarily excreted in urine. **Half-life:** 10–20 min.

AVAILABILITY
Injection: 20 units/ml.

INDICATIONS AND DOSAGES
▸ **Cardiac arrest**
IV
Adults, Elderly. 40 units as a one-time bolus dose.
▸ **Diabetes insipidus**
IM/Subcutaneous
Adults, Elderly. 5–10 units, 2–4 times/day. Range: 5–60 units/day.
Children. 2.5–10 units, 2–4 times/day.
IV infusion
Adults, Children. 0.5 mUnits/kg/hr. May double dose q30min. Maximum: 10 mUnits/kg/hr.
▸ **Abdominal distention**
IM
Adults, Elderly. Initially, 5 units. Subsequent doses of 10 units q3–4h.
▸ **GI hemorrhage**
IV infusion
Adults, Elderly. Initially, 0.2–0.4 units/min progressively increased to 0.9 units/min.
Children. 0.002–0.005 units/kg/min. Titrate as needed. Maximum: 0.01 units/kg/min.

UNLABELED USES
Adjunct in treatment of acute, massive hemorrhage

CONTRAINDICATIONS
None known

INTERACTIONS
Drug
Carbamazepine, chlorpropamide, clofibrate: May increase the effects of vasopressin.
Demeclocycline, lithium, nor-

epinephrine: May decrease the effects of vasopressin.

Herbal
None known.

Food
None known.

DIAGNOSTIC TEST EFFECTS
None known.

IV INCOMPATIBILITIES
Amphotericin B complex (Abelcet, AmBisome, Amphotec), diazepam (Valium), etomidate (Amidate), furosemide (Lasix), thiopentothal

IV COMPATIBILITIES
Dobutamine (Dobutrex), dopamine (Intropin), heparin, lorazepam (Ativan), midazolam (Versed), milrinone (Primacor), verapamil (Calan, Isoptin)

SIDE EFFECTS
Frequent
Pain at injection site with vasopressin tannate
Occasional
Stomach cramps, nausea, vomiting, diarrhea, dizziness, diaphoresis, paleness, circumoral pallor, trembling, headache, eructation, flatulence
Rare
Chest pain, confusion
Allergic reaction: Rash or hives; pruritus; wheezing or difficulty breathing; swelling of face and extremities. Sterile abscess with vasopressin tannate.

SERIOUS REACTIONS
• Anaphylaxis, myocardial infarction (MI), and water intoxication have occurred.
• The elderly and very young are at higher risk for water intoxication.

NURSING CONSIDERATIONS

Baseline Assessment
• Establish the patient's baselines for blood pressure (B/P), serum electrolyte levels, pulse, urine specific gravity, and weight.

Lifespan Considerations
• Be aware that vasopressin should be used cautiously in breast-feeding women.
• Be aware that vasopressin should be used cautiously in children and the elderly due to the risk of water intoxication and hyponatremia.

Precautions
• Use cautiously in patients with arteriosclerosis, asthma, cardiac disease, goiter with cardiac complications, migraine, nephritis, renal disease, seizures, and vascular disease.

Administration and Handling
◀ALERT▶ May administer intranasally on cotton pledgets, by nasal spray; individualize dosage.
Subcutaneous/IM
• Give with 1 to 2 glasses of water to reduce side effects.
IV
• Store at room temperature.
• Dilute with D_5W or 0.9% NaCl to concentration of 0.1 to 1 unit/ml.
• Give as IV infusion.

Intervention and Evaluation
• Monitor the patient's fluid intake and output closely, and restrict the patient's intake as ordered, to prevent water intoxication.
• Weigh the patient daily, if indicated.
• Check the patient's B/P and pulse 2 times a day.
• Monitor the patient's serum electrolyte levels and urine specific gravity.
• Evaluate the patient's injection site for abscess, erythema, and pain.

• Report side effects experienced by the patient to the physician for dose reduction.
• Be alert for early signs of water intoxication, such as drowsiness, headache, and listlessness.
• Withhold the medication, as prescribed, and report immediately if the patient experiences any allergic symptoms or chest pain.

Patient Teaching
• Warn the patient to notify the physician if he or she experiences any chest pain, headache, shortness of breath, or other symptoms.
• Stress to the patient the importance of monitoring his or her fluid intake and output.
• Urge the patient to avoid alcohol during vasopressin therapy.

HORMONAL AGENTS

levothyroxine
liothyronine
methimazole
propylthiouracil

Uses: Two *thyroid hormones*—levothyroxine and liothyronine—are used to treat primary or secondary hypothyroidism, myxedema, cretinism, or simple goiter. Levothyroxine is also used in thyroid cancer management. Levothyroxine and liothyronine are used in thyroid suppression tests.

Propylthiouracil and *methimazole* are used to treat hyperthyroidism, especially before thyroid surgery or radioactive iodine therapy.

Action: *Thyroid hormones* are essential for normal growth, development, and energy metabolism. They promote growth and development by controlling deoxyribonucleic acid transcription and protein synthesis, which are required for nervous system development. These agents stimulate energy use by increasing the basal metabolic rate, which increases oxygen consumption and heat production. They also act as cardiac stimulants by increasing the heart rate, force of cardiac contractions, and cardiac output.

Propylthiouracil blocks the oxidation of iodine in the thyroid gland, thereby preventing the synthesis of thyroid hormones.

COMBINATION PRODUCTS

THYROLAR: levothyroxine/liothyronine 12.5 mcg/3.1 mcg; 25 mcg/6.25 mcg; 50 mcg/12.5 mcg; 100 mcg/25 mcg; 150 mcg/37.5 mcg.

levothyroxine
lee-voe-thye-**rox**-een
(Droxine[AUS], Eltroxin[CAN], Levothroid, Levoxyl, Novothyrox[CAN], Oroxine[AUS], Synthroid, Unithroid)
Do not confuse with liothyronine.

CATEGORY AND SCHEDULE
Pregnancy Risk Category: A

MECHANISM OF ACTION
A synthetic isomer of thyroxine involved in normal metabolism, growth, and development, especially the central nervous system (CNS) of infants. Possesses catabolic and anabolic effects. *Therapeutic Effect:* Increases basal metabolic rate, enhances gluconeogenesis, stimulates protein synthesis.

PHARMACOKINETICS
Variable, incomplete absorption from the gastrointestinal (GI) tract. Protein binding: greater than 99%. Widely distributed. Deiodinated in peripheral tissues, minimal metabolism in liver. Eliminated by biliary excretion. **Half-life:** 6–7 days.

AVAILABILITY

Tablets: 0.025 mg, 0.05 mg, 0.075 mg, 0.088 mg, 0.1 mg, 0.112 mg, 0.125 mg, 0.137 mg, 0.15 mg, 0.175 mg, 0.2 mg, 0.3 mg.
Injection: 200 mcg, 500 mcg.

INDICATIONS AND DOSAGES
▸ **Hypothyroidism**
PO

Adults, Elderly. Initially, 12.5–50 mcg. May increase by 25–50 mcg/day q2–4wks. Maintenance: 100–200 mcg/day.
Children older than 12 yrs. 150 mcg/day.
Children 6–12 yrs. 100–125 mcg/day.
Children older than 1–5 yrs. 75–100 mcg/day.
Children older than 6–12 mos. 50–75 mcg/day.
Children older than 3–6 mos. 25–50 mcg/day.
Children 3 mos. and younger. 10–15 mcg/day.
▸ **Myxedema coma or stupor (medical emergency)**
IV

Adults, Elderly. 200–500 mcg once, then 75–300 mcg/day
▸ **Thyroid suppression therapy**
PO

Adults, Elderly. 2–6 mcg/kg/day for 7–10 days.
▸ **Thyroid stimulating hormone (TSH) suppression in thyroid cancer, nodules, euthyroid goiters**
PO

Adults, Elderly. 2–6 mcg/kg/day for 7–10 days.
IV

Adults, Elderly, Children. Initial dosage approximately half the previously established oral dosage.

CONTRAINDICATIONS
Hypersensitivity to any component of tablets, such as tartrazine, allergy to aspirin, lactose intolerance, myocardial infarction (MI) and thyrotoxicosis uncomplicated by hypothyroidism, treatment of obesity

INTERACTIONS
Drug

Cholestyramine, colestipol: May decrease the absorption of levothyroxine.
Oral anticoagulants: May alter the effects of oral anticoagulants
Sympathomimetics: May increase the effects and coronary insufficiency of levothyroxine.
Herbal
None known.
Food
None known.

DIAGNOSTIC TEST EFFECTS
None known.

IV INCOMPATIBILITIES
Do not use or mix with other IV solutions.

SIDE EFFECTS
Occasional
Children may have reversible hair loss upon initiation
Rare
Dry skin, GI intolerance, skin rash, hives, pseudotumor cerebri or severe headache in children

SERIOUS REACTIONS
• Excessive dosage produces signs and symptoms of hyperthyroidism including weight loss, palpitations, increased appetite, tremors, nervousness, tachycardia, hypertension, headache, insomnia, and menstrual irregularities.
• Cardiac arrhythmias occur rarely.

NURSING CONSIDERATIONS

Baseline Assessment
• Determine if the patient is hypersensitive to aspirin, lactose, and tartrazine.
• Obtain the patient's baseline weight and vital signs.
• Know that the signs and symptoms of adrenal insufficiency, diabetes insipidus, diabetes mellitus, and hypopituitarism may become intensified.
• Treat the patient with adrenocortical steroids, as prescribed, before thyroid therapy in coexisting hypoadrenalism and hypothyroidism.

Lifespan Considerations
• Be aware that levothyroxine does not cross the placenta and is minimally excreted in breast milk.
• There are no age-related precautions noted in children.
• Be aware that levothyroxine should be used cautiously in neonates in interpreting thyroid function tests.
• Be aware that the elderly may be more sensitive to thyroid effects. Individualized dosages are recommended for this patient population.

Precautions
• Use cautiously in elderly patients and patients with angina pectoris, hypertension, or other cardiovascular disease.

Administration and Handling
◄ALERT► Do not interchange brands because there have been problems with bioequivalence between manufacturers.
◄ALERT► Begin therapy with small doses and increase the dosage gradually, as prescribed.

PO
• Give at same time each day to maintain hormone levels.
• Administer before breakfast to prevent insomnia.
• Crush tablets as needed

IV
• Store vials at room temperature.
• Reconstitute 200-mcg or 500-mcg vial with 5 ml 0.9% NaCl to provide a concentration of 40 or 100 mcg/ml, respectively; shake until clear.
• Use immediately, and discard unused portions.
• Give each 100 mcg or less over 1 minute.

Intervention and Evaluation
• Monitor the patient's pulse for rate and rhythm. Report a marked increase in pulse rate or one that exceeds of 100 beats per minute (bpm).
• Assess the patient for nervousness and tremors.
• Evaluate the patient's appetite and sleep pattern.

Patient Teaching
• Caution the patient against discontinuing the drug. Explain to the patient that replacement for hypothyroidism is life-long.
• Stress to the patient that follow-up office visits and thyroid function tests are essential.
• Instruct the patient to take the drug at the same time each day, preferably in the morning.
• Teach the patient to monitor his or her pulse, and advise the patient to notify the physician if there is a change in rhythm, a marked increase in rate, or a pulse of 100 beats or more.
• Instruct the patient not to change brands of the drug.
• Warn the patient to notify the physician promptly if he or she experiences chest pain, insomnia, nervousness, tremors, or weight loss.
• Tell the pediatric patient and his or her caregiver that children may have reversible hair loss or increased aggressiveness during the first few months of therapy.
• Warn the patient that the full therapeutic effect of the drug may take 1 to 3 weeks to appear.

liothyronine

lye-oh-**thigh**-roe-neen
(Cytomel, Tertroxin[AUS],
Triostat)
**Do not confuse with
levothyroxine.**

CATEGORY AND SCHEDULE
Pregnancy Risk Category: A

MECHANISM OF ACTION
A synthetic form thyroid hormone
T_3 involved in normal metabolism,
growth, and development, especially
the central nervous system (CNS) of
infants. Possesses catabolic and
anabolic effects. *Therapeutic Effect:*
Increases basal metabolic rate,
enhances gluconeogenesis, stimulates protein synthesis.

AVAILABILITY
Tablets: 5 mcg, 25 mcg, 50 mcg.
Injection: 10 mcg/ml.

INDICATIONS AND DOSAGES
▸ **Hypothyroidism**
PO
Adults, Elderly. Initially, 25 mcg/
day. May increase in 12.5–25 mcg/
day increments q1–2wks. Maximum
100 mcg/day.
Children. Initially, 5 mcg/day. May
increase by 5 mcg/day q3–4wks.
Maintenance: *Infants.* 20 mcg/day.
Children 1–3 yrs. 50 mcg/day.
Children older than 3 yrs. 100 mcg/
day.
▸ **Myxedema**
PO
Adults, Elderly. Initially, 5 mcg/day.
Increase by 5–10 mcg q1–2wks
(after 25 mcg/day reached, may
increase by 12.5-mcg increments).
Maintenance: 50–100 mcg/day.

▸ **Nontoxic goiter**
PO
Adults, Elderly. Initially, 5 mcg/day.
Increase by 5–10 mcg/day
q1–2wks. When 25 mcg/day ob-
tained, may increase by
12.5–25 mcg/day q1–2wks.
Maintenance: 75 mcg/day.
Children. 5 mcg/day. May increase
by 5 mcg q1–2wks. Maintenance:
15–20 mcg/day.
▸ **Congenital hypothyroidism**
PO
Children. Initially, 5 mcg/day.
Increase by 5 mcg/day q3–4 days.
Maintenance: *Infants.* 20 mcg/day.
Children 1–3 yrs. 50 mcg/day.
Children older than 3 yrs. Full adult
dosage.
▸ **T_3 suppression test**
PO
Adults, Elderly. 75–100 mcg/day for
7 days, then repeat I^{131} thyroid
uptake test.
▸ **Myxedema coma, precoma**
IV
Adults, Elderly. Initially, 25–50 mcg
(10–20 mcg in patients with cardio-
vascular disease). Total dose at least
65 mcg/day.

CONTRAINDICATIONS
Myocardial infarction (MI) and
thyrotoxicosis uncomplicated by
hypothyroidism, treatment of obesity

INTERACTIONS
Drug
Cholestyramine, colestipol: May
decrease the absorption of liothyronine.
Oral anticoagulants: May alter the
effects of these drugs.
Sympathomimetics: May increase
the effects and coronary insufficiency of liothyronine.
Herbal
None known.

Food
None known.

DIAGNOSTIC TEST EFFECTS
None known.

SIDE EFFECTS
Occasional
Children may have reversible hair loss upon initiation
Rare
Dry skin, gastrointestinal (GI) intolerance, skin rash, hives, pseudotumor cerebri or severe headache in children

SERIOUS REACTIONS
• Excessive dosage produces signs and symptoms of hyperthyroidism including weight loss, palpitations, increased appetite, tremors, nervousness, tachycardia, increased blood pressure (B/P), headache, insomnia, and menstrual irregularities.
• Cardiac arrhythmias occur rarely.

NURSING CONSIDERATIONS
Baseline Assessment
• Determine if the patient is hypersensitive to aspirin and tartrazine.
• Obtain the patient's baseline weight and vital signs.
• Know that the signs and symptoms of adrenal insufficiency, diabetes insipidus, diabetes mellitus, and hypopituitarism may become intensified.
• Treat the patient with adrenocortical steroids before thyroid therapy in coexisting hypoadrenalism and hypothyroidism.
Precautions
• Use cautiously in patients with adrenal insufficiency, cardiovascular disease, coronary artery disease, diabetes insipidus, and diabetes mellitus.

Administration and Handling
◀ALERT▶ Initial and subsequent dosage based on patient's clinical status, response. Administer IV dose over 4 hours but no longer than 12 hours apart.
Intervention and Evaluation
• Monitor the patient's pulse for rate and rhythm (report pulse of 100 or marked increase).
• Assess the patient for nervousness and tremors.
• Evaluate the patient's appetite and sleep pattern.
Patient Teaching
• Caution the patient against discontinuing the drug. Explain to the patient that replacement for hypothyroidism is life-long.
• Stress to the patient that follow-up office visits and thyroid function tests are essential.
• Instruct the patient to take the drug at the same time each day, preferably in the morning.
• Teach the patient to monitor his or her pulse and advise the patient to notify the physician if there is a change in rhythm, a marked increase in rate, or a pulse of 100 beats or more.
• Tell the patient not to change brands of the drug.
• Warn the patient to notify the physician promptly if he or she experiences chest pain, insomnia, nervousness, tremors, or weight loss.
• Explain to the pediatric patient and his or her caregiver that children may have reversible hair loss or increased aggressiveness during the first few months of therapy.

methimazole
meth-**im**-ah-zole
(Tapazole)

CATEGORY AND SCHEDULE
Pregnancy Risk Category: D

MECHANISM OF ACTION
A thiomidazole derivative that inhibits synthesis of thyroid hormone by interfering with incorporation of iodine into tyrosyl residues. *Therapeutic Effect:* Effective in the treatment of hyperthyroidism.

AVAILABILITY
Tablets: 5 mg, 10 mg.

INDICATIONS AND DOSAGES
▶ **Hyperthyroidism**
PO
Adults, Elderly. Initially, 15–60 mg/day in 3 divided doses. Maintenance: 5–15 mg/day.
Children. Initially, 0.4 mg/kg/day in 3 divided doses. Maintenance: One-half the initial dose.

CONTRAINDICATIONS
None known

INTERACTIONS
Drug
Amiodarone, iodinated glycerol, iodine, potassium iodide: May decrease response.
Digoxin: May increase the blood concentration of digoxin as patient becomes euthyroid.
I^{131}: May decrease thyroid uptake of I^{131}.
Oral anticoagulants: May decrease the effects of oral anticoagulants.
Herbal
None known.
Food
None known.

DIAGNOSTIC TEST EFFECTS
May increase LDH concentrations, prothrombin time, serum alkaline phosphatase, bilirubin, SGOT (AST), and SGPT (ALT) levels. May decrease prothrombin level, white blood cell (WBC) count.

SIDE EFFECTS
Frequent (5%–4%)
Fever, rash, pruritus
Occasional (3%–1%)
Dizziness, loss of taste, nausea, vomiting, stomach pain, peripheral neuropathy or numbness in fingers, toes, face
Rare (less than 1%)
Swollen lymph nodes or salivary glands

SERIOUS REACTIONS
• Agranulocytosis, which may occur as long as 4 mos after therapy, pancytopenia, and hepatitis have occurred.

NURSING CONSIDERATIONS
Baseline Assessment
• Obtain the patient's baseline pulse and weight.
• Expect to perform baseline thyroid function studies.
Precautions
• Use cautiously in patients older than 40 years of age, in patients taking methimazole in combination with other agranulocytosis-inducing drugs, and in patients with impaired liver function.
Intervention and Evaluation
• Monitor the patient's pulse and weight daily.
• Assess the patient's skin for rash, pruritus, and swollen lymph glands.
• Monitor the patient's complete blood count (CBC), prothrombin time, and serum hepatic enzymes.

- Evaluate the patient for signs and symptoms of bleeding and infection.

Patient Teaching

- Caution the patient against exceeding the ordered dose.
- Instruct the patient to space drug doses evenly around the clock.
- Teach the patient to take his or her resting pulse daily to monitor therapeutic results.
- Urge the patient to restrict his or her consumption of iodine products and seafood.
- Warn the patient to notify the physician immediately if he or she experiences illness and unusual bleeding or bruising.

propylthiouracil
pro-pill-thye-oh-**your**-ah-sill
(Propylthiouracil, Propyl-Thyracil[CAN])

CATEGORY AND SCHEDULE
Pregnancy Risk Category: D

MECHANISM OF ACTION
A thiourea derivative that blocks oxidation of iodine in the thyroid gland, blocks synthesis the thyroxine and triiodothyronine. *Therapeutic Effect:* Inhibits synthesis of thyroid hormone.

AVAILABILITY
Tablets: 50 mg.

INDICATIONS AND DOSAGES
▸ **Hyperthyroidism**
PO
Adults, Elderly. Initially: 300–450 mg/day in divided doses q8h. Maintenance: 100–150 mg/day in divided doses q8–12h.
Children. Initially: 5–7 mg/kg/day in divided doses q8h. Maintenance:

1/3 to 2/3 of initial dose in divided doses q8–12h.
Neonates. 5–10 mg/kg/day in divided doses q8h.

CONTRAINDICATIONS
None known

INTERACTIONS
Drug
Amiodarone, iodinated glycerol, iodine, potassium iodide: May decrease response.
Digoxin: May increase the blood concentration of this drug as patient becomes euthyroid.
I^{131}: May decrease thyroid uptake of I^{131}.
Oral anticoagulants: May decrease the effects of oral anticoagulants.
Herbal
None known.
Food
None known.

DIAGNOSTIC TEST EFFECTS
May increase LDH concentrations, prothrombin time, serum alkaline phosphatase, bilirubin, SGOT (AST), and SGPT (ALT) levels.

SIDE EFFECTS
Frequent
Urticaria, rash, pruritus, nausea, skin pigmentation, hair loss, headache, paresthesia
Occasional
Drowsiness, lymphadenopathy, vertigo
Rare
Drug fever, lupus-like syndrome

SERIOUS REACTIONS
- Agranulocytosis may occur as long as 4 mos after therapy; pancytopenia and fatal hepatitis have occurred.

NURSING CONSIDERATIONS

Baseline Assessment
• Obtain the patient's baseline pulse and weight.
• Expect to obtain baseline lab tests, including LDH concentrations, prothrombin time, serum alkaline phosphatase, bilirubin, SGOT (AST), and SGPT (ALT) levels.

Precautions
• Use cautiously in patients older than 40 years of age, in patients taking methimazole in combination with other agranulocytosis-inducing drugs.

Intervention and Evaluation
• Monitor the patient's pulse and weight daily.
• Assess the patient's skin for eruptions, itching, and swollen lymph glands.
• Monitor the patient's hematology results for bone marrow suppression.
• Be alert to signs and symptoms of hepatitis including drowsiness, jaundice, nausea, and vomiting.
• Evaluate the patient for signs and symptoms of bleeding and infection.

Patient Teaching
• Instruct the patient to space drug doses evenly around the clock.
• Teach the patient to take his or her resting pulse daily to monitor therapeutic results.
• Urge the patient to restrict his or her consumption of iodine products and seafood.
• Warn the patient to notify the physician immediately if he or she experiences cold intolerance, depression, or weight gain.

agalsidase beta
calcitonin
dutasteride
finasteride
glucagon
  hydrochloride
imiglucerase
laronidase
miglustat
octreotide acetate
pegvisomant
raloxifene
teriparatide acetate
testosterone,
  testosterone
  cypionate,
  testosterone
  enanthate,
  testosterone
  propionate,
  testosterone
  transdermal

Uses: Miscellaneous hormonal agents have a wide variety of indications. *Agalsidase beta* is an enzyme used to treat Fabry disease, an X-linked genetic disorder. *Calcitonin* is used to treat Paget's disease, osteoporosis in postmenopausal women, and (as an adjunct) hypercalcemia. *Dutasteride* and *finasteride* are prescribed to treat benign prostatic hyperplasia (BPH). *Glucagon* is used as treatment of severe hypoglycemia in diabetic patients and as an aid in x-rays of the gastrointestinal (GI) tract. *Imiglucerase* and *miglustat* are helpful in managing Gaucher's disease. *Laronidase* is used to improve pulmonary function and walking capacity in patients with Hurler and Hurler-Scheie forms of mucopolysaccharidosis I (MPS I) and for patients with the Scheie form who have moderate to severe symptoms. *Octreotide* is prescribed to control the symptoms of metastatic carcinoid tumors, vasoactive intestinal peptic-secreting tumors, secretory diarrhea, and acromegaly. *Pegvisomant* is used to normalize the serum level of insulin-like growth factor-I (IGF-I) in patients with acromegaly who've had an inadequate response to surgery or radiation therapy or other medical treatments. *Raloxifene* is used to prevent and treat osteoporosis in postmenopausal women: *teriparatide* is indicated to treat osteoporosis in anyone at high risk for fractures. *Testosterone* is used to treat male hypogonadism, delayed male puberty, and inoperable breast cancer.

Action: Because miscellaneous hormonal agents belong to different subclasses, their actions vary widely. *Agalsidase beta* provides an exogenous source of alpha-galactosidase A, an enzyme missing in patients with Fabry disease. This drug catalyzes the hydrolysis of glycosphingolipid, reducing deposits in the capillary endothelium of kidney and other cells. *Calcitonin* decreases osteoclast activity, decreases sodium and calcium reabsorption in the kidneys, and increases calcium absorption in the GI tract. *Dutasteride* and *finasteride* inhibit the enzyme that converts testosterone into dihydrotestosterone (DHT) in the prostate gland, which reduces the serum DHT level. *Glucagon* promotes hepatic glycogenolysis and gluconeogenesis. *Imiglucerase* catalyzes the hydrolysis of glycolipid glucocerebrosidase to glucose and ceramide. *Miglustat* reduces the formation of glucosylceramide, which isn't broken down effectively in patients with Gaucher's disease. *Laronidase* provides exogenous lysosomal enzymes, which are needed for catabolism of glycosaminoglycans. *Octreotide* suppresses the secretion of serotonin and gastroenteropancreatic peptides, which enhances fluid and electrolyte absorption from the GI tract. *Pegvisomant* selectively binds to growth hormone (GH) receptors on cell surfaces, where it blocks the binding and action of endogenous GH and decreases the serum level of IGF-I and other GH-responsive serum proteins. *Raloxifene* affects some receptors as estrogen, thereby preventing bone loss. *Teriparatide* acts on bone to mobilize calcium and on the kidneys to decrease calcium clearance and increase phosphate excretion. *Testosterone* mimics the endogenous androgen, promoting the development of male sex organs and maintaining secondary sex characteristics in androgen-deficient men.

agalsidase beta
ah-**gull**-sigh-dase
(Fabrazyme)

CATEGORY AND SCHEDULE
Pregnancy Risk Category: B

MECHANISM OF ACTION
An enzyme that treats Fabry disease, an X-linked genetic disorder. Agalsidase beta catalyzes the hydrolysis of glycosphingolipid metabolism, reducing the deposits in capillary endothelium of the kidney and other cell types. *Therapeutic Effect:* Provides a exogenous source of alpha-galactosidase A, an enzyme, missing in those with Fabry disease.

AVAILABILITY
Powder for Injection: 37 mg (5 mg/ml when reconstituted).

INDICATIONS AND DOSAGES
▸ **Fabry disease**
IV infusion
Adults, Elderly. Give no more than 0.25 mg/min (15 mg/hr). May slow infusion rate if infusion-related reaction occurs. If no reaction,

infusion rate may be increased by increments of 0.05 to 0.08 mg/min (increments of 3 to 5 mg/hr).

CONTRAINDICATIONS
None known

INTERACTIONS
Drug
None known.
Herbal
None known.
Food
None known.

DIAGNOSTIC TEST EFFECTS
None known.

IV INCOMPATIBILITIES
Do not mix with any other medications.

SIDE EFFECTS
Expected infusion reaction (52%–45%)
Rigors, fever, headache
Frequent (38%–21%)
Rhinitis, nausea, anxiety, pharyngitis, edema, skeletal pain
Occasional (17%–14%)
Temperature change sensation, hypotension, pallor, paresthesia, pruritus, urticaria, bronchitis
Rare (10%–7%)
Bronchitis, depression, arthralgia, dyspepsia, including epigastric discomfort and heartburn, laryngitis, sinusitis

SERIOUS REACTIONS
• Frequently occurring serious infusion reactions include tachycardia, hypertension, throat tightness, chest pain, dyspnea, vomiting, lip edema, and rash.
• Other adverse events are characterized by bradycardia, arrhythmias, vertigo, nephritic syndrome, stroke, and cardiac arrest.

NURSING CONSIDERATIONS
Baseline Assessment
• Give antipyretics prior to IV infusion, as prescribed.
Precautions
• Use cautiously in febrile patients and patients with compromised cardiac function, moderate to severe hypertension, and renal impairment.
Administration and Handling
◀ALERT▶ Pretreat with antipyretics prior to infusion, as prescribed.
IV
• Store vials in refrigerator.
• Use reconstituted and diluted solution immediately; if this is not possible, solution is stable for 24 hours if refrigerated.
• Allow vial to reach room temperature before reconstitution, about 30 minutes.
• Reconstitute each vial by slowly injecting 7.2 ml sterile water for injection.
• Roll and tilt gently.
• Before adding reconstituted solution to 500 ml 0.9% NaCl, remove an equal volume from the 500 ml infusion bag, and then add to 500 ml 0.9% NaCl infusion bag.
• Administer at a rate of no more than 0.25 mg/minute (15 mg/hour). May slow infusion rate if infusion-related reaction occurs. If no reaction, infusion rate may be increased by increments of 0.05 to 0.08 mg/minute or increments of 3 to 5 mg/hour.
Intervention and Evaluation
• Monitor the patient for infusion reaction. Plan to decrease the infusion rate or temporarily stop the infusion if the patient experiences infusion reaction. As prescribed, give additional antipyretics, antihistamines, or steroids to alleviate these symptoms.

• Closely monitor patients with compromised cardiac function as these patients are at an increased risk of severe complications from infusion reactions.

Patient Teaching

• Tell the patient to let you know as soon as adverse reactions occur.

• Inform patients a registry has been established in order to better understand Fabry disease and to evaluate long-term treatment effects of agalsidase.

---

calcitonin
kal-sih-**toe**-nin
(Caltine[CAN], Miacalcin)

CATEGORY AND SCHEDULE
Pregnancy Risk Category: C

MECHANISM OF ACTION
A synthetic hormone that acts on bone to decrease osteoclast activity, decreases tubular reabsorption of sodium and calcium in kidneys, increases absorption of calcium in the gastrointestinal (GI) tract. *Therapeutic Effect:* Regulates serum calcium concentrations.

PHARMACOKINETICS
Injection: Rapidly metabolized (primarily in kidney). Primarily excreted in urine. **Half-life:** 70–90 min. Nasal: Rapid absorption. **Half-life:** 43 min.

AVAILABILITY
Injection: 200 units/ml.
Nasal Spray: 200 units/activation.

INDICATIONS AND DOSAGES
▸ **Skin testing**
Adults, Elderly. Prepare a 10 units/ml dilution; withdraw 0.05 ml from 200 units/ml vial solution in tuberculin syringe; fill up to 1 ml with 0.9% NaCl. Take 0.1 ml and inject intracutaneously on inner aspect of forearm. Observe after 15 min; a positive response is the appearance of more than mild erythema or wheal.

▸ **Paget's disease**
Subcutaneous/IM
Adults, Elderly. Initially, 100 units/day, improvement in biochemical abnormalities, bone pain seen in first few months; in neurologic lesion, often longer than 1 yr. Maintenance: 50 units/day or 50–100 units every other day.
Intranasal
Adults, Elderly. 200–400 units/day.

▸ **Osteoporosis imperfecta**
IM/Subcutaneous
Adults. 2 units/kg 3 times/wk.

▸ **Postmenopausal osteoporosis**
Subcutaneous/IM
Adults, Elderly. 100 units/day with adequate calcium and vitamin D intake.
Intranasal
Adults, Elderly. 200 units as single daily spray, alternating nostrils daily.

▸ **Hypercalcemia**
Subcutaneous/IM
Adults, Elderly. Initially, 4 units/kg q12h; may increase to 8 units/kg q12h if no response in 2 days; may further increase to 8 units/kg q6h if no response in 2 days.

UNLABELED USES
Treatment of secondary osteoporosis due to drug therapy or hormone disturbance

CONTRAINDICATIONS
Hypersensitivity to gelatin desserts and salmon protein

INTERACTIONS
Drug
None known.
Herbal
None known.
Food
None known.

DIAGNOSTIC TEST EFFECTS
None known.

SIDE EFFECTS
Frequent
Subcutaneous/IM (10%): Nausea may occur 30 min after injection, usually diminishes with continued therapy, inflammation at injection site
Nasal (12%–10%): Rhinitis, nasal irritation, redness, sores
Occasional
Subcutaneous/IM (5%–2%): Flushing of face or hands
Nasal (5%–3%): Back pain, arthralgia, epistaxis, headache
Rare
Subcutaneous/IM: Epigastric discomfort, dry mouth, diarrhea, flatulence
Nasal: Itching of earlobes, edema of feet, rash, increased sweating

SERIOUS REACTIONS
• Potential hypersensitivity reaction with protein allergy.

NURSING CONSIDERATIONS
Baseline Assessment
• Check the patient's baseline electrolyte levels.
• Perform a skin test on the patient before beginning calcitonin therapy in patients suspected of sensitivity to calcitonin.
Lifespan Considerations
• Be aware that calcitonin does not cross the placenta and it is unknown if the drug is distributed in breast milk.
• Be aware that calcitonin's safe usage during breast-feeding has not been established; the drug inhibits lactation in animals.
• Be aware the safety and efficacy of this drug have not been established in children.
• There are no age-related precautions noted in the elderly.
Precautions
• Use cautiously in patients with a history of allergy and renal dysfunction.
Administration and Handling
Intranasal
• Refrigerate. Nasal preparation can be stored at room temperature once pump is activated.
• Have the patient clear his or her nasal passages as much as possible.
• Tilt the patient's head slightly forward and insert spray tip into nostril, pointing toward nasal passages, away from nasal septum.
• Spray into the patient's nostril while holding other nostril closed and instruct the patient to concurrently inspire through nose to permit medication as high into nasal passage as possible.
IM/Subcutaneous
• May be administered subcutaneous or IM. No more than 2-ml dose should be given IM at any one site.
• Keep in mind that bedtime administration may reduce flushing and nausea.
Intervention and Evaluation
• Ensure rotation of injection sites. Check injection sites for inflammation.
• Assess the patient's vertebral bone mass and document its improvement or stabilization.
• Assess the patient for allergic response, hypotension, rash, short-

ness of breath, swelling, tachycardia, and urticaria.

Patient Teaching
- Instruct the patient and family on aseptic technique and proper injection of the medication, including rotation of injection sites.
- Tell the patient that nausea is transient, and usually decreases with continued therapy.
- Warn the patient to notify the physician immediately if he or she experiences itching, rash, shortness of breath, or significant nasal irritation.

dutasteride
do-tah-**stir**-eyed
(Avodart)

CATEGORY AND SCHEDULE
Pregnancy Risk Category: X

MECHANISM OF ACTION
An androgen hormone inhibitor that inhibits steroid 5-alpha reductase, an intracellular enzyme that converts testosterone into dihydrotestosterone (DHT) in the prostate gland, providing a reduction in serum DHT. *Therapeutic Effect:* Regresses enlarged prostate gland.

PHARMACOKINETICS

Route	Onset	Peak	Duration
PO	24 hrs	–	3–8 wks

Moderately absorbed after PO administration. Widely distributed. Protein binding: 99%. Metabolized in the liver. Primarily excreted via the feces. **Half-life:** Up to 5 wks.

AVAILABILITY
Tablets: 0.5 mg.

INDICATIONS AND DOSAGES
▸ **Benign prostatic hyperplasia (BPH)**
PO
Adults, Elderly. 0.5 mg once a day.

UNLABELED USES
Treatment of hair loss

CONTRAINDICATIONS
Females, physical handling of tablet in those who may become or are pregnant

INTERACTIONS
Drug
None known.
Herbal
None known.
Food
None known.

DIAGNOSTIC TEST EFFECTS
Produces decrease in serum prostate-specific antigen (PSA) levels

SIDE EFFECTS
Occasional
Gynecomastia, sexual dysfunction, including decreased libido, impotence, and ejaculatory disturbances

SERIOUS REACTIONS
- Toxicity manifested as rash, diarrhea, abdominal pain

NURSING CONSIDERATIONS
Baseline Assessment
- Expect to perform serum PSA determinations in those with BPH before therapy begins and periodically thereafter.

Administration and Handling
PO
• Do not crush or break film-coated tablets.
• Give dutasteride without regards to meals.
Precautions:
• Use cautiously in patients with impaired liver disease, preexisting sexual dysfunction, such as impotence and reduced male libido, and presence of obstructive uropathy.
Intervention and Evaluation
• Diligently monitor the patient's fluid intake and output.
• Assess the patient for signs and symptoms of BPH including hesitancy, post-void dribbling, reduced force of urinary stream, and sensation of incomplete bladder emptying.
Patient Teaching
• Discuss the potential for impotence with the patient. Explain that the volume of ejaculate may be decreased during treatment.
• Tell the patient that he may not notice improved urinary flow for up to 6 months after treatment.
• Warn the patient that women who may be or are pregnant should not handle dutasteride tablets. Explain that the drug is pregnancy risk category X.

finasteride
fin-**ah**-stir-eyd
(Propecia, Proscar)
Do not confuse with Posicor, ProSom, Prozac, or Psorcon.

CATEGORY AND SCHEDULE
Pregnancy Risk Category: X

MECHANISM OF ACTION
An androgen hormone inhibitor that inhibits steroid 5-alpha reductase, an intracellular enzyme that converts testosterone into dihydrotestosterone (DHT) in the prostate gland, providing a reduction in serum DHT. *Therapeutic Effect:* Regresses the enlarged prostate gland.

PHARMACOKINETICS

Route	Onset	Peak	Duration
PO	24 hrs	1–2 days	5–7 days

Protein binding: 90%. Rapidly absorbed from the gastrointestinal (GI) tract. Widely distributed. Metabolized in liver. **Half-life:** 6–8 hrs. Onset of clinical effect: 3–6 mos of continued therapy.

AVAILABILITY
Tablets: 1 mg, 5 mg.

INDICATIONS AND DOSAGES
▸ **Benign prostatic hypertrophy**
PO
Adults, Elderly. 5 mg once a day (minimum 6 mos).
▸ **Hair loss**
PO
Adults. 1 mg a day.

UNLABELED USES
Adjuvant monotherapy after radical prostatectomy in treatment of prostate cancer

CONTRAINDICATIONS
Exposure to semen in those who may become pregnant, physical handling of tablet in those who may become or are pregnant

INTERACTIONS
Drug
None known.
Herbal
None known.

Food
None known.

DIAGNOSTIC TEST EFFECTS
Produces decrease in serum prostate-specific antigen (PSA) levels even in presence of prostate cancer

SIDE EFFECTS
Rare (4%–2%)
Impotence, decreased libido, gynecomastia, decreased volume of ejaculate

SERIOUS REACTIONS
• None known.

NURSING CONSIDERATIONS
Baseline Assessment
• Expect to perform a digital rectal exam, and serum PSA determination in patients with BPH before beginning finasteride therapy and periodically thereafter.
• Plan to obtain hepatic enzyme levels before initiation of therapy.
Lifespan Considerations
• Be aware that physical handling of finasteride tablets should be avoided in females who may become or are pregnant. Finasteride may produce abnormalities of external genitalia of male fetus.
• Be aware that this drug is not indicated in children.
• Be aware that the efficacy of this drug has not been established in the elderly.
Precautions
• Use cautiously in patients with liver function impairment.
Administration and Handling
PO
• Do not break or crush film-coated tablets.
• Give finasteride without regard to meals.

Intervention and Evaluation
• Diligently monitor the patient's fluid intake and output, especially in patients with large residual urinary volume or severely diminished urinary flow for obstructive uropathy.
Patient Teaching
• Instruct the patient that the drug may, in rare cases, cause impotence.
• Explain to the patient that he may not notice improved urinary flow even if prostate gland shrinks.
• Stress to the patient that he needs to take the drug longer than 6 months.
• Explain to the patient that it is unknown if taking this drug decreases the need for surgery.
• Warn the patient that because of the potential risk to a male fetus, a woman who is or may become pregnant should not handle finasteride tablets or be exposed to his semen.
• Tell the patient that the volume of his ejaculate may decrease during treatment.

glucagon hydrochloride
glue-ka-gon
(Glucagen[AUS], Glucagon Emergency Kit)
Do not confuse with Glaucon.

CATEGORY AND SCHEDULE
Pregnancy Risk Category: B

MECHANISM OF ACTION
A glucose elevating agent that promotes hepatic glycogenolysis, gluconeogenesis. Stimulates enzyme to increase production of cyclic adenosine monophosphate (cAMP).

Therapeutic Effect: Increases plasma glucose concentration, relaxant effect on smooth muscle, and exerts inotropic myocardial effect.

AVAILABILITY
Powder for Injection: 1 mg.

INDICATIONS AND DOSAGES
▸ **Hypoglycemia**
Subcutaneous/IM/IV
Adults, Elderly, Children weighing greater than 20 kg. 0.5–1 mg. May repeat 1–2 additional doses if response is delayed.
Children weighing 20 kg or less. 0.5 mg.
▸ **Diagnostic aid**
IM/IV
Adults, Elderly. 0.25–2 mg.

UNLABELED USES
Esophageal obstruction due to foreign bodies, treatment of toxicity associated with beta-blockers, calcium channel blockers

CONTRAINDICATIONS
Hypersensitivity to glucagon protein, pheochromocytoma

INTERACTIONS
Drug
Anticoagulants: May increase the effects of these drugs.
Herbal
None known.
Food
None known.

DIAGNOSTIC TEST EFFECTS
May decrease serum potassium levels.

IV INCOMPATIBILITIES
Do not mix with any other medications.

SIDE EFFECTS
Occasional
Nausea, vomiting
Rare
Allergic reaction, such as urticaria, respiratory distress, and hypotension

SERIOUS REACTIONS
• Overdose may produce persistent nausea or vomiting, and hypokalemia, marked by severe weakness, decreased appetite, irregular heartbeat, and muscle cramps.

NURSING CONSIDERATIONS
Baseline Assessment
• Obtain an immediate assessment of the patient, including clinical signs and symptoms and history.
• Give glucagon immediately, as prescribed, if hypoglycemic coma is established.
Precautions
• Use cautiously in patients with history of insulinoma or pheochromocytoma.
Administration and Handling
◂**ALERT**▸ Place the patient on his or her side to avoid potential aspiration because glucagon, as well as hypoglycemia, may produce nausea and vomiting.
◂**ALERT**▸ Administer IV dextrose if the patient fails to respond to glucagon.
Subcutaneous/IM/IV
• Store vial at room temperature.
• Remember that after reconstitution, the solution is stable for 48 hours if refrigerated. If reconstituted with sterile water for injection, use immediately. Do not use glucagon solution unless clear.
• Reconstitute powder with manufacturer's diluent when preparing doses of 2 mg or less. For doses greater than 2 mg, dilute with Sterile Water for Injection.

• To provide 1 mg glucagon/ml, use 1 ml diluent. For 1-mg vial of glucagon, use 10 ml diluent for 10-mg vial.
• Patient will usually awaken in 5 to 20 minutes. Although 1–2 additional doses may be administered, the concern for effects of continuing cerebral hypoglycemia requires consideration of parenteral glucose.
• When the patient awakens, give supplemental carbohydrate to restore hepatic glycogen stores and prevent secondary hypoglycemia. If the patient fails to respond to glucagon, give IV glucose as prescribed.

Intervention and Evaluation
• Monitor the patient's response time carefully.
• Have IV dextrose readily available in the event the patient does not awaken within 5 to 20 minutes.
• Assess the patient for possible allergic reaction, including hypotension, respiratory difficulty, and urticaria.
• Give oral carbohydrates when the patient is conscious.

Patient Teaching
• Teach the patient to recognize the significance of identifying symptoms of hypoglycemia, including anxiety, diaphoresis, difficulty concentrating, headache, hunger, nausea, nervousness, pale and cool skin, shakiness, unconsciousness, unusual tiredness, and weakness.
• Instruct the patient, family, or friends to give sugar form first, such as hard candy, honey, orange juice, sugar cubes, or table sugar dissolved in water or juice, followed by a protein source, such as cheese and crackers or half a sandwich or glass of milk if symptoms of hypoglycemia develop.
• Urge the patient to wear a medical identification bracelet.

imiglucerase
im-ih-**gloo**-sir-ace
(Cerezyme)
Do not confuse with Cerebyx or Ceredase.

CATEGORY AND SCHEDULE
Pregnancy Risk Category: C

MECHANISM OF ACTION
An enzyme analogue of enzyme beta-glucocerebrosidase, which catalyzes hydrolysis of glycolipid glucocerebroside to glucose and ceramide. *Therapeutic Effect:* Minimizes conditions associated with Gaucher's disease, such as anemia and bone disease.

AVAILABILITY
Powder for Injection: 200 units, 424 units.

INDICATIONS AND DOSAGES
▸ **Gaucher's disease**
IV infusion (over 1–2 hrs)
Adults, Elderly, Children. Initially, 2.5 units/kg 3 times/wk up to 60 units/kg/wk. Maintenance: Progressive reduction in dosage while monitoring patient response.

CONTRAINDICATIONS
None known

INTERACTIONS
Drug
None known.
Herbal
None known.
Food
None known.

DIAGNOSTIC TEST EFFECTS
None known.

IV INCOMPATIBILITIES
Do not mix with any other medication.

SIDE EFFECTS
Frequent (3%)
Headache
Occasional (less than 3%–1%)
Nausea, abdominal discomfort, dizziness, pruritus, rash, small decrease in blood pressure (B/P) or urinary frequency

NURSING CONSIDERATIONS
Baseline Assessment
• Expect to perform baseline lab tests, including complete blood count (CBC), serum hepatic enzyme levels, and platelets.
Administration and Handling
IV
• Refrigerate.
• Once reconstituted, the solution is stable for 24 hours if refrigerated.
• Reconstitute with 5.1 ml sterile water to provide concentration of 40 units/ml.
• Further dilute with 100 to 200 ml 0.9% NaCl.
• Infuse over 1 to 2 hours.
Intervention and Evaluation
• Monitor the patient's complete blood count (CBC), hepatic enzymes, and platelets.
Patient Teaching
• Let the patient know about any required follow-up tests.
• Instruct the patient to tell you about any side effects, such as headache.

laronidase
lar-**on**-ih-dase
(Aldurazyme)

CATEGORY AND SCHEDULE
Pregnancy Risk Category: B

MECHANISM OF ACTION
An enzyme that increases the catabolism of glycosaminoglycans in those who are deficient of lysosomal enzymes required for glycosaminoglycan catabolism.
Therapeutic Effect: Prevents glycosaminoglycans from causing widespread cellular, tissue, and organ dysfunction.

AVAILABILITY
Injection: 2.9 mg/5 ml vial.

INDICATIONS AND DOSAGES
▸ **Mucopolysaccharidosis**
IV infusion
Adults, Elderly. 0.58 mg/kg once weekly.

CONTRAINDICATIONS
None known

INTERACTIONS
Drug
None known.
Herbal
None known.
Food
None known.

DIAGNOSTIC TEST EFFECTS
None known.

SIDE EFFECTS
Frequent (36%–18%)
Infusion related reactions, such as facial flushing, rash, fever, and headache
Occasional (9%)
Cough, bronchospasm, urticaria, pruritus, angioedema, dependent edema, hypotension, hyperreflexia

SERIOUS REACTIONS
• Upper respiratory tract infection occurs commonly.

• Anaphylactic reaction, such as angioedema, severe bronchospasm, and dyspnea, occurs rarely.

NURSING CONSIDERATIONS
Baseline Assessment
• Pre-treat the patient with antipyretics and antihistamines 60 minutes prior to starting the IV infusion.
Administration and Handling
• Refrigerate. Do not shake.
• Once reconstituted, use solution immediately. If this isn't possible, store the solution in the refrigerator no longer than 36 hours from the time of preparation to completion of administration.
• Pre-treat the patient with antipyretics and antihistamines, as prescribed, 60 minutes prior to the start of the IV infusion.
• Total volume of the infusion is determined by the patient's body weight. Patients with a body weight of 20 kg or less should receive a total volume of 100 ml. Patients with a body weight of more than 20 kg should receive a total volume of 250 ml.
• Dilute with 0.1% albumin (human) in 0.9% NaCl. Administer using a 0.2 micrometer filter.
• Begin initial infusion rate at 10 mcg/kg/hr, and increase incrementally every 15 minutes to 20 mcg/kg/hr, then 50 mcg/kg/hr, and then 100 mcg/kg/hr during the first hour, as prescribed.
• Give the remainder of the infusion at 200 mcg/kg/hr over 2 to 3 hours for a total infusion time of 3 to 4 hours.
Intervention and Evaluation
• Assess the patient's skin for evidence of facial flushing and rash.
• Monitor the patient carefully for infusion-related reactions. Slowing the infusion rate, temporarily stopping the infusion, or administering additional antipyretics and antihistamines will reduce or impede infusion related reactions.
Patient Teaching
• Tell the patient that a registry for patients with mucopolysaccharides has been established to monitor and evaluate treatments. Explain that information regarding the registry program can be obtained by his or her physician.
• Instruct the patient or the patient's parent to report side effects immediately.

miglustat
mig-**lew**-stat
(Zavesca)

CATEGORY AND SCHEDULE
Pregnancy Risk Category: X

MECHANISM OF ACTION
A Gaucher disease agent that inhibits the enzyme, glucosylceramide synthase, reducing the rate of synthesis of most glycosphingolipids. *Therapeutic Effect:* Allows the residual activity of the deficient enzyme, glucocerebrosidase, to be more effective in degrading lysosomal storage within tissue, minimizing conditions, such as anemia and bone disease, associated with Gaucher's disease.

AVAILABILITY
Capsules: 100 mg.

INDICATIONS AND DOSAGES
▸ **Gaucher's disease**
PO
Adults, Elderly. One 100 mg capsule three times/day at regular intervals.

▶ **Dosage in renal impairment**
Mild renal impairment, creatinine
clearance 50–70 ml/min
Adults, Elderly. 100 mg twice a day.
Moderate renal impairment, creati-
nine clearance 30–49 ml/min
Adults, Elderly. 100 mg a day.

CONTRAINDICATIONS
Women who are or may become
pregnant

INTERACTIONS
Drug
Imiglucerase: May decrease the
effects of imiglucerase.
Herbal
None known.
Food
None known.

DIAGNOSTIC TEST EFFECTS
None known.

SIDE EFFECTS
Expected (89%–65%)
Diarrhea, weight loss
Frequent (39%–11%)
Hand tremor, flatulence, headache,
abdominal pain, nausea
Occasional (7%–4%)
Paresthesia, anorexia, dyspepsia,
including heartburn and epigastric
distress, leg cramps, vomiting

SERIOUS REACTIONS
• Thrombocytopenia occurs in 7%
of patients.
• Overdose produces dizziness and
neutropenia

NURSING CONSIDERATIONS
Baseline Assessment
• Plan to perform a baseline neurological evaluation and with
follow-up neurological evaluations
at 6-month intervals throughout
treatment.

Precautions
• Use cautiously in patients with
fertility impairment and renal func-
tion impairment.
Administration and Handling
• Give miglustat without regard to
food.
• Do not open, crush, or break
capsule.
Intervention and Evaluation
• Encourage the patient to maintain
adequate fluid intake.
• Assess the patient's bowel sounds
for peristalsis.
• Assess the patient's daily pattern
of bowel activity and stool consistency.
• Weigh the patient weekly.
• Evaluate the patient for evidence
of hand tremor.
Patient Teaching
• Instruct the patient to avoid high
carbohydrate foods during miglustat
treatment if he or she experiences
diarrhea.
• Teach patients to maintain reliable
contraceptive methods during miglustat treatment.
• Warn the patient that he must notify the physician and plan to stop
miglustat therapy before trying to
conceive and maintain contraceptive
methods for 3 months thereafter.

octreotide acetate
ock-**tree**-oh-tide
(Sandostatin, Sandostatin LAR)
**Do not confuse with
OctreoScan, Sandimmune, or
Sandoglobulin.**

CATEGORY AND SCHEDULE
Pregnancy Risk Category: B

MECHANISM OF ACTION
A secretory inhibitory, growth hormone suppressant that suppresses secretion of serotonin, gastroentero-pancreatic peptides. Enhances fluid and electrolyte absorption from the gastrointestinal (GI) tract. *Therapeutic Effect:* Prolongs intestinal transit time.

PHARMACOKINETICS

Route	Onset	Peak	Duration
Subcutaneous	N/A	N/A	Up to 12 hrs

Rapidly, completely absorbed from injection site. Excreted in urine. Removed by hemodialysis. **Half-life:** 1.5 hrs.

AVAILABILITY
Injection: 0.05 mg/ml, 0.1 mg/ml, 0.2 mg/ml, 0.5 mg/ml, 1 mg/ml.
Suspension for Injection: 10-mg, 20-mg, 30-mg vials.

INDICATIONS AND DOSAGES
▸ **Diarrhea (Sandostatin)**
Subcutaneous
Adults, Elderly. 50 mcg 1–2 times/day.
IV
Adults, Elderly. Initially, 50–100 mcg q8h. May increase by 100 mcg/dose q48h. Maximum: 500 mcg q8h.
Subcutaneous/IV
Children. 1–10 mcg/kg q12h.
▸ **Carcinoid Tumors (Sandostatin)**
Subcutaneous/IV
Adults, Elderly. 100–600 mcg/day in 2–4 divided doses.
▸ **Vipomas (Sandostatin)**
Subcutaneous/IV
Adults, Elderly. 200–300 mcg/day in 2–4 divided doses.

▸ **Esophageal Varices (Sandostatin)**
IV
Adults, Elderly. Bolus of 25–50 mcg followed by IV infusion of 25–50 mcg/hr.
▸ **Acromegaly (Sandostatin)**
Subcutaneous/IV
Adults, Elderly. 50 mcg 3 times/day. Increase as needed. Maximum: 500 mcg 3 times/day.
▸ **Acromegaly (Sandostatin LAR)**
IM
Adults, Elderly. 20 mg q4wks for 3 mos. Maximum: 40 mg q4wks.
▸ **Vipomas, Carcinoid Tumors (Sandostatin LAR)**
IM
Adults, Elderly. 20 mg q4wks.

UNLABELED USES
AIDS-associated secretory diarrhea, chemotherapy-induced diarrhea, control of bleeding of esophageal varices, insulinomas, small bowel fistulas

CONTRAINDICATIONS
None known

INTERACTIONS
Drug
Glucagon, growth hormone, insulin, oral hypoglycemics: May alter glucose concentrations with glucagon, growth hormone, insulin, and oral hypoglycemics.
Herbal
None known.
Food
None known.

DIAGNOSTIC TEST EFFECTS
May decrease T_4 concentration.

SIDE EFFECTS
Frequent (10%–6%, 58%–30% in acromegalics)
Diarrhea, nausea, abdominal dis-

comfort, headache, pain at injection site
Occasional (5%–1%)
Vomiting, flatulence, constipation, alopecia, flushing, itching, dizziness, fatigue, arrhythmias, bruising, blurred vision
Rare (less than 1%)
Depression, decreased libido, vertigo, palpitations, shortness of breath

SERIOUS REACTIONS
• There is an increased risk of cholelithiasis.
• There is a potential for hypothyroidism with prolonged high therapy.
• Gastrointestinal (GI) bleeding, hepatitis, and seizures occur rarely.

NURSING CONSIDERATIONS
Baseline Assessment
• Establish the patient's baseline blood glucose levels, blood pressure (B/P), electrolytes, and weight.
Lifespan Considerations
• Be aware that it is unknown if octreotide is excreted in breast milk.
• Be aware that the dosage is not established in children.
• There are no age-related precautions noted in the elderly.
Precautions
• Use cautiously in patients with insulin-dependent diabetes and renal failure.
Administration and Handling
◄ALERT► Sandostatin may be given IV, IM, subcutaneous. Sandostatin LAR may be given only IM.
Subcutaneous
• Do not use if particulates or discoloration is noted.
• Avoid multiple injections at the same site within short periods of time.

IM
• Give immediately after mixing.
• Administer intragluteally at 4-week intervals.
• Avoid deltoid injections.
Intervention and Evaluation
• Monitor the patient's blood glucose levels, fecal fat, fluid and electrolyte balance, and thyroid function tests.
• Monitor growth hormone levels in acromegaly patients.
• Weigh the patient every 2 to 3 days, report more than 5 lbs gain a week.
• Monitor the patient's B/P, pulse, and respirations periodically during treatment.
• Be alert for decreased urinary output and edema of the ankles and fingers in the patient.
• Assess the patient's daily pattern of bowel frequency and stool consistency.
Patient Teaching
• Therapy should provide significant improvement of symptoms.
• Tell the patient to weigh himself or herself daily, and to report a weight gain of greater than 5 lbs per week.

pegvisomant
peg-**vis**-oh-mant
(Somavert)

CATEGORY AND SCHEDULE
Pregnancy Risk Category: B

MECHANISM OF ACTION
A protein that selectively binds to growth hormone receptors on cell surfaces, blocking the binding of endogenous growth hormones, interfering with growth hormone signal transduction. *Therapeutic Effect:* Decreases serum concentrations of insulin-like growth factor

(IGF)-1 serum protein, normalizing serum insulin-like growth factor-1 GF-1 levels.

PHARMACOKINETICS

Following subcutaneous administration, does not distribute extensively into tissues, and less than 1% is excreted in the urine. **Half-life:** 6 days.

AVAILABILITY

Powder for Injection: 10 mg, 15 mg, 20 mg vials.

INDICATIONS AND DOSAGES
▸ **Acromegaly**
Subcutaneous
Adults, Elderly. Initially, 40 mg, given as a loading dose, and then 10 mg daily. After 4–6 weeks, adjust dosage in 5-mg increments if the serum IGF-1 concentration is still elevated, or 5-mg decrements if the IGF-1 levels has decreased below the normal range. Do not exceed maximum daily dose of 30 mg.

CONTRAINDICATIONS

Latex allergy because the stopper on the vial contains latex

INTERACTIONS
Drug
Insulin and oral hypoglycemic agents: Dosing of these drugs should be reduced at the initiation of pegvisomant therapy.
Opioid therapy patients: May require higher dosage of pegvisomant.
Herbal
None known.
Food
None known.

DIAGNOSTIC TEST EFFECTS

Interferes with measurement of serum growth hormone concentration. May increase SGOT (AST), SGPT (ALT), and transaminase levels. Decreases effect of insulin on carbohydrate metabolism.

SIDE EFFECTS
Frequent (23%)
Infection characterized as cold symptoms, upper respiratory infection, blister, ear infection.
Occasional (8%–5%)
Back pain, dizziness, injection site reaction, peripheral edema, sinusitis, nausea
Rare (less than 4%)
Diarrhea, paresthesia

SERIOUS REACTIONS
• May produce marked elevation of liver enzymes, including serum transaminase levels.
• Substantial weight gain occurs rarely.

NURSING CONSIDERATIONS

Baseline Assessment
• Expect to obtain the patient's baseline serum alkaline phosphatase, bilirubin, SGOT (AST), and SGPT (ALT) levels.
Lifespan Considerations
• Be aware that it is unknown if pegvisomant is excreted in breast milk.
• Be aware that the safety and efficacy of pegvisomant have not been established in children.
• Be aware that in the elderly, treatment should begin at the low end of the dosage range.
Precautions
• Use cautiously in elderly patients and patients with diabetes mellitus.
Administration and Handling
Subcutaneous
• Store unreconstituted vials in refrigerator.

• Administer within 6 hours following reconstitution.
• Be aware that the solution normally appears clear after reconstitution. Discard if particulate is present or if solution appears cloudy.
• Withdraw 1 ml sterile water for injection and inject into the vial of pegvisomant, aiming the stream against the glass wall.
• Hold the vial between the palms of both hands and roll to dissolve the powder; do not shake.
• Administer subcutaneously only 1 dose from each vial.

Intervention and Evaluation
• Monitor all patients with tumors that secrete growth hormone with periodic imaging scans of sella turcica for progressive tumor growth, as ordered.
• Monitor diabetic patients for hypoglycemia.
• Plan to obtain the patient's IGF-1 serum concentrations 4 to 6 weeks after therapy begins, and periodically thereafter. Adjust drug dosage based on these results, not on growth hormone assays, as prescribed.

Patient Teaching
• Stress to the patient that routine monitoring of serum hepatic enzyme tests is essential during pegvisomant treatment.
• Warn the patient to notify the physician if he or she experiences a yellowing of the skin or sclera of eyes, or any other adverse effects.
• Make sure that patients with diabetes mellitus are aware of the signs and symptoms of hypoglycemia, and know how to treat it.

raloxifene
rah-**lock**-sih-feen
(Evista)

CATEGORY AND SCHEDULE
Pregnancy Risk Category: X

MECHANISM OF ACTION
A selective estrogen receptor modulator that affects some receptors as estrogen. *Therapeutic Effect:* Like estrogen, prevents bone loss and improves lipid profiles.

PHARMACOKINETICS
Rapidly absorbed after PO administration. Highly bound to plasma proteins (greater than 95%) and albumin. Undergoes extensive first-pass metabolism in liver. Excreted mainly in feces with a lesser amount in urine. Unknown if removed by hemodialysis. **Half-life:** 27.7 hrs.

AVAILABILITY
Tablets: 60 mg.

INDICATIONS AND DOSAGES
▶ **Prevention or treatment of osteoporosis**
PO
Adults, Elderly. 60 mg a day.

UNLABELED USES
Breast cancer in postmenopausal women, prevents fractures

CONTRAINDICATIONS
Active or history of venous thromboembolic events, such as deep vein thrombosis, pulmonary embolism, and retinal vein thrombosis, pregnancy, those who may become pregnant

INTERACTIONS
Drug
Ampicillin, Cholestyramine: Reduces raloxifene peak levels and extent of absorption.
Hormone replacement therapy, systemic estrogen: Do not use concurrently hormone replacement therapy or systemic estrogen.
Warfarin: May decrease the effects of warfarin, decreases prothrombin time.
Herbal
None known.
Food
None known.

DIAGNOSTIC TEST EFFECTS
Lowers serum total and LDL cholesterol, but does not affect HDL cholesterol or triglycerides. Slight decrease in inorganic phosphate, platelet count, serum albumin, total calcium, and total protein.

SIDE EFFECTS
Frequent (25%–10%)
Hot flashes, flu syndrome, arthralgia, sinusitis
Occasional (9%–5%)
Weight gain, nausea, myalgia, pharyngitis, cough, dyspepsia, leg cramps, rash, depression
Rare (4%–3%)
Vaginitis, urinary tract infection, peripheral edema, flatulence, vomiting, fever, migraine, diaphoresis

SERIOUS REACTIONS
• Pneumonia, gastroenteritis, chest pain, vaginal bleeding, and breast pain occur rarely.

NURSING CONSIDERATIONS
Baseline Assessment
• Determine if the patient is pregnant.
• Discontinue the drug 72 hours before and during prolonged immobilization, such as postoperative recovery and prolonged bed rest. Resume therapy, as prescribed, only after the patient is fully ambulatory.
• Expect to establish the patient's total and LDL cholesterol serum blood levels before beginning raloxifene therapy and routinely thereafter.
Lifespan Considerations
• Be aware that it is unknown if raloxifene is distributed in breast milk. Raloxifene use is not recommended for nursing mothers.
• Be aware that raloxifene is not used in children.
• There are no age-related precautions noted in the elderly.
Precautions
• Use cautiously in patients with cardiovascular disease, history of cervical or uterine cancer, and liver or renal impairment.
Administration and Handling
PO
• Give raloxifene at any time of day without regard to meals.
Intervention and Evaluation
• Monitor the patient's bone mineral density, inorganic phosphate, platelet count, serum total calcium levels, total and LDL cholesterol concentrations, and total serum protein levels.
Patient Teaching
• Warn the patient to avoid prolonged restriction of movement during travel. Explain that limited movement increases the risk of venous thromboembolic events.
• Instruct the patient to take supplemental calcium and vitamin D if his or her daily dietary intake is inadequate.
• Encourage the patient to discontinue alcohol consumption and cigarette smoking during raloxifene therapy.

• Instruct the patient to engage in regular exercise.

teriparatide acetate
tear-ee-**pear**-ah-tide
(Forteo)

CATEGORY AND SCHEDULE
Pregnancy Risk Category: C

MECHANISM OF ACTION
A synthetic hormone that acts on bone to mobilize calcium; also acts on kidney to reduce calcium clearance, increase phosphate excretion. *Therapeutic Effect:* Promotes an increased rate of release of calcium from bone into blood, stimulates new bone formation.

AVAILABILITY
Injection: 3-ml prefilled pen containing 750 mcg teriparatide.

INDICATIONS AND DOSAGES
▸ **Osteoporosis**
Subcutaneous
Adults, Elderly. 20 mcg once a day into the thigh or abdominal wall.

CONTRAINDICATIONS
Hypercalcemic disorders, such as hyperparathyroidism, serum calcium above normal level, those at increased risk for osteosarcoma, including Paget's disease, unexplained elevations of alkaline phosphatase, open epiphyses, and prior radiation therapy that includes the skeleton

INTERACTIONS
Drug
Digoxin: May increase serum concentrations of digoxin

Herbal
None known.
Food
None known.

DIAGNOSTIC TEST EFFECTS
May increase serum calcium levels.

SIDE EFFECTS
Occasional
Leg cramps, nausea, dizziness, headache, orthostatic hypotension, tachycardia

SERIOUS REACTIONS
• None known.

NURSING CONSIDERATIONS
Baseline Assessment
• Expect to check the patient's blood parathyroid hormone levels and urinary serum calcium levels.
Precautions
• Use cautiously in patients with bone metastases, history of skeletal malignancies, and metabolic bone diseases other than osteoporosis.
• Use cautiously in patients on concurrent therapy with digoxin.
Administration and Handling
Subcutaneous
• Refrigerate, minimizing the time out of the refrigerator. Do not freeze; discard if frozen.
• Administer into the thigh or abdominal wall.
Intervention and Evaluation
• Plan to monitor the patient's bone mineral density, parathyroid hormone levels, hypercalcemia, and urinary and serum calcium levels.
• Monitor the patient's blood pressure (B/P) for hypotension and pulse for tachycardia.
Patient Teaching
• Instruct the patient to immediately sit or lie down if he or she experi-

ences symptoms of orthostatic hypotension.
• Warn the patient to notify the physician if he or she experiences persistent symptoms of hypercalcemia, including asthenia or loss of energy or strength, constipation, lethargy, nausea, and vomiting.

testosterone
tess-**toss**-ter-own
(Andronaq, Delatestryl[CAN], Histerone, Striant)
testosterone cypionate
(Depotest, Depo-Testosterone)
testosterone enanthate
(Delatest)
testosterone propionate
(Testex)
testosterone transdermal
(Androderm, Testim, Testoderm, Testoderm TTS)
Do not confuse with testolactone.

CATEGORY AND SCHEDULE
Pregnancy Risk Category: X

MECHANISM OF ACTION
A primary endogenous androgen that promotes growth and development of male sex organs, maintains secondary sex characteristics in androgen-deficient males.

PHARMACOKINETICS
Well absorbed after IM administration. Protein binding: 98%. Metabolized in liver (undergoes first-pass metabolism). Primarily excreted in urine. Unknown if removed by hemodialysis. **Half-life:** 10–20 min.

AVAILABILITY
Injection: 50 mg/ml (Aqueous suspension), 100 mg/ml (aqueous suspension, Cypionate, Propionate), 200 mg/ml (Cypionate and Enanthate).
Pellets for subcutaneous implantation: 75 mg.
Transdermal Gel: 25 mg (2.5 g gel/pack), 50 mg (5 g gel/pack).
Transdermal System: 2.5 mg/day, 4 mg/day, 5 mg/day, 6 mg/day.
Buccal System: 30 mg.

INDICATIONS AND DOSAGES
▶ **Male hypogonadism**
IM
Adults, Elderly. 10–25 mg 2–3 times/wk (Aqueous/propionate), 50–400 mg q2–4wks (Cypionate/enanthate).
Children. 40–50 mg/m^2/dose qmo (Cypionate or enanthate, Initial pubertal growth), 100 mg/m^2/dose qmo (Terminal growth phase).
Maintenance virilizing dose: 100 mg/m^2/dose 2 times/mo.
Transdermal (patches)
Adults, Elderly. Start Testoderm therapy with 6 mg/day patch. Apply Testoderm patch to scrotal skin. Apply Testoderm TTS patch to arm, back or upper buttocks. Start Androderm therapy with 5 mg/day patch applied at night. Apply Androderm patch to abdomen, back, thighs, or upper arms.
Transdermal (gel)
Adults, Elderly. Initial Androgel dose of 5 mg delivers 50 mg testosterone and is applied once daily to the abdomen, shoulders, or upper arms. May increase to 7.5 g then to 10 g Androgel if necessary. Initial Testim dose of 5 g delivers 50 mg testosterone and is applied once a day to the shoulders or upper arms. May increase to 10 g Testim.
Subcutaneous (pellets)
Adults, Elderly: 150-450 mg q3–6mos.

▶ **Delayed Puberty**
IM
Children. 40–50 mg/m^2/dose qmo for 6 mos.
▶ **Breast carcinoma**
IM
Adults. 50–100 mg 3 times/wk (Aqueous), 200–400 mg q2–4wks (Cypionate or enanthate), 50–100 mg 3 times/wk (Propionate).

CONTRAINDICATIONS
Cardiac impairment, hypercalcemia, pregnancy, prostatic or breast cancer in males, severe liver or renal disease

INTERACTIONS
Drug
Liver toxic medications: May increase liver toxicity.
Oral anticoagulants: May increase the effects of oral anticoagulants.
Herbal
None known.
Food
None known.

DIAGNOSTIC TEST EFFECTS
May increase blood Hgb and Hct, LDL concentrations, serum alkaline phosphatase, bilirubin, calcium, potassium, SGOT (AST) levels, and sodium levels. May decrease HDL concentrations.

SIDE EFFECTS
Frequent
Gynecomastia, acne, amenorrhea or other menstrual irregularities
Females: Hirsutism, deepening of voice, clitoral enlargement that may not be reversible when drug is discontinued
Occasional
Edema, nausea, insomnia, oligospermia, priapism, male pattern of baldness, bladder irritability, hypercalcemia in immobilized patients or those with breast cancer, hypercholesterolemia, inflammation and pain at IM injection site
Transdermal: Itching, erythema, skin irritation
Rare
Polycythemia with high dosage, hypersensitivity

SERIOUS REACTIONS
• Peliosis hepatitis or liver, spleen replaced with blood-filled cysts, hepatic neoplasms and hepatocellular carcinoma have been associated with prolonged high-dosage, anaphylactic reactions.

<hr>

NURSING CONSIDERATIONS

Baseline Assessment
• Establish the patient's baseline blood Hgb and Hct, blood pressure (B/P), and weight.
• Check the patient's serum cholesterol and electrolyte levels, and hepatic enzyme test results, if ordered.
• Know that wrist x-rays may be ordered to determine bone maturation in children.
Precautions
• Use cautiously in patients with diabetes and liver or renal impairment.
Lifespan Considerations
• Be aware that testosterone use is contraindicated during lactation.
• Be aware that the safety and efficacy of testosterone have not been established in children, so use with caution.
• Be aware that testosterone use in the elderly may increase the risk of hyperplasia or stimulate growth of occult prostate carcinoma.
Administration and Handling
IM
• Give deep in gluteal muscle.
• Do not give IV.
• Warming and shaking re-dissolves

crystals that may form in long-acting preparations.

* A wet needle may cause solution to become cloudy; this does not affect potency.

Transdermal

* Apply Testoderm to clean, dry scrotal skin that has been dry-shaved for optimal skin contact. Testoderm TTS may be applied to arm, back, or upper buttock.

* Apply Androderm to clean, dry area on skin on back, abdomen, upper arms, or thighs. Do not apply to bony prominences, such as the shoulder, or oily, damaged, irritated skin. Do not apply to scrotum.

* Rotate Androderm application site with 7-day interval to same site.

Transdermal Gel (Androgel, Testim)

* Apply (morning preferred) to clean, dry, intact skin of shoulder or upper arms. Androgel may also be applied to the abdomen.

* Open packet(s), squeeze entire contents into the palm of the hand and immediately apply to the application site.

* Allow to dry.

* Do not apply to genitals.

Buccal (Striant)

* Apply to gum area above incisor tooth.

* Not affected by consumption of alcohol or food, gum chewing, or tooth brushing.

* Remove prior to placing the new system.

Intervention and Evaluation

* Weigh the patient daily and report weekly gains of more than 5 lbs.

* Evaluate the patient for edema.

* Monitor the patient's intake and output and sleep patterns.

* Check the patient's B/P at least 2 times a day.

* Assess the patient's blood Hgb and Hct periodically when giving

high dosages, as ordered. Also plan to check serum cholesterol and electrolyte levels, as well as liver function test results.

* Expect to perform radiological exam of hand or wrist when using in prepubertal children.

* Monitor patients with breast cancer or immobility for hypercalcemia, confusion, irritability, lethargy, muscle weakness.

* Ensure the patient consumes adequate calories and protein.

* Assess the patient for signs of virilization, such as deepening of the voice.

* Examine the patient's injection site for pain, redness, or swelling.

Patient Teaching

* Stress to the patient the importance of monitoring tests and regular visits to the physician.

* Warn the patient not to take any other medications, including over-the-counter drugs, without first consulting the physician.

* Instruct the patient to apply the patch to a clean, dry, hairless part of the skin, avoiding bony prominences.

* Teach the patient to consume a diet high in calories and protein. Tell the patient that food may be better tolerated if he or she takes in small, frequent meals.

* Instruct the patient to weigh himself or herself each day and to report to the physician weight gains of 5 lbs or more per week.

* Warn the patient to notify the physician if he or she experiences acne, nausea, pedal edema, or vomiting. Tell female patients to also promptly report deepening of voice, hoarseness, and menstrual irregularities. Tell male patients to report difficulty urinating, frequent erections, and gynecomastia.

auranofin
aurothioglucose
gold sodium
  thiomalate
hydroxychloroquine
  sulfate
leflunomide
methotrexate sodium
sulfasalazine

Uses: Antirheumatic agents are used to relieve symptoms of rheumatoid arthritis, especially in patients with insufficient therapeutic response to nonsteroidal anti-inflammatory drugs. Specific antirheumatic agents may be used to treat malaria (hydroxychloroquine), trophoblastic neoplasms and other cancers (methotrexate), and ulcerative colitis and inflammatory bowel disease (sulfasalazine).

Action: Disease-modifying antirheumatic drugs include gold compounds and immunosuppressive and antimalarial agents. *Gold compounds,* such as auranofin, aurothioglucose, and gold sodium thiomalate, depress leukocyte migration and suppress prostaglandin activity. They may also inhibit the destructive lysosomal enzymes in leukocytes, which are released at joints. Some *immunosuppressive agents,* such as methotrexate, suppress the inflammatory process of rheumatoid arthritis; others, such as leflunomide, inhibit enzymes in the pathway of pyrimidine synthesis. *Antimalarial agents,* such as hydroxychloroquine, act by an unknown mechanism in rheumatoid arthritis.

auranofin
aur-an-**oh**-fin
(Ridaura)
Do not confuse with Cardura.

aurothioglucose
ah-row-thigh-oh-**glue**-cose
(Gold-50[AUS], Solganal)

CATEGORY AND SCHEDULE
Pregnancy Risk Category: C

MECHANISM OF ACTION
A gold compound that alters cellular mechanisms, collagen biosynthesis, enzyme systems, and immune responses. *Therapeutic Effect:* Suppresses synovitis of the active stage of rheumatoid arthritis.

PHARMACOKINETICS
Auranofin (29% gold): Moderately absorbed from the gastrointestinal (GI) tract. Protein binding: 60%. Rapidly metabolized. Primarily excreted in urine. **Half-life:** 21–31 days. Aurothioglucose (50% gold): Slow, erratic absorption after IM administration. Protein binding: 95%–99%. Primarily excreted in urine. **Half-life:** 3–27 days (half-life increased with increased number of doses).

AVAILABILITY
Capsules: 3 mg.
Injection: 50 mg/ml suspension.

INDICATIONS AND DOSAGES
▸ **Rheumatoid arthritis**
IM
Adults, Elderly. Initially, 10 mg, then 25 mg for 2 doses, then 50 mg weekly thereafter until total dose of 0.8–1 g given. If patient is improved and there are no signs of toxicity, may give 50 mg at 3- to 4-wk intervals for many months.
Children. 0.25 mg/kg, may increase by 0.25 mg/kg each week. Maintenance: 0.75–1 mg/kg/dose. Maximum: 25-mg dose for total of 20 doses, then q2–4wks.
PO
Adults, Elderly. 6 mg/day in 1 or 2 divided doses. If there is no response in 6 mos, may increase to 9 mg/day (in 3 divided doses). If response is still inadequate, discontinue.
Children. 0.1 mg/kg/day in 1–2 divided doses. Maintenance: 0.15 mg/kg/day. Maximum: 0.2 mg/kg/day.

UNLABELED USES
Treatment of pemphigus, psoriatic arthritis

CONTRAINDICATIONS
Bone marrow aplasia, history of gold-induced pathologies, including blood dyscrasias, exfoliative dermatitis, necrotizing enterocolitis, and pulmonary fibrosis, serious adverse effects with previous gold therapy, severe blood dyscrasias

INTERACTIONS
Drug
Bone marrow depressants; hepatotoxic, nephrotoxic medications: May increase risk of aurothioglucose toxicity.
Penicillamine: May increase risk of hematologic or renal adverse effects of aurothioglucose.

Herbal
None known.
Food
None known.

DIAGNOSTIC TEST EFFECTS
May decrease Hgb, Hct, platelets, white blood cell (WBC) count. May alter liver function tests. May increase urine protein.

SIDE EFFECTS
Frequent
Auranofin: Diarrhea (50%), pruritic rash (26%), abdominal pain (14%), stomatitis (13%), nausea (10%)
Aurothioglucose: Rash (39%), stomatitis (19%), diarrhea (13%).
Occasional
Nausea, vomiting, anorexia, abdominal cramps

SERIOUS REACTIONS
• Gold toxicity is the primary serious reaction. Signs and symptoms of gold toxicity include decreased hemoglobin, leukopenia (WBC count less than 4,000/mm^3), reduced granulocyte counts (less than 150,000/mm^3), proteinuria, hematuria, stomatitis (sores, ulcers and white spots in the mouth and throat), blood dyscrasias (anemia, leukopenia, thrombocytopenia and eosinophilia), glomerulonephritis, nephritic syndrome, and cholestatic jaundice.

NURSING CONSIDERATIONS
Baseline Assessment
• Determine if the patient is pregnant before beginning treatment.
• Check the results of the patient's complete blood count (CBC), particularly BUN, Hct, Hgb, platelet count, serum alkaline phosphatase, creatinine, SGOT (AST), and SGPT (ALT) levels to assess renal and liver function and urinalysis, before therapy begins.

Lifespan Considerations
• Be aware that aurothioglucose crosses the placenta and is distributed in breast milk. Use only when the drug's benefits outweigh the possible hazard to the fetus.
• There are no age-related precautions noted in children.
• Use cautiously in the elderly, who may have age-related decreased renal function.

Precautions
• Use cautiously in patients with blood dyscrasias, compromised cerebral or cardiovascular circulation, eczema, a history of sensitivity to gold compounds, marked hypertension, renal or liver impairment, severe debilitation, Sjögren's syndrome in rheumatoid arthritis, and systemic lupus erythematosus.

Administration and Handling
PO
• Give without regard to food.
IM
◀ALERT▶ Give as weekly injections.
• Give in upper outer quadrant of gluteus maximus.

Intervention and Evaluation
• Assess the patient's pattern of daily bowel activity and stool consistency.
• Test the patient's urine for hematuria and proteinuria.
• Monitor the results of blood chemistries, CBC, and renal and liver function studies.
• Assess the patient for pruritus which may be the first sign of an impending rash.
• Assess the patient's skin daily for ecchymoses, purpura, and rash.
• Examine the patient's oral mucous membranes, palate, pharynx, and tongue borders for ulceration. Investigate any patient complaints of a metallic taste in the mouth as this is a sign of stomatitis.

• Evaluate the patient for the expected therapeutic response, including improved grip strength, increased joint mobility, reduced joint tenderness, and relief of pain, stiffness, and swelling.

Patient Teaching
• Advise the patient that the therapeutic response of the drug may be expected in 3 to 6 months.
• Warn the patient to avoid exposure to sunlight. Explain that sun exposure may cause a gray to blue pigment to appear on the skin.
• Urge the patient to notify the physician if indigestion, metallic taste, pruritus, rash, or sore mouth occurs.
• Stress to the patient that he or she maintain diligent oral hygiene to help prevent stomatitis.

gold sodium thiomalate
gold sodium thigh-oh-**mal**-ate
(Myochrysine, Myocrisin[AUS])

CATEGORY AND SCHEDULE
Pregnancy Risk Category: C

MECHANISM OF ACTION
A gold compound whose mechanism of action is unknown. May decrease prostaglandin synthesis or alter cellular mechanisms by inhibiting sulfhydryl systems. *Therapeutic Effect:* Decreases synovial inflammation, retards cartilage and bone destruction, suppresses or prevents but does not cure, arthritis, synovitis.

AVAILABILITY
Injection: 50 mg/ml.

INDICATIONS AND DOSAGES
▶ **Rheumatoid arthritis**
IM
Adults, Elderly. Initially, 10 mg, then 25 mg for second dose. Follow with 25–50 mg/wk until improvement noted or total of 1 g administered. Maintenance: 25–50 mg q2wks for 2–20 wks; if stable, may increase to q3–4wk intervals.
Children. Initially, 10 mg, then 1 mg/kg/wk. Maximum single dose: 50 mg. Maintenance: 1 mg/kg/dose at 2- to 4-wk intervals.
▶ **Dosage in renal impairment**

Creatinine Clearance	Dosage
50–80 ml/min	50% of usual dosage
less than 50 ml/min	not recommended

UNLABELED USES
Treatment of psoriatic arthritis

CONTRAINDICATIONS
Colitis, concurrent use of antimalarials, immunosuppressive agents, penicillamine, or phenylbutazone, congestive heart failure (CHF), exfoliative dermatitis, history of blood dyscrasias, severe liver or renal impairment, systemic lupus erythematosus

INTERACTIONS
Drug
Bone marrow depressants, liver toxic, nephrotoxic medications: May increase the risk of toxicity.
Penicillamine: May increase the risk of adverse hematologic or renal effects.
Herbal
None known.
Food
None known.

DIAGNOSTIC TEST EFFECTS
May decrease blood Hgb and Hct, platelet and white blood cell (WBC) counts. May alter liver function tests. May increase urine protein.

SIDE EFFECTS
Frequent
Pruritic dermatitis, stomatitis, marked by erythema, redness, shallow ulcers of oral mucous membranes, sore throat, and difficulty swallowing, diarrhea or loose stools, abdominal pain, nausea
Occasional
Vomiting, anorexia, flatulence, dyspepsia, conjunctivitis, photosensitivity
Rare
Constipation, urticaria, rash

SERIOUS REACTIONS
• Signs of gold toxicity including decreased Hgb, leukopenia (WBC less than 4,000 mm^3), reduced granulocyte counts (less than 150,000/mm^3), proteinuria, hematuria, blood dyscrasias, including anemia, leukopenia, thrombocytopenia, and eosinophilia, glomerulonephritis, nephrotic syndrome, and cholestatic jaundice may occur.

NURSING CONSIDERATIONS
Baseline Assessment
• Determine if the patient is pregnant before beginning treatment.
• Plan to perform a complete blood count (CBC), particularly BUN, Hct, Hgb, platelet count, serum alkaline phosphatase, creatinine, SGOT (AST), and SGPT (ALT) levels, and white blood cell (WBC) count to assess liver and renal function and a urinalysis of the patient before beginning therapy.
Administration and Handling
◀ALERT▶ Give gold sodium thioma-

late as weekly injections, as prescribed.

Intervention and Evaluation
• Assess the patient's daily pattern of
bowel activity and stool consistency.
• Assess the patient's urine tests for
hematuria or proteinuria.
• Monitor the patient's CBC and
liver and renal function studies.
• Assess the patient's skin daily for
ecchymoses, purpura, and rash.
• Assess the patient's borders of
tongue, oral mucous membranes,
palate, and pharynx for ulceration.
• Evaluate any patient complaints of
metallic taste sensation, sign of
stomatitis.
• Evaluate the patient for therapeutic response, improved grip strength,
increased joint mobility, reduced
joint tenderness, and relief of pain,
stiffness, and swelling.

Patient Teaching
• Tell the patient that the drug's
therapeutic response may take
6 months or more to appear.
• Warn the patient to avoid exposure to sunlight. Explain that a gray
to blue skin pigment may appear.
• Stress to the patient that he or she
must maintain diligent oral hygiene
during gold sodium thiomalate
therapy.

hydroxychloroquine sulfate
See miscellaneous anti-infective
agents

leflunomide
lee-**flew**-no-mide
(Arava)

CATEGORY AND SCHEDULE
Pregnancy Risk Category: X

MECHANISM OF ACTION
An immunomodulatory agent that
extends the immune response exhibited in rheumatoid synovium,
hinders proliferation of lymphocytes,
possesses anti-inflammatory action.
Therapeutic Effect: Reduces signs
and symptoms of rheumatoid arthritis and retards structural damage.

PHARMACOKINETICS
Well absorbed after PO administration. Protein binding: greater than
99%. Metabolized to active metabolite in gastrointestinal (GI) wall and
liver. Mechanisms of excretion include both renal and biliary systems.
Not removed by hemodialysis. **Half-
life:** 16 days.

AVAILABILITY
Tablets: 10 mg, 20 mg.

INDICATIONS AND DOSAGES
▸ **Rheumatoid arthritis**
PO
Adults, Elderly. Initially, 100 mg
daily for 3 days, then 10–20 mg
daily.

CONTRAINDICATIONS
Pregnancy or plans to become
pregnant

INTERACTIONS
Drug
Rifampin: Increases the blood
concentration of leflunomide.
Warfarin: May increase the effects
of warfarin.
Herbal
None known.
Food
None known.

DIAGNOSTIC TEST EFFECTS
May increase liver enzymes, espe-
cially SGOT (AST), and SGPT
(ALT).

SIDE EFFECTS
Frequent (20%–10%)
Diarrhea, respiratory tract infection, hair loss, rash, nausea

SERIOUS REACTIONS
• Transient thrombocytopenia and leukopenia occur rarely.

NURSING CONSIDERATIONS
Baseline Assessment
• Determine if the patient is pregnant.
• Assess the patient's limitations in activities of daily living due to rheumatoid arthritis.
Lifespan Considerations
• Be aware that leflunomide can cause fetal harm and it is unknown if the drug is excreted in breast milk. Avoid using with breast-feeding women.
• Be aware that the safety and efficacy of leflunomide have not been established in children younger than 18 years of age.
• There are no age-related precautions noted in the elderly.
Precautions
• Use cautiously in breast-feeding mothers and patients with immuno-deficiency or bone marrow dysplasias, impaired liver or renal function, and positive hepatitis B or C serology.

Administration and Handling
PO
• Give leflunomide without regard to food.
Intervention and Evaluation
• Monitor the patient's tolerance to the medication.
• Assess the patient for symptom-atic relief of rheumatoid arthritis.
• Monitor the patient's liver function tests.
Patient Teaching
• Teach the patient that leflunomide may be taken without regard to food.
• Explain to the patient that the drug's therapeutic effect may take longer than 8 weeks to appear.
• Warn the patient to avoid becoming pregnant during leflunomide therapy. Explain to the patient that this drug is pregnancy risk category X.

methotrexate sodium
See antimetabolites

sulfasalazine
See miscellaneous anti-infective agents

hepatitis B immune globulin (human)

immune globulin IV (IGIV)

lymphocyte immune globulin N

respiratory syncytial immune globulin

Rh$_o$(D) immune globulin

Uses: Immune globulins are primarily used to immunize patients against infectious diseases, such as hepatitis B virus and respiratory syncytial virus infections. In addition, *antithymocyte globulin* is used to prevent and treat allograft rejection, to treat aplastic anemia, and to prevent graft-vs-host disease after bone marrow transplantation. *Immune globulin IV* is used to treat primary immunodeficiency syndromes, Kawasaki disease, and idiopathic thrombocytopenic purpura; to prevent bacterial infections in patients with hypogammaglobulinemia; and as an adjunct in bone marrow transplantation. *Rh$_o$(D) immune globulin* is used to prevent isoimmunization in Rh-negative patients exposed to Rh-positive blood.

Action: These immune globulins provide passive immunization, which involves administration of preformed antibodies. Passive immunity isn't permanent and doesn't last as long as active immunity, which results from immunization with an antigen to develop defenses against a future exposure.

hepatitis B immune globulin (human)
(Bayhep B, Nabi-HB)

CATEGORY AND SCHEDULE
Pregnancy Risk Category: C

MECHANISM OF ACTION
An immune globulin of inactivated hepatitis B virus that provides passive immunization against hepatitis B virus.

AVAILABILITY
Injection: 5-ml vial.

INDICATIONS AND DOSAGES
▸ **Acute exposure**

IM
Adults, Elderly. 0.06 ml/kg usual dose; 3–5 ml for postexposure prophylaxis. Repeat at 28–30 days after exposure.

CONTRAINDICATIONS
Allergies to gamma globulin or thimerosal, IgA deficiency, IM injections in patients with coagulation disorders or thrombocytopenia

INTERACTIONS
Drug
None known.
Herbal
None known.
Food
None known.

DIAGNOSTIC TEST EFFECTS
None known.

SIDE EFFECTS
Frequent
Headache (26%), local pain
(12%)
Occasional (5%)
Malaise, nausea, myalgia

SERIOUS REACTIONS
• None significant.

NURSING CONSIDERATIONS

Baseline Assessment
• Ask the patient if he or she has a
known allergy to thimerosal, eggs
or chicken products before administering.
• Expect to obtain baseline hepatic
enzyme levels and hepatitis B
antibodies.
Lifespan Considerations
• None known.
Precautions
• Use cautiously in patients with
coagulation disorders and thrombo-
cytopenia.
• Know that the drug is contraindicated in patients with allergies to
gamma globulin or thimerosal, and
IgA deficiency.
Administration and Handling
◀ ALERT ▶ Avoid giving IM injections in patients with coagulation disorders or thrombocyto-
penia
IM
• Refrigerate, do not freeze.
• Give via IM injection only in
gluteal or deltoid area.
Intervention and Evaluation
◀ ALERT ▶ This drug is for IM injection only.
• Use care when administering to
patients with bleeding disorders and
thrombocytopenia.

• Plan to obtain periodic liver
function studies and hepatitis B
antibody levels.
Patient Teaching
• Advise the patient to complete the full course of immunization.
• Tell the patient to report any
side effects, as soon as possible,
including headache or injection site
pain.
• Teach the patient how hepatitis B
is transmitted, such as by blood and
body fluid.

immune globulin IV (IGIV)
(Baygam, Gamimune N,
Gammagard, Gammar-IV,
Gammunex, Polygam,
Sandoglobulin, Venoglobulin-I)
**Do not confuse with
Sandimmune or Sandostatin.**

CATEGORY AND SCHEDULE
Pregnancy Risk Category: C

MECHANISM OF ACTION
An immune serum that increases
antibody titer and antigen-antibody
reaction. *Therapeutic Effect:* Provides passive immunity against
infection. Induces rapid increase in
platelet counts. Produces anti-
inflammatory effect.

PHARMACOKINETICS
Evenly distributed between intravas-
cular and extravascular space.
Half-life: 21–23 days.

AVAILABILITY
Injection: 5%, 10%.
Powder for Injection: 0.5 g, 2.5 g,
6 g, 10 g, 20 g.

INDICATIONS AND DOSAGES
▸ **Primary immunodeficiency syndrome**
IV infusion
Adults, Elderly, Children.
200–400 mg/kg q1mo.
▸ **Idiopathic thrombocytopenia purpura (ITP)**
IV infusion
Adults, Elderly, Children.
400–1,000 mg/kg/day for 2–5 days.
▸ **Kawasaki disease**
IV infusion
Adults, Elderly, Children. 2 g/kg as a single dose.
▸ **Chronic lymphocytic leukemia (CLL)**
IV infusion
Adults, Elderly, Children.
400 mg/kg q3–4wks.

UNLABELED USES
Control and prevention of infections in infants and children immunosuppressed in association with acquired immune deficiency syndrome (AIDS) or AIDS related complex (ARC), prevention of acute infections in immunosuppressed patients, prophylaxis and treatment of infections in high-risk, preterm, low-birth-weight neonates, treatment of chronic inflammatory demyelinating polyneuropathies, multiple sclerosis

CONTRAINDICATIONS
Allergic response to thimerosal, any coagulation disorder for IM administration, history of allergic response to gamma globulin or anti-immunoglobulin A (IgA) antibodies, isolated immunoglobulin A (IgA) deficiency, severe thrombocytopenia for IM administration

INTERACTIONS
Drug
Live virus vaccines: May decrease the patient's antibody response to the vaccine, increase vaccine side effects, and potentiate virus replication.
Herbal
None known.
Food
None known.

DIAGNOSTIC TEST EFFECTS
None known.

IV INCOMPATIBILITIES
Do not mix with any other medications.

SIDE EFFECTS
Frequent
Tachycardia, backache, headache, joint or muscle pain
Occasional
Fatigue, wheezing, rash or pain at injection site, leg cramps, hives, bluish color of lips and nailbeds, lightheadedness

SERIOUS REACTIONS
• Anaphylactic reactions occur rarely but there is increased incidence when repeated injections of immune globulin are given. Epinephrine should be readily available.
• Overdose may produce chest tightness, chills, diaphoresis, dizziness, flushed face, nausea, vomiting, fever, and hypotension.

NURSING CONSIDERATIONS

Baseline Assessment
• Determine the patient's history and patient's family history of exposure to the disease.
• Have epinephrine readily available in case of an anaphylactic reaction.
• Make sure the patient is well hydrated before giving immune globulin IV.

Lifespan Considerations
• Be aware that it is unknown if immune globulin IV crosses the placenta or is distributed in breast milk.
• There are no age-related precautions noted in children or the elderly.

Precautions
• Use cautiously in patients with cardiovascular disease, diabetes mellitus, history of thrombosis, impaired renal function, sepsis, and volume depletion.
• Use cautiously in patients who concomitantly use nephrotoxic drugs.

Administration and Handling
IV
• Refer to individual IV preparations for storage requirements, stability after reconstitution.
• Reconstitute only with diluent provided by manufacturer.
• Discard partially used or turbid preparations.
• Give by infusion only.
• After reconstituted, administer through separate tubing.
• Avoid mixing with other medication or IV infusion fluids.
• Remember that the rate of infusion varies among products.
• Monitor the patient's blood pressure (B/P) and vital signs diligently during and immediately after IV administration. Be aware that a precipitous fall in B/P may indicate anaphylactic reaction.
• Stop patient infusion immediately if anaphylactic reaction is suspected. Epinephrine should be readily available.

Intervention and Evaluation
• Control the rate of IV infusion carefully. Too rapid of an infusion increases the risk of a precipitous fall in B/P, and signs of anaphylaxis such as chest tightness, chills, diaphoresis, facial flushing, fever, nausea, and vomiting. Stop infusion temporarily if aforementioned signs noted.
• Assess the patient closely during infusion, especially in the first hour.
• Monitor the patient's vital signs continuously.
• Monitor the patient's platelets for treatment of ITP.

Patient Teaching
• Explain to the patient the rationale for therapy.
• Explain to the patient that he or she should have a rapid response to therapy, lasting 1 to 3 months.
• Warn the patient to notify the physician if he or she experiences decreased urine output, edema, fluid retention, shortness of breath, or sudden weight gain.

lymphocyte immune globulin N
lym-phow-site
(Atgam)
Do not confuse with Ativan.

CATEGORY AND SCHEDULE
Pregnancy Risk Category: C

MECHANISM OF ACTION
A biologic response modifier that acts as a lymphocyte selective immunosuppressant, reducing the number of circulating thymus-dependent lymphocytes (T lymphocytes) and altering the function of T lymphocytes, which are responsible for cell-mediated and humoral immunity. Antithymocyte also stimulates the release of hematopoietic growth factors. *Therapeutic Effect:* Prevents allograft rejection, treats aplastic anemia.

AVAILABILITY
Injection: 250 mg/5 ml.

INDICATIONS AND DOSAGES
▶ **Prevent or treat renal allograft rejection**
IV infusion
Adults. Usual dosage: 10–30 mg/kg/day.
Children. Usual dosage: 5–25 mg/kg/day.
▶ **Delay of onset of rejection**
IV infusion
Adults, Children. 15 mg/kg/day for 14 days, then 15 mg/kg/day every other day for 14 days. Give first dose within 24 hrs before or after transplant.
▶ **Treatment of rejection**
IV infusion
Adults, Children. 10–15 mg/kg/day for 14 days. May continue with alternate-day therapy up to 21 doses.
▶ **Aplastic anemia**
IV infusion
Adults. 10–20 mg/kg/day for 8–14 days. May continue alternate-day therapy up to 21 doses.

UNLABELED USES
Immunosuppressant in bone marrow, heart, and liver transplants, treatment of pure red cell aplasia, multiple sclerosis, myasthenia gravis, and scleroderma

CONTRAINDICATIONS
Systemic hypersensitivity reaction to previous injection of antithymocyte globulin

INTERACTIONS
Drug
None known.
Herbal
None known.
Food
None known.

DIAGNOSTIC TEST EFFECTS
May alter renal function tests.

IV INCOMPATIBILITIES
No information is available via Y-site administration.

SIDE EFFECTS
Frequent
Fever (51%), thrombocytopenia (30%), rash (2%), chills (16%), leukopenia (14%), systemic infection (13%).
Occasional (10%–5%)
Serum sickness–like symptoms, dyspnea, apnea, arthralgia, chest pain, back pain, flank pain, nausea, vomiting, diarrhea, phlebitis.

SERIOUS REACTIONS
• Thrombocytopenia occurs but is generally transient.
• Severe hypersensitivity reaction, including anaphylaxis, occurs rarely.

NURSING CONSIDERATIONS
Baseline Assessment
• To prevent chemical phlebitis, avoid using a peripheral vein for IV infusion. Instead, expect to use a central venous catheter, Groshong catheter, or peripherally inserted central catheter (PICC).
Precautions
• Use cautiously in patients receiving concurrent immunosuppressive therapy.
Administration and Handling
IV
• Keep refrigerated before and after dilution.
• Discard diluted solution after 24 hours.
• Further dilute the total daily dose with 0.9% NaCl, as prescribed, to a final concentration that doesn't exceed 4 mg/ml.

• Gently rotate diluted solution; avoid shaking solution.
• Use a 0.2- to 1-micron filter. Give the total daily dose over a minimum of 4 hours.
Intervention and Evaluation
• Expect to monitor the patient frequently for chills, erythema, fever, and itching. Obtain an order for prophylactic antihistamines or corticosteroids to treat these possible side effects.
Patient Teaching
• Stress the importance of avoiding exposure to colds or infections and to notify the physician as soon as signs or symptoms develop.
• Explain that during the IV infusion, the patient should immediately report chest pain, rapid or irregular heartbeats, shortness of breath or wheezing, or swelling of the face or throat.

respiratory syncytial immune globulin
(RespiGam)

CATEGORY AND SCHEDULE
Pregnancy Risk Category: C

MECHANISM OF ACTION
An immune serum with a high concentration of neutralizing and protective antibodies specific for respiratory syncytial virus (RSV).

AVAILABILITY
Injection: 2,500 mcg RSV immune globulin.

INDICATIONS AND DOSAGES
▸ **Prevents RSV in children with bronchopulmonary dysplasia (BPD) and history of premature birth**

IV infusion
Children younger than 24 mos.
750 mg/kg (15 ml/kg). Initially, 1.5 ml/kg/hr for first 15 min, then 3.6 ml/kg/hr for remainder of infusion. Administer monthly for total of 5 doses beginning in September or October.

CONTRAINDICATIONS
IgA deficiency

INTERACTIONS
Drug
Live virus vaccines: May reduce antibody response, may not replicate successfully.
Herbal
None known.
Food
None known.

DIAGNOSTIC TEST EFFECTS
None known.

SIDE EFFECTS
Occasional (6%–2%)
Fever, vomiting, wheezing.
Rare (less than 1%)
Diarrhea, rash, tachycardia, hypertension, hypoxia, injection site inflammation

NURSING CONSIDERATIONS
Baseline Assessment
• Assess the patient's routine arterial blood gases, blood chemistry, electrolytes, osmolality, and total protein.
• Determine the patient's cardiopulmonary status and vital signs before giving the drug, before each dosage or rate increase, and at 30-minute intervals during the infusion and ending 30 minutes after the infusion is completed.
• Record the child's body weight in kilograms.

• Perform a baseline pulmonary assessment, including lung sounds, presence of intercostal retraction, and respiratory rate.

Precautions
• Use cautiously in patients with pulmonary disease.

Administration and Handling
IV
• Refrigerate vials. Do not freeze.
• Do not shake.
• Start infusion within 6 hours and completed within 12 hours of vial entry.
• Initial infusion rate of 1.5 ml/kg/hr for first 15 minutes, then increase to 3 ml/kg/hr next 15 minutes. Infusion rate of 6 ml/kg/hr 30 minutes to end of infusion. Maximum infusion rate is 6 ml/kg/hr.

Intervention and Evaluation
• Monitor the patient's arterial blood gases, blood pressure (B/P), heart rate, respiratory rates, RSV antibody titers, and temperature.
• Observe the patient for rales, intercostals or supraventricular retractions, and wheezing.

Patient Teaching
• Advise the patient to notify the physician if he or she has any heart disease or lung impairment.
• Warn the patient to notify the physician if he or she experiences any allergic reactions (e.g., chest tightness, facial swelling, itching, tingling in the mouth or throat), drowsiness, fever, muscle stiffness, nausea, or vomiting.
• Teach parents how to minimize their child's exposure to infected individuals.
• Encourage the parents to have their child immunized, as recommended.
• Tell the parents to monitor the child for signs infection, including fever.

Rh$_o$(D) immune globulin
(BayRho-D full dose, BayRho Minidose, MICRhogam, RhoGAM, WinRho SDF)

CATEGORY AND SCHEDULE
Pregnancy Risk Category: C

MECHANISM OF ACTION
An immune globulin that is responsible for most cases of Rh sensitization (occurs when Rh-positive fetal red blood cells [RBCs] enter the maternal circulation of an Rh-negative woman). Injection of anti-D globulin results in opsonization of the fetal RBCs, which are then phagocytized in the spleen, preventing immunization of the mother. Injection of anti-D into an Rh-positive patient with idiopathic thrombocytopenic purpura (ITP) coats the patient's own D-positive RBCs with antibody and, as they are cleared by the spleen, they saturate the capacity of the spleen to clear antibody-coated cells, sparing antibody-coated platelets.

AVAILABILITY
Injection, Powder for Reconstitution (WinRho SDF): 120 mcg, 300 mcg, 1000 mcg.
Injection Solution: 50 mcg, 300 mcg.

INDICATIONS AND DOSAGES
▶ **ITP**
IV
Adults, Elderly, Children. (WinRho SDF): Initially, 50 mcg/kg as single dose (reduce to 25–40 mcg/kg if Hgb less than 10 g/dl) Maintenance: 25–60 mcg/kg based on platelet and Hgb levels.

▸ **Pregnancy**
IM (BayRho-D Full Dose,
RhoGAM)
Adults. 300 mcg preferably within
72 hrs of delivery.
IV/IM (WinRho SDF)
Adults. 300 mcg at 28 wks. Follow-
ing delivery: 120 mcg preferably
within 72 hrs.
▸ **Threatened abortion**
IM (BayRho-D Full Dose,
RhoGAM)
Adults. 300 mcg as soon as
possible.
▸ **Abortion, miscarriage, termination
of ectopic pregnancy**
IM (BayRho-D, RhoGAM)
Adults. 300 mcg if greater than
13 wks gestation, 50 mcg if less
than 13 wks gestation.
IM/IV (WinRho SDF)
Adults. 120 mcg after 34 wks gesta-
tion.
▸ **Transfusion incompatibility**
IV
Adults. 3,000 units (600 mcg) q8h
until total dose given.
IM
Adults. 6,000 units (1,200 mcg)
q12h until total dose given.

CONTRAINDICATIONS
Hypersensitivity of any component,
IgA deficiency, $Rh_o(D)$-positive
mother or pregnant woman, transfusion of $Rh_o(D)$-positive blood in
previous 3 months, prior sensitization to $Rh_o(D)$, mothers whose Rh
group or immune status is uncertain

INTERACTIONS
Drug
Live virus vaccines: May interfere
with immune response to live virus
vaccines.
Herbal
None known.
Food
None known.

DIAGNOSTIC TEST EFFECTS
None known.

SIDE EFFECTS
Hypotension, pallor, vasodilation
(IV formulation), fever, headache,
chills, dizziness, somnolence, lethargy, rash, pruritus, abdominal pain,
diarrhea, discomfort and swelling at
injection site, back pain, myalgia,
arthralgia, weakness

SERIOUS REACTIONS
• None known.

NURSING CONSIDERATIONS
Baseline Assessment
• Assess the patient for bleeding
disorders.
• Assess the patient's Hgb levels.
Administer this drug cautiously in
patients with an Hgb level less than
8 g/dl.
Precautions
• Use cautiously in patients with
bleeding disorders, particularly
thrombocytopenia, and blood Hgb
less than 8 g/dl.
Administration and Handling
◂ALERT▸ Must give this drug within
72 hours after exposure of incom-
patible blood transfusion or massive
fetal hemorrhage.
IV
• Refrigerate vials (do not freeze).
• Once reconstituted, solution is stable for 12 hours at room temperature.
• Reconstitute 120 mcg and 300
mcg with 2.5 ml NaCl (8.5 ml for
1,000-mcg vial).
• Gently swirl; do not shake.
• Infuse over 3 to 5 minutes.
IM
• Reconstitute 120 mcg and 300
mcg with 2.5 ml NaCl (8.5 ml for
1,000-mcg vial).
• Administer into deltoid muscle of
upper arm or anterolateral aspect of
upper thigh.

Intervention and Evaluation

• Monitor the patient's complete blood count (CBC), especially BUN, Hgb, platelet count, and serum creatinine, reticulocyte count, and urinalysis.

• Assess the patient for signs and symptoms of hemolysis.

Patient Teaching

• Teach the patient that this drug is given only by injection. Advise the patient that he or she may experience pain at the injection site.

• Warn the patient to notify the physician if he or she experiences chills, dizziness, fever, headache, or rash.

73 Immunologic Agents

adalimumab
alefacept
anakinra
azathioprine
basiliximab
cyclosporine
daclizumab
efalizumab
etanercept
glatiramer
interferon alfa-2a
interferon alfa-2b
interferon alfacon-1
interferon alfa-n3
interferon beta-1a
interferon beta-1b
interferon gamma-1b
muromonab-CD3
mycophenolate
  mofetil
peginterferon alfa-2a
peginterferon alfa-2b
sirolimus
tacrolimus
thalidomide

Uses: Immunologic agents can stimulate or suppress immune function. *Immunostimulants,* such as inteferons and peginterferons, are used to treat infection, immunodeficiency disorders, and cancer. *Immunosuppressants,* such as basiliximab and tacrolimus, are used to inhibit the immune response in autoimmune diseases and to improve short-term and long-term allograft survival. For additional uses, see the specific entries in this chapter.

Action: *Immunostimulants* enhance immune activity, including increased phagocytosis by macrophages and augmentation of specific cytotoxicity by T-lymphocytes. *Immunosuppressants* dampen the immune response; most of them do this by affecting interleukin-2, others by affecting inosine monophosphate dehydrogenase. For additional actions, see the specific entries in this chapter.

COMBINATION PRODUCTS
REBETRON: interferon alfa-2b/ribavirin (an antiviral) 3 million units/200 mg.

adalimumab
ah-dah-**lim**-you-mab
(Humira)

CATEGORY AND SCHEDULE
Pregnancy Risk Category: B

MECHANISM OF ACTION
A monoclonal antibody that binds specifically to tumor necrosis factor (TNF) alpha cell, blocking its action with the cell surface of TNF receptors. *Therapeutic Effect:* Reduces inflammation, tenderness; swelling of joints slows or prevents progressive destruction of joints in those with rheumatoid arthritis.

PHARMACOKINETICS
Half-life: 10–20 days.

AVAILABILITY
Injection: Syringe 40 mg/0.8 ml.

INDICATIONS AND DOSAGES
▶ **Rheumatoid arthritis**
Subcutaneous
Adults, Elderly. 40 mg every other week.

CONTRAINDICATIONS
Active infections

INTERACTIONS
Drug
Methotrexate: Reduces the absorption of adalimumab by 29%–40%, but no adjustments to drug dose is necessary if given concurrently with methotrexate.
Herbal
None known.
Food
None known.

DIAGNOSTIC TEST EFFECTS
May increase blood cholesterol and other components of the lipid profile, and serum alkaline phosphatase levels

SIDE EFFECTS
Frequent (20%)
Injection site reactions, including erythema, itching, pain, and swelling
Occasional (12%–9%)
Headache, rash, sinusitis, nausea
Rare (7%–5%)
Abdominal pain, back pain, hypertension

SERIOUS REACTIONS
• Infection consisting primarily of upper respiratory tract infections, bronchitis, and urinary tract infections occurs rarely.
• More serious infection such as pneumonia, hypersensitivity reaction, tuberculosis, cellulitis, pyelonephritis, and septic arthritis also rarely occurs.

NURSING CONSIDERATIONS
Baseline Assessment
• Assess the duration, location, onset, and type of inflammation or pain.
• Inspect the appearance of the patient's affected joints for deformities, immobility, and skin condition.
• Expect to obtain baseline lab values, including hepatic enzyme levels and a lipid profile.
Lifespan Considerations
• Be aware that it is unknown if adalimumab is excreted in breast milk.
• Be aware that the safety and efficacy of adalimumab have not been established in children.
• Be aware that cautious use in the elderly is necessary due to increased risk of serious infection and malignancy.
Precautions
• Use cautiously in elderly patients, pregnant patients, and patients with cardiovascular disease, demyelinating disorders, history of sensitivity to monoclonal antibodies, and preexisting or recent onset of central nervous system (CNS) disturbances.
Administration and Handling
Subcutaneous
• Refrigerate. Do not freeze.
• Discard unused portion.
• Rotate injection sites.
• Give new injection at least 1 inch from an old site and never into area when skin is bruised, hard, red, or tender.
Intervention and Evaluation
• Monitor the patient's lab values, particularly serum alkaline phosphatase.

• Assess the patient for therapeutic response, improved grip strength, increased joint mobility, reduced joint tenderness, and relief of pain, stiffness, and swelling.

Patient Teaching

• Instruct the patient on how to administer subcutaneous injections, including injection sites.

• Tell the patient that injection site reaction generally occurs in the first month of treatment and decreases in frequency during continued therapy.

• Warn the patient against receiving live vaccines during treatment.

---

alefacept
ale-fah-cept
(Amevive)

CATEGORY AND SCHEDULE
Pregnancy Risk Category: B

MECHANISM OF ACTION
An immunologic agent that interferes with lymphocyte activation by binding to the lymphocyte antigen, inhibiting interaction of T lymphocytes. *Therapeutic Effect:* Reduces the number of circulating total lymphocytes, predominant in psoriatic lesions.

PHARMACOKINETICS
Half-life: 270 hrs.

AVAILABILITY
Powder for Injection: 7.5 mg, 15 mg.

INDICATIONS AND DOSAGES
▸ **Plaque psoriasis**
IM
Adults, Elderly. 15 mg once weekly for 12 wks

IV
Adults, Elderly. 7.5 mg once weekly for 12 wks.

CONTRAINDICATIONS
History of systemic malignancy, concurrent immunosuppressive agents or phototherapy

INTERACTIONS
Drug
None known.
Herbal
None known.
Food
None known.

DIAGNOSTIC TEST EFFECTS
Decreases serum T lymphocyte levels. May increase serum transaminase levels.

IV INCOMPATIBILITIES
Do not mix with any other medications. Do not reconstitute with other diluents other than that supplied by the manufacturer.

SIDE EFFECTS
Frequent (16%)
Injection site reactions with IM administration, including pain and inflammation
Occasional (5%)
Chills
Rare (2% or less)
Pharyngitis, dizziness, cough, nausea, myalgia, injection site pain or inflammation

SERIOUS REACTIONS
• Lymphopenia, malignancies, serious infections requiring hospitalization, including cellulitis, abscess, pneumonia, and postoperative wound infection, and hypersensitivity reactions occur rarely.

• Coronary artery disorder and

myocardial infarction occur in less than 1% of patients.

NURSING CONSIDERATIONS

Baseline Assessment

• Obtain the patient's baseline CD_{4+} lymphocyte counts prior to treatment and weekly during the 12-week dosing period.

Lifespan Considerations

• Be aware that it is unknown if alefacept crosses the placenta or is distributed in breast milk.

• Be aware that the safety and efficacy of this drug have not been established in children.

• Be aware that cautious use is necessary in the elderly due to a higher incidence of infections and certain malignancies.

Precautions

• Use cautiously in elderly patients and patients at high risk for malignancy.

• Use cautiously in patients with chronic infections and a history of recurrent infection.

Administration and Handling

◀ALERT▶ May re-treat, as prescribed, for an additional 12 weeks if a minimum of a 12-week interval has passed since previous course of therapy and CD_{4+} T lymphocyte counts are within normal limits.

◀ALERT▶ For both IM/IV administration, withdraw 0.6 ml of the supplied diluent with the needle pointed at the sidewall of the vial, slowly inject the diluent into the vial of alefacept. Although some foaming will occur, avoid excessive foaming by not shaking or vigorously agitating the vial; swirl gently to dissolve.

IM/IV

• Store unopened vials at room temperature. Following reconstitu-

tion, use immediately or if refrigerated, within 4 hours.

• Discard unused portion within 4 hours of reconstitution.

• Reconstituted solution normally appears clear and colorless to slightly yellow. Do not use if discolored or cloudy or if undissolved material remains.

IM

• Reconstitute 15 mg with 0.6 ml of supplied diluent, sterile water for injection; 0.5 mg of reconstituted solution contains 15 mg alefacept.

• Inject the full 0.5 ml of solution.

• Use a different IM site for each new injection. Give injections at least 1 inch from the old site.

• Avoid areas where the skin is tender, bruised, red, or hard.

IV

• Reconstitute 7.5 mg with 0.6 ml of supplied diluent, sterile water for injection; 0.5 mg of reconstituted solution contains 7.5 mg alefacept.

• Prepare 2 syringes with 3 ml 0.9% NaCl for pre- and post-administration flush.

• Prime the winged infusion set with 3 ml 0.9% NaCl and insert the set into the vein.

• Attach the medication-filled syringe to the infusion set and give over no more than 5 seconds.

• Flush with 3 ml 0.9% NaCl.

Intervention and Evaluation

• Closely monitor CD_{4+} lymphocyte counts.

• Withhold dose if CD_{4+} T lymphocyte counts are below 250 cells/mcL. Discontinue treatment if the patient's levels remain below 250 cells/mcL.

Patient Teaching

• Stress to the patient that regular monitoring of white blood cell (WBC) count during therapy is necessary.

• Warn the patient to notify the physician if he or she experiences

any signs of infection or evidence of malignancy.

• Tell the patient to avoid situations that might place him or her at risk for infection, including contact with infected individuals.

anakinra
ana-**kin**-rah
(Kineret)

CATEGORY AND SCHEDULE
Pregnancy Risk Category: B

MECHANISM OF ACTION
An interleukin-1 receptor antagonist that blocks the binding of interleukin-1 (IL-1), a protein that is a major mediator of joint disease and is present in excess in patients with rheumatoid arthritis. *Therapeutic Effect:* Inhibits inflammatory response.

PHARMACOKINETICS
No accumulation of anakinra in tissues or organs was observed following daily subcutaneous doses. Excreted in the urine. **Half-life:** 4–6 hrs.

AVAILABILITY
Solution: 100-mg syringe.

INDICATIONS AND DOSAGES
▶ **Rheumatoid arthritis**
Subcutaneous
Adults, Children older than 18 yrs, Elderly. 100 mg/day, given at same time each day.

CONTRAINDICATIONS
Known hypersensitivity to *E. coli*–derived proteins, serious infection

INTERACTIONS
Drug
Live virus vaccines: May cause live virus vaccines to be ineffective.
Herbal
None known.
Food
None known.

DIAGNOSTIC TEST EFFECTS
May decrease absolute neutrophil count (ANC), platelet count, and white blood cell (WBC) count. May increase eosinophil count.

SIDE EFFECTS
Occasional
Injection site reactions, including ecchymosis, erythema, and inflammation
Rare
Headache, nausea, diarrhea, abdominal pain

SERIOUS REACTIONS
• Infections, including upper respiratory tract infection, sinusitis, influenza-like symptoms, and cellulitis have been noted.
• Neutropenia may occur, particularly when used in combination with tumor necrosis factor (TNF)-blocking agents.

NURSING CONSIDERATIONS
Baseline Assessment
• Do not give live virus vaccines concurrently with anakinra because the vaccination may not be effective.
Lifespan Considerations
• Be aware that it is unknown if anakinra is distributed in breast milk.
• Be aware that the safety and efficacy of anakinra have not been established in children.

• Use anakinra cautiously in the elderly, who may experience age-related decreased renal function.
Precautions
• Use cautiously in patients with asthma or renal function impairment. Asthmatic patients taking anakinra have a higher incidence of serious infection occurrence. Patients with renal function impairment have an increased risk of toxic reaction.
Administration and Handling
Subcutaneous
• Store in refrigerator. Do not freeze or shake.
• Do not use if particulate or discoloration is noted.
• Give by subcutaneous injection.
Intervention and Evaluation
• Expect to monitor the patient's neutrophil count before therapy begins, monthly for 3 months while receiving therapy, and then quarterly for up to 1 year.
• Evaluate the patient for any inflammatory reactions, especially during first 4 weeks of therapy. Inflammation is uncommon after the first month of therapy.
Patient Teaching
• Teach the patient the proper drug dosage and the correct procedure to administer the subcutaneous dosage.
• Explain the importance of proper disposal of syringes and needles to the patient.

azathioprine
asia-**thigh**-oh-preen
(Alti-Azathioprine[CAN], Azasan, Imuran, Thioprine[AUS])
Do not confuse with Azulfidine, Elmiron, or Imferon.

CATEGORY AND SCHEDULE
Pregnancy Risk Category: D

MECHANISM OF ACTION
An immunologic agent that antagonizes purine metabolism and inhibits DNA, protein, and RNA synthesis. *Therapeutic Effect:* Suppresses cell-mediated hypersensitivities; alters antibody production, immune response in transplant recipients. Reduces arthritis severity.

AVAILABILITY
Tablets: 50 mg, 75 mg, 100 mg.
Injection: 100-mg vial.

INDICATIONS AND DOSAGES
▶ **Kidney transplantation**
IV/PO
Adults, Elderly, Children. Initially, 2–5 mg/kg/day on day of transplant, then 1–3 mg/kg/day as maintenance dose.
▶ **Rheumatoid arthritis**
PO
Adults. Initially, 1 mg/kg/day as single or in 2 divided doses. May increase by 0.5 mg/kg/day after 6–8 wks at 4-wk intervals up to maximum dose of 2.5 mg/kg/day. Maintenance: Lowest effective dosage. May decrease dose by 0.5 mg/kg or 25 mg/day q4wks (other therapy maintained).
Elderly. Initially, 1 mg/kg/day (50–100 mg); may increase by 25 mg/day until response or toxicity.

▸ **Dosage in renal impairment**

Creatinine Clearance	Dose
10–50 ml/min	75%
less than 10 ml/min	50%

UNLABELED USES
Treatment of biliary cirrhosis, chronic active hepatitis, glomerulonephritis, inflammatory bowel disease, inflammatory myopathy, multiple sclerosis, myasthenia gravis, nephrotic syndrome, pemphigoid, pemphigus, polymyositis, systemic lupus erythematosus

CONTRAINDICATIONS
Pregnant rheumatoid arthritis patients

INTERACTIONS
Drug
Allopurinol: May increase azathioprine's activity and risk for azathioprine toxicity.
Bone marrow depressants: May increase the bone marrow depression of these drugs.
Live virus vaccines: May potentiate virus replication, increase the vaccine's side effects, and decrease the patient's antibody response to the vaccine.
Other immunosuppressants: May increase the risk of infection or development of neoplasms.
Herbal
None known.
Food
None known.

DIAGNOSTIC TEST EFFECTS
May decrease serum albumin, Hgb, and serum uric acid levels. May increase serum alkaline phosphatase, serum amylase, serum bilirubin, SGOT (AST), and SGPT (ALT) levels.

IV INCOMPATIBILITIES
Methyl and propyl parabens, phenol

SIDE EFFECTS
Frequent
Nausea, vomiting, anorexia, particularly during early treatment and with large doses
Occasional
Rash
Rare
Severe nausea, vomiting with diarrhea, stomach pain, hypersensitivity reaction

SERIOUS REACTIONS
• There is an increased risk of neoplasia, new, abnormal growth tumors.
• Significant leukopenia and thrombocytopenia may occur, particularly in those undergoing kidney rejection.
• Hepatotoxicity occurs rarely.

NURSING CONSIDERATIONS
Baseline Assessment
• If azathioprine is being given for arthritis, assess the duration, location, onset, and type of fever, inflammation, or pain. Inspect the appearance of affected joints for deformities, immobility, and skin condition.
Precautions
• Use cautiously in immunosuppressed patients.
• Use cautiously in patients previously treated for rheumatoid arthritis with alkylating agents such as chlorambucil, cyclophosphamide, and melphalan.
• Use cautiously in patients with chickenpox currently or who've recovered recently, and those with decreased liver or renal function, gout, herpes zoster, or infection.

Administration and Handling
PO
• Give during or after meals to reduce the potential for GI disturbances.
• Store the oral form at room temperature.
IV
• Store the parenteral form at room temperature.
• After reconstitution, the IV solution is stable for 24 hours.
• Reconstitute 100-mg vial with 10 ml Sterile Water for Injection to provide a concentration of 10 mg/ml.
• Swirl the vial gently and dissolve the solution.
• May further dilute solution in 50 ml D_5W or 0.9% NaCl.
• Infuse the solution over 30 to 60 minutes. Range: 5 minutes to 8 hours.

Intervention and Evaluation
• Perform and monitor complete blood count (CBC), especially platelet count and serum hepatic enzyme levels weekly during the first month of therapy, twice monthly during the second and third months of treatment, then monthly thereafter.
• Expect to reduce or discontinue the drug dose if a rapid fall in white blood cell (WBC) count occurs.
• Assess the patient for delayed bone marrow suppression. Routinely watch for any change from normal.
• In patients receiving azathioprine to treat arthritis, evaluate for signs of a therapeutic response including improved grip strength, increased joint mobility, reduced joint tenderness, and relief of pain, stiffness, and swelling.

Patient Teaching
• Warn the patient to notify the physician if abdominal pain, fever, mouth sores, sore throat, or unusual bleeding occurs.

• Explain to the rheumatoid arthritis patient that the drug's therapeutic response may take up to 12 weeks to manifest.
• Caution women of childbearing age to avoid pregnancy.

basiliximab
bay-zul-**ix**-ah-mab
(Simulect)

CATEGORY AND SCHEDULE
Pregnancy Risk Category: B

MECHANISM OF ACTION
This monoclonal antibody binds to interleukin-2 (IL-2) receptor complex and inhibits IL-2 binding. *Therapeutic Effect:* Prevents lymphocytic activity and impairs response of the immune system to antigens.

PHARMACOKINETICS
Half-life: Adults: 4–10 days; children: 5–17 days.

AVAILABILITY
Powder for Injection: 10 mg, 20 mg.

INDICATIONS AND DOSAGES
▶ **Prophylaxis of organ rejection**
IV
Adults, Elderly, Children weighing 35 kg or more. Two doses of 20 mg each in reconstituted volume of 50 ml given as IV infusion over 20–30 min. Give first dose of 20 mg within 2 hrs before transplant surgery and the second dose of 20 mg 4 days after transplant. *Children weighing less than 35 kg.* 10 mg dose as above.

CONTRAINDICATIONS
None known

INTERACTIONS
Drug
None known.
Herbal
None known.
Food
None known.

DIAGNOSTIC TEST EFFECTS
Alters serum calcium and potassium, blood glucose, Hgb, and Hct levels. Increases BUN and serum cholesterol, creatinine, and uric acid levels. Decreases serum magnesium, serum phosphate, and platelet count.

IV INCOMPATIBILITIES
Specific information not available. Other medications should not be added simultaneously through same IV line.

SIDE EFFECTS
Frequent (greater than 10%)
GI disturbances, as evidenced by constipation, diarrhea, and dyspepsia, central nervous system (CNS) effects, manifested as dizziness, headache, insomnia, and tremor, respiratory infection, dysuria, acne, leg or back pain, peripheral edema, hypertension
Occasional (10%–3%)
Angina, neuropathy, abdominal distention, tachycardia, rash, hypotension, urinary disturbances as evidenced by frequent micturition, genital edema, and hematuria, joint pain, increased hair growth, muscle pain

SERIOUS REACTIONS
• None known.

NURSING CONSIDERATIONS
Baseline Assessment
• Expect to obtain the patient's baseline BUN, blood glucose, and serum calcium, creatinine, phosphatase, potassium, and uric acid levels.
• Obtain the patient's vital signs, particularly blood pressure (B/P) and pulse rate before beginning therapy.
• Breast-feeding is not recommended in female patients receiving basiliximab.
Lifespan Considerations
• Be aware that it is unknown if basiliximab crosses the placenta or is distributed in breast milk.
• There are no age-related precautions noted in children or the elderly.
Precautions
• Use cautiously in patients with a history of malignancy or who have an infection.
Administration and Handling
IV
• Refrigerate the drug. After reconstitution, use within 4 hours (24 hours if refrigerated).
• Discard the solution if a precipitate forms.
• Reconstitute with 5 ml Sterile Water for Injection.
• Shake gently to dissolve.
• Further dilute with 50 ml 0.9% NaCl or D_5W. Gently invert to avoid foaming.
• Infuse over 20 to 30 minutes.
Intervention and Evaluation
• Diligently monitor all of the patient's laboratory test results, especially the patient's complete blood count (CBC).
• Assess the patient's B/P for signs of hypertension or hypotension.
• Assess the patient's pulse for evidence of tachycardia.
• Determine if the patient is experiencing adverse CNS effects, GI disturbances, and urinary changes.
• Monitor the patient for signs or symptoms of a wound infection or

systemic infection, including fever, sore throat, and unusual bleeding or bruising.

Patient Teaching

• Warn the patient to report difficulty in breathing or swallowing, itching, rapid heartbeat, rash, swelling of lower extremities, or weakness to the physician.

• Caution women of childbearing age to avoid pregnancy while taking basiliximab.

cyclosporine

sigh-klo-**spore**-in
(Neoral, Restasis, Sandimmune Neoral[AUS], Sandimmune)
Do not confuse with cycloserine or Cyklokapron.

CATEGORY AND SCHEDULE

Pregnancy Risk Category: C

MECHANISM OF ACTION

A cyclic polypeptide that inhibits interleukin-2, a proliferative factor needed for T-cell activity. *Therapeutic Effect:* Inhibits both cellular and humoral immune responses.

PHARMACOKINETICS

Variably absorbed from the gastrointestinal (GI) tract. Widely distributed. Protein binding: 90%. Metabolized in liver. Eliminated primarily by biliary or fecal excretion. Not removed by hemodialysis. **Half-life:** adults 10–27 hrs, children 7–19 hrs.

AVAILABILITY

Capsules: 25 mg, 100 mg.
Oral Solution: 100 mg/ml in a 50-ml calibrated liquid measuring device.
IV Solution: 50 mg/ml (5-ml amps).
Ophthalmic Emulsion: 0.05%.

INDICATIONS AND DOSAGES

▸ **Prevention of allograft rejection**
PO
Adults, Elderly, Children. Initially, 15 mg/kg as single dose 4–12 hrs prior to transplantation, continue daily dose of 10–14 mg/kg/day for 1–2 wks. Taper dose by 5%/wk over 6–8 wks. Maintenance: 5–10 mg/kg/day.
IV
Adults, Elderly, Children. Give one third of oral dose: 5–6 mg/kg as single dose 4–12 hrs prior to transplantation, continue this daily single dose until patient is able to take oral medication.

▸ **Psoriasis, rheumatoid arthritis**
PO
Adults. 2.5 mg/kg daily in 2 divided doses.

▸ **Dry eye**
Ophthalmic
Adults, Elderly. Apply 2 times/day.

UNLABELED USES

Treatment of alopecia areata, aplastic anemia, atopic dermatitis, Behçet's disease, biliary cirrhosis, corneal transplantation

CONTRAINDICATIONS

History of hypersensitivity to cyclosporine or polyoxyethylated castor oil

INTERACTIONS

Drug
Angiotensin-converting enzyme (ACE) inhibitors, potassium-sparing diuretics, potassium supplements: May cause hyperkalemia.
Cimetidine, danazol, diltiazem, erythromycin, ketoconazole: May increase blood concentration and risk of liver toxicity and nephrotoxicity.
Immunosuppressants: May increase risk of infection and lymphoproliferative disorders.

Live virus vaccines: May decrease the patient's antibody response to the vaccine, increase vaccine side effects, and potentiate virus replication.

Lovastatin: May increase the risk of acute renal failure and rhabdomyolysis.

Herbal

St. John's wort: May alter the absorption of cyclosporine.

Food

Grapefruit and grapefruit juice: May increase the absorption and risk of toxicity of cyclosporine.

DIAGNOSTIC TEST EFFECTS

May increase BUN, serum alkaline phosphatase, amylase, bilirubin, creatinine, potassium, uric acid, SGOT (AST), and SGPT (ALT) levels. May decrease magnesium. Therapeutic blood peak serum level is 50–300 ng/ml; toxic blood serum level is greater than 400 ng/ml.

IV INCOMPATIBILITIES

Amphotericin B complex (AmBisome, Amphotec, Abelcet), magnesium

IV COMPATIBILITIES

Propofol (Diprivan)

SIDE EFFECTS

Frequent

Mild to moderate hypertension (26%), increased hair growth or hirsutism (21%), tremor (12%)

Occasional (4%–2%)

Acne, cramping, gingival hyperplasia, marked by red, bleeding and tender gums, paresthesia, diarrhea, nausea, vomiting, headache

Rare (less than 1%)

Hypersensitivity reaction, abdominal discomfort, gynecomastia, sinusitis

SERIOUS REACTIONS

• Mild nephrotoxicity occurs in 25% of renal transplants after transplantation, 38% in cardiac transplants, and 37% of liver transplants.

• Liver toxicity occurs in 4% of renal, 7% of cardiac, and 4% of liver transplant patients. Both toxicities are usually responsive to dosage reduction.

• Severe hyperkalemia and hyperuricemia occur occasionally.

NURSING CONSIDERATIONS

Baseline Assessment

• Note that if nephrotoxicity occurs, mild toxicity is generally noted 2 to 3 months after transplantation, and more severe toxicity is generally noted early after transplantation.

• Know that liver toxicity may be noted during first month after transplantation.

Lifespan Considerations

• Be aware that cyclosporine readily crosses the placenta and is distributed in breast milk. Breast-feeding should be avoided in this patient population.

• There are no age-related precautions noted in pediatric transplant patients.

• Be aware that in the elderly there is an increased risk of hypertension and an increased serum creatinine level.

Precautions

• Use cautiously in pregnant patients and patients with cardiac impairment, chickenpox, herpes zoster infection, hypokalemia, liver impairment, malabsorption syndrome, and renal impairment.

• Use cautiously in ophthalmic patients with active eye infection.

Administration and Handling

◀ALERT▶ Remember that oral solution is available in bottle form with calibrated liquid measuring device. Expect to begin therapy with oral form as soon as possible.

◄**ALERT**► Expect to give with adrenal corticosteroids. Know that administering other immunosuppressive agents with cyclosporine increases the susceptibility to infection and the development of lymphoma.

PO

• Oral solution may be mixed in glass container with chocolate milk, milk, or orange juice, preferably at room temperature. Stir well. Drink immediately. Avoid using Styrofoam containers, because the liquid form of the drug can adhere to the wall of the container.

• Add more diluent to glass container and mix with remaining solution to ensure total amount is given.

• Dry outside of calibrated liquid measuring device before replacing in cover. Do not rinse with water.

• Avoid refrigeration of oral solution because separation of solution may occur. Discard oral solution after 2 months once bottle is opened.

IV

• Store parenteral form at room temperature.

• Protect IV solution from light.

• After diluted, solution is stable for 24 hours.

• Dilute each ml concentrate with 20 to 100 ml 0.9% NaCl or D_5W.

• Infuse over 2 to 6 hours.

• Monitor the patient continuously for the first 30 minutes after instituting infusion, and frequently thereafter for hypersensitivity reaction, including facial flushing and dyspnea.

Intervention and Evaluation

• Diligently monitor the patient's BUN, LDH concentrations, serum bilirubin, creatinine, SGOT (AST), and SGPT (ALT) levels for liver toxicity or nephrotoxicity. Mild toxicity noted by slow rise in serum levels; more overt toxicity noted by rapid rise in levels. Hematuria is also noted in nephrotoxicity.

• Monitor the patient's serum potassium level for hyperkalemia.

• Encourage the patient to maintain diligent oral hygiene to prevent gum hyperplasia.

• Monitor the patient's blood pressure (B/P) for hypertension.

• Know that the therapeutic serum level of cyclosporine is peak of 50 to 300 ng/ml and that the toxic serum level of cyclosporine is over 400 ng/ml.

Patient Teaching

• Instruct the patient to take the drug at the same times each day, and to notify the physician for further instructions if he or she forgets to take a dose.

• Tell the patient to take his or her dose after a trough level has been drawn.

• Stress to the patient that routine blood testing while receiving cyclosporine is essential to therapy.

• Tell the patient that he or she may experience headache and tremor as a response to the medication.

• Warn the patient to avoid consuming grapefruit and grapefruit juice as these foods increase the blood concentration and side effects of cyclosporine.

• Tell the patient to maintain good oral hygiene to prevent gingivitis caused by gingival hyperplasia.

• Tell the patient to keep the gelcaps in a dry, cool environment, away from direct light.

Keep the gelcaps in their original foil wrapping. Keep the liquid form in the amber-colored glass container.
• Instruct the patient to avoid prolonged exposure to the sun, and to wear sunscreen.

daclizumab
day-**cly**-zu-mab
(Zenapax)

CATEGORY AND SCHEDULE
Pregnancy Risk Category: C

MECHANISM OF ACTION
A monoclonal antibody that binds to and inhibits interleukin-2–mediated lymphocyte activation, a critical pathway in cellular immune response involved in allograft rejection. *Therapeutic Effect:* Prevents organ rejection.

PHARMACOKINETICS
Half-life: 20 days (adults).

AVAILABILITY
Injection: 25 mg/5 ml.

INDICATIONS AND DOSAGES
▶ **Prophylaxis of acute organ rejection in patients receiving renal transplants, in combination with an immunosuppressive regimen**
IV
Adults, Children. 1 mg/kg over 15 min. First dose no more than 24 hrs before transplantation, then q14 days for total of 5 doses. Maximum: 100 mg.

UNLABELED USES
Graft vs. host disease

CONTRAINDICATIONS
None known

INTERACTIONS
Drug
None known.
Herbal
None known.
Food
None known.

DIAGNOSTIC TEST EFFECTS
None known.

IV INCOMPATIBILITIES
Do not mix with any other medication.

SIDE EFFECTS
Occasional (greater than 2%)
Constipation, nausea, diarrhea, vomiting, abdominal pain, edema, headache, dizziness, fever, pain, fatigue, insomnia, weakness, arthralgia, myalgia, increased sweating

SERIOUS REACTIONS
• None known.

NURSING CONSIDERATIONS
Baseline Assessment
• Expect to obtain the patient's baseline lab values, including a complete blood count (CBC), and vital signs, particularly blood pressure (B/P) and pulse rate.
Lifespan Considerations
• Be aware that it is unknown if daclizumab crosses the placenta or is distributed in breast milk.
• There are no age-related precautions noted in children or the elderly.
Precautions
• Use cautiously in patients with a history of malignancy and infection.

Administration and Handling
IV
• Protect from light; refrigerate vials.
• Once reconstituted, solution is stable for 4 hours at room temperature, 24 hours if refrigerated.
• Dilute in 50 ml 0.9% NaCl.
• Invert gently. Avoid shaking.
• Infuse over 15 minutes.

Intervention and Evaluation
• Diligently monitor all blood serum levels and complete blood count (CBC).
• Assess the patient's blood pressure (B/P) for hypertension and hypotension and pulse for evidence of tachycardia.
• Determine if the patient is experiencing gastrointestinal (GI) disturbances and urinary changes.
• Monitor the patient for signs and symptoms of systemic infection such as fever or sore throat, unusual bleeding or bruising, and wound infection.

Patient Teaching
• Warn the patient to notify the physician if he or she experiences difficulty in breathing or swallowing, itching or swelling of the lower extremities, rash, tachycardia, and weakness.
• Caution the patient to avoid pregnancy during daclizumab therapy.
• Tell the patient to avoid circumstances that place him or her at risk for infection, such as crowded areas.

efalizumab
ef-ah-**liz**-ewe-mab
(Raptiva)
CATEGORY AND SCHEDULE
Pregnancy Risk Category: C

MECHANISM OF ACTION
A monoclonal antibody that interferes with lymphocyte activation by binding to the lymphocyte antigen, inhibiting the adhesion of leukocytes to other cell types. *Therapeutic Effect:* Prevents release of cytokines and growth and migration of circulating total lymphocytes, predominant in psoriatic lesions.

AVAILABILITY
Powder for Injection: 150 mg, designed to deliver 125 mg/1.25 ml.

INDICATIONS AND DOSAGES
▸ **Psoriasis**
Subcutaneous
Adults, Elderly. Initially, 0.7 mg/kg followed by weekly subcutaneous doses of 1 mg/kg. Maximum: Single dose not to exceed 200 mg.

CONTRAINDICATIONS
Concurrent use of immunosuppressive agents

INTERACTIONS
Drug
Immunosuppressive agents: Increase the risk of infection.
Live virus vaccines: Decrease the immune response.
Herbal
None known.
Food
None known.

DIAGNOSTIC TEST EFFECTS
Increases lymphocyte count.

SIDE EFFECTS
Frequent (32%–10%)
Headache, chills, nausea, pain at injection site
Occasional (8%–7%)
Myalgia, flu syndrome, fever
Rare (4%)
Back pain, acne

SERIOUS REACTIONS
• Thrombocytopenia, malignancies, serious infections, including cellulitis, abscess, pneumonia, and post-operative wound infection, and hypersensitivity reactions occur rarely.

NURSING CONSIDERATIONS
Baseline Assessment
• Plan to perform baseline lab studies, including a lymphocyte count.
• Examine the patient's skin before beginning therapy and document the extent and location of psoriasis lesions.
Precautions
• Use cautiously in patients with asthma, chronic infections, a history of allergic reactions, a history of malignancy, and recurrent infections.
Administration and Handling
Subcutaneous
• Store unopened vial in refrigerator.
• Reconstituted solution may be stored at room temperature for up to 8 hours.
• Use syringe and needles that are provided.
• Inject the 1.3 ml of Sterile water for Injection into the vial using the provided prefilled diluent syringe.
• Swirl to dissolve; do not shake. Dissolution takes approximately 5 minutes.
Patient Teaching
• Make sure the patient and caregiver know about preparing and injecting the drug, if the patient is to take it at home.
• Tell the patient about potential side effects, including headache, chills, nausea, and pain at the injection site.

etanercept
ee-**tan**-er-cept
(Enbrel)

CATEGORY AND SCHEDULE
Pregnancy Risk Category: B

MECHANISM OF ACTION
A protein that binds to tumor necrosis factor (TNF), blocking its interaction with cell surface receptors. TNF is involved in inflammatory and immune responses; elevated TNF is found in synovial fluid of rheumatoid arthritis patients. *Therapeutic Effect:* Reduces rheumatoid arthritis effects.

PHARMACOKINETICS
Well absorbed after subcutaneous administration. Blocks interactions with cell surface tumor necrosis factor receptors (TNFR). **Half-life:** 115 hrs.

AVAILABILITY
Powder for Injection: 25 mg.

INDICATIONS AND DOSAGES
▶ **Rheumatoid arthritis (RA)**
Subcutaneous
Adults, Elderly. 25 mg twice weekly given 72–96 hrs apart.
Children 4–17 yrs. 0.4 mg/kg (Maximum: 25 mg dose) twice weekly given 72–96 hrs apart.

UNLABELED USES
Crohn's disease

CONTRAINDICATIONS
Serious active infection or sepsis

INTERACTIONS
Drug
None known.

Herbal
None known.
Food
None known.

DIAGNOSTIC TEST EFFECTS
None known.

SIDE EFFECTS
Frequent (37%)
Injection site reaction, including erythema, itching, pain, and swelling, incidence of abdominal pain, vomiting—more common in children than adults
Occasional (16%–4%)
Headache, rhinitis, dizziness, pharyngitis, cough, asthenia, abdominal pain, dyspepsia
Rare (less than 3%)
Sinusitis, allergic reaction

SERIOUS REACTIONS
• Infection, including pyelonephritis, cellulitis, osteomyelitis, wound infection, leg ulcer, septic arthritis, and diarrhea and upper respiratory tract infection, including bronchitis and pneumonia, occur frequently (29%–38%).
• Formation of autoimmune antibodies may occur.
• Serious adverse effects occur rarely, such as heart failure, hypertension, hypotension, pancreatitis, gastrointestinal (GI) hemorrhage, and dyspnea.

NURSING CONSIDERATIONS

Baseline Assessment
• Assess the duration, location, onset, and type of inflammation or pain the patient is experiencing.
• Temporarily discontinue therapy and expect to treat the patient with varicella-zoster immune globulin, as prescribed, if the patient experiences significant exposure to varicella virus during treatment.

Lifespan Considerations
• Be aware that it is unknown if etanercept is excreted in breast milk.
• There are no age-related precautions noted in children older than 4 years of age.
• There are no age-related precautions noted in the elderly.

Precautions
• Use cautiously in patients with a history of recurrent infections or illnesses that predispose to infection, such as diabetes mellitus.

Administration and Handling
◀ALERT▶ Do not add other medications to solution. Do not use filter during reconstitution or administration.
Subcutaneous
• Refrigerate.
• Once reconstituted, may be stored under refrigeration for up to 6 hours.
• Reconstitute with 1 ml of sterile bacteriostatic water for injection (0.9% benzyl alcohol). Do not reconstitute with other diluents.
• Slowly inject the diluent into the vial. Some foaming will occur. To avoid excessive foaming, slowly swirl contents until powder is dissolved over less than 5 minutes.
• Inspect solution for particles or discoloration. Reconstituted solution normally appears clear and colorless. If discolored, cloudy, or particles remain, discard solution; do not use.
• Withdraw all the solution into syringe. Final volume should be approximately 1 ml.
• Inject into the patient's abdomen, thigh, or upper arm. Rotate injection sites.
• Give new injection at least 1 inch from an old site and never into area

when skin is tender, bruised, hard, or red.

Intervention and Evaluation
• Assess the patient for joint swelling, pain, and tenderness.
• Obtain the patient's complete blood count (CBC) and erythrocyte sedimentation rate (ESR) or C-reactive protein level.

Patient Teaching
• Instruct the patient in subcutaneous injection technique, including areas of the body acceptable as injection sites.
• Explain to the patient that injection site reaction generally occurs in first month of treatment and decreases in frequency during continued etanercept therapy.
• Caution the patient against receiving live vaccines during treatment.
• Warn the patient to notify the physician if he or she experiences bleeding, bruising, pallor, or persistent fever.

glatiramer
glah-**tie**-rah-mir
(Copaxone)
Do not confuse with Compazine.

CATEGORY AND SCHEDULE
Pregnancy Risk Category: B

MECHANISM OF ACTION
An immunosuppressive whose exact mechanism is unknown. May act by modifying immune processes thought to be responsible for pathogenesis of multiple sclerosis. *Therapeutic Effect:* Slows progression of multiple sclerosis.

PHARMACOKINETICS
Substantial fraction of glatiramer is hydrolyzed locally. Some fraction of injected material enters lymphatic circulation, reaching regional lymph nodes; some may enter systemic circulation intact.

AVAILABILITY
Injection: 20 mg/ml, prefilled syringes.

INDICATIONS AND DOSAGES
▸ **Multiple sclerosis**
Subcutaneous
Adults, Elderly. 20 mg once a day.

CONTRAINDICATIONS
Hypersensitivity to glatiramer or mannitol

INTERACTIONS
Drug
None known.
Herbal
None known.
Food
None known.

DIAGNOSTIC TEST EFFECTS
None known.

SIDE EFFECTS
Expected (73%–40%)
Pain, erythema, inflammation, pruritus at injection site, asthenia or loss of strength and energy
Frequent (27%–18%)
Arthralgia, vasodilation, anxiety, hypertonia, nausea, transient chest pain, dyspnea, flu syndrome, rash, pruritus
Occasional (17%–10%)
Palpitations, back pain, diaphoresis, rhinitis, diarrhea, urinary urgency
Rare (8%–6%)
Anorexia, fever, neck pain, peripheral edema, ear pain, facial edema, vertigo, vomiting

SERIOUS REACTIONS
• Infection occurs commonly.
• Lymphadenopathy occurs occasionally.

NURSING CONSIDERATIONS
Baseline Assessment
• Obtain baseline vital signs, including temperature.
• Assess the patient's baseline knowledge about administering subcutaneous injections.
Lifespan Considerations
• Be aware that it is unknown if glatiramer is distributed in breast milk.
• Be aware that the safety and efficacy of glatiramer have not been established in children.
• Be aware that there is no information on glatiramer use in the elderly available.
Precautions
• Use cautiously in patients with immediate post injection reaction, including anxiety, chest pain, dyspnea, flushing, palpitations, and urticaria.
Administration and Handling
Subcutaneous
• Refrigerate syringes.
Intervention and Evaluation
• Assess the patient's injection site for reaction.
• Monitor the patient for chills and fever, or other evidence of infection, and treat accordingly.
Patient Teaching
• Warn the patient to notify the physician if he or she experiences difficulty in breathing or swallowing, itching or swelling of the lower extremities, rash, and weakness.
• Caution the patient to avoid pregnancy during glatiramer therapy.
• Instruct the patient in the correct administration of subcutaneous injections.
• Teach the patient about proper disposal of needles.

interferon alfa-2a
inn-ter-**fear**-on
(Roferon-A)
Do not confuse with interferon alfa-2b.

CATEGORY AND SCHEDULE
Pregnancy Risk Category: C

MECHANISM OF ACTION
A biologic response modifier that inhibits viral replication in virus-infected cells. *Therapeutic Effect:* Suppresses cell proliferation; increases phagocytic action of macrophages; augments specific lymphocytic cell toxicity.

PHARMACOKINETICS
Well absorbed after IM, subcutaneous administration. Undergoes proteolytic degradation during reabsorption in kidney. **Half-life:** IM: 2 hrs; Subcutaneous: 3 hrs.

AVAILABILITY
Injection: 3 million units, 6 million units, 9 million units, 36 million units.

INDICATIONS AND DOSAGES
▸ **Hairy cell leukemia**
Subcutaneous/IM
Adults. Initially, 3 million units/day for 16–24 wks. Maintenance: 3 million units 3 times/wk. Do not use 36-million-unit vial.
▸ **Chronic myelocytic leukemia (CML)**
Subcutaneous/IM
Adults. 9 million units daily.

▶ **Melanoma**
Subcutaneous/IM
Adults, Elderly. 12 million units/m^2 3 times/wk for 3 mos.
▶ **AIDS-related Kaposi's sarcoma**
Subcutaneous/IM
Adults. Initially, 36 million units/day for 10–12 wks, may give 3 million units on day 1; 9 million units on day 2; 18 million units on day 3; then begin 36 million units/day for remainder of 10–12 wks. Maintenance: 36 million units/day 3 times/wk.
▶ **Chronic hepatitis C**
Subcutaneous/IM
Adults. Initially, 6 million units once a day for 3 wks, then 3 million units 3 times/wk for 6 mos.

UNLABELED USES
Treatment of active, chronic hepatitis, bladder or renal carcinoma, malignant melanoma, multiple myeloma, mycosis fungoides, non-Hodgkin's lymphoma

CONTRAINDICATIONS
None known

INTERACTIONS
Drug
Bone marrow depressants: May have additive effect.
Herbal
None known.
Food
None known.

DIAGNOSTIC TEST EFFECTS
May increase LDH concentration, serum alkaline phosphatase, SGOT (AST), and SGPT (ALT) levels. May decrease blood Hgb and Hct, and leukocyte and platelet counts.

SIDE EFFECTS
Frequent (greater than 20%)
Flu-like symptoms, including fever, fatigue, headache, aches, pains, anorexia, and chills, nausea, vomiting, coughing, dyspnea, hypotension, edema, chest pain, dizziness, diarrhea, weight loss, taste change, abdominal discomfort, confusion, paresthesia, depression, visual and sleep disturbances, diaphoresis, lethargy
Occasional (20%–5%)
Partial alopecia, rash, dry throat or skin, pruritus, flatulence, constipation, hypertension, palpitations, sinusitis
Rare (less than 5%)
Hot flashes, hypermotility, Raynaud's syndrome, bronchospasm, earache, ecchymosis

SERIOUS REACTIONS
• Arrhythmias, stroke, transient ischemic attacks, congestive heart failure (CHF), pulmonary edema, and myocardial infarction (MI) occur rarely.

NURSING CONSIDERATIONS
Baseline Assessment
• Plan to perform blood chemistries, BUN, complete blood count (CBC), platelet counts, serum alkaline phosphatase, creatinine, SGOT (AST), and SGPT (ALT) levels, and urinalysis before beginning therapy, and routinely thereafter.
Lifespan Considerations
• Be aware that interferon alfa-2a use should be avoided during pregnancy. Breast-feeding is not recommended in this patient population.
• Be aware that the safety and efficacy of interferon alfa-2a have not been established in children.
• Be aware that in the elderly, cardiotoxicity and neurotoxicity may occur more frequently.
• In the elderly, age-related renal impairment may require cautious use of interferon alfa-2a.

Precautions
• Use cautiously in patients with cardiac diseases, compromised central nervous system (CNS) function, history of cardiac abnormalities, liver or renal impairment, myelosuppression, and seizure disorders.

Administration and Handling
◀ALERT▶ Be aware that the subcutaneous route of administration is preferred for thrombocytopenic patients and other patients at risk for bleeding.

◀ALERT▶ Remember that the drug dosage is individualized based on the patient's clinical response and tolerance of the drug's adverse effects. When used in combination therapy, expect to consult specific protocols for optimum dosage, and sequence of drug administration. If severe adverse reactions occur, modify the drug dosage or temporarily discontinue the medication, as prescribed.

Subcutaneous/IM
• Refrigerate.
• Do not shake vial. Do not use if precipitate or discoloration occurs; solution normally appears colorless.

Intervention and Evaluation
• Offer the patient emotional support.
• Monitor all levels of the patient's clinical function, as well as for the numerous side effects.
• Encourage the patient to drink ample fluids, particularly during early therapy.

Patient Teaching
• Tell the patient that the drug's clinical response may take 1 to 3 months to appear.
• Instruct the patient that flu-like symptoms tend to diminish with continued therapy.

• Urge the patient not to consume alcohol during drug therapy.
• Caution the patient to use caution when performing tasks that require mental alertness or motor skills.
• Warn the patient to notify the physician if he or she experiences nausea or vomiting that continues at home.
• Tell female patients to use contraception, and to notify the physician if she suspects pregnancy.

interferon alfa-2b
inn-ter-**fear**-on
(Intron-A)
Do not confuse with interferon alfa-2b.

CATEGORY AND SCHEDULE
Pregnancy Risk Category: C

MECHANISM OF ACTION
A biologic response modifier that inhibits viral replication in virus-infected cells, suppresses cell proliferation. *Therapeutic Effect:* Increases phagocytic action of macrophages, augments specific cytotoxicity of lymphocytes.

PHARMACOKINETICS
Well absorbed after IM, subcutaneous administration. Undergoes proteolytic degradation during reabsorption in kidney. **Half-life:** 2–3 hrs.

AVAILABILITY
Injection Powder for Reconstitution: 3 million units, 5 million units, 6 million units, 10 million units, 18 million units, 25 million units, 50 million units.
Injection, Prefilled Syringes: 3 million units, 5 million units, 6 million

units, 10 million units, 18 million units, 25 million units, 50 million units.

INDICATIONS AND DOSAGES
▸ **Hairy cell leukemia**
IM/Subcutaneous
Adults. 2 million units/m^2 3 times/wk. If severe adverse reactions occur, modify dose or temporarily discontinue.
▸ **Condylomata acuminata**
Intralesional
Adults. 1 million units/lesion 3 times/wk for 3 wks. Use only 10-million-units vial, reconstitute with no more than 1 ml diluent. Use tuberculin (TB) syringe with 25- or 26-gauge needle. Give in evening with acetaminophen, which alleviates side effects.
▸ **AIDS-related Kaposi's sarcoma**
IM/Subcutaneous
Adults. 30 million units/m^2 3 times/wk. Use only 50 million units vials. If severe adverse reactions occur, modify dose or temporarily discontinue.
▸ **Chronic hepatitis C**
IM/Subcutaneous
Adults. 3 million units 3 times/wk for up to 6 mos, for up to 18–24 mos for chronic hepatitis C.
▸ **Chronic hepatitis B**
IM/Subcutaneous
Adults. 30–35 million units/wk, 5 million units/day or 10 million units 3 times/wk.
▸ **Malignant melanoma**
IV
Adults. Initially, 20 million units/m^2 5 times/wk for 4 wks. Maintenance: 10 million units IM/Subcutaneous for 48 wks.

UNLABELED USES
Treatment of bladder, cervical, renal carcinoma, chronic myelocytic leukemia, laryngeal papillomatosis, multiple myeloma, mycosis fungoides

CONTRAINDICATIONS
None known

INTERACTIONS
Drug
Bone marrow depressants: May have additive effect.
Herbal
None known.
Food
None known.

DIAGNOSTIC TEST EFFECTS
May increase LDH concentration, activated partial thromboplastin time, prothrombin time, serum alkaline phosphatase, SGOT (AST), and SGPT (ALT) levels. May decrease blood Hgb and Hct and leukocyte and platelet counts.

IV INCOMPATIBILITIES
No information available. Do not mix with other medications via Y-site administration.

SIDE EFFECTS
Frequent
Flu-like symptoms, including fever, fatigue, headache, aches, pains, anorexia, and chills, rash with hairy cell leukemia (Kaposi's sarcoma only)
Kaposi's sarcoma: All previously mentioned side effects plus depression, dyspepsia, dry mouth or thirst, alopecia, rigors
Occasional
Dizziness, pruritus, dry skin, dermatitis, alteration in taste
Rare
Confusion, leg cramps, back pain, gingivitis, flushing, tremor, nervousness, eye pain

SERIOUS REACTIONS
• Hypersensitivity reaction occurs rarely.
• Severe adverse reactions of flu-like symptoms appear dose related.

NURSING CONSIDERATIONS

Baseline Assessment
• Perform blood chemistries, BUN, complete blood count (CBC), serum alkaline phosphatase, creatinine, SGOT (AST), and SGPT (ALT) levels, and urinalysis before beginning therapy and routinely thereafter.

Lifespan Considerations
• Be aware that interferon alfa-2b use should be avoided during pregnancy. Breast-feeding is not recommended in this patient population.
• Be aware that the safety and efficacy of interferon alfa-2b have not been established in children.
• Be aware that in the elderly, cardiotoxicity and neurotoxicity may occur more frequently.
• In the elderly, age-related renal impairment may require cautious use of interferon alfa-2b.

Precautions
• Use cautiously in patients with cardiac diseases, compromised central nervous system (CNS) function, history of cardiac abnormalities, liver or renal impairment, myelosuppression, and seizure disorders.

Administration and Handling
◀ALERT▶ Know that the drug dosage is individualized based on the patient's clinical response and tolerance of the drug's adverse effects. When used in combination therapy, consult specific protocols for optimum dosage and sequence of drug administration, as prescribed.
◀ALERT▶ Remember that side effects are dose-related.

Subcutaneous/IM
• Do not give IM if the patient's platelet count is less than 50,000/m³; instead give subcutaneous.
• For hairy cell leukemia patients, reconstitute each 3-million-unit vial with 1 ml bacteriostatic water for injection to provide concentration of 3 million units/ml, 1-ml to 5-million-units vial; 2-ml to 10-million-units vial; 5-ml to 25-million-units vial provides concentration of 5 million units/ml.
• For condylomata acuminata, reconstitute each 10-million-unit vial with 1 ml bacteriostatic water for injection to provide concentration of 10 million units/ml.
• For acquired immune deficiency syndrome (AIDS)-related Kaposi's sarcoma patients, reconstitute 50-million-unit vial with 1 ml bacteriostatic water for injection to provide concentration of 50 million units/ml.
• Agitate the vial gently and withdraw solution with sterile syringe.
IV
• Refrigerate unopened vials, stable for 7 days at room temperature.
• Prepare immediately before use.
• Reconstitute with diluent provided by manufacturer.
• Withdraw desired dose and further dilute with 100 ml 0.9% NaCl to provide final concentration at least 10 million units/100 ml.
• Administer over 20 minutes.

Intervention and Evaluation
• Offer the patient emotional support.
• Monitor all levels of the patient's clinical function, as well as the numerous side effects.
• Encourage the patient to drink ample fluids, particularly during early therapy.

Patient Teaching
• Explain to the patient that the drug's clinical response may take 1 to 3 months to appear.
• Tell the patient that flu-like symptoms tend to diminish with continued therapy. Explain to the patient that some symptoms may be alleviated or minimized by bedtime doses.
• Caution the patient against receiving immunizations without the physician's approval as interferon alfa-2b lowers the body's resistance.
• Warn the patient to avoid contact with those who have recently received live virus vaccine.
• Warn the patient to avoid tasks that require mental alertness or motor skills until his or her response to the drug is established.
• Suggest to the patient that sips of tepid water may relieve dry mouth.

interferon alfacon-1
inn-ter-**fear**-on
(Infergen)

CATEGORY AND SCHEDULE

MECHANISM OF ACTION
A biologic response modifier that stimulates the immune system. *Therapeutic Effect:* Inhibits hepatitis C virus.

AVAILABILITY
Injection: 15-mcg vials, 9-mcg vials.

INDICATIONS AND DOSAGES
▸ **Chronic hepatitis C**
Subcutaneous
Adults. 9 mcg 3 times/wk for 24 wks. May increase to 15 mcg in patients tolerating 9-mcg dose and not responding adequately.

SIDE EFFECTS
Frequent (greater than 50%)
Headache, fatigue, fever, depression

NURSING CONSIDERATIONS
Baseline Assessment
• Expect to obtain baseline serum alkaline phosphatase, SGOT (AST), and SGPT (ALT) levels to assess liver function, hepatitis C virus (HCV) serum antibodies, and HCV-RNA.
Administration and Handling
◂**ALERT**▸ At least 48 hours should elapse between doses of interferon alfacon-1.
Intervention and Evaluation
• Plan to obtain periodic HCV antibody and serum hepatic enzyme levels.
Patient Teaching
• Tell the patient to report any side effects as soon as possible, including headache or injection site pain.
• Teach the patient how hepatitis C is thought to be transmitted, such as by blood and body fluid.

interferon alfa-n3
inn-ter-**fear**-on
(Alferon N)

CATEGORY AND SCHEDULE
Pregnancy Risk Category: C

MECHANISM OF ACTION
A biologic response modifier that inhibits viral replication in virus-infected cells. *Therapeutic Effect:* Suppresses cell proliferation, increases phagocytic action of macrophages, augments specific cytotoxicity of lymphocytes.

AVAILABILITY
Injection: 5 million units.

INDICATIONS AND DOSAGES
▸ **Condylomata acuminata**
Intralesional
Adults, Children older than 18 yrs.
0.05 ml (250,000 units) per wart
2 times/wk up to 8 wks. Maximum
dose/treatment session: 0.5 ml
(2.5 million units). Do not repeat
for 3 mos after initial 8 wks unless
warts enlarge or new warts appear.

UNLABELED USES
Treatment of active chronic hepatitis, bladder carcinoma, chronic
myelocytic leukemia, laryngeal
papillomatosis, malignant melanoma, multiple myeloma, mycosis
fungoides, non-Hodgkin's lymphoma

CONTRAINDICATIONS
Previous history of anaphylactic
reaction to egg protein, mouse
immunoglobulin (IgG), or neomycin

INTERACTIONS
Drug
Bone marrow depressants: May
have additive effect.
Herbal
None known.
Food
None known.

DIAGNOSTIC TEST EFFECTS
May increase LDH concentration,
serum alkaline phosphatase, SGOT
(AST), and SGPT (ALT) levels.
May decrease blood Hgb and Hct
and leukocyte and platelet counts.

SIDE EFFECTS
Frequent
Flu-like symptoms, including fever,
fatigue, headache, aches, pains,
anorexia, and chills

Occasional
Dizziness, pruritus, dry skin, dermatitis, alteration in taste
Rare
Confusion, leg cramps, back pain,
gingivitis, flushing, tremor, nervousness, eye pain

SERIOUS REACTIONS
• Hypersensitivity reaction occurs
rarely.
• Severe adverse reactions of flu-like symptoms appear dose related.

NURSING CONSIDERATIONS
Precautions
• Use cautiously in patients with
diabetes mellitus with ketoacidosis,
hemophilia, pulmonary embolism,
seizure disorders, severe myelosuppression, severe pulmonary disease,
thrombophlebitis, uncontrolled
congestive heart failure (CHF), and
unstable angina.
Administration and Handling
Intralesional
• Refrigerate vial. Do not freeze or
shake.
• Inject into base of each wart with
30-gauge needle.
Intervention and Evaluation
• Monitor all levels of the patient's
clinical function, as well as the
numerous side effects.
• Encourage the patient to drink
ample fluids, particularly during
early therapy.
Patient Teaching
• Warn the patient that flu-like
symptoms tend to diminish with
continued therapy. Explain to the
patient that some symptoms may be
alleviated or minimized by bedtime
doses.
• Let the patient know about any
follow-up testing.

interferon beta-1a
inn-ter-**fear**-on
(Avonex, Rebif)
Do not confuse with Avelox or interferon beta-1b.

CATEGORY AND SCHEDULE
Pregnancy Risk Category: C

MECHANISM OF ACTION
A biologic response modifier that interacts with specific cell receptors found on surface of human cells. *Therapeutic Effect:* Possesses antiviral and immuno-regulatory activities.

PHARMACOKINETICS
After IM administration, peak serum levels attained in 3–15 hrs. Biologic markers increase within 12 hrs and remain elevated for 4 days. **Half-life:** 10 hrs (IM).

AVAILABILITY
Prefilled Syringes Powder for Injection: 22 mcg (Rebif), 30 mcg (Avonex), 44 mcg (Rebif).

INDICATIONS AND DOSAGES
▸ **Relapsing-remitting multiple sclerosis**
IM
Adults. 30 mcg Avonex once weekly.
Subcutaneous
Adults. Initially 8.8 mcg Rebif 3 times/wk, may increase over 4–6 wks to 44 mcg Rebif 3 times/wk.

UNLABELED USES
Treatment of acquired immune deficiency syndrome (AIDS), AIDS-related Kaposi's sarcoma, malignant melanoma, renal cell carcinoma

CONTRAINDICATIONS
Hypersensitivity to albumin, interferon

INTERACTIONS
Drug
None known.
Herbal
None known.
Food
None known.

DIAGNOSTIC TEST EFFECTS
May increase blood glucose levels, BUN, serum alkaline phosphatase, bilirubin, calcium, SGOT (AST), and SGPT (ALT) levels. May decrease blood Hgb, neutrophil, platelet, and white blood cell (WBC) counts.

SIDE EFFECTS
Frequent
Headache (67%), flu-like symptoms (61%), myalgia (34%), upper respiratory infection (31%), pain (24%), asthenia, chills (21%), sinusitis (18%), infection (11%)
Occasional
Abdominal pain, arthralgia (9%), chest pain, dyspnea (6%), malaise, syncope (4%)
Rare
Injection site reaction, hypersensitivity reaction (3%)

SERIOUS REACTIONS
• Anemia occurs in 8% of patients.

NURSING CONSIDERATIONS
Baseline Assessment
• Obtain blood chemistries, including complete blood count (CBC), serum alkaline phosphatase, SGOT (AST), and SGPT (ALT) levels.
• Assess the patient's home situation for support of therapy.

Lifespan Considerations
• Be aware that interferon beta-1a has abortifacient potential.
• Be aware that it is unknown if interferon beta-1a is distributed in breast milk.
• Be aware that the safety and efficacy of interferon beta-1a have not been established in children.
• Be aware that there is no information on interferon beta-1a use in the elderly.

Precautions
• Use cautiously in pediatric patients younger than 18 years of age and patients with chronic progressive multiple sclerosis.

Administration and Handling
IM
• Refrigerate vials.
• Following reconstitution, use within 6 hours if refrigerated. Discard if discolored or contains a precipitate.
• Reconstitute 33-mcg (6.6-million-unit) vial with 1.1 ml diluent, which is supplied by the manufacturer.
• Gently swirl to dissolve medication; do not shake.
• Discard unused portion because it contains no preservative.
Subcutaneous
• Administer drug at the same time of day 3 days each week. Doses to be separated by at least 48 hours.

Intervention and Evaluation
• Assess for the patient for flu-like symptoms, headache, and muscle aches.
• Periodically monitor the patient's lab results and reevaluate injection technique.
• Evaluate the patient for depression and suicidal ideation.

Patient Teaching
• Caution the patient against changing the drug dose schedule or drug dosage without consultation with the physician.
• Instruct the patient on the correct reconstitution of the product and its administration, including aseptic technique. Explain to the patient that he or she must dispose of needles and syringes in the provided puncture-resistant container.
• Tell the patient that he or she may experience injection site reactions. Teach the patient to document the type and severity of injection site reactions. Explain to the patient that these reactions will not require discontinuation of therapy.
• Warn the patient to immediately notify the physician if he or she experiences depression or suicidal ideation.

interferon beta-1b
inn-ter-**fear**-on
(Betaferon, Betaseron)
Do not confuse with interferon beta-1a.

CATEGORY AND SCHEDULE
Pregnancy Risk Category: C

MECHANISM OF ACTION
A biologic response modifier that interacts with specific cell receptors found on surface of human cells. *Therapeutic Effect:* Possesses antiviral and immunoregulatory activities.

PHARMACOKINETICS
Half-life: 8 min–4.3 hrs.

AVAILABILITY
Powder for Injection: 0.3 mg (9.6 million units).

INDICATIONS AND DOSAGES
▶ **Relapsing-remitting multiple sclerosis**
Subcutaneous
Adults. 0.25 mg (8 million units) every other day.

UNLABELED USES
Treatment of acquired immune deficiency syndrome (AIDS), AIDS-related Kaposi's sarcoma, acute non-A and non-B hepatitis, malignant melanoma, renal cell carcinoma malignant melanoma

CONTRAINDICATIONS
Hypersensitivity to albumin, interferon

INTERACTIONS
Drug
None known.
Herbal
None known.
Food
None known.

DIAGNOSTIC TEST EFFECTS
May increase blood glucose, BUN, serum alkaline phosphatase, bilirubin, calcium, SGOT (AST), and SGPT (ALT) levels. May decrease blood Hgb, neutrophils, platelets, and white blood cell (WBC) counts.

SIDE EFFECTS
Frequent
Injection site reaction (85%), headache (84%), flu-like symptoms (76%), fever (59%), pain (52%), asthenia (49%), myalgia (44%), sinusitis (36%), diarrhea, dizziness (35%), mental status changes (29%), constipation (24%), diaphoresis (23%), vomiting (21%)
Occasional
Malaise (15%), somnolence (6%), alopecia (4%)

SERIOUS REACTIONS
• Seizures occur rarely.

NURSING CONSIDERATIONS
Baseline Assessment
• Obtain blood chemistries, including complete blood count (CBC), serum alkaline phosphatase, SGOT (AST), and SGPT (ALT) levels.
• Assess the patient's home situation for support of therapy.
Lifespan Considerations
• Be aware that it is unknown if interferon beta-1b is distributed in breast milk.
• Be aware that the safety and efficacy of interferon beta-1b have not been established in children.
• Be aware that there is no information available on interferon beta-1b use in the elderly.
Precautions
• Use cautiously in pediatric patients younger than 18 years of age and patients with chronic progressive multiple sclerosis.
Administration and Handling
Subcutaneous
• Store vials at room temperature.
• After reconstitution the solution is stable for 3 hours if refrigerated.
• Use within 3 hours of reconstitution.
• Discard the solution if it is discolored or contains a precipitate.
• Reconstitute 0.3-mg (9.6-million-unit) vial with 1.2 ml diluent, which is supplied by manufacturer, to provide concentration of 0.25 mg/ml (8 million units/ml).
• Gently swirl to dissolve medication; do not shake.
• Withdraw 1 ml solution and inject subcutaneous into the patient's abdomen, arms, hips, or thighs using a 27-gauge needle.
• Discard unused portion because it contains no preservative.

Intervention and Evaluation
• Periodically monitor lab results and reevaluate injection technique.
• Assess the patient for nausea because there is a high incidence of this side effect.
• Monitor the patient's sleep pattern.
• Assess the patient's daily pattern of bowel activity and stool consistency.
• Assist the patient with ambulation if he or she experiences dizziness.
• Determine if the patient experiences epigastric discomfort and heartburn.
• Monitor the patient's food intake.
• Evaluate the patient for depression and suicidal ideation.

Patient Teaching
• Tell the patient to notify the physician if he or she experiences flu-like symptoms. Explain to the patient that flu-like symptoms occur commonly but decrease as therapy continues.
• Warn the patient to immediately notify the physician if he or she experiences depression or suicidal ideation.
• Tell the patient to avoid pregnancy.

---

interferon gamma-1b
inn-ter-*fear*-on
(Actimmune, Imukin[AUS])

CATEGORY AND SCHEDULE
Pregnancy Risk Category: C

MECHANISM OF ACTION
A biologic response modifier that induces activation of macrophages in blood monocytes to phagocytes, which is necessary in cellular immune response to intracellular and extracellular pathogens. *Therapeutic Effect:* Enhances phagocytic function, antimicrobial activity of monocytes.

PHARMACOKINETICS
Slowly absorbed after subcutaneous administration.

AVAILABILITY
Injection: 100 mcg (3 million units).

INDICATIONS AND DOSAGES
▸ **Chronic granulomatous disease, severe, malignant osteopetrosis**
Subcutaneous
Adults, Children older than 1 yr.
50 mcg/m^2 (1.5 million units/m^2) in patients with body surface area (BSA) greater than 0.5 m^2; 1.5 mcg/kg/dose in patients with BSA 0.5 m^2 or less. Give 3 times/wk.

CONTRAINDICATIONS
Hypersensitivity to *Escherichia coli* products

INTERACTIONS
Drug
Bone marrow depressants:
May increase bone marrow depression.
Herbal
None known.
Food
None known.

DIAGNOSTIC TEST EFFECTS
None known.

SIDE EFFECTS
Frequent
Fever (52%); headache (33%); rash (17%); chills, fatigue, diarrhea (14%)
Occasional (13%–10%)
Vomiting, nausea

Rare (6%–3%)
Weight loss, myalgia, anorexia

SERIOUS REACTIONS
• May exacerbate preexisting central nervous system (CNS) disturbances, including decreased mental status, gait disturbance, and dizziness, as well as cardiac disorders.

NURSING CONSIDERATIONS
Baseline Assessment
• Plan to perform blood chemistries, including BUN, serum alkaline phosphatase, creatinine, SGOT (AST), SGPT (ALT) levels, to assess hepatic and renal function, complete blood count (CBC), and urinalysis before beginning drug therapy, and at 3-month intervals during course of treatment.
Lifespan Considerations
• Be aware that it is unknown if interferon gamma-1b crosses the placenta or is distributed in breast milk.
• Be aware that the safety and efficacy of interferon gamma-1b have not been established in children younger than 1 year of age.
• Be aware that children experience flu-like symptoms may frequently.
• Be aware that there is no information available on interferon gamma-1b use in the elderly.
Precautions
• Use cautiously in patients with compromised central nervous system (CNS) function, myelosuppression, preexisting cardiac diseases, including arrhythmias, congestive heart failure (CHF), and myocardial ischemia, and seizure disorders.
Administration and Handling
◀ALERT▶ Avoid excessive agitation of vial; do not shake.
Subcutaneous
• Refrigerate vials. Do not freeze.

• Do not keep at room temperature longer than 12 hours; discard after 12 hours.
• Vials are single dose; discard unused portion.
• Do not use if discolored or precipitate forms; solution normally appears clear, colorless.
• When given 3 times a week, administer in left deltoid, right deltoid, and anterior thigh.
Intervention and Evaluation
• Monitor the patient for flu-like symptoms, including chills, fatigue, fever, and muscle aches.
• Assess the patient's skin for rash.
Patient Teaching
• Tell the patient that flu-like symptoms, such as chills, fatigue, fever, and muscle aches, are generally mild and tend to disappear as treatment continues. Explain to the patient that symptoms may be minimized with bedtime administration.
• Warn the patient to avoid performing tasks that require mental alertness or motor skills until his or her response to the drug is established.
• Instruct the patient the proper technique of administration and disposal of needles and syringes.
• Teach the patient that vials should remain refrigerated.

muromonab-CD3
meur-oh-**mon**-ab
(Orthoclone, OKT3)

CATEGORY AND SCHEDULE
Pregnancy Risk Category: C

MECHANISM OF ACTION
An antibody derived from purified IgG_2 immune globulin that

reacts with T3 (CD3) antigen of human T-cell membranes. Blocks function of T cells, which has major role in acute renal rejection. *Therapeutic Effect:* Reverses graft rejection.

AVAILABILITY
Injection: 1 mg/ml.

INDICATIONS AND DOSAGES
▸ **Treat acute allograft rejection**
IV
Adults, Elderly, Children weighing more than 30 kg. 5 mg/day for 10–14 days. Begin when acute renal rejection is diagnosed.
Children younger than 12 yrs. 0.1 mg/kg/day for 10–14 days.

CONTRAINDICATIONS
History of hypersensitivity to muromonab-CD3 or any murine origin product, patients with fluid overload evidenced by chest x-ray or a greater than 3% weight gain within the week before initial treatment

INTERACTIONS
Drug
Live virus vaccines: May decrease the patient's response to the vaccine, increase the vaccine's side effects, and potentiate virus replication.
Other immunosuppressants: May increase the risk of infection or development of lymphoproliferative disorders.
Herbal
Echinacea: May decrease the effects of muromonab.
Food
None known.

DIAGNOSTIC TEST EFFECTS
None known.

IV INCOMPATIBILITIES
Do not mix with any other medications.

SIDE EFFECTS
Frequent
First-dose reaction: Fever, chills, dyspnea, malaise occurs 30 min– 6 hrs after first dose reaction and will markedly diminish with subsequent dosing after first 2 days of treatment.
Occasional
Chest pain, nausea, vomiting, diarrhea, tremor

SERIOUS REACTIONS
• Cytokine release syndrome (CRS) may range from flu-like illness to life-threatening shock-like reaction.
• Occasionally fatal hypersensitivity reactions occur.
• Severe pulmonary edema occurs in less than 2% of those treated with muromonab-CD3.
• Infection, caused by immunosuppression generally occurs within 45 days after initial treatment, cytomegalovirus occurs in 19% of patients, and herpes simplex occurs in 27% of patients.
• Severe and life-threatening infection occurs in less than 4.8% of patients.

NURSING CONSIDERATIONS
Baseline Assessment
• Plan to obtain a chest x-ray within 24 hours of beginning muromonab therapy to ensure the patient's lungs are clear of fluid.
• Know that the patient's weight should be 3% or less above minimum weight the week before beginning treatment; pulmonary edema occurs when fluid overload is present before muromonab treatment.

• Have resuscitative drugs and equipment immediately available.

Precautions

• Use cautiously in patients with impaired cardiac, liver, or renal function.

Administration and Handling

IV

• Refrigerate ampoule. If left out of refrigerator for longer than 4 hours, do not use.

• Do not shake ampoule before using.

• Fine translucent particles may develop, but does not affect potency.

• Draw solution into syringe through 0.22-micron filter. Discard filter; use needle for IV administration.

• Administer IV push over less than 1 minute.

• Give methylprednisolone 1 mg/kg before and 100 mg hydrocortisone 30 minutes after drug dose, as prescribed to decrease adverse reactions to the first dose.

Intervention and Evaluation

• Monitor the patient's immunologic tests, including plasma levels and quantitative T lymphocyte surface phenotyping, liver and renal function tests, and white blood cell (WBC) count, before beginning and during therapy.

• Give antipyretics to patients experiencing fevers exceeding 100°F.

• Expect to monitor the patient for fluid overload by chest x-ray, and monitor the patient's weight. Observe the patient for any weight gain of more than 3% over his or her pre-therapy weight.

• Assess the patient's lung sounds for fluid overload.

• Monitor the patient's intake and output.

• Assess the patient's daily pattern of bowel activity and stool consistency.

Patient Teaching

• Tell the patient he or she may experience first-dose reaction, including chest tightness, chills, diarrhea, fever, nausea, vomiting, and wheezing.

• Warn the patient to avoid receiving immunizations during therapy.

• Caution the patient to avoid crowds and those with known infections during muromonab therapy.

mycophenolate mofetil

my-koe-**phen**-oh-late
(CellCept)

CATEGORY AND SCHEDULE

Pregnancy Risk Category: C

MECHANISM OF ACTION

An immunologic agent that inhibits inosine monophosphate dehydrogenase, an enzyme that deprives lymphocytes of nucleotides necessary for DNA and RNA synthesis. Inhibits proliferation of T and B lymphocytes. Suppresses immunologically mediated inflammatory response. *Therapeutic Effect*: Prevents transplant rejection.

PHARMACOKINETICS

Rapidly, extensively absorbed after PO administration (food does not alter the extent of absorption, but plasma concentration decreased in presence of food). Protein binding: 97%. Completely hydrolyzed to active metabolite mycophenolic acid (MPA). Primarily excreted in urine. Not removed by hemodialysis. **Half-life:** 17.9 hrs.

AVAILABILITY
Capsules: 250 mg.
Tablets: 500 mg.
Oral Suspension: 200 mg/ml.
Injection: 500 mg.

INDICATIONS AND DOSAGES
▸ **Renal transplant**
IV/PO
Adults, Elderly. 1 g 2 times/day.
▸ **Cardiac transplant**
IV/PO
Adults, Elderly. 1.5 g 2 times/day.
▸ **Liver transplant**
IV
Adults, Elderly. 1 g 2 times/day.
PO
Adults, Elderly. 1.5 g 2 times/day.
▸ **Usual pediatric dosage**
PO: 600 mg/m²/dose 2 times/day.
Maximum: 2 g/dose.

UNLABELED USES
Prevents organ rejection in patients
undergoing heart transplant

CONTRAINDICATIONS
Mycophenolic acid

INTERACTIONS
Drug
Acyclovir, ganciclovir: Competes
with MPA, an active metabolite for
renal excretion; may increase
plasma concentration of each in
presence of renal impairment.
*Antacids (aluminum, magnesium-
containing), cholestyramine:* May
decrease the absorption of mycophenolate.
Live virus vaccines: May decrease
the patient's antibody response to
vaccine, increase the vaccine's side
effects, and potentiate virus replication.
Other immunosuppressants: May
increase the risk of infection or
development of lymphomas.

Probenecid: May increase myco-
phenolate blood concentration.
Herbal
Echinacea: May decrease the ef-
fects of mycophenolate.
Food
May decrease plasma concentration
of the drug.

DIAGNOSTIC TEST EFFECTS
May increase serum cholesterol,
phosphate, serum alkaline phosphatase, creatinine, SGOT (AST), and
SGPT (ALT) levels. Alters blood
glucose and lipid levels, serum
calcium, potassium, and uric acid.

IV INCOMPATIBILITIES
Compatible only with D_5W. Do not
infuse concurrently with other drugs
or IV solutions.

SIDE EFFECTS
Frequent (37%–20%)
Urinary tract infection (UTI), hypertension, peripheral edema, diarrhea,
constipation, fever, headache,
nausea
Occasional (18%–10%)
Dyspepsia, including heartburn,
indigestion, and epigastric pain,
dyspnea, cough, hematuria, asthenia
or loss of strength and energy,
vomiting, edema, tremors, abdominal, chest, or back pain, oral moniliasis, acne
Rare (9%–6%)
Insomnia, respiratory infection,
rash, dizziness

SERIOUS REACTIONS
• Significant anemia, leukopenia,
thrombocytopenia, neutropenia, and
leukocytosis may occur, particularly
in those undergoing kidney rejection.
• Sepsis and infection occur occasionally.
• Gastrointestinal (GI) tract hemorrhage occurs rarely.

• There is an increased risk of neoplasia or new, abnormal growth tumor.

NURSING CONSIDERATIONS

Baseline Assessment

• Plan to perform a negative serum or urine pregnancy test in female patients of childbearing potential within 1 week before beginning mycophenolate therapy.

• Assess the patient's medical history, especially for active digestive disease, drug history, including use of other immunosuppressants, and renal function.

Lifespan Considerations

• Be aware that it is unknown if mycophenolate crosses the placenta or is distributed in breast milk. Breast-feeding should be avoided in this patient population.

• Be aware that the safety and efficacy of mycophenolate have not been established in children.

• In the elderly, age-related renal impairment may require dosage adjustments.

Precautions

• Use cautiously in female patients of childbearing potential and in patients with active serious digestive disease, neutropenia, and renal impairment.

Administration and Handling

PO

• Give mycophenolate on an empty stomach.

• Do not open or crush capsules.

• Avoid inhalation of powder in capsules and avoid direct contact of powder on skin or mucous membranes. If contact occurs, wash thoroughly with soap and water, rinse eyes profusely with plain water.

• Store reconstituted suspension in refrigerator or at room temperature.

• Suspension is stable for 60 days after reconstitution.

• Suspension can be administered orally or via a nasogastric tube (minimum size: 8 French).

IV

• Store at room temperature.

• Reconstitute each 500-mg vial with 14 ml D_5W. Gently agitate.

• For 1-g dose, further dilute with 140 ml D_5W; for 1.5-g dose further dilute with 210 ml D_5W, providing a concentration of 6 mg/ml.

• Infuse over at least 2 hours.

Intervention and Evaluation

• Plan to obtain a complete blood count (CBC) of the patient weekly during the first month of therapy, twice monthly during second and third months of treatment, then monthly throughout the first year.

• Reduce or discontinue the drug dosage if the patient experiences a rapid fall in white blood cell (WBC) count.

• Assess the patient for delayed bone marrow suppression.

• Report any major changes in assessment of the patient. Routinely monitor for any change from normal.

Patient Teaching

• Tell the female patient to use effective contraception before, during, and for 6 weeks after discontinuing mycophenolate therapy, even if there has been a history of infertility, other than hysterectomy. Instruct the patient that two forms of contraception must be used concurrently unless abstinence is absolute.

• Warn the patient to notify the physician if he or she experiences abdominal pain, fever, sore throat, or unusual bleeding or bruising.

• Stress to the patient the need for laboratory tests while taking this medication.

• Inform patients that there is a risk that malignancies will occur.

peginterferon alfa-2a
peg-inn-ter-**fear**-on
(Pegasys)

CATEGORY AND SCHEDULE
Pregnancy Risk Category: C

MECHANISM OF ACTION
An immunomodulator that inhibits viral replication in virus-infected cells by binding to specific membrane receptors on cell surface. *Therapeutic Effect:* Suppresses cell proliferation, produces reversible decreases in leukocyte and platelet counts.

PHARMACOKINETICS
Readily absorbed after subcutaneous administration. Excreted by the kidneys. **Half-life:** 80 hrs.

AVAILABILITY
Injection: 180 mcg/ml.

INDICATIONS AND DOSAGES
▸ **Hepatitis C**
Subcutaneous
Adults 18 yrs and older, Elderly. 180 mcg (1 ml) once weekly for 48 wks; given in the abdomen or thigh.
▸ **Renal function impairment requiring hemodialysis**
Adults, Elderly. 135 mcg.
▸ **Liver function impairment, including a progressive increase in SGPT (ALT) above baseline**
Adults, Elderly. 90 mcg.

CONTRAINDICATIONS
Autoimmune hepatitis, decompensated liver disease, infants, neonates

INTERACTIONS
Drug
Bone marrow depressants: May have additive effect.
Theophylline: May increase the serum level of theophylline.
Herbal
None known.
Food
None known.

DIAGNOSTIC TEST EFFECTS
May increase SGPT (ALT) level. May decrease absolute neutrophil count (ANC), platelet count, and white blood cell (WBC) counts. May cause a slight decrease in blood Hgb and Hct.

SIDE EFFECTS
Frequent (54%)
Headache
Occasional (23%–13%)
Alopecia, nausea, insomnia, anorexia, dizziness, diarrhea, abdominal pain, flu-like symptoms, such as fever, body ache, and fatigue, psychiatric reactions, including depression, irritability, and anxiety, injection site reaction
Rare (8%–5%)
Impaired concentration, diaphoresis, dry mouth, nausea, vomiting

SERIOUS REACTIONS
• Serious, acute hypersensitivity reactions, including urticaria, angioedema, bronchoconstriction, and anaphylaxis, pancreatitis, colitis, hyperthyroidism or hypothyroidism, ophthalmologic disorders, and pulmonary abnormalities occur rarely.

NURSING CONSIDERATIONS

Baseline Assessment
• Plan to perform blood chemistries, including BUN, serum alkaline phosphatase, creatinine, SGOT

(AST), and SGPT (ALT) levels to assess hepatic and renal function, complete blood count (CBC), electrocardiogram (EKG), and urinalysis of the patient before beginning therapy and routinely thereafter.

• Ensure that patients with diabetes mellitus or hypertension have an ophthalmologic exam before beginning therapy.

Lifespan Considerations

• Be aware that peginterferon alfa-2a may have abortifacient potential.

• Be aware that it is unknown if peginterferon alfa-2a is distributed in breast milk.

• Be aware that the safety and efficacy of peginterferon alfa-2a have not been established in children younger than 18 years of age.

• Be aware that cardiac, central nervous system (CNS), and systemic effects may be more severe in the elderly, particularly in patients with impaired renal function.

Precautions

• Use extremely cautiously in patients with a history of neuropsychiatric disorders.

• Use cautiously in elderly patients and in patients with autoimmune disorders, cardiac diseases, colitis, compromised CNS function, endocrine abnormalities, myelosuppression, ophthalmic disorders, pulmonary disorders, and renal impairment with a creatinine clearance less than 50 ml/min.

Administration and Handling

◄ **ALERT** ► If the patient experiences moderate to severe adverse reactions, modify the dose to 135 mcg (0.75 ml); dose reduction to 90 mcg (0.5 ml) may be necessary. Reduce dose to 135 mcg (0.75 ml) if neutrophil count is less than 750 cells/mm^3. In those with ANC less than 500 cells/mm^3, discontinue treatment until

ANC returns to 1,000 cells/mm^3. Reduce dose to 90 mcg if platelet count is less than 50,000 cells/mm^3.

Subcutaneous

• Refrigerate.

• Vials are for single use only; discard unused portion.

• Give subcutaneous in the abdomen or thigh.

Intervention and Evaluation

• Monitor the patient for depression.

• Offer the patient emotional support.

• Monitor the patient for abdominal pain and bloody diarrhea, evidence of colitis.

• Monitor the patient for chest x-ray for pulmonary infiltrates.

• Assess the patient for hyperglycemia and pulmonary function impairment.

• Encourage the patient to drink ample fluids, particularly during early therapy.

• Assess the patient's serum hepatitis C virus RNA levels after 24 weeks of treatment.

Patient Teaching

• Tell the patient that the drug's therapeutic effect should appear in 1 to 3 months.

• Explain to the patient that flu-like symptoms tend to diminish with continued therapy.

• Warn the patient to immediately notify the physician if he or she experiences depression or suicidal ideation.

• Caution the patient to avoid performing tasks requiring mental alertness or motor skills until his or her response to the drug is established.

peginterferon alfa-2b
peg-inn-ter-**fear**-on
(PEG-Intron)

CATEGORY AND SCHEDULE
Pregnancy Risk Category: C

MECHANISM OF ACTION
An immunomodulator that inhibits viral replication in virus-infected cells, suppresses cell proliferation by binding to specific membrane receptors on cell surface. *Therapeutic Effect:* Increases phagocytic action of macrophages, augmenting specific cytotoxicity of lymphocytes.

AVAILABILITY
Injection: 50 mcg/0.5 ml; 80 mcg/0.5 ml; 120 mcg/0.5 ml; 150 mcg/0.5 ml.

INDICATIONS AND DOSAGES
▸ **Chronic Hepatitis C**
Subcutaneous
Adults 18 yrs and older, Elderly.
Administer once weekly for 1 yr on the same day each wk.

Vial Strength (mcg/ml)	Weight (kg)	mcg*	ml*
100	37–45	40	0.4
	46–56	50	0.5
160	57–72	64	0.4
	73–88	80	0.5
240	89–106	96	0.4
	107–136	120	0.5
300	137–160	150	0.5

*of peginterferon alpha-2b to administer

CONTRAINDICATIONS
Autoimmune hepatitis, decompensated liver disease, history of psychiatric disorders

INTERACTIONS
Drug
Bone marrow depressants: May have additive effect.
Herbal
None known.
Food
None known.

DIAGNOSTIC TEST EFFECTS
May increase blood glucose levels and SGPT (ALT) levels. May decrease blood neutrophil and platelet counts.

SIDE EFFECTS
Frequent (50%–47%)
Flu-like symptoms, including fever, headache, rigors, body ache, fatigue, and nausea, may decrease in severity as treatment continues; injection site disorders, including inflammation, bruising, itchiness, and irritation
Occasional (29%–18%)
Depression, anxiety, emotional lability, irritability, insomnia, alopecia, diarrhea
Rare
Rash, increased diaphoresis, dry skin, dizziness, flushing, vomiting, dyspepsia, such as heartburn, epigastric pain

SERIOUS REACTIONS
• Serious, acute hypersensitivity reactions, such as urticaria, angioedema, bronchoconstriction, and anaphylaxis and pancreatitis occur rarely.
• Ulcerative colitis may occur within 12 weeks of the initiation of treatment.
• Pulmonary disorders and hypothyroidism or hyperthyroidism may occur.

NURSING CONSIDERATIONS

Baseline Assessment
• Perform blood chemistries, including BUN, serum alkaline phosphatase, creatinine, SGOT (AST), and SGPT (ALT) levels to assess hepatic and renal function, complete blood count (CBC), electrocardiogram (EKG), and urinalysis before beginning therapy and routinely thereafter.
• Ensure patients with diabetes mellitus or hypertension have an ophthalmologic exam before beginning therapy.

Precautions
• Use cautiously in elderly patients and patients with autoimmune disorders, cardiac diseases, compromised central nervous system (CNS) function, endocrine disorders, myelosuppression, ophthalmic disorders, pulmonary disorders, and renal impairment with a creatinine clearance less than 50 ml/min.

Administration and Handling
◄ALERT► If severe adverse reactions occur, modify the drug dose or temporarily discontinue the drug, as prescribed. Know that the dosage is based on weight.
◄ALERT► Remember that the drug's side effects are dose-related.
Subcutaneous
• Store at room temperature.
• Reconstitute with supplied diluent (5-ml vial). Use immediately or after reconstituted; may be refrigerated for 24 hours or less before use.

Intervention and Evaluation
• Monitor the patient for depression.
• Offer the patient emotional support.
• Monitor the patient for abdominal pain and bloody diarrhea as evidence by colitis.
• Monitor the patient for pulmonary infiltrates by chest x-ray.

• Assess the patient for hyperglycemia and pulmonary function impairment.
• Encourage the patient to drink ample fluids, particularly during early therapy.
• Assess the patient's serum hepatitis C virus RNA levels after 24 weeks of treatment.

Patient Teaching
• Instruct the patient to consume adequate fluids and to avoid alcohol.
• Advise the patient that he or she may experience flu-like syndrome including body aches, headache, and nausea.
• Warn the patient to notify the physician if he or she experiences bloody diarrhea, fever, persistent abdominal pain, signs of depression or infection, and unusual bruising or bleeding.

sirolimus
sigh-row-**lie**-mus
(Rapamune)

CATEGORY AND SCHEDULE
Pregnancy Risk Category: C

MECHANISM OF ACTION
An immunosuppressant that inhibits T-lymphocyte proliferation induced by stimulation of cell surface receptors, mitogens, alloantigens, lymphokines. Prevents activation of an enzyme called target of rapamycin (TOR) a key regulatory kinase in cell cycle progression. *Therapeutic Effect:* Inhibits T- and B-cell proliferation, essential components of immune response.

AVAILABILITY
Oral Solution: 1 mg/ml.
Tablets: 1 mg, 2 mg.

INDICATIONS AND DOSAGES
▶ **Prophylaxis of organ rejection**
PO
Adults. Loading dose: 6 mg.
Maintenance: 2 mg/day.
Children 13 yrs and older weighing less than 40 kg. 3 mg/m^2 loading dose; then, 1 mg/m^2/day.

CONTRAINDICATIONS
Current malignancy, hypersensitivity to sirolimus, current malignancy

INTERACTIONS
Drug
Cyclosporine, diltiazem, ketoconazole: May increase blood concentration and risk of toxicity of sirolimus.
Rifampin: May decrease the blood concentration and effects of sirolimus.
Herbal
None known.
Food
Grapefruit juice: May decrease the metabolism of sirolimus.

DIAGNOSTIC TEST EFFECTS
May decrease blood Hgb, Hct, and platelet count. May increase serum cholesterol, creatinine, and triglyceride levels.

SIDE EFFECTS
Occasional
Hypercholesterolemia, hyperlipidemia, hypertension, rash
High dose (5 mg/day): Anemia, arthralgia, diarrhea, hypokalemia, thrombocytopenia

SERIOUS REACTIONS
• None known.

NURSING CONSIDERATIONS
Baseline Assessment
• Determine if the female patient is pregnant or breast-feeding.
• Determine if the patient is taking

other medications, especially cyclosporine, diltiazem, ketoconazole, and rifampin.
• Determine if the patient has chickenpox, herpes zoster, infection, or malignancy.
• Expect to perform baseline lab tests, including a CBC and lipid profile.
Precautions
• Use cautiously in patients with chickenpox, herpes zoster, impaired liver function, and infection.
Intervention and Evaluation
• Monitor the patient's serum hepatic enzyme levels function periodically.
Patient Teaching
• Tell the patient to avoid consuming grapefruit or grapefruit juice.
• Caution the patient against contact with those with colds or other infections.
• Stress to the patient that close monitoring by the physician is an important part of sirolimus therapy.
• Tell the patient to take the drug at the same each day, and to notify the physician if he or she misses a dose.

tacrolimus
tack-row-**lee**-mus
(Prograf, Protopic)

CATEGORY AND SCHEDULE
Pregnancy Risk Category: C

MECHANISM OF ACTION
An immunologic agent that binds to intracellular protein, forming a complex, inhibiting phosphatase activity. Inhibits T-lymphocyte activation. *Therapeutic Effect:* Suppresses immunologically mediated inflammatory response. Assists

in preventing organ transplant rejection.

PHARMACOKINETICS

Variably absorbed after PO administration (food reduces absorption). Protein binding: 75%–97%. Extensively metabolized in the liver. Excreted in urine. Not removed by hemodialysis. **Half-life:** 11.7 hrs.

AVAILABILITY

Capsules: 0.5 mg, 1 mg, 5 mg.
Injection: 5 mg/ml.
Ointment: 0.03%, 0.1%.

INDICATIONS AND DOSAGES
▸ **Prophylaxis of transplant rejection**
IV infusion
Adults, Elderly. 0.03–0.1 mg/kg/day.
Children. 0.03–0.15 mg/kg/day.
PO
Adults, Elderly. 0.15–0.3 mg/kg/day in 2 divided doses 12 hrs apart.
Children. 0.15–0.4 mg/kg/day in 2 divided doses 12 hrs apart.
IV infusion
Children (without preexisting liver or renal dysfunction). 0.05–1.5 mg/kg/day.
PO
Children (without preexisting liver or renal dysfunction). 0.3 mg/kg/day.
▸ **Atopic dermatitis**
Topical
Adults, Elderly, Children 2 yrs and older. 0.03% ointment to affected area 2 times/day. Continue for 1 wk after symptoms have cleared.

UNLABELED USES

Prophylaxis of organ rejection in patients receiving allogeneic bone marrow, cardiac, pancreas, pancreatic island cell, and small bowel transplantation, treatment of autoimmune disease, severe recalcitrant psoriasis

CONTRAINDICATIONS

Concurrent use with cyclosporine increases the risk of ototoxicity, hypersensitivity to HCO-60 polyoxyl 60 hydrogenated castor oil used in solution for injection, hypersensitivity to tacrolimus

INTERACTIONS
Drug
Aminoglycosides, amphotericin B, cisplatin: Increases the risk of renal dysfunction.
Antacids: Decrease the absorption of the drug.
Antifungals, bromocriptine, calcium channel blockers, cimetidine, clarithromycin, cyclosporine, danazol, diltiazem, erythromycin, methylprednisolone, metoclopramide: Increase tacrolimus blood concentration.
Carbamazepine, phenobarbital, phenytoin, rifamycin: Decreases tacrolimus blood concentrations.
Cyclosporine: Increases the risk of nephrotoxicity.
Live virus vaccines: May decrease the patient's antibody response to the vaccine, increase the patient's antibody response to the vaccine, and potentiate virus replication.
Other immunosuppressants: May increase risk of infection or development of lymphomas.
Herbal
Echinacea: May decrease the effects of tacrolimus.
Food
Grapefruit, grapefruit juice: May alter the effects of the drug.

DIAGNOSTIC TEST EFFECTS

May increase blood glucose levels, BUN, serum creatinine, and white blood cell (WBC) count. May decrease serum magnesium, red blood cell (RBC), and thrombocyte counts. Alters serum potassium level.

IV INCOMPATIBILITIES

No known specific drug incompatibilities. Do not mix with other medications if possible.

IV COMPATIBILITIES

Calcium gluconate, dexamethasone (Decadron), diphenhydramine (Benadryl), dobutamine (Dobutrex), dopamine (Intropin), furosemide (Lasix), heparin, hydromorphone (Dilaudid), insulin, leucovorin, lorazepam (Ativan), morphine, nitroglycerin, potassium chloride

SIDE EFFECTS

Frequent (greater than 30%)
Headache, tremor, insomnia, paresthesia, diarrhea, nausea, constipation, vomiting, abdominal pain, hypertension
Occasional (29%–10%)
Rash, pruritus, anorexia, asthenia, peripheral edema, photosensitivity

SERIOUS REACTIONS

• Nephrotoxicity and pleural effusion occur frequently.
• Overt nephrotoxicity characterized by increasing serum creatinine and a decrease in urine output.
• Thrombocytopenia, leukocytosis, anemia, and atelectasis occur occasionally.
• Neurotoxicity, including tremor, headache, and mental status changes, occurs commonly.
• Sepsis and infection occur occasionally.
• Significant anemia, thrombocytopenia and leukocytosis may occur.

NURSING CONSIDERATIONS

Baseline Assessment

• Assess the patient's drug history, especially for other immunosuppressants, and medical history, especially renal function.
• Prepare an aqueous solution of epinephrine 1:1,000 available at bedside as well as oxygen (O_2) before beginning IV infusion.
• Assess the patient continuously for the first 30 minutes following start of infusion and at frequent intervals thereafter.
• Plan to obtain baseline lab tests, including BUN, CBC, hepatic enzyme levels, serum creatinine, and serum electrolytes.

Lifespan Considerations

• Be aware that tacrolimus crosses the placenta and is distributed in breast milk. Breast-feeding should be avoided in this patient population.
• Be aware that hyperkalemia and renal dysfunction are noted in neonates.
• Be aware that children may require higher drug dosages due to decreased bioavailability and increased clearance.
• Be aware that post-transplant lymphoproliferative disorder is more common in children, especially children younger than 3 years of age.
• In the elderly, age-related renal impairment may require dosage adjustment.

Precautions

• Use cautiously in patients with immunosuppression, liver and renal function impairment.

Administration and Handling

◀ALERT▶ In patients unable to take capsules, initiate therapy with IV infusion. Give oral dose 8 to 12 hours after discontinuing IV infusion. Titrate dosing based on clinical assessments of rejection and patient tolerance. In patients with liver or renal function impairment, give lowest IV and oral dosing range, as prescribed. Plan to delay dosing up to 48 hours or longer in patients with postoperative oliguria.

PO
• Administer tacrolimus on an empty stomach.
• Use polyethylene oral syringe or glass container when giving oral solution, avoid plastic or Styrofoam.
• Do not give with grapefruit or grapefruit juice or within 2 hours of antacids.

Topical
• For external use only.
• Do not cover with occlusive dressing.
• Rub in gently and completely onto clean, dry skin.

IV
• Store diluted infusion solution in glass or polyethylene containers and discard after 24 hours.
• Do not store in a container made from polyvinyl chloride (PVC) because the drug is less stable, and there's a risk of drug absorption into the container.
• Dilute with an appropriate amount, 250 to 1,000 ml, depending on desired dose, 0.9% NaCl or D_5W to provide a concentration between 0.004 and 0.02 mg/ml.
• Give tacrolimus as continuous IV infusion.
• Continuously monitor the patient for anaphylaxis for at least 30 minutes after start of infusion.
• Stop the infusion immediately at first sign of hypersensitivity reaction.

Intervention and Evaluation
• Closely monitor patients with impaired renal function.
• Monitor the patient's lab values, especially complete blood count (CBC), hepatic enzyme levels, and serum creatinine and potassium levels.

• Monitor the patient's intake and output closely.
• Perform a CBC of the patient weekly during the first month of therapy, twice monthly during second and third months of treatment, then monthly throughout the first year.
• Report any major change in the assessment of the patient.

Patient Teaching
• Instruct the patient to take the drug dose at the same time each day. Tell the patient to notify the physician if he or she misses a dose.
• Caution the patient to avoid crowds and those with infection.
• Warn the patient to notify the physician if he or she experiences chest pain, dizziness, headache, decreased urination, rash, respiratory infection, or unusual bleeding or bruising.
• Urge the patient to avoid exposure to sunlight and artificial light as this may cause photosensitivity reaction.
• Instruct the patient on the proper administration of the drug. Instruct him or her to avoid grapefruit, and to take the oral solution in the oral syringe or glass container on an empty stomach.

thalidomide
thah-**lid**-owe-mide
(Thalomid)

CATEGORY AND SCHEDULE
Pregnancy Risk Category: X

MECHANISM OF ACTION
An immunomodulator whose exact mechanism is unknown. Has sedative, anti-inflammatory, and immunosuppressive activity. Action may

be due to selective inhibition of the production of tumor necrosis factor alpha.
Therapeutic Effect: Reduces local and systemic effects of leprosy.

AVAILABILITY
Capsules: 50 mg, 100 mg, 200 mg.

INDICATIONS AND DOSAGES
▶ **Acquired immune deficiency syndrome (AIDS)-related muscle wasting**
Adults. 100–300 mg a day.

UNLABELED USES
Crohn's disease, recurrent aphthous ulcers in human immunodeficiency virus (HIV) patients, wasting syndrome of HIV or cancer

CONTRAINDICATIONS
Neutropenia, peripheral neuropathy; pregnancy, sensitivity to thalidomide

INTERACTIONS
Drug
Alcohol, central nervous system (CNS) depressants: May increase sedative effects.
Medication associated with peripheral neuropathy, such as INH, lithium, metronidazole, phenytoin: May increase peripheral neuropathy.
Medications decreasing effectiveness of hormonal contraceptives, such as carbamazepine, protease inhibitors, rifampin: May decrease the effectiveness of the contraceptive; must use 2 other methods of contraception.
Herbal
None known.
Food
None known.

DIAGNOSTIC TEST EFFECTS
None known.

SIDE EFFECTS
Frequent
Drowsiness, dizziness, mood changes, constipation, xerostomia, peripheral neuropathy
Occasional
Increased appetite, weight gain, headache, loss of libido, edema of face and limbs, nausea, hair loss, dry skin, skin rash, hypothyroidism

SERIOUS REACTIONS
• Neutropenia, peripheral neuropathy, and thromboembolism occur rarely.

NURSING CONSIDERATIONS
Baseline Assessment
• Determine if the female patient is pregnant. Thalidomide use is contraindicated in pregnant women.
• Determine if the patient is using other medications.
• Assess the patient for hypersensitivity to thalidomide.
Precautions
• Use cautiously in patients with a history of seizures.
Intervention and Evaluation
• Monitor the patient's HIV viral load, nerve conduction studies, and white blood cell (WBC) count.
• Observe the patient for signs and symptoms of peripheral neuropathy.
Patient Teaching
• Urge the patient to avoid consuming alcohol or using other drugs that cause drowsiness during thalidomide therapy.
• Instruct female patients of childbearing age to perform a pregnancy test within 24 hours before beginning thalidomide therapy, then every 2 to 4 weeks.
• Warn the patient to discontinue the drug and notify the physician if he or she experiences symptoms of peripheral neuropathy.

black cohosh
chamomile
DHEA
dong quai
echinacea
feverfew
garlic
ginger
ginkgo biloba
ginseng
glucosamine/
  chondroitin
kava kava
melatonin
St. John's wort
saw palmetto
valerian
yohimbe

Uses: Many patients take herbal supplements because they believe these natural medicines are safer and healthier than conventional drugs, because cultural influences and recommendations from family members and friends make these remedies attractive, or because herbal preparations offer convenience and relatively low cost. Herbals are used for various purposes, ranging from menopausal symptom relief and immune system stimulation to memory enhancement and sleep promotion. For specific uses, see the entries in this chapter.

Action: Herbal supplements are plant-derived products that promote health and relieve disease symptoms. Although some are effective, many aren't and a few can be harmful. Their actions vary greatly. For example, *black cohosh* is a phytoestrogen that may have estrogen-like effects. However, its exact mechanism is unknown. *Echinacea* may increase phagocytosis and lymphocyte activity, possibly by releasing tumor necrosis factor, interleukin-I, and interferon. *Ginkgo biloba* possesses antioxidant and free radical scavenging properties, which protect tissues from oxidative damage. *Melatonin* is a pineal hormone that interacts with melatonin receptors in the brain to regulate the body's circadian rhythm and sleep patterns. For additional mechanisms of action, see the entries in this chapter.

black cohosh
Also known as baneberry, bugbane, bugwort, fairy candles (Black Cohosh Softgel, Remifemin)

CATEGORY AND SCHEDULE
Pregnancy Risk Category: N/A
OTC

MECHANISM OF ACTION
An herb whose mechanism of action is unknown. A phytoestrogen that may have estrogen-like effects. *Therapeutic Effect:* Reduces symptoms of menopause, such as hot flashes.

AVAILABILITY
Softgel Capsules: 40 mg.
Tablets: 20 mg.

INDICATIONS AND DOSAGES
▸ **To treat symptoms of menopause, to induce labor, to reduce lipids and blood pressure, sedative**
PO
Adults, Elderly. 20–80 mg 2 times/day.

CONTRAINDICATIONS
Pregnancy (has menstrual and uterine stimulant effects that may increase risk of miscarriage); therapy use 6 mo or longer

INTERACTIONS
Drug
Antihypertensives: May increase the action of these drugs.
Tamoxifen: May have additive antiproliferative effect.
Herbal
None known.
Food
None known.

DIAGNOSTIC TEST EFFECTS
May decrease serum LH concentration.

SIDE EFFECTS
Nausea, headache, dizziness, increase in weight, visual changes, migraines

SERIOUS REACTIONS
• Overdosage may cause nausea or vomiting, decreased heart rate, and diaphoresis.

NURSING CONSIDERATIONS
Baseline Assessment
• Determine if the patient is pregnant or breast-feeding.
Lifespan Considerations
• Be aware that the use of black cohosh in pregnant and breast-feeding women is contraindicated.

• Be aware that the safety and efficacy of this herb have not been established in children.
• There are no age-related precautions noted in the elderly.
Precautions
• Use cautiously in patients with breast, ovarian, or uterine cancer, endometriosis, and uterine fibroids.
Intervention and Evaluation
• Monitor the patient's blood pressure (B/P) and serum lipid levels.
Patient Teaching
• Warn the patient to notify the physician immediately if she becomes pregnant, breast-feeds, or plans to become pregnant.
• Advise the patient not to take black cohosh for longer than 6 months.

chamomile
(**ka**-mow-meal)
Also known as German chamomile, pinheads
(Blossom 120/jar, 45/jar, 30/jar)

CATEGORY AND SCHEDULE
Pregnancy Risk Category: N/A
OTC

MECHANISM OF ACTION
An herb with antiallergic and anti-inflammatory action due to inhibiting release of histamine. Possesses antiallergic, antiflatulent, antispasmodic, mild sedative, anti-inflammatory action.

AVAILABILITY
Whole Flowers: 120/jar; 45/jar, 30/jar (chamomile whole flowers) 120 g, 45 g, 30 g.

INDICATIONS AND DOSAGES
▸ **Treat symptoms of flatulence, travel sickness, diarrhea, insomnia, gastrointestinal (GI) spasms**
PO
Adults, Elderly. 2–8 g of dried flower heads 3 times/day or 1 cup of tea 3–4 times/day.

CONTRAINDICATIONS
Pregnancy

INTERACTIONS
Drug
Aspirin, clopidogrel, dalteparin, enoxaparin, heparin, warfarin: May increase anticoagulation and risk of bleeding.
Benzodiazepines: May cause additive effects.
Herbal
Ginseng, kava, St. John's wort, valerian: May increase sedative effects.
Feverfew, garlic, ginger, ginkgo, licorice: May increase the risk of bleeding.
Food
None known.

DIAGNOSTIC TEST EFFECTS
None known.

SIDE EFFECTS
Allergic reaction (e.g., contact dermatitis, severe hypersensitivity reaction, anaphylactic reaction), eye irritation

SERIOUS REACTIONS
• Anaphylactic reaction (bronchospasm, severe pruritus, angioedema) may occur.

NURSING CONSIDERATIONS

Baseline Assessment
• Determine if the patient is asthmatic, breast-feeding, or pregnant.

• Determine if the patient is taking other medications, such as those that increase risk of bleeding or have sedative properties.
• Assess the patient for allergies to aster, daisies, chrysanthemums, or ragweed.
Lifespan Considerations
• Be aware that chamomile use is contraindicated in pregnancy and breast-feeding. Chamomile is a teratogen, affects the menstrual cycle, and has uterine stimulant effects.
• Be aware that the safety and efficacy of chamomile have not been established in children.
• There are no age-related precautions noted in the elderly.
Precautions
• Use cautiously in patients with asthma because this herb may exacerbate the condition, and in patients allergic to aster, daisies, chrysanthemums, or ragweed.
Intervention and Evaluation
• Monitor the patient for signs and symptoms of an allergic reaction.
Patient Teaching
• Warn the patient to notify the physician immediately if she becomes pregnant, breast-feeds, or plans to become pregnant.
• Advise the patient that chamomile may cause mild sedation. Advise the patient not to perform activities requiring motor skills until his or her response to the herb is established.
• Urge the patient to avoid alcohol, anticoagulants, and other sedatives during chamomile therapy.

DHEA
Also known as prasterone

CATEGORY AND SCHEDULE
Pregnancy Risk Category: N/A
OTC

MECHANISM OF ACTION
An herb that is produced in the adrenal glands and liver and is metabolized to androstenedione, a major precursor to androgens and estrogens. Also produced in the central nervous system (CNS) and concentrated in the limbic regions; may function as an excitatory neuroregulator. *Therapeutic Effect:* Androgen or estrogen-like hormonal effects may be responsible for DHEA benefits.

AVAILABILITY
Capsules: 25 mg.
Tablets: 25 mg.

INDICATIONS AND DOSAGES
▶ **To improve depressed mood and fatigue in HIV patients**
PO
Adults, Elderly. 30–90 mg/day.
▶ **Improvement of cognitive function and memory, increase bone mineral density, energy, muscle mass, strength, stimulate immune system, prevention of osteoporosis, treatment of atherosclerosis, cancer, hyperglycemia, prevention of osteoporosis**
PO
Adults, Elderly. 25–50 mg/day.

CONTRAINDICATIONS
None known

INTERACTIONS
Drug
Androgen and Estrogen therapy: May interfere with these therapies.

Triazolam: May increase blood concentration of triazolam.
Herbal
None known.
Food
None known.

DIAGNOSTIC TEST EFFECTS
None known.

SIDE EFFECTS
Acne, hair loss, hirsutism, voice deepening, insulin resistance, altered menstrual pattern, hypertension, abdominal pain, fatigue, headache, nasal congestion.

SERIOUS REACTIONS
• None known.

NURSING CONSIDERATIONS
Baseline Assessment
• Assess the patient for hormone-sensitive tumors because DHEA may stimulate their growth.
• Avoid use of hormone replacement therapy.
Lifespan Considerations
• Be aware that DHEA may adversely effect pregnancy by increasing androgen levels and that its use should be avoided during pregnancy.
• Be aware that the safety and efficacy of DHEA have not been established in children.
• In the elderly, age-related liver impairment may require caution.
Precautions
• DHEA use may increase the risk of breast, hormone-sensitive, and prostate cancers.
• Avoid DHEA use in patients with breast, ovarian, or uterine cancer, diabetes mellitus (can increase insulin resistance or sensitivity), depression (may increase risk of

adverse psychiatric effects), endometriosis, and uterine fibroids.

Intervention and Evaluation
• Assess the patient for changes in mood and sleep pattern.
• Monitor the patient for aggressiveness, irritability, and restlessness.

Patient Teaching
• Warn patients to avoid DHEA use during breast-feeding, concurrent hormone replacement therapy, and pregnancy.
• Advise the patient that if he or she experiences acne, a lower DHEA dosage may provide relief from the condition.

dong quai
Also known as Chinese angelica, dang gui, tang kuei, toki

CATEGORY AND SCHEDULE
Pregnancy Risk Category: N/A
OTC

MECHANISM OF ACTION
An herb that competitively inhibits estradiol binding to estrogen receptors. Has vasodilation, antispasmodic, and central nervous system (CNS) stimulant activity. *Therapeutic Effect:* Reduces symptoms of menopause.

AVAILABILITY
Softgel: 200 mg, 530 mg, 565 mg.

INDICATIONS AND DOSAGES
▸ **Gynecologic ailments, including menstrual cramps and menopause symptoms; uterine stimulant; control hypertension; as an antiinflammatory, vasodilator, immunosuppressant, analgesic, and antipyretic**

PO
Adults, Elderly. 3–4 g/day in divided doses with meals.

CONTRAINDICATIONS
Bleeding disorders, excessive menstrual flow, pregnancy due to uterine stimulant effect

INTERACTIONS
Drug
Warfarin: Increases anticoagulant effect and risk of bleeding with this drug.
Herbal
Feverfew, garlic, ginger, ginkgo, ginseng: May increase the risk of bleeding.
Food
None known.

DIAGNOSTIC TEST EFFECTS
May increase prothrombin time and international normalized ratio (INR).

SIDE EFFECTS
Diarrhea, photosensitivity, nausea, vomiting, anorexia, increased menstrual flow

SERIOUS REACTIONS
• None known.

NURSING CONSIDERATIONS
Baseline Assessment
• Determine if the patient is breast-feeding, pregnant, or plans to become pregnant.
• Determine if the patient is taking other medications, especially those that increase risk of bleeding.
Lifespan Considerations
• Be aware that dong quai use is contraindicated in pregnancy and breast-feeding.

• Be aware that the safety and efficacy of dong quai have not been established in children.
• There are no age-related precautions noted in the elderly.

Precautions
• Use cautiously in patients who are breast-feeding and patients with breast, ovarian, and uterine cancer.

Intervention and Evaluation
• Assess the patient for hypersensitivity reaction.

Patient Teaching
• Warn the patient to notify the physician immediately if she becomes or plans to become pregnant.
• Caution the patient not to breast-feed during dong quai therapy.
• Advise the patient that dong quai use may cause a photosensitivity reaction. Instruct the patient to wear protective clothing and sunscreen to protect against a photosensitivity reaction.

echinacea
Also known as black susans, comb flower, red sunflower, scurvy root

CATEGORY AND SCHEDULE
Pregnancy Risk Category: N/A
OTC

MECHANISM OF ACTION
An herb that stimulates the immune system. Possesses antiviral and immune stimulatory effects. Increases phagocytosis and lymphocyte activity, possibly by releasing tumor necrosis factor, interleukin-1, and interferon. *Therapeutic Effect:* Prevents or reduces symptoms associated with upper respiratory infections.

AVAILABILITY
Capsules: 200 mg, 380 mg, 400 mg, 500 mg.
Powder: 25 g, 100 g, 500 g.
Liquid.

INDICATIONS AND DOSAGES
▶ **Prevention and treatment of the common cold, other upper respiratory infections, urinary tract infections, vaginal candidiasis**
PO
Adults, Elderly. 6–9 ml herbal juice for up to a maximum of 8 wks.

CONTRAINDICATIONS
Autoimmune disease, children younger than 2 yrs, breast-feeding, history of allergic conditions, pregnancy, tuberculosis

INTERACTIONS
Drug
Immunosuppressant therapy, such as, corticosteroids, cyclosporine, mycophenolate: May interfere with this therapy.
Topical econazole: May reduce recurring vaginal candida infections.
Herbal
None known.
Food
None known.

DIAGNOSTIC TEST EFFECTS
None known.

SIDE EFFECTS
Well tolerated. May cause allergic reaction (urticaria, acute asthma or dyspnea, angioedema), fever, nausea, vomiting, diarrhea, unpleasant taste, abdominal pain, dizziness.

SERIOUS REACTIONS
• None known.

NURSING CONSIDERATIONS

Baseline Assessment
• Determine if the patient is breast-feeding, pregnant, has a history of autoimmune disease, and is currently receiving immunosuppressant therapy.

Lifespan Considerations
• Be aware that echinacea use is contraindicated during breast-feeding and pregnancy.
• Be aware that the safety and efficacy of echinacea have not been established in children younger than 2 years of age.
• There are no age-related precautions noted in the elderly.

Precautions
• Use cautiously in patients with diabetes mellitus because this herb may alter control of blood glucose.
• Do not use echinacea for more than 8 weeks because this may decrease the herb's effectiveness.

Administration and Handling
◀ ALERT ▶ A variety of doses have been used depending on the preparation.

Intervention and Evaluation
• Assess the patient for improvement in infection and hypersensitivity reaction.

Patient Teaching
• Warn the patient not to use echinacea during breast-feeding or pregnancy.
• Caution the patient against administering echinacea to children younger than 2 years of age.
• Advise the patient not to use echinacea longer than 8 weeks without at least a 1-week rest period.

feverfew
Also known as bachelor's button, featherfew, midsummer daisy, Santa Maria

CATEGORY AND SCHEDULE
Pregnancy Risk Category: N/A
OTC

MECHANISM OF ACTION
An herb whose exact mechanism is unknown. May inhibit platelet aggregation and serotonin release from platelets and leukocytes. Also inhibits or blocks prostaglandin synthesis. *Therapeutic Effect:* Reduces pain intensity, vomiting, noise sensitivity with severe migraine headaches.

AVAILABILITY
Capsules: 100 mg.
Feverfew Leaf: 380 mg.

INDICATIONS AND DOSAGES
▸ **Migraine headache**
PO
Adults, Elderly. 50–100 mg extract/day. Leaf: 50–125 mg/day.

CONTRAINDICATIONS
Allergies to chrysanthemums, daisies, marigolds, ragweed, lactation, pregnancy (may cause uterine contraction or abortion)

INTERACTIONS
Drug
Anticoagulants, antiplatelets: May increase the risk of bleeding with these drugs.
NSAIDs: May decrease the effectiveness of feverfew.
Herbal
Garlic, ginger, ginkgo biloba: May increase the risk of bleeding.

Food
None known.

DIAGNOSTIC TEST EFFECTS
None known.

SIDE EFFECTS
Oral: Abdominal pain, muscle stiffness, pain, indigestion, diarrhea, flatulence, nausea, vomiting
Chewing leaf: Mouth ulceration, inflammation of oral mucosa and tongue, swelling of lips, loss of taste

SERIOUS REACTIONS
• Hypersensitivity reaction may occur.

NURSING CONSIDERATIONS

Baseline Assessment
• Determine if the patient is breast-feeding or pregnant.
Lifespan Considerations
• Be aware that feverfew use during lactation and pregnancy is contraindicated.
• Be aware that the safety and efficacy of feverfew have not been established in children. Feverfew use should be avoided in children.
• There are no age-related precautions noted in the elderly.
Intervention and Evaluation
• Assess the patient for hypersensitivity reaction.
• Evaluate the patient for joint or muscle pain and mouth ulcers.
Patient Teaching
• Warn the patient not to use feverfew while breast-feeding or pregnant.
• Caution the patient to avoid using feverfew in children.

garlic
Also known as ail, allium, nectar of the gods, poor man's treacle, stinking rose

CATEGORY AND SCHEDULE
Pregnancy Risk Category: N/A
OTC

MECHANISM OF ACTION
An herb that possesses antithrombotic properties, can increase fibrinolytic activity, decrease platelet aggregation, and increase prothrombin time. Acts as an HMG-CoA reductase inhibitor.
Therapeutic Effect: Lowers cholesterol levels. Causes smooth muscle relaxation or vasodilation, reducing blood pressure (B/P). Reduces oxidative stress and LDL oxidation, preventing age-related vascular changes and atherosclerosis. Prevents endothelial cell depletion, producing antioxidant effect.

AVAILABILITY
Capsules: 100 mg, 300 mg, 500 mg, 1,000 mg, 1.5 g.
Tablets: 400 mg, 1,250 mg.
Tea.
Extract.
Oil.
Powder.

INDICATIONS AND DOSAGES
▸ **Hyperlipidemia, hypertension**
PO (capsules, powder, tea)
Adults, Elderly. 600–1,200 mg/ day in divided doses 3 times/ day.

CONTRAINDICATIONS
Patients with bleeding disorders

INTERACTIONS
Drug
Anticoagulants, antiplatelets, such as warfarin, aspirin, clopidogrel, enoxaparin: May enhance the effects of these drugs.
Cyclosporine, oral contraceptives: May decrease the effects of these drugs.
Insulin, oral antidiabetic agents: May increase the hypoglycemic effect of these drugs.
Other HIV antiretrovirals, saquinavir: May decrease the blood concentration and effects of these drugs.
Herbal
Feverfew, ginger, ginkgo, ginseng: May increase the risk of bleeding.
Food
None known.

DIAGNOSTIC TEST EFFECTS
May decrease blood glucose and cholesterol levels and increase international normalized ratio (INR).

SIDE EFFECTS
Breath or body odor, mouth or gastrointestinal (GI) burning, heartburn, nausea, vomiting, diarrhea, allergic reactions (e.g., rhinitis, urticaria, angioedema).

SERIOUS REACTIONS
• None known.

NURSING CONSIDERATIONS
Baseline Assessment
• Assess the patient's blood serum lipid levels and determine whether the patient is taking anticoagulants or antiplatelets before beginning therapy.
• Determine if the patient is a diabetic or taking insulin or oral hypoglycemic agents.

Lifespan Considerations
• Be aware that garlic use may stimulate labor and cause colic in infants.
• Be aware that the safety and efficacy of garlic have not been established in children and also that it may be beneficial in children with hypercholesterolemia.
• There are no age-related precautions noted in the elderly.
Precautions
• Use cautiously in patients with diabetes mellitus because garlic may decrease blood glucose levels; in hypothyroidism because garlic may reduce iodine uptake; and in inflammatory gastrointestinal (GI) conditions, because garlic may irritate the GI tract.
• Use garlic with caution because it may prolong bleeding time. Have the patient discontinue its use 1 to 2 weeks before surgery.
Administration and Handling
◀ALERT▶ Appropriate doses for other conditions vary depending on the preparation used.
Intervention and Evaluation
• Monitor the patient's blood glucose levels, coagulation studies, complete blood count (CBC), and serum lipid levels.
• Assess the patient for contact dermatitis and hypersensitivity reaction.
Patient Teaching
• Warn the patient to avoid garlic use during breast-feeding and pregnancy.
• Advise the patient to inform all of his or her health care providers of garlic use.
• Instruct the patient to discontinue garlic use 1 to 2 weeks before any procedure in which bleeding may occur.

ginger
Also known as black ginger, race ginger, zingiber

CATEGORY AND SCHEDULE
Pregnancy Risk Category: N/A
OTC

MECHANISM OF ACTION
An herb that possesses antipyretic, analgesic, antitussive, and sedative properties. Increases gastrointestinal (GI) motility; may act on serotonin receptors, primarily 5-HT$_3$. *Therapeutic Effect:* Reduces nausea and vomiting.

AVAILABILITY
Capsules: 470 mg, 550 mg.
Root: 470 mg, 550 mg.
Extract.
Powder.
Tablets.
Tea.
Tincture.

INDICATIONS AND DOSAGES
▶ **Prevention of nausea and vomiting in early pregnancy**
PO
Adults. 250 mg 4 times/day. Maximum: 4 g/day.
▶ **Prevention of nausea and vomiting from motion sickness**
PO
Adults. 1 g (dried powder root) 30 min before travel.
▶ **Nausea**
PO
Adults. 550–1,100 mg 3 times/day.

CONTRAINDICATIONS
None known

INTERACTIONS
Drug
Anticoagulants, antiplatelets: Large amounts may increase risk of bleeding with these drugs.
Herbal
Feverfew, garlic, ginkgo, ginseng: May increase the risk of bleeding.
Food
None known.

DIAGNOSTIC TEST EFFECTS
None known.

SIDE EFFECTS
Abdominal discomfort, heartburn, diarrhea, hypersensitivity reaction, nausea

SERIOUS REACTIONS
• Central nervous system (CNS) depression and arrhythmias may occur.

NURSING CONSIDERATIONS
Baseline Assessment
• Determine if the patient is taking anticoagulants and antiplatelets before beginning therapy because these agents may increase the risk of bleeding.
Lifespan Considerations
• Be aware that ginger use during pregnancy is controversial and that large amounts of ginger may cause abortion.
• Be aware that the safety and efficacy of ginger have not been established in children.
• There are no age-related precautions noted in the elderly.
Precautions
• Use cautiously in pregnant patients and patients with bleeding conditions and diabetes mellitus (may cause hypoglycemia).
Intervention and Evaluation
• Monitor the patient for hypersensitivity reaction.
Patient Teaching
• Advise patients to use ginger

cautiously during breast-feeding and pregnancy.

ginkgo biloba
Also known as fossil tree, maidenhair tree, tanakan

CATEGORY AND SCHEDULE
Pregnancy Risk Category: N/A
OTC

MECHANISM OF ACTION
An herb that possesses antioxidant and free radical scavenging properties. *Therapeutic Effect:* Protects tissues from oxidative damage and may prevent progression of tissue degeneration in patients with dementia. Inhibits platelet-activating factor bonding at numerous cells, decreasing platelet aggregation, smooth muscle contraction; may also increase cardiac contractility and coronary blood flow. Decreases blood viscosity, improving circulation by relaxing vascular smooth muscle. Increases cerebral and peripheral blood flow and reduces vascular permeability. May influence neurotransmitter system and act as a cholinergic agent.

AVAILABILITY
Capsules: 40 mg, 60 mg.
Tablets: 40 mg, 60 mg.
Fluid Extract.
Tincture.

INDICATIONS AND DOSAGES
▸ **Dementia syndromes, including Alzheimer's**
PO
Adults, Elderly. 120–240 mg/day (extract) in 2–3 doses.

▸ **Vertigo, tinnitus**
PO
Adults, Elderly. 120–160 mg/day.

CONTRAINDICATIONS
Lactation, pregnancy

INTERACTIONS
Drug
Anticoagulants, antiplatelets, such as warfarin, aspirin, heparin, clopidogrel: May increase bleeding with these drugs.
MAOIs: May increase the effects of these drugs.
Herbal
Feverfew, garlic, ginger, ginseng: May increase the risk of bleeding.
Food
None known.

DIAGNOSTIC TEST EFFECTS
May alter blood glucose levels.

SIDE EFFECTS
Headache, dizziness, palpitations, constipation, allergic skin reactions. Large doses may cause nausea, vomiting, diarrhea, weakness, lack of muscle tone.

SERIOUS REACTIONS
• None known.

NURSING CONSIDERATIONS
Baseline Assessment
• Determine if the patient is taking anticoagulants, antiplatelets, or MAOIs.
• Assess the patient for history of bleeding disorders, diabetes mellitus, and seizures.
Lifespan Considerations
• Be aware that ginkgo biloba use in breast-feeding and pregnancy is contraindicated.
• Be aware that the safety and efficacy of ginkgo biloba have not

been established in children. Ginkgo biloba use should be avoided in children.
• There are no age-related precautions noted in the elderly.
Precautions
• Use cautiously in patients with bleeding disorders, diabetes mellitus, epilepsy, and patients prone to seizures.
• Avoid ginkgo biloba use in couples having difficulty conceiving.
Intervention and Evaluation
• Monitor the patient's blood glucose levels.
• Assess the patient for signs and symptoms of a hypersensitivity reaction.
Patient Teaching
• Warn the patient not to use ginkgo biloba while taking anticoagulants and antiplatelets.
• Advise the patient that it may take up to 6 months before the herb becomes effective.
• Warn the patient not to use ginkgo biloba during breast-feeding and pregnancy.
• Caution the patient to avoid ginkgo biloba use in children.

ginseng
Also known as Asian ginseng, Chinese ginseng, red ginseng

CATEGORY AND SCHEDULE
Pregnancy Risk Category: N/A
OTC

MECHANISM OF ACTION
An herb that affects the hypothalamic-pituitary-adrenal axis. Appears to stimulate natural killer cell action. *Therapeutic Effect:*

Reduces stress. Affects immune function.

AVAILABILITY
Capsules: 100 mg, 250 mg, 410 mg, 500 mg.
Tablets: 250 mg, 1,000 mg.
Dried Root.
Extract.
Powder.
Tea (usually 1,500 mg/bag).
Tincture.

INDICATIONS AND DOSAGES
▸ **Aids in blood glucose control, boosts energy level, enhances brain activity, improves cognitive function, concentration, memory, and work efficiency, increases physical endurance and resistance to stress**
PO
Adults, Elderly. Tablets or capsules: 200–600 mg/day. Powder root: 0.6–3 g 1–3 times/day. Tea: 1,500 mg 1–3 times/day.

CONTRAINDICATIONS
Bleeding tendencies or thrombosis, lactation, pregnancy

INTERACTIONS
Drug
Anticoagulants, antiplatelets, such as aspirin, clopidogrel, enoxaparin, heparin, warfarin: May increase bleeding with these drugs.
Furosemide: May decrease the effects of furosemide.
Immunosuppressant drugs, such as cyclosporine and prednisone: May interfere with these drugs.
Insulin, oral antidiabetic agents: May increase the effects of these drugs.
Herbal
Chamomile, feverfew, garlic, ginger, ginkgo: May increase the risk of bleeding.

Food
Coffee, tea: May increase the effects of ginseng.

DIAGNOSTIC TEST EFFECTS
May prolong activated partial thromboplastin time (aPTT). May decrease blood glucose levels.

SIDE EFFECTS
Frequent
Insomnia
Occasional
Vaginal bleeding, amenorrhea, palpitations, hypertension, diarrhea, headache, allergic reactions

SERIOUS REACTIONS
• None known.

NURSING CONSIDERATIONS
Baseline Assessment
• Determine if the patient is breast-feeding, pregnant, and taking anti-coagulants and immunosuppressants.
• Determine if the patient has diabetes mellitus or is taking insulin or other oral hypoglycemic agents.
• Establish the patient's baseline blood glucose level.
Lifespan Considerations
• Be aware that ginseng should not be used in breast-feeding or pregnant women. There is insufficient information on this herb to determine its safety in these patient populations.
• Be aware that the safety and efficacy of this herb have not been established in children.
• There are no age-related precautions noted in the elderly.
Precautions
• Use cautiously in patients with cardiac disorders, diabetes mellitus, endometriosis, hormone-sensitive cancers,

including breast, ovarian, and uterine cancer, and uterine fibroids.
Intervention and Evaluation
• Monitor the patient's blood glucose levels and coagulation studies.
• Assess the patient for signs and symptoms of a hypersensitivity reaction, including a rash.
Patient Teaching
• Warn the patient to avoid ginseng use while breast-feeding and pregnant.
• Warn the patient to avoid ginseng use in children.
• Caution the patient to avoid continuous ginseng use for longer than 3 months.

glucosamine/ chondroitin

CATEGORY AND SCHEDULE
Pregnancy Risk Category: N/A
OTC

MECHANISM OF ACTION
Glucosamine: Necessary for synthesis of mucopolysaccharides, which comprise the body's tendons, ligaments, cartilage, synovial fluid. May decrease glucose-induced insulin secretion. *Therapeutic Effect:* Relieves symptoms of osteoarthritis. Chondroitin: Endogenously found in cartilage tissue, substrate for forming joint matrix structure. May have some anticoagulant properties. *Therapeutic Effect:* Relieves symptoms of osteoarthritis.

AVAILABILITY
Glucosamine
Capsules: 500 mg.
Tablets: 500 mg.
Chondroitin
Capsules: 250 mg.

INDICATIONS AND DOSAGES
▶ **Osteoarthritis**
PO
Adults, Elderly. (Glucosamine):
500 mg 3 times/day or 1–2 g/day.
(Chondroitin): 200–400 mg
2–3 times/day.

CONTRAINDICATIONS
None known

INTERACTIONS
Drug
Chondroitin: Monitor anticoagulant
therapy
Glucosamine: None known.
Herbal
None known.
Food
None known.

DIAGNOSTIC TEST EFFECTS
Glucosamine: May increase blood
glucose levels. Chondroitin: May
increase antifactor Xa level.

SIDE EFFECTS
Glucosamine: Mild gastrointestinal
(GI) symptoms, such as gas, bloating, and cramps
Chondroitin: Well tolerated. May
cause nausea, diarrhea, constipation,
edema, alopecia, allergic reactions

SERIOUS REACTIONS
• None known.

NURSING CONSIDERATIONS
Baseline Assessment
• Determine if the patient is taking
anticoagulants, antidiabetics, and
antiplatelets drugs.
• Determine if the patient is breast-
feeding or pregnant.
Lifespan Considerations
• Be aware that glucosamine or
chondroitin use should be avoided

in breast-feeding and pregnant
women.
• Be aware that the safety and
efficacy of glucosamine/chondroitin
have not been established in children.
• There are no age-related precautions noted in the elderly.
Precautions
• Use glucosamine cautiously in
patients with diabetes mellitus
because it may increase insulin
resistance.
Administration and Handling
◀**ALERT**▶ Many combination products are available.
Intervention and Evaluation
• Monitor the patient to determine
the effectiveness of herb therapy in
altering blood glucose levels and
relieving osteoarthritis symptoms.
Patient Teaching
• Warn the patient to avoid glucosamine or chondroitin use during
breast-feeding and pregnancy.
• Warn the patient to avoid glucosamine or chondroitin use in children.
• Advise the patient that it may take
several months of therapy to be
effective.
• Advise the patient that glucosamine may alter blood glucose
levels.

kava kava
Also known as ava, kew, sakau,
tonga, yagona

CATEGORY AND SCHEDULE
Pregnancy Risk Category: N/A
OTC

MECHANISM OF ACTION
An herb whose exact mechanism of
action is unknown, but possesses

central nervous system (CNS) effects. *Therapeutic Effect:* Anxiolytic, sedative, analgesic effects.

AVAILABILITY

Capsules: 140 mg, 150 mg, 250 mg, 300 mg, 425 mg, 500 mg.
Liquid.
Extract.
Tincture.

INDICATIONS AND DOSAGES
▶ **Treatment of anxiety disorders**
PO
Adults, Elderly. 100 mg 3 times/day or 1 cup of the tea 3 times/day.

CONTRAINDICATIONS
Breast-feeding, pregnancy (may cause loss of uterine tone)

INTERACTIONS
Drug
Alcohol, benzodiazepines: May increase the risk of drowsiness.
Herbal
Chamomile, ginseng, goldenseal, melatonin, St. John's wort, valerian: May increase the risk of excessive drowsiness.
Food
None known.

DIAGNOSTIC TEST EFFECTS
May increase liver function tests.

SIDE EFFECTS
Gastrointestinal (GI) upset, headache, dizziness, vision changes (blurred vision, red eyes), allergic skin reactions, dermopathy (dry, flaky skin, yellowing of the eyes, skin, hair, nails), nausea, vomiting, weight loss, shortness of breath

SERIOUS REACTIONS
• None known.

NURSING CONSIDERATIONS
Baseline Assessment
• Determine if the patient is breast-feeding, pregnant, or using other CNS depressants.
• Establish the patient's baseline hepatic enzyme levels to assess liver function.
Lifespan Considerations
• Be aware that kava kava use in breast-feeding and pregnant women is contraindicated.
• Be aware that the safety and efficacy of kava kava have not been established in children.
• There are no age-related precautions noted in the elderly.
Precautions
• Use cautiously in patients with depression and history of recurrent hepatitis.
Administration and Handling
◀ALERT▶ Be aware that kava kava may be removed from the market.
Intervention and Evaluation
• Monitor the patient's hepatic enzyme levels.
• Examine the patient for allergic skin reactions.
Patient Teaching
• Warn the patient to avoid kava kava use if she is breast-feeding, pregnant, or planning to become pregnant.
• Advise the patient that kava kava is not for use in children younger than 12 years of age because it may be habit-forming.
• Caution the patient to avoid tasks that require mental alertness or motor skills until his or her response to the herb is established.

melatonin
Also known as pineal hormone

CATEGORY AND SCHEDULE
Pregnancy Risk Category: N/A
OTC

MECHANISM OF ACTION
A hormone synthesized endogenously by the pineal gland. Interacts with melatonin receptors in the brain. *Therapeutic Effect:* Regulates the body's circadian rhythm, sleep patterns. Acts as an antioxidant, protecting cells from oxidative damage by free radicals.

AVAILABILITY
Lozenges: 3 mg.
Powder.
Tablets: 0.5 mg, 3 mg.

INDICATIONS AND DOSAGES
▸ **Insomnia**
PO
Adults, Elderly. 0.5–5 mg at bedtime.
▸ **Jet lag**
PO
Adults, Elderly. 5 mg/day beginning 3 days before flight and 3 days after flight.

CONTRAINDICATIONS
Breast-feeding, pregnancy

INTERACTIONS:
Drug
Alcohol, benzodiazepines: May be additive with these drugs.
Immunosuppressants: May interfere with these drugs.
Isoniazid: May enhance the effects of isoniazid.
Herbal
Chamomile, ginseng, goldenseal,

kava kava, valerian: May increase sedative effects.
Food
None known.

DIAGNOSTIC TEST EFFECTS
May increase human growth hormone levels. May decrease luteinizing hormone (LH) levels.

SIDE EFFECTS
Headache, transient depression, fatigue, drowsiness, dizziness, abdominal cramps or irritability, decreased alertness, hypersensitivity reaction, tachycardia, nausea, vomiting, anorexia, changes in sleep patterns, confusion

SERIOUS REACTIONS
• None known.

NURSING CONSIDERATIONS
Baseline Assessment
• Determine if the patient is breast-feeding, pregnant, and using other medications, especially central nervous system (CNS) depressants.
• Establish the patient's history of depression or seizures.
• Assess the patient's sleep pattern if used for insomnia.
Lifespan Considerations
• Be aware that melatonin use in breast-feeding and pregnant women is contraindicated.
• Be aware that the safety and efficacy of melatonin have not been established in children.
• There are no age-related precautions noted in the elderly.
Precautions
• Use cautiously in patients with cardiovascular disease, depression (may worsen dysphoria), liver disease, and seizures (may increase incidence).

Intervention and Evaluation

• Monitor the herb's effectiveness in improving the patient's insomnia.

• Assess the patient for CNS effects and hypersensitivity reactions.

Patient Teaching

• Warn the patient not to take melatonin if breast-feeding, pregnant, or planning to become pregnant.

• Encourage an environment conducive to sleep (low lighting, quiet).

• Caution the patient to avoid performing tasks that require mental alertness or motor skills, such as driving, during melatonin therapy.

St. John's wort

Also known as amber, demon chaser, goatweed, hardhay, rosin rose, tipton weed

CATEGORY AND SCHEDULE

Pregnancy Risk Category: N/A
OTC

MECHANISM OF ACTION

An herb that inhibits catechol-*O*-methyl transferase (COMT) and monoamine oxidase (MAO); modulates effects of serotonin by inhibiting serotonin reuptake and 5-HT$_3$ and 5-HT$_4$ antagonism. *Therapeutic Effect:* Produces antidepressant effect.

AVAILABILITY

Capsules: 150 mg, 300 mg,
Liquid Extract.
Tincture.

INDICATIONS AND DOSAGES
▸ **Depression**
PO

Adults, Elderly. 300 mg 3 times/day is the most common.

CONTRAINDICATIONS

Breast-feeding (may cause increased muscle tone of uterus, infants may experience colic, drowsiness, lethargy), pregnancy

INTERACTIONS
Drug

Angiotensin-converting enzyme (ACE) inhibitors: May cause hypertension.

Antidepressants: May increase the therapeutic effect of St. John's wort.

Cyclosporine: May cause organ rejection.

Digoxin: May cause exacerbation of congestive heart failure (CHF).

Indinavir: May decrease the blood concentration and effects of indinavir.

Herbal

Chamomile, ginseng, goldenseal, kava kava, valerian: May increase the therapeutic and adverse effects of St. John's wort.

Food

Tyramine-containing foods: Large doses with these foods may cause a hypertensive crisis.

DIAGNOSTIC TEST EFFECTS

May increase international normalized ratio (INR) and prothrombin time (PT) in patients treated with warfarin.

SIDE EFFECTS

Abdominal cramps, insomnia, vivid dreams, restlessness, anxiety, agitation, irritability, fatigue, dry mouth, headache, dizziness, photosensitivity, confusion

SERIOUS REACTIONS
• None known.

NURSING CONSIDERATIONS
Baseline Assessment
• Determine if the patient is breast-feeding, pregnant, and taking other medications.
• Determine the patient's history of psychiatric disease.
• Assess the patient's anxiety level, memory, mental status, and mood.
Lifespan Considerations
• Be aware that St. John's wort use is contraindicated in breast-feeding and pregnant women.
• Be aware that the safety and efficacy of St. John's wort have not been established in children.
• There are no age-related precautions noted in the elderly.
Precautions
• Use cautiously in patients with bipolar disorder and schizophrenia.
Intervention and Evaluation
• Monitor changes in the patient's behavior and depressive state.
• Monitor the patient for signs of side effects.
Patient Teaching
• Caution the patient against abruptly discontinuing St. John's wort.
• Warn the patient not to take any medications, including over-the-counter drugs, without first notifying the physician.
• Urge the patient to avoid foods high in tyramine, such as aged cheese, pickled products, beer, and wine.
• Advise the patient that the herb's therapeutic effect may take 4 to 6 weeks to appear.
• Urge the patient to wear protective clothing and sunscreen and to avoid overexposure to sunlight while taking St. John's wort.

saw palmetto
Also known as American dwarf palm tree, cabbage palm, sabal, zu-zhong

CATEGORY AND SCHEDULE
Pregnancy Risk Category: N/A
OTC

MECHANISM OF ACTION
An herb that appears to inhibit 5-alpha-reductase and prevent conversion of testosterone to dihydrotestosterone (DHT). *Therapeutic Effect:* Reduces prostate growth. Contains antiandrogenic, antiproliferative, and anti-inflammatory properties.

AVAILABILITY
Capsules: 80 mg, 160 mg, 500 mg.
Berries.
Fluid Extract.
Tea.

INDICATIONS AND DOSAGES
▸ **Benign prostate hyperplasia (BPH)**
PO
Adults, Elderly. 160 mg 2 times/day or 320 mg once/day.

CONTRAINDICATIONS
Lactation due to antiandrogenic and estrogenic activity, pregnancy

INTERACTIONS
Drug
Hormone therapy, oral contraceptives: May interfere with these drugs.
Herbal
None known.
Food
None known.

DIAGNOSTIC TEST EFFECTS
None known.

SIDE EFFECTS
Mild anorexia, dizziness, nausea, vomiting, constipation, diarrhea, headache, impotence, hypersensitivity reactions, back pain

SERIOUS REACTIONS
• None known.

NURSING CONSIDERATIONS
Baseline Assessment
• Determine if the patient uses oral contraceptives or is taking part in hormone replacement therapy because saw palmetto may interfere with these therapies.
• Assess the patient's urinary patterns.
Lifespan Considerations
• Be aware that saw palmetto use is contraindicated in breast-feeding and pregnant women.
• Be aware that the safety and efficacy of saw palmetto have not been established in children.
• There are no age-related precautions noted in the elderly.
Intervention and Evaluation
• Assess the patient for signs and symptoms of hypersensitivity reactions.
• Monitor the patient for symptoms of benign prostatic hyperplasia, including frequent or painful urination, hesitancy, and urgency. Assess the patient for decreased nocturia, decreased residual urine volume, and improved urinary flow.
Patient Teaching
• Instruct the patient to take saw palmetto with food.
• Advise the male patient to be tested and obtain a prostate-specific antigen (PSA) test before using saw palmetto.

valerian
Also known as all-heal, amantilla, garden heliotrope, valeriana.

CATEGORY AND SCHEDULE
Pregnancy Risk Category: N/A
OTC

MECHANISM OF ACTION
An herb that appears to inhibit enzyme system responsible for catabolism of gamma-aminobutyric acid (GABA), increasing GABA concentration and decreasing central nervous system (CNS) activity. *Therapeutic Effect:* Produces sedative effects. Also has anxiolytic, antidepressant, anticonvulsant effects.

AVAILABILITY
Capsules.
Tablets.
Extract.
Tea.
Tincture.

INDICATIONS AND DOSAGES
▸ **Sedation for insomnia, sleeping disorders associated with anxiety, and restlessness**
PO
Adults, Elderly. Extract: 400–900 mg ½–1 hr before bedtime. Tea: 1 cup taken several times/day.

CONTRAINDICATIONS
Liver disease, lactation, pregnancy

INTERACTIONS
Drug
Alcohol, barbiturates, benzodiazepines: May cause additive effect and increase adverse effects of valerian.

Herbal

Chamomile, ginseng, kava kava, melatonin, St. John's wort: May enhance the therapeutic effect and adverse effects of valerian.

Food

None known.

DIAGNOSTIC TEST EFFECTS

None known.

SIDE EFFECTS

Headache, hangover, cardiac disturbances

SERIOUS REACTIONS

• Difficulty walking, excitability, hypothermia, increased muscle relaxation, and insomnia may occur.

NURSING CONSIDERATIONS

Baseline Assessment

• Determine if the patient is using other central nervous system (CNS) depressants, especially a benzodiazepine.

• Assess the patient's baseline serum hepatic enzyme levels to assess liver function.

Lifespan Considerations

• Be aware that valerian use is contraindicated in breast-feeding and pregnant women.

• Be aware that the safety and efficacy of valerian have not been established in children. Valerian use should be avoided in children.

• There are no age-related precautions noted in the elderly.

Intervention and Evaluation

• Monitor the herb's effectiveness in decreasing the patient's insomnia.

• Assess the patient for hypersensitivity reaction.

• Monitor the patient's liver function tests.

Patient Teaching

• Advise the patient that it may take up to 4 weeks of valerian administration before he or she feels significant relief.

• Caution the patient to avoid performing tasks that require mental alertness or motor skills while taking valerian.

• Warn the female patient to notify the physician if she starts breast-feeding or becomes pregnant.

• Instruct the patient to taper off valerian doses slowly and caution the patient not to abruptly discontinue the herb.

yohimbe

Also known as aphrodien, corynine, johimbi

CATEGORY AND SCHEDULE

Pregnancy Risk Category: N/A
OTC

MECHANISM OF ACTION

An herb that produces genital blood vessel dilation, improves nerve impulse transmission to genital area. Increases penile blood flow, central sympathetic excitation impulses to genital tissues. *Therapeutic Effect:* Improves sexual vigor, affects impotence.

AVAILABILITY

Tablets: 5 mg.
Liquid: 5 mg/5 ml.

INDICATIONS AND DOSAGES

▸ **Impotence**
PO
Adults, Elderly. 15–30 mg/day in divided doses.

CONTRAINDICATIONS

Angina, heart disease, benign prostatic hypertrophy, depression, heart disease, lactation, liver disease, pregnancy (may have uterine relaxant effect, cause fetal toxicity), renal disease

INTERACTIONS
Drug
Antidiabetics, antihypertensives: May interfere with the effects of these drugs.
Clonidine: May antagonize the effects of clonidine.
MAOIs, sympathomimetics, tricyclic antidepressants: Has additive effects with these drugs.
Herbal
Ephedra: May increase the risk of hypertensive crises.
Ginkgo biloba, St. John's wort: May have additive therapeutic and adverse effects.
Food
Caffeine-containing products (such as coffee, tea, and chocolate), tyramine-containing foods (such as aged cheese and chianti wine): May increase the risk of hypertensive crises.

DIAGNOSTIC TEST EFFECTS
None known.

SIDE EFFECTS
Excitement, tremors, insomnia, anxiety, hypertension, tachycardia, dizziness, headache, irritability, salivation, dilated pupils, nausea, vomiting, hypersensitivity reaction

SERIOUS REACTIONS
• Paralysis, severe hypotension, irregular heartbeats, and cardiac failure may occur. Overdose can be fatal.

NURSING CONSIDERATIONS

Baseline Assessment
• Determine if the patient is breast-feeding or pregnant.

• Determine the patient's other medical conditions, especially angina, heart disease, and benign prostatic hyperplasia, and medication history.
• Assess the patient's baseline blood serum chemistries, especially BUN, serum alkaline phosphatase, creatinine, SGOT (AST) and SGPT (ALT) levels to assess liver and renal function.

Lifespan Considerations
• Be aware that yohimbe use is contraindicated in breast-feeding and pregnant women.
• Be aware that the safety and efficacy of yohimbe have not been established in children.
• Be aware that yohimbe use should be avoided in breast-feeding women, children, and pregnant women.
• In the elderly, age-related liver and renal impairment may require discontinuation of yohimbe.

Precautions
• Use cautiously in patients with anxiety, diabetes mellitus, hypertension, post-traumatic stress disorder, and schizophrenia.

Intervention and Evaluation
• Monitor the patient's blood pressure (B/P) and liver and renal function tests.
• Assess the patient for signs and symptoms of a hypersensitivity reaction.

Patient Teaching
• Warn the patient not to take any other medications, including over-the-counter drugs, without first notifying the physician.
• Warn the female patient to immediately notify the physician if she starts breast-feeding or becomes pregnant.

aluminum hydroxide

calcium acetate,
  calcium carbonate,
  calcium chloride,
  calcium citrate,
  calcium glubionate,
  calcium gluconate

citrates
  potassium citrate,
  potassium citrate
  and citric acid,
  sodium citrate
  and citric acid,
  tricitrates

fluoride

magnesium,
  magnesium chloride,
  magnesium citrate,
  magnesium
  hydroxide,
  magnesium oxide,
  magnesium protein
  complex,
  magnesium sulfate

phosphate

potassium acetate,
  potassium
  bicarbonate-citrate,
  potassium chloride,
  potassium gluconate

sodium bicarbonate

sodium chloride

zinc oxide, zinc
  sulfate

Uses: Minerals and electrolytes are used as replacements to correct specific electrolyte imbalances, such as hypokalemia, hyponatremia, and hypermagnesemia. Additional uses vary greatly. *Aluminum* is used to treat hyperacidity and gastroesophageal reflux disease (GERD) and to prevent gastrointestinal (GI) bleeding and phosphate calculi formation. *Calcium* is also prescribed to treat hyperacidity. *Citrates* treat metabolic acidosis. *Fluoride* prevents dental caries in children. *Magnesium* is also used to treat hypertension, torsades de pointes, encephalopathy, constipation, hyperacidity, and seizures from acute nephritis. *Phosphates* are used to prevent and treat hypophosphatemia, to treat constipation, to evacuate the colon for examination, and to acidify the urine and reduce calcium calculi formation. *Sodium bicarbonate* is used to manage metabolic acidosis and hyperacidity, alkalinize urine, stabilize acid-base balance, and treat cardiac arrest. *Sodium chloride* is also used to promote hydration, assess renal function, and manage hyperosmolar diabetes; in addition, it has nasal and ophthalmic uses. *Zinc oxide* is used to protect the skin from mild irritation and abrasions and to promote the healing of chapped skin and diaper rash. *Zinc sulfate* helps prevent zinc deficiency and is used to promote wound healing.

Action: Minerals are needed for normal body function. Electrolytes are substances that carry a positive or negative charge. Their functions include transmission of nerve impulses to contract skeletal and smooth muscles. Additional specific actions vary with the agent. *Aluminum* reduces gastric acid, binds with phosphate, and may increase calcium absorption. (See illustration, *Sites of Action: Drugs Used to Treat GERD,* page 932.) *Calcium* neutralizes or reduces gastric acid. *Citrates* increase urinary pH and citrate, decrease calcium activity, increase plasma bicarbonate, and buffer excess hydrogen ions. *Fluoride*

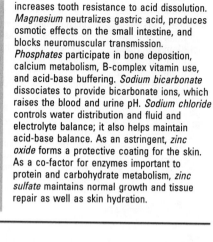

increases tooth resistance to acid dissolution. *Magnesium* neutralizes gastric acid, produces osmotic effects on the small intestine, and blocks neuromuscular transmission. *Phosphates* participate in bone deposition, calcium metabolism, B-complex vitamin use, and acid-base buffering. *Sodium bicarbonate* dissociates to provide bicarbonate ions, which raises the blood and urine pH. *Sodium chloride* controls water distribution and fluid and electrolyte balance; it also helps maintain acid-base balance. As an astringent, *zinc oxide* forms a protective coating for the skin. As a co-factor for enzymes important to protein and carbohydrate metabolism, *zinc sulfate* maintains normal growth and tissue repair as well as skin hydration.

COMBINATION PRODUCTS
GAVISCON: (oral suspension) aluminum hydroxide/magnesium carbonate (an antacid) 31.7 mg/119.3 mg.
GAVISCON: (tablets) aluminum hydroxide/magnesium trisilicate (an antacid) 80 mg/20 mg.
GELUSIL: aluminum hydroxide/magnesium hydroxide (an antacid)/simethicone (an antiflatulent) 200 mg/200 mg/25 mg.
HALEY'S M-O: magnesium/mineral oil (a laxative) 300 mg/1.25 ml.
MAALOX: aluminum hydroxide/magnesium hydroxide (an antacid) 200 mg/200 mg (oral suspension); 225 mg/200 mg (tablets).
MAALOX PLUS: aluminum hydroxide/magnesium hydroxide (an antacid)/simethicone (an antiflatulent) 200 mg/200 mg/25 mg.
MYLANTA: aluminum hydroxide/magnesium hydroxide (an antacid)/simethicone (an antiflatulent) 200 mg/200 mg/20 mg; 400 mg/400 mg/40 mg.
PEPCID COMPLETE: calcium chloride/magnesium hydroxide (an antacid)/famotidine (a histamine [H$_2$] antagonist) 800 mg/165 mg/10 mg.
SILAIN-GEL: aluminum hydroxide/magnesium hydroxide (an antacid)/simethicone (an antiflatulent).

aluminum hydroxide
(Alternagel, Alu-Cap, Alu-Tab, Amphojel, Basaljel[CAN])

CATEGORY AND SCHEDULE
Pregnancy Risk Category: C
Considered safe unless chronic, high-dose usage.
OTC

MECHANISM OF ACTION
An antacid that reduces gastric acid by binding with phosphate in the intestine, and then is excreted as aluminum carbonate in feces. Aluminum carbonate may increase the absorption of calcium due to decreased serum phosphate levels. The drug also has astringent and adsorbent properties. *Therapeutic Effect:*

Neutralizes or increases gastric pH; reduces phosphates in urine, preventing formation of phosphate urinary stones; reduces serum phosphate levels; decreases fluidity of stools.

AVAILABILITY
Aluminum hydroxide
Capsules: 475 mg.
Suspension: 320 mg/5 ml, 600 mg/5 ml.

INDICATIONS AND DOSAGES
▸ **Peptic ulcer disease**
PO
Adults, Elderly. 15–45 ml q3–6h or 1 and 3 hrs after meals and at bedtime.
Children. 5–15 ml as above.
▸ **Antacid**
PO
Adults, Elderly. 30 ml 1 and 3 hrs after meals and at bedtime.
▸ **Gastrointestinal (GI) bleeding prevention**
PO
Adults, Elderly. 30–60 ml/hr.
Children. 5–15 ml. q1–2h.
▸ **Hyperphosphatemia**
PO
Adults, Elderly. 500–1800 mg 1 and 3 hrs after meals and at bedtime.
Children. 50–150 mg/kg/24 hrs q4–6h.

CONTRAINDICATIONS
Children age 6 yrs or younger, intestinal obstruction

INTERACTIONS
Drug
Anticholinergics, quinidine: May decrease excretion of aluminum hydroxide.
Iron preparations, isoniazid, ketoconazole, quinolones, tetracyclines: May decrease absorption of aluminum hydroxide.

Methenamine: May decrease effects of methenamine.
Salicylate: May increase salicylate excretion.
Herbal
None known.
Food
None known.

DIAGNOSTIC TEST EFFECTS
May increase serum gastrin levels and systemic and urinary pH. May decrease serum phosphate levels.

SIDE EFFECTS
Frequent
Chalky taste, mild constipation, stomach cramps
Occasional
Nausea, vomiting, speckling or whitish discoloration of stools

SERIOUS REACTIONS
• Prolonged constipation may result in intestinal obstruction.
• Excessive or chronic use may produce hypophosphatemia manifested as anorexia, malaise, muscle weakness or bone pain and resulting in osteomalacia and osteoporosis.
• Prolonged use may produce urinary calculi.

NURSING CONSIDERATIONS
Baseline Assessment
• Do not give other oral medications within 1 to 2 hours of antacid administration.
Precautions
• Use cautiously in patients with Alzheimer's disease, advanced age, chronic diarrhea, constipation, dehydration, fecal impaction, fluid restrictions, gastric outlet obstruction, gastrointestinal or rectal bleeding, impaired renal function, or symptoms of appendicitis.

Administration and Handling

PO

◀ALERT▶ Usual dose is 30 to 60 ml.

• Administer 1 to 3 hours after meals.

• Expect the dosage to be individualize based on the neutralizing capacity of the antacid.

• For chewable tablets, instruct the patient to thoroughly chew tablets before swallowing and then to drink a glass of water or milk.

• If administering a suspension, shake well before use.

Intervention and Evaluation

• Assess the patient's pattern of daily bowel activity and stool consistency.

• Expect to monitor the patient's serum aluminum, serum calcium, serum phosphate, and uric acid levels.

• Evaluate and document the patient's relief from gastric distress.

Patient Teaching

• Instruct the patient to chew tablets thoroughly before swallowing and to then drink a glass of water or milk.

• Explain to the patient that the tablets may discolor his or her stool and provide reassurance that this is expected and will resolve when the medication is discontinued.

• Stress to the patient that he or she maintain adequate fluid intake.

calcium acetate
(PhosLo)
calcium carbonate
(Apo-Cal[CAN], Calsan[CAN], Caltrate[CAN], Dicarbosil, OsCal, Titralac, Tums)
calcium chloride
(Calcijex[CAN])
calcium citrate
(Citracal, Calcitrate)
calcium glubionate
(Calcione, Calciquid)
calcium gluconate
Do not confuse with Asacol, Citrucel, or PhosChol.

CATEGORY AND SCHEDULE
Pregnancy Risk Category: C
OTC (acetate, carbonate, citrate, glubionate, gluconate [tablets only])

MECHANISM OF ACTION
An electrolyte replenisher that is essential for the function and integrity of nervous, muscular, and skeletal systems. These agents play an important role in normal cardiac and renal function, respiration, blood coagulation, and cell membrane and capillary permeability. Assists in regulating release and storage of neurotransmitters and hormones. Neutralizes or reduces gastric acid (increase pH). Calcium Acetate: Combines with dietary phosphate, forming insoluble calcium phosphate. *Therapeutic Effects:* Replaces calcium in deficiency states, controls hyperphosphatemia in end-stage renal disease.

PHARMACOKINETICS
Moderately absorbed from small intestine (dependent on presence of

vitamin D metabolites, pH). Primarily eliminated in feces.

AVAILABILITY

Calcium Acetate
Tablets: 667 mg.
Capsules: 667 mg.
Calcium Carbonate
Tablets: 500 mg, 650 mg, 1,250 mg, 1,500 mg.
Tablets (chewable): 350 mg, 500 mg, 750 mg, 1,250 mg.
Capsules: 1,250 mg.
Calcium Chloride
Injection: 10%.
Calcium Citrate
Tablets: 950 mg.
Calcium Glubionate
Syrup.
Calcium Gluconate
Tablets: 500 mg, 650 mg, 975 mg, 1,000 mg.
Injection: 10%.

INDICATIONS AND DOSAGES
▸ **Hypophosphatemia (calcium acetate)**
PO
Adults, Elderly. 2 tablets calcium acetate 3 times/day with meals.
▸ **Hypocalcemia (calcium carbonate)**
PO
Adults, Elderly. 1–2 g of calcium carbonate/day in 3–4 divided doses.
Children. 45–65 mg/kg/day of calcium carbonate in 3–4 divided doses.
▸ **Antacid (calcium carbonate)**
PO
Adults, Elderly. 1–2 tabs (5–10 ml) calcium carbonate q2h as needed.
▸ **Osteoporosis (calcium carbonate)**
PO
Adults, Elderly. 1200 mg calcium carbonate/day.

▸ **Antihypocalcemic (calcium glubionate)**
PO
Adults, Elderly. 15 ml calcium glubionate 3–4 times/day.
Children 1–4 yrs. 10 ml calcium glubionate 3 times/day.
Children younger than 1 yr. 5 ml calcium glubionate 5 times/day.
▸ **Cardiac arrest (calcium chloride)**
IV
Adults, Elderly. 2–4 mg/kg of calcium chloride. May repeat q10min.
Children. 20 mg/kg calcium chloride. May repeat in 10 min.
▸ **Hypocalcemia (calcium chloride)**
IV
Adults, Elderly. 0.5–1 g calcium chloride repeated q4–6h as needed.
Children. 2.5–5 mg/kg/dose of calcium chloride q4–6h.
▸ **Hypocalcemia tetany (calcium chloride)**
IV
Adults, Elderly. 1 g calcium chloride may repeat in 6 hours.
Children. 10 mg/kg of calcium chloride over 5–10 min. May repeat in 6–8 hrs.
▸ **Hypocalcemia (calcium gluconate)**
IV
Adults, Elderly. 2–15 g of calcium gluconate/24 hrs.
Children. 200–500 mg/kg/day of calcium gluconate.
▸ **Hypocalcemia tetany (calcium gluconate)**
IV
Adults, Elderly. 1–3 g calcium gluconate until therapeutic response.
Children. 100–200 mg/kg/dose of calcium gluconate q6–8h.

UNLABELED USES
Calcium Carbonate: Treatment of hyperphosphatemia

CONTRAINDICATIONS

Calcium renal calculi, hypercalcemia, hypercalciuria, sarcoidosis, digoxin toxicity, sarcoidosis, ventricular fibrillation

Calcium acetate: Hypoparathyroidism, decreased renal function

INTERACTIONS
Drug

Digoxin: May increase the risk of arrhythmias.

Etidronate, gallium: May antagonize the effects of these drugs.

Ketoconazole, phenytoin, tetracyclines: May decrease the absorption of these drugs.

Methenamine, parenteral magnesium:. May decrease the effects of these drugs.

Herbal
None known.
Food
None known.

DIAGNOSTIC TEST EFFECTS

May increase blood gastrin, blood pH, and serum calcium. May decrease serum phosphate and potassium.

IV INCOMPATIBILITIES

Calcium chloride: amphotericin B complex (Ambisone, abelcet), propofol (Diprivan), sodium bicarbonate

Calcium gluconate: amphotericin c complex (AmBisome, Abelcet), fluconazole (Diflucan)

IV COMPATIBILITIES

Calcium chloride: Amikacin (Amikin), dobutamine (Dobutrex), lidocaine, milrinone (Primacor), morphine, norepinephrine (Levophed)

Calcium gluconate: Ampicillin, aztreonam (Azactam), cefazolin (Ancef), cefepime (Maxipime), ciprofloxacin (Cipro), dobutamine (Dobutrex), enalapril (Vasotec), famotidine (Pepcid), furosemide (Lasix), heparin, lidocaine, magnesium sulfate, meropenem (Merrem IV), midazolam (Versed), milrinone (Primacor), norepinephrine (Levophed), piperacillin tazobactam (Zosyn), potassium chloride, propofol (Diprivan)

SIDE EFFECTS
Frequent
Parenteral: Hypotension, flushing, feeling of warmth, nausea, vomiting; pain, rash, redness, burning at injection site; sweating, decreased blood pressure (B/P)
PO: Chalky taste
Occasional
PO: Mild constipation, fecal impaction, swelling of hands and feet, metabolic alkalosis (muscle pain, restlessness, slow breathing, poor taste)
Calcium carbonate: Milk-alkali syndrome (headache, decreased appetite, nausea, vomiting, unusual tiredness)
Rare
Difficult or painful urination

SERIOUS REACTIONS

• Hypercalcemia is a serious reaction of calcium acetate use. The early signs of hypercalcemia are constipation, headache, dry mouth, increased thirst, irritability, decreased appetite, metallic taste, fatigue, weakness, and depression. Later signs of hypercalcemia are confusion, drowsiness, increased blood pressure (B/P), increased light sensitivity, irregular heartbeat, nausea, vomiting, and increased urination.

NURSING CONSIDERATIONS

Baseline Assessment

• Assess the patient's B/P, electrocardiogram (EKG), and serum magnesium, potassium and phosphate levels as well as BUN and serum creatinine to assess renal function tests.

Lifespan Considerations

• Be aware that calcium acetate is distributed in breast milk and it is unknown whether calcium chloride or gluconate are distributed in breast milk.

• Be aware that children experience extreme irritation and possible tissue necrosis or sloughing with IV form. Restrict IV use in children due to small vasculature.

• Be aware that in the elderly oral absorption may be decreased.

Precautions

• Use cautiously in patients with chronic renal impairment, decreased cardiac function, dehydration, history of renal calculi, and ventricular fibrillation during cardiac resuscitation.

Administration and Handling

PO

• Give tablets with a full glass of water 0.5 to 1 hour after meals.

• Give syrup before meals to increase absorption, diluted in juice or water.

• Chewable tablets must be well chewed before swallowing.

IV

• Store at room temperature.

• May give calcium chloride undiluted or may dilute with equal amount 0.9% NaCl or Sterile Water for Injection.

• May give calcium gluconate undiluted or may dilute in up to 1,000 ml NaCl.

• Give calcium chloride by slow IV push: 0.5 to 1 ml/min. Rapid administration may produce bradycardia, chalky or metallic taste, drop in B/P, peripheral vasodilation, and sensation of heat.

• Give calcium gluconate by IV push: 0.5 to 1 ml/min. Rapid administration may produce arrhythmias, drop in B/P, myocardial infarction (MI), and vasodilation.

• Maximum rate for intermittent IV calcium gluconate infusion is 200 mg/min (e.g., 10 ml/min when 1 g diluted with 50 ml diluent).

Intervention and Evaluation

• Monitor the patient's B/P, electrocardiogram (EKG), and serum magnesium, phosphate, and potassium levels as well as renal function tests and urine calcium concentrations.

• Monitor the patient for signs and symptoms of hypercalcemia.

Patient Teaching

• Stress to the patient the importance of diet.

• Instruct the patient to take tablets with a full glass of water, one half to 1 hour after meals.

• Teach the patient to consume liquid before meals.

• Advise the patient not to take the vitamin within 1 to 2 hours of other fiber-containing foods and oral medications.

• Urge the patient to avoid consuming excessive amounts of alcohol, caffeine, and tobacco.

citrates (potassium citrate, potassium citrate and citric acid, sodium citrate and citric acid, tricitrates)

(Bicitra, Oracit, Polycitra, Urocit-K)

CATEGORY AND SCHEDULE
Pregnancy Risk Category: C (potassium citrate) Other forms not expected to cause fetal harm.

MECHANISM OF ACTION
This alkalinizer increases urinary pH and increases the solubility of cystine in urine and the ionization of uric acid to urate ion. Increasing urinary pH and urinary citrate decreases calcium ion activity and decreases saturation of calcium oxalate. Increases plasma bicarbonate, buffers excess hydrogen ion concentration. *Therapeutic Effect:* Increases blood pH and reverses acidosis.

AVAILABILITY
Tablets: 5 mEq, 10 mEq.
Syrup.
Oral Solution.

INDICATIONS AND DOSAGES
▶ **Treatment of metabolic acidosis**
PO
Adults, Elderly. 15–30 ml after meals and at bedtime. Urocit K: 30–60 mEq/day in 3–4 divided doses.
Children. 5–15 ml after meals and at bedtime or 2–3 mEq/kg/day in 3–4 divided doses.

CONTRAINDICATIONS
Acute dehydration, anuria, azotemia, heat cramps, hypersensitivity to citrate, patients with sodium-restricted diet, severe myocardial damage, severe renal impairment, untreated Addison's disease
Urocit K: anticholinergics, intestinal obstruction or stricture, patients with delayed gastric emptying, severe peptic ulcer disease

INTERACTIONS
Drug
Angiotensin-converting enzyme (ACE) inhibitors, NSAIDs, potassium-containing medication, potassium-sparing diuretics: May increase the risk of hyperkalemia.
Antacids: May increase the risk of systemic alkalosis.
Methenamine: May decrease the effects of methenamine.
Quinidine: May increase the excretion of quinidine.
Herbal
None known.
Food
None known.

DIAGNOSTIC TEST EFFECTS
None known.

SIDE EFFECTS
Occasional
Diarrhea, mild abdominal pain, nausea, vomiting

SERIOUS REACTIONS
• Metabolic alkalosis, bowel obstruction or perforation, hyperkalemia, and hypernatremia occur rarely.

NURSING CONSIDERATIONS
Precautions
• Use cautiously in patients with congestive heart failure (CHF), hypertension, and pulmonary edema.
• Use cautiously because citrate

use may increase the risk of urolithiasis.

Intervention and Evaluation
• Assess the electrocardiogram (EKG) and urinary pH in patients with cardiac disease.
• Assess the patient's complete blood count (CBC), particularly blood Hct and Hgb, serum acid-base balance, and serum creatinine.

Patient Teaching
• Instruct the patient to take citrates after meals.
• Teach the patient to mix citrates in juice or water and to follow citrate consumption with additional liquid.

---

fluoride
flur-eyd
(Fluor-A-Day, Fluoritab, Fluotic[CAN], Luride)

CATEGORY AND SCHEDULE
Pregnancy Risk Category: N/A

MECHANISM OF ACTION
A trace element that increases tooth resistance to acid dissolution. *Therapeutic Effect:* Promotes remineralization of decalcified enamel, inhibits dental plaque bacteria, increases resistance to development of caries. Maintains bone strength.

AVAILABILITY
Topical Cream: 1.1%.
Gel-Drops: 1.1%.
Topical Gel: 0.4%, 1.1%.
Lozenge: 2.2 mg.
Oral Solution Drops: 1.1 mg/ml.
Oral Solution Rinse: 0.05%, 0.2%, 0.44%.
Tablets (chewable): 0.58 mg, 1.1 mg, 2.2 mg.

INDICATIONS AND DOSAGES
▸ **Dietary supplement for the prevention of dental caries in children**

Water Fluoride	Age	mg/day
less than 0.3 ppm	less than 2 yrs	0.25 mg/day
	2–3 yrs	0.5 mg/day
	3–13 yrs	1 mg/day
0.3–0.7 ppm	less than 2 yrs	None
	2–3 yrs	0.25 mg/day
	3–13 yrs	0.5 mg/day
greater than 0.7 ppm	None	None

CONTRAINDICATIONS
Arthralgia, gastrointestinal (GI) ulceration, severe renal insufficiency

INTERACTIONS
Drug
Aluminum hydroxide, calcium: May decrease the absorption of fluoride.
Herbal
None known.
Food
None known.

DIAGNOSTIC TEST EFFECTS
May increase serum alkaline phosphatase and SGOT (AST) levels.

SIDE EFFECTS
Rare
Oral mucous membrane ulceration

SERIOUS REACTIONS
• Hypocalcemia, tetany, bone pain (especially of the ankles and feet), electrolyte disturbances, and arrhythmias occur rarely.
• Fluoride use may cause skeletal fluorosis, osteomalacia, and osteosclerosis.

NURSING CONSIDERATIONS

Patient Teaching
* Instruct the patient not to take fluoride with dairy products as these foods decrease absorption.
* Teach the patient to apply gels and rinses at bedtime after brushing or flossing. Stress to the patient that he or she should expectorate excess fluoride, not swallow it.
* Advise the patient not to drink, eat, or rinse mouth after application.

magnesium
See laxatives

phosphates
(Fleet enema, Fleet Phosphosoda, K-Phosphate, Neutra-Phos K, Uro KP)

CATEGORY AND SCHEDULE
Pregnancy Risk Category: C

MECHANISM OF ACTION
An electrolyte that participates in bone deposition, calcium metabolism, utilization of B complex vitamins, buffer in acid-base equilibrium. Laxative: Exerts osmotic effect in small intestine. *Therapeutic Effect:* Produces distention; promotes peristalsis, evacuation of bowel.

PHARMACOKINETICS
Poorly absorbed after PO administration. PO form excreted in feces, IV forms excreted in urine.

AVAILABILITY
Injection: 3 mM/ml.
Tablets.
Oral Solution.
Enema.
Powder.

INDICATIONS AND DOSAGES
▶ **Hypophosphatemia**
IV
Adults, Elderly. 50–70 mmol/day.
Children. 0.5–1.5 mmol/kg/day.
PO
Adults, Elderly. 50–150 mmol/day.
Children. 2–3 mmol/kg/day.
▶ **Laxative**
PO
Adults, Elderly, Children older than 4 yrs. 1–2 capsules/packets 4 times/day.
Children 4 yrs and younger. 1 capsule/packet 4 times/day.
Rectal
Adults, Elderly, Children 12 years and older. 4.5-oz enema as single dose. May repeat.
Children younger than 12 yrs. 2.25-oz enema as single dose. May repeat.
▶ **Urinary acidification**
PO
Adults, Elderly. 2 tablets 4 times/day.

UNLABELED USES
Prevention of calcium renal calculi

CONTRAINDICATIONS
Abdominal pain (from rectal dosage form, congestive heart failure [CHF], fecal impaction) from rectal dosage form, hypocalcemia, hyperkalemia, hypomagnesemia, hypernatremia, hyperphosphatemia, phosphate kidney stones, severe renal function impairment

INTERACTIONS
Drug
Angiotensin-converting enzyme (ACE) inhibitors, NSAIDs, potassium-containing medications, potassium-sparing diuretics, salt

substitutes with potassium phosphate: May increase potassium blood concentration.

Antacids: May decrease the absorption of phosphate.

Calcium-containing medications: May increase the risk of calcium deposition in soft tissues, and decrease phosphate absorption.

Digoxin, potassium phosphate: May increase the risk of heart block caused hyperkalemia.

Glucocorticoids: May cause edema with sodium phosphate.

Phosphate-containing medications: May increase the risk of hyperphosphatemia.

Sodium-containing medication with sodium phosphate: May increase the risk of edema.

Herbal
None known.

Food
None known.

DIAGNOSTIC TEST EFFECTS
None known.

IV INCOMPATIBILITIES
Dobutamine (Dobutrex)

IV COMPATIBILITIES
Diltiazem (Cardizem), enalapril (Vasotec), famotidine (Pepcid), magnesium sulfate, metoclopramide (Reglan)

SIDE EFFECTS
Frequent
Mild laxative effect first few days of therapy
Occasional
Gastrointestinal (GI) upset, including diarrhea, nausea, abdominal pain, and vomiting
Rare
Headache, dizziness, mental confusion, heaviness of legs, fatigue, muscle cramps, numbness or tingling of hands, feet, around lips, peripheral edema, irregular heartbeat, weight gain, thirst

SERIOUS REACTIONS
• High phosphate levels may produce extra skeletal calcification.

NURSING CONSIDERATIONS
Baseline Assessment
• Assess for the presence of gastrointestinal (GI) pain. Note its pattern, duration, quality, intensity, location, and areas of radiation, as well as factors that relieve or worsen the pain.
• Assess the amount, color, and consistency of the stool of the patient taking phosphates as a laxative.
• Assess the daily pattern of bowel activity and evaluate the bowel sounds for peristalsis of the patient taking phosphates as a laxative.
• Assess the patient for history of recent abdominal surgery, nausea, vomiting, and weight loss.
• Assess the results of baseline phosphate levels and urine pH.
Lifespan Considerations
• Be aware that it is unknown if phosphates cross the placenta or are distributed in breast milk.
• There are no age-related precautions noted in children or the elderly.
Precautions
• Use cautiously in patients with adrenal insufficiency, cirrhosis, and renal impairment.
• Use cautiously in patients concurrently receiving potassium-sparing drugs.
Administration and Handling
PO
• Dissolve tablets in water.
• Give after meals or with food to decrease GI upset.

• Maintain high fluid intake to prevent kidney stones.
IV
• Store at room temperature.
• Dilute before using.
• Infuse at a maximum rate of 0.06 mmol phosphate/kg/hr, as prescribed.

Intervention and Evaluation
• Monitor the patient's serum alkaline phosphatase, bilirubin, calcium, phosphorus, potassium, sodium, SGOT (AST), and SGPT (ALT) levels routinely.

Patient Teaching
• Warn the patient to notify the physician if he or she experiences diarrhea, nausea, or vomiting.

---

potassium acetate
(Potassium acetate)
potassium bicarbonate/citrate
(K-Lyte)
potassium chloride
(Apo-K[CAN], Kaochlor, K-Dur, K-Lor, K-Lor-Con M 15, Klotrix, K-Lyte-Cl, Micro-K, Slow-K)
potassium gluconate
(Kaon)
Do not confuse with Cardura or Slow-FE.

CATEGORY AND SCHEDULE
Pregnancy Risk Category: C
(A for potassium chloride)

MECHANISM OF ACTION
An electrolyte that is necessary for multiple cellular metabolic processes. Primary action is intracellular. *Therapeutic Effect:* Is necessary for nerve impulse conduction, contraction of cardiac, skeletal, and smooth muscle; maintains normal renal function and acid-base balance.

PHARMACOKINETICS
Well absorbed from the gastrointestinal (GI) tract. Enters cells via active transport from extracellular fluid. Primarily excreted in urine.

AVAILABILITY
Acetate
Injection: 2 mEq/ml.
Bicarbonate and Citrate
Effervescent Tablets: 25 mEq, 50 mEq.
Chloride
Tablets: 6.7 mEq, 8 mEq, 10 mEq, 20 mEq.
Liquid: 20 mEq/15 ml, 30 mEq/ 15 ml, 40 mEq/15 ml.
Oral Powder: 20 mEq, 25 mEq.
Injection: 2 mEq/ml.
Gluconate
Liquid: 20 mEq/15 ml.

INDICATIONS AND DOSAGES
▶ **Prevention of hypokalemia (on diuretic therapy)**
PO
Adults, Elderly. 20–40 mEq/day in 1–2 divided doses.
Children. 1–2 mEq/kg in 1–2 divided doses.
▶ **Treatment of hypokalemia**
IV
Adults, Elderly. 5–10 mEq/hr. Maximum: 400 mEq/day.
Children. 1 mEq/kg over 1–2 hrs.
PO
Adults, Elderly. 40–80 mEq/day further doses based on laboratory values.
Children. 1–2 mEq/day, further doses based on laboratory values.

CONTRAINDICATIONS
Digitalis toxicity, heat cramps, hyperkalemia, patients receiving

potassium-sparing diuretics, postoperative oliguria, severe burns, severe renal impairment, shock with dehydration or hemolytic reaction, untreated Addison's disease

INTERACTIONS
Drug
Anticholinergics: May increase the risk of gastrointestinal (GI) lesions. *Angiotensin-converting enzyme inhibitors (ACE) inhibitors, beta-adrenergic blockers, heparin, NSAIDs, potassium-containing medications, potassium-sparing diuretics, salt substitutes:* May increase potassium blood concentration.
Herbal
None known.
Food
None known.

DIAGNOSTIC TEST EFFECTS
None known.

IV INCOMPATIBILITIES
Amphotericin B complex (Abelcet, AmBisome, Amphotec), methylprednisolone (Solu-Medrol), phenytoin (Dilantin)

IV COMPATIBILITIES
Aminophylline, amiodarone (Cordarone), atropine, aztreonam (Azactam), calcium gluconate, cefepime (Maxipime), ciprofloxacin (Cipro), clindamycin (Cleocin), dexamethasone (Decadron), digoxin (Lanoxin), diltiazem (Cardizem), diphenhydramine (Benadryl), dobutamine (Dobutrex), dopamine (Intropin), enalapril (Vasotec), famotidine (Pepcid), fluconazole (Diflucan), furosemide (Lasix), granisetron (Kytril), heparin, hydrocortisone (Solu-Cortef), insulin, lidocaine, lorazepam (Ativan), magnesium sulfate, methylprednisolone (Solu-Medrol), midazolam (Versed), milrinone (Primacor), metoclopramide (Reglan), morphine, norepinephrine (Levophed), ondansetron (Zofran), oxytocin (Pitocin), piperacillin/tazobactam (Zosyn), procainamide (Pronestyl), propofol (Diprivan), propranolol (Inderal)

SIDE EFFECTS
Occasional
Nausea, vomiting, diarrhea, flatulence, abdominal discomfort with distention, phlebitis with IV administration (particularly when potassium concentration of greater than 40 mEq/L is infused).
Rare
Rash

SERIOUS REACTIONS
• Hyperkalemia (observed particularly in elderly or in patients with impaired renal function) manifested as paresthesia of extremities, heaviness of legs, cold skin, grayish pallor, hypotension, mental confusion, irritability, flaccid paralysis, and cardiac arrhythmias.

NURSING CONSIDERATIONS
Baseline Assessment
• Give the patient oral doses after meals or with food with a full glass of fruit juice or water to minimize gastrointestinal (GI) irritation.
Lifespan Considerations
• Be aware that it is unknown if potassium crosses the placenta and is distributed in breast milk.
• There are no age-related precautions noted in children.
• Be aware that the elderly may be at increased risk for hyperkalemia.
• In the elderly, age-related ability to excrete potassium is reduced.
Precautions
• Use cautiously in patients with

cardiac disease and tartrazine sensitivity, which is most common in those with aspirin hypersensitivity.

Administration and Handling

◀ALERT▶ Know that potassium dosage is individualized.

PO

• Give with or after meals and with full glass of water to decrease GI upset.

• Mix, dissolve with juice or water before administering effervescent tablets, liquids, and powder.

• Instruct the patient to swallow the tablets whole and avoid chewing or crushing the tablets.

IV

• Store at room temperature.

• For IV infusion only, must dilute before administration, mix well.

• Avoid adding potassium to hanging IV.

• Infuse slowly at rate no more than 40 mEq/L; no faster than 20 mEq/hr.

• Check the patient's IV site closely during infusion for phlebitis as evidenced by hardness of vein, heat, pain, and red streaking of skin over vein, and extravasation manifested as cool skin, little or no blood return, pain, and swelling.

Intervention and Evaluation

• Monitor the patient's serum potassium level, particularly those with renal function impairment.

• Dilute the preparation further or give with meals if the patient experiences GI disturbance.

• Be alert to a decrease in the patient's urinary output, which may be an indication of renal insufficiency.

• Assess the patient's daily pattern of bowel activity and stool consistency.

• Monitor the patient's intake and output diligently for diuresis and IV site for extravasation and phlebitis.

• Be alert to signs and symptoms of hyperkalemia, including cold skin, feeling of heaviness of legs, paresthesia of extremities and tongue, and skin pallor.

Patient Teaching

• Give the patient a list of foods rich in potassium including apricots, avocados, bananas, beans, beef, broccoli, brussel sprouts, cantaloupe, chicken, dates, fish, ham, lentils, milk, molasses, potatoes, prunes, raisins, spinach, turkey, watermelon, veal, and yams.

• Warn the patient to notify the physician if he or she experiences a feeling of heaviness in the legs or numbness of extremities or tongue.

sodium bicarbonate

CATEGORY AND SCHEDULE

Pregnancy Risk Category: C

OTC

MECHANISM OF ACTION

An alkalinizing agent that dissociates to provide bicarbonate ion. *Therapeutic Effect:* Neutralizes hydrogen ion concentration, raises blood and urinary pH.

PHARMACOKINETICS

Route	Onset	Peak	Duration
PO	15 min	N/A	1–3 hrs
IV	Immediate	N/A	8–10 min

After administration, sodium bicarbonate dissociates to sodium and bicarbonate ions. Forms or excretes carbon dioxide (CO_2). With increased hydrogen ions, combines to form carbonic acid and then dissociates to CO_2, which is excreted by the lungs. Plasma concentration regulated by the kidneys, which have the ability to excrete or make bicarbonate.

AVAILABILITY
Tablets: 325 mg, 650 mg.
Injection: 0.5 mEq/ml (4.2%), 0.6 mEq/ml (5%), 0.9 mEq/ml (7.5%), 1 mEq/ml (8.4%).

INDICATIONS AND DOSAGES
▸ **Cardiac arrest**
IV
Adults, Elderly. Initially, 1 mEq/kg (as 7.5%–8.4% solution). May repeat with 0.5 mEq/kg q10min during continued cardiopulmonary arrest. Use in the postresuscitation phase based on arterial blood pH, $PaCO_2$ base deficit.
Children, Infants. Initially, 1 mEq/kg.
▸ **Metabolic acidosis (less severe)**
IV infusion
Adults, Elderly, Children. 2–5 mEq/kg over 4–8 hrs. May repeat based on laboratory values.
▸ **Acidosis (associated with chronic renal failure)**
PO
Adults, Elderly. Initially, 20–36 mEq/day in divided doses.
▸ **Renal tubular acidosis (Distal)**
PO
Adults, Elderly. 0.5–2 mEq/kg/day in 4–6 divided doses.
Children. 2–3 mEq/kg/day in divided doses.
▸ **Renal tubular acidosis (Proximal)**
PO
Adults, Elderly, Children. 5–10 mEq/kg/day in divided doses.
▸ **Alkalinization of urine**
PO
Adults, Elderly. Initially, 4 g, then 1–2 g q4h. Maximum: 16 g/day.

Children. 84–840 mg/kg/day in divided doses.
▸ **Antacid**
PO
Adults, Elderly. 300 mg–2 g 1–4 times/day.

CONTRAINDICATIONS
Excessive chloride loss due to diarrhea or gastrointestinal (GI) suction or vomiting, hypocalcemia, metabolic or respiratory alkalosis

INTERACTIONS
Drug
Calcium-containing products: May result in milk-alkali syndrome.
Lithium, salicylates: May increase the excretion of these drugs.
Methenamine: May decrease the effects of methenamine.
Quinidine, ketoconazole, tetracyclines: May decrease the excretion of these drugs.
Herbal
None known.
Food
Milk, milk products: May result in milk-alkali syndrome.

DIAGNOSTIC TEST EFFECTS
May increase serum, urinary pH.

IV INCOMPATIBILITIES
Ascorbic acid, diltiazem (Cardizem), dobutamine (Dobutrex), dopamine (Intropin), hydromorphone (Dilaudid), magnesium sulfate, midazolam (Versed), morphine, norepinephrine (Levophed)

IV COMPATIBILITIES
Aminophylline, calcium chloride, furosemide (Lasix), heparin, insulin, lidocaine, mannitol, milrinone (Primacor), morphine, phenylephrine (Neo-Synephrine), phenytoin (Dilantin), potassium chloride,

propofol (Diprivan), vancomycin (Vancocin)

SIDE EFFECTS
Frequent
Abdominal distention, flatulence, belching

SERIOUS REACTIONS
• Excessive or chronic use may produce metabolic alkalosis (irritability, twitching, numbness or tingling of extremities, cyanosis, slow or shallow respirations, headache, thirst, nausea).
• Fluid overload results in headache, weakness, blurred vision, behavioral changes, incoordination, muscle twitching, rise in blood pressure (B/P), decrease in pulse rate, rapid respirations, wheezing, coughing, and distended neck veins.
• Extravasation may occur at IV site, resulting in necrosis and ulceration.

NURSING CONSIDERATIONS
Baseline Assessment
• Do not give other oral medication within 1 to 2 hours of antacid administration.
Lifespan Considerations
• Be aware that sodium bicarbonate use may produce hypernatremia, increase tendon reflexes in neonate or fetus whose mother is a chronic, high-dose user.
• Be aware that sodium bicarbonate may be distributed in breast milk.
• There are no age-related precautions noted in children.
• Be aware that sodium bicarbonate should not be used as an antacid in children younger than 6 years of age.
• In the elderly, age-related renal impairment may require caution.

Precautions
• Use cautiously in patients with congestive heart failure (CHF), receiving corticosteroid therapy, in edematous states, and with renal insufficiency.
Administration and Handling
◀ALERT▶ May give by IV push, IV infusion, or orally. Drug doses are individualized and based on laboratory values, patient age, clinical conditions, weight, and severity of acidosis. Know that metabolic alkalosis may result if the bicarbonate deficit is fully corrected during the first 24 hours.
PO
• Give 1 to 3 hours after meals.
IV
◀ALERT▶ If sodium bicarbonate is being given for acidosis, give when plasma bicarbonate is less than 15 mEq/L.
• Store at room temperature.
• May give undiluted.
◀ALERT▶ For direct IV administration in neonates and infants, use 0.5 mEq/ml concentration.
• For IV push, give up to 1 mEq/kg over 1 to 3 minutes for myocardial infarction (MI).
• For IV infusion, do not exceed rate of infusion of 50 mEq/hr. For children younger than 2 years, premature infants, neonates, administer by slow infusion, up to 8 mEq/min.
Intervention and Evaluation
• Monitor the patient's blood and urine pH, CO_2 level, plasma bicarbonate, partial pressure of carbon dioxide in arterial blood ($PaCO_2$) levels, and serum electrolytes.
• Observe the patient for signs and symptoms of fluid overload and metabolic alkalosis.
• Assess the patient for clinical improvement of metabolic acidosis,

including relief from disorientation, hyperventilation, and weakness.
• Assess the patient's pattern of daily bowel activity and stool consistency.
• Monitor the patient's serum calcium, phosphate, and uric acid levels.
• Assess the patient for relief of gastric distress.

Patient Teaching
• Advise the patient who is considering breast-feeding to first consult with her physician before taking sodium bicarbonate.
• Encourage the patient to check with the physician before taking any over-the-counter medications, which may contain sodium.

---

sodium chloride
(Ocean Mist, Salinex, Sodium chloride[CAN])

CATEGORY AND SCHEDULE
Pregnancy Risk Category: C
OTC (tablets, nasal solution, ophthalmic solution, ophthalmic ointment)

MECHANISM OF ACTION
Sodium is a major cation of extracellular fluid that controls water distribution, fluid and electrolyte balance, osmotic pressure of body fluids; maintains acid-base balance.

PHARMACOKINETICS
Well absorbed from the gastrointestinal (GI) tract. Widely distributed. Primarily excreted in urine.

AVAILABILITY
Tablets: 1 g

Nasal Solution (OTC): 0.4%, 0.6%, 0.75%.
Ophthalmic Solution (OTC): 2%, 5%.
Ophthalmic Ointment (OTC): 5%.
Injection (concentrate): 14.6%, 23.4%.
Injection (infusion): 0.45%, 0.9%, 3%, 5%.
Irrigation: 0.45%, 0.9%.

INDICATIONS AND DOSAGES
▸ **Prevention and treatment of sodium and chloride deficiencies; source of hydration**
IV infusion
Adults, Elderly. (0.9% or 0.45%): 1–2 L/day. (3% or 5%): 100 ml over 1 hr; assess serum electrolyte concentration before giving additional fluid.
▸ **Prevention of heat prostration and muscle cramps from excessive perspiration**
PO
Adults, Elderly. 1–2 g 3 times/day.
▸ **Relieves dry and inflamed nasal membranes, restores moisture**
Intranasal
Adults, Elderly. Take as needed.
▸ **Diagnostic aid in ophthalmoscopic exam, therapy in reduction of corneal edema**
Ophthalmic solution
Adults, Elderly. 1–2 drops q3–4h.
Ophthalmic ointment
Adults, Elderly. Once a day or as directed.

CONTRAINDICATIONS
Fluid retention, hypernatremia

INTERACTIONS
Drug
Hypertonic saline and oxytocics: May cause uterine hypertonus, possible uterine ruptures or lacerations.

Herbal
None known.
Food
None known.

DIAGNOSTIC TEST EFFECTS
None known.

SIDE EFFECTS
Frequent
Facial flushing
Occasional
Fever, irritation or phlebitis or
extravasation at injection site
Ophthalmic: Temporary burning or
irritation

SERIOUS REACTIONS
• Too rapid administration may
produce peripheral edema, congestive heart failure (CHF), and pulmonary edema.
• Excessive dosage produces hypokalemia, hypervolemia, and hypernatremia.

NURSING CONSIDERATIONS

Baseline Assessment
• Assess the patient's fluid balance, including daily weight,
edema, intake and output, and
lung sounds.
Lifespan Considerations
• There are no age-related precautions noted in children or the elderly.
Precautions
• Use cautiously in patients with
cirrhosis, congestive heart failure
(CHF), hypertension, and renal
impairment.
• Do not use NaCl preserved with
benzyl alcohol in neonates.
Administration and Handling
◀ALERT▶ Drug dosage based on the
patient's acid-base status, age,
clinical condition, fluid and electrolyte status, and weight.

PO
• Do not crush or break enteric-
coated or extended-release
tablets.
• Administer with a full glass of
water.
Nasal
• Instruct patient to begin inhaling
slowly just before releasing medication into nose.
• Teach the patient to inhale slowly,
then release air gently through
mouth.
• Continue technique for 20 to
30 seconds.
Ophthalmic
• Place a gloved finger on the
patient's lower eyelid and pull it out
until a pocket is formed between
the patient's eye and lower lid.
• Hold the dropper above the pocket
and place the prescribed number of
drops (or apply thin strip of ointment) in pocket.
• Instruct the patient to close eyes
gently so that medication will not
be squeezed out of sac.
• When lower lid is released, have
the patient keep the affected eye
open without blinking for at least
30 seconds for solution; for ointment, have patient close the affected eye and roll eyeball around
to distribute medication.
• When using drops, apply gentle
finger pressure to lacrimal sac
(bridge of the nose, inside corner of
the eye) for 1 to 2 minutes after
administration of solution to reduce
systemic absorption.
IV
• Hypertonic solutions (3% or 5%)
are administered via large vein;
avoid infiltration; do not exceed
100 ml/hr.
• Vials containing 2.5 to 4 mEq/ml
(concentrated NaCl) must be diluted
with D_5W or $D_{10}W$ before administration.

Intervention and Evaluation
• Monitor the patient's fluid balance and IV site for extravasation.
• Monitor the patient's acid-base balance, blood pressure (B/P), and serum electrolytes.
• Assess the patient for hypernatremia associated with edema, elevated B/P, and weight gain and hyponatremia associated with dry mucous membranes, muscle cramps, nausea, and vomiting.

Patient Teaching
• Advise the patient that he or she may experience temporary burning or irritation upon instillation of ophthalmic medication.
• Instruct the patient to discontinue ophthalmic medication and notify the physician if he or she experiences acute redness of eyes, double vision, headache, pain on exposure to light, rapid change in vision (side and straight ahead), severe pain, or the sudden appearance of floating spots.

zinc oxide
(Balmex, Desitin)
zinc sulfate
(Orazinc)

CATEGORY AND SCHEDULE
Pregnancy Risk Category: C

MECHANISM OF ACTION
A mineral that acts as an enzyme co-factor and skin protectant. Oxide: Mild astringent, protector. *Therapeutic Effect:* Protective coating for skin. Sulfate: Co-factor for enzymes important for protein and carbohydrate metabolism. *Therapeutic Effect:* Maintains normal growth and tissue repair, as well as skin hydration.

AVAILABILITY
Oxide
Ointment: 10%, 20%, 40%.
Sulfate
Capsules: 110 mg, 220 mg.
Tablets: 110 mg.
Injection: 1 mg/ml.

INDICATIONS AND DOSAGES
▶ **Oxide: Protective for mild skin irritation and abrasions. Promotes healing of chapped skin, diaper rash.**
Topical
Adults, Elderly, Children. Apply as needed.
▶ **Sulfate: Treatment and prevention of zinc deficiency states, promotes wound healing.**
PO
Adults, Elderly. 220 mg 3 times a day.

CONTRAINDICATIONS
None known

INTERACTIONS
Drug
H-2 blockers, such as famotidine: May decrease zinc absorption.
Quinolones, such as ciprofloxacin, tetracycline: May decrease the absorption of quinolones and tetracycline.
Herbals
None known.
Food
Coffee, dairy products: May decrease zinc absorption.

DIAGNOSTIC TEST EFFECTS
None known.

SIDE EFFECTS
None available

SERIOUS REACTIONS
• None available

NURSING CONSIDERATIONS

Baseline Assessment
• Assess the skin for signs of infection prior to application of topical zinc.

Lifespan Considerations
• Avoid using during pregnancy, unless prescribed.

Administration and Handling
Topical
• For external use only.

• Avoid use in the eyes.
PO
• Take zinc oxide with food.

Patient Teaching
• Explain that coffee and dairy products may decrease the absorption of zinc oxide.
• If nausea occurs, instruct the patient to take zinc oxide with food.
• Instruct the patient to notify the physician if the skin condition doesn't improve after using zinc oxide for 7 days.

ascorbic acid
  (vitamin C)
cyanocobalamin
  (vitamin B_{12})
folic acid, sodium
  folate (vitamin B_9)
leucovorin calcium
  (folinic acid,
  citrovorum factor)
niacin, nicotinic acid
  (vitamin B_3)
pyridoxine
  hydrochloride
  (vitamin B_6)
thiamine
  hydrochloride
  (vitamin B_1)
vitamin A
vitamin D, calcitriol,
  dihydrotachysterol,
  ergocalciferol
vitamin E
vitamin K,
  phytonadione

Uses: Vitamins are primarily used to supplement the diet to meet the body's need for the organic substances required for growth, reproduction, and maintenance of health. The need for vitamin supplementation may result from inadequate dietary intake, increased physiologic need (such as during pregnancy), or certain disorders or conditions, such as Crohn's disease, renal disease, and gastrectomy. Some vitamins have additional uses. *Vitamin C* is used to prevent and treat scurvy. *Leucovorin* is used to prevent and treat methotrexate, pyrimethamine, and trimethoprim toxicity. As an adjunct, *niacin* is used to treat hyperlipidemias and peripheral vascular disease. *Pyridoxine* is used to treat isoniazid poisoning, seizures in neonates who don't respond to conventional therapy, and sideroblastic anemia caused by increased serum iron concentrations. *Thiamine* is helpful in treating alcoholic patients with altered sensorium. *Vitamin K* is used to prevent and treat hemorrhagic states in neonates and to act as the antidote for hemorrhage caused by oral anticoagulants.

Action: Vitamins are essential for energy transformation and regulation of metabolic processes. They're catalysts for all reactions using proteins, fats, and carbohydrates for energy, growth, and cell maintenance.

Water-soluble vitamins, such as folic acid and vitamins C, B_1, B_2, B_3, B_6, and B_{12}, act as coenzymes for almost every cellular reaction in the body. B-complex vitamins differ from one another in structure and function, but are grouped together because they were first isolated from the same source (yeast and liver).

Fat-soluble vitamins, such as vitamins A, D, E, and K, are soluble in lipids, are stored in body tissue when excessive quantities are consumed, and may be toxic when taken in large quantities. Vitamin A is needed for normal retinal function, night vision, bone growth, gonadal function, embryonic

development and epithelial cell integrity. Vitamin D is essential for calcium absorption and use and for normal calcification of bone. Vitamin E prevents oxidation and protects fatty acids from free radicals. Vitamin K is required for hepatic formation of coagulation factors II, VII, IX, and X.

ascorbic acid (vitamin C)
(Apo-C[CAN], Cecon, Cenolate, Pro-C[AUS], Redoxon[CAN])

CATEGORY AND SCHEDULE
Pregnancy Risk Category: A (C if used in doses above the recommended daily allowance [RDA])
OTC

MECHANISM OF ACTION
This vitamin assists in collagen formation and tissue repair and is involved in oxidation reduction reactions and other metabolic reactions. *Therapeutic Effect:* Involved in carbohydrate utilization, metabolism, and synthesis of carnitine, lipids, and proteins. Preserves blood vessel integrity.

PHARMACOKINETICS
Readily absorbed from the gastrointestinal (GI) tract. Protein binding: 25%. Metabolized in liver. Excreted in urine. Removed by hemodialysis.

AVAILABILITY
Tablets: 100 mg, 250 mg, 500 mg, 1 g.
Tablets (chewable): 60 mg, 100 mg, 250 mg, 500 mg.
Tablets (controlled-release): 500 mg, 1 g, 1,500 mg.
Capsules (controlled-release): 500 mg.
Liquid: 500 mg/5 ml.
Syrup: 500 mg/5 ml.
Injection: 250 mg/ml, 500 mg/ml.

INDICATIONS AND DOSAGES
▸ **Dietary supplement**
PO
Adults, Elderly. 45–60 mg/day.
Children older than 4 yrs. 30–40 mg/day.
▸ **Deficiency**
PO/IM/IV
Adults, Elderly. 75–150 mg/day.
▸ **Scurvy**
PO
Adults, Elderly. 300 mg–1 g/day.
▸ **Burns**
PO
Adults, Elderly. Up to 2 g/day.
▸ **Enhance wound healing**
PO
Adults, Elderly. 300–500 mg/day for 7–10 days.

UNLABELED USES
Prevention of common cold, control of idiopathic methemoglobinemia, urinary acidifier

CONTRAINDICATIONS
None known.

INTERACTIONS
Drug
Deferoxamine: May increase iron toxicity.

Herbal
None known.
Food
None known.

DIAGNOSTIC TEST EFFECTS
May decrease serum bilirubin and urinary pH. May increase uric acid and urine oxalate.

IV INCOMPATIBILITIES
No information available via Y-site administration.

IV COMPATIBILITIES
Calcium gluconate, heparin

SIDE EFFECTS
Rare
Abdominal cramps, nausea, vomiting, diarrhea, increased urination with doses exceeding 1 g.
Parenteral: Flushing, headache, dizziness, sleepiness or insomnia, soreness at injection site.

SERIOUS REACTIONS
• Ascorbic acid may produce urine acidification, leading to crystalluria.
• Large doses of ascorbic acid given IV may lead to deep vein thrombosis.
• Prolonged use of large doses of ascorbic acid may result in scurvy when dosage is reduced to normal.

NURSING CONSIDERATIONS
Lifespan Considerations
• Be aware that ascorbic acid crosses the placenta and is excreted in breast milk.
• Be aware that large doses of ascorbic acid during pregnancy may produce scurvy in neonates.
• There are no age-related precautions noted in children and the elderly.

Precautions
• Use cautiously in patients who receive daily doses of a salicylate and those with diabetes mellitus, history of renal stones, sodium restrictions, and receiving warfarin therapy.
Administration and Handling
PO
• May give without regard to food.
IV
• Refrigerate and protect from freezing and sunlight.
• May give undiluted or dilute in D_5W, 0.9% NaCl, or lactated Ringer's.
• For IV push, dilute with equal volume of D_5W or 0.9% NaCl and infuse over 10 minutes. For IV solution, infuse over 4 to 12 hours.
Intervention and Evaluation
• Assess the patient for signs of clinical improvement, such as an improved sense of well-being and improved sleep patterns.
• Monitor for signs and symptoms of the recurrence of vitamin C deficiency, including bleeding gums, digestive difficulties, gingivitis, poor wound healing, and joint pain.
Patient Teaching
• Alert the patient that abrupt vitamin C withdrawal may produce rebound deficiency. Instruct the patient to reduce ascorbic acid dosage gradually, as prescribed.
• Inform the patient to eat foods rich in vitamin C, including black currant jelly, brussel sprouts, citrus fruits, guava, green peppers, rose hips, spinach, strawberries, and watercress.

cyanocobalamin (vitamin B₁₂)
sye-ah-no-koe-**bal**-a-min
(Bedoz[CAN], Cytamen[AUS])

CATEGORY AND SCHEDULE
Pregnancy Risk Category: A
(C if used at dosages greater than RDA)

MECHANISM OF ACTION
A coenzyme for metabolic functions, including fat and carbohydrate metabolism and protein synthesis. *Therapeutic Effect:* Necessary for growth, cell replication, hematopoiesis, and myelin synthesis.

PHARMACOKINETICS
Absorbed in lower half of ileum in presence of calcium. Initially, bound to intrinsic factor; this complex passes down intestine, binding to receptor sites on ileal mucosa. In presence of calcium, absorbed systemically. Protein binding: High. Metabolized in liver. Primarily eliminated in urine unchanged. **Half-life:** 6 days.

AVAILABILITY
Tablets: 50 mcg, 100 mcg, 250 mcg, 500 mcg, 660 mcg, 1 mg, 2 mg, 2.5 mg.
Tablet (controlled-release): 1,000 mcg, 1,500 mcg.
Injection: 1,000 mcg/ml.
Intranasal gel: 500 mcg per actuation of 0.1 ml

INDICATIONS AND DOSAGES
▸ **Severe vitamin B₁₂ deficiency, pernicious anemia**
IM/Subcutaneous
Adults, Elderly. 1,000 mcg with folic acid 15 mg (IV or IM) once, then 1,000 mcg and 5 mg folic acid (oral) each day for 1 week.
▸ **Uncomplicated vitamin B₁₂ deficiency**
IM/Subcutaneous
Adults, Elderly. 100 mcg/day for 5–10 days then 100–200 mcg monthly.
PO
Adults, Elderly. 1,000–2,000 mcg/day
Intranasal
Adults, Elderly. 500 mcg (1 spray) every week (after deficiency corrected).
▸ **Supplement**
PO
Adults, Elderly. 2–6 mcg/day.
Children. 0.3–2 mcg/day.

CONTRAINDICATIONS
Folate deficient anemia, hereditary optic nerve atrophy, history of allergy to cobalamin

INTERACTIONS
Drug
Alcohol, colchicines: May decrease the absorption of cyanocobalamin.
Ascorbic acid: May destroy vitamin B₁₂.
Folic acid (large doses): May decrease cyanocobalamin blood concentration.
Herbal
None known.
Food
None known.

DIAGNOSTIC TEST EFFECTS
None known.

SIDE EFFECTS
Occasional
Diarrhea, itching

SERIOUS REACTIONS
• Rare allergic reaction generally

due to impurities in preparation, may occur.
• May produce peripheral vascular thrombosis, pulmonary edema, hypokalemia, and congestive heart failure (CHF).

NURSING CONSIDERATIONS

Lifespan Considerations
• Be aware that cyanocobalamin crosses the placenta and is excreted in breast milk.
• There are no age-related precautions noted in children or the elderly.
Administration and Handling
PO
• Give cyanocobalamin with meals to increase absorption.
Intervention and Evaluation
• Assess the patient for signs and symptoms of CHF and hypokalemia, especially in those receiving cyanocobalamin by the subcutaneous or IM route, and pulmonary edema.
• Monitor the patient's serum potassium levels, which normally ranges between 3.5 to 5 mEq/L, and serum B_{12} levels, which normally range between 200 to 800 mcg/ml. Also monitor the patient for a rise in the blood reticulocyte count, which peaks in 5 to 8 days.
• Evaluate the patient for reversal of deficiency symptoms including anorexia, ataxia, fatigue, hyporeflexia, insomnia, irritability, loss of positional sense, pallor, and palpitations on exertion.
• Know that the patient's therapeutic response to treatment is usually dramatic and occurs within 48 hours.
Patient Teaching
• Stress to the pernicious anemia patient that lifetime treatment may be necessary.
• Warn the patient to notify the physician if he or she experiences symptoms of an infection.

• Suggest to the patient that he or she eat foods rich in vitamin B_{12} including clams, dairy products, egg yolks, fermented cheese, herring, muscle meats, organ meats, oysters, and red snapper.

folic acid (vitamin B₉)
foe-lick
(Apo-Folic[CAN], Folvite, Megafol[AUS])
Do not confuse with Florvite.

sodium folate
(Folvite-parenteral)

CATEGORY AND SCHEDULE
Pregnancy Risk Category: A
(C if more than RDA)
OTC (0.4 mg and 0.8 mg tablets only)

MECHANISM OF ACTION
A coenzyme that stimulates production of platelets, red blood cells (RBCs), and white blood cells (WBCs). *Therapeutic Effect:* Essential for nucleoprotein synthesis, maintenance of normal erythropoiesis.

PHARMACOKINETICS
Oral form almost completely absorbed from the gastrointestinal (GI) tract (upper duodenum). Protein binding: High. Metabolized in liver, plasma to active form. Excreted in urine. Removed by hemodialysis.

AVAILABILITY
Tablets: 0.4 mg, 0.8 mg, 1 mg.
Injection: 5 mg/ml.

INDICATIONS AND DOSAGES
▸ **Vitamin B$_9$ deficiency**
IV/IM/Subcutaneous/PO
Adults, Elderly, Children older than 10 yrs. Initially, 1 mg/day.
Maintenance: 0.5 mg/day.
Children 1–10 yrs. Initially 1 mg/day. Maintenance: 0.1–0.4 mg/day.
Infants. 50 mcg/day.
▸ **Supplement**
PO/IM/IV/Subcutaneous
Adults, Elderly, Children older than 4 yrs. 0.4 mg/day.
Children 1–4 yrs. 0.3 mg/day.
Children younger than 1 yr. 0.1 mg/day.
Pregnancy. 0.8 mg/day.

UNLABELED USES
Decreases risk of colon cancer

CONTRAINDICATIONS
Anemias (aplastic, normocytic, pernicious, refractory)

INTERACTIONS
Drug
Analgesics, anticonvulsants, carbamazepine, estrogens: May increase folic acid requirements.
Antacids, cholestyramine: May decrease the absorption of folic acid.
Hydantoin anticonvulsants: May decrease the effects of these drugs.
Methotrexate, triamterene, trimethoprim: May antagonize the effects of folic acid.
Herbal
None known.
Food
None known.

DIAGNOSTIC TEST EFFECTS
May decrease vitamin B$_{12}$ concentration.

SIDE EFFECTS
None known

SERIOUS REACTIONS
• Allergic hypersensitivity occurs rarely with parenteral form. Oral folic acid is nontoxic.

NURSING CONSIDERATIONS
Baseline Assessment
• Know that the physician will rule out pernicious anemia with a Schilling test and vitamin B$_{12}$ blood level before beginning folic acid therapy because the signs of pernicious anemia may be masked while irreversible neurologic damage progresses.
• Know that resistance to treatment may occur if alcoholism, antimetabolic drugs, decreased hematopoiesis, or deficiency of vitamin B$_6$, B$_{12}$, C, or E is evident.
Lifespan Considerations
• Be aware that folic acid is distributed in breast milk.
• There are no age-related precautions noted in children or the elderly.
Administration and Handling
◂ALERT▸ Know that the parenteral form is used in acutely ill, enteral or parenteral alimentation, and patients unresponsive to oral route in gastrointestinal (GI) malabsorption syndrome and that folic acid dosages greater than 0.1 mg a day may conceal signs of pernicious anemia.
Intervention and Evaluation
• Assess the patient for therapeutic improvement, improved sense of well-being and relief from iron deficiency symptoms, which include fatigue, headache, pallor, shortness of breath, and sore tongue.
Patient Teaching
• Encourage the patient to eat foods rich in folic acid including fruits, organ meats, and vegetables.

leucovorin calcium (folinic acid, citrovorum factor)

lou-koe-vor-in
(Calcium Leucovorin[AUS],
Lederle, Leucovorin,
Wellcovorin)
**Do not confuse with Wellbutrin
or Wellferon.**

CATEGORY AND SCHEDULE
Pregnancy Risk Category: C

MECHANISM OF ACTION
A folic acid antagonist that competes with methotrexate for same transport processes into cells; limits methotrexate action on normal cells. *Therapeutic Effect:* Allows purine, DNA, RNA, protein synthesis.

PHARMACOKINETICS
Readily absorbed from the gastrointestinal (GI) tract. Widely distributed. Primarily concentrated in liver. Metabolized in liver, intestinal mucosa to active metabolite. Primarily excreted in urine. **Half-life:** 15 min (metabolite: 30–35 min).

AVAILABILITY
Tablets: 5 mg, 10 mg, 15 mg, 25 mg.
Injection: 10 mg/ml.
Powder for Injection: 50 mg, 100 mg, 200 mg, 350 mg, 500 mg.

INDICATIONS AND DOSAGES
▸ **Conventional rescue dosage**
Adults, Elderly, Children. 10 mg/m^2 parenterally one time then q6h orally until serum methotrexate less than 10^{-8} M. If 24-hr serum creatinine increased by 50% or more over baseline or methotrexate greater

than 5×10^{-6} M or 48-hr level greater than 9×10^{-7} M, increase to 100 mg/m^2 IV q3h until methotrexate level less than 10^{-8} M.
▸ **Folic acid antagonist overdosage**
PO
Adults, Elderly, Children. 2–15 mg/day for 3 days or 5 mg q3 days.
▸ **Folate deficient megaloblastic anemia**
IM
Adults, Elderly, Children. 1 mg/day.
▸ **Megaloblastic anemia**
IM
Adults, Elderly, Children. 3–6 mg/day.
▸ **Prevention of hematologic toxicity (for toxoplasmosis)**
IV/PO
Adults, Elderly, Children. 5–10 mg/day, repeat q3 days.
▸ **Prevention of hematologic toxicity, PCP**
IV/PO
Adults, Children. 25 mg once weekly.

UNLABELED USES
Ewing's sarcoma, gestational trophoblastic neoplasms, non-Hodgkin's lymphoma, treatment adjunct for head and neck carcinoma

CONTRAINDICATIONS
Pernicious anemia, other megaloblastic anemias secondary to vitamin B_{12} deficiency.

INTERACTIONS
Drug
5-fluorouracil: May increase the effects and toxicity of 5-fluorouracil.
Anticonvulsants: May decrease the effects of anticonvulsants.
Herbal
None known.

Food
None known.

DIAGNOSTIC TEST EFFECTS
None known.

IV INCOMPATIBILITIES
Amphotericin B complex (Abelcet, AmBisome, Amphotec), droperidol (Inapsine), foscarnet (Foscavir)

IV COMPATIBILITIES
Cisplatin (Platinol AQ), cyclophosphamide (Cytoxan), doxorubicin (Adriamycin), etoposide (VePesid), filgrastim(Neupogen), fluorouracil, gemcitabine (Gemzar), granisetron (Kytril), heparin, methotrexate, metoclopramide (Reglan), mitomycin (Mutamycin), piperacillin-tazobactam (Zosyn), vinblastine (Velban), vincristine (Oncovin)

SIDE EFFECTS
Frequent
With 5-fluorouracil: Diarrhea, stomatitis, nausea, vomiting, lethargy or malaise or fatigue, alopecia, anorexia
Occasional
Urticaria, dermatitis

SERIOUS REACTIONS
• Excessive dosage may negate chemotherapeutic effect of folic acid antagonists.
• Anaphylaxis occurs rarely.
• Diarrhea may cause rapid clinical deterioration and death.

NURSING CONSIDERATIONS
Baseline Assessment
• Give leucovorin, as prescribed, as soon as possible, preferably within 1 hour, for treatment of accidental overdosage of folic acid antagonists.
Lifespan Considerations
• Be aware that it is unknown if leucovorin crosses the placenta or is distributed in breast milk.
• Be aware that leucovorin use in children may increase the risk of seizures by counteracting anticonvulsant effects of barbiturate and hydantoins.
• In the elderly, age-related renal impairment may require dosage adjustment when used in rescue from effects of high-dose methotrexate therapy.
Precautions
• Use cautiously in patients with bronchial asthma and a history of allergies.
• Use leucovorin with 5-fluorouracil cautiously in patients with GI toxicities.
Administration and Handling
◄ALERT► For rescue therapy in cancer chemotherapy, refer to specific protocol being used for optimal dosage and sequence of leucovorin administration.
PO
• Scored tablets may be crushed.
IV
• Store vials for parenteral use at room temperature.
• Injection normally appears as clear, yellowish solution.
• Use immediately if reconstituted with Sterile Water for Injection; is stable for 7 days if reconstituted with Bacteriostatic Water for Injection.
• Reconstitute each 50-mg vial with 5 ml Sterile Water for Injection or Bacteriostatic Water for Injection containing benzyl alcohol to provide concentration of 10 mg/ml.
• Due to benzyl alcohol in 1-mg ampoule and in Bacteriostatic Water for Injection, reconstitute doses greater than 10 mg/m^2 with Sterile Water for Injection.
• Further dilute with D_5W or 0.9% NaCl.
• Do not exceed 160 mg/min if

given by IV infusion (because of calcium content).

Intervention and Evaluation
• Monitor the patient for vomiting, which may require a change from oral to parenteral therapy.
• Observe elderly and debilitated patients closely because of risk of severe toxicities.
• Assess the patient's BUN, complete blood count (CBC), and serum creatinine to assess renal function (important in leukovorin rescue).
• Assess electrolytes and liver function tests of patients also taking 5-fluorouracil in combination with leucovorin.

Patient Teaching
• Explain to the patient the purpose of medication in the treatment of cancer.
• Warn the patient to notify the physician if he or she experiences allergic reaction or vomiting.

---

niacin, nicotinic acid
See antihyperlipidemics

---

pyridoxine hydrochloride (vitamin B₆)
pie-rih-**docks**-in
(Hexa-Betalin[CAN], Pyridoxine, Pyroxin[AUS])
Do not confuse with paroxetine, pralidoxime, or Pyridium.

CATEGORY AND SCHEDULE
Pregnancy Risk Category: A
OTC

MECHANISM OF ACTION
A coenzyme for various metabolic functions that maintains metabolism of proteins, carbohydrates, and fats. Aids in release of liver and muscle glycogen and in the synthesis of gamma-aminobutyric acid (GABA) in the central nervous system (CNS).

PHARMACOKINETICS
Readily absorbed primarily in jejunum. Stored in liver, muscle, brain. Metabolized in liver. Primarily excreted in urine. Removed by hemodialysis. **Half-life:** 15–20 days.

AVAILABILITY
Capsules: 100 mg, 150 mg, 200 mg, 250 mg, 500 mg.
Injection: 100 mg/ml.
Tablets: 10 mg, 25 mg, 50 mg, 100 mg, 250 mg, 500 mg.
Tablets (time release): 500 mg.

INDICATIONS AND DOSAGES
▸ **Pyridoxine deficiency**
PO
Adults, Elderly. (Caused by inadequate diet) 2.5–10 mg/day; after signs of deficiency decrease, 2.5–5 mg/day for several wks. (Drug-induced) 10–50 mg/day (INH, penicillamine); 100–300 mg/day (cyclosporine). (Inborn error of metabolism) 100–500 mg/day.
Children. 5–25 mg/day for 3 wks, then 1.5–2.5 mg/day.
▸ **Seizures in neonates**
IM/IV
Neonates. 10–100 mg/day; then oral therapy of 50–100 mg/day for life.
▸ **Drug-induced neuritis**
PO
Adults. 100–300 mg/day in divided doses for 3 wks, then 25–100 mg/day.

Children. 50–100 mg/day as treatment, then 1–2 mg/kg/day as prophylaxis.

▸ **Sideroblastic anemia**
PO
Adults, Elderly. 200–600 mg/day. After adequate response, 30–50 mg/day for life.

CONTRAINDICATIONS
None known

INTERACTIONS
Drug
Immunosuppressants, isoniazid, penicillamine: May antagonize pyridoxine (may cause anemia or peripheral neuritis).
Levodopa: Reverses the effects of levodopa.
Herbal
None known.
Food
None known.

DIAGNOSTIC TEST EFFECTS
None known.

IV INCOMPATIBILITIES
Do not mix with any other medications.

SIDE EFFECTS
Occasional
Stinging at IM injection site
Rare
Headache, nausea, somnolence, high dosages cause sensory neuropathy (paresthesia, unstable gait, clumsiness of hands)

SERIOUS REACTIONS
• Long-term megadoses (2 to 6 g over longer than 2 mos) may produce sensory neuropathy (reduced deep tendon reflex, profound impairment of sense of position in distal limbs, gradual sensory ataxia).

Toxic symptoms reverse with drug discontinuance.
• Seizures have occurred following IV megadoses.

NURSING CONSIDERATIONS
Lifespan Considerations
• Be aware that pyridoxine crosses the placenta and is excreted in breast milk.
• Be aware that high dosages of pyridoxine in utero may produce seizures in neonates.
• There are no age-related precautions noted in children or the elderly.
Administration and Handling
◀ALERT▶ Give orally unless malabsorption, nausea, or vomiting occurs. Avoid IV use in cardiac patients.
IV
• Give undiluted or may be added to IV solutions and given as infusion.
Intervention and Evaluation
• Observe the patient for improvement of deficiency symptoms, including nervous system abnormalities (anxiety, depression, insomnia, motor difficulty, peripheral numbness and tremors) and skin lesions (glossitis, seborrhea-like lesions around eyes, mouth, nose).
• Evaluate the patient for nutritional adequacy.
Patient Teaching
• Advise the patient that he or she may experience discomfort with IM injection.
• Encourage the patient to eat foods rich in pyridoxine, including avocados, bananas, bran, carrots, eggs, hazelnuts, legumes, organ meats, shrimp, soybeans, sunflower seeds, tuna, and wheat germ.

thiamine hydrochloride (vitamin B₁)

thigh-ah-min
(Betalin, Betaxin[CAN])

CATEGORY AND SCHEDULE

Pregnancy Risk Category: A
(C if used in doses above RDA)
OTC (tablets)

MECHANISM OF ACTION

A water-soluble vitamin that combines with adenosine triphosphate (ATP) in liver, kidney, and leukocytes to form thiamine diphosphate. *Therapeutic Effect:* Is necessary for carbohydrate metabolism.

PHARMACOKINETICS

Readily absorbed from the gastrointestinal (GI) tract, primarily in duodenum, after IM administration. Widely distributed. Metabolized in liver. Primarily excreted in urine.

AVAILABILITY

Tablets: 50 mg, 100 mg, 250 mg.
Injection: 100 mg/ml.

INDICATIONS AND DOSAGES

▶ **Dietary supplement**
PO
Adults, Elderly. 1–2 mg/day.
Children. 0.5–1 mg/day.
Infants. 0.3–0.5 mg/day.
▶ **Thiamine deficiency**
PO
Adults, Elderly. 5–30 mg/day, in single or 3 divided doses, for 1 mo.
Children. 10–50 mg/day in 3 divided doses.

▶ **Critically ill or malabsorption syndrome**
IM/IV
Adults, Elderly. 5–100 mg, 3 times/day.
Children. 10–25 mg/day.
▶ **Metabolic disorders**
PO
Adults, Elderly, Children. 10–20 mg/day; up to 4 g in divided doses/day.

CONTRAINDICATIONS

None known.

INTERACTIONS

Drug
None known.
Herbal
None known.
Food
None known.

DIAGNOSTIC TEST EFFECTS

None known.

IV COMPATIBILITIES

Famotidine (Pepcid), multivitamins

SIDE EFFECTS

Frequent
Pain, induration, tenderness at IM injection site

SERIOUS REACTIONS

• Rare, severe hypersensitivity reaction with IV administration may result in feeling of warmth, pruritus, urticaria, weakness, diaphoresis, nausea, restlessness, tightness in throat, angioedema (swelling of face or lips), cyanosis, pulmonary edema, gastrointestinal (GI) tract bleeding, and cardiovascular collapse.

NURSING CONSIDERATIONS

Lifespan Considerations
• Be aware that thiamine crosses the placenta and it is unknown if thiamine is excreted in breast milk.
• There are no age-related precautions noted in children or the elderly.

Administration and Handling
◀ALERT▶ Know that the IM and IV routes of administration are used only in the acutely ill or those who are unresponsive to the PO route, such as with GI malabsorption syndrome. Be aware that the IM route is preferred to the IV route. Give by IV push, or add to most IV solutions and give as infusion.

Intervention and Evaluation
• Monitor the patient's electrocardiogram (EKG) and laboratory values for erythrocyte count.
• Assess the patient for signs and symptoms of improvement, including an improved sense of well-being and weight gain.
• Observe the patient for reversal of deficiency symptoms. For neurologic signs and symptoms, expect a decrease in peripheral neuropathy, ataxia, hyporeflexia, muscle weakness, nystagmus, ophthalmoplegia, and peripheral neuropathy. For cardiac signs and symptoms, assess for a decrease in peripheral edema, bounding arterial pulse, tachycardia, and venous hypertension. Also assess for a decreased confused state.

Patient Teaching
• Advise the patient that he or she may experience discomfort with IM injection.
• Encourage the patient to consume foods rich in thiamine including legumes, nuts, organ meats, pork, rice bran, seeds, wheat germ, whole grain and enriched cereals, and yeast.

• Advise the patient that his or her urine may appear bright yellow during thiamine therapy.

vitamin A
(Aquasol A)
Do not confuse with Anusol.

CATEGORY AND SCHEDULE
Pregnancy Risk Category: A
(X if doses above RDA)

MECHANISM OF ACTION
A fat-soluble vitamin that may be a cofactor in biochemical reactions. *Therapeutic Effect:* Is essential for normal function of retina. Necessary for visual adaptation to darkness, bone growth, testicular and ovarian function, embryonic development; preserves integrity of epithelial cells.

PHARMACOKINETICS
Absorption dependent on bile salts, pancreatic lipase, dietary fat. Transported in blood to liver, stored in parenchymal liver cells, then transported in plasma as retinol, as needed. Metabolized in liver. Excreted in bile and, to a lesser amount, in urine.

AVAILABILITY
Capsules: 8,000 units, 10,000 units, 25,000 units.
Injection: 50,000 units/ml.
Tablets: 5,000 units, 10,000 units, 15,000 units.

INDICATIONS AND DOSAGES
▶ **Severe deficiency with xerophthalmia**
IM
Adults, Elderly, Children older than 8 yrs. 50,000–100,000 units/day for

3 days, then 50,000 units/day for 14 days.
Children 1–8 yrs. 5,000–15,000 units/day for 10 days.
PO
Adults, Elderly, Children older than 8 yrs. 500,000 units/day for 3 days, then 50,000 units/day for 14 days, then 10,000–20,000 units/day for 2 mo.
Children 1–8 yrs. 5,000 units/kg/day for 5 days or until recovery occurs.

‣ **Malabsorption syndrome**
PO
Adults, Elderly, Children older than 8 yrs. 50,000 units/day.

‣ **Dietary supplement**
PO
Adults, Elderly. 4,000–5,000 units/day.
Children 7–10 yrs. 3,300–3,500 units/day.
Children 4–6 yrs. 2,500 units/day.
Children 6 mos–3 yrs. 1,500–2,000 units/day.
Neonates younger than 6 mos. 1,500 units/day.

CONTRAINDICATIONS
Hypervitaminosis A, oral use in malabsorption syndrome

INTERACTIONS
Drug
Cholestyramine, colestipol, mineral oil: May decrease the absorption of vitamin A.
Isotretinoin: May increase the risk of toxicity.
Herbal
None known.
Food
None known.

DIAGNOSTIC TEST EFFECTS
May increase BUN, serum cholesterol, serum calcium, and serum triglyceride levels. May decrease blood erythrocyte and leukocyte counts.

SIDE EFFECTS
None known.

SERIOUS REACTIONS
• Chronic overdosage produces malaise, nausea, vomiting, drying or cracking of skin or lips, inflammation of tongue or gums, irritability, loss of hair, and night sweats.
• Bulging fontanelles in infants have been noted.

NURSING CONSIDERATIONS
Lifespan Considerations
• Be aware that vitamin A crosses the placenta and is distributed in breast milk.
• Use vitamin A with caution at higher doses in children and the elderly.
Precautions
• Use cautiously in patients with renal impairment.
Administration and Handling
◀ALERT▶ Know that the IM route of administration is used only in the acutely ill or patients unresponsive to oral route, such as those with gastrointestinal (GI) malabsorption syndrome.
PO
• Do not crush, open, or break capsule form.
• Give vitamin A without regard to food.
IM
• For IM injection in adults, if dosage is 1 ml (50,000 units), may give in deltoid muscle; if dosage is greater than 1 ml, give in gluteus maximus muscle. Know that the anterolateral thigh is site of choice for infants and children younger than 7 months.

Intervention and Evaluation
• Closely assess the patient for overdosage symptoms during prolonged daily administration greater than 25,000 units.
• Monitor the patient for therapeutic serum vitamin A levels, valued at 80 to 300 units/ml.

Patient Teaching
• Encourage the patient to consume foods rich in vitamin A, including cod, halibut, tuna, and shark. Explain to the patient that naturally occurring vitamin A is found only in animal sources.
• Warn the patient to avoid taking cholestyramine (Questran) and mineral oil during vitamin A therapy.

---

vitamin D
calcitriol
(Calcijex[AUS], Rocaltrol)
dihydrotachysterol
(DHT, Hytakerol)
ergocalciferol
(Calciferol, Deltalin, Drisdol, Ostelin[AUS])
paricalcitol
(Zemplar)

CATEGORY AND SCHEDULE
Pregnancy Risk Category: A
(D if used in doses above RDA)

MECHANISM OF ACTION
A fat-soluble vitamin that is essential for absorption, utilization of calcium phosphate, and normal calcification of bone. *Therapeutic Effect:* Stimulates calcium and phosphate absorption from small intestine, promotes secretion of calcium from bone to blood, promotes renal tubule phosphate resorption, acts on bone cells to stimulate skeletal growth and on parathyroid gland to suppress hormone synthesis and secretion.

PHARMACOKINETICS
Readily absorbed from small intestine. Concentrated primarily in liver, fat deposits. Activated in liver, kidney. Eliminated via biliary system; excreted in urine. **Half-life:** calcifediol: 10–22 days; calcitriol: 3–6 hrs; ergocalciferol: 19–48 hrs.

AVAILABILITY
Calcitriol (Calcijex, Rocaltrol)
Capsule: 0.25 mcg, 0.5 mcg.
Injection: 1 mcg/ml, 2 mcg/ml.
Oral Solution: 1 mcg/ml.
Dihydrotachysterol (DHT)
Oral Solution: 0.2 mg/ml.
Capsule: 0.125 mg.
Tablets: 0.125 mg, 0.2 mg, 0.4 mg.
Ergocalciferol (Calciferol, Drisdol)
Capsules: 50,000 units.
Liquid Drops: 8,000 units/ml.
Tablet: 400 units.
Paricalcitol (Zemplar)
Injection: 2 mcg/ml, 5 mcg/ml.

INDICATIONS AND DOSAGES
▸ **Dietary supplement**
PO
Adults, Elderly, Children. 10 mcg (400 units)/day.
Neonates. 10–20 mcg (400–800 units)/day.
▸ **Renal failure**
PO
Adults, Elderly. 0.5 mg/day.
Children. 0.1–1 mg/day.
▸ **Hypoparathyroidism**
PO
Adults, Elderly. 625 mcg–5 mg/day (with calcium supplements).
Children. 1.25–5 mg/day (with calcium supplements).
▸ **Vitamin D–dependent rickets**
PO
Adults, Elderly. 250 mcg–1.5 mg/day.

Children. 75–125 mcg/day. Maximum: 1,500 mcg/day.
▸ **Nutritional rickets and osteomalacia**
PO
Adults, Elderly, Children. 25–125 mcg/day for 8–12 wks.
Adults, Elderly (malabsorption). 250–7,500 mcg/day.
Children (malabsorption). 250–625 mcg/day.
▸ **Vitamin D–resistant rickets**
PO
Adults, Elderly. 250–1,500 mcg/day (with phosphate supplements).
Children. Initially 1,000–2,000 mcg/day (with phosphate supplements). May increase at 3- to 4-mo intervals in 250- to 600-mcg increments.

CONTRAINDICATIONS
Hypercalcemia, malabsorption syndrome, vitamin D toxicity

INTERACTIONS
Drug
Aluminum-containing antacid (long-term use): May increase aluminum concentration and aluminum bone toxicity.
Calcium-containing preparations, thiazide diuretics: May increase the risk of hypercalcemia.
Magnesium-containing antacids: May increase magnesium concentration.
Herbal
None known.
Food
None known.

DIAGNOSTIC TEST EFFECTS
May increase serum cholesterol, calcium, magnesium, and phosphate levels. May decrease serum alkaline phosphatase.

SIDE EFFECTS
None known.

SERIOUS REACTIONS
• Early signs of overdosage are manifested as weakness, headache, somnolence, nausea, vomiting, dry mouth, constipation, muscle and bone pain, and metallic taste sensation.
• Later signs of overdosage are evidenced by polyuria, polydipsia, anorexia, weight loss, nocturia, photophobia, rhinorrhea, pruritus, disorientation, hallucinations, hyperthermia, hypertension, and cardiac arrhythmias.

NURSING CONSIDERATIONS
Baseline Assessment
• Know that vitamin D therapy should begin at the lowest possible dosage.
Lifespan Considerations
• Be aware that it is unknown if vitamin D crosses the placenta or is distributed in breast milk.
• Be aware that children may be more sensitive to the effects of vitamin D.
• There are no age-related precautions noted in the elderly.
Precautions
• Use cautiously in patients with contrary artery disease, kidney stones, and renal impairment.
Administration and Handling
◂ALERT▸ 1 mcg = 40 units.
PO
• Give vitamin D without regard to food.
• Have the patient swallow the vitamin whole and avoid crushing, chewing, or opening the capsules.
Intervention and Evaluation
• Monitor the patient's BUN, serum alkaline phosphatase, serum calcium, serum creatinine, serum magnesium, serum phosphate, and urinary calcium levels. Know that

the therapeutic serum calcium level is 9 to 10 mg/dl.
• Estimate the patient's daily dietary calcium intake.
• Encourage the patient to maintain adequate fluid intake.

Patient Teaching
• Encourage the patient to consume foods rich in vitamin D including eggs, leafy vegetables, margarine, meats, milk, vegetable oils, and vegetable shortening.
• Warn the patient not to take mineral oil during vitamin D therapy.
• Advise the patient receiving chronic renal dialysis not to take magnesium-containing antacids during vitamin D therapy.
• Encourage the patient to drink plenty of liquids.

vitamin E
(Aquasol E)
Do not confuse with Anusol.

CATEGORY AND SCHEDULE
Pregnancy Risk Category: A
(C if used in doses above RDA)
OTC

MECHANISM OF ACTION
An antioxidant that prevents oxidation of vitamins A and C, protects fatty acids from attack by free radicals, protects red blood cells (RBCs) from hemolysis by oxidizing agents.

PHARMACOKINETICS
Variably absorbed from the gastrointestinal (GI) tract (requires bile salts, dietary fat, normal pancreatic function). Primarily concentrated in adipose tissue. Metabolized in liver. Primarily eliminated via biliary system.

AVAILABILITY
Capsules: 100 units, 200 units, 400 units, 600 units, 800 units, 1,000 units.
Oral Drops: 15 units/0.3 ml.

INDICATIONS AND DOSAGES
▶ **Vitamin E deficiency**
PO
Adults, Elderly. 60–75 units/day.
Children. 1 unit/kg/day.

UNLABELED USES
Decreases severity of tardive dyskinesia

CONTRAINDICATIONS
None known

INTERACTIONS
Drug
Cholestyramine, colestipol, mineral oil: May decrease the absorption of vitamin E.
Iron (large doses): May increase vitamin E requirements.
Herbal
None known.
Food
None known.

DIAGNOSTIC TEST EFFECTS
None known.

SIDE EFFECTS
None known.

SERIOUS REACTIONS
• Chronic overdosage produces fatigue, weakness, nausea, headache, blurred vision, flatulence, and diarrhea.

NURSING CONSIDERATIONS

Lifespan Considerations
• Be aware that it is unknown if vitamin E crosses the placenta or is distributed in breast milk.

• There are no age-related precautions noted in normal dosages in children or the elderly.

Precautions

• Vitamin E use may impair hematologic response in patients with iron deficiency anemia.

Administration and Handling

PO

• Do not crush, open, or break capsules or tablets.

• Give vitamin E without regard to food.

Patient Teaching

• Instruct the patient to swallow capsules whole, not to chew, open, or crush them.

• Warn the patient to notify the physician if he or she experiences signs and symptoms of toxicity including blurred vision, diarrhea, dizziness, flu-like symptoms, headache, and nausea.

• Encourage the patient to consume foods rich in vitamin E, including eggs, leafy vegetables, margarine, meats, milk, vegetable oils, and vegetable shortening.

vitamin K phytonadione (vitamin K₁)

fy-toe-na-dye-own
(AquaMEPHYTON, Mephyton)
Do not confuse with melphalan or mephenytoin.

CATEGORY AND SCHEDULE

Pregnancy Risk Category: C

MECHANISM OF ACTION

A fat-soluble vitamin that is necessary for hepatic formation of coagulation factors II, VII, IX, and X. *Therapeutic Effect:* Is essential for normal clotting of blood.

PHARMACOKINETICS

Readily absorbed from the gastrointestinal (GI) tract (duodenum), after IM, subcutaneous administration. Metabolized in liver. Excreted in urine, eliminated via biliary system. Parenteral: Controls hemorrhage within 3–6 hrs, normal prothrombin time in 12–14 hrs. PO: Effect in 6–10 hrs.

AVAILABILITY

Tablets: 5 mg.
Injection: 2 mg/ml, 10 mg/ml.

INDICATIONS AND DOSAGES

▶ **Oral anticoagulant overdose**

IV/Subcutaneous/PO
Adults, Elderly. 2.5–10 mg/dose. May repeat in 6–8 hrs if given IV/ subcutaneous or 12–48 hrs if given orally.
Children. 0.5–5 mg depending on need for further anticoagulation, severity of bleeding.

▶ **Vitamin K deficiency**

IV/IM/Subcutaneous
Adults, Elderly. 10 mg.
Children. 1–2 mg/dose.
PO
Adults, Elderly. 2.5–25 mg/24 hrs.
Children. 2.5–5 mg/24 hrs.

▶ **Hemorrhagic disease in newborn**

IM/Subcutaneous
Neonate. Treatment: 1–2 mg/dose/ day. Prophylaxis: 0.5–1 mg within 1 hr of birth. May repeat in 6–8 hrs if necessary.

CONTRAINDICATIONS

None known

INTERACTIONS

Drug

Broad-spectrum antibiotics, high-dose salicylates: May increase vitamin K requirements.
Cholestyramine, colestipol, mineral oil, sucralfate: May decrease the absorption of vitamin K.

Oral anticoagulants: May decrease the effects of these drugs.
Herbal
None known.
Food
None known.

DIAGNOSTIC TEST EFFECTS
None known.

IV INCOMPATIBILITIES
No known incompatibility noted via Y-site administration.

IV COMPATIBILITIES
Heparin, potassium chloride

SIDE EFFECTS
Occasional
Pain; soreness; swelling at IM injection site; repeated injections, pruritic erythema, flushed face, unusual taste

SERIOUS REACTIONS
• May produce hyperbilirubinemia in newborn (especially premature infants).
• Rarely, severe reaction occurs immediately after IV administration (cramplike pain, chest pain, dyspnea, facial flushing, dizziness, rapid or weak pulse, rash, diaphoresis, hypotension that may progress to shock, and cardiac arrest).

NURSING CONSIDERATIONS
Lifespan Considerations
• Be aware that vitamin K crosses the placenta and is distributed in breast milk.
• There are no age-related precautions noted in children or the elderly.
Administration and Handling
◄ALERT► Subcutaneous route is preferred. IV/IM restricted for emergency situations.

◄ALERT► Know that the PO or subcutaneous route of administration is less likely to produce side effects than the IM or IV route.
PO
• Scored tablets may be crushed.
Subcutaneous/IM
• Inject into anterolateral aspect of thigh or deltoid region.
IV
• Store at room temperature.
• May dilute with preservative-free NaCl or D_5W immediately before use. Do not use other diluents. Discard unused portions.
• Administer slow IV at rate of 1 mg/minute.
• Monitor the patient continuously for signs and symptoms of hypersensitivity.
• Monitor the patient for an anaphylactic reaction during and immediately after IV administration.
Intervention and Evaluation
• Monitor the international normalized ratio (INR) and prothrombin time (PT) routinely in patients taking anticoagulants.
• Examine the patient's skin for bruises and petechiae.
• Assess the patient's gums for erythema and gingival bleeding.
• Test the patient's urine for hematuria.
• Assess the patient's blood Hct, platelet count, and stool and urine samples for occult blood.
• Monitor the patient for abdominal or back pain, decrease in blood pressure (B/P), increase in pulse rate, and severe headache, which may indicate hemorrhage.
• Determine if the patient has an increase in the amount of discharge during menses.
• Assess the patient's peripheral pulses.

- Examine the patient for excessive bleeding from minor cuts and scratches.

Patient Teaching

- Advise the patient that he or she may experience discomfort with parenteral administration.
- Instruct adult patients to use an electric razor and soft toothbrush to prevent bleeding.
- Warn the patient to notify the physician if he or she experiences black or red stool, coffee-ground vomitus, red or dark urine, or red-speckled mucus from cough.
- Caution the patient against taking any other medications, including over-the-counter preparations, without physician approval because they may interfere with platelet aggregation.
- Encourage the patient to consume foods rich in vitamin K, including cow's milk, egg yolks, leafy green vegetables, meat, tomatoes, and vegetable oil.

bethanechol chloride
cevimeline
neostigmine
physostigmine
pilocarpine
  hydrochloride
pyridostigmine
  bromide

Uses: Cholinergics are primarily used to treat urine retention and myasthenia gravis and to reverse non-depolarizing neuromuscular blockade. Additionally, cevimeline is used to treat dry mouth in Sjögren's syndrome. Neostigmine is used to prevent postoperative urine retention and to diagnose myasthenia gravis. Physostigmine and pilocarpine are used to treat glaucoma Physostigmine is also used to reverse anticholinergic and tricyclic antidepressant toxicity.

Action: Some cholinergics, such as bethanechol and pilocarpine, directly bind to cholinergic (muscarinic) receptors and activate them, mimicking the action of acetylcholine. Others, such as neostigmine and physostigmine, inhibit the enzyme acetylcholinesterase, preventing the destruction of acetylcholine. Cholinergic agents mainly affect the heart, exocrine glands, and smooth muscle. In the heart, they can lead to bradycardia. In the exocrine glands, they may increase sweating, salivation, and bronchial secretions. In smooth muscle, they promote contraction. Several also stimulate ciliary muscles, leading to miosis.

bethanechol chloride
be-than-eh-coal
(Duvoid[CAN], Myotonachol[CAN], Urecholine)
Do not confuse with betaxolol.

CATEGORY AND SCHEDULE
Pregnancy Risk Category: C

MECHANISM OF ACTION
A cholinergic that acts directly at cholinergic receptors of smooth muscle of urinary bladder and gastrointestinal (GI) tract. Increases tone of detrusor muscle. *Therapeutic Effect:* May initiate micturition, bladder emptying. Stimulates gastric, intestinal motility.

AVAILABILITY
Tablets: 5 mg, 10 mg, 25 mg, 50 mg.
Injection: 5 mg/ml.

INDICATIONS AND DOSAGES
▶ **Postoperative and postpartum urinary retention, atony of bladder**
PO
Adults, Elderly. 10–50 mg 3–4 times/day. Minimum effective dose determined by initially giving 5–10 mg, and repeating same amount at 1-hr intervals until de-

sired response achieved, or maximum of 50 mg reached.
Children. 0.6 mg/kg/day in 3–4 divided doses.
Subcutaneous
Adults, Elderly. Initially, 2.5–5 mg. Minimum effective dose determined by giving 2.5 mg (0.5 ml), repeating same amount at 15- to 30-min intervals up to a maximum of 4 doses. Minimum dose repeated 3–4 times/day.
Children. 0.2 mg/kg/day in 3–4 divided doses.

UNLABELED USES
Treatment of congenital megacolon, gastroesophageal reflux, postoperative gastric atony

CONTRAINDICATIONS
Active or latent bronchial asthma, acute inflammatory GI tract conditions, anastomosis, bladder wall instability, cardiac disease, coronary artery disease, epilepsy, hypertension, hyperthyroidism, hypotension, mechanical GI and urinary obstruction or recent GI resection, parkinsonism, peptic ulcer, pronounced bradycardia, vasomotor instability

INTERACTIONS
Drug
Cholinesterase inhibitors: May increase the effects and risk of toxicity of bethanechol.
Procainamide, quinidine: May decrease the effects of bethanechol.
Herbal
None known.
Food
None known.

DIAGNOSTIC TEST EFFECTS
May increase serum amylase, lipase, and SGOT (AST) levels.

SIDE EFFECTS
Occasional
Belching, change in vision, blurred vision, diarrhea, frequent urinary urgency
Rare
Subcutaneous: Shortness of breath, chest tightness, bronchospasm

SERIOUS REACTIONS
• Overdosage produces central nervous system (CNS) stimulation, including insomnia, nervousness, and orthostatic hypotension, and cholinergic stimulation, such as headache, increased salivation and sweating, nausea, vomiting, flushed skin, stomach pain, and seizures.

NURSING CONSIDERATIONS
Baseline Assessment
• Avoid giving IM or IV because it will precipitate a violent cholinergic reaction if bethanechol is given, including bloody diarrhea, circulatory collapse, myocardial infarction (MI), severe hypotension, and shock. The antidote is 0.6–1.2 mg atropine sulfate.
Administration and Handling
◀ALERT▶ Realize that the side effects are more noticeable with subcutaneous administration.
Intervention and Evaluation
• Assess the patient for cholinergic reaction manifested as blurred vision, excessive salivation and sweating, feeling of facial warmth, GI cramping or discomfort, lacrimation, pallor, and urinary urgency.
• Observe the patient for difficulty chewing or swallowing and progressive muscle weakness.
• Measure and record fluid intake and output.
Patient Teaching
• Tell the patient to notify the physician if he or she experiences

diarrhea, difficulty breathing, increased salivary secretions, irregular heartbeat, muscle weakness, nausea, severe abdominal pain, sweating, and vomiting.

cevimeline
sev-ee-**me**-line
(Evoxac)
Do not confuse with Eurax.

CATEGORY AND SCHEDULE
Pregnancy Risk Category: C

MECHANISM OF ACTION
A cholinergic agonist that binds to muscarinic receptors. *Therapeutic Effect:* Increases secretion of exocrine glands, such as the salivary glands, relieving dry mouth symptoms.

AVAILABILITY
Capsules: 30 mg.

INDICATIONS AND DOSAGES
▶ **Dry mouth**
PO
Adults. 30 mg 3 times/day.

CONTRAINDICATIONS
Acute iritis, narrow-angle glaucoma, uncontrolled asthma

INTERACTIONS
Drug
Amiodarone, diltiazem, erythromycin, fluoxetine, itraconazole, ketoconazole, paroxetine, quinidine, ritonavir, verapamil: May increase the effects of cevimeline.
Atropine, phenothiazines, tricyclic antidepressants: May decrease the effects of cevimeline.
Beta-blockers: May increase the potential for conduction disturbances.

Herbal
None known.
Food
Food: Decreases the absorption rate of cevimeline.

DIAGNOSTIC TEST EFFECTS
None known.

SIDE EFFECTS
Frequent (19%–11%)
Excessive sweating, headache, nausea, sinusitis, rhinitis, upper respiratory tract infections, diarrhea
Occasional (10%–3%)
Dyspepsia, abdominal pain, coughing, urinary tract infection, vomiting, back pain, rash, dizziness, fatigue
Rare (2%–1%)
Skeletal pain, insomnia, hot flashes, excessive salivation, rigors, anxiety

SERIOUS REACTIONS
• May produce decreased visual acuity, especially at night, and impairment of depth perception.

NURSING CONSIDERATIONS
Baseline Assessment
• Before beginning therapy, ask about a history of acute iritis, narrow-angle glaucoma, and uncontrolled asthma.
• Tell the patient that taking this drug may alter visual acuity, so he or she should not plan to drive.
Precautions
• Use cautiously in patients with cardiovascular disease, chronic bronchitis, cholelithiasis, congestive heart failure (CHF), and a history of nephrolithiasis.
Patient Teaching
• Warn the patient to use caution while driving at night or performing hazardous duties in reduced lighting.

- Encourage the patient to drink extra fluids to prevent the possibility of dehydration.
- Instruct the patient that cevimeline may be taken without regard to food.
- Tell the patient that cevimeline may cause decreased visual acuity, especially at night, and impaired depth perception.

neostigmine
nee-oh-**stig**-meen
(Prostigmin)
Do not confuse with physostigmine.

CATEGORY AND SCHEDULE
Pregnancy Risk Category: C

MECHANISM OF ACTION
A cholinergic that prevents destruction of acetylcholine by attaching to enzyme, anticholinesterase. *Therapeutic Effect:* Improves intestinal and skeletal muscle tone; increases secretions, salivation.

AVAILABILITY
Injection: 0.5 mg/ml, 1 mg/ml.
Tablets: 15 mg.

INDICATIONS AND DOSAGES
▶ **Myasthenia gravis**
PO
Adults, Elderly. Initially, 15–30 mg 3–4 times/day. Increase as necessary. Usual maintenance dose: 150 mg/day (range of 15–375 mg).
Children. 2 mg/kg/day or 60 mg/m^2/day divided q3–4h.
Subcutaneous/IM/IV
Adults. 0.5–2.5 mg as needed.
Children. 0.01–0.04 mg/kg q2–4h.

▶ **Diagnosis of myasthenia gravis**
IM
Adults, Elderly. 0.022 mg/kg. If cholinergic reaction occurs, discontinue tests and administer 0.4–0.6 mg or more atropine sulfate IV.
Children. 0.025–0.04 mg/kg IM preceded by atropine sulfate 0.011 mg/kg subcutaneous.
▶ **Prevention of postoperative urinary retention**
Subcutaneous/IM
Adults, Elderly. 0.25 mg q4–6h for 2–3 days.
▶ **Postop distention, urinary retention**
Subcutaneous/IM
Adults, Elderly. 0.5–1 mg. Catheterize if voiding does not occur within 1 hr. After voiding, continue 0.5 mg q3h for 5 injections.
▶ **Reversal of neuromuscular blockade**
IV
Adults, Elderly. 0.5–2.5 mg given slowly.
Children. 0.025–0.08 mg/kg/dose.
Infants. 0.025–0.1 mg/kg/dose.

CONTRAINDICATIONS
Gastrointestinal (GI) and genitourinary (GU) obstruction, peritonitis

INTERACTIONS
Drug
Anticholinergics: Reverse or prevent the effects of neostigmine.
Cholinesterase inhibitors: May increase the risk of toxicity.
Neuromuscular blocking agents: Antagonizes neuromuscular blocking agents.
Procainamide, quinidine: May antagonize the action of neostigmine.
Herbal
None known.

Food
None known.

DIAGNOSTIC TEST EFFECTS
None known.

IV INCOMPATIBILITIES
None known.

IV COMPATIBILITIES
Glycopyrrolate (Robinul), heparin, ondansetron (Zofran), potassium chloride, thiopental (Pentothal)

SIDE EFFECTS
Frequent
Muscarinic effects, including diarrhea, increased sweating or watering of mouth, nausea, vomiting, and stomach cramps or pain
Occasional
Muscarinic effects, including increased frequency or urge to urinate, increased bronchial secretions, and unusually small pupils or watering of eyes

SERIOUS REACTIONS
• Overdose produces a cholinergic reaction manifested as abdominal discomfort or cramping, nausea, vomiting, diarrhea, flushing, feeling of warmth or heat about face, excessive salivation and sweating, lacrimation, pallor, bradycardia or tachycardia, hypotension, urinary urgency, blurred vision, bronchospasm, pupillary contraction, and involuntary muscular contraction visible under the skin.

NURSING CONSIDERATIONS

Baseline Assessment
• Expect to give larger doses at the time of the patient's greatest fatigue.
• Avoid giving large doses to pa-

tients with megacolon or reduced GI motility.
Precautions
• Use cautiously in patients with arrhythmias, asthma, bradycardia, epilepsy, hyperthyroidism, peptic ulcer disease, and recent coronary occlusion.
Administration and Handling
◀ALERT▶ Discontinue all anticholinesterase therapy at least 8 hours before testing, as prescribed. Plan to give 0.011 mg/kg atropine sulfate IV simultaneously with neostigmine or IM 30 minutes before administering neostigmine to prevent adverse effects.
Intervention and Evaluation
• Monitor the patient's muscle strength and vital signs.
• Monitor the patient for therapeutic response to the drug, decreased fatigue, improved chewing and swallowing, and increased muscle strength.
• Monitor the patient's fluid intake and output.
• Palpate the patient's bladder for signs of distension.
Patient Teaching
• Warn the patient to notify the physician if he or she experiences diarrhea, difficulty breathing, increased salivary secretions, irregular heartbeat, muscle weakness, nausea, severe abdominal pain, sweating, and vomiting.
• Tell the patients to keep a log of his or her energy levels and muscle strength to get a better idea of drug dosing.

physostigmine
(Antilirium)
Do not confuse with Prostigmin or pyridostigmine.

CATEGORY AND SCHEDULE
Pregnancy Risk Category: C

MECHANISM OF ACTION
A parasympathomimetic (cholinergic) that inhibits destruction of acetylcholine by enzyme acetylcholinesterase. *Therapeutic Effect:* Improves skeletal muscle tone, stimulates salivary and sweat gland secretion.

AVAILABILITY
Injection: 1 mg/ml.

INDICATIONS AND DOSAGES
▸ **Antidote**
IM/IV
Adults, Elderly. Initially, 0.5–2 mg. If no response, repeat q20min until response occurs or adverse cholinergic effects occur. If initial response occurs, may give additional doses of 1–4 mg at 30- to 60-min intervals as life-threatening signs recur, such as arrhythmias, seizures, and deep coma.
Children. 0.01–0.03 mg/kg. May give additional doses at 5- to 10-min intervals until response occurs, adverse cholinergic effects occur, or total dose of 2 mg given.

UNLABELED USES
Systemic: Treatment of hereditary ataxia

CONTRAINDICATIONS
Active uveal inflammation, angle-closure (narrow-angle) glaucoma before iridectomy, asthma, cardiovascular disease, diabetes, gangrene, glaucoma associated with iridocyclitis, hypersensitivity to cholinesterase inhibitors or any component of the preparation, mechanical obstruction of intestinal and urogenital tract, patients receiving ganglionic-blocking agents, vagotonic state

INTERACTIONS
Drug
Cholinesterase agents, including bethanechol and carbachol: May increase the effects cholinesterase agents.
Succinylcholine: May prolong the action of succinylcholine.
Herbal
None known.
Food
None known.

DIAGNOSTIC TEST EFFECTS
None known.

SIDE EFFECTS
Expected
Miosis, increased gastrointestinal (GI) and skeletal muscle tone, reduced pulse rate
Occasional
Hypertensive patients may react with marked fall in blood pressure (B/P)
Rare
Allergic reaction

SERIOUS REACTIONS
• Parenteral overdosage produces a cholinergic reaction manifested as abdominal discomfort or cramping, nausea, vomiting, diarrhea, flushing, feeling of warmth or heat about face, excessive salivation, diaphoresis, urinary urgency, and blurred vision. Requires a withdrawal of all anticholinergic drugs and immediate use of 0.6–1.2 mg atropine sulfate IM/IV for adults, 0.01 mg/kg in

infants and children younger than 12 yrs.

NURSING CONSIDERATIONS

Baseline Assessment
• Have tissues readily available at patient's bedside.
• Plan to discontinue ophthalmic physostigmine at least 3 weeks before ophthalmic surgery.

Precautions
• Use cautiously in patients with bradycardia, bronchial asthma, disorders that may respond adversely to vagotonic effects, epilepsy, GI disturbances, hypotension, parkinsonism, peptic ulcer disease, and recent myocardial infarction (MI).
• Expect to use ophthalmic physostigmine only when shorter acting miotics are not adequate, except in aphakics.

Intervention and Evaluation
• Assess the patient's vital signs immediately before and every 15 to 30 minutes after parenteral physostigmine administration.
• Monitor the patient for cholinergic reaction, such as abdominal pain, dyspnea, hypotension, irregular heartbeat, muscle weakness, and sweating, after parenteral physostigmine administration.

Patient Teaching
• Tell the patient that the drug's adverse effects often subside after the first few days of therapy.
• Warn the patient to avoid night driving and activities requiring visual acuity in dim light during physostigmine therapy.

pilocarpine hydrochloride

pie-low-car-pine
(Adsorbocarpine, Akarpine, Carpine, Isopto, Ocu-Carpine, Ocusert Pilo-20[AUS], Ocusert Pilo-40 [AUS], Pilocar, Pilopine, Pilopt Eye Drops[AUS], Piloptic, Pilostat, PV Carpine Liquifilm Ophthalmic Solution[AUS], Salagen)

CATEGORY AND SCHEDULE
Pregnancy Risk Category: C

MECHANISM OF ACTION
A cholinergic parasympathomimetic that increases secretion by the exocrine glands by stimulating cholinergic receptors. *Therapeutic Effect:* Produces salivary gland production.

PHARMACOKINETICS

Route	Onset	Peak	Duration
PO	20 min	1 hr	3–5 hrs

Inactivation of pilocarpine thought to occur at neuronal synapses and probably in plasma. Excreted in the urine. Absorption is decreased if taken with a high-fat meal. **Half-life:** 4–12 hrs.

AVAILABILITY
Tablets: 5 mg.

INDICATIONS AND DOSAGES
▶ **Head and neck cancer**
PO
Adults, Elderly. 5 mg three times a day. Range: 15–30 mg/day, do not exceed 2 tablets/dose.

▶ **Sjögren's syndrome**
PO
Adults, Elderly. 5 mg four times a
day. Range: 20–40 mg/day.
▶ **Dosage in hepatic impairment**
PO
Adults, Elderly. 5 mg two times a
day.

CONTRAINDICATIONS

Uncontrolled asthma, when miosis
is undesirable, such as with acute
iritis, narrow-angle (angle-closure)
glaucoma

INTERACTIONS
Drug

Anticholinergics: May antagonize
the effects of anticholinergics.
Beta blockers: May produce conduction disturbances.
Herbal
None known.
Food
High-fat meals: May decrease
the absorption rate of pilocarpine.

DIAGNOSTIC TEST EFFECTS
None known.

SIDE EFFECTS

Frequent (29%)
Diaphoresis
Occasional (11%–05%)
Headache, dizziness, urinary frequency, flushing, dyspepsia, including heartburn and epigastric distress, nausea, asthenia or feeling of
fatigue, weakness, lacrimation,
visual disturbances
Rare (less than 4%)
Diarrhea, abdominal pain, peripheral
edema, chills

SERIOUS REACTIONS

• Dehydration may develop if the
patient sweats excessively and does
not drink enough fluids.

• There is a 2 to 3 times higher
increase in urinary frequency, diarrhea, and dizziness in patients
65 yrs and older than compared to
patients younger than 65 yrs.

NURSING CONSIDERATIONS
Baseline Assessment
• Assess the patient's oral mucosa
for evidence of dryness.
• Encourage the patient to maintain
adequate daily fluid intake.
Lifespan Considerations
• Be aware that pilocarpine use may
impair reproductive function.
• Be aware that the safety and
efficacy of pilocarpine have not
been established in children.
• Be aware that the elderly have
an increased incidence of diarrhea, dizziness, and urinary frequency.
Precautions
• Use cautiously in patients with
liver function impairment, pulmonary disease, and significant cardiovascular disease.
Administration and Handling
• May give pilocarpine without
regard to food.
Intervention and Evaluation
• Assess the patient's daily pattern
of bowel activity and stool consistency.
• Monitor the patient for dehydration, such as decreased skin turgor
and tenting, and dizziness.
• Monitor the patient's urinary
frequency.
Patient Teaching
• Instruct the patient to drink
several glasses of water between
meals.
• Caution the patient that he or she
may experience visual changes,
especially at night.
• Warn the patient to avoid tasks
that require mental alertness and

motor skills until his or her response to the drug is established.

pyridostigmine bromide

pier-id-oh-**stig**-meen
(Mestinon, Regonol)
Do not confuse with Mesantoin, Metatensin, physostigmine, Renagel, Reglan, or Regroton.

CATEGORY AND SCHEDULE
Pregnancy Risk Category: C

MECHANISM OF ACTION
An anticholinesterase that prevents destruction of acetylcholine by enzyme, anticholinesterase. *Therapeutic Effect:* Produces miosis; increases tone of intestinal, skeletal muscles; stimulates salivary, sweat gland secretions.

AVAILABILITY
Tablets: 60 mg.
Tablets (sustained-release): 180 mg.
Syrup: 60 mg/5 ml.
Injection: 5 mg/ml.

INDICATIONS AND DOSAGES
▸ **Myasthenia gravis**
PO
Adults, Elderly. Initially, 60 mg 3 times/day. Increase dose at intervals of 48 hrs or more until therapeutic response is achieved. When increased dosage does not produce further increase in muscle strength, reduce dose to previous dosage level. Maintenance: 60–1,500 mg/day.
Children. Initially, 7 mg/kg/day in 5–6 divided doses.
Neonates. 5 mg q4–6h.

PO (extended-release)
Adults, Elderly. 180–540 mg 1–2 times/day (must maintain at least 6 hrs between doses).
IM/IV
Adults, Elderly. 2 mg q2–3h.
IM
Neonates. 0.05–0.15 mg/kg q4–6h.
▸ **Reversal of nondepolarizing muscle relaxants**
IV
Adults, Elderly. 10–20 mg with, or shortly after, 0.6–1.2 mg atropine sulfate or 0.3–0.6 mg glycopyrrolate.
Children. 0.1–0.25 mg/kg/dose preceded by atropine or glycopyrrolate.

CONTRAINDICATIONS
Mechanical gastrointestinal (GI) and urinary obstruction

INTERACTIONS
Drug
Anticholinergics: Prevents or reverses the effects of pyridostigmine.
Cholinesterase inhibitors: May increase the risk of toxicity.
Neuromuscular blocking agents: Antagonizes neuromuscular blocking agents.
Procainamide, quinidine: May antagonize the action of pyridostigmine.
Herbal
None known.
Food
None known.

DIAGNOSTIC TEST EFFECTS
None known.

IV INCOMPATIBILITIES
Do not mix with any other medications.

SIDE EFFECTS

Frequent

Miosis, increased GI and skeletal muscle tone, reduced pulse rate, constriction of bronchi and ureters, salivary and sweat gland secretion

Occasional

Headache, rash, slight temporary decrease in diastolic blood pressure (B/P) with mild reflex tachycardia, short periods of atrial fibrillation in hyperthyroid patients, marked fall in B/P with hypertensive patients

SERIOUS REACTIONS

• Overdosage may produce a cholinergic crisis, manifested by increasingly severe muscle weakness that appears first in muscles involving chewing, swallowing, followed by muscular weakness of shoulder girdle and upper extremities, and respiratory muscle paralysis followed by pelvis girdle and leg muscle paralysis. Requires withdrawal of all cholinergic drugs and immediate use of 1–4 mg atropine sulfate IV for adults, 0.01 mg/kg in infants and children younger than 12 yrs.

NURSING CONSIDERATIONS

Baseline Assessment

• Give larger doses at time of the patient's greatest fatigue.

• Assess the patient's muscle strength before testing for diagnosis of myasthenia gravis and after drug administration.

• Avoid giving large doses in patients with megacolon or reduced GI motility.

Precautions

• Use cautiously in patients with bradycardia, bronchial asthma, cardiac arrhythmias, epilepsy, hyperthyroidism, peptic ulcer disease, recent coronary occlusion, and vagotonia.

Administration and Handling

◀ALERT▶ Remember that drug dosage and frequency of administration are dependent on daily clinical patient response, including exacerbations, physical and emotional stress, and remissions.

PO

• Give pyridostigmine with food or milk.

• Crush tablets as needed. Instruct patients that extended-release tablets may be broken, but not to chew or crush them.

• Give larger doses at times of increased fatigue, for example for patients with difficulty in chewing, 30 to 45 minutes before meals.

IM/IV

• Give large parenteral doses concurrently with 0.6 to 1.2 mg atropine sulfate IV, as prescribed, to minimize side effects.

Intervention and Evaluation

• Monitor the patient's respirations closely during myasthenia gravis testing or if dosage is increased.

• Assess the patient diligently for cholinergic reaction, as well as bradycardia in the myasthenic patient in crisis.

• Coordinate dosage time vs. periods of patient fatigue and increased or decreased muscle strength.

• Monitor the patient for therapeutic response to medication, decreased fatigue, improved chewing and swallowing, and increased muscle strength.

• Have tissues available at the patient's bedside.

Patient Teaching
• Warn the patient to notify the physician if he or she experiences diarrhea, difficulty breathing, increased salivary secretions, irregular heartbeat, muscle weakness, nausea, severe abdominal pain, sweating, or vomiting.
• Tell the patients to keep a log of his or her energy levels and muscle strength to get a better idea of drug dosing.

amiloride
  hydrochloride
bumetanide
chlorthalidone
furosemide
hydrochlorothiazide
indapamide
mannitol
metolazone
spironolactone
torsemide
triamterene

Uses: Several subclasses of diuretics have slightly different indications. *Thiazide diuretics,* such as hydrochlorothiazide and metolazone, are used to manage edema caused by various disorders, including congestive heart failure (CHF) and hepatic cirrhosis. They're also used alone or with other antihypertensives to control hypertension. *Loop diuretics,* such as bumetanide and furosemide, are prescribed to manage edema caused by CHF, hepatic cirrhosis, and renal disease. Whether used alone or with other antihypertensives, furosemide is also administered to treat hypertension. *Potassium-sparing diuretics,* such as amiloride and spironolactone, are used as adjuncts to thiazide or loop diuretics in treating CHF and hypertension. *Osmotic diuretics,* such as mannitol, are used to prevent and treat the oliguric phase of acute renal failure, to reduce increased intracranial pressure, and to promote the urinary excretion of certain toxic substances.

Action: Diuretics act to increase the excretion of water, sodium, and other electrolytes by the kidneys. Although their exact mechanism in hypertension is unknown, these agents may act by reducing plasma volume or decreasing peripheral vascular resistance. They're subclassified based on their mechanism and site of action. *Thiazide diuretics* act at the cortical diluting segment of the nephron, blocking sodium, chloride, and water reabsorption and promoting the excretion of sodium, chloride, potassium, and water. *Loop diuretics* act primarily at the thick ascending limb of the loop of Henle to inhibit sodium, chloride, and water absorption. Among the *potassium-sparing diuretics,* amiloride and triamterene act on the distal nephron, decreasing sodium reuptake and reducing potassium excretion; spironolactone blocks aldosterone from acting on the distal nephron, which causes potassium retention and sodium excretion. *Osmotic diuretics* work in the proximal convoluted tubule by increasing the

osmotic pressure of the glomerular filtrate and inhibiting the passive reabsorption of water, sodium, and chloride. (See illustration, *Sites of Action: Diuretics,* page 1326.)

COMBINATION PRODUCTS

ACCURETIC: hydrochlorothiazide/quinapril (an ACE inhibitor) 12.5 mg/10 mg; 12.5 mg/20 mg; 25 mg/20 mg.

ALDACTAZIDE: hydrochlorothiazide/spironolactone (a potassium-sparing diuretic) 25 mg/25 mg; 50 mg/50 mg.

ALDORIL: hydrochlorothiazide/methyldopa (an antihypertensive) 15 mg/250 mg; 25 mg/250 mg; 30 mg/500 mg; 50 mg/500 mg.

APRESAZIDE: hydrochlorothiazide/hydralazine (a vasodilator) 25 mg/25 mg; 50 mg/50 mg; 50 mg/100 mg.

ATACAND HCT: hydrochlorothiazide/candesartan (an angiotensin II receptor antagonist) 12.5 mg/16 mg; 12.5 mg/32 mg.

AVALIDE: hydrochlorothiazide/irbesartan (an angiotensin II receptor antagonist) 12.5 mg/150 mg; 12.5 mg/300 mg.

BENICAR HCT: hydrochlorothiazide/olmesartan (an angiotensin II receptor antagonist) 12.5 mg/20 mg; 12.5 mg/40 mg; 25 mg/40 mg.

CAPOZIDE: hydrochlorothiazide/captopril (an ACE inhibitor) 15 mg/25 mg; 15 mg/50 mg; 25 mg/25 mg; 25 mg/50 mg.

COMBIPRES: chlorthalidone/clonidine (an antihypertensive) 15 mg/0.1 mg; 15 mg/0.2; 15 mg/0.3 mg.

DIOVAN HCT: hydrochlorothiazide/valsartan (an angiotensin II receptor antagonist) 12.5 mg/80 mg; 12.5 mg/160 mg.

DYAZIDE: hydrochlorothiazide/triamterene (a potassium-sparing diuretic) 25 mg/37.5 mg; 25 mg/50 mg; 50 mg/75 mg.

HYZAAR: hydrochlorothiazide/losartan (an angiotensin II receptor antagonist) 12.5 mg/50 mg; 25 mg/100 mg.

INDERIDE: hydrochlorothiazide/propranolol (a beta-blocker) 25 mg/40 mg; 25 mg/80 mg; 50 mg/80 mg; 50 mg/120 mg; 50 mg/160 mg.

INDERIDE LA: hydrochlorothiazide/propranolol (a beta-blocker) 50 mg/80 mg; 50 mg/120 mg; 50 mg/160 mg.

LOPRESSOR HCT: hydrochlorothiazide/metoprolol (a beta-blocker) 25 mg/50 mg; 25 mg/100 mg; 50 mg/100 mg.

LOTENSIN HCT: hydrochlorothiazide/benazepril (an ACE inhibitor) 6.25 mg/5 mg; 12.5 mg/10 mg; 12.5 mg/20 mg; 25 mg/20 mg.

MAXZIDE: hydrochlorothiazide/triamterene (a potassium-sparing diuretic) 25 mg/37.5 mg; 25 mg/50 mg; 50 mg/75 mg.

MICARDIS HCT: hydrochlorothiazide/telmisartan (an angiotensin II receptor antagonist) 12.5 mg/40 mg; 12.5 mg/80 mg.

MODURETIC: hydrochlorothiazide/amiloride (a potassium-sparing diuretic) 50 mg/5 mg.

NORMOZIDE: hydrochlorothiazide/labetalol (a beta-blocker) 25 mg/100 mg; 25 mg/300 mg.

PRINZIDE: hydrochlorothiazide/lisinopril (an ACE inhibitor)

12.5 mg/10 mg; 12.5 mg/20 mg; 25 mg/20 mg.

TENORETIC: chlorthalidone/atenolol (a beta-blocker) 25 mg/50 mg; 25 mg/100 mg.

TEVETEN HCT: hydrochlorothiazide/eprosartan (an angiotensin II receptor antagonist) 12.5 mg/600 mg; 25 mg/600 mg.

TIMOLIDE: hydrochlorothiazide/timolol (a beta-blocker) 25 mg/10 mg.

UNIRETIC: hydrochlorothiazide/moexipril (an ACE inhibitor) 12.5 mg/7.5 mg; 25 mg/15 mg.

VASERETIC: hydrochlorothiazide/enalapril (an ACE inhibitor) 12.5 mg/5 mg; 25 mg/10 mg.

ZESTORETIC: hydrochlorothiazide/lisinopril (an ACE inhibitor) 12.5 mg/10 mg; 12.5 mg/20 mg; 25 mg/20 mg.

ZIAC: hydrochlorothiazide/bisoprolol (a beta-blocker) 6.25 mg/5 mg; 6.25 mg/10 mg.

---

amiloride hydrochloride

ah-**mill**-or-ride
(Kaluril[AUS], Midamor)
Do not confuse with amiodarone or amlodipine.

CATEGORY AND SCHEDULE

Pregnancy Risk Category: B (D if used in pregnancy-induced hypertension)

MECHANISM OF ACTION

A guanidine derivative that acts as a potassium-sparing diuretic, antihypertensive, and antihypokalemic by directly interfering with sodium reabsorption in the distal tubule. *Therapeutic Effect:* Increases sodium and water excretion and decreases potassium excretion.

PHARMACOKINETICS

Route	Onset	Peak	Duration
PO	2 hrs	6–10 hrs	24 hrs

Incompletely absorbed from gastrointestinal (GI) tract. Protein binding: Minimal. Primarily excreted in urine; partially eliminated in feces. **Half-life:** 6–9 hrs.

AVAILABILITY

Tablets: 5 mg.

INDICATIONS AND DOSAGES

▸ **To counteract potassium loss induced by other diuretics**
PO
Adults, Children weighing more than 20 kg. 5–10 mg/day up to 20 mg.
Elderly. Initially, 5 mg/day or every other day.
Children weighing 6–20 kg. 0.625 mg/kg/day. Maximum: 10 mg/day.
▸ **Dosage in renal impairment**

Creatinine Clearance	Dosage
10–50 ml/min	50% of normal
less than 10 ml/min	avoid use

UNLABELED USES

Treatment of edema associated with congestive heart failure (CHF), liver cirrhosis, and nephrotic syndrome; treatment of hypertension, reduces lithium-induced polyuria, slows pulmonary function reduction in cystic fibrosis

CONTRAINDICATIONS

Acute or chronic renal insufficiency, anuria, diabetic nephropathy, patients on other potassium-sparing diuretics, serum potassium greater than 5.5 mEq/L

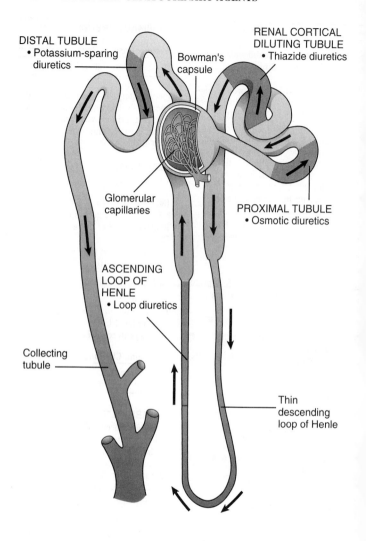

Sites of Action: Diuretics

Diuretics act primarily to increase water and sodium excretion by the kidneys, thereby increasing urine output. In the process, chloride, potassium, and other electrolytes may also be excreted. Generally, most diuretics act by blocking sodium, water, and chloride reabsorption by peritubular capillaries in the nephrons. As a result, water and electrolytes remain in the convoluted tubules to be excreted as urine. The increased water and electrolyte excretion reduces blood volume—and ultimately blood pressure.

Diuretics belong to four major subclasses: thiazide, loop, potassium-sparing, and osmotic diuretics. Although similar in action, drugs in each subclass act at different sites along the nephron. Also, because the solute concentration decreases as the filtrate passes through the nephron's tubules, drugs that act earlier in the process can block more water and electrolytes, promoting greater diuresis.

Thiazide diuretics, such as hydrochlorothiazide, act in the early portion of the distal convoluted tubule, called the cortical diluting segment. These drugs block sodium, chloride, and water reabsorption and promote their excretion along with potassium.

Loop diuretics, such as furosemide, act primarily in the thick ascending limb of the loop of Henle, blocking sodium, water, and chloride reabsorption. Then these substances are excreted along with potassium.

Potassium-sparing diuretics, such as spironolactone, act in the late portion of the distal convoluted tubule and collecting tubule. Here, they inhibit the action of aldosterone, leading to sodium excretion and potassium retention. Although triamterene and amiloride, two other potassium-sparing diuretics, act at the same site, they don't affect aldosterone. Instead, these drugs directly block the exchange of sodium and potassium, leading to decreased sodium reabsorption and decreased potassium excretion.

Osmotic diuretics, such as mannitol, work in the proximal convoluted tubule. As their name implies, these diuretics increase the osmotic pressure of the glomerular filtrate, inhibiting the passive reabsorption of water, sodium, and chloride.

INTERACTIONS
Drug
ACE inhibitors, including captopril, and potassium-containing diuretics: May increase potassium levels.
Anticoagulants, including heparin: May decrease effect of anticoagulants, including heparin.
Lithium: May decrease lithium clearance and increase risk of amiloride toxicity.
NSAIDs: May decrease antihypertensive effect.
Herbal
None known.
Food
None known.

DIAGNOSTIC TEST EFFECTS
May increase BUN, calcium excretion, and glucose, serum creatinine, serum magnesium, serum potassium, and uric acid levels. May decrease serum sodium levels.

SIDE EFFECTS
Frequent (8%–3%)
Headache, nausea, diarrhea, vomiting, decreased appetite
Occasional (3%–1%)
Dizziness, constipation, abdominal pain, weakness, fatigue, cough, impotence
Rare (less than 1%)
Tremors, vertigo, confusion, nervousness, insomnia, thirst, dry mouth, heartburn, shortness of breath, increased urination, hypotension, rash

SERIOUS REACTIONS
• Severe hyperkalemia may produce irritability, anxiety, a feeling of heaviness in the legs, paresthesia of

hands, face, and lips, hypotension, bradycardia, tented T waves, widening of QRS, and ST depression.

NURSING CONSIDERATIONS

Baseline Assessment

* As appropriate, assess the patient's serum electrolyte levels, especially for low potassium.
* Monitor the patient's renal function tests and serum hepatic enzyme levels.
* Determine the location and extent of edema and assess the patient's skin turgor. Note the skin temperature and moisture level.
* Check the patient's mucous membranes to determine his or her hydration status.
* Assess the patient's muscle strength and mental status.
* Determine the patient's baseline weight.
* Initiate strict intake and output procedures and document.
* Obtain a baseline 12-lead EKG.
* Assess the patient's pulse rate and rhythm.

Lifespan Considerations

* Be aware that it is unknown if amiloride crosses the placenta or is distributed in breast milk.
* There are no age-related precautions noted in children.
* In the elderly, age-related decreased renal function increases the risk of hyperkalemia and may require caution.

Precautions

* Use cautiously in patients with a BUN greater than 30 mg/dl or serum creatinine greater than 1.5 mg/dl.
* Use cautiously in the debilitated and elderly.
* Use cautiously in those with cardiopulmonary disease, diabetes mellitus, or liver insufficiency.

Administration and Handling

PO
* Give with food to avoid GI distress.

Intervention and Evaluation

* Expect to monitor the patient's blood pressure (B/P), vital signs, electrolytes, intake and output, and weight. Note the extent of diuresis.
* Watch for changes from the initial assessment. Hyperkalemia may result in cardiac arrhythmias, a change in mental status, muscle cramps, muscle strength changes, or tremor.
* Monitor the patient's serum potassium level, particularly during initial therapy.
* Weigh the patient each day.
* Assess lung sounds for rales, rhonchi, or wheezing.

Patient Teaching

* Advise the patient to expect an increase in the volume and frequency of urination.
* Explain to the patient that the therapeutic effect of the drug takes several days to begin and can last for several days after the drug is discontinued.
* Warn the patient that a high-potassium diet and potassium supplements can be dangerous, especially if he or she has liver or kidney problems. Caution the patient to avoid foods high in potassium such as apricots, bananas, legumes, meat, orange juice, raisins, whole grains, including cereals, and white and sweet potatoes.
* Instruct the patient to notify the physician if he or she experiences the signs and symptoms of hyperkalemia: confusion, difficulty breathing, irregular heartbeat, nervousness, numbness of the hands, feet, or lips, unusual tiredness, and weakness in the legs.

bumetanide
byew-**met**-ah-nide
(Bumex, Burinex[CAN])

CATEGORY AND SCHEDULE
Pregnancy Risk Category: C
(D if used in pregnancy-induced
hypertension)

MECHANISM OF ACTION
A loop diuretic that enhances excretion of sodium, chloride, and to lesser degree, potassium, by direct action at ascending limb of loop of Henle and in the proximal tubule. *Therapeutic Effect:* Produces diuresis.

PHARMACOKINETICS

Route	Onset	Peak	Duration
PO	30–60 min	60–120 min	4–6 hrs
IM	40 min	60–120 min	4–6 hrs
IV	Rapid	15–30 min	2–3 hrs

Completely absorbed from the gastrointestinal (GI) tract (absorption decreased in congestive heart failure [CHF], nephrotic syndrome). Protein binding: 94%–96%. Partially metabolized in liver. Primarily excreted in urine. Not removed by hemodialysis. **Half-life:** 1–1.5 hrs.

AVAILABILITY
Tablets: 0.5 mg, 1 mg, 2 mg.
Injection: 0.25 mg/ml.

INDICATIONS AND DOSAGES
▸ **Edema**
PO
Adults, Children older than 18 yrs.
0.5–2 mg given as single dose in AM. May repeat at 4- to 5-hr intervals.
Elderly. 0.5 mg/day, increase as needed.

IM/IV
Adults, Elderly. 0.5–2 mg/dose.
May repeat in 2–3 hrs.
Continuous IV
Adults, Elderly. 0.5–1 mg/hr.
IV/IM/PO
Children. 0.15–0.1 mg/kg/dose
q6–24h.
▸ **Hypertension**
PO
Adults, Elderly. Initially, 0.5 mg/day. Range: 1–4 mg/day. Maximum: 5 mg/day. For larger doses may divide into 2–3 doses/day.
IV/IM/PO
Children. 0.015–0.1 mg/kg/dose
q6–24h.

UNLABELED USES
Treatment of hypercalcemia, hypertension

CONTRAINDICATIONS
Anuria, hepatic coma, severe electrolyte depletion

INTERACTIONS
Drug
Amphotericin, nephrotoxic agents, ototoxic agents: May increase the risk of toxicity.
Anticoagulants, heparin: May decrease the effects of anticoagulants and heparin.
Hypokalemia-causing agents: May increase the risk of hypokalemia.
Lithium: May increase the risk of toxicity of lithium.
Herbal
None known.
Food
None known.

DIAGNOSTIC TEST EFFECTS
May increase blood glucose levels, BUN, uric acid, and urinary phosphate levels. May decrease serum calcium, chloride, magnesium, potassium, and sodium levels.

IV INCOMPATIBILITIES
Midazolam (Versed)

IV COMPATIBILITIES
Aztreonam (Azactam), cefepime (Maxipime), diltiazem (Cardizem), dobutamine (Dobutrex), furosemide (Lasix), lorazepam (Ativan), milrinone (Primacor), morphine, piperacillin tazobactam (Zosyn), propofol (Diprivan)

SIDE EFFECTS
Expected
Increase in urine frequency and volume
Frequent
Orthostatic hypotension, dizziness
Occasional
Blurred vision, diarrhea, headache, anorexia, premature ejaculation, impotence, GI upset
Rare
Rash, urticaria, pruritus, weakness, muscle cramps, nipple tenderness

SERIOUS REACTIONS
• Vigorous diuresis may lead to profound water and electrolyte depletion, resulting in hypokalemia, hyponatremia, dehydration, coma, and circulatory collapse.
• Acute hypotensive episodes may occur.
• Ototoxicity manifested as deafness, vertigo, and tinnitus or ringing in ears may occur, especially in patients with severe renal impairment or who are on other ototoxic drugs.
• Blood dyscrasias have been reported.

NURSING CONSIDERATIONS
Baseline Assessment
• Check the patient's vital signs, especially blood pressure (B/P) for hypotension, prior to administration.
• Assess the patient's baseline electrolytes, particularly for low potassium.
• Evaluate the patient for edema.
• Determine the patient's hydration status.
• Measure and record the patient's fluid intake and output.
Lifespan Considerations
• Be aware that it is unknown if bumetanide is distributed in breast milk.
• Be aware that the safety and efficacy of bumetanide have not been established in children.
• Be aware that the elderly may be more sensitive to hypotension and electrolyte effects.
• Be aware that the elderly are at an increased risk for circulatory collapse or thrombolic episode.
• In the elderly, age-related renal impairment may require reduced or extended dosage interval.
Precautions
• Use cautiously in elderly and debilitated patients.
• Use cautiously in patients with diabetes mellitus, hypersensitivity to sulfonamides, and impaired liver or renal function.
Administration and Handling
PO
• Give bumetanide with food to avoid GI upset, preferably with breakfast to help prevent nocturia.
IV
• Store at room temperature.
• Stable for 24 hours if diluted.
• May give undiluted but is compatible with D_5W, 0.9% NaCl, or lactated Ringer's.
• Administer IV push over 1 to 2 minutes.
• May give as continuous infusion.
Intervention and Evaluation
• Continue to monitor the patient's B/P, electrolytes, intake and output, vital signs, and weight.
• Note the extent of patient diuresis.

- Observe the patient for changes from his or her initial assessment. Hypokalemia may result in cardiac arrhythmias, change in mental status, muscle cramps, muscle strength changes, and tremor. Hyponatremia may result in clammy or cold skin, confusion, and thirst.

Patient Teaching

- Tell the patient to expect to have hearing abnormalities, such as a sense of fullness or ringing in ears, and increased frequency and volume of urination.
- Encourage the patient to consume foods high in potassium such as apricots, bananas, legumes, meat, orange juice, white and sweet potatoes, raisins, and whole grains, including cereals.
- Instruct the patient to rise slowly from a sitting or lying position.
- Tell the patient to take the drug with food to avoid GI distress.

chlorthalidone
klor-**thal**-ih-doan
(Apo-Chlorthalidone[CAN], Thalitone)

CATEGORY AND SCHEDULE
Pregnancy Risk Category: B
(D if used in pregnancy-induced hypertension)

MECHANISM OF ACTION
A thiazide diuretic that blocks reabsorption of sodium, potassium, and chloride at distal convoluted tubule of the kidney's nephron. As an antihypertensive, reduces plasma, extracellular fluid volume, peripheral vascular resistance. *Therapeutic Effect:* As diuretic, promotes renal excretion of sodium and water. As antihypertensive, lowers blood pressure (B/P).

PHARMACOKINETICS

Route	Onset	Peak	Duration
PO (diuretic)	2 hrs	2–6 hrs	Up to 36 hrs

Rapidly absorbed from the gastrointestinal (GI) tract. Excreted unchanged in urine. **Half-life:** 35–50 hrs. Onset antihypertensive effect: 3–4 days; optimal therapeutic effect: 3–4 wks.

AVAILABILITY
Tablets: 15 mg, 25 mg, 50 mg, 100 mg.

INDICATIONS AND DOSAGES
▸ **Hypertension, edema**
PO
Adults. 25–100 mg/day or 100 mg 3 times/wk.
Elderly. Initially, 12.5–25 mg/day or every other day.

CONTRAINDICATIONS
Anuria, history of hypersensitivity to sulfonamides or thiazide diuretics, renal decompensation

INTERACTIONS
Drug
Cholestyramine, colestipol: May decrease the absorption and effects of chlorthalidone.
Digoxin: May increase the risk of toxicity of digoxin, if hypokalemia occurs.
Lithium: May increase the risk of toxicity of lithium.
Herbal
None known.
Food
None known.

DIAGNOSTIC TEST EFFECTS

May increase blood glucose levels, serum cholesterol, LDL, bilirubin, calcium, creatinine, uric acid, and triglyceride levels. May decrease urinary calcium levels, and serum magnesium, potassium, sodium levels.

SIDE EFFECTS

Expected
Increase in urine frequency and volume
Frequent
Potassium depletion that rarely produces symptoms
Occasional
Anorexia, impotence, diarrhea, orthostatic hypotension, GI upset, photosensitivity
Rare
Rash

SERIOUS REACTIONS

• Vigorous diuresis may lead to profound water loss and electrolyte depletion, resulting in hypokalemia, hyponatremia, and dehydration.
• Acute hypotensive episodes may occur.
• Hyperglycemia may be noted during prolonged therapy.
• Overdosage can lead to lethargy and coma without changes in electrolytes or hydration.

NURSING CONSIDERATIONS

Baseline Assessment

• Monitor the patient's blood pressure (B/P) for hypotension before chlorthalidone administration.
• Assess the patient's baseline electrolytes, particularly serum potassium levels.
• Assess the patient's edema, mucous membranes, and skin turgor for hydration status.

• Evaluate the patient's mental status and muscle strength.

Lifespan Considerations

• Be aware that chlorthalidone crosses the placenta and a small amount of the drug is distributed in breast milk. Breast-feeding is not recommended in this patient population.
• There are no age-related precautions noted in children.
• Be aware that the elderly may be more sensitive to hypotensive and electrolyte effects.

Precautions

• Use cautiously in elderly and debilitated patients.
• Use cautiously in patients with diabetes mellitus, gout, hypercholesterolemia, impaired hepatic function, and severe renal disease.

Administration and Handling

PO
• Give chlorthalidone with food or milk if GI upset occurs, preferably with breakfast to help prevent nocturia.
• Crush scored tablets as needed.

Intervention and Evaluation

• Monitor the patient for electrolyte disturbances. Know that hypokalemia may result in changes in mental status, muscle cramps, nausea, tachycardia, tremor, vomiting, and weakness; hyponatremia may result in clammy and cold skin, confusion, and thirst.
• Periodically check the patient's blood glucose levels, as ordered, for hyperglycemia during prolonged therapy.

Patient Teaching

• Instruct the patient to rise slowly from lying to sitting position and to permit his or her legs to dangle momentarily before standing to reduce the drug's hypotensive effect.
• Encourage the patient to eat foods

high in potassium, such as apricots, bananas, legumes, meat, orange juice, white and sweet potatoes, raisins, and whole grains, including cereals.
• Warn the patient to avoid prolonged exposure to sunlight.
• Tell the patient to take the drug with food to avoid GI distress, and early in the day to avoid nocturia.

furosemide

feur-**oh**-sah-mide
(Apo-Furosemide[CAN], Lasix, Uremide[AUS], Urex-M[AUS])
Do not confuse with Torsemide.

CATEGORY AND SCHEDULE

Pregnancy Risk Category: C
(D if used in pregnancy-induced hypertension)

MECHANISM OF ACTION

A loop diuretic that enhances excretion of sodium, chloride, potassium by direct action at ascending limb of loop of Henle. *Therapeutic Effect:* Produces diuretic effect.

PHARMACOKINETICS

Route	Onset	Peak	Duration
PO	30–60 min	1–2 hrs	6–8 hrs
IM	30 min	N/A	N/A
IV	5 min	20–60 min	2 hrs

Well absorbed from the gastrointestinal (GI) tract. Protein binding: 91%–97%. Partially metabolized in liver. Primarily excreted in urine in severe renal impairment, nonrenal clearance increases. Not removed by hemodialysis. **Half-life:** 30–90 min, half-life is increased in patients with impaired renal, liver function and in neonates.

AVAILABILITY

Tablets: 20 mg, 40 mg, 80 mg.
Oral Solution: 10 mg/ml, 40 mg/ 5 ml.
Injection: 10 mg/ml.

INDICATIONS AND DOSAGES
▶ **Edema and hypertension**
PO
Adults, Elderly. Initially, 20–80 mg/ dose, may increase by 20–40 mg/ dose at 6- to 8-hr intervals. May titrate up to 600 mg/day in severe edematous states.
Children. 1–6 mg/kg/day in divided doses q6–12h.
IM/IV
Adults, Elderly. 20–40 mg/dose; may repeat in 1–2 hrs and increase by 20 mg/dose.
Children. 1–2 mg/kg/dose q6–12h.
Neonates. 1–2 mg/kg/dose q12–24h.
IV infusion
Adults, Elderly. Bolus of 0.1 mg/kg, then 0.1 mg/kg/hr; may double q2h. Maximum: 0.4 mg/kg/hr.
Children. 0.05 mg/kg/hr; titrate to desired effect.

UNLABELED USES

Treatment of hypercalcemia

CONTRAINDICATIONS

Anuria, liver coma, severe electrolyte depletion

INTERACTIONS
Drug

Amphotericin, nephrotoxic and ototoxic agents: May increase the risk of toxicity.
Anticoagulants, heparin: May decrease the effects of anticoagulants and heparin.
Hypokalemia-causing agents: May increase the risk of hypokalemia.
Lithium: May increase the risk of toxicity of lithium.

Probenecid: May increase furosemide blood concentration.

Herbal
None known.

Food
None known.

DIAGNOSTIC TEST EFFECTS
May increase blood glucose, BUN, and serum uric acid levels. May decrease serum calcium, chloride, magnesium, potassium, and sodium levels.

IV INCOMPATIBILITIES
Ciprofloxacin (Cipro), diltiazem (Cardizem), dobutamine (Dobutrex), dopamine (Intropin), doxorubicin (Adriamycin), droperidol (Inapsine), esmolol (Brevibloc), famotidine (Pepcid), filgrastim (Neupogen), fluconazole (Diflucan), gemcitabine (Gemzar), gentamicin (Garamycin), idarubicin (Idamycin), labetalol (Trandate), meperidine (Demerol), metoclopramide (Reglan), midazolam (Versed), milrinone (Primacor), nicardipine (Cardene), ondansetron (Zofran), quinidine, thiopental (Pentothal), vecuronium (Norcuron), vinblastine (Velban), vincristine (Oncovin), vinorelbine (Navelbine)

IV COMPATIBILITIES
Aminophylline, amiodarone (Cordarone), bumetanide (Bumex), calcium gluconate, cimetidine (Tagamet), heparin, hydromorphone (Dilaudid), lidocaine, morphine, nitroglycerin, norepinephrine (Levophed), potassium chloride, propofol (Diprivan)

SIDE EFFECTS
Expected
Increase in urinary frequency and volume

Frequent
Nausea, gastric upset with cramping, diarrhea, or constipation, electrolyte disturbances
Occasional
Dizziness, lightheadedness, headache, blurred vision, paresthesia, photosensitivity, rash, weakness, urinary frequency or bladder spasm, restlessness, diaphoresis
Rare
Flank pain, loin pain

SERIOUS REACTIONS
• Vigorous diuresis may lead to profound water loss and electrolyte depletion, resulting in hypokalemia, hyponatremia, and dehydration.
• Sudden volume depletion may result in increased risk of thrombosis, circulatory collapse, and sudden death.
• Acute hypotensive episodes may also occur, sometimes several days after the beginning of therapy.
• Ototoxicity manifested as deafness, vertigo, and tinnitus or ringing and roaring in ears may occur, especially in patients with severe renal impairment.
• Furosemide use can exacerbate diabetes mellitus, systemic lupus erythematosus, gout, and pancreatitis.
• Blood dyscrasias have been reported.

NURSING CONSIDERATIONS
Baseline Assessment
• Monitor the patient's vital signs, especially blood pressure (B/P) for hypotension before giving furosemide.
• Assess the patient's baseline electrolytes, particularly for low potassium.

- Evaluate the patient's edema, mucous membranes, and skin turgor for hydration status.
- Evaluate the patient's mental status and muscle strength.
- Record the patient's skin moisture and temperature.
- Obtain the patient's baseline weight.
- Begin monitoring the patient's fluid intake and output.

Lifespan Considerations
- Be aware that furosemide crosses the placenta and is distributed in breast milk.
- Be aware that the drug's half-life is increased in neonates and may require increased dosage interval.
- Be aware that the elderly may be more sensitive to the drug's electrolyte and hypotensive effects, developing circulatory collapse, or thromboembolic effect.
- In the elderly, age-related renal function impairment may require dosage adjustment.

Precautions
- Use cautiously in patients with liver cirrhosis.

Administration and Handling
PO
- Give furosemide with food to avoid GI upset, preferably with breakfast to help prevent nocturia.
IM
- Monitor the patient for temporary pain at injection site.
IV
- Solution normally appears clear, colorless.
- Discard yellow solutions.
- May give undiluted but is compatible with D_5W, 0.9% normal saline, or lactated Ringer's solutions.
- Administer each 40 mg or fraction by IV push over 1 to 2 minutes. Do not exceed administration rate of 4 mg a minute in patients with renal impairment.

Intervention and Evaluation
- Monitor the patient's B/P, electrolytes, fluid intake and output, vital signs, and weight.
- Note the extent of patient diuresis.
- Observe the patient for changes from the initial assessment. Hypokalemia may result in cardiac arrhythmias, changes in mental status and muscle strength, muscle cramps, and tremor. Hyponatremia may result in clammy and cold skin, confusion, and thirst.

Patient Teaching
- Tell the patient to expect an increase in the frequency and volume of urination.
- Warn the patient to notify the physician if he or she experiences hearing abnormalities, such as ringing or roaring in the ears, or a sense of fullness in the ears, irregular heartbeat, or signs of electrolyte imbalances.
- Encourage the patient to eat foods high in potassium such as apricots, bananas, legumes, meat, orange juice, white or sweet potatoes, raisins, and whole grains, such as cereals.
- Urge the patient to avoid overexposure to artificial lights, such as sun lamps, and sunlight.

---

hydrochlorothiazide
high-drow-chlor-oh-**thigh**-ah-zide
(Apo-Hydro[CAN], Dichlotride[AUS], Esidrix, HydroDIURIL, Microzide, Oretic)

CATEGORY AND SCHEDULE
Pregnancy Risk Category: B, D if used in pregnancy-induced hypertension

MECHANISM OF ACTION

A sulfonamide derivative that acts as a thiazide diuretic and antihypertensive. As a diuretic blocks reabsorption of water, the electrolytes sodium and potassium at cortical diluting segment of distal tubule. As an antihypertensive reduces plasma, extracellular fluid volume, decreases peripheral vascular resistance (PVR) by direct effect on blood vessels. *Therapeutic Effect:* Promotes diuresis, reduces blood pressure (B/P).

PHARMACOKINETICS

Route	Onset	Peak	Duration
PO (diuretic)	2 hrs	4–6 hrs	6–12 hrs

Variably absorbed from the gastrointestinal (GI) tract. Primarily excreted unchanged in urine. Not removed by hemodialysis. **Half-life:** 5.6–14.8 hrs.

AVAILABILITY

Capsules: 12.5 mg.
Tablets: 25 mg, 50 mg, 100 mg.
Oral Solution: 50 mg/5 ml.

INDICATIONS AND DOSAGES
▸ **Edema, hypertension**
PO
Adults. 12.5–100 mg/day. Maximum: 200 mg/day.
Children 6 mos–12 yrs. 2 mg/kg/day. Maximum: 200 mg/day.
Children younger than 6 mos. 2–4 mg/kg/day. Maximum: 37.5 mg/day.

UNLABELED USES

Treatment of diabetes insipidus, prevention of calcium-containing renal stones

CONTRAINDICATIONS

Anuria, history of hypersensitivity to sulfonamides or thiazide diuretics, renal decompensation

INTERACTIONS
Drug
Cholestyramine, colestipol: May decrease the absorption and effects of hydrochlorothiazide.
Digoxin: May increase the risk of toxicity of digoxin caused by hypokalemia.
Lithium: May increase the risk of toxicity of lithium.
Herbal
None known.
Food
None known.

DIAGNOSTIC TEST EFFECTS

May increase blood glucose levels, serum cholesterol, LDL, bilirubin, calcium, creatinine, uric acid, and triglyceride levels. May decrease urinary calcium, and serum magnesium, potassium, and sodium levels.

SIDE EFFECTS

Expected
Increase in urine frequency and volume
Frequent
Potassium depletion
Occasional
Postural hypotension, headache, gastrointestinal (GI) disturbances, photosensitivity reaction

SERIOUS REACTIONS

• Vigorous diuresis may lead to profound water loss and electrolyte depletion, resulting in hypokalemia, hyponatremia, and dehydration.
• Acute hypotensive episodes may occur.
• Hyperglycemia may be noted during prolonged therapy.
• GI upset, pancreatitis, dizziness,

paresthesias, headache, blood dys-crasias, pulmonary edema, allergic pneumonitis, and dermatologic reactions occur rarely.
• Overdosage can lead to lethargy and coma without changes in electrolytes or hydration.

NURSING CONSIDERATIONS

Baseline Assessment
• Monitor the patient's vital signs, especially blood pressure (B/P) for hypotension before giving hydrochlorothiazide.
• Plan to assess the patient's baseline electrolytes, particularly for hypokalemia.
• Evaluate the patient's mucous membranes, peripheral edema, and skin turgor for hydration status.
• Evaluate the patient's mental status and muscle strength.
• Record the patient's skin moisture and temperature.
• Obtain and record the patient's baseline weight.
• Begin monitoring the patient's fluid intake and output.

Lifespan Considerations
• Be aware that hydrochlorothiazide crosses the placenta and a small amount is distributed in breast milk. Breast-feeding is not recommended in this patient population.
• There are no age-related precautions noted in children, except that jaundiced infants may be at risk for hyperbilirubinemia.
• Be aware that the elderly may be more sensitive to the drug's electrolyte and hypotensive effects.
• In the elderly, age-related renal impairment may require caution.

Precautions
• Use cautiously in debilitated and elderly patients.
• Use cautiously in patients with diabetes mellitus, impaired liver function, severe renal disease, and thyroid disorders.

Administration and Handling
PO
• May give hydrochlorothiazide with food or milk if GI upset occurs, preferably with breakfast to help prevent nocturia.

Intervention and Evaluation
• Continue to monitor the patient's B/P, electrolytes, intake and output, vital signs, and weight daily.
• Record the extent of patient diuresis.
• Observe the patient for changes from the initial assessment. Hypokalemia may result in change in mental status, muscle cramps, nausea, tachycardia, tremor, vomiting, and weakness. Hyponatremia may result in clammy and cold skin, confusion, and thirst.
• Be especially alert for potassium depletion in patients taking digoxin, such as cardiac arrhythmias.
• Give the patient potassium supplements, if ordered.
• Assess the patient for constipation, which may occur with exercise diuresis.

Patient Teaching
• Tell the patient to expect an increase in the frequency and volume of urination.
• Instruct the patient to rise slowly from lying to sitting position and to permit legs to dangle momentarily before standing to reduce the drug's hypotensive effect.
• Encourage the patient to eat foods high in potassium such as apricots, bananas, legumes, meat, orange juice, white and sweet potatoes, raising, and whole grains, such as cereals.
• Urge the patient to protect his or her skin from sunlight and ultraviolet rays as a photosensitivity reaction may occur.

indapamide
in-**dap**-ah-myd
(Dapa-tabs[AUS], Indahexal[AUS], Insig[AUS], Lozide[CAN], Lozol, Natrilix[AUS], Natrilix SR[AUS])
Do not confuse with iodamide or iopamidol.

CATEGORY AND SCHEDULE
Pregnancy Risk Category: B
(D if used in pregnancy-induced hypertension)

MECHANISM OF ACTION
A thiazide that acts as a diuretic and antihypertensive. As a diuretic, blocks reabsorption of water and the electrolytes sodium and potassium at cortical diluting segment of distal tubule. *Therapeutic Effect:* Promotes renal excretion of sodium and water. As an antihypertensive, reduces plasma, extracellular fluid volume; decreases peripheral vascular resistance (PVR) by direct effect on blood vessels. *Therapeutic Effect:* Reduces blood pressure (B/P).

AVAILABILITY
Tablets: 1.25 mg, 2.5 mg.

INDICATIONS AND DOSAGES
▸ **Edema**
PO
Adults. Initially, 2.5 mg/day, may increase to 5 mg/day in 1 wk.
▸ **Hypertension**
PO
Adults, Elderly. Initially, 1.25 mg, may increase to 2.5 mg/day in 4 wks or 5 mg/day after additional 4 wks.

CONTRAINDICATIONS
None known

INTERACTIONS
Drug
Digoxin: May increase the risk of digoxin toxicity caused by hypokalemia.
Lithium: May decrease clearance and increase the toxicity of lithium.
Herbal
None known.
Food
None known.

DIAGNOSTIC TEST EFFECTS
May increase plasma renin activity. May decrease protein-bound iodine, serum calcium, potassium, and sodium levels.

SIDE EFFECTS
Frequent (5% and greater)
Fatigue, numbness of extremities, tension, irritability, agitation, headache, dizziness, lightheadedness, insomnia, muscle cramping
Occasional (less than 5%)
Tingling of extremities, frequent urination, polyuria, hives, rhinorrhea, flushing, weight loss, orthostatic hypotension, depression, blurred vision, nausea, vomiting, diarrhea or constipation, dry mouth, impotence, rash, pruritus

SERIOUS REACTIONS
• Vigorous diuresis may lead to profound water loss and electrolyte depletion, resulting in hypokalemia, hyponatremia, and dehydration.
• Acute hypotensive episodes may occur.
• Hyperglycemia may be noted during prolonged therapy.
• Gastrointestinal (GI) upset, pancreatitis, dizziness, paresthesias, headache, blood dyscrasias, pulmonary edema, allergic pneumonitis, and dermatologic reactions occur rarely.
• Overdosage can lead to lethargy

and coma without changes in electrolytes or hydration.

Baseline Assessment
• Assess the patient's blood pressure (B/P) for hypotension before giving indapamide.
• Assess the patient's baseline serum electrolyte levels, particularly for hypokalemia.
• Evaluate the patient's mucous membranes, peripheral edema, and skin turgor for hydration status.
• Evaluate the patient's mental status and muscle strength.
• Assess the patient's skin moisture and temperature.
• Obtain and record the patient's baseline weight.
• Begin monitoring the patient's fluid intake and output.
Precautions
• Use cautiously in patients with anuria, diabetes mellitus, a history of hypersensitivity to sulfonamides or thiazide diuretics, impaired liver function, renal decompensation, severe renal disease, and thyroid disorders.
• Use cautiously in debilitated and elderly patients.
Administration and Handling
PO
• Give indapamide with food or milk if GI upset occurs, preferably with breakfast to help prevent nocturia.
• Do not crush or break tablets.
Intervention and Evaluation
• Continue to monitor the patient's B/P, electrolytes, intake and output, vital signs, and weight.
• Record the extent of patient diuresis.
• Observe the patient for changes from the initial assessment. Hypo-

kalemia may result in change in mental status, muscle cramps, nausea, tachycardia, tremor, vomiting, and weakness. Hyponatremia may result in clammy and cold skin, confusion, and thirst.
Patient Teaching
• Tell the patient to expect an increase in the frequency and volume of urination.
• Instruct the patient to rise slowly from lying to sitting position and to permit legs to dangle momentarily before standing to reduce the drug's hypotensive effect.
• Teach the patient to take indapamide early in the day to avoid nocturia.
• Encourage the patient to eat foods high in potassium such as apricots, bananas, legumes, meat, orange juice white and sweet, potatoes, raising, and whole grains, such as cereals.

mannitol
man-ih-toll
(Osmitrol)

CATEGORY AND SCHEDULE
Pregnancy Risk Category: C

MECHANISM OF ACTION
An osmotic diuretic, antiglaucoma, and antihemolytic agent that elevates osmotic pressure of glomerular filtrate; increases flow of water into interstitial fluid and plasma, inhibiting renal tubular reabsorption of sodium, chloride. Enhances flow of water from eye into plasma. *Therapeutic Effect:* Produces diuresis, reduces intraocular pressure (IOP).

PHARMACOKINETICS

Indication	Onset	Peak	Duration
diuresis	1–3 hrs	N/A	N/A
reduced IOP	15 min	N/A	3–6 hrs

Remains in extracellular fluid. Primarily excreted in urine. Removed by hemodialysis. **Half-life:** 100 min. Onset diuresis occurs in 1–3 hrs, decreases IOP in 0.5–1 hr, duration 4–6 hrs. Decreases cerebrospinal fluid (CSF) pressure in 15 min, duration 3–8 hrs.

AVAILABILITY

Injection: 5%, 10%, 15%, 20%, 25%.

INDICATIONS AND DOSAGES

▸ **Prevention, treatment of oliguric phase of acute renal failure, before evidence of permanent renal failure, promotes urinary excretion of toxic substances, such as aspirin, barbiturates, bromides, and imipramine, reduces increased intracranial pressure due to cerebral edema, edema of injured spinal cord, IOP due to acute glaucoma**
IV
Adults, Elderly, Children. Initially, 0.5–1 g/kg, then 0.25–0.5 g/kg q4–6h.

CONTRAINDICATIONS

Dehydration, intracranial bleeding, severe pulmonary edema and congestion, severe renal disease

INTERACTIONS
Drug
Digoxin: May increase the risk of toxicity of digoxin caused by hypokalemia.
Herbal
None known.

Food
None known.

DIAGNOSTIC TEST EFFECTS

May decrease serum phosphate, potassium, and sodium levels.

IV INCOMPATIBILITIES

Cefepime (Maxipime), doxorubicin liposome (Doxil), filgrastim (Neupogen)

IV COMPATIBILITIES

Cisplatin (Platinol), ondansetron (Zofran), propofol (Diprivan)

SIDE EFFECTS
Frequent
Dry mouth, thirst
Occasional
Blurred vision, increased urination, headache, arm pain, backache, nausea, vomiting, urticaria or hives, dizziness, hypotension or hypertension, tachycardia, fever, angina-like chest pain

SERIOUS REACTIONS

• Fluid and electrolyte imbalance may occur because of rapid administration of large doses or inadequate urinary output resulting in overexpansion of extracellular fluid.
• Circulatory overload may produce pulmonary edema and congestive heart failure (CHF).
• Excessive diuresis may produce hypokalemia and hyponatremia.
• Fluid loss in excess of electrolyte excretion may produce hypernatremia and hyperkalemia.

NURSING CONSIDERATIONS

Baseline Assessment
• Monitor the patient's vital signs, especially blood pressure (B/P) for hypotension before giving mannitol.
• Evaluate the patient's mucous

membranes, peripheral edema, and skin turgor for hydration status.
• Obtain and record the patient's baseline weight.
• Begin monitoring the patient's fluid intake and output.

Lifespan Considerations
• Be aware that it is unknown if mannitol crosses the placenta or is distributed in breast milk.
• Be aware that the safety and efficacy of mannitol have not been established in children younger than 12 years of age.
• In the elderly, age-related renal impairment may require caution.

Administration and Handling
◀ALERT▶ Assess the patient's IV site for patency before each dose. Pain and thrombosis are noted with extravasation.
◀ALERT▶ Test dose of 12.5 g for adults (200 mg/kg for children) over 3 to 5 minutes to produce a urine flow of at least 30 to 50 ml/hr over 2 to 3 hours (1 ml/kg/hr for children).

IV
• Store at room temperature.
• If crystals are noted in solution, warm bottle in hot water and shake vigorously at intervals. Do not use if crystals remain after warming procedure.
• Cool to body temperature before administration.
• Use an in-line filter (less than 5 microns) for drug concentrations greater than 20%.
• Test dose for oliguria is IV push over 3 to 5 minutes. Test dose for cerebral edema or elevated intracranial pressure is IV over 20 to 30 minutes. Maximum concentration: 25%.
• Do not add potassium chloride (KCl) or sodium chloride (NaCl) to mannitol 20% or greater.

• Do not add to whole blood for transfusion.

Intervention and Evaluation
• Monitor the patient's urine output to ascertain therapeutic response.
• Monitor the results of the patient's BUN, electrolytes, and serum hepatic enzyme level test results.
• Weigh the patient daily.
• Observe the patient for changes from the initial assessment. Know that hypokalemia may result in cardiac arrhythmias, change in mental status, muscle cramps, nausea, tachycardia, tremor, vomiting, and weakness; hyperkalemia may result in arrhythmias, colic, diarrhea, and muscle twitching followed by paralysis or weakness; hyponatremia may result in clammy and cold skin, confusion, drowsiness, and thirst.

Patient Teaching
• Tell the patient to expect an increase in the frequency and volume of urination.
• Explain to the patient that mannitol may cause dry mouth.
• Tell the patient to weigh himself or herself daily.

metolazone
me-**toh**-lah-zone
(Mykrox, Zaroxolyn)
Do not confuse with methazolamide, metoprolol, or Zarontin.

CATEGORY AND SCHEDULE
Pregnancy Risk Category: B, D if used in pregnancy-induced hypertension

MECHANISM OF ACTION
A thiazide-like diuretic and antihypertensive. As a diuretic, blocks

reabsorption of sodium, potassium, and chloride at distal convoluted tubule, promoting delivery of sodium to potassium side, increasing potassium excretion, (Na-K) exchange. *Therapeutic Effect:* Produces renal excretion of sodium and water. As an antihypertensive, reduces plasma, extracellular fluid volume. *Therapeutic Effect:* Decreases peripheral vascular resistance, reduced blood pressure (B/P) by direct effect on blood vessels.

PHARMACOKINETICS

Route	Onset	Peak	Duration
PO (diuretic)	1 hr	2 hrs	12–24 hrs

Incompletely absorbed from the gastrointestinal (GI) tract. Protein binding: 95%. Primarily excreted unchanged in urine. Not removed by hemodialysis. **Half-life:** 14 hrs.

AVAILABILITY

Tablets: 2.5 mg, 5 mg, 10 mg.
Tablets (Mykrox): 0.5 mg.

INDICATIONS AND DOSAGES
▸ **Edema (Zaroxolyn)**
PO
Adults. 5–10 mg once a day in morning. Reduce dosage to lowest maintenance level when dry weight is achieved, in nonedematous state.
▸ **Edema due to renal disease (Zaroxolyn)**
PO
Adults. 5–20 mg once a day in morning. Reduce dosage to lowest maintenance level when dry weight is achieved, in nonedematous state.
▸ **Hypertension (Zaroxolyn)**
PO
Adults. 2.5–5 mg once a day in morning.

▸ **Usual elderly dosage (Zaroxolyn)**
PO
• *Elderly.* Initially, 2.5 mg/day or every other day.
▸ **Hypertension (Mykrox)**
PO
Adults. 0.5 mg once daily in morning. Dosage may be increased to 1 mg once daily if blood pressure (B/P) response is insufficient.
▸ **Usual pediatric dosage (Mykrox)**
PO
Children. 0.2–0.4 mg/kg/day in divided doses q12–24h.

CONTRAINDICATIONS

Anuria, history of hypersensitivity to sulfonamides or thiazide diuretics, liver coma or precoma, renal decompensation

INTERACTIONS
Drug
Cholestyramine, colestipol: May decrease the absorption and effects of metolazone.
Digoxin: May increase the risk of toxicity of digoxin caused by hypokalemia.
Lithium: May increase the risk of toxicity of lithium.
Herbal
None known.
Food
None known.

DIAGNOSTIC TEST EFFECTS

May increase blood glucose levels, serum cholesterol, LDL, bilirubin, calcium, creatinine, uric acid, and triglyceride levels. May decrease urinary calcium, and serum magnesium, potassium, and sodium levels.

SIDE EFFECTS
Expected
Increase in urine frequency and volume
Frequent (10%–9%)
Dizziness, lightheadedness, headache
Occasional (6%–4%)
Muscle cramps and spasm, fatigue, lethargy
Rare (less than 2%)
Weakness, palpitations, depression, nausea, vomiting, abdominal bloating, constipation, diarrhea, urticaria

SERIOUS REACTIONS
• Vigorous diuresis may lead to profound water loss and electrolyte depletion, resulting in hypokalemia, hyponatremia, and dehydration.
• Acute hypotensive episodes may occur.
• Hyperglycemia may be noted during prolonged therapy.
• Gastrointestinal (GI) upset, pancreatitis, dizziness, paresthesias, headache, blood dyscrasias, pulmonary edema, allergic pneumonitis, and dermatologic reactions occur rarely.
• Overdosage can lead to lethargy and coma without changes in electrolytes or hydration.

NURSING CONSIDERATIONS
Baseline Assessment
• Monitor the patient's blood pressure (B/P) for hypotension before giving metolazone.
• Assess the patient's baseline electrolytes, particularly for hypokalemia.
• Evaluate the patient's mucous membranes, peripheral edema, and skin turgor for hydration status.
• Evaluate the patient's mental status and muscle strength.
• Assess the patients' skin moisture and temperature.

• Obtain and record the patient's baseline weight.
• Begin monitoring the patient's fluid intake and output.
Lifespan Considerations
• Be aware that metolazone crosses the placenta and a small amount is distributed in breast milk. Breast-feeding is not recommended in this patient population.
• There are no age-related precautions noted in children.
• Be aware that the elderly may be more sensitive to the drug's electrolyte and hypotensive effects.
• In the elderly, age-related renal impairment may require caution.
Precautions
• Use cautiously in patients with diabetes, elevated cholesterol and triglycerides, gout, impaired liver function, lupus erythematosus, and severe renal disease.
Administration and Handling
PO
• May give metolazone with food or milk if GI upset occurs, preferably with breakfast to help prevent nocturia.
Intervention and Evaluation
• Continue to monitor the patient's B/P, electrolytes, intake and output, vital signs, and weight.
• Record the extent of patient diuresis.
• Observe the patient for changes from the initial assessment. Hypokalemia may result in change in mental status, muscle cramps, nausea, tachycardia, tremor, vomiting, and weakness. Hyponatremia may result in clammy and cold skin, confusion, and thirst.
Patient Teaching
• Tell the patient to expect an increase in the frequency and volume of urination.
• Instruct the patient to rise slowly from lying to sitting position and to

permit legs to dangle momentarily before standing to reduce the drug's hypotensive effect.
• Encourage the patient to eat foods high in potassium such as apricots, bananas, legumes, meat, orange juice, white and sweet potatoes, raising, and whole grains, such as cereals.

spironolactone
spear-own-oh-**lak**-tone
(Aldactone, Novospiroton[CAN], Spiractin[AUS])

CATEGORY AND SCHEDULE
Pregnancy Risk Category: C
(D if used in pregnancy-induced hypertension)

MECHANISM OF ACTION
An aldosterone antagonist that competitively inhibits action of aldosterone. Interferes with sodium reabsorption in distal tubule. *Therapeutic Effect:* Increases potassium retention while promoting sodium and water excretion.

PHARMACOKINETICS

Route	Onset	Peak	Duration
PO	24–48 hrs	48–72 hrs	48–72 hrs

Well absorbed from the gastrointestinal (GI) tract (increased with food). Protein binding: 91%–98%. Metabolized in liver to active metabolite. Primarily excreted in urine. Unknown if removed by hemodialysis. **Half-life:** 0–24 hrs (metabolite: 13–24 hrs).

AVAILABILITY
Tablets: 25 mg, 50 mg, 100 mg.

INDICATIONS AND DOSAGES
▸ **Diuretic, hypertension**
PO
Adults, Elderly. 25–200 mg/day in 1–2 divided doses.
Children. 1.5–3.3 mg/kg/day in divided doses q6– 12h.
Neonates. 1–3 mg/kg/day q12–24h.
▸ **Congestive heart failure (CHF)**
PO
Adults, Elderly. 25 mg/day.
▸ **Diagnosis of primary aldosteronism**
PO
Adults, Elderly. 100–400 mg/day in 1–2 divided doses.
Children. 100–400 mg/m^2/day in 1–2 divided doses.
▸ **Dosage in renal impairment**

Creatinine Clearance	Interval
10–50 ml/min	12–24 hrs
less than 10 ml/min	Avoid use

UNLABELED USES
Treatment of female hirsutism, polycystic ovary syndrome

CONTRAINDICATIONS
Acute renal insufficiency and impairment, anuria, hyperkalemia, BUN and serum creatinine over twice normal values levels

INTERACTIONS
Drug
Angiotensin-converting enzyme (ACE) inhibitors, such as captopril, potassium-containing medications, potassium supplements: May increase serum potassium levels.
Anticoagulants, heparin: May decrease the effects of anticoagulants and heparin
Digoxin: May increase the half-life of digoxin.
Lithium: May decrease the clear-

ance and increase the risk of toxicity of lithium.
NSAIDs: May decrease the antihypertensive effect.
Herbal
None known.
Food
None known.

DIAGNOSTIC TEST EFFECTS

May increase blood glucose levels, BUN, calcium excretion, serum creatinine, magnesium, potassium, and uric acid levels. May decrease serum sodium levels.

SIDE EFFECTS

Frequent
Hyperkalemia for patients on potassium supplements or with renal insufficiency, dehydration, hyponatremia, lethargy
Occasional
Nausea, vomiting, anorexia, cramping, diarrhea, headache, ataxia, drowsiness, confusion, fever
Male: Gynecomastia, impotence, decreased libido
Female: Menstrual irregularities or amenorrhea, postmenopausal bleeding, breast tenderness
Rare
Rash, urticaria, hirsutism

SERIOUS REACTIONS

• Severe hyperkalemia may produce arrhythmias, bradycardia, EKG changes (tented T waves, widening QRS), and depression. These may proceed to cardiac standstill or ventricular fibrillation.
• Cirrhosis patients are at risk for hepatic decompensation if dehydration or hyponatremia occurs.
• Patients with primary aldosteronism may experience rapid weight loss and severe fatigue during high-dose therapy.

NURSING CONSIDERATIONS
Baseline Assessment
• Monitor the patient's baseline vital signs and note the patient's pulse rate and quality.
• Assess the patient's baseline BUN, serum creatinine, serum electrolyte levels, and serum hepatic enzyme levels to assess renal function and urinalysis results. Also expect to perform a baseline EKG.
• Evaluate the patient's mucous membranes and skin turgor for hydration status.
• Evaluate the patient for edema and note its extent and location.
• Obtain and record the patient's baseline weight.
• Begin monitoring the patient's fluid intake and output.
Lifespan Considerations
• Be aware that an active metabolite of spironolactone is excreted in breast milk. Breast-feeding is not recommended in this patient population.
• There are no age-related precautions noted in children.
• Be aware that the elderly may be more susceptible to hyperkalemia development.
• In the elderly, age-related renal impairment may require cautious use.
Precautions
• Use cautiously in patients who concurrently use supplemental potassium and who are dehydrated.
• Use cautiously in patients with hyponatremia and impaired liver or renal function.
Administration and Handling
PO
• Oral suspension containing crushed tablets in cherry syrup is stable for up to 30 days if refrigerated.
• Drug absorption enhanced if taken with food.
• Crush scored tablets as needed.

Intervention and Evaluation

• Monitor the patient's B/P and electrolytes values, particularly for hyperkalemia. Hyperkalemia may result in arrhythmias, colic, diarrhea, and muscle twitching followed by paralysis and weakness.
• Obtain an EKG, as ordered, if hyperkalemia is severe.
• Observe the patient for hyponatremia. Hyponatremia may result in clammy and cold skin, confusion, drowsiness, dry mouth, and thirst.
• Obtain and record the patient's daily weight.
• Record changes in the patient's edema and skin turgor.

Patient Teaching

• Tell the patient to expect an increase in the frequency and volume of urination.
• Caution the patient to avoid consuming foods high in potassium such as apricots, bananas, legumes, meat, orange juice, white and sweet potatoes, raising, and whole grains, such as cereals.
• Warn the patient that the therapeutic effect of spironolactone takes several days to begin and can last for several days once the drug is discontinued. Explain that this time frame may not apply if he or she is on a potassium-losing drug concomitantly. Expect the physician to help establish the patient's diet and use of supplements.
• Warn the patient to notify the physician if he or she experiences electrolyte imbalance or an irregular or slow pulse.
• Inform the patient that spironolactone may cause drowsiness. Warn the patient to avoid performing tasks that require mental alertness or motor skills until his or her response to the drug is established.

torsemide
tore-seh-mide
(Demadex)

CATEGORY AND SCHEDULE
Pregnancy Risk Category: B

MECHANISM OF ACTION
A loop diuretic that acts as an antiedema and antihypertensive agent. As a diuretic enhances excretion of sodium, chloride, potassium, water at ascending limb of loop of Henle. *Therapeutic Effect:* Produces diuretic effect. As an antihypertensive reduces plasma, extracellular fluid volume. *Therapeutic Effect:* Lowers blood pressure (B/P).

PHARMACOKINETICS

Route	Onset	Peak	Duration
PO	1 hr	1–2 hrs	6–8 hrs
IV	10 min	1 hr	6–8 hrs

Rapidly, well absorbed from the gastrointestinal (GI) tract. Protein binding: 97%–99%. Metabolized in liver. Primarily excreted in urine. Not removed by hemodialysis. **Half-life:** 3.3 hrs.

AVAILABILITY
Tablets: 5 mg, 10 mg, 20 mg, 100 mg.
Injection: 10 mg/ml.

INDICATIONS AND DOSAGES
▸ **Hypertension**
PO
Adults, Elderly. Initially, 5 mg/day. May increase to 10 mg/day if no response in 4–6 wks. If no response, additional antihypertensive added.

▸ **Congestive heart failure (CHF)**
IV/PO
Adults, Elderly. Initially, 10–20 mg/day. May increase by approximately doubling dose until desired diuretic dose attained. Doses greater than 200 mg have not been adequately studied.

▸ **Chronic renal failure**
IV/PO
Adults, Elderly. Initially, 20 mg/day. May increase by approximately doubling dose until desired diuretic dose attained. Doses greater than 200 mg have not been adequately studied.

▸ **Cirrhosis of the liver**
IV/PO
Adults, Elderly. Initially, 5 mg/day given with aldosterone antagonist or potassium-sparing diuretic. May increase by approximately doubling dose until desired diuretic dose attained. Doses greater than 40 mg have not been adequately studied.

CONTRAINDICATIONS
Anuria, liver coma, severe electrolyte depletion

INTERACTIONS
Drug
Amphotericin: May increase the risk of nephrotoxicity.
Anticoagulants, heparin, thrombolytics: May decrease the effects of anticoagulants, heparin, and thrombolytics.
Digoxin: May increase the risk of arrhythmias induced by digoxin and hypokalemia.
Hypokalemia-causing medications: May increase the risk of hypokalemia.
Lithium: May increase the risk of toxicity of lithium.
Nephrotoxic and ototoxic medications: May increase nephrotoxicity and ototoxicity.
NSAIDs, probenecid: May decrease the effects of torsemide.
Other antihypertensives: May increase the antihypertensive effect of other antihypertensives.
Herbal
None known.
Food
None known.

DIAGNOSTIC TEST EFFECTS
May increase BUN, serum creatinine, and uric acid levels. May decrease serum calcium, chloride, magnesium, potassium, and sodium levels.

IV INCOMPATIBILITIES
Do not mix with any other medications.

IV COMPATIBILITIES
Milrinone (Primacor)

SIDE EFFECTS
Frequent (10%–4%)
Headache, dizziness, rhinitis
Occasional (3%–1%)
Asthenia, insomnia, nervousness, diarrhea, constipation, nausea, dyspepsia, edema, electrocardiogram (EKG) changes, sore throat, cough, arthralgia, myalgia
Rare (less than 1%)
Syncope, hypotension, arrhythmias

SERIOUS REACTIONS
• Ototoxicity may occur with a too rapid IV rate or with high dosages, torsemide must be administered slowly.
• Overdosage produces acute, profound water loss, volume and electrolyte depletion, dehydration, decreased blood volume, and circulatory collapse.

NURSING CONSIDERATIONS

Baseline Assessment
• Monitor the patient's electrolyte levels, especially potassium levels.
• Obtain and record the patient's baseline weight.
• Evaluate the patient for rhonchi and crackles in lungs.

Lifespan Considerations
• Be aware that it is unknown if torsemide is excreted in breast milk.
• Be aware that the safety and efficacy of this drug have not been established in children.
• There are no age-related precautions noted in the elderly.

Precautions
• Use extremely cautiously in patients with a hypersensitivity to sulfonamides.
• Use cautiously in cardiac patients, elderly patients, and patients with ascites, cirrhosis of the liver, history of ventricular arrhythmias, renal impairment, and systemic lupus erythematosus.
• Use cautiously in pediatric patients because the safety of torsemide use in children is unknown.

Administration and Handling
PO
• Give torsemide without regard to food. Give torsemide with food to avoid GI upset, preferably with breakfast to help prevent nocturia.
IV
◀ALERT▶ Flush IV line with 0.9% NaCl before and after torsemide administration.
• Store torsemide at room temperature.
• May give undiluted as IV push over 2 minutes.
• For continuous IV infusion, dilute with 0.9% or 0.45% NaCl or D_5W and infuse over 24 hours.
• Know that a too rapid IV rate and high dosages may cause ototoxicity. Administer IV push slowly.

Intervention and Evaluation
• Monitor the patient's blood pressure (B/P), serum electrolytes, especially potassium levels, intake and output, and weight.
• Notify the physician of any hearing abnormality experienced by the patient.
• Note the extent of patient diuresis.
• Assess the patient's lungs for crackles and rhonchi.
• Evaluate the patient for edema, particularly of dependent areas.
• Assess the patient for signs of hypokalemia, including cardiac arrhythmias, change in mental status and muscle strength, or tremor. Know that less potassium is lost with torsemide than with furosemide.

Patient Teaching
• Instruct the patient to take torsemide in the morning to prevent nocturia.
• Tell the patient to expect an increase in the frequency and volume of urination.
• Warn the patient to notify the physician if he or she experiences cramps, dizziness, irregular heartbeats, muscle weakness, or nausea.
• Caution the patient against taking other medications, including over-the-counter drugs, without first consulting the physician.
• Encourage the patient to eat foods high in potassium such as apricots, bananas, legumes, meat, orange juice, white or sweet potatoes, raising, and whole grains, such as cereals.

triamterene

try-**am**-tur-een
(Dyrenium)
Do not confuse with diazoxide, Maxidex, and trimipramine.

CATEGORY AND SCHEDULE

Pregnancy Risk Category: C
(D if used in pregnancy-induced hypertension)

MECHANISM OF ACTION

A potassium-sparing diuretic that inhibits sodium, potassium, ATPase. Interferes with sodium and potassium exchange in distal tubule, cortical collecting tubule, and collecting duct. *Therapeutic Effect:* Increases sodium and decreases potassium excretion. Also increases magnesium, decreases calcium loss.

PHARMACOKINETICS

Route	Onset	Peak	Duration
PO	2–4 hrs	N/A	7–9 hrs

Incompletely absorbed from the gastrointestinal (GI) tract. Widely distributed. Metabolized in liver. Primarily eliminated in feces via biliary route. **Half-life:** 1.5–2.5 hrs (half-life is increased in patients with impaired renal function).

AVAILABILITY

Capsules: 50 mg, 100 mg.

INDICATIONS AND DOSAGES

▶ **Edema, hypertension**
PO
Adults, Elderly. 25–100 mg/day in 1 or 2 divided doses. Maximum: 300 mg/day.
Children. 2–4 mg/kg/day in 1 or 2 divided doses. Maximum: 6 mg/kg/day or 300 mg/day.

UNLABELED USES

Treatment adjunct for hypertension, prophylaxis and treatment of hypokalemia

CONTRAINDICATIONS

Drug-induced or preexisting hyperkalemia, progressive or severe renal disease, severe liver disease

INTERACTIONS
Drug

Angiotensin-converting enzyme (ACE) inhibitors, such as captopril, potassium-containing medications, potassium supplements: May increase serum potassium levels.
Anticoagulants, heparin: May decrease the effects of anticoagulants and heparin.
Lithium: May decrease the clearance and increase the risk of toxicity of lithium.
NSAIDs: May decrease the antihypertensive effect.
Herbal
None known.
Food
None known.

DIAGNOSTIC TEST EFFECTS

May increase blood glucose, BUN, calcium, serum creatinine, potassium, and uric acid. May decrease serum magnesium and sodium.

SIDE EFFECTS

Occasional
Fatigue, nausea, diarrhea, abdominal distress, leg aches, headache
Rare
Anorexia, weakness, rash, dizziness

SERIOUS REACTIONS

• May produce hyponatremia (drowsiness, dry mouth, increased

thirst, lack of energy) or severe hyperkalemia (irritability, anxiety, heaviness of legs, paresthesia, hypotension, bradycardia, EKG changes [tented T waves, widening QRS, ST depression]).
• Agranulocytosis, nephrolithiasis, and thrombocytopenia occur rarely.

NURSING CONSIDERATIONS

Baseline Assessment
• Assess the patient's baseline electrolytes, particularly for low serum potassium levels.
• Assess the patient's BUN, serum creatinine, and serum hepatic enzyme levels to assess renal function.
• Examine the patient for edema and note its extent and location.
• Evaluate the patient's mucous membranes and skin turgor for hydration status.
• Evaluate the patient's mental status and muscle strength.
• Assess the patient's skin moisture and temperature.
• Obtain and record the patient's baseline weight.
• Begin monitoring the patient's fluid intake and output.
• Assess the patient's pulse rate and rhythm.

Lifespan Considerations
• Be aware that triamterene crosses the placenta and is distributed in breast milk. Breast-feeding is not recommended in this patient population.
• Be aware that the safety and efficacy of this drug have not been established in children.
• Be aware that the elderly may be at increased risk for developing hyperkalemia.

Precautions
• Use cautiously in patients with diabetes mellitus, history of renal calculi, and impaired liver and renal functions.
• Use cautiously in patients receiving other potassium-sparing diuretics or potassium supplements.

Administration and Handling
PO
• Give triamterene with food if GI disturbances occur.
• Do not crush or break capsules.

Intervention and Evaluation
• Monitor the patient's B/P, electrolytes, particularly potassium levels, fluid intake and output, vital signs, and daily weight.
• Record the amount of patient diuresis.
• Observe the patient for changes from the initial assessment. Hypokalemia may result in change in mental status, muscle cramps, nausea, tachycardia, tremor, vomiting, and weakness.
• Assess the patient's lung sounds for rhonchi and wheezing.

Patient Teaching
• Tell the patient to expect an increase in the frequency and volume of urination.
• Instruct the patient to take triamterene in the morning to help prevent nocturia.
• Inform the patient that the drug's therapeutic effect takes several days to begin and can last for several days after the drug is discontinued.
• Warn the patient to notify the physician if he or she experiences dry mouth, fever, headache, nausea, persistent or severe weakness, sore throat, unusual bleeding or bruising, and vomiting.
• Encourage the patient to avoid excessive intake of foods high in potassium and to avoid salt substitutes.

79 Spasmolytics

flavoxate
oxybutynin
phenazopyridine
  hydrochloride
tolterodine tartrate

Uses: Spasmolytic agents are used to treat urinary frequency and urgency, or urge incontinence. Flavoxate also relieves other symptoms of cystitis, proctatitis, urethritis, and related disorders. Oxybutynin also minimizes other symptoms of neurogenic bladder. Phenazopyridine also relieves other symptoms of urinary mucosal irritation, which may be caused by infection, trauma, or surgery. Tolterodine also reduces other symptoms of overactive bladder.

Action: Most spasmolytics competitively block the actions of acetylcholine at muscarinic receptors. Because of this cholinergic blockade, flavoxate, oxybutynin, and tolterodine relax detrusor and other smooth muscle, counteracting muscle spasms in the urinary tract. Phenazopyridine exerts a topical analgesic effect on the urinary mucosa.

COMBINATION PRODUCTS

ZOTRIM: phenazopyridine/ trimethoprim (an anti-infective)/ sulfamethoxazole (a sulfonamide) 200 mg/160 mg/800 mg.

---

flavoxate

flay-**vocks**-ate
(Urispas)
Do not confuse with Urised.

CATEGORY AND SCHEDULE

Pregnancy Risk Category: B

MECHANISM OF ACTION

An anticholinergic that relaxes detrusor and other smooth muscle by cholinergic blockade, counteracting muscle spasm of urinary tract. *Therapeutic Effect:* Produces anticholinergic, local anesthetic, analgesic effect, relieving urinary symptoms.

AVAILABILITY

Tablets: 100 mg.

INDICATIONS AND DOSAGES
▸ **Urinary antispasmodic**
PO
Adults, Elderly, Adolescents.
100–200 mg 3–4 times/day.

CONTRAINDICATIONS

Duodenal or pyloric obstruction, gastrointestinal (GI) hemorrhage, GI obstruction, ileus, obstructions of the lower urinary tract

INTERACTIONS
Drug
None known.
Herbal
None known.
Food
None known.

DIAGNOSTIC TEST EFFECTS
None known.

SIDE EFFECTS

Generally well tolerated. Side effects usually mild and transient.
Frequent
Drowsiness, dry mouth, throat
Occasional
Constipation, difficult urination, blurred vision, dizziness, headache, increased light sensitivity, nausea, vomiting, stomach pain
Rare
Confusion—primarily in elderly, hypersensitivity, increase intraocular pressure, leukopenia

SERIOUS REACTIONS

• Anticholinergic effect may occur with overdose, including unsteadiness, severe dizziness, drowsiness, fever, flushed face, shortness of breath, nervousness, and irritability.

NURSING CONSIDERATIONS

Baseline Assessment
• Assess the patient's dysuria, urinary frequency, incontinence, suprapubic pain, and urinary urgency.
• Plan to obtain a urine sample for culture and sensitivity testing and urinalysis.
Precautions
• Use cautiously in patients with glaucoma.
Intervention and Evaluation
• Monitor the patient for symptomatic relief.
• Observe elderly patients for mental confusion.
Patient Teaching
• Warn the patient to avoid performing tasks that require mental alertness or motor skills until his or her response to the drug is established.
• Teach the patient about the drug's adverse side effects that are related to overdose, including unsteadiness, severe dizziness, drowsiness, fever,

flushed face, shortness of breath, nervousness, and irritability.

oxybutynin

ox-ee-**byoo**-tih-nin
(Ditropan, Ditropan XL, Oxytrol)
Do not confuse with diazepam or Oxycontin.

CATEGORY AND SCHEDULE

Pregnancy Risk Category: B

MECHANISM OF ACTION

An anticholinergic that exerts antispasmodic (papaverine-like) and antimuscarinic or atropine-like action on detrusor smooth muscle of bladder. *Therapeutic Effect:* Increases bladder capacity, diminishes frequency of uninhibited detrusor muscle contraction, delays desire to void.

PHARMACOKINETICS

Route	Onset	Peak	Duration
PO	0.5–1 hr	3–6 hrs	6–10 hrs

Rapid absorption from the gastrointestinal (GI) tract. Metabolized in liver. Primarily excreted in urine. Unknown if removed by hemodialysis. **Half-life:** 1–2.3 hrs.

AVAILABILITY

Tablets: 5 mg.
Syrup: 5 mg/5 ml.
Tablets (extended-release): 5 mg, 10 mg, 15 mg.
Transdermal: 3.9 mg.

INDICATIONS AND DOSAGES

‣ **Neurogenic bladder**
PO
Adults. 5 mg 2–3 times/day up to 5 mg 4 times/day.

Elderly. 2.5–5 mg 2 times/day. May increase by 2.5 mg/day q1–2 days.
Children older than 5 yrs. 5 mg 2 times/day up to 5 mg 4 times/day.
Children 1–5 yrs. 0.2 mg/kg/dose 2–4 times/day.
PO (extended release)
Adults. 5–10 mg/day up to 30 mg/day.
Transdermal
Adults. 3.9 mg/day 2 times/wk. Apply q3–4 days.

CONTRAINDICATIONS

GI obstruction, genitourinary (GU) obstruction, glaucoma, myasthenia gravis, partial or complete GU obstruction, toxic megacolon, ulcerative colitis

INTERACTIONS
Drug
Medications with anticholinergic effects, such as antihistamines: May increase the effects of oxybutynin.
Herbal
None known.
Food
None known.

DIAGNOSTIC TEST EFFECTS

None known.

SIDE EFFECTS

Frequent
Constipation, dry mouth, drowsiness, decreased sweating
Occasional
Decreased lacrimation, salivary or sweat gland secretion, sexual ability, urinary hesitancy and retention, suppressed lactation, blurred vision, mydriasis, nausea or vomiting, insomnia

SERIOUS REACTIONS

• Overdosage produces central nervous system (CNS) excitation, including nervousness, restlessness, hallucinations, and irritability, hypotension or hypertension, confusion, fast heartbeat or tachycardia, flushed or red face, and respiratory depression, such as shortness of breath or troubled breathing.

NURSING CONSIDERATIONS

Baseline Assessment
• Assess the patient's dysuria, urinary frequency, incontinence, and urinary urgency.
Lifespan Considerations
• Be aware that it is unknown if oxybutynin crosses the placenta or is distributed in breast milk.
• There are no age-related precautions noted in children older than 5 years of age.
• Be aware that the elderly may be more sensitive to the drug's anticholinergic effects, such as dry mouth, and urinary retention.
Precautions
• Use cautiously in patients with cardiovascular disease, hypertension, hyperthyroidism, liver or renal impairment, neuropathy, prostatic hypertrophy, and reflux esophagitis.
Administration and Handling
PO
• Give oxybutynin without regard to meals.
Intervention and Evaluation
• Monitor the patient for symptomatic relief.
• Monitor the patient's intake and output and palpate the patient's bladder for signs of urinary retention.
• Assess the patient's daily pattern of bowel activity and stool consistency.
Patient Teaching
• Urge the patient to avoid alcohol during oxybutynin therapy.
• Warn the patient to avoid performing tasks requiring mental

alertness or motor skills until his or her response to the drug is established.
• Tell the patient that oxybutynin may cause drowsiness and dry mouth.

phenazopyridine hydrochloride

feen-ah-zoe-**peer**-ih-deen
(Azo-Gesic, Azo-Standard, Phenazo[CAN], Prodium, Pyridium, Pyronium[CAN], Uristat)
Do not confuse with pyridoxine.

CATEGORY AND SCHEDULE
Pregnancy Risk Category: B

MECHANISM OF ACTION
An interstitial cystitis agent that exerts topical analgesic effect on urinary tract mucosa. *Therapeutic Effect:* Provides relief of urinary pain, burning, urgency, frequency.

PHARMACOKINETICS
Well absorbed from the gastrointestinal (GI) tract. Partially metabolized in liver. Primarily excreted in urine.

AVAILABILITY
Tablets: 95 mg, 100 mg, 200 mg.

INDICATIONS AND DOSAGES
▶ **Analgesic**
PO
Adults. 100–200 mg 3–4 times/day.
Children older than 6 yrs. 12 mg/kg/day in 3 divided doses for 2 days.

▶ **Dose interval in renal impairment**

Creatinine Clearance	Interval
50–80 ml/min	q8–16h
less than 50 ml/min	Avoid use

CONTRAINDICATIONS
Liver and renal insufficiency

INTERACTIONS
Drug
None known.
Herbal
None known.
Food
None known.

DIAGNOSTIC TEST EFFECTS
May interfere with urinalysis color reactions, such as urinary glucose, ketone tests, urinary protein, or determination of urinary steroids.

SIDE EFFECTS
Occasional
Headache, GI disturbance, rash, pruritus

SERIOUS REACTIONS
• Overdosage levels or patients with impaired renal function or severe hypersensitivity may develop renal toxicity, hemolytic anemia, and liver toxicity.
• Methemoglobinemia generally occurs as result of massive and acute overdosage.

NURSING CONSIDERATIONS
Lifespan Considerations
• Be aware that it is unknown if phenazopyridine crosses the placenta or is distributed in breast milk.
• There are no age-related precautions noted in children older than 6 years of age.

• In the elderly, age-related renal impairment may increase toxicity.
Administration and Handling
PO
• Give phenazopyridine with meals.
Intervention and Evaluation
• Assess the patient for therapeutic response, relief of burning, frequency of urination, pain, burning, and urgency.
Patient Teaching
• Tell the patient that his or her urine will turn a reddish orange color during phenazopyridine therapy.
• Explain to the patient that this drug may stain fabric.
• Instruct the patient to take phenazopyridine with meals to reduce the possibility of GI upset.

---

tolterodine tartrate
toll-**tear**-oh-deen
(Detrol, Detrol LA)

CATEGORY AND SCHEDULE
Pregnancy Risk Category: C

MECHANISM OF ACTION
An antispasmodic that exhibits potent antimuscarinic activity by interceding via cholinergic muscarinic receptors, thereby relaxing urinary bladder contraction. *Therapeutic Effect:* Decreases urinary frequency, urgency.

PHARMACOKINETICS
Rapidly, well absorbed after PO administration. Protein binding: 96%. Extensive first-pass hepatic metabolism to active metabolite. Primarily excreted in urine. Unknown if removed by hemodialysis.
Half-life: 1.9–3.7 hrs.

AVAILABILITY
Tablets: 1 mg, 2 mg.
Capsules (extended-release): 2 mg, 4 mg.

INDICATIONS AND DOSAGES
▸ **Overactive bladder**
PO
Adults, Elderly. 1–2 mg twice a day.
▸ **Severe liver impairment**
Adults, Elderly. 1 mg twice a day.
PO (extended-release)
Adults, Elderly. 2–4 mg once a day.

CONTRAINDICATIONS
Uncontrolled narrow-angle glaucoma, urinary retention

INTERACTIONS
Drug
Clarithromycin, erythromycin, itraconazole, ketoconazole, miconazole: May increase tolterodine blood concentration.
Fluoxetine: May inhibit the metabolism of tolterodine.
Herbal
None known.
Food
None known.

DIAGNOSTIC TEST EFFECTS
None known.

SIDE EFFECTS
Frequent (40%)
Dry mouth
Occasional (11%–4%)
Headache, dizziness, fatigue, constipation, dyspepsia, including heartburn, indigestion, and epigastric discomfort, upper respiratory infection, urinary tract infection, abnormal vision caused by altered accommodation and dry eyes, nausea, diarrhea
Rare (3%)
Somnolence, chest or back pain,

arthralgia, rash, weight gain, dry skin

SERIOUS REACTIONS

• Overdosage can result in severe anticholinergic effects, including gastrointestinal (GI) cramping, feeling of facial warmth, excessive salivation, diaphoresis, lacrimation, pallor, urinary urgency, blurred vision, and QT interval prolongation.

NURSING CONSIDERATIONS

Lifespan Considerations

• Be aware that it is unknown if tolterodine is distributed in breast milk. Breast-feeding is not recommended in this patient population.

• Be aware that the safety and efficacy of this drug have not been established in children.

• There are no age-related precautions noted in the elderly.

Precautions

• Use cautiously in patients with clinically significant bladder outflow obstruction because of a risk of urinary retention, GI obstructive disorders, such as pyloric stenosis, which raises the risk of gastric retention, renal function impairment, and treated narrow-angle glaucoma.

Administration and Handling

PO

• May give tolterodine without regard to food.

Intervention and Evaluation

• Assist the patient with ambulation if he or she experiences dizziness.

• Determine if the patient experiences a change in vision.

• Monitor the patient for incontinence and postvoid residuals.

Patient Teaching

• Tell the patient that tolterodine use may cause blurred vision, constipation, and dry eyes and mouth.

• Warn the patient to notify the physician if he or she experiences changes in mental status or confusion.

80 Miscellaneous Renal and Genitourinary Agents

sevelamer hydrochloride
sildenafil citrate
tadalafil
vardenafil

Uses: Miscellaneous renal and genitourinary agents are used for two different disorders. Sevelamer is prescribed to reduce the serum phosphorus level in patients with end-stage renal disease. Sildenafil, tadalafil, and vardenafil are used to treat male erectile dysfunction.

Action: Miscellaneous renal and genitourinary agents have distinct actions. Sevelamer binds with dietary phosphorus in the gastrointestinal tract, allowing it to be removed by normal digestive processes. Sildenafil, tadalafil, and vardenafil selectively inhibit phosphodiesterase type 5, the enzyme that normally degrades cyclic guanosine monophosphate in the corpus cavernosum of the penis. This action relaxes smooth muscle, increases blood flow, and facilitates erection.

sevelamer hydrochloride
seh-**vell**-ah-mur
(Renagel)
Do not confuse with Reglan or Regonol.

CATEGORY AND SCHEDULE
Pregnancy Risk Category: C

MECHANISM OF ACTION
An antihyperphosphatemia that binds and removes dietary phosphorus in the gastrointestinal (GI) tract and eliminates phosphorus through normal digestive process. *Therapeutic Effect:* Decreases incidence of hypercalcemic episodes in patients receiving calcium acetate treatment.

PHARMACOKINETICS
Not absorbed systemically. Unknown if removed by hemodialysis.

AVAILABILITY
Capsules: 403 mg.
Tablets: 400 mg, 800 mg.

INDICATIONS AND DOSAGES
▸ **Hyperphosphatemia**
PO
Adults, Elderly. 800–1600 mg with each meal depending on severity of hyperphosphatemia.

CONTRAINDICATIONS
Bowel obstruction, hypophosphatemia

INTERACTIONS
Drug
None known.
Herbal
None known.
Food
None known.

DIAGNOSTIC TEST EFFECTS
None known.

SIDE EFFECTS
Frequent (20%–11%)
Infection, pain, hypotension, diarrhea, dyspepsia, nausea, vomiting
Occasional (10%–1%)
Headache, constipation, hypertension, thrombosis, increased coughing

SERIOUS REACTIONS
• None known.

NURSING CONSIDERATIONS
Baseline Assessment
• Obtain the patient's baseline serum phosphorus level.
• Assess the patient for signs of bowel obstruction, including absent bowel sounds, abdominal distension, and pain.
Lifespan Considerations
• Be aware that sevelamer is not distributed in breast milk.
• Be aware that the safety and efficacy of sevelamer have not been established in children.
• There are no age-related precautions noted in the elderly.
Precautions
• Use cautiously in patients with dysphagia, major GI tract surgery, severe GI tract motility disorders, and swallowing disorders.
Administration and Handling
PO
• Give sevelamer with meals.
• Do not break capsules apart before administration because contents expand in water.
• Space other medications by 1 hour or more before or 3 hours after sevelamer.
Intervention and Evaluation
• Monitor the patient's serum bicarbonate, chloride, serum calcium, and phosphorus levels.
Patient Teaching
• Instruct the patient to take sevelamer with meals and to swallow sevelamer capsules or tablets whole.
• Tell the patient to take other medications 1 hour or more before or 3 hours after sevelamer.
• Warn the patient to notify the physician if he or she experiences diarrhea, hypotension, nausea, persistent headache, or vomiting.

sildenafil citrate
sill-**den**-ah-fill
(Viagra)
Do not confuse with Vaniqa.

CATEGORY AND SCHEDULE
Pregnancy Risk Category: B

MECHANISM OF ACTION
An erectile dysfunction adjunct that inhibits type V cyclic GMP, a specific phosphodiesterase, the predominant isoenzyme in human corpus cavernosum in the penis. *Therapeutic Effect:* Relaxes smooth muscle, and increases blood flow, facilitating an erection.

AVAILABILITY
Tablets: 25 mg, 50 mg, 100 mg.

INDICATIONS AND DOSAGES
▶ **Erectile dysfunction**
PO
Adults. 50 mg (30 minutes–4 hrs before sexual activity). Range: 25–100 mg.

UNLABELED USES
Diabetic gastroparesis, treatment of sexual dysfunction from SSRI antidepressants

CONTRAINDICATIONS
Concurrent use of organic nitrates or sodium nitroprusside in any form

INTERACTIONS
Drug
Cimetidine, erythromycin, itraconazole, ketoconazole: May increase sildenafil plasma concentration.
Nitrates: Potentiates the hypotensive effects of nitrates.
Herbal
None known.
Food
High-fat meals: When taken concurrently, reduces the absorption rate of absorption and time to maximum effectiveness by 1 hour.

DIAGNOSTIC TEST EFFECTS
None known.

SIDE EFFECTS
Occasional
Headache, flushing (16%–10%), dyspepsia, such as heartburn, indigestion, and epigastric pain, nasal congestion, urinary tract infection, abnormal vision, diarrhea (7%–3%)
Rare (2%)
Dizziness, rash

SERIOUS REACTIONS
• None known.

NURSING CONSIDERATIONS
Baseline Assessment
• Expect to assess the patient's cardiovascular status before beginning sildenafil treatment for erectile dysfunction.
Precautions
• Use cautiously in patients with anatomic deformation of the penis, cardiac, liver and renal function impairment, and predisposition to priapism, including leukemia, multiple myeloma, and sickle cell anemia.
Administration and Handling
PO
• May take approximately 1 hour before sexual activity but may

be taken anywhere from 4 hours to 30 minutes before sexual activity.
Patient Teaching
• Tell the patient that sildenafil has no effect in the absence of sexual stimulation.
• Explain to the patient that high fat meals reduce the absorption rate and time to maximum effectiveness by 1 hour.

tadalafil
tah-**dal**-ah-fil
(Cialis)

CATEGORY AND SCHEDULE
Pregnancy Risk Category: not applicable

MECHANISM OF ACTION
A phosphodiesterase inhibitor that increases cyclic guanosine monophosphate in smooth muscle cells by inhibiting a specific enzyme, phosphodiesterase type 5, the predominant isoenzyme in human corpus cavernosum in the penis. *Therapeutic Effect:* Relaxes smooth muscle, increases blood flow, resulting in penile rigidity.

PHARMACOKINETCS

Route	Onset	Peak	Duration
PO	16 min	2 hrs	36 hrs

Rapidly absorbed following PO administration. No effect on penile blood flow without sexual stimulation. **Half-life:** 17.5 hours.

AVAILABILITY
Tablets: 5 mg, 10 mg, 20 mg.

INDICATIONS AND DOSAGES
▶ **Erectile dysfunction**
PO
Adults, Elderly. 10 mg prior to sexual activity. Dose may be increased to 20 mg or decreased to 5 mg, based on tolerability. Maximum dosing frequency is once daily.
▶ **Moderate renal function impairment, serum creatinine 31–50 ml/min**
PO
Adults, Elderly. 5 mg prior to sexual activity. Maximum dose: 10 mg not more than once every 48 hours.
▶ **Mild or moderate hepatic function impairment (Child-Pugh class A or B)**
PO
Adults, Elderly. No more than 10 mg once a day.

CONTRAINDICATIONS
Patients concurrently using any alpha blocker other than 0.4 mg once a day tamsulosin, and nitrates or sodium nitroprusside in any form because it potentiates hypotensive effects of these medications, severe liver impairment

INTERACTIONS
Drug
Alcohol: Increases the potential for postural hypotension.
Doxazosin: May produce additive hypotensive effects.
Erythromycin, indinavir, itraconazole, ketoconazole, ritonavir: May increase tadalafil blood concentration.
Nitrates: Potentiates hypotensive effects of nitrates. Concurrent use of nitrates is contraindicated.
Herbal
None known.
Food
None known.

DIAGNOSTIC TEST EFFECTS
None known.

SIDE EFFECTS
Occasional
Headache, dyspepsia, including heartburn, indigestion, and epigastric pain, back pain, myalgia, nasal congestion, flushing

SERIOUS REACTIONS
• Prolonged erections (over 4 hours) and priapism or painful erections over 6 hours in duration, occur rarely.

NURSING CONSIDERATIONS
Baseline Assessment
• Assess the patient's cardiovascular status before beginning treatment for erectile dysfunction.
Lifespan Considerations
• There are no age-related precautions noted in the elderly.
• Be aware that this drug is not indicated for use in women and children.
Precautions
• Use cautiously in patients with anatomical deformation of the penis, liver or renal function impairment, and patients that may be predisposed to priapism such as those with leukemia, multiple myeloma, and sickle cell anemia.
Administration and Handling
PO
• May give without regard to food.
• Do not crush or break film-coated tablets.
Patient Teaching
• Explain to the patient that the drug has no effect in the absence of sexual stimulation.
• Warn the patient to seek treatment immediately if he experiences an erection longer than 4 hours.

vardenafil
var-**den**-ah-fill
(Levitra)

CATEGORY AND SCHEDULE
Pregnancy Risk Category: not
applicable

MECHANISM OF ACTION
An erectile dysfunction adjunct that
inhibits a specific enzyme, phosphodiesterase type 5, the predominant
isoenzyme in human corpus cavernosum in the penis. *Therapeutic
Effect:* Relaxes smooth muscle,
increases blood flow, resulting in
penile rigidity.

PHARMACOKINETICS
Rapidly absorbed following oral
administration. Extensive tissue
distribution. Protein binding: 95%.
Metabolized in the liver. Excreted
predominately in the feces with a
lesser amount eliminated in the
urine. No effect on penile blood
flow without sexual stimulation.
Half-life: 4–5 hrs.

AVAILABILITY
Tablets: 2.5 mg, 5 mg, 10 mg,
20 mg.

INDICATIONS AND DOSAGES
▸ **Erectile dysfunction**
PO
Adults. 10 mg approximately
60 min prior to sexual activity.
Dose may be increased to 20 mg or
decreased to 5 mg, based on tolera-
bility. Maximum dosing frequency
is once daily.
Elderly older than 65 yrs. 5 mg.
▸ **Moderate hepatic function impair-
ment (Child-Pugh B)**
PO
Adults. 5 mg prior to sexual activity.

▸ **Concurrent ritonavir**
PO
Adults. 2.5 mg in a 72-hour period.
▸ **Concurrent ketoconazole and itra-
conazole at 400 mg/day, indinavir**
PO
Adults. 2.5 mg in a 24-hour period.
▸ **Concurrent ketoconazole and
itraconazole at 200 mg/day, erythro-
mycin**
PO
Adults. 5 mg in a 24-hour period.

CONTRAINDICATIONS
Patients concurrently using alpha-
blocking agents, and nitrates or
sodium nitroprusside in any form
because it potentiates hypotensive
effects of these medications

INTERACTIONS
Drug
*Erythromycin, indinavir, itracona-
zole, ketoconazole, ritonavir:* May
increase vardenafil concentration.
Nitrates: Potentiates the hypotensive
effects of nitrates. Concurrent use of
nitrates is contraindicated.
Herbal
None known.
Food
High-fat meals: Time to maximum
effectiveness is delayed briefly
when taken with a high-fat meal.

DIAGNOSTIC TEST EFFECTS
None known.

SIDE EFFECTS
Occasional
Headache, flushing, rhinitis, indiges-
tion
Rare (less than 2%)
Dizziness, changes in color vision,
blurred vision

SERIOUS REACTIONS
• Prolonged erections for over
4 hours and priapism or painful

erections over 6 hours in duration occur rarely.

NURSING CONSIDERATIONS

Baseline Assessment
• Assess the patient's cardiovascular status before beginning treatment for erectile dysfunction.

Lifespan Considerations
• There are no age-related precautions noted in the elderly, but the initial drug dose should be 5 mg.

Precautions
• Use cautiously in patients with anatomical deformation of the penis, liver or renal function impairment, and patients that may be predisposed to priapism, including patients with leukemia, multiple myeloma, and sickle cell anemia.

Administration and Handling
PO
• May take approximately 1 hour before sexual activity.
• Do not crush or break film-coated tablets.

Patient Teaching
• Explain to the patient that the drug has no effect in the absence of sexual stimulation.
• Warn the patient to seek treatment immediately if he experiences an erection for longer than 4 hours.
• Explain that the time to maximum effectiveness is delayed briefly when taken with a high-fat meal.

azelastine
cetirizine
clemastine fumarate
desloratidine
diphenhydramine
hydrochloride
fexofenadine
hydrochloride
hydroxyzine
loratadine
promethazine
hydrochloride

Uses: Antihistamines are chiefly used to relieve symptoms of upper respiratory allergic disorders. They're also used to manage allergic reactions to other drugs as well as blood transfusion reactions. These agents are used as a second choice in treating angioneurotic edema. Some can be used to provide preoperative and postoperative sedation, to manage insomnia, to relieve anxiety and tension, and to control muscle spasms. They also may be used to treat acute urticaria, other dermatologic conditions, motion sickness, and Parkinson's disease.

Action: As histamine (H_1) antagonists, antihistamines cause vasoconstriction, which helps decrease edema, bronchodilation, and mucus secretion. These agents also block the increased capillary permeability and formation of edema and wheals caused by histamine. Many antihistamines can bind to receptors in the central nervous system, causing primarily depression (with decreased alertness, slowed reaction times, and somnolence), but also stimulation (with restlessness, nervousness, and inability to sleep). Some may counter motion sickness. (See illustration, *Sites of Action: Respiratory Agents*, page 1364.)

COMBINATION PRODUCTS

ALLEGRA-D: fexofenadine/pseudo-ephedrine (a nasal decongestant) 60 mg/120 mg.

CALADRYL: diphenhydramine/calamine (an astringent)/camphor (a counterirritant).

CLARITIN-D: loratadine/pseudo-ephedrine (a nasal decongestant) 5 mg/ 120 mg; 10 mg/240 mg.

PHENERGAN WITH CODEINE: promethazine/codeine (a cough suppressant) 6.25 mg/10 mg per 5 ml.

PHENERGAN VC: promethazine/phenylephrine (a vasopressor) 6.25 mg/5 mg per 5 ml.

PHENERGAN VC WITH CODEINE: promethazine/phenylephrine (a vasopressor)/codeine (a cough suppressant) 6.25 mg/5 mg/10 mg per 5 ml.

ZYRTEC D-12 HOUR TABLETS: cetirizine/pseudoephedrine (a nasal decongestant) 5 mg/120 mg.

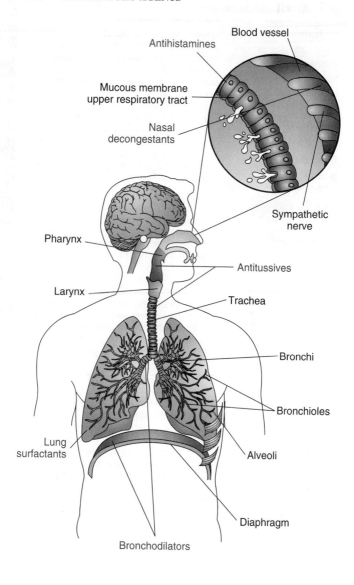

Sites of Action: Respiratory Agents

Drugs from several classes are used to manage respiratory disorders. Each class of drugs—and individual drugs within each class—can act at different sites in the respiratory tract.

Antihistamines, such as diphenhydramine, help relieve symptoms of upper respiratory allergic disorders by blocking the stimulation of histamine$_1$ (H_1 receptors primarily in the mucous membranes of the upper respiratory tract. Normally, H_1-receptor stimulation results in vasodilation, increased capillary permeability and mucous secretion, and bronchoconstriction. When antihistamines block H_1 receptors, vasoconstriction occurs, which decreases edema, capillary permeability, and mucous secretion. The drugs also cause bronchodilation, improving airflow to and from the lungs. Unlike first-generation antihistamines, such as diphenhydramine, which cross the blood-brain barrier and cause sedation, second-generation antihistamines, such as loratidine, don't cross the blood-brain barrier and produce little or no sedation.

Non-narcotic antitussives, such as benzonatate, act on the stretch and cough receptors in the respiratory tract, including the pharynx, larynx and tracheobronchial tree. Because benzonatate also has local anesthetic properties, it anesthetizes irritated tissues and suppresses cough. Another antitussive, guaifenesin, has an expectorant action that alters respiratory tract secretions, making mucous more viscous and less adhesive and making the cough more productive.

All bronchodilators open the bronchioles to improve airflow. However, subclasses of bronchodilators work in different ways. Beta$_2$-adrenergic agonists may be short-acting, such as albuterol, and long-acting, such as salmeterol. Both types stimulate beta$_2$ receptors in the lungs, resulting in relaxation of bronchial smooth muscle, increased vital capacity, and decreased airway resistance. These agents also block histamine release from mast cells, decreasing capillary permeability and mucous secretion. Anticholinergics, such as ipratropium, block muscarinic cholinergic receptors in the bronchi, leading to bronchodilation. These drugs exert more action on larger airways, whereas beta$_2$-adrenergic agonists act primarily on smaller airways, Methylxanthines, such as aminophylline, work by inhibiting phosphodiesterase and adenosine, relaxing bronchial smooth muscle and promoting bronchodilation. These drugs also increase the contractility of the diaphragm and may enhance mucous clearance.

Lung surfactants, such as beractant, restore pulmonary surfactant in infants who have a deficiency of it. They work by lowering the surface tension on alveoli. As a result, the alveoli become more stable and less likely to collapse. These actions lead to improved lung compliance and respiratory gas exchange.

Nasal decongestants, such as pseudoephedrine, constrict blood vessels in the nose by mimicking the actions of the sympathetic nervous system. They directly stimulate alpha$_1$-adrenergic receptors in the smooth muscle of nasal blood vessels, which shrinks swollen mucous membranes and decreases mucous production by reducing fluid exudation.

azelastine
aye-zeh-**las**-teen
(Astelin, Optivar)

CATEGORY AND SCHEDULE
Pregnancy Risk Category: C

MECHANISM OF ACTION
An antihistamine that competes with histamine for histamine receptor sites on cells in the blood vessels, gastrointestinal (GI) tract, and respiratory tract. *Therapeutic Effect:* Inhibits symptoms associated with seasonal allergic rhinitis such as increased mucus production and sneezing.

PHARMACOKINETICS

Route	Onset	Peak	Duration
Nasal spray	0.5–1 hr	2–3 hrs	12 hrs
Ophthalmic	N/A	3 min	8 hrs

Well absorbed through nasal mucosa. Primarily excreted in feces.
Half-life: 22 hrs.

AVAILABILITY
Nasal Spray: 137 mcg.
Ophthalmic Solution: 0.05%.

INDICATIONS AND DOSAGES
▸ **Allergic rhinitis**
Nasal
Adults, Elderly, Children 12 yrs or older. 2 sprays 2 times a day.
Children 5–11 yrs. 1 spray 2 times a day.
▸ **Vasomotor rhinitis**
Nasal
Adults, Elderly, Children 12 yrs or older. 2 sprays twice a day.
▸ **Allergic conjunctivitis**
Ophthalmic
Adults, Elderly, Children 3 yrs or older. 1 drop into affected eye twice a day.

CONTRAINDICATIONS
History of hypersensitivity to antihistamines, newborn or premature infants, nursing mothers, third trimester of pregnancy

INTERACTIONS
Drug
Alcohol, central nervous system (CNS) depressants: May increase CNS depression.
Cimetidine: May increase azelastine blood concentration.
Herbal
None known.
Food
None known.

DIAGNOSTIC TEST EFFECTS
May suppress flare and wheal reaction to antigen skin testing unless drug is discontinued 4 days before testing. May increase SGPT (AST) levels.

SIDE EFFECTS
Frequent (20%–15%)
Headache, bitter taste
Rare
Nasal burning, paroxysmal sneezing
Ophthalmic: Transient eye burning or stinging, bitter taste, headache

SERIOUS REACTIONS
• Epistaxis or nosebleed occurs rarely.

NURSING CONSIDERATIONS

Baseline Assessment
• Determine if the patient has a hypersensitivity to antihistamines.
Lifespan Considerations
• Be aware that it is unknown if azelastine crosses the placenta or is distributed in breast milk.

• Do not use azelastine in patients during the third trimester of pregnancy.
• Be aware that the safety and efficacy of azelastine have not been established in children younger than 12 years old.
• There are no age-related precautions noted in the elderly.

Precautions
• Use cautiously in patients with renal function impairment.

Administration and Handling
Nasal
• Clear the patient's nasal passages as much as possible before use.
• Tilt the patient's head slightly forward.
• Insert the spray tip into one of the patient's nostrils, pointing the spray toward the nasal passage, away from nasal septum.
• Spray into the patient's nostril while holding the patient's other nostril closed and instruct the patient to inhale at the same time through his or her nose to deliver the medication as high into the nasal passages as possible.
Ophthalmic
• Tilt the patient's head back; place solution in conjunctival sac.
• Have the patient close his or her eyes, then press gently on the lacrimal sac for 1 minute.

Intervention and Evaluation
• Assess the patient's therapeutic response to the medication.

Patient Teaching
• Advise the patient to clear his or her nasal passages before using azelastine.
• Teach the patient that before using the medication the first time, he or she should prime the pump with 4 sprays or until a fine mist appears. After the first use and if the pump hasn't been used for 3 or more days, tell the patient to prime the pump with 2 sprays or until a fine mist appears.
• Teach the patient to wipe the tip of the applicator with a clean, damp tissue and to replace the cap immediately after use.
• Warn the patient to avoid spraying the medication in the eyes.

cetirizine
sih-**tier**-eh-zeen
(Reactine[CAN], Zyrtec)
Do not confuse with Zyprexa.

CATEGORY AND SCHEDULE
Pregnancy Risk Category: B

MECHANISM OF ACTION
A second-generation piperazine that competes with histamine for H_1-receptor sites on effector cells in the gastrointestinal (GI) tract, blood vessels, and respiratory tract. *Therapeutic Effect:* Prevents allergic response, produces mild bronchodilation, blocks histamine-induced bronchitis.

PHARMACOKINETICS

Route	Onset	Peak	Duration
PO	less than 1 hr	4–8 hr	less than 24 hrs

Rapidly, almost completely absorbed from GI tract. Protein binding: 93%. Food has no effect on absorption. Undergoes low first-pass metabolism; not extensively metabolized. Primarily excreted in urine (greater than 80% as unchanged drug). **Half-life:** 6.5–10 hrs.

AVAILABILITY
Tablets: 5 mg, 10 mg.
Syrup: 5 mg/5 ml.

INDICATIONS AND DOSAGES
▶ **Allergic rhinitis, hives**
PO
Adults. 5–10 mg/day. May increase up to 20 mg/day.
Elderly. Initially, 5 mg/day. May increase to 10 mg/day.
Children 6–11 yrs. 5–10 mg once a day.
Children 2–5 yrs. Initially, 2.5 mg once a day. Maximum: 5 mg once a day or 2.5 mg q12h.
▶ **Renal impairment, creatinine clearance 11–31 ml/min, hemodialysis, creatinine clearance less than 7 ml/min, hepatic impairment**
PO
Adults, Elderly. 5 mg once a day.

UNLABELED USES
Treatment of bronchial asthma

CONTRAINDICATIONS
Hypersensitivity to cetirizine, hydroxyzine

INTERACTIONS
Drug
Alcohol, central nervous system (CNS) depressants: May increase CNS depression.
Herbal
None known.
Food
None known.

DIAGNOSTIC TEST EFFECTS
May suppress wheal and flare reactions to antigen skin testing, unless antihistamines are discontinued 4 days before testing.

SIDE EFFECTS
Minimal anticholinergic effects
Occasional (10%–2%)
Pharyngitis, dry mouth, nose, throat, nausea, vomiting, abdominal pain, headache, dizziness, fatigue, thickening mucus, drowsiness, increased sensitivity of skin to sun

SERIOUS REACTIONS
• Children may experience dominant paradoxical reaction, including restlessness, insomnia, euphoria, nervousness, and tremors.
• Dizziness, sedation, and confusion more likely to occur in elderly patients.

NURSING CONSIDERATIONS
Baseline Assessment
• Assess the patient's lung sounds.
• Assess the severity of the patient's rhinitis, urticaria, or other symptoms.
• Expect to obtain the patient's baseline serum hepatic enzyme levels to assess liver function.
Lifespan Considerations
• Be aware that cetirizine use is not recommended during the early months of pregnancy.
• Be aware that it is unknown if cetirizine is excreted in breast milk. Breast-feeding is not recommended in this patient population.
• Be aware that cetirizine is less likely to cause anticholinergic effects in children.
• Be aware that the elderly are more sensitive to the drug's anticholinergic effects, such as dry mouth and urinary retention. Dizziness, sedation, and confusion are more likely to occur in the elderly.
Precautions
• Use cautiously in patients with impaired liver or renal function.
• Remember that cetirizine may cause drowsiness at dosages greater than 10 mg/day.

Administration and Handling
PO
• Give cetirizine without regard to meals.
Intervention and Evaluation
• Ensure that the patient with upper respiratory allergies increases fluid intake to maintain thin secretions and offset thirst.
• Monitor the patient's symptoms for therapeutic response.
Patient Teaching
• Warn the patient to avoid performing tasks that require motor skills if he or she experiences drowsiness during cetirizine therapy.
• Tell the patient to avoid alcohol during cetirizine therapy.
• Urge the patient to avoid prolonged exposure to sunlight.

clemastine fumarate
kleh-**mass**-teen
(Dayhistol, Tavist, Tavist-1)

CATEGORY AND SCHEDULE
Pregnancy Risk Category: B

MECHANISM OF ACTION
An ethanolamine that competes with histamine on effector cells in the gastrointestinal (GI) tract, blood vessels, and respiratory tract. *Therapeutic Effect:* Relieves allergic conditions, including urticaria and pruritus. Anticholinergic effects cause drying of nasal mucosa.

PHARMACOKINETICS

Route	Onset	Peak	Duration
PO	15–60 min	5–7 hrs	10–12 hrs

Well absorbed from GI tract. Metabolized in liver. Excreted primarily in urine.

AVAILABILITY
Tablets: 1.34 mg, 2.68 mg.
Syrup: 0.67 mg/5 ml, 0.5 mg/5 ml.
Elixir: 0.5 mg/ml.

INDICATIONS AND DOSAGES
▸ **Allergic rhinitis**
PO
Adults, Children older than 12 yrs. 1.34–2.68 mg 3 times/day. Maximum: 8.04 mg/day.
Children 6–12 yrs. 0.67–1.34 mg 2 times/day. Maximum: 4.02 mg/day.
Children younger than 6 yrs. 0.335–0.67 mg/day in 2–3 divided doses Maximum: 1.34 mg.
Elderly. 1.34 mg 1–2 times/day.
▸ **Allergic urticaria, angioedema**
PO
Adults, Children older than 12 yrs. 2.68 mg 1–3 times/day. Do not exceed 8.04 mg/day.
Children 6–12 yrs. 1.34 mg 2 times/day. Do not exceed 4.02 mg/day.
Elderly. 1.34 mg 1–2 times/day.

CONTRAINDICATIONS
Hypersensitivity to clemastine, narrow-angle glaucoma, patients receiving MAOIs

INTERACTIONS
Drug
Alcohol, central nervous system (CNS) depressants: May increase CNS depressant effects.
MAOIs: May increase anticholinergic and CNS depressant effects.
Herbal
None known.
Food
None known.

DIAGNOSTIC TEST EFFECTS
May suppress wheal, flare reactions to antigen skin testing, unless antihistamines discontinued 4 days prior to testing.

SIDE EFFECTS
Frequent
Drowsiness, dizziness, dry mouth, nose, or throat, urinary retention, thickening of bronchial secretions
Elderly
Frequent
Sedation, dizziness, hypotension
Occasional
Epigastric distress, flushing, blurred vision, tinnitus, paresthesia, sweating, chills

SERIOUS REACTIONS
• Children may experience dominant paradoxical reaction, including restlessness, insomnia, euphoria, nervousness, and tremors.
• Overdosage in children may result in hallucinations, convulsions, and death.
• Hypersensitivity reaction, marked by eczema, pruritus, rash, cardiac disturbances, angioedema, and photosensitivity, may occur.
• Overdosage may vary from CNS depression, including sedation, apnea, cardiovascular collapse, or death to severe paradoxical reaction, such as hallucinations, tremor, and seizures.

NURSING CONSIDERATIONS

Baseline Assessment
• Obtain the history of recently ingested drugs and foods, environmental exposure, and emotional stress of the patient undergoing allergic reaction.
• Monitor the depth, quality, rate, and rhythm of the patient's pulse.
• Monitor the patient's respirations. Assess the patient's lung sounds for crackles, rhonchi, and wheezing.

Lifespan Considerations
• Be aware that clemastine is excreted in breast milk.
• Be aware that the safety and

efficacy of clemastine have not been established in children younger than 6 years of age.
• In the elderly, age-related renal impairment may require dosage adjustment.

Precautions
• Use cautiously in patients with asthma, GI or genitourinary (GU) obstruction, peptic ulcer disease, and prostatic hypertrophy.

Administration and Handling
◀ALERT▶ Be aware that the fixed-combination form (Tavist-D) may produce mild CNS stimulation.
PO
• Give clemastine without regard to meals.
• Crush scored tablets as needed. Do not crush extended-release or film-coated forms.

Intervention and Evaluation
• Monitor the patient's blood pressure (B/P), especially in elderly patients who are at increased risk of hypotension development.
• Monitor pediatric patients closely for paradoxical reaction.

Patient Teaching
• Tell the patient that he or she will develop tolerance to the drug's antihistaminic effect.
• Explain to the patient that he or she may develop tolerance to the drug's sedative effect.
• Warn the patient to avoid performing tasks that require mental alertness or motor skills until his or her response to the drug is established.
• Inform the patient that dizziness, drowsiness, and dry mouth are expected side effects of clemastine. Explain to the patient that consuming coffee and tea may help reduce his or her drowsiness.
• Urge the patient to avoid alcohol during antihistamine therapy.

desloratidine
des-low-**rah**-tah-deen
(Clarinex)

CATEGORY AND SCHEDULE
Pregnancy Risk Category: C

MECHANISM OF ACTION
A nonsedating antihistamine that exhibits selective peripheral histamine H_1 receptor blocking action. Competes with histamine at receptor site. Desloratidine has 2.5–4 times greater potency than its parent compound, loratadine. *Therapeutic Effect:* Prevents allergic response mediated by histamine, such as rhinitis and urticaria.

PHARMACOKINETICS
Rapidly, almost completely absorbed from the gastrointestinal (GI) tract. Distributed mainly in liver, lungs, GI tract, bile. Metabolized in liver to active metabolite and undergoes extensive first-pass metabolism. Excreted in urine, eliminated in feces. **Half-life:** 27 hrs, half-life is increased in the elderly and patients with liver or renal disease.

AVAILABILITY
Tablets: 5 mg.
Reditabs: 5 mg.

INDICATIONS AND DOSAGES
▶ **Allergic rhinitis, hives**
PO
Adults, Elderly, Children older than 12 yrs. 5 mg once a day.
▶ **Liver or renal impairment**
Adults, Elderly, Children older than 12 yrs. 5 mg every other day.

CONTRAINDICATIONS
None known.

INTERACTIONS
Drug
Erythromycin, ketoconazole: May increase desloratidine blood concentrations.
Herbal
None known.
Food
None known.

DIAGNOSTIC TEST EFFECTS
May suppress wheal and flare reactions to antigen skin testing, unless antihistamines are discontinued 4 days before testing.

SIDE EFFECTS
Frequent (12%)
Headache
Occasional (3%)
Dry mouth, somnolence
Rare (less than 3%)
Fatigue, dizziness, diarrhea, nausea

SERIOUS REACTIONS
• None known.

NURSING CONSIDERATIONS
Baseline Assessment
• Assess the patient's lung sounds for wheezing and skin for urticaria.
• Plan to discontinue the drug 4 days before antigen skin testing.
Lifespan Considerations
• Be aware that desloratidine is excreted in breast milk.
• Be aware that children and the elderly are more sensitive to anticholinergic effects, such as dry mouth, nose, and throat.
Precautions
• Use cautiously in patients with liver impairment.
• Be aware that desloratidine's safety in children younger than 6 years of age is unknown.

Administration and Handling
PO
• Do not crush or break film-coated tablets.

Intervention and Evaluation
• Increase the fluid intake in patients with upper respiratory allergies to decrease the viscosity of secretions, offset thirst, and replace lost fluids from diaphoresis.
• Monitor the patient for therapeutic response.

Patient Teaching
• Tell the patient that desloratidine does not cause drowsiness.
• Warn the patient to avoid driving and performing tasks that require visual acuity if he or she experiences blurred vision or eye pain.
• Urge the patient to avoid consuming alcohol during desloratidine therapy.

diphenhydramine hydrochloride
dye-phen-**high**-dra-meen
(Allerdryl[CAN], Benadryl, Nytol[CAN], Unisom Sleepgels[AUS])
Do not confuse with benazepril, Bentyl, Benylin, calamine, or dimenhydrinate.

CATEGORY AND SCHEDULE
Pregnancy Risk Category: B
OTC (capsules, tablets, chewable tablets, syrup, elixir, cream, spray)

MECHANISM OF ACTION
An ethanolamine that competes with histamine at histaminic receptor sites. Inhibits central acetylcholine. *Therapeutic Effect:* Results in anticholinergic, antipruritic, antitus-sive, antiemetic effects. Produces antidyskinetic, sedative effect.

PHARMACOKINETICS

Route	Onset	Peak	Duration
PO	15–30 min	1–4 hrs	4–6 hrs
IM/	less than	1–4 hrs	4–6 hrs
IV	15 min		

Well absorbed after PO, parenteral administration. Widely distributed. Protein binding: 98%–99%. Metabolized in liver. Primarily excreted in urine. **Half-life:** 1–4 hrs.

AVAILABILITY
Capsules: 25 mg, 50 mg.
Tablets: 25 mg, 50 mg.
Tablets (chewable): 12.5 mg.
Syrup: 12.5 mg/5 ml.
Elixir: 12.5 mg/5 ml.
Injection: 50 mg/ml.
Cream: 2%
Spray: 2%.

INDICATIONS AND DOSAGES
▸ **Moderate to severe allergic reaction, dystonic reaction**
PO/IM/IV
Adults, Elderly. 25–50 mg q4h.
Maximum: 400 mg/day.
Children. 5 mg/kg/day in divided doses q6–8h. Maximum: 300 mg/day.
▸ **Motion sickness, minor allergic rhinitis**
PO/IM/IV
Adults, Elderly, Children 12 yrs and older. 25–50 mg q4–6h. Maximum: 300 mg/day.
Children 6–11 yrs. 12.5–25 mg q4–6h. Maximum: 150 mg/day.
Children 2–5 yrs. 6.25 mg q4–6h. Maximum: 37.5 mg/day.
▸ **Antitussive**
PO
Adults, Elderly, Children 12 yrs and

older. 25 mg q4h. Maximum:
150 mg/day.
Children 6–11 yrs. 12.5 mg q4h.
Maximum: 75 mg/day.
Children 2–5 yrs. 6.25 mg q4h.
Maximum: 37.5 mg/day.
▸ **Nighttime sleep aid**
PO
*Adults, Elderly, Children 12 yrs and
older.* 50 mg qhs.
Children 2–11 yrs. 1 mg/kg/dose.
Maximum: 50 mg.
▸ **Pruritus relief**
Topical
*Adults, Elderly, Children 12 yrs and
older.* 1% or 2% strength: Apply
3–4 times/day.
Children 2–11 yrs. 1% strength:
Apply 3–4 times/day.

CONTRAINDICATIONS

Acute asthmatic attack, patients
receiving MAOIs

INTERACTIONS
Drug
*Alcohol, central nervous system
(CNS) depressants:* May increase
CNS depressant effects.
Anticholinergics: May increase
anticholinergic effects.
MAOIs: May increase anticholiner-
gic and CNS depressant effects.
Herbal
None known.
Food
None known.

DIAGNOSTIC TEST EFFECTS

May suppress wheal and flare reactions to antigen skin testing unless
antihistamines are discontinued
4 days before testing.

IV INCOMPATIBILITIES

Allopurinol (Aloprim), amphotericin
B complex (Abelcet, AmBisome,
Amphotec), cefepime (Maxipime),

dexamethasone (Decadron), foscarnet (Foscavir)

IV COMPATIBILITIES

Atropine, cisplatin (Platinol), cyclophosphamide (Cytoxan), cytarabine
(ARA-C), droperidol (Inapsine),
fentanyl, glycopyrrolate (Robinul),
heparin, hydrocortisone (Solu-
Cortef), hydromorphone (Dilaudid), hydroxyzine (Vistaril), lidocaine, metoclopramide (Reglan),
ondansetron (Zofran), potassium chloride,
propofol (Diprivan)

SIDE EFFECTS
Frequent
Drowsiness, dizziness, muscular
weakness, hypotension, dry mouth,
nose, throat, and lips, urinary reten-
tion, thickening of bronchial secre-
tions
Elderly
Frequent
Sedation, dizziness, hypotension
Occasional
Epigastric distress, flushing, visual
or hearing disturbances, paresthesia,
diaphoresis, chills

SERIOUS REACTIONS

• Children may experience dominant paradoxical reactions, including restlessness, insomnia, euphoria,
nervousness, and tremors.
• Overdosage in children may result
in hallucinations, seizures, and
death.
• Hypersensitivity reaction, such as
eczema, pruritus, rash, cardiac
disturbances, and photosensitivity,
may occur.
• Overdosage may vary from CNS
depression, including sedation,
apnea, hypotension, cardiovascular
collapse, or death to severe paradoxical reaction, such as hallucinations, tremor, and seizures.

NURSING CONSIDERATIONS

Baseline Assessment

• Obtain the history of recently ingested drugs and food, emotional stress, and environmental exposure in patients having acute allergic reaction.

• Monitor the depth, rate, rhythm, and type of patient respirations and the quality and rate of the patient's pulse.

• Assess the patient's lung sounds for crackles, rhonchi, and wheezing.

• Plan to discontinue drug 4 days prior to antigen skin testing.

Lifespan Considerations

• Be aware that diphenhydramine crosses the placenta and is detected in breast milk. Also know that diphenhydramine use may inhibit lactation, and that diphenhydramine use in breast-feeding women may produce irritability in breast-feeding infants.

• Be aware that there is an increased risk of seizures in neonates and premature infants if the drug is used during the third trimester of pregnancy.

• Be aware that diphenhydramine use is not recommended in newborns or premature infants as these groups are at an increased risk of experiencing paradoxical reaction.

• Be aware that the elderly are at an increased risk of developing confusion, dizziness, hyperexcitability, hypotension, and sedation.

Precautions

• Use cautiously in patients with asthma, cardiovascular disease, chronic obstructive pulmonary disease (COPD), hypertension, hyperthyroidism, narrow-angle glaucoma, increased intraocular pressure (IOP), peptic ulcer disease, prostatic hypertrophy, pyloro-duodenal or bladder neck obstruction, and seizure disorders.

Administration and Handling

PO

• Give diphenhydramine without regard to meals.

• Crush scored tablets as needed.

• Do not crush, break, or open capsules or film-coated tablets.

IM

• Give deep IM into large muscle mass.

IV

• May be given undiluted.

• Give IV injection over at least 1 minute.

Intervention and Evaluation

• Monitor the patient's blood pressure (B/P), especially in the elderly because of increased risk of hypotension.

• Monitor pediatric patients closely for paradoxical reaction.

Patient Teaching

• Explain to the patient that he or she will not develop a tolerance to the drug's antihistaminic effects but may develop tolerance to the drug's sedative effects.

• Warn the patient to avoid performing tasks that require mental alertness or motor skills until his or her response to the drug is established.

• Warn the patient that expected responses to the drug include dizziness, drowsiness, and dry mouth.

• Urge the patient to avoid consuming alcohol during diphenhydramine therapy.

fexofenadine hydrochloride
fecks-**oh**-fen-ah-deen
(Allegra, Telfast[AUS])

CATEGORY AND SCHEDULE
Pregnancy Risk Category: C

MECHANISM OF ACTION
A piperidine that prevents and antagonizes most histamine effects, such as urticaria and pruritus. *Therapeutic Effect:* Relieves allergic rhinitis symptoms.

PHARMACOKINETICS
Rapidly absorbed after PO administration. Does not cross blood-brain barrier. Protein binding: 60%–70%. Minimally metabolized. Eliminated in feces, excreted in urine. Not removed by hemodialysis. **Half-life:** 14.4 hrs, half-life is increased in patients with impaired renal function.

AVAILABILITY
Capsules: 60 mg.
Tablets: 30 mg, 60 mg, 180 mg.

INDICATIONS AND DOSAGES
▶ **Allergic rhinitis**
PO
Adults, Elderly, Children 12 yrs and older. 60 mg 2 times/day or 180 mg once a day.
Children 6–11 yrs. 30 mg 2 times/day.
▶ **Dosage in renal impairment**
PO
Adults, Elderly, Children 12 yrs and older. 60 mg once a day.
Children 6–11 yrs. 30 mg once a day.

CONTRAINDICATIONS
None known

INTERACTIONS
Drug
None known.
Herbal
None known.
Food
None known.

DIAGNOSTIC TEST EFFECTS
May suppress wheal and flare reactions to antigen skin testing. Discontinue at least 4 days before testing.

SIDE EFFECTS
Rare (less than 2%)
Drowsiness, headache, fatigue, nausea, vomiting, abdominal distress, dysmenorrhea

SERIOUS REACTIONS
• None known.

NURSING CONSIDERATIONS
Baseline Assessment
• Obtain the history of recently ingested drugs and foods, emotional stress, and environmental exposure in patients undergoing an allergic reaction.
• Monitor depth, rate, rhythm, and type of patient respirations and the quality and rate of the patient's pulse.
• Assess the patient's lung sounds for crackles, rhonchi, and wheezing.
• Plan to discontinue drug 4 days before antigen skin testing.
Lifespan Considerations
• Be aware that it is unknown if fexofenadine crosses the placenta or is distributed in breast milk.
• Be aware that the safety and efficacy of fexofenadine have not been established in children younger than 12 years of age.
• There are no age-related precautions noted in the elderly.

Precautions
• Use cautiously in patients with severe renal impairment.
Administration and Handling
PO
• Give fexofenadine without regard to food.
Intervention and Evaluation
• Assess the patient for therapeutic response relief from allergy symptoms including itching, red, watery eyes, rhinorrhea, and sneezing.
Patient Teaching
• Warn the patient to avoid performing tasks that require mental alertness or motor skills until his or her response to the drug is established.
• Urge the patient to avoid alcohol during antihistamine therapy.
• Tell the patient that drinking coffee or tea may help reduce drowsiness.

---

hydroxyzine
See antianxiety agents

---

loratadine
low-**rah**-tah-deen
(Claratyne[AUS], Claritin, Claritin Reditabs)

CATEGORY AND SCHEDULE
Pregnancy Risk Category: B

MECHANISM OF ACTION
An antihistamine that is long acting with selective peripheral histamine H_1 receptor antagonist action. Competes with histamine for receptor site. *Therapeutic Effect:* Prevents allergic responses mediated by histamine, such as urticaria and pruritus.

PHARMACOKINETICS

Route	Onset	Peak	Duration
PO	1–3 hrs	8–12 hrs	longer than 24 hrs

Rapidly, almost completely absorbed from the gastrointestinal (GI) tract. Protein binding: 97% (metabolite: 73%–77%). Distributed mainly in liver, lungs, GI tract, bile. Metabolized in liver to active metabolite, undergoes extensive first-pass metabolism. Excreted in urine, eliminated in feces. Not removed by hemodialysis. **Half-life:** 8.4 hrs; metabolite: 28 hrs, half-life increased in elderly, liver disease.

AVAILABILITY
Tablets: 10 mg.
Rapid Dissolution Tablet: 10 mg.
Syrup: 10 mg/10 ml.

INDICATIONS AND DOSAGES
▶ **Allergic rhinitis, hives**
PO
Adults, Elderly, Children 6 yrs and older. 10 mg once a day.
Children 2–5 yrs. 5 mg once a day.
▶ **Dosage in hepatic impairment**
Adults, Elderly, Children. 10 mg every other day.

UNLABELED USES
Adjunct treatment of bronchial asthma

CONTRAINDICATIONS
Hypersensitivity to loratadine or any ingredient

INTERACTIONS
Drug
Clarithromycin, erythromycin, fluconazole, ketoconazole: May increase loratadine blood concentrations.

Herbal
None known.
Food
Food: Delays the absorption of loratadine.

DIAGNOSTIC TEST EFFECTS

May suppress wheal and flare reactions to antigen skin testing, unless antihistamines are discontinued 4 days before testing.

SIDE EFFECTS

Frequent (12%–8%)
Headache, fatigue, drowsiness
Occasional (3%)
Dry mouth, nose, throat
Rare
Photosensitivity

SERIOUS REACTIONS

• None known.

NURSING CONSIDERATIONS

Baseline Assessment
• Assess the patient for allergy symptoms.
• Assess the patient's lung sounds for crackles, rhonchi, and wheezing, and skin for urticaria.
• Expect to discontinue the drug 4 days prior to antigen skin testing.
Lifespan Considerations
• Be aware that loratadine is excreted in breast milk.
• Be aware that children and the elderly are more sensitive to the drug's anticholinergic effects, such as dry mouth, nose, and throat.
Precautions
• Use cautiously in breast-feeding women, children, and patients with liver impairment.
Administration and Handling
PO
• Give on an empty stomach as food delays drug absorption.

Intervention and Evaluation
• Increase the fluid intake to maintain thin secretions and offset thirst and loss of fluids from increased sweating in patients with upper respiratory allergies.
• Monitor the patient for therapeutic response.
Patient Teaching
• Instruct the patient to drink plenty of water to help prevent dry mouth.
• Urge the patient to avoid consuming alcohol during antihistamine therapy.
• Explain to the patient that loratadine use may cause drowsiness.
• Warn the patient to avoid tasks requiring mental alertness or motor skills until his or her response to the drug is established.
• Tell the patient that loratadine use may cause photosensitivity reactions. Stress to the patient that he or she should avoid direct exposure to sunlight and should wear sunscreen.

---

promethazine hydrochloride
pro-**meth**-ah-zeen
(Histantil[CAN], Insomn-Eze[AUS], Phenergan)
Do not confuse with promazine.

CATEGORY AND SCHEDULE
Pregnancy Risk Category: C

MECHANISM OF ACTION

A phenothiazine that acts as an antiemetic, antihistamine, and sedative-hypnotic. As an antihistamine, inhibits histamine at histamine receptor sites. *Therapeutic Effect:* Prevents, antagonizes most allergic effects, such as urticaria and pruritus. As an antiemetic, diminishes vestibular stimulation, depresses labyrinthine function, acts on chemoreceptor trigger zone. *Therapeutic Effect:* Produces antiemetic effect. As a sedative-hypnotic, decreases stimulation to brainstem reticular formation. *Therapeutic Effect:* Produces central nervous system (CNS) depression.

PHARMACOKINETICS

Route	Onset	Peak	Duration
PO	20 min	N/A	2–8 hrs
IM	20 min	N/A	2–8 hrs
Rectal	20 min	N/A	2–8 hrs
IV	3–5 min	N/A	2–8 hrs

Well absorbed from the gastrointestinal (GI) tract after IM administration. Widely distributed. Metabolized in liver. Primarily excreted in urine. Not removed by hemodialysis. **Half-life:** 16–19 hrs.

AVAILABILITY

Tablets: 12.5 mg, 25 mg, 50 mg.
Syrup: 6.25 mg/5 ml.
Suppository: 12.5 mg, 25 mg, 50 mg.
Injection: 25 mg/ml, 50 mg/ml.

INDICATIONS AND DOSAGES
▸ **Allergic symptoms**
IV/IM
Adults, Elderly. 25 mg. May repeat in 2 hrs.
PO
Adults, Elderly. 6.25–12.5 mg 3 times/day plus 25 mg at bedtime.
Children. 0.1 mg/kg/dose (Maximum: 12.5 mg) 3 times/day plus 0.5 mg/kg/dose (maximum: 25 mg) at bedtime.
▸ **Motion sickness**
PO
Adults, Elderly. 25 mg 30–60 min before departure; may repeat in 8–12 hrs, then every morning on rising and before evening meal.

Children. 0.5 mg/kg (same regimen).
▸ **Prevention of nausea, vomiting**
PO/IM/IV/Rectal
Adults, Elderly. 12.5–25 mg q4–6h as needed.
Children. 0.25–1 mg/kg q4–6h as needed.
▸ **Preoperative and postoperative sedation; adjunct to analgesics**
IM/IV
Adults, Elderly. 25–50 mg.
Children. 12.5–25 mg.

CONTRAINDICATIONS
GI or genitourinary (GU) obstruction, narrow-angle glaucoma, severe CNS depression or coma

INTERACTIONS
Drug
Alcohol, central nervous system (CNS) depressants: May increase CNS depressant effects.
Anticholinergics: May increase anticholinergic effects.
MAOIs: May intensify and prolong anticholinergic and CNS depressant effects.
Herbal
None known.
Food
None known.

DIAGNOSTIC TEST EFFECTS
May suppress wheal and flare reactions to antigen skin testing, unless discontinued 4 days before testing.

IV INCOMPATIBILITIES
Allopurinol (Aloprim), amphotericin B complex (Abelcet, AmBisome, Amphotec), heparin, ketorolac (Toradol), nalbuphine (Nubain), piperacillin tazobactam (Zosyn)

IV COMPATIBILITIES
Atropine, diphenhydramine (Benadryl), glycopyrrolate

(Robinul), hydromorphone (Dilaudid), hydroxyzine (Vistaril), midazolam (Versed), morphine

SIDE EFFECTS

Expected
Drowsiness, disorientation
Elderly
Expected
Hypotension, confusion, syncope
Frequent
Dry mouth, urinary retention, thickening of bronchial secretions
Occasional
Epigastric distress, flushing, visual disturbances, hearing disturbances, wheezing, paresthesia, sweating, chills
Rare
Dizziness, urticaria, photosensitivity, nightmares
Fixed-combination form with pseudoephedrine: mild CNS stimulation

SERIOUS REACTIONS

• Paradoxical reaction, particularly in children, manifested as excitation, nervousness, tremor, hyperactive reflexes, and convulsions.
• CNS depression has occurred in infants and young children, such as respiratory depression, sleep apnea, and SIDS.
• Long-term therapy may produce extrapyramidal symptoms noted as dystonia or abnormal movements, pronounced motor restlessness, which most frequently occurs in children, and parkinsonian symptoms in elderly patient.
• Blood dyscrasias, particularly agranulocytosis, have occurred.

NURSING CONSIDERATIONS

Baseline Assessment
• Assess the patient's blood pressure (B/P) and pulse rate if the patient is given the parenteral form of promethazine.
• Assess the patient for dehydration, including dry mucous membranes, longitudinal furrows in tongue, and poor skin turgor, if promethazine is used as an antiemetic.
• Expect to discontinue drug 4 days before antigen skin testing.

Lifespan Considerations
• Be aware that promethazine readily crosses the placenta and it is unknown if the drug is excreted in breast milk.
• Be aware that promethazine use may inhibit platelet aggregation in neonates if taken within 2 weeks of birth.
• Be aware that promethazine use may produce extrapyramidal symptoms and jaundice in neonates if taken during pregnancy.
• Be aware that children may experience increased excitement.
• Be aware that promethazine use is not recommended for children younger than 2 years of age.
• Be aware that the elderly are more sensitive to the drug's anticholinergic effects, such as dry mouth, confusion, dizziness, hyperexcitability, hypotension, and sedation.

Precautions
• Use cautiously in patients with asthma, history of seizures, impaired cardiovascular disease, liver function impairment, patients suspected of Reye's syndrome, peptic ulcer disease, and sleep apnea.

Administration and Handling
PO
• Give promethazine without regard to meals.
• Crush scored tablets as needed.
IM
◄ALERT► Avoid giving subcutaneously because significant tissue necrosis may occur. Inject carefully because inadvertent intra-arterial

injection may produce severe arteriospasm, resulting in severe circulation impairment.
- Give injection deep IM.

IV
- Store at room temperature.
- May be given undiluted or dilute with 0.9% NaCl; final dilution should not exceed 25 mg/ml.
- Administer at 25 mg/min rate through IV infusion tube, as prescribed.
- Inject slowly because a too rapid rate of infusion may result in transient fall in B/P, producing orthostatic hypotension and reflex tachycardia.
- If the patient complains of pain at the IV site, stop injection immediately because of the possibility of intra-arterial needle placement and perivascular extravasation.

Rectal
- Refrigerate suppository.
- Moisten suppository with cold water before inserting well into rectum.

Intervention and Evaluation
- Monitor the serum electrolytes in patients with severe vomiting.
- Assist the patient with ambulation if he or she experiences drowsiness and lightheadedness.

Patient Teaching
- Instruct the patient that drowsiness and dry mouth are expected responses to the drug.
- Suggest to the patient sips of tepid water and sugarless gum may relieve dry mouth.
- Tell the patient that drinking coffee or tea may help reduce drowsiness.
- Warn the patient to notify the physician if he or she experiences visual disturbances.
- Warn the patient to avoid performing tasks that require mental alertness or motor skills until his or her response to the drug is established.
- Urge the patient to avoid alcohol and other CNS depressants during promethazine therapy.

benzonatate
guaifenesin (glyceryl guaiacolate)

Uses: Antitussives are used to suppress cough. Specifically, *benzonatate* is used to relieve nonproductive cough, including acute cough caused by minor throat and bronchial irritation. *Guaifenesin* is used to relieve cough when mucus is present in the respiratory tract.

Action: Antitussives act in different ways to relieve cough. *Benzonatate* decreases the sensitivity of stretch receptors in the respiratory tract, which reduces cough production. *Guaifenesin* stimulates respiratory tract secretions by decreasing the adhesiveness and viscosity or phlegm, which promotes the removal of viscous mucus. (See illustration, *Sites of Action: Respiratory Agents,* page 1364.)

COMBINATION PRODUCTS
ROBITUSSIN AC: guaifenesin/codeine (a narcotic analgesic) 100 mg/ 10 mg; 75 mg/2.5 mg per 5 ml.
ROBITUSSIN DM: guaifenesin/ dextromethorphan (a cough suppressant) 100 mg/10 mg per 5 ml.

benzonatate
ben-**zow**-nah-tate
(Tessalon Perles)

CATEGORY AND SCHEDULE
Pregnancy Risk Category: C

MECHANISM OF ACTION
A non-narcotic antitussive that anesthetizes stretch receptors in respiratory passages, lungs, and pleura. *Therapeutic Effect:* Reduces cough production.

AVAILABILITY
Capsules: 100 mg, 200 mg.

INDICATIONS AND DOSAGES
▸ **Antitussive**
PO
Adults, Elderly, Children older than 10 yrs. 100 mg 3 times/day, up to 600 mg/day.

CONTRAINDICATIONS
None known

INTERACTIONS
Drug
Central nervous system (CNS) depressants: May increase the effects of benzonatate.
Herbal
None known.
Food
None known.

DIAGNOSTIC TEST EFFECTS
None known.

SIDE EFFECTS
Occasional
Mild drowsiness, mild dizziness, constipation, gastrointestinal (GI) upset, skin eruptions, nasal congestion

SERIOUS REACTIONS
• Paradoxical reaction, including restlessness, insomnia, euphoria, nervousness, and tremors has been noted.

NURSING CONSIDERATIONS
Baseline Assessment
• Assess the frequency, severity, and type of patient cough.
• Monitor the amount, color, and consistency of the patient's sputum.
Precautions
• Use cautiously in patients with productive cough.
Administration and Handling
PO
• Give benzonatate without regard to meals.
• Swallow whole, do not chew or dissolve in mouth because it may produce temporary local anesthesia or choking.
Intervention and Evaluation
• Have the patient begin deep breathing and coughing exercises, particularly in patients with impaired pulmonary function.
• Monitor the patient for paradoxical reaction.
• Increase the patient's environmental humidity and fluid intake to lower the viscosity of his or her lung secretions.
• Assess the patient for clinical improvement and record onset of relief of patient cough.
Patient Teaching
• Tell the patient to avoid tasks that require mental alertness or motor skills until his or her response to the drug is established.
• Explain to the patient that dizziness, drowsiness, and dry mouth occur often.
• Instruct the patient to swallow the pill whole, not to chew or allow it to dissolve in the mouth.

guaifenesin (glyceryl guaiacolate)
guay-**fen**-ah-sin
(Balminil[CAN], Benylin E[CAN], Humibid, Mucinex, Robitussin)

CATEGORY AND SCHEDULE
Pregnancy Risk Category: C
OTC

MECHANISM OF ACTION
An expectorant that stimulates respiratory tract secretion by decreasing phlegm adhesiveness, viscosity, fluid volume. *Therapeutic Effect:* Promotes removal of viscous mucus.

PHARMACOKINETICS
Well absorbed from the gastrointestinal (GI) tract. Metabolized in liver. Excreted in urine.

AVAILABILITY
Tablets: 100 mg, 200 mg.
Tablets (sustained-release): 600 mg.
Capsules: 200 mg.
Capsules (sustained-release): 300 mg.
Syrup: 100 mg/5 ml.
Liquid: 200 mg/5 ml, 100 mg/5 ml.

INDICATIONS AND DOSAGES
▶ **Expectorant**
PO
Adults, Elderly, Children older than 12 yrs. 200–400 mg q4h.
Maximum: 2.4 g/day.
Children 6–12 yrs. 100–200 mg q4h. Maximum: 1.2 g/day.
Children 2–5 yrs. 50–100 mg q4h.
Maximum: 600 mg/day.
Children younger than 2 yrs.
12 mg/kg/day in 6 divided doses.

CONTRAINDICATIONS
None known

INTERACTIONS
Drug
None known.
Herbal
None known.
Food
None known.

DIAGNOSTIC TEST EFFECTS
None known.

SIDE EFFECTS
Rare
Dizziness, headache, rash, diarrhea, nausea, vomiting, stomach pain

SERIOUS REACTIONS
• Excessive dosage may produce nausea and vomiting.

NURSING CONSIDERATIONS
Baseline Assessment
• Assess the frequency, severity, and type of patient cough.
• Increase the patient's environmental humidity and fluid intake to lower the viscosity of the patient's lung secretions.
• Ask about a history of cigarette smoking, asthma, emphysema, and chronic bronchitis because the drug is not recommended for use with coughs caused by these conditions.
Lifespan Considerations
• Be aware that it is unknown if guaifenesin crosses the placenta or is distributed in breast milk.
• There are no age-related precautions noted in children and the elderly.

• Be aware that guaifenesin should be used cautiously in patients younger than 2 years of age with persistent cough.
Administration and Handling
◀ALERT▶ Give extended-release capsules at 12-hour intervals, as prescribed.
PO
• Store syrup, liquid, or capsules at room temperature.
• Give guaifenesin without regard to meals.
• Do not crush or break sustained-release capsule. May sprinkle contents on soft food, then swallow without chewing or crushing.
Intervention/Evaluation
• Have the patient begin deep breathing and coughing exercises, particularly in patients with impaired pulmonary function.
• Assess the patient for clinical improvement and record the onset of relief of the patient's cough.
Patient Teaching
• Caution the patient to avoid performing tasks that require mental alertness or motor skills until his or her response to the drug is established.
• Tell the patient not to take guaifenesin for chronic cough.
• Urge the patient to maintain adequate hydration by drinking plenty of fluids.
• Warn the patient to notify the physician if his or her cough persists or if fever, rash, headache, or sore throat is present with cough.

83 Bronchodilators

albuterol
aminophylline
  (theophylline
  ethylenediamine),
  theophylline
formoterol fumarate
ipratropium bromide
levalbuterol
metaproterenol sulfate
salmeterol
terbutaline sulfate

Uses: Bronchodilators are used to relieve bronchospasm that occurs during anesthesia and in bronchial asthma, bronchitis, emphysema, and chronic obstructive pulmonary disease. Some may also be prescribed to prevent bronchospasm. Terbutaline is also used to delay premature labor.

Action: Each bronchodilator subclass works by a different mechanism of action. *Beta₂-adrenergic agonists,* such as albuterol and formoterol, stimulate beta receptors in the lungs, resulting in relaxed bronchial smooth muscle, increased vital capacity, and decreased airway resistance. Terbutaline also relaxes uterine muscle, inhibiting labor contractions. *Anticholinergics,* such as ipratropium, inhibit cholinergic receptors on bronchial smooth muscle, blocking the action of acetylcholine. This causes bronchodilation and inhibits secretions from glands in the nasal mucosa. *Methylxanthines,* such as aminophylline, directly relax smooth muscle in the bronchial airways and pulmonary blood vessels, relieving bronchospasm and increasing vital capacity. They also produce cardiac and skeletal muscle stimulation. (See illustration, *Sites of Action: Respiratory Agents,* page 1364.)

COMBINATION PRODUCTS

ADVAIR: salmeterol/fluticasone (a corticosteroid) 50 mcg/100 mcg; 50 mcg/250 mcg; 50 mcg/500 mcg.
COMBIVENT: ipratropium/albuterol (a bronchodilator) 18 mcg/103 mcg per actuation from the mouthpiece.
DUONEB: ipratropium/albuterol base (a bronchodilator) 0.5 mg/2.5 ml per 3 ml.

albuterol
ale-**beut**-er-all
(Airomir[AUS], Asmol CFC-Free[AUS], Epaq Inhaler[AUS], Novosalmol[CAN], Proventil, Respax[AUS], Ventolin, Ventolin CFC-Free[AUS], Volmax, Vospire ER)
Do not confuse with atenolol or Prinivil.

CATEGORY AND SCHEDULE
Pregnancy Risk Category: C

MECHANISM OF ACTION

A sympathomimetic (adrenergic agonist) that stimulates beta$_2$-adrenergic receptors in the lungs, resulting in relaxation of bronchial smooth muscle. *Therapeutic Effect:* Relieves bronchospasm, reduces airway resistance.

PHARMACOKINETICS

Route	Onset	Peak	Duration
PO	15–30 min	2–3 hrs	4–6 hrs
PO extended release	30 min	2–4 hrs	12 hrs
Inhalation	5–15 min	0.5–2 hrs	2–5 hrs

Rapidly, well absorbed from the gastrointestinal (GI) tract; gradual absorption from bronchi following inhalation. Metabolized in liver. Primarily excreted in urine. **Half-life:** Oral, 2.7–5 hrs; inhalation, 3.8 hrs.

AVAILABILITY

Tablets: 2 mg, 4 mg.
Tablets (extended-release): 4 mg, 8 mg.
Syrup: 2 mg/5 ml.
Aerosol: Metered dose inhaler.
Solution for Inhalation: 0.83 mg/ml, 5 mg/ml.
Capsules for Inhalation: 200 mcg.

INDICATIONS AND DOSAGES

▶ **Bronchospasm**
PO
Adults. 2–4 mg 3–4 times/day. Maximum: 8 mg 4 times/day. Sustained-release: 1–2 tabs q12h.
Elderly. 2 mg 3–4 times/day. Maximum: 8 mg 4 times/day.
Children 7–12 yrs. 2 mg 3–4 times/day. Repeatabs: 4 mg 2 times/day.
Children 2–6 yrs. 0.1–0.2 mg/kg 3–4 times/day. Maximum: 4 mg 3 times/day.
Inhalation
Adults, Elderly, Children 12 yrs and older. Metered dose inhaler: 1–2 inhalations q4–6h. Maximum: 12 inhalations/day.
Children younger than 12 yrs. 1–2 inhalations 4 times a day.
Nebulization
Adults, Elderly. 2.5–10 mg q1-4h as needed or continuous infusion of 10–15 mg/hr.
Children. 0.15–0.3 mg/kg (Maximum: 10 mg) q1-4h as needed or continuous infusion of 0.5 mg/kg/hr.
▶ **Exercise-induced bronchospasm**
Inhalation
Adults, Elderly, Children older than 12 yrs. 2 inhalations 30 min before exercise.

CONTRAINDICATIONS

History of hypersensitivity to sympathomimetics

INTERACTIONS

Drug
Beta-adrenergic blocking agents (beta-blockers): Antagonizes effects of albuterol.
Digoxin: May increase risk of arrhythmias with digoxin.
MAOIs, tricyclic antidepressants: May potentiate cardiovascular effects.
Herbal
None known.
Food
None known.

DIAGNOSTIC TEST EFFECTS

May increase blood glucose levels. May decrease serum potassium levels.

SIDE EFFECTS

Frequent

Headache (27%); nausea (15%); restlessness, nervousness, trembling (20%); dizziness (less than 7%); throat dryness and irritation, pharyngitis (less than 6%); blood pressure (B/P) changes including hypertension (5%–3%); heartburn, transient wheezing (less than 5%)

Occasional (3%–2%)

Insomnia, weakness, unusual or bad taste or taste or smell change. Inhalation: Dry, irritated mouth or throat; coughing; bronchial irritation.

Rare

Drowsiness, diarrhea, dry mouth, flushing, sweating, anorexia

SERIOUS REACTIONS

• Excessive sympathomimetic stimulation may produce palpitations, extrasystoles, tachycardia, chest pain, a slight increase in B/P followed by a substantial decrease, chills, sweating, and blanching of skin.

• Too frequent or excessive use may lead to loss of bronchodilating effectiveness and severe, paradoxical bronchoconstriction.

NURSING CONSIDERATIONS

Baseline Assessment

• Offer emotional support. Patients receiving this drug may become anxious because of their difficulty in breathing and also from the sympathomimetic response to the drug.

Lifespan Considerations

• Be aware that albuterol appears to cross the placenta and it is unknown if albuterol is distributed in breast milk.

• Albuterol may inhibit uterine contractility.

• Be aware that safety and efficacy have not been established in children less than 2 years of age (syrup) or less than 6 years of age (tablets).

• The elderly may be more likely to develop tremors or tachycardia because of the age-related increased sympathetic sensitivity.

Precautions

• Use cautiously in patients with cardiovascular disease, diabetes mellitus, hypertension, or hyperthyroidism.

Administration and Handling

PO

• Do not crush or break extended-release tablets.

• May give without regard to food.

Inhalation

• Shake container well and have the patient exhale completely through the mouth. Have the patient place the mouthpiece into the mouth and close the lips while holding the inhaler upright.

• Ask the patient to inhale deeply through the mouth while fully depressing the top of the canister, and to hold his or her breath as long as possible before exhaling slowly.

• Have the patient wait 2 minutes before inhaling the second dose because this allows for deeper bronchial penetration.

• Have the patient rinse his or her mouth with water immediately after inhalation to prevent mouth and throat dryness.

Nebulization

• Dilute 0.5 ml of 0.5% solution to a final volume of 3 ml with 0.9% NaCl to provide 2.5 mg.

• Administer over 5 to 15 minutes.

• The nebulizer should be used with compressed air or oxygen (O_2) at a rate of 6 to 10 L/min.

Intervention and Evaluation
• Monitor the 12-lead EKG, ABG determinations, quality and rate of pulse; the rate, depth, rhythm, and type of respirations; and serum potassium levels.
• Assess the patient's lung sounds for signs of bronchoconstriction, such as wheezing, and for rales.

Patient Teaching
• Instruct the patient on the proper use of an inhaler.
• Encourage the patient to increase fluid intake to decrease the viscosity of his or her pulmonary secretions.
• Inform the patient not to take more than 2 inhalations at any one time (excessive use may produce paradoxical bronchoconstriction or a decreased bronchodilating effect).
• Advise the patient that rinsing his or her mouth with water immediately after inhalation may prevent mouth and throat dryness.
• Urge the patient to avoid excessive use of caffeine derivatives, such as chocolate, cocoa, coffee, cola, and tea.

aminophylline (theophylline ethylenediamine)
am-in-ah-phil-lin
(Aminophylline)
Do not confuse with amitriptyline or ampicillin.

theophylline
(SloBid, Theo-Dur, Theolair, Uniphyl)
Immediate-release: Aerolate, Theolair. Extended-release: Theo-24, Uniphyl.
Do not confuse with Dolobid.

CATEGORY AND SCHEDULE
Pregnancy Risk Category: C

MECHANISM OF ACTION
A xanthine derivative that acts as a bronchodilator by directly relaxing smooth muscle of the bronchial airway and pulmonary blood vessels. *Therapeutic Effect:* Relieves bronchospasm, increases vital capacity. Produces cardiac, skeletal muscle stimulation.

AVAILABILITY
Capsules: 125 mg.
Capsules (sustained release): 65 mg, 125 mg, 130 mg, 200 mg, 260 mg, 300 mg.
Capsules (sustained release 24 hrs): 100 mg, 200 mg, 300 mg, 400 mg.
Elixir: 80 mg/15 ml.
Injection: 25 mg/ml, 800 mg/ 500 ml.
Liquid: 80 mg/15 ml.
Tablet: 125 mg, 250 mg, 300 mg.
Tablet (controlled release): 100 mg, 200 mg, 300 mg, 400 mg, 450 mg, 600 mg.
Tablet (controlled release 12 hrs): 100 mg, 200 mg, 300 mg.

INDICATIONS AND DOSAGES
▸ **Chronic bronchospasm**
PO
Adults, Elderly, Children. 16 mg/kg or 400 mg/day (whichever is less) in 2–4 divided doses (6-to 12-hr intervals). May increase by 25% every 2–3 days up to maximum of 24 mg/kg/day.
Children (1–8 yrs). 20 mg/kg/day.
Children (9–12 yrs). 18 mg/kg/day.
Children (older than 12–16 yrs). 13 mg/kg/day.
Children (older than 16 yrs). Doses above maximum based on serum theophylline concentrations, clinical condition, presence of toxicity.
▸ **Acute bronchospasm in patients not currently taking theophylline**
IV loading dose
Adults, Children older than 1 yr.

Initially, 6 mg/kg (aminophylline), then begin maintenance aminophylline dosage based on patient group.
Neonates. 5 mg/kg.

Patient Group	Maintenance Aminophylline Dosage
Neonates	5 mg/kg q12h
Children (6 wks–6 mos)	0.5 mg/kg/hr
Children (older than 6 mos–1 yr)	0.6–0.7 mg/kg/hr
Children (1–8 yrs)	1–1.2 mg/kg/hr
Children (9–12 yrs), young adult smokers	0.9 mg/kg/hr
Children (older than 12–16 yrs)	0.7 mg/kg/hr
Adult, non-smoker	0.7 mg/kg/hr
Older patients, patients with cor pulmonale, congestive heart failure (CHF) or liver impairment	0.25 mg/kg/hr

PO/loading dose
Adults, children older than 1 yr.
Initially, 5 mg/kg (theophylline), then begin maintenance theophylline dosage based on patient group.

Patient Group	Maintenance Theophylline Dosage
Children (1–8 yrs)	4 mg/kg q6h
Children (9–16 yrs), young adult smokers	3 mg/kg q6h
Healthy, nonsmoking adults	3 mg/kg q8h
Older patients, patients with cor pulmonale	2 mg/kg q8h
Patients with CHF or liver disease	1–2 mg/kg q12h

▸ **Acute bronchospasm in patients currently taking theophylline**
PO/IV
Adults, children older than 1 yr.
Obtain serum theophylline level. If not possible and patient is in respiratory distress and not experiencing toxicity, may give 2.5 mg/kg dose. Maintenance: Dosage based on peak serum theophylline concentrations, clinical condition, and presence of toxicity.

UNLABELED USES
Treatment of apnea in neonates

CONTRAINDICATIONS
History of hypersensitivity to caffeine or xanthine

INTERACTIONS
Drug
Beta-blockers: May decrease effects of aminophylline.
Cimetidine, ciprofloxacin, erythromycin, norfloxacin: May increase aminophylline blood concentration and risk of aminophylline toxicity.
Glucocorticoids: May produce hypernatremia.
Phenytoin, primidone, rifampin: May increase aminophylline metabolism.
Smoking: May decrease aminophylline blood concentration.
Herbal
None known.
Food
None known.

DIAGNOSTIC TEST EFFECTS
None known.

IV INCOMPATIBILITIES
Amiodarone (Cordarone), ciprofloxacin (Cipro), dobutamine (Dobutrex), ondansetron (Zofran)

IV COMPATIBILITIES
Aztreonam (Azactam), ceftazidime (Fortaz), fluconazole (Diflucan), heparin, morphine, potassium chloride

SIDE EFFECTS
Frequent
Momentary change in sense of smell during IV administration, shakiness, restlessness, tachycardia, trembling
Occasional
Heartburn, vomiting, headache, mild diuresis, insomnia, nausea

SERIOUS REACTIONS
• Too rapid a rate of IV administration may produce a marked fall in blood pressure (B/P) with accompanying faintness and lightheadedness, palpitations, tachycardia, hyperventilation, nausea, vomiting, angina-like pain, seizures, ventricular fibrillation, and cardiac standstill.

NURSING CONSIDERATIONS

Baseline Assessment
• Offer the patient emotional support. Anxiety may occur because of difficulty in breathing and from the sympathomimetic response to the drug.
• As ordered, obtain the peak serum concentration 1 hour after IV dose, 1 to 2 hours after immediate-release dose, and 3 to 8 hours after extended-release dose. Obtain the serum trough level just before next dose.
Precautions
• Use cautiously in patients with diabetes mellitus, glaucoma, hypertension, hyperthyroidism, impaired cardiac, renal or liver function, peptic ulcer disease, or a seizure disorder.
Administration and Handling
PO
• Give with food to avoid gastrointestinal (GI) distress.
• Do not crush or break extended-release forms.

IV
• Store at room temperature.
• Discard if solution contains a precipitate.
• Give loading dose diluted in 100 to 200 ml of D_5W or 0.9% NaCl. Prepare maintenance dose in larger volume parenteral infusion.
• Do not exceed flow rate of 1 ml/min (25 mg/min) for either piggyback or infusion
• Administer loading dose over 20 to 30 minutes.
• Use infusion pump or microdrip to regulate IV administration.
Intervention and Evaluation
◀ALERT▶ Aminophylline dosage is calculated based on lean body weight. The dosage is also based on peak serum theophylline concentrations, the patient's clinical condition, and the absence of theophylline toxicity.
• Expect to monitor the rate, depth, rhythm, and type of breathing as well as to assess the lung sounds for rhonchi, wheezing, or rales.
• Expect to monitor the patient's arterial blood gases (ABGs) and the quality and rate of the pulse.
• Examine the patient's lips and fingernails for evidence of oxygen depletion such as blue or gray lips, blue or dusky colored fingernails in light-skinned patients; and gray fingernails in dark-skinned patients.
• Assess the patient for clavicular retractions and hand tremor.
• Evaluate the patient for signs of clinical improvement such as cessation of clavicular retractions, quieter and slower respirations, and a relaxed facial expression.
• Monitor serum theophylline levels. The therapeutic serum level range is 10 to 20 mcg/ml.
Patient Teaching
• Encourage the patient to increase his or her fluid intake to

decrease the thickness of lung secretions.
• Urge the patient to avoid excessive use of caffeine derivatives such as chocolate, coffee, cola, cocoa, and tea.
• Explain to the patient that smoking, charcoal-broiled food, and a high-protein, low-carbohydrate diet may decrease theophylline level.

formoterol fumarate
four-**moh**-tur-all
(Foradil Aerolizer, Foradile[AUS], Oxis[AUS])

CATEGORY AND SCHEDULE
Pregnancy Risk Category: C

MECHANISM OF ACTION
A long-acting bronchodilator that stimulates beta$_2$-adrenergic receptors in the lungs, resulting in relaxation of bronchial smooth muscle. Also inhibits release of mediators from various cells in the lungs, including mast cells, with little effect on heart rate. *Therapeutic Effect:* Relieves bronchospasm, reduces airway resistance. Produces improved bronchodilation, nighttime improved asthma control, improved peak flow rates.

PHARMACOKINETICS

Route	Onset	Peak	Duration
Inhalation	1–3 min	0.5–1 hr	12 hrs

Absorbed from bronchi following inhalation. Metabolized in liver. Primarily excreted in urine. Unknown if removed by hemodialysis.
Half-life: 10 hrs.

AVAILABILITY
Inhalation Powder in Capsules: 12 mcg.

INDICATIONS AND DOSAGES
▸ **Maintenance treatment of asthma**
Inhalation
Adults, Elderly, Children older than 5 yrs. Inhale contents of 1 capsule every 12 hrs.
▸ **Exercise-induced asthma**
Inhalation
Adults, Elderly, Children older than 12 yrs. Inhale contents of 1 capsule at least 15 min before exercise.

CONTRAINDICATIONS
None known

INTERACTIONS
Drug
Beta-adrenergic blocking agents: May antagonize bronchodilating effects.
Diuretics, steroids, xanthine derivatives: May increase the risk of hypokalemia.
Drugs that can prolong QT interval, including erythromycin, quinidine, and thioridazine, MAOIs, tricyclic antidepressants: May potentiate cardiovascular effects with drugs that can prolong QT interval.
Herbal
None known.
Food
None known.

DIAGNOSTIC TEST EFFECTS
May decrease serum potassium levels. May increase blood glucose levels.

SIDE EFFECTS
Occasional
Tremor, cramps, tachycardia, insomnia, headache, irritability, irritation of mouth or throat

SERIOUS REACTIONS
• Excessive sympathomimetic stimulation may produce palpitations, extrasystoles, and chest pain.

NURSING CONSIDERATIONS

Baseline Assessment
• Ask the patient about a history of cardiovascular disease, convulsive disorder, hypertension, and thyrotoxicosis.
• Check the patient's baseline EKG, and measure the QT interval.
• Check the patient's baseline peak flow readings.

Lifespan Considerations
• Be aware that it is unknown if formoterol crosses the placenta or is distributed in breast milk.
• Be aware that the safety and efficacy of formoterol have not been established in children younger than 5 years of age.
• Be aware that the elderly may be more sensitive to tachycardia or tremor due to age-related increased sympathetic sensitivity.

Precautions
• Use cautiously in patients with cardiovascular disease, convulsive disorder, hypertension, and thyrotoxicosis.

Administration and Handling
• Maintain capsules in individual blister pack until immediately before use. Do not swallow capsules. Do not use with a spacer.
Inhalation
• Pull off aerolizer inhaler cover, twisting mouthpiece in direction of the arrow to open.
• Place capsule in chamber. Capsule is pierced by pressing and releasing buttons on the side of the aerolizer, once only.

• Have the patient exhale completely; place mouthpiece into the patient's mouth and have the patient close his or her lips.
• Instruct the patient to inhale quickly and deeply through mouth because this causes capsule to spin and dispense the drug. Next tell the patient to hold his or her breath as long as possible before exhaling slowly.
• Check capsule to make sure all the powder is gone. If not, instruct the patient to inhale again to receive the rest of the dose.
• Have the patient rinse his or her mouth with water immediately after inhalation to prevent mouth and throat dryness.

Intervention and Evaluation
• Monitor the depth, rate, rhythm, and type of patient respirations.
• Monitor the quality and rate of the patient's pulse.
• Monitor the patient's arterial blood gases (ABGs), electrocardiogram (EKG), and serum potassium levels.
• Assess the patient's lung sounds for rhonchi and wheezing, signs of bronchoconstriction.

Patient Teaching
• Instruct the patient on the proper use of the inhaler.
• Teach the patient to increase his or her fluid intake to decrease lung secretion viscosity.
• Tell the patient that rinsing his or her mouth with water immediately after inhalation may prevent mouth and throat irritation.
• Urge the patient to avoid excessive use of caffeine derivatives such as chocolate, coffee, cola, and tea.
• Teach the patient how to measure peak flow readings, and keep a log of measurements.

ipratropium bromide
ih-prah-**trow**-pea-um
(Aproven[AUS], Atrovent)
Do not confuse with Alupent.

CATEGORY AND SCHEDULE
Pregnancy Risk Category: B

MECHANISM OF ACTION
An anticholinergic that blocks the action of acetylcholine at parasympathetic sites in bronchial smooth muscle. *Therapeutic Effect:* Causes bronchodilation, inhibits secretions from the glands lining the nasal mucosa.

PHARMACOKINETICS

Route	Onset	Peak	Duration
Inhalation	1–3 min	1–2 hrs	4–6 hrs

Minimal systemic absorption. Metabolized in liver (systemic absorption). Primarily eliminated in feces. **Half-life:** 1.5–4 hrs.

AVAILABILITY
Oral Inhalation: 18 mcg/actuation.
Aerosol Solution for Inhalation: 0.02% (500-mcg vial).
Nasal Spray: 0.03%, 0.06%.

INDICATIONS AND DOSAGES
▶ **Bronchospasm**
Inhalation
Adults, Elderly. 2 inhalations 4 times/day. Wait 1–10 min before administering second inhalation. Maximum: 12 inhalations/24 hrs.
Children 3–12 yrs. 1–2 inhalations 3 times/day. Maximum: 6 inhalations/24 hrs.
Nebulization
Adults, Elderly. 500 mcg 3–4 times/day.

Children. 125–250 mcg 3 times/day.
Neonates. 25 mcg/kg/dose 3 times/day.
▶ **Rhinorrhea**
Intranasal
Adults, Children 6–12 yrs (0.03%). 2 sprays 2–3 times/day.
Adults, Children older than 12 yrs (0.06%). 2 sprays 3–4 times/day.

CONTRAINDICATIONS
History of hypersensitivity to atropine

INTERACTIONS
Drug
Cromolyn inhalation solution: Avoid mixing these drugs because they form a precipitate.
Herbal
None known.
Food
None known.

DIAGNOSTIC TEST EFFECTS
None known.

SIDE EFFECTS
Frequent
Inhalation (6%–3%): Cough, dry mouth, headache, nausea
Nasal: Dry nose and mouth, headache, nasal irritation
Occasional
Inhalation (2%): Dizziness, transient increased bronchospasm
Rare (less than 1%)
Hypotension, insomnia, metallic and unpleasant taste, palpitations, urinary retention
Nasal: Diarrhea or constipation, dry throat, stomach pain, stuffy nose

SERIOUS REACTIONS
• Worsening of narrow-angle glaucoma, acute eye pain, and hypotension occur rarely.

NURSING CONSIDERATIONS

Baseline Assessment
• Offer the patient emotional support because of the high incidence of anxiety caused by breathing difficulty and the sympathomimetic response to drug.

Lifespan Considerations
• Be aware that it is unknown if ipratropium is distributed in breast milk.
• There are no age-related precautions noted in children and the elderly.

Precautions
• Use cautiously in patients with bladder neck obstruction, narrow-angle glaucoma, and prostatic hypertrophy.

Administration and Handling
Inhalation
• Shake container well, have the patient exhale completely through his or her mouth; place mouthpiece into the patient's mouth and have the patient close his or her lips, holding inhaler upright.
• Instruct the patient to inhale deeply through the mouth while fully depressing the top of the canister. Tell the patient to hold his or her breath as long as possible before exhaling slowly.
• Wait 2 minutes before inhaling second dose to allow for deeper bronchial penetration.
• Have the patient rinse his or her mouth with water immediately after inhalation to prevent mouth and throat dryness.

Intervention and Evaluation
• Monitor the depth, rate, rhythm, and type of patient respirations.
• Monitor the quality and rate of the patient's pulse.
• Assess the patient's lung sounds for crackles, rhonchi, and wheezing.
• Monitor the patient's arterial blood gases (ABGs).
• Observe the patient's fingernails and lips for blue or dusky color in light-skinned patients; gray in dark-skinned patients.
• Observe the patient for clavicular, intercostals, and sternal retractions, and hand tremor.
• Evaluate the patient for clinical improvement, cessation of retractions, quieter, slower respirations, and relaxed facial expression.

Patient Teaching
• Instruct the patient to increase his or her fluid intake to decrease the viscosity of his or her lung secretions.
• Teach the patient not to take more than 2 inhalations at any one time. Explain to the patient that excessive use may produce paradoxical bronchoconstriction or a decreased bronchodilating effect.
• Suggest to the patient that rinsing mouth with water immediately after inhalation may prevent mouth and throat dryness.
• Urge the patient to avoid excessive use of caffeine derivatives such as chocolate, cocoa, coffee, and tea.

levalbuterol
lee-val-**bwet**-err-all
(Xopenex)
Do not confuse with Xanax.

CATEGORY AND SCHEDULE
Pregnancy Risk Category: C

MECHANISM OF ACTION
A sympathomimetic that stimulates beta$_2$-adrenergic receptors in the lungs resulting in relaxation of bronchial smooth muscle. *Therapeu-*

tic Effect: Relieves bronchospasm, reduces airway resistance.

PHARMACOKINETICS

Route	Onset	Peak	Duration
Inhalation	10–17 min	1.5 hrs	5–6 hrs

Metabolized in the liver to inactive metabolite. **Half-life:** 3.3–4 hrs.

AVAILABILITY

Solution for Nebulization: 0.31 in 3-ml vials, 0.63 mg in 3-ml vials; 1.25 mg in 3-ml vials.

INDICATIONS AND DOSAGES
▸ **Treatment and prevention of bronchospasm**
Nebulization
Adults, Elderly, Children 12 yrs and older. Initially, 0.63 mg 3 times/day 6–8 hrs apart. May increase to 1.25 mg 3 times/day with dose monitoring.
Children 3–11 yrs. Initially 0.31 mg 3 times/day. Maximum: 0.63 mg 3 times/day

CONTRAINDICATIONS

History hypersensitivity to sympathomimetics

INTERACTIONS
Drug
Beta-adrenergic blocking agents (beta-blockers): Antagonize the effects of levalbuterol.
Digoxin: May increase the risk of arrhythmias with digoxin.
MAOIs, tricyclic antidepressants: May potentiate cardiovascular effects.
Herbal
None known.
Food
None known.

DIAGNOSTIC TEST EFFECTS
May increase serum potassium levels.

SIDE EFFECTS
Frequent
Tremor, nervousness, headache, throat dryness and irritation
Occasional
Dry, irritated mouth or throat, coughing, bronchial irritation
Rare
Drowsiness, diarrhea, dry mouth, flushing, diaphoresis, anorexia

SERIOUS REACTIONS
• Excessive sympathomimetic stimulation may produce palpitations, extrasystoles, tachycardia, chest pain, and a slight increase in blood pressure (B/P) followed by substantial decrease, chills, diaphoresis, and blanching of skin.
• Too frequent or excessive use may lead to loss of bronchodilating effectiveness and severe, paradoxical bronchoconstriction.

NURSING CONSIDERATIONS
Baseline Assessment
• Offer the patient emotional support because of a high incidence of anxiety because of difficulty in breathing and sympathomimetic response to drug.
Lifespan Considerations
• Be aware that levalbuterol crosses the placenta and it is unknown if the drug is distributed in breast milk.
• Be aware that the safety and efficacy of levalbuterol have not been established in patients younger than 12 years of age.
• Be aware that in the elderly a lower initial dosage is recommended.

Precautions
• Use cautiously in patients with cardiovascular disorders, such as cardiac arrhythmias, diabetes mellitus, hypertension, and seizures.

Administration and Handling
Nebulization
• Do not dilute.
• Protect from light and excessive heat. Store at room temperature.
• Once foil is opened, use within 2 weeks.
• Discard if solution is not colorless.
• Do not mix with other medications.
• Give over 5 to 15 minutes.

Intervention and Evaluation
• Monitor the depth, rate, rhythm, and type of patient respirations.
• Monitor the patient's arterial blood gases (ABG), electrocardiogram (EKG), quality and rate of the pulse, and serum potassium levels.
• Assess the patient's lung sounds for crackles and wheezing, signs of bronchoconstriction.

Patient Teaching
• Instruct the patient to increase his or her fluid intake to decrease the viscosity of his or her lung secretions.
• Tell the patient that rinsing his or her mouth with water immediately after inhalation may prevent mouth and throat dryness.
• Urge the patient to avoid excessive use of caffeine derivatives such as chocolate, coffee, cola, and tea.
• Warn the patient to notify the physician if he or she experiences chest pain, dizziness, headache, palpitations, tachycardia, or tremors.

metaproterenol sulfate
met-ah-pro-**tair**-in-all
(Alupent)
Do not confuse with Atrovent, metipranolol, or metoprolol.

CATEGORY AND SCHEDULE
Pregnancy Risk Category: C

MECHANISM OF ACTION
A sympathomimetic or adrenergic agonist that stimulates beta$_2$-adrenergic receptors, resulting in relaxation of bronchial smooth muscle. *Therapeutic Effect:* Relieves bronchospasm; reduces airway resistance.

AVAILABILITY
Solution for Oral Inhalation: 0.4%, 0.6%, 5%.
Syrup: 10 mg/5 ml.
Tablets: 10 mg, 20 mg.

INDICATIONS AND DOSAGES
▸ **Treatment of bronchospasm**
PO
Adults, Children older than 9 yrs. 20 mg 3–4 times/day.
Elderly. 10 mg 3–4 times/day. May increase to 20 mg/dose.
Children 6–9 yrs. 10 mg 3–4 times/ day.
Children 2–5 yrs. 1.3–2.6 mg/kg/ day in 3–4 divided doses.
Children younger than 2 yrs. 0.4 mg/kg 3–4 times/day.
Inhalation
Adults, Elderly, Children older than 12 yrs. 2–3 inhalations q3–4h.
Maximum: 12 inhalations/24 hrs.
Nebulization
Adults, Elderly, Children 12 yrs and older. 10–15 mg (0.2–0.3 ml) of 5% q4–6h.

Children younger than 12 yrs, Infants. 0.5–1 mg/kg (0.01–0.02 ml/kg) of 5% q4–6h.

CONTRAINDICATIONS

Narrow angle glaucoma, preexisting cardiac arrhythmias associated with tachycardia

INTERACTIONS
Drug

Beta-blockers: May decrease the effects of beta-blockers.
Digoxin, other sympathomimetics: May increase the risk of arrhythmias.
MAOIs: May increase the risk of hypertensive crises.
Tricyclic antidepressants: May increase cardiovascular effects.
Herbal
None known.
Food
None known.

DIAGNOSTIC TEST EFFECTS

May decrease serum potassium levels.

SIDE EFFECTS

Frequent (10% or greater)
Shakiness, nervousness, nausea, dry mouth
Occasional (9%–1%)
Dizziness, vertigo, weakness, headache, gastrointestinal (GI) distress, vomiting, cough, dry throat
Rare (less than 1%)
Drowsiness, diarrhea, unusual taste

SERIOUS REACTIONS

• Excessive sympathomimetic stimulation may cause palpitations, extrasystoles, tachycardia, chest pain, and a slight increase in blood pressure (B/P) followed by a substantial decrease, chills, diaphoresis, and blanching of skin.

• Too frequent or excessive use may lead to loss of bronchodilating effectiveness and severe, paradoxical bronchoconstriction.

NURSING CONSIDERATIONS
Baseline Assessment

• Offer the patient emotional support because of the high incidence of anxiety caused by breathing difficulty and the sympathomimetic response to drug.
Precautions

• Use cautiously in patients with arrhythmias, congestive heart failure (CHF), diabetes mellitus, hypertension, hyperthyroidism, ischemic heart disease, and seizure disorder.
Intervention and Evaluation

• Monitor the depth, rate, rhythm, and type of patient respirations.
• Monitor the patient's arterial blood gases (ABGs) and pulmonary function tests.
• Assess the patient's lung sounds for rhonchi and wheezing, signs of bronchoconstriction.
• Observe the patient's fingernails and lips for a blue or dusky color in light-skinned patients, gray in dark-skinned patients, signs of hypoxemia.
• Evaluate the patient for clinical improvement, cessation of clavicular, inter-costal, and sternal retractions, quieter, slower respirations, and relaxed facial expression.
Patient Teaching

• Instruct the patient to increase his or her fluid intake to decrease the viscosity of his or her lung secretions.
• Teach the patient not to exceed the recommended dosage.
• Tell the patient that metaproterenol may cause inability to

sleep, nervousness, and restlessness.
• Warn the patient to notify the physician if he or she experiences chest pain, difficulty breathing, dizziness, flushing, headache, palpitations, tachycardia, and tremors.
• Urge the patient to avoid excessive use of caffeine derivatives such as chocolate, cocoa, coffee, cola, and tea.

salmeterol
sal-**met**-er-all
(Serevent Diskus)
Do not confuse with Serentil.

CATEGORY AND SCHEDULE
Pregnancy Risk Category: C

MECHANISM OF ACTION
An adrenergic agonist that stimulates beta$_2$-adrenergic receptors in the lungs resulting in relaxation of bronchial smooth muscle. *Therapeutic Effect:* Relieves bronchospasm, reducing airway resistance.

PHARMACOKINETICS

Route	Onset	Peak	Duration
Inhalation	10–20 min	3 hrs	12 hrs

Primarily acts in lung; low systemic absorption. Protein binding: 95%. Metabolized by hydroxylation. Primarily eliminated in feces.
Half-life: 3–4 hrs.

AVAILABILITY
Aerosol Powder: 50 mcg.

INDICATIONS AND DOSAGES
▸ **Maintenance and prevention of asthma**
Inhalation
Adults, Elderly, Children older than 4 yrs. (Diskus) 1 activation (50 mcg) q12h. Prevention of exercise-induced bronchospasm
Inhalation
Adults, Elderly, Children older than 4 yrs. 1 inhalation at least 30 minutes before exercise.
▸ **Chronic obstructive pulmonary disease (COPD) Inhalation**
Adults, Elderly. 1 inhalation q12h.

CONTRAINDICATIONS
History of hypersensitivity to sympathomimetics

INTERACTIONS
Drug
Beta-adrenergic blockers: May decrease the effects of beta-adrenergic blockers.
Herbal
None known.
Food
None known.

DIAGNOSTIC TEST EFFECTS
May decrease serum potassium levels.

SIDE EFFECTS
Frequent (28%)
Headache
Occasional (7%–3%)
Cough, tremor, dizziness, vertigo, throat dryness or irritation, pharyngitis
Rare (less than 3%)
Palpitations, tachycardia, shakiness, nausea, heartburn, gastrointestinal (GI) distress, diarrhea

SERIOUS REACTIONS
• May prolong QT interval, which may lead to ventricular arrhythmias.

• May cause hypokalemia and hyperglycemia.

NURSING CONSIDERATIONS

Baseline Assessment

• Ask the patient about a history of sensitivity to sympathomimetics.
• Assess a baseline electrocardiogram (EKG), and measure the QT interval.
• Check the patient's baseline peak flow readings.

Lifespan Considerations

• Be aware that it is unknown if salmeterol is excreted in breast milk.
• There are no age-related precautions noted in children older than 4 years of age.
• Be aware that in the elderly lower dosages may be needed due to increased sympathetic sensitivity and increased susceptibility to tachycardia or tremors.

Precautions

• Use cautiously in patients with cardiovascular disorders, such as coronary insufficiency, arrhythmias, and hypertension, seizure disorder, and thyrotoxicosis.
• Salmeterol use is not for acute symptoms and may cause paradoxical bronchospasm.

Administration and Handling

Inhalation

• Shake container well. Instruct the patient to exhale completely through the mouth. Place mouthpiece into the patient's mouth and have the patient close his or her lips, holding inhaler upright.
• Have the patient inhale deeply through mouth while fully depressing the top of canister. Instruct the patient to hold his or her breath as long as possible before exhaling slowly.

• Teach the patient to wait 2 minutes before inhaling a second dose to allow for deeper bronchial penetration.
• Instruct the patient to rinse his or her mouth with water immediately after inhalation to prevent mouth and throat dryness.

Intervention and Evaluation

• Monitor the depth, rate, rhythm, and type of patient respirations.
• Monitor the patient's blood pressure (B/P) and the quality and rate of the patient's pulse.
• Assess the patient's lungs for crackles, rhonchi, and wheezing.
• Periodically evaluate the patient's serum potassium levels.

Patient Teaching

• Explain to the patient that salmeterol use is not for relief of acute episodes.
• Teach the patient to keep the drug canister at room temperature. Inform the patient that cold decreases the drug's effects.
• Caution the patient against abruptly discontinuing the drug or exceeding the recommended dosage.
• Warn the patient to notify the physician if he or she experiences chest pain or dizziness.
• Instruct the patient to wait at least 1 full minute before the second inhalation.
• Teach the patient to administer the dose 30 to 60 minutes before exercising when the drug is used to prevent exercise-induced bronchospasm.
• Urge the patient to avoid excessive consumption of caffeine derivatives such as chocolate, coffee, colas, and tea.
• Teach the patient how to measure peak flow readings, and keep a log of measurements.

terbutaline sulfate
tur-byew-ta-leen
(Brethine)
Do not confuse with Brethaire, terbinafine, or tolbutamide.

CATEGORY AND SCHEDULE
Pregnancy Risk Category: B

MECHANISM OF ACTION
A sympathomimetic or adrenergic agonist that stimulates beta$_2$-adrenergic receptors. *Therapeutic Effect:* Bronchospasm: Relaxes bronchial smooth muscle, relieves bronchospasm, reduces airway resistance. Labor: Relaxes uterine muscle, inhibiting uterine contractions.

AVAILABILITY
Tablets: 2.5 mg, 5 mg.
Injection: 1 mg/ml.

INDICATIONS AND DOSAGES
▶ **Bronchospasm**
PO
Adults, Elderly, Children older than 15 yrs. Initially, 2.5 mg 3–4 times/day. Maintenance: 2.5–5 mg 3 times/day q6h while awake. Maximum: 15 mg/day.
Children 12–15 yrs. 2.5 mg 3 times/day. Maximum: 7.5 mg/day.
Children younger than 12 yrs. Initially, 0.05 mg/kg/dose q8h. May increase up to 0.15 mg/kg/dose. Maximum: 5 mg.
Subcutaneous
Adults, Children 12 yrs and older. Initially, 0.25 mg. Repeat in 15–30 min if substantial improvement does not occur. Maximum: No more than 0.5 mg/4 hrs.
Children younger than 12 yrs. 0.005–0.01 mg/kg/dose to a maxi-

mum of 0.4 mg/dose q15–20min for 2 doses.
▶ **Preterm labor**
IV
Adults. 2.5–10 mcg/min. May increase gradually q15-20 min up to 17.5–30 mcg/min.
PO
Adults. 2.5–10 mg q4-6h.

CONTRAINDICATIONS
History of hypersensitivity to sympathomimetics

INTERACTIONS
Drug
Beta-blockers: May decrease the effects of beta-blockers.
Digoxin, sympathomimetics: May increase the risk of arrhythmias.
MAOIs: May increase the risk of hypertensive crises.
Tricyclic antidepressants: May increase cardiovascular effects.
Herbal
None known.
Food
None known.

DIAGNOSTIC TEST EFFECTS
May decrease serum potassium levels.

SIDE EFFECTS
Frequent (23%–18%)
Tremor, shakiness, nervousness
Occasional (11%–10%)
Drowsiness, headache, nausea, heartburn, dizziness
Rare (3%–1%)
Flushing, weakness, drying or irritation of oropharynx noted with inhalation therapy

SERIOUS REACTIONS
• Too frequent or excessive use may lead to loss of bronchodilating effectiveness and severe, paradoxical bronchoconstriction.

• Excessive sympathomimetic stimulation may cause palpitations, extrasystoles, tachycardia, chest pain, and a slight increase in blood pressure (B/P) followed by a substantial decrease, chills, sweating, and blanching of skin.

NURSING CONSIDERATIONS

Baseline Assessment
• Offer emotional support to the patient taking terbutaline for bronchospasm because these patients have a high incidence of anxiety due to difficulty in breathing and sympathomimetic response to drug.
• Assess the baseline maternal B/P and pulse, the duration and frequency of contractions, and the fetal heart rate in the patient taking terbutaline for preterm labor.

Precautions
• Use cautiously in patients with diabetes mellitus, history of seizures, hypertension, hyperthyroidism, and impaired cardiac function.

Administration and Handling
PO
• Give terbutaline without regard to food. May give terbutaline with food if the patient experiences gastrointestinal (GI) upset.
• Crush tablets as needed.
Subcutaneous
• Do not use if solution appears discolored.
• Inject subcutaneously into lateral deltoid region.

Intervention and Evaluation
• Monitor the depth, rate, rhythm, and type of patient respirations.

• Monitor the quality and rate of the patient's pulse.
• Assess the patient's lungs for rhonchi and wheezing.
• Periodically evaluate the patient's serum potassium levels.
• Monitor the patient's arterial blood gases (ABGs).
• Observe the patient's fingernails and lips for a blue or dusky color in light-skinned patients, gray in dark-skinned patients, signs of hypoxemia.
• Observe the patient for clavicular retractions and hand tremor.
• Evaluate the patient for clinical improvement, cessation of clavicular retractions, quieter, slower respirations, and relaxed facial expression.
• Monitor the duration and frequency of the patient's contractions when the drug is used for preterm labor.
• Diligently monitor the pregnant patient's fetal heart rate.

Patient Teaching
• Warn the patient to notify the physician if he or she experiences chest pain, difficulty breathing, dizziness, flushing, headache, muscle tremors, or palpitations.
• Tell the patient that terbutaline may cause nervousness and shakiness.
• Urge the patient to avoid excessive consumption of caffeine derivatives such as chocolate, coffee, colas, and tea.

beractant
calfactant
poractant alfa

Uses: Lung surfactants are used to prevent and treat respiratory distress syndrome (RDS) in premature neonates, often improving oxygenation within minutes of administration.

Action: By replenishing pulmonary surfactant, which is deficient in premature neonates, lung surfactants lower the surface tension on alveolar surfaces during respiration. These agents also stabilize the alveoli to prevent the collapse that may occur with resting transpulmonary pressures. Their actions improve lung compliance and respiratory gas exchange. (See illustration, *Sites of Action: Respiratory Agents,* page 1364.)

beractant
burr-**act**-ant
(Survanta)
Do not confuse with Sufenta.

CATEGORY AND SCHEDULE
Pregnancy Risk Category: This drug is not indicated for use in pregnant women.

MECHANISM OF ACTION
A natural bovine lung extract that lowers surface tension on alveolar surfaces during respiration, stabilizes alveoli vs. collapse that may occur at resting transpulmonary pressures. *Therapeutic Effect:* Replenishes surfactant, restores surface activity to lungs.

PHARMACOKINETICS
Not absorbed systemically.

AVAILABILITY
Suspension: 25 mg/ml vial.

INDICATIONS AND DOSAGES
▸ **Prevention and rescue treatment of respiratory distress syndrome**

(RDS) or hyaline membrane disease in premature infants
Intratracheal
Infants. 100 mg of phospholipids/ kg birth weight (4 ml/kg). Give within 15 min of birth if infant weighs less than 1,250 g with evidence of surfactant deficiency; give within 8 hrs when RDS confirmed by x-ray and requiring mechanical ventilation. May repeat 6 hrs or longer after preceding dose. As many as 4 doses may be given during the first 48 hrs of life.

CONTRAINDICATIONS
None known

INTERACTIONS
Drug
None known.
Herbal
None known.
Food
None known.

DIAGNOSTIC TEST EFFECTS
None known.

SIDE EFFECTS
Frequent
Transient bradycardia, oxygen (O_2) desaturation; increased carbon dioxide (CO_2) retention
Occasional
Endotracheal tube reflux
Rare
Apnea, endotracheal tube blockage, hypotension/hypertension, pallor, vasoconstriction

SERIOUS REACTIONS
• Nosocomial sepsis may occur and is associated with increased mortality.

<hr>

NURSING CONSIDERATIONS
Baseline Assessment
• Administer the drug in a highly supervised setting. Clinicians in care of the neonate must be experienced with intubation and ventilator management.
• Offer emotional support to the patient's parents.
Lifespan Considerations
• There are no age-related precautions noted for neonates.
Precautions
• Use cautiously in patients at risk for circulatory overload.
Administration and Handling
Intratracheal
• Refrigerate vials.
• Warm by standing vial at room temperature for 20 minutes or warm in hand 8 minutes.
• If settling occurs, gently swirl vial—do not shake—to disperse.
• After warming, may return to refrigerator within 8 hours one time only.
• Each vial should be injected with a needle only one time; discard unused portions.
• Color normally appears off-white to light brown.

• Instill through catheter inserted into infant's endotracheal tube. Do not instill into main stem bronchus.
• Monitor for bradycardia, decreased O_2 saturation during administration. Stop dosing procedure, as prescribed, if the patient experiences these effects, then begin appropriate measures before reinstituting therapy.
Intervention and Evaluation
• Monitor the infant with arterial or transcutaneous measurement of systemic O_2 and CO_2.
• Assess the patient's lung sounds for crackles, rales, and rhonchi.
Patient Teaching
• Tell parents the purpose of treatment and the expected outcome.
• Limit visitors during treatment, and monitor for hand washing and other infection control measures to minimize the risk of nosocomial infections.

calfactant
cal-**fak**-tant
(Infasurf)

CATEGORY AND SCHEDULE
Pregnancy Risk Category: This drug is not indicated for use in pregnant women.

MECHANISM OF ACTION
A natural lung extract that modifies alveolar surface tension, stabilizing the alveoli. *Therapeutic Effect:* Restores surface activity to infant lungs, improves lung compliance and respiratory gas exchange.

PHARMACOKINETICS
No studies have been performed.

AVAILABILITY
Intratracheal Suspension: 35 mg/ml vials.

INDICATIONS AND DOSAGES
▶ **Respiratory distress syndrome (RDS)**
Intratracheal
Neonates. Instill 3 ml/kg of birth weight as soon as possible after birth, administered as 2 doses of 1.5 ml/kg. Repeat doses of 3 ml/kg of birth weight, up to a total of 3 doses, 12 hrs apart.

CONTRAINDICATIONS
None known

INTERACTIONS
Drug
None known.
Herbal
None known.
Food
None known.

DIAGNOSTIC TEST EFFECTS
None known.

SIDE EFFECTS
Frequent
Cyanosis (65%), airway obstruction (39%), bradycardia (34%), reflux of surfactant into endotracheal tube (21%), requirement of manual ventilation (16%)
Occasional (3%)
Reintubation

SERIOUS REACTIONS
• Complications may occur as apnea, patent ductus arteriosus, intracranial hemorrhage, sepsis, pulmonary air leaks, pulmonary hemorrhage, and necrotizing entero-colitis.

NURSING CONSIDERATIONS
Baseline Assessment
• Administer drug in a highly super-vised setting. Clinicians in care of the neonate must be experienced with intubation and ventilator man-agement.
• Offer emotional support to the patient's parents.
Lifespan Considerations
• There are no age-related precau-tions noted in neonates.
• This drug is only for use in neo-nates.
Precautions
• Use cautiously in patients with a hypersensitivity to calfactant.
Administration and Handling
Intratracheal
• Refrigerate.
• Unopened, unused vials may be returned to refrigerator only once after having been warmed to room temperature.
• Do not shake.
• Enter only once, discard unused suspension.
Intervention and Evaluation
• Monitor the neonate with arterial or transcutaneous measurement of systemic oxygen (O_2) and carbon dioxide (CO_2).
• Assess the patient's lung sounds for crackles, rales, and rhonchi.
Patient Teaching
• Tell parents the purpose of treat-ment and the expected outcome.
• Limit visitors during treatment, and monitor for hand washing and other infection control measures to minimize the risk of nosocomial infections.

poractant alfa
pour-**act**-tant
(Curosurf, Curosurg[CAN])

CATEGORY AND SCHEDULE
Pregnancy Risk Category: This drug is not indicated for use in pregnant women.

MECHANISM OF ACTION
A pulmonary surfactant that reduces surface tension of alveoli during ventilation; stabilizes alveoli against collapse that may occur at resting transpulmonary pressures. *Therapeutic Effect:* Prevents alveoli from collapsing during expiration by lowering surface tension between air and alveolar surfaces.

AVAILABILITY
Intratracheal Suspension: 1.5 ml (120 mg), 3 ml (240 mg).

INDICATIONS AND DOSAGES
▸ **Respiratory distress syndrome (RDS)**
Endotracheal
Infants. Initially, 2.5 ml/kg birth weight (BW). Up to 2 subsequent doses of 1.25 ml/kg BW at 12-hr intervals. Maximum Total Dose: 5 ml/kg.

UNLABELED USES
Adult RDS due to viral pneumonia, HIV-infected infants with *Pneumocystis carinii* pneumonia, prophylaxis for RDS, treatment in adult RDS following near-drowning

CONTRAINDICATIONS
None known.

INTERACTIONS
Drug
None known.

Herbal
None known.
Food
None known.

DIAGNOSTIC TEST EFFECTS
None known.

SIDE EFFECTS
Frequent
Transient bradycardia, oxygen (O_2) desaturation, increased carbon dioxide (CO_2) tension
Occasional
Endotracheal tube reflux
Rare
Apnea, endotracheal tube blockage, hypotension/hypertension, pallor, vasoconstriction

SERIOUS REACTIONS
• Pneumonia (17%), septicemia (14%), bronchopulmonary dysplasia (18%), intracranial hemorrhage (51%), patent ductus arteriosus (60%), pneumothorax (21%), and pulmonary interstitial emphysema (21%) may occur.

NURSING CONSIDERATIONS
Baseline Assessment
• Plan to correct acidosis, anemia, hypoglycemia, hypotension, and hypothermia before beginning poractant alfa administration.
• Change ventilator settings, as prescribed, to 40 to 60 breaths a minute, inspiratory time 0.5 sec, and supplemental O_2 sufficient to maintain SaO_2 greater than 92% immediately before poractant alfa administration.
• Administer drug in a highly supervised setting. Clinicians in care of the neonate must be experienced with intubation and ventilator management.
• Offer emotional support to the neonate patient's parents.

Lifespan Considerations
• There are no age-related precautions noted for the neonate.

Precautions
• Use cautiously in patients at risk for circulatory overload.

Administration and Handling
Intrathecal
• Refrigerate vials.
• Warm by standing vial at room temperature for 20 minutes or warm in hand 8 minutes.
• To obtain uniform suspension, turn upside down gently, swirl vial, but do not shake.
• After warming, may return to refrigerator one time only.
• Withdraw entire contents of vial into a 3- or 5-ml plastic syringe through large-gauge needle (20 gauge or larger).
• Attach syringe to catheter and instill through catheter inserted into infant's endotracheal tube.

• Monitor the infant for bradycardia and decreased O_2 saturation during administration. Stop the dosing procedure if the infant experiences these effects, then begin appropriate measures before reinstituting therapy.

Intervention and Evaluation
• Monitor the infant with arterial or transcutaneous measurement of systemic O_2 and CO_2.
• Assess the patient's lung sounds for crackles, rales, and rhonchi.
• Monitor the patient's heart rate.

Patient Teaching
• Tell parents the purpose of treatment and the expected outcome.
• Limit visitors during treatment, and monitor for hand washing and other infection control measures to minimize the risk of nosocomial infections.

naphazoline
phenylephrine
  hydrochloride
pseudoephedrine
  hydrochloride,
  pseudoephedrine
  sulfate
sodium chloride

Uses: Nasal decongestants are used to relieve stuffiness caused by such conditions as common cold, acute or chronic rhinitis, hay fever, and other allergies. Sodium chloride is administered nasally to restore moisture and relieve dry, inflamed nasal membranes.

Action: Most nasal decongestants stimulate alpha$_1$-adrenergic receptors on nasal blood vessels, causing vasoconstriction that shrinks swollen membranes and allows nasal drainage. As a major extracellular cation, sodium chloride soothes the nasal passages. (See illustration, *Sites of Action: Respiratory Agents,* page 1364.)

COMBINATION PRODUCTS

ALLEGRA-D: pseudoephedrine/fexofenadine (an antihistamine) 120 mg/ 60 mg.

CHILDREN'S ADVIL COLD: pseudoephedrine/ibuprofen (an NSAID) 15 mg/100 mg per 5 ml.

CLARITIN-D: pseudoephedrine/loratadine (an antihistamine) 120 mg/ 5 mg; 240 mg/10 mg.

NAPHCON-A: naphazoline/pheniramine (an antihistamine) 0.25%/0.3%.

PHENERGAN VC: phenylephrine/promethazine (an antihistamine) 5 mg/6.25 mg per 5 ml.

PHENERGAN VC WITH CODEINE: phenylephrine/promethazine (an antihistamine)/codeine (a narcotic analgesic) 5 mg/6.25 mg/10 mg per 5 ml.

ZYRTEC D-12 HOUR TABLETS: pseudoephedrine/cetirizine (an antihistamine) 120 mg/5 mg.

naphazoline

na-**faz**-oh-leen
(Albalon Liquifilm[AUS], AK-Con, Clear Eyes[AUS], Naphcon, Privine, Vasocon)

CATEGORY AND SCHEDULE
Pregnancy Risk Category: C

MECHANISM OF ACTION
A sympathomimetic that directly acts on alpha-adrenergic receptors in arterioles of conjunctiva. *Therapeutic Effect:* Causes vasoconstriction, with subsequent decreased congestion to area.

AVAILABILITY
Ophthalmic Solution: 0.012%, 0.1%.
Nasal Drops: 0.05%.
Nasal Spray: 0.05%.

INDICATIONS AND DOSAGES
▸ **Relief of nasal congestion due to acute or chronic rhinitis, common cold, hayfever or other allergies**
Intranasal

Adults, Elderly, Children older than 12 yrs. 1–2 drops/sprays (0.05%) in each nostril q3–6h.
Children 6–12 yrs. 1 spray/drop q6h as needed.

▸ **Control of hyperemia in patients with superficial corneal vascularity, relief of congestion, itching, and minor irritation, may be used during some ocular diagnostic procedures**
Ophthalmic
Adults, Elderly, Children older than 6 yrs. 1–2 drops q3–4h for 3–4 days.

CONTRAINDICATIONS
Before peripheral iridectomy, eyes capable of angle closure, narrow-angle glaucoma, or patients with a narrow angle who do not have glaucoma

INTERACTIONS
Drug
Maprotiline, tricyclic antidepressants: May increase the effects of naphazoline.
Herbal
None known.
Food
None known.

DIAGNOSTIC TEST EFFECTS
None known.

SIDE EFFECTS
Occasional
Nasal: Burning, stinging, drying nasal mucosa, sneezing, rebound congestion
Ophthalmic: Blurred vision, large pupils, increased eye irritation

SERIOUS REACTIONS
• Large doses may produce tachycardia, palpitations, lightheadedness, nausea, and vomiting.
• Overdosage in patients older than 60 years of age may produce hallucinations, CNS depression, and seizures.

NURSING CONSIDERATIONS
Baseline Assessment
• Ask the patient if he or she takes tricyclic antidepressants before administering drug.
Precautions
• Use cautiously in patients with cerebral arteriosclerosis, coronary artery disease, diabetes, heart disease, hypertension, hypertensive cardiovascular disease, hyperthyroidism, and long-standing bronchial asthma.
Administration and Handling
◀ALERT▶ Be aware that if naphazoline is systemically absorbed, the patient may experience fast, irregular, and pounding heartbeat, headache, insomnia, lightheadedness, nausea, nervousness, and trembling.
Patient Teaching
• Caution the patient not to use naphazoline longer than 72 hours without consulting a physician.
• Warn the patient to use caution when performing tasks that require visual acuity during naphazoline therapy.
• Tell the patient to discontinue the drug and contact the physician if he or she experiences acute eye redness, dizziness, eye pain, floating spots, headache, insomnia, irregular heartbeat, pain with light exposure, tremor, vision changes, or weakness.
• Explain to the patient that if naphazoline is used too frequently he or she may experience rebound effects.

phenylephrine hydrochloride

See vasopressors

pseudoephedrine hydrochloride

su-do-eh-**fed**-rin
(Dimetapp sinus liquid caps[AUS], Eltor[CAN], Sudafed)

pseudoephedrine sulfate

(Afrinol Repetabs)

CATEGORY AND SCHEDULE

Pregnancy Risk Category: C
OTC

MECHANISM OF ACTION

A sympathomimetic that directly stimulates alpha-adrenergic and beta-adrenergic receptors. *Therapeutic Effect:* Produces vasoconstriction of respiratory tract mucosa; shrinks nasal mucous membranes; reduces edema, nasal congestion.

PHARMACOKINETICS

Route	Onset	Peak	Duration
PO Tablets, syrup	15–30 min	N/A	4–6 hrs
PO Extended release	N/A	N/A	8–12 hrs

Well absorbed from the gastrointestinal (GI) tract. Partially metabolized in liver. Primarily excreted in urine. Not removed by hemodialysis. **Half-life:** 9–16 hrs (Children: 3.1 hrs).

AVAILABILITY

Gelcaps: 30 mg.
Liquid: 15 mg/5 ml.
Oral Drops: 7.5 mg/0.8 ml.
Syrup: 30 mg/5 ml.
Tablets: 30 mg, 60 mg.
Tablets (chewable): 15 mg.
Tablets (extended-release): 120 mg, 240 mg.

INDICATIONS AND DOSAGES
▶ **Decongestant**
PO
Adults, Children older than 12 yrs. 60 mg q4–6h. Maximum: 240 mg/day.
Children 6–12 yrs. 30 mg q6h. Maximum: 120 mg/day.
Children 2–5 yrs. 15 mg q6h. Maximum: 60 mg/day.
Children younger than 2 yrs. 4 mg/kg/day in divided doses q6h.
Elderly. 30–60 mg q6h as needed.
PO (extended release)
Adults, Children older than 12 yrs. 120 mg q12h.

CONTRAINDICATIONS

Coronary artery disease, lactating women, MAOI therapy, severe hypertension

INTERACTIONS
Drug
Antihypertensive, beta-adrenergic blockers, diuretics: May decrease the effects of antihypertensives, beta-adrenergic blockers, and diuretics.
MAOIs: May increase cardiac stimulant and vasopressor effects.
Herbal
None known.
Food
None known.

DIAGNOSTIC TEST EFFECTS

None known.

SIDE EFFECTS
Occasional (10%–5%)
Nervousness, restlessness, insomnia, trembling, headache
Rare (4%–1%)
Increased sweating, weakness

SERIOUS REACTIONS
• Large doses may produce tachycardia, palpitations—particularly in those with cardiac disease, lightheadedness, nausea, and vomiting.
• Overdosage in patients older than 60 years of age may result in hallucinations, CNS depression, and seizures.

NURSING CONSIDERATIONS

Baseline Assessment
• Ask the patient if he or she takes antihypertensive, beta-adrenergic blockers, diuretics, or MAOIs before administering drug.

Lifespan Considerations
• Be aware that pseudoephedrine crosses the placenta and is distributed in breast milk.
• Be aware that the safety and efficacy of pseudoephedrine have not been established in children younger than 2 years of age.
• In the elderly, age-related prostatic hypertrophy may require dosage adjustment.

Precautions
• Use cautiously in elderly patients and patients with diabetes, heart disease, hyperthyroidism, ischemic heart disease, and prostatic hypertrophy.

Administration and Handling
PO
• Do not chew or crush extended-release tablets; swallow whole.

Patient Teaching
• Tell the patient to discontinue the drug if he or she experiences adverse reactions.
• Warn the patient to notify the physician if he or she experiences dizziness, insomnia, irregular or rapid heartbeat, or tremors.

---

sodium chloride
See minerals/electrolytes

86 Respiratory Inhalants and Intranasal Steroids

acetylcysteine
  (*N*-acetylcysteine)
beclomethasone
  dipropionate
budesonide
cromolyn sodium
flunisolide
fluticasone propionate
mometasone furoate
  monohydrate
nedocromil sodium
triamcinolone,
  triamcinolone
  acetonide,
  triamcinolone
  diacetate,
  triamcinolone
  hexacetonide

Uses: Most respiratory inhalants and intranasal steroids are used to treat seasonal and perennial rhinitis, to prevent all major symptoms of rhinitis, and to manage bronchial asthma. Acetylcysteine is prescribed as an adjunct to treat bronchopulmonary disease and pulmonary complications of cystic fibrosis. It's also used in tracheostomy care and the treatment of acetaminophen overdose. Beclomethasone is also used to prevent nasal polyp recurrence after surgery.

Action: Several mechanisms of action account for the effects of respiratory inhalants and intranasal steroids. *Acetylcysteine* splits the disulfide linkages between mucoproteins, reducing the viscosity of pulmonary secretions. *Intranasal steroids,* such as beclomethasone and fluticasone, prevent the inflammatory response to allergens. *Cromolyn* and *nedocromil* prevent the release of inflammatory mediators from mast cells.

COMBINATION PRODUCTS

ADVAIR: fluticasone/salmeterol (a bronchodilator) 100 mcg/50 mcg; 250 mcg/50 mcg; 500 mcg/50 mcg.
MYCO-II: triamcinolone/nystatin (an antifungal) 0.1%/100,000 units/g.
MYCOLOG II: triamcinolone/nystatin (an antifungal) 0.1%/100,000 units/g.
MYCO-TRIACET: triamcinolone/nystatin (an antifungal) 0.1%/100,000 units/g.

acetylcysteine (*N*-acetylcysteine)

ah-sea-tyl-**sis**-teen
(Mucomyst, Parvolex[CAN])
Do not confuse with acetylcholine.

CATEGORY AND SCHEDULE

Pregnancy Risk Category: B

MECHANISM OF ACTION

An intratracheal respiratory inhalant that splits the linkage of mucoproteins. *Therapeutic Effect:* Reduces viscosity of pulmonary secretions, facilitates removal by coughing, postural drainage, mechanical means. Protects against acetaminophen overdose–induced liver toxicity.

AVAILABILITY
Solution: 10%, 20%.

INDICATIONS AND DOSAGES
▸ **Adjunctive treatment for viscid mucus secretions from chronic bronchopulmonary disease and for pulmonary complications of cystic fibrosis.**
Nebulization
Adults, Elderly, Children (20% solution). 3–5 ml 3–4 times/day. Range: 1–10 ml q2–6h.
Adults, Elderly, Children (10% solution). 6–10 ml 3–4 times/day. Range: 2–20 ml q2–6h.
Infants. 1–2 ml (20%) or 2–4 ml (10%) 3–4 times/day.
▸ **To treat viscid mucus secretions in patients with a tracheostomy**
Intratracheal instillation
Adults, Children. 1–2 ml of 10%–20% solution instilled into tracheostomy q1–4h.
▸ **Acetaminophen overdose**
Oral solution (5%)
Adults, Elderly, Children. Loading dose of 140 mg/kg, followed in 4 hrs by maintenance dose of 70 mg/kg q4h for 17 additional doses (unless acetaminophen assay reveals nontoxic level).
▸ **To prevent renal damage from dyes used during certain diagnostic tests**
PO
Adults, Elderly. 600 mg 2 times/day for 4 doses starting the day before the procedure.

UNLABELED USES
Prevention of renal damage from dyes given during certain diagnostic tests (e.g., CT scans)

CONTRAINDICATIONS
None known

INTERACTIONS
Drug
None known.
Herbal
None known.
Food
None known.

DIAGNOSTIC TEST EFFECTS
None known.

SIDE EFFECTS
Frequent
Inhalation: Stickiness on face, transient unpleasant odor
Occasional
Inhalation: Increased bronchial secretions, irritated throat, nausea, vomiting, rhinorrhea
Rare
Inhalation: Skin rash
Oral: Facial edema, bronchospasm, wheezing

SERIOUS REACTIONS
• Large dosage may produce severe nausea and vomiting.

NURSING CONSIDERATIONS
Baseline Assessment
• Assess pretreatment respirations for their rate, depth, and rhythm when this drug is used as a mucolytic.
Precautions
• Use cautiously in patients with bronchial asthma or who are elderly or debilitated with severe respiratory insufficiency.
Intervention and Evaluation
• Discontinue treatment and notify the physician if bronchospasm occurs. Expect to administer a bronchodilator as needed.
• Monitor the rate, depth, rhythm, and type of respirations, such as abdominal or thoracic.

• Check the sputum for its color, consistency, and amount.

Patient Teaching

• Explain to the patient that a slight, disagreeable odor from the solution may be noticed during initial administration but that the odor disappears quickly.

• Stress to the patient the importance of drinking plenty of fluids to maintain adequate hydration.

• Teach the patient proper coughing and deep breathing activities.

beclomethasone dipropionate

beck-low-**meth**-ah-sewn
(Aqueous Nasal Spray[AUS], Beclodisk[CAN], Becloforte inhaler[CAN], Beconase AQ, Becotide[AUS], Qvar)
Do not confuse with baclofen.

CATEGORY AND SCHEDULE

Pregnancy Risk Category: C

MECHANISM OF ACTION

An adrenocorticosteroid that controls the rate of protein synthesis; depresses migration of polymorphonuclear leukocytes and fibroblasts; prevents or controls inflammation; and reverses capillary permeability. *Therapeutic Effect:* Inhalation: Inhibits bronchoconstriction, produces smooth muscle relaxation, decreases mucus secretion. Intranasal: Decreases response to seasonal and perennial rhinitis.

PHARMACOKINETICS

Rapidly absorbed from pulmonary, nasal, and GI tissue. Protein binding: 87%. Metabolized in liver, undergoes extensive first-pass effect.

Primarily eliminated in feces. **Half-life:** 15 hrs.

AVAILABILITY

Aerosol for Inhalation. Intranasal: 42 mcg, 84 mcg per spray.

INDICATIONS AND DOSAGES

▸ **Control of bronchial asthma in patients requiring chronic steroid therapy**
Oral inhalation
Adults, Elderly Children older than 12 yrs. 2 puffs 3–4 times a day. Maximum: 20 puffs a day.
Children 6–12 yrs. 1–2 puffs 3–4 times/day. Maximum: 10 puffs a day.
▸ **Relief of seasonal or perennial rhinitis, prevention of nasal polyps from recurring after surgical removal, treatment of nonallergic rhinitis**
Nasal inhalation
Adults, Children 12 yrs and older. 1–2 sprays in each nostril 2 times a day.
Children 6–11 yrs. 1 spray in each nostril 2 times a day. May increase up to 2 sprays 2 times/day into each nostril.

UNLABELED USES

Nasal: Prophylaxis of seasonal rhinitis

CONTRAINDICATIONS

Hypersensitivity to beclomethasone, status asthmaticus

INTERACTIONS

Drug
None known.
Herbal
None known.
Food
None known.

DIAGNOSTIC TEST EFFECTS
None known.

SIDE EFFECTS
Frequent
Inhalation (14%–4%): Throat irritation, dry mouth, hoarseness, cough
Intranasal: Burning, dryness inside nose
Occasional
Inhalation (3%–2%): Localized fungal infection (thrush)
Intranasal: Nasal-crusting nosebleed, sore throat, ulceration of nasal mucosa
Rare
Inhalation: Transient bronchospasm, esophageal candidiasis
Intranasal: Nasal and pharyngeal candidiasis, eye pain

SERIOUS REACTIONS
• Acute hypersensitivity reaction as evidenced by urticaria, angioedema, and severe bronchospasm occurs rarely.
• Any transfer from systemic to local steroid therapy may unmask previously suppressed bronchial asthma condition.

NURSING CONSIDERATIONS
Baseline Assessment
• Determine if the patient has any hypersensitivity to corticosteroids.
Lifespan Considerations
• Be aware that it is unknown if beclomethasone crosses the placenta or is distributed in breast milk.
• In children, prolonged treatment and high dosages may decrease the patient's short-term growth rate and cortisol secretion.
• There are no age-related precautions noted in the elderly.
Precautions
• Use cautiously in patients with cirrhosis, glaucoma, hypothyroidism, osteoporosis, tuberculosis, and untreated systemic infections.
Administration and Handling
Inhalation
• Shake the container well, instruct the patient to exhale completely, and place the mouthpiece between the patient's lips. Have the patient inhale and hold his or her breath as long as possible before exhaling.
• Allow at least 1 minute between inhalations.
• Have the patient rinse his or her mouth after each use to decrease dry mouth and hoarseness.
Intranasal
• Have the patient clear his or her nasal passages as much as possible.
• Insert the spray tip into the patient's nostril, pointing toward the nasal passages, away from the nasal septum.
• Spray beclomethasone into the nostril while holding the patient's other nostril closed and at the same time, have the patient inhale through nose to deliver the medication as high into the nasal passages as possible.
Intervention and Evaluation
• In those patients receiving bronchodilators by inhalation concomitantly with inhalation of steroid therapy, advise the patient to use a bronchodilator several minutes before taking the corticosteroid aerosol to enhance the penetration of the steroid into the bronchial tree.
Patient Teaching
• Advise the patient not to change the dose schedule or stop taking beclomethasone. Explain to the patient that he or she must taper off beclomethasone use gradually under medical supervision.
• Encourage the patient receiving beclomethasone by inhalation to maintain careful mouth hygiene.

Instruct the patient to rinse his or her mouth with water immediately after inhalation to prevent mouth or throat dryness and fungal infection of mouth. Urge the patient to notify the physician or nurse if he or she develops a sore throat or mouth.
• In patients receiving beclomethasone intranasally, warn the patient to notify the physician if nasal irritation occurs or there is no improvement in symptoms, such as sneezing.
• Teach the patient to clear his or her nasal passages prior to intranasal beclomethasone use.
• Advise the patient that he or she should notice symptom improvement in several days.

budesonide
byew-**des**-oh-nyd
(Entocort, Pulmicort, Rhinocort, Rhinocort Aqua, Rhinocort Aqueous[AUS], Rhinocort Hayfever[AUS])

CATEGORY AND SCHEDULE
Pregnancy Risk Category: B

MECHANISM OF ACTION
A glucocorticosteroid that decreases and prevents tissue response to inflammatory process. *Therapeutic Effect:* Inhibits accumulation of inflammatory cells.

PHARMACOKINETICS
Minimally absorbed from nasal tissue, moderately absorbed from inhalation. Protein binding: 88%. Primarily metabolized in liver. **Half-life:** 2–3 hrs.

AVAILABILITY
Capsule: 3 mg (Entocort EC).
Powder for oral inhalation: 200 mcg (Pulmicort Turbuhaler).
Suspension for nasal inhalation: 50 mcg/inhalation (Pulmicort).
Suspensions for oral inhalation: 0.25 mg/2 ml; 0.5 mg/2 mg (Pulmicort Respules).
Nasal spray suspension: 32 mcg/spray (Rhinocort Aqua).

INDICATIONS AND DOSAGES
▶ **Allergic rhinitis**
Intranasal
Adults, Elderly, Children 6 yrs and older. Rhinocort: 2 sprays to each nostril 2 times/day or 4 sprays to each nostril in morning. Rhinocort Aqua: 1 spray to each nostril once a day. Maximum: Adults, Children older than 12 yrs: 8 sprays/day. Children younger than 12 yrs: 4 sprays/day.
Nebulization
Children 6 mos–8 yrs. 0.25–1 mg/day titrated to lowest effective dosage.
Inhalation
Adults, Elderly, Children 6 yrs and older. Initially, 200–400 mcg 2 times/day. Maximum: Adults: 800 mcg 2 times/day. Children: 400 mcg 2 times/day.
▶ **Crohn's disease**
PO
Adults, Elderly. 9 mg once a day for up to 8 wks.

UNLABELED USES
Treatment of vasomotor rhinitis

CONTRAINDICATIONS
Hypersensitivity to any corticosteroid or components, persistently positive sputum cultures for *Candida albicans*, primary treatment of status asthmaticus, systemic fungal

infections, untreated localized infection involving nasal mucosa

INTERACTIONS
Drug
None known.
Herbal
None known.
Food
None known.

DIAGNOSTIC TEST EFFECTS
None known.

SIDE EFFECTS
Frequent (greater than 3%)
Nasal: Mild nasopharyngeal irritation, burning, stinging, dryness, headache, cough
Inhalation: Flu-like syndrome, headache, pharyngitis
Occasional (3%–1%)
Nasal: Dry mouth, dyspepsia, rebound congestion, rhinorrhea, loss of sense of taste
Inhalation: Back pain, vomiting, altered taste and voice, abdominal pain, nausea, dyspepsia

SERIOUS REACTIONS
• Acute hypersensitivity reaction, including urticaria, angioedema, and severe bronchospasm, occurs rarely.

NURSING CONSIDERATIONS
Baseline Assessment
• Determine if the patient is hypersensitive to any corticosteroids or components of the drug.
Lifespan Considerations
• Be aware that it is unknown if budesonide crosses the placenta or is distributed in breast milk.
• Be aware that prolonged treatment and high dosages may decrease the cortisol secretion and short-term growth rates in children.

• There are no age-related precautions noted in the elderly.
Precautions
• Use cautiously in patients with adrenal insufficiency, cirrhosis, glaucoma, hypothyroidism, osteoporosis, tuberculosis, and untreated infection.
Administration and Handling
Inhalation
• Shake the container well. Instruct the patient to exhale completely, then place the mouthpiece between the patient's lips, have the patient inhale, and instruct the patient to hold his or her breath as long as possible before exhaling.
• Allow at least 1 minute between inhalations.
• Have the patient rinse his or her mouth after each use to decrease dry mouth and hoarseness.
Intranasal
• Have the patient clear his or her nasal passages before using budesonide.
• Tilt the patient's head slightly forward.
• Insert the spray tip into the patient's nostril, pointing toward nasal passages, away from nasal septum.
• Spray into 1 nostril while holding the patient's other nostril closed. Concurrently have the patient inspire through the nostril to allow medication as high into nasal passages as possible.
Intervention and Evaluation
• Monitor the patient for relief of symptoms.
Patient Teaching
• Tell the patient that he or she may experiences symptomatic improvement in 24 hours, but the drug's full effect may take 3 to 7 days to appear.
• Warn the patient to notify the physician if he or she experiences

nasal irritation, no symptomatic improvement, or sneezing.

cromolyn sodium
krom-oh-lin
(Apo-Cromolyn[CAN], Crolom, Gastrocom, Intal, Nasalcrom, Opticrom, Rynacrom[AUS])

CATEGORY AND SCHEDULE
Pregnancy Risk Category: B

MECHANISM OF ACTION
An antiasthmatic and antiallergic agent that prevents mast cell release of histamine, leukotrienes, and slow-reacting substances of anaphylaxis by inhibiting degranulation after contact with antigens. *Therapeutic Effect:* Prevents release histamine from mast cells after exposure to allergens.

PHARMACOKINETICS
Minimal absorption after PO, inhalation, or nasal administration. Absorbed portion excreted in urine or via biliary elimination. **Half-life:** 80–90 min.

AVAILABILITY
Aerosol: 800 mcg.
Liquid: 100 mg/5 ml.
Nasal Spray: 4%.
Nebulization: 20 mg/2 ml.
Ophthalmic Drops: 4%.

INDICATIONS AND DOSAGES
▸ **Asthma**
Inhalation (nebulization)
Adults, Elderly, Children older than 2 yrs. 20 mg 3–4 times/day.
Aerosol spray
Adults, Elderly, Children 12 yrs and older. Initially, 2 sprays 4 times/day.

Maintenance: 2–4 sprays 3–4 times/day.
Children 5–11 yrs. Initially, 2 sprays 4 times/day, then 1–2 sprays 3–4 times/day.
▸ **Prevention of bronchospasm**
Inhalation (nebulization)
Adults, Elderly, Children older than 2 yrs. 20 mg not longer than 1 hr prior to exercise or allergic exposure.
Aerosol spray
Adults, Elderly, Children older than 5 yrs. 2 sprays not longer than 1 hr prior to exercise or allergic exposure.
▸ **Food allergy, inflammatory bowel disease (IBD)**
PO
Adults, Elderly, Children older than 12 yrs. 200–400 mg 4 times/day.
Children 2–12 yrs. 100–200 mg 4 times/day. Maximum: 40 mg/kg/day.
▸ **Allergic rhinitis**
Intranasal
Adults, Elderly, Children older than 6 yrs. 1 spray each nostril 3–4 times/day. May increase up to 6 times/day.
▸ **Systemic mastocytosis**
PO
Adults, Elderly, Children older than 12 yrs. 200 mg 4 times/day.
Children 2–12 yrs. 100 mg 4 times/day. Maximum: 40 mg/kg/day.
Children younger than 2 yrs. 20 mg/kg/day in 4 divided doses. Maximum (children 6 mos–2 yrs): 30 mg/kg/day.
▸ **Conjunctivitis**
Ophthalmic
Adults, Elderly, Children older than 4 yrs. 1–2 drops in both eyes 4–6 times/day.

CONTRAINDICATIONS
Status asthmaticus

INTERACTIONS
Drug
None known.
Herbal
None known.
Food
None known.

DIAGNOSTIC TEST EFFECTS
None known.

SIDE EFFECTS
Frequent
Inhalation: Cough, dry mouth and throat, stuffy nose, throat irritation, unpleasant taste
Nasal: Burning, stinging, irritation of nose, increased sneezing
Ophthalmic: Burning, stinging of eye
PO: Headache, diarrhea
Occasional
Inhalation: Bronchospasm, hoarseness, watering eyes
Nasal: Cough, headache, unpleasant taste, postnasal drip
Ophthalmic: Increased watering and itching of eye
PO: Skin rash, abdominal pain, joint pain, nausea, insomnia
Rare
Inhalation: Dizziness, painful urination, muscle and joint pain, skin rash
Nasal: Nosebleeds, skin rash
Ophthalmic: Chemosis or edema of conjunctiva, eye irritation

SERIOUS REACTIONS
• Anaphylaxis occurs rarely when cromolyn is given via inhalation, nasal, and PO.

NURSING CONSIDERATIONS
Baseline assessment
• Perform baseline assessment of lung sounds, auscultating for adventitious sounds.

• Determine the patient's baseline exercise and activity tolerance.
• Measure baseline peak flow readings, and if ordered, pulmonary function testing.
Lifespan Considerations
• Be aware that it is unknown if cromolyn crosses the placenta or is distributed in breast milk.
• There are no age-related precautions noted in children.
• In the elderly, age-related liver and renal impairment may require dosage adjustment.
Precautions
• Use cautiously in patients with arrhythmias and coronary artery disease.
• Discontinue and taper doses cautiously as symptoms may recur.
Administration and Handling
Inhalation
• Shake container well. Instruct the patient to exhale completely. Place the mouthpiece fully into the patient's mouth and have the patient inhale deeply and slowly while depressing the canister. Instruct the patient to hold his or her breath as long as possible before exhaling.
• Wait 1 to 10 minutes before inhaling second dose to allow for deeper bronchial penetration.
• Have the patient rinse his or her mouth with water immediately after inhalation to prevent mouth and throat dryness.
• Instruct the patient on the use of a spinhaler if he or she is to receive cromolyn by nebulization or inhalation capsules.
Ophthalmic
• Place a gloved finger on the patient's lower eyelid and pull it down until a pocket is formed between the patient's eye and lower lid.
• Hold the dropper above the pocket

and place the prescribed number of drops in the patient's pocket.
• Instruct the patient to close his or her eyes gently so that medication will not be squeezed out of the lacrimal sac.
• Apply gentle finger pressure to the patient's lacrimal sac at the inner canthus for 1 minute after installation to lessen the risk of systemic absorption.
PO
• Give cromolyn at least 30 minutes before meals.
• Pour contents of capsule in hot water, stirring until completely dissolved; add equal amount cold water while stirring.
• Do not mix with food, fruit juice, or milk.
Nasal
• Nasal passages should be clear, which may require nasal decongestant.
• Inhale through nose.
Intervention and Evaluation
• Monitor the depth, rate, rhythm, and type of patient respirations.
• Monitor the quality and rate of the patient's pulse.
• Assess the patient's lung sounds for crackles, rhonchi, and wheezing.
• Observe the patient's fingernails and lips for blue or dusky color in light-skinned patients; gray in dark-skinned patients.
Patient Teaching
• Instruct the patient to increase his or her fluid intake to decrease the viscosity of his or her lung secretions.
• Teach the patient to rinse his or her mouth with water immediately after inhalation to prevent mouth and throat dryness.
• Tell the patient that the effects of therapy are dependent on administering the drug at regular intervals.
• Instruct the patient on the use of a spinhaler if he or she is to receive cromolyn by nebulization or inhalation capsules.

flunisolide
flew-**nis**-oh-lide
(AeroBid, Nasalide, Nasarel, Rhinalar[CAN])
Do not confuse with fluocinonide or Nasalcrom.

CATEGORY AND SCHEDULE
Pregnancy Risk Category: C

MECHANISM OF ACTION
An adrenocorticosteroid that controls the rate of protein synthesis, depresses migration of polymorphonuclear leukocytes, reverses capillary permeability, stabilizes lysosomal membranes. *Therapeutic Effect:* Prevents or controls inflammation.

AVAILABILITY
Aerosol: 250 mcg/activation.
Nasal Spray: 25 mcg/activation.

INDICATIONS AND DOSAGES
▶ **Control of bronchial asthma in those requiring chronic steroid therapy**
Inhalation
Adults, Elderly. 2 inhalations 2 times/day, morning and evening. Maximum: 4 inhalations 2 times/day.
Children 6–15 yrs. 2 inhalations 2 times/day.
▶ **Relief of symptoms of perennial and seasonal rhinitis**
Intranasal
Adults, Elderly. Initially, 2 sprays each nostril 2 times/day, may increase to 2 sprays 3 times/day. Maximum: 8 sprays each nostril/day.

Children 6–14 yrs. Initially, 1 spray 3 times/day or 2 sprays 2 times/day. Maximum: 4 sprays each nostril/day. Maintenance: Smallest amount to control symptoms.

UNLABELED USES

Prevents recurrence of postsurgical nasal polyps

CONTRAINDICATIONS

Hypersensitivity to any corticosteroid, persistently positive sputum cultures for *Candida albicans,* primary treatment of status asthmaticus, systemic fungal infections

INTERACTIONS

Drug
None known.
Herbal
None known.
Food
None known.

DIAGNOSTIC TEST EFFECTS

None known.

SIDE EFFECTS

Frequent
Inhalation (25%–10%): Unpleasant taste, nausea, vomiting, sore throat, diarrhea, upset stomach, cold symptoms, nasal congestion
Occasional
Inhalation (9%–3%): Dizziness, irritability, nervousness, shakiness, abdominal pain, heartburn, fungal infection in mouth, pharynx, larynx, edema
Intranasal: Mild nasopharyngeal irritation, dryness, rebound congestion, bronchial asthma, rhinorrhea, loss of sense of taste

SERIOUS REACTIONS

• Acute hypersensitivity reaction, including urticaria, angioedema, and severe bronchospasm, occurs rarely.

• Transfer from systemic to local steroid therapy may unmask previously suppressed bronchial asthma condition.

NURSING CONSIDERATIONS

Baseline Assessment
• Establish if the patient has a history of asthma and rhinitis.
Precautions
• Use cautiously in patients with adrenal insufficiency.
Administration and Handling
◀ALERT▶ Expect to see improvement of the patient's symptoms within a few days, or relief of symptoms within 3 weeks. Prepare to discontinue the drug beyond 3 weeks if the patient doesn't experience any significant improvement.
Inhalant
• Shake container well. Have the patient exhale as completely as possible.
• Place the mouthpiece fully into the patient's mouth, then while holding the inhaler upright, have the patient inhale deeply and slowly while pressing the top of the canister. Instruct the patient to hold his or her breath as long as possible before exhaling, then to exhale slowly.
• Wait 1 minute between inhalations when multiple inhalations are ordered to allow for deeper bronchial penetration.
• Have the patient rinse his or her mouth with water immediately after inhalation to prevent mouth and throat dryness and oral candidiasis.
Intranasal
• Ensure that the patient clears his or her nasal passages before using flunisolide. The patient may need topical nasal decongestants 5 to 15 minutes before flunisolide use.

• Tilt the patient's head slightly forward.

• Insert spray tip up in one patient nostril, pointing toward inflamed nasal turbinates, away from nasal septum.

• Pump medication into one of the patient's nostrils while holding his or her other nostril closed. Instruct the patient to concurrently inspire through the nose.

• Discard opened nasal solution after 3 months.

Intervention and Evaluation

• Tell patients receiving bronchodilators by inhalation concomitantly with steroid inhalation therapy to use the bronchodilator several minutes before corticosteroid aerosol to enhance penetration of the steroid into the bronchial tree.

• Monitor the depth, rate, rhythm, and type of patient's respirations.

• Monitor the patient's arterial blood gases (ABGs) and the quality and rate of the patient's pulse.

• Assess the patient's lung sounds for rales, rhonchi, and wheezing.

Patient Teaching

• Caution the patient against abruptly discontinuing the drug or changing the drug's dose schedule. Explain to the patient that he or she must taper off drug doses gradually under medical supervision.

• Urge the patient to maintain careful oral hygiene.

• Instruct the patient to rinse his or her mouth with water immediately after inhalation to prevent mouth and throat dryness and oral candidiasis.

• Instruct the patient to increase his or her fluid intake to decrease the viscosity of his or her lung secretions.

• Teach patients taking flunisolide intranasally the proper use of nasal spray. Instruct the patient to

clear his or her nasal passages before use.

• Warn the patient to notify the physician if he or she experiences nasal irritation, no improvement in symptoms, or sneezing.

• Explain to the patient that he or she should notice symptomatic improvement in several days.

fluticasone propionate
flew-**tih**-cah-sewn
(Cutivate, Flixotide Disks[AUS], Flixotide Inhaler [AUS], Flonase, Flovent)

CATEGORY AND SCHEDULE
Pregnancy Risk Category: C

MECHANISM OF ACTION
A corticosteroid that controls the rate of protein synthesis, depresses migration of polymorphonuclear leukocytes, reverses capillary permeability, stabilizes lysosomal membranes. *Therapeutic Effect:* Prevents or controls inflammation.

PHARMACOKINETICS
Inhalation/intranasal: Protein binding: 91%. Undergoes extensive first-pass metabolism in liver. Excreted in urine. **Half-life:** 3–7.8 hrs. Topical: Amount absorbed depends on drug, area, skin condition (absorption increased with elevated skin temperature, hydration, inflamed or denuded skin).

AVAILABILITY
Aerosol for Oral Inhalation (Flovent): 44 mcg/inhalation, 110 mcg/inhalation, 220 mcg/inhalation.
Topical Cream (Cutivate): 0.05%.

Topical Ointment (Cutivate):
0.005%.
*Powder for Oral Inhalation
(Flovent Diskus, Flovent Rotadisk):*
50 mcg, 100 mcg, 250 mcg.
Intranasal Spray (Flonase):
50 mcg/inhalation.

INDICATIONS AND DOSAGES
▸ **Allergic rhinitis**
Intranasal
Adults, Elderly. Initially, 200 mcg
(2 sprays each nostril once daily or
1 spray each nostril q12h).
Maintenance: 1 spray each nostril
once daily. Maximum: 200 mcg/
day.
Children older than 4 yrs. Initially, 100 mcg (1 spray each nostril once daily). Maximum: 200
mcg/day.
▸ **Relief of inflammation and pruritus associated with steroid-responsive disorders, such as contact dermatitis and eczema**
Topical
*Adults, Elderly, Children older than
3 mos.* Apply sparingly to affected
area 1–2 times/day.
▸ **Maintenance treatment of asthma for those requiring oral corticosteroid therapy using dry powder formulation**
Inhalation
Children 4–11 yrs. 50–100 mcg
twice a day.
▸ **Previous treatment: bronchodilators**
Inhalation
*Adults, Elderly, Children older than
12 yrs.* Initially, 100 mcg q12h.
Maximum: 500 mcg/day.
▸ **Previous treatment inhaled steroids**
Inhalation
*Adults, Elderly, Children older than
12 yrs.* Initially, 100–250 mcg q12h.
Maximum: 500 mcg q12h.

▸ **Previous treatment with oral steroids**
Inhalation
*Adults, Elderly, Children older than
12 yrs.* Diskus: 500–1,000 mcg
2 times/day. Rotadisk: 1,000 mcg
2 times/day.

CONTRAINDICATIONS
Untreated localized infection of
nasal mucosa
Inhalation: Primary treatment of
status asthmaticus or other acute
asthma episodes

INTERACTIONS
Drug
None known.
Herbal
None known.
Food
None known.

DIAGNOSTIC TEST EFFECTS
None known.

SIDE EFFECTS
Frequent
Inhalation: Throat irritation, hoarseness, dry mouth, coughing, temporary wheezing, localized fungal infection in mouth, pharynx, and larynx—particularly if mouth is not rinsed with water after each administration
Intranasal: Mild nasopharyngeal irritation; nasal irritation, burning, stinging, dryness, rebound congestion, rhinorrhea, loss of sense of taste
Occasional
Intranasal: Nasal and pharyngeal candidiasis, headache
Inhalation: Oral candidiasis
Topical: Burning and itching of skin

SERIOUS REACTIONS
• None known.

NURSING CONSIDERATIONS

Baseline Assessment
• Establish the patient's baseline history of asthma, rhinitis, and skin disorder.

Lifespan Considerations
• Be aware that it is unknown if fluticasone crosses the placenta or is distributed in breast milk.
• Be aware that the safety and efficacy of fluticasone have not been established in children younger than 4 years of age.
• Be aware that children older than 4 years of age may experience growth suppression with prolonged or high doses.
• There are no age-related precautions noted in the elderly.

Precautions
• Use cautiously in patients with active or quiescent tuberculosis, untreated fungal, bacterial, or systemic ocular herpes simplex, and viral infection

Administration and Handling
Inhalation
• Shake container well. Have the patient exhale as completely as possible.
• Place the mouthpiece fully into the patient's mouth, then while holding the inhaler upright, have the patient inhale deeply and slowly while pressing the top of the canister. Instruct the patient to hold his or her breath as long as possible before exhaling, then to exhale slowly.
• Wait 1 minute between inhalations when multiple inhalations ordered to allow for deeper bronchial penetration.
• Have the patient rinse his or her mouth with water immediately after inhalation to prevent mouth and throat dryness.

Intranasal
• Ensure that the patient clears his or her nasal passages before using fluticasone. The patient may need topical nasal decongestants 5 to 15 minutes before fluticasone use.
• Tilt the patient's head slightly forward.
• Insert spray tip up in one patient nostril, pointing toward inflamed nasal turbinates, away from nasal septum.
• Pump medication into one of the patient's nostrils while holding his or her other nostril closed. Instruct the patient to concurrently inspire through the nose.

Intervention and Evaluation
• Monitor the depth, rate, rhythm, and type of patient respirations.
• Monitor the patient's arterial blood gases (ABGs) and the quality and rate of the patient's pulse.
• Assess the patient's lung sounds for rales, rhonchi, and wheezing.
• Evaluate the patient's oral mucous membranes for evidence of candidiasis.
• Monitor growth in pediatric patients.
• Examine the involved area for therapeutic response to irritation in patients using topical fluticasone.

Patient Teaching
• Tell patients receiving bronchodilators by inhalation concomitantly with steroid inhalation therapy to use the bronchodilator several minutes before corticosteroid aerosol to enhance penetration of the steroid into the bronchial tree.
• Caution the patient against abruptly discontinuing the drug or changing the drug's dose schedule. Explain to the patient that he or she must taper off drug doses gradually under medical supervision.
• Urge the patient to maintain careful oral hygiene.

• Instruct the patient to rinse his or her mouth with water immediately after inhalation to prevent mouth and throat dryness and oral candidiasis.

• Instruct the patient to increase his or her fluid intake to decrease the viscosity of his or her lung secretions.

• Teach patients taking fluticasone intranasally the proper use of nasal spray. Instruct the patient to clear his or her nasal passages before use.

• Warn the patient to notify the physician if he or she experiences nasal irritation, no improvement in symptoms, or sneezing.

• Tell the patient that he or she should notice symptomatic improvement in several days.

• Instruct the patient using topical fluticasone to rub a thin film gently onto affected area.

• Teach patients to use topical fluticasone only for the prescribed area and not longer than prescribed. Warn the patient to avoid topical fluticasone contact with eyes.

mometasone furoate monohydrate
(Nasonex)

CATEGORY AND SCHEDULE
Pregnancy Risk Category: C

MECHANISM OF ACTION
An adrenocorticosteroid that acts as an anti-inflammatory. Inhibits early activation of allergic reaction, release of inflammatory cells into nasal tissue. *Therapeutic Effect:* Decreases response to seasonal and perennial rhinitis.

PHARMACOKINETICS
Undetectable in plasma. Protein binding: 98%–99%. The portion of the dose that is swallowed undergoes extensive metabolism. Excreted vial bile, and to a lesser extent, into the urine.

AVAILABILITY
Nasal Spray.

INDICATIONS AND DOSAGES
▸ **Allergic rhinitis**
Nasal spray
Adults, Elderly, Children older than 12 yrs. 2 sprays in each nostril once a day.
Children 2–12 yrs. 1 spray in each nostril once a day. Improvement occurs within 11 hrs to 2 days following first dose. Maximum benefit achieved within 1–2 wks.

CONTRAINDICATIONS
Hypersensitivity to any corticosteroid, persistently positive sputum cultures for *Candida albicans*, systemic fungal infections, untreated localized infection involving nasal mucosa.

INTERACTIONS
Drug
None known.
Herbal
None known.
Food
None known.

DIAGNOSTIC TEST EFFECTS
None known.

SIDE EFFECTS
Occasional
Nasal irritation, stinging
Rare
Nasal or pharyngeal candidiasis

SERIOUS REACTIONS
• Acute hypersensitivity reaction, including urticaria, angioedema, and severe bronchospasm, occurs rarely.

• Transfer from systemic to local steroid therapy may unmask previously suppressed bronchial asthma condition.

NURSING CONSIDERATIONS

Baseline Assessment
• Determine if the patient is hypersensitive to any corticosteroids.
Lifespan Considerations
• Be aware that it is unknown if mometasone crosses the placenta or is distributed in breast milk.
• Be aware that high dosages and prolonged treatment may decrease cortisol secretion and short-term growth rate in children.
• There are no age-related precautions noted in the elderly.
Precautions
• Use cautiously in patients with adrenal insufficiency, cirrhosis, glaucoma, hypothyroidism, osteoporosis, tuberculosis, and untreated infection.
Administration and Handling
Intranasal
• Shake well before each use. Ensure that the patient clears his or her nasal passages before using mometasone.
• Insert spray tip up in one patient nostril, pointing toward inflamed nasal turbinates, away from nasal septum.
• Pump medication into one of the patient's nostrils while holding his or her other nostril closed. Instruct the patient to concurrently inspire through the nose to permit the medication as high into nasal passages as possible.
Patient Teaching
• Teach the patient the proper use of mometasone nasal spray.
• Instruct the patient to clear his or her nasal passages before using mometasone.

• Caution the patient against abruptly discontinuing the drug or changing the drug's dose schedule. Explain to the patient that he or she must taper off drug doses gradually under medical supervision.
• Warn the patient to notify the physician if he or she experiences nasal irritation, no improvement in symptoms, or sneezing.

nedocromil sodium
ned-oh-**crow**-mul
(Alocril, Mireze[CAN], Tilade)

CATEGORY AND SCHEDULE
Pregnancy Risk Category: B

MECHANISM OF ACTION
A mast cell stabilizer that prevents activation, release of mediators of inflammation, such as histamine, leukotrienes, mast cells, eosinophils, and monocytes. *Therapeutic Effect:* Prevents both early and late asthmatic responses.

AVAILABILITY
Aerosol for Inhalation: 1.75 mg/ activation.
Ophthalmic Solution: 2%.

INDICATIONS AND DOSAGES
▶ **Mild to moderate asthma**
Oral inhalation
Adults, Elderly, Children 6 yrs and older. 2 inhalations 4 times/day. May decrease to 3 times/day then 2 times/day as control of asthma occurs.
▶ **Allergic conjunctivitis**
Ophthalmic
Adults, Elderly, Children 3 yrs and older. 1–2 drops in each eye 2 times/day.

UNLABELED USES
Prevention of bronchospasm in patients with reversible obstructive airway disease

CONTRAINDICATIONS
None known

INTERACTIONS
Drug
None known.
Herbal
None known.
Food
None known.

DIAGNOSTIC TEST EFFECTS
None known.

SIDE EFFECTS
Frequent (10%–6%)
Cough, pharyngitis, bronchospasm, headache, unpleasant taste
Occasional (5%–1%)
Rhinitis, upper respiratory tract infection, abdominal pain, fatigue
Rare (less than 1%)
Diarrhea, dizziness

SERIOUS REACTIONS
• None known.

NURSING CONSIDERATIONS

Baseline assessment
• Perform baseline assessment of lung sounds, auscultating for adventitious sounds.

• Determine the patient's baseline exercise and activity tolerance.
• Measure baseline peak flow readings, and if ordered, pulmonary function testing.
Precautions
• Remember that nedocromil is not used for reversing acute bronchospasm.
Intervention and Evaluation
• Evaluate the patient for therapeutic response, less frequent or severe asthmatic attacks and reduced dependence on antihistamines.
Patient Teaching
• Instruct the patient to increase his or her fluid intake to decrease the viscosity of his or her lung secretions.
• Explain to the patient that the drug must be administered at regular intervals, even when symptom-free, to achieve optimal results of therapy.
• Tell the patient that the unpleasant taste he or she experiences after nedocromil inhalation may be relieved by rinsing his or her mouth with water immediately after inhalation.
• Teach the patient how to use a peak flow meter and to record the values in a log.

triamcinolone
See adrenocortical steroids

87 Miscellaneous Respiratory Agents

dornase alfa
montelukast
omalizumab
zafirlukast

Uses: Because they belong to separate subclasses, miscellaneous respiratory agents have different indications. Along with standard therapy, *dornase alfa* is used to reduce the frequency of respiratory infections and improve pulmonary function in patients with advanced cystic fibrosis. *Montelukast* and *zafirlukast* are used for prophylaxis and long-term treatment of asthma. *Omalizumab* is prescribed to treat moderate to severe persistent asthma triggered by year-round allergens.

Action: Miscellaneous respiratory agents act by various mechanisms. *Dornase alfa* selectively splits and hydrolyzed deoxyribonucleic acid in sputum, reducing sputum viscidity and elasticity. *Montelukast* and *zafirlukast* act on leukotriene receptors. This decreases the effects of leukotrienes, which increase eosinophil migration, producing mucus and edema of the airway wall and causing bronchoconstriction. *Omalizumab* works by blocking immunoglobulin E, an underlying cause of allergic asthma.

dornase alfa
door-naze al-fah
(Pulmozyme)

CATEGORY AND SCHEDULE
Pregnancy Risk Category: B

MECHANISM OF ACTION
A respiratory inhalant, enzyme that selectively splits, hydrolyzes DNA in sputum. *Therapeutic Effect*: Reduces sputum viscid elasticity.

AVAILABILITY
Inhalation: 2.5 mg ampoules for nebulization.

INDICATIONS AND DOSAGES
▸ **Management of pulmonary function in cystic fibrosis**
Nebulization
Adults, Children older than 5 yrs.
2.5 mg (1 ampoule) once daily via recommended nebulizer. May increase to twice daily dosing.

CONTRAINDICATIONS
Sensitivity to dornase alfa, epoetin alfa

INTERACTIONS
Drug
None known.
Herbal
None known.
Food
None known.

DIAGNOSTIC TEST EFFECTS
None known.

SIDE EFFECTS
Frequent (greater than 10%)
Pharyngitis, chest pain or discomfort, sore throat, changes in voice
Occasional (10%–3%)
Conjunctivitis, hoarseness, skin rash

SERIOUS REACTIONS
• None significant.

NURSING CONSIDERATIONS

Baseline Assessment
• Assess the patient's arterial blood gases (ABGs), dyspnea, fatigue, lung sounds, and pulmonary secretions for amount, color, and viscosity.
Administration and Handling
Nebulization
• Refrigerate, protect from light.
• Do not expose to room temperature longer than 24 hours.
• Do not mix with other medications in nebulizer.
Intervention and Evaluation
• Provide emotional support to the patient as well as to his or her family and parents.
• Assess the patient for relief of dyspnea and fatigue.
• Examine the patient for decreased viscosity of pulmonary secretions.
• Encourage the patient to increase his or her fluid intake.
Patient Teaching
• Instruct the patient not to dilute or mix dornase alfa with other medications. Teach the patient to refrigerate the drug.
• Explain to the patient that he or she may have hoarseness or other upper airway irritation during dornase alfa therapy.
• Teach the patient how to use and clean the nebulizer.

montelukast
mon-**tee**-leu-cast
(Singulair)

CATEGORY AND SCHEDULE
Pregnancy Risk Category: B

MECHANISM OF ACTION
An antiasthmatic that inhibits cysteinyl leukotriene receptors, producing inhibition of the effects on bronchial smooth muscle. *Therapeutic Effect:* Attenuates bronchoconstriction, decreases vascular permeability, mucosal edema, mucus production.

PHARMACOKINETICS

Route	Onset	Peak	Duration
PO	N/A	N/A	24 hrs
PO, chewable	N/A	N/A	24 hrs

Rapidly absorbed from the gastrointestinal (GI) tract. Protein binding: 99%. Extensively metabolized in the liver. Excreted almost exclusively in the feces. **Half-life:** 2.7–5.5 hrs (half-life is slightly longer in the elderly).

AVAILABILITY
Tablets: 10 mg.
Tablets (chewable): 4 mg, 5 mg.
Oral Granules: 4 mg.

INDICATIONS AND DOSAGES
▸ **Bronchial asthma**
PO
Adults, Elderly, Adolescents older than 14 yrs. One 10-mg tablet a day, taken in the evening.
Children 6–14 yrs. One 5-mg chewable tablet a day, taken in the evening.
Children 1–5 yrs. One 4-mg chew-

able tablet a day, taken in the evening.

CONTRAINDICATIONS
None known

INTERACTIONS
Drug
Phenobarbital, rifampin: May reduce the duration of action of montelukast.
Herbal
None known.
Food
None known.

DIAGNOSTIC TEST EFFECTS
May increase SGOT (AST) and SGPT (ALT) levels.

SIDE EFFECTS
Adults, Adolescents older than 14 yrs
Frequent (18%)
Headache
Occasional (4%)
Influenza
Rare (3%–2%)
Abdominal pain, cough, dyspepsia, dizziness, fatigue, dental pain
Children 6–14 yrs
Rare (less than 2%)
Diarrhea, laryngitis, pharyngitis, nausea, otitis media, sinusitis, viral infection

SERIOUS REACTIONS
• None known.

NURSING CONSIDERATIONS

Baseline Assessment
• Inform parents of phenylketonuric patients that the montelukast chewable tablet contains phenylalanine, a component of aspartame.
• Do not abruptly substitute montelukast for inhaled or oral corticosteroids.

Lifespan Considerations
• Be aware that it is unknown if montelukast is excreted in breast milk. Use montelukast during pregnancy only if necessary.
• There are no age-related precautions noted in children older than 6 years of age and the elderly.

Precautions
• Use cautiously in patients with impaired liver function and on systemic corticosteroid treatment reduction during montelukast therapy.

Administration and Handling
PO
• Administer montelukast in the evening without regard to food ingestion.

Intervention and Evaluation
• Monitor the depth, rate, rhythm, and type of patient respirations.
• Monitor the quality and rate of the patient's pulse.
• Assess the patient's lung sounds for crackles, rhonchi, and wheezing.
• Observe the patient's fingernails and lips for blue or dusky color in light-skinned patients; gray in dark-skinned patients (signs of hypoxemia).

Patient Teaching
• Instruct the patient to increase his or her fluid intake to decrease the viscosity of his or her lung secretions.
• Teach the patient to take the drug as prescribed, even during symptom-free periods as well as during exacerbations of asthma.
• Caution the patient not to alter the dosage or abruptly discontinue his or her other asthma medications.
• Explain to the patient that montelukast is not for the treatment of acute asthma attacks.
• Tell patients with aspirin sensitivity to avoid aspirin and NSAIDs while taking montelukast.

omalizumab
oh-mah-**liz**-uw-mab
(Xolair)

CATEGORY AND SCHEDULE
Pregnancy Risk Category: B

MECHANISM OF ACTION
A monoclonal antibody that selectively binds to human immunoglobulin E (IgE). Inhibits the binding of IgE on the surface of mast cells and basophiles. *Therapeutic Effect:* Reduction of surface-bound IgE limits the degree of release of mediators of the allergic response, reducing or preventing asthmatic attacks.

PHARMACOKINETICS
Following subcutaneous administration, absorbed slowly, with peak concentration in 7–8 days. Excreted in the liver reticuloendothelial system and endothelial cells. **Half-life:** 26 days.

AVAILABILITY
Powder for Injection: 202.5 mg or 150 mg/1.2 ml following reconstitution.

INDICATIONS AND DOSAGES
▶ **Treatment of moderate to severe, persistent asthma in those reactive to a perennial allergen and inadequately controlled asthma symptoms with inhaled corticosteroids**
Subcutaneous
Adults, Elderly, Children older than 12 yrs. 150–375 mg every 2–4 wks, dosing and frequency depending on immunoglobulin E (IgE) level and body weight.

▶ **Subcutaneous dosage given every 4 weeks**

Pretreatment IgE serum levels (units/ml)	Body Weight (kg) 30–60	Body Weight (kg) 61–70	Body Weight (kg) 71–90	Body Weight (kg) 91–150
greater than 30 to 100	150	150	150	300
greater than 100-200	300	300	300	See next table
greater than 200–300	300	See next table	See next table	See next table

▶ **Subcutaneous dosage given every 2 weeks:**

Pretreatment IgE serum levels (units/ml)	Body Weight (kg) 30–60	Body Weight (kg) 61–70	Body Weight (kg) 71–90	Body Weight (kg) 91–150
greater than 201–300	See previous table	225	225	300
greater than 301–400	225	225	300	Do not dose
greater than 401–500	300	300	375	Do not dose
greater than 501–600	300	375	Do not dose	Do not dose
greater than 601–700	375	Do not dose	Do not dose	Do not dose

UNLABELED USES
Treatment of seasonal allergic rhinitis

CONTRAINDICATIONS
None known

INTERACTIONS
Drug
None known.
Herbal
None known.
Food
None known.

DIAGNOSTIC TEST EFFECTS
Total IgE levels do not return to pretreatment levels for up to 1 year following omalizumab discontinuation.

SIDE EFFECTS
Frequent (45%–11%)
Injection site reaction, including bruising, redness, warmth, stinging, hive formation, and stinging, viral infections, sinusitis, headache, pharyngitis
Occasional (8%–3%)
Arthralgia, leg pain, fatigue, dizziness
Rare (2%)
Arm pain, earache, dermatitis, pruritus

SERIOUS REACTIONS
• Anaphylaxis, occurring within 2 hrs of the first or subsequent administration, occurs in 0.1% of patients.
• Malignant neoplasms occur in 0.5% of patients.

NURSING CONSIDERATIONS

Baseline Assessment
• Obtain the patient's baseline serum total IgE levels before beginning omalizumab therapy because the omalizumab dosage is based on these pretreatment levels.
• Remember that omalizumab is not for the treatment of acute exacerbations of asthma, acute bronchospasm, or status asthmaticus.

Lifespan Considerations
• Be aware that since IgE is present in breast milk, it is assumed that omalizumab is present in breast milk. Use omalizumab only if clearly needed.
• Be aware that the safety and efficacy of omalizumab have not been established in children younger than 12 years of age.
• There are no age-related precautions noted in the elderly.

Precautions
• Be aware that omalizumab is not for use in reversing acute bronchospasm or status asthmaticus.

Administration and Handling
◀ALERT▶ Remember that testing of IgE levels during omalizumab treatment cannot be used as a guide for omalizumab dose determination because IgE levels remain elevated for up to 1 year after discontinuation of omalizumab treatment. Expect to base omalizumab dosage on IgE levels obtained before beginning omalizumab treatment.
• Use only clear or slightly opalescent solution; solution is slightly viscous.
• Store in refrigerator.
• Reconstituted solution is stable for 8 hours if refrigerated or within 4 hours after reconstitution when stored at room temperature.
• Use only sterile water for injection to prepare for subcutaneous administration.
• Medication takes 15 to 20 minutes to dissolve.
• Draw 1.4 ml sterile water for injection into a 3 ml syringe with a 1 inch, 18-gauge needle and inject contents into powdered vial.
• Swirl vial for approximately 1 minute but do not shake. Then swirl vial again for 5 to 10 seconds

every 5 minutes until no gel-like particles appear in the solution. Do not use if contents do not dissolve completely by 40 minutes.
• Invert the vial for 15 seconds to allow the solution to drain toward the stopper.
• Using a new 3 ml syringe with a 1 inch 18-gauge needle, withdraw the required 1.2 ml dose and replace 18-gauge needle with a 25-gauge needle for subcutaneous administration.
• Subcutaneous administration may take 5 to 10 seconds to administer due to omalizumab's viscosity.

Intervention and Evaluation
• Monitor the depth, rate, rhythm, and type of patient respirations, and the quality and rate of the patient's pulse.
• Assess the patient's lung sounds for rales, rhonchi, and wheezing.
• Observe the patient's fingernails and lips for a blue or dusky color in light-skinned patients, gray in dark-skinned patients.

Patient Teaching
• Instruct the patient to increase his or her fluid intake to decrease lung secretion viscosity.
• Warn the patient not to alter the dosage of or discontinue other asthma medications.

---

zafirlukast
zay-**fur**-leu-cast
(Accolate)
Do not confuse with Accupril or Aclovate.

CATEGORY AND SCHEDULE
Pregnancy Risk Category: B

MECHANISM OF ACTION
An antiasthma agent that binds to leukotriene receptors. Inhibits bronchoconstriction due to sulfur dioxide, cold air, specific antigens, such as grass, cat dander, and ragweed. *Therapeutic Effect:* Reduces airway edema, smooth muscle constriction, alters cellular activity associated with inflammatory process.

PHARMACOKINETICS
Rapidly absorbed after PO administration (food reduces absorption). Protein binding: 99%. Extensively metabolized in liver. Primarily excreted in feces. Unknown if removed by hemodialysis. **Half-life:** 10 hrs.

AVAILABILITY
Tablets: 10 mg, 20 mg.

INDICATIONS AND DOSAGES
▶ **Bronchial asthma**
PO
Adults, Elderly, Children older than 12 yrs. 20 mg twice a day.
Children 5–12 yrs. 10 mg twice a day.

CONTRAINDICATIONS
None known

INTERACTIONS
Drug
Aspirin: Increases zafirlukast blood concentration.
Erythromycin, theophylline: Decreases zafirlukast blood concentration.
Warfarin: Coadministration of warfarin increases prothrombin time (PT).
Herbal
None known.
Food
None known.

DIAGNOSTIC TEST EFFECTS
May increase SGPT (ALT) levels.

SIDE EFFECTS
Frequent (13%)
Headache
Occasional (3%)
Nausea, diarrhea
Rare (less than 3%)
Generalized pain, asthenia, myalgia,
fever, dyspepsia, vomiting, dizziness

SERIOUS REACTIONS
• Coadministration of inhaled corticosteroids increases the risk of
upper respiratory infection.

NURSING CONSIDERATIONS

Baseline Assessment
• Obtain the patient's medication
history.
• Assess the patient's hepatic enzyme levels.

Lifespan Considerations
• Be aware that zafirlukast is distributed in breast milk. Zafirlukast
use is not recommended in breast-
feeding women.
• Be aware that the safety and
efficacy of this drug have not been
established in children younger than
5 years of age.
• There are no age-related precautions noted in the elderly.

Precautions
• Use cautiously in patients with
impaired liver function.

Administration and Handling
PO
• Give zafirlukast 1 hour before or
2 hours after meals.
• Do not crush or break tablets.

Intervention and Evaluation
• Monitor the depth, rate, rhythm,
and type of patient respirations.
• Monitor the quality and rate of the
patient's pulse.
• Monitor the patient's liver function test results.
• Assess the patient's lung sounds
for crackles, rhonchi, and wheezing.
• Observe the patient's fingernails
and lips for blue or dusky color in
light-skinned patients; gray in
dark-skinned patients (signs of
cyanosis).

Patient Teaching
• Instruct the patient to increase his
or her fluid intake to decrease the
viscosity of his or her lung secretions.
• Teach the patient to take the drug
as prescribed, even during
symptom-free periods.
• Caution the patient not to alter the
dosage or abruptly discontinue his
or her other asthma medications.
• Explain to the patient that
zafirlukast is not for the treatment
of acute asthma episodes.
• Warn breast-feeding mothers not
to breast-feed during zafirlukast
therapy.
• Warn the patient to notify the
physician if he or she experiences
abdominal pain, flu-like symptoms,
jaundice, nausea, or worsening of
asthma.

Appendixes

ANESTHETICS: GENERAL

USES

IV anesthetic agents are used to induce general anesthesia. The general anesthetic state consists of unconsciousness, amnesia, analgesia, immobility, and attenuation of autonomic responses to noxious stimuli.

Volatile inhalation agents produce all the components of the anesthetic state but are administered through the lungs via an anesthesia machine. Agents for use include desflurane, enflurane, halothane, isoflurane, and sevoflurane. They're used in practice to maintain general anesthesia.

ACTION

IV anesthetic agents act on the gamma-aminobutyric acid (GABA) receptor complex to produce central nervous system (CNS) depression. GABA is the primary inhibitory neurotransmitter in the CNS. Ketamine produces dissociation between the thalamus and the limbic system.

Volatile inhalation agents aren't fully understood, but may disrupt neuronal transmission throughout the CNS. These agents may either block excitatory or enhance inhibitory transmission through axons or synapses.

ANESTHETICS: GENERAL

Name	Availability	Uses	Dosage Range	Side Effects
Etomidate (Amidate)	I: 2 mg/ml	IV induction	0.2–0.6 mg/kg	Myoclonus, pain on injection, nausea, vomiting, respiratory depression
Ketamine (Ketalar)	I: 10 mg/ml, 50 mg/ml, 100 mg/ml	Analgesia, sedation, IV induction	1–4.5 mg/kg	Delirium, euphoria, nausea, vomiting
Methohexital (Brevital)	Powder for injection: 500 mg	IV induction, sedation	50–120 mg	Cardiovascular depression, myoclonus, nausea, vomiting, respiratory depression

Midazolam (Versed)	I: 1 mg/ml, 5 mg/ml	Anxiolytic, amnesic, sedation	1-5 mg titrated slowly	Respiratory depression
Propofol (Diprivan)	I: 10 mg/ml	Sedation IV induction Maintenance	0.5 mg/kg 2-2.5 mg/kg 100-200 mcg/kg/min	Cardiovascular depression, delirium, euphoria, pain on injection, respiratory depression
Thiopental (Pentothal)	**Powder for injection:** 2.5% (25 mg/ml)	IV induction	Titrate vs. pt response. **Average:** 50-75 mg	Cardiovascular depression, nausea, vomiting, respiratory depression

I, Injection.

Appendix B

ANESTHETICS: LOCAL

USES	ACTION
Local anesthetics are used to prevent the initiation of electrical impulses needed for spinal and peripheral nerve conduction. Local or regional anesthesia is selective for the surgical site. Epidural, spinal (intrathecal), IV regional, peripheral nerve block, or topical or local infiltration can be selected. **Alert:** Most side effects are manifestations of excessive plasma concentrations.	Local anesthetics provide anesthesia by reversibly binding to and blocking sodium channels, which slows the rate of depolarization of the nerve action potential and prevents the propagation of the electrical impulses needed for nerve conduction. Most local anesthetics fall into one of two groups: esters or amides.

ANESTHETICS: LOCAL

Name	Uses	Maximum Recommended Dosage (mg)	Onset/Duration	Side Effects*
Esters				
Chloroprocaine (Nesacaine)	Local infiltrate Nerve block Spinal	600–800	Fast/Short	Excitation (for example, convulsions) followed by depression (drowsiness to unconsciousness), bradycardia, heart block, decreased contractile force, hypotension, hypersensitivity reaction
Procaine (Novocain)	Local infiltrate Nerve block Spinal	400–500	Fast/Short	Same as above

		100 (topical)	Slow/Long	Same as above
Tetracaine (Pontocaine)	Topical Spinal			Same as above
Amides				
Bupivacaine (Marcaine, Sensorcaine)	Local infiltrate Nerve block Epidural Spinal	175	Moderate/Long	Same as above
Etidocaine (Duranest)	Local infiltrate Nerve block Epidural	300	Fast/Long	Same as above
Levobupivacaine (Chirocaine)	Nerve block Epidural	–	Moderate/Long	Same as above
Lidocaine (Lidoderm, Xylocaine)	Local infiltrate Nerve block Spinal Epidural Topical IV regional	300	Fast/Moderate	Same as above
Mepivacaine (Carbocaine, Polocaine)	Local infiltrate Nerve block Epidural	300	Moderate/Moderate	Same as above
Ropivacaine (Naropin)	Local infiltrate Nerve block Epidural Spinal	200	Moderate/Long	Same as above

*Most side effects are manifestations of excessive plasma concentrations.
Fast, less than 1 hour; *moderate*, 1–3 hours; *long*, 3–12 hours.

Appendix C

ANOREXIANTS

USES

Anorexiants are used for obesity management. *Noradrenergic agents* are prescribed for short-term treatment of obesity. *Orlistat and sibutramine* are used for long-term treatment.

ACTIONS

Noradrenergic agents, such as benzphetamine, diethylpropion, phendimetrazine, and phentermine, activate central beta-receptors in the hypothalamus.

Orlistat inhibits pancreatic lipase, resulting in decreased fat absorption. It also inhibits digestion of dietary triglycerides and decreases absorption of cholesterol and fat-soluble vitamins.

Sibutramine inhibits serotonin, dopamine, and norepinephrine reuptake, which stimulates thermogenesis.

ANOREXIANTS

Name	Availability	Dosage	Side Effects
Benzphetamine (Didrex)	T: 50 mg	25–50 mg 1–3 times/day	Headache, insomnia, nervousness, irritability, dry mouth, constipation, euphoria, palpitations, hypertension
Diethylpropion (Tenuate)	T: 25 mg, 75 mg	25 mg 3 times/day or 75 mg sustained-release once daily	Headache, insomnia, nervousness, irritability, dry mouth, constipation, euphoria, palpitations, hypertension

Orlistat (Xenical) (See Miscellaneous GI Agents.)	C: 120 mg	120 mg 3 times/day before meals	Flatulence, rectal incontinence, oily stools
Phendimetrazine (Bontril)	C: 105 mg T: 35 mg	17.5–70 mg 2–3 times/day or 105 mg sustained-release once daily	Headache, insomnia, nervousness, irritability, dry mouth, constipation, euphoria, palpitations, hypertension
Phentermine (Ionamin)	C: 15 mg, 30 mg, 37.5 mg	18.75–37.5 mg once daily	Headache, insomnia, nervousness, irritability, dry mouth, constipation, euphoria, palpitations, hypertension
Sibutramine (Meridia)	C: 5 mg, 10 mg, 15 mg	10 mg initially, then increase to 15 mg/day or decrease to 5 mg/day	Increased B/P, heart rate, headache, dry mouth, loss of appetite, insomnia, constipation

C, Capsules; *T,* tablets.

Appendix D

CALCULATION OF DOSES

Frequently, dosages ordered do not correspond exactly to what is available and must therefore be calculated.

Ratio/proportions: Most important in setting up this calculation is that the units of measure are the same on both sides of the equation.

Problem: Patient A is to receive 65 mg of a medication only available in an 80 mg/2 ml vial. What volume (ml) needs to be administered to the patient?

STEP 1: Set up ratio.

$$\frac{80}{2 \text{ ml}} = \frac{65}{x(\text{ml})}$$

STEP 2: Cross multiply.

$$(80 \text{ mg})(x \text{ ml}) = (65 \text{ mg})(2 \text{ ml})$$
$$80 \text{ x} = 130$$

STEP 3: Divide each side of equation by number with x.

$$\frac{80 \text{ x}}{80} = \frac{130}{80}$$

STEP 4: Volume to be administered for correct dose.

$$x = 130 \div 80 \text{ or } 1.625 \text{ ml}$$

Calculations in micrograms per kilogram per minute: Frequently, medications given by IV infusion are ordered as micrograms per kilogram per minute.

Problem: 63-year-old patient (weight 165 lbs) is to receive Medication A at a rate of 8 micrograms per kilogram per minute (mcg/kg/min). Given a solution containing Medication A in a concentration of 500 mg/250 ml, at what rate (ml/hr) would you infuse this medication?

STEP 1: Convert to same units. In this problem, the dose is expressed in mcg/kg; therefore convert patient weight to kg (1 kg = 2.2 lbs) and drug concentration to mcg (1 mg = 1,000 mcg).

$$165 \text{ lbs} \times \frac{1 \text{ kg}}{2.2 \text{ lbs}} = \frac{165 \text{ kg}}{2.2} = 75 \text{ kg}$$

$$\frac{500 \text{ mg}}{250 \text{ ml}} \text{ or } \frac{2 \text{ mg}}{\text{ml}} \times \frac{1,000 \text{ mcg}}{1 \text{ mg}} = \frac{2,000 \text{ mcg}}{1 \text{ ml}} \text{ or } \frac{1 \text{ ml}}{2,000 \text{ mcg}}$$

STEP 2: Number of micrograms per minute (mcg/min).

$$\frac{8 \text{ mcg}}{\text{kg}} \times 75 \text{ kg(patient wt)} = \frac{600 \text{ mcg}}{1 \text{ min}} \text{ or } \frac{1 \text{ min}}{600 \text{ mcg}}$$

STEP 3: Number of milliliters per minute (ml/min).

$$\frac{600 \text{ mcg}}{1 \text{ min}} \times \frac{1 \text{ ml}}{2,000 \text{ mcg}} = \frac{600(\text{ml})}{2,000(\text{min})} = \frac{0.3 \text{ ml}}{\text{min}}$$

STEP 4: Number of milliliters per hour (ml/hr).

$$\frac{0.3 \text{ ml}}{\text{min}} \times \frac{60 \text{ min}}{1 \text{ hr}} = \frac{18 \text{ ml}}{\text{hr}}$$

STEP 5: If the number of drops per minute (gtts/min) were desired, and if the IV set delivered 60 drops per milliliter (gtts/ml) (varies with IV set, information provided by manufacturer), then:

$$\frac{0.3 \text{ ml}}{\text{min}} \times \frac{60 \text{ drops}}{\text{ml}} = \frac{18 \text{ drops}}{\text{min}}$$

Appendix E

COMBINATION DRUGS BY TRADE NAME

Many drugs are available in fixed combinations of two or more medications. Some of the most common trade names for combination drugs in the United States are listed below, along with their generic components and classifications.

Combination Product Name	Generic Components
AC Gel	cocaine (an anesthetic)/epinephrine (a vasopressor)
Accuretic	quinapril (an ACE inhibitor)/hydrochlorothiazide (a diuretic)
Activella	estradiol (an estrogen)/norethindrone (a hormone)
Advair	fluticasone (a corticosteroid)/salmeterol (a bronchodilator)
Aggrenox	aspirin (an antiplatelet and non-narcotic analgesic)/dipyridamole (an antiplatelet)
Aldactazide	spironolactone(a potassium-sparing diuretic)/hydrochlorothiazide (a diuretic)
Aldoril	methyldopa (an antihypertensive)/hydrochlorothiazide (a diuretic)
Allegra-D	fexofenadine (an antihistamine)/pseudoephedrine (a nasal decongestant)
Anexsia	hydrocodone (a narcotic analgesic)/acetaminophen (a non-narcotic analgesic)
Apresazide	hydralazine (a vasodilator)/hydrochlorothiazide (a diuretic)
Arthrotec	diclofenac (an NSAID)/misoprostol (an antisecretory gastric protectant)
Atacand HCT	candesartan (an angiotensin II receptor antagonist)/hydrochlorothiazide (a diuretic)
Avalide	irbesartan (an angiotensin II receptor antagonist)/hydrochlorothiazide (a diuretic)
Avandamet	rosiglitazone (an antidiabetic)/metformin (an antidiabetic)
Bactrim	sulfamethoxazole (a sulfonamide)/trimethoprim (an anti-infective)
Bellergal-S	ergotamine (an antimigraine)/belladonna (an anticholinergic)/phenobarbital (an anticonvulsant)
Benicar HCT	olmesartan (an angiotensin II receptor antagonist)/hydrochlorothiazide (a diuretic)

Bicillin CR	penicillin G benzathine (a penicillin)/penicillin procaine (a penicillin)
Blephamide	sulfacetamide (an anti-infective)/prednisolone (an adrenocortical steroid)
Caladryl	calamine (an astringent)/ diphenhydramine (an antihistamine)/camphor (a counterirritant)
Capital with Codeine	acetaminophen (a non-narcotic analgesic)/codeine (a narcotic analgesic)
Capozide	captopril (an ACE inhibitor)/hydrochlorothiazide (a diuretic)
Children's Advil Cold	ibuprofen (an NSAID)/pseudoephedrine (a nasal decongestant)
CiproDex Otic	ciprofloxacin (an anti-infective)/dexamethasone (an adrenocortical steroid)
Cipro HC Otic	ciprofloxacin (an anti-infective)/hydrocortisone (and adrenocortical steroid)
Claritin-D	loratadine (an antihistamine)/pseudoephedrine (a nasal decongestant)
Combipatch	estradiol (an estrogen)/norethindrone (a hormone)
Combipres	clonidine (an antihypertensive)/chlorthalidone (a diuretic)
Combivent	ipratropium (a bronchodilator)/albuterol (a bronchodilator)/
Combivir	lamivudine (an antiretroviral)/zidovudine (an antiretroviral)
Cortisporin	neomycin (and anti-infective)/polymyxin B (an anti-infective)/hydrocortisone (an adrenocortical steroid)
Corzide	nadolol (a beta-blocker)/bendroflumethiazide (a diuretic)
Cosopt	dorzolamide (a carbonic anhydrase inhibitor)/ timolol (a beta-blocker)/
Darvocet A 500	propoxyphene (a narcotic analgesic)/ acetaminophen (a non-narcotic analgesic)
Darvocet-N	propoxyphene (a narcotic analgesic)/ acetaminophen (a non-narcotic analgesic)
Dexacidin	neomycin (an anti-infective)/polymyxin (an anti-infective)/dexamethasone (an adrenocortical steroid)
Dilantin with PB	phenobarbital (an anticonvulsant)/phenytoin (an anticonvulsant)
Diovan HCT	valsartan (an angiotensin II receptor antagonist)/ hydrochlorothiazide (a diuretic)
Duoneb	ipratropium (a bronchodilator)/albuterol base (a bronchodilator)

(continued)

Combination Product Name	Generic Components
Dyazide	triamterene (a potassium-sparing diuretic)/ hydrochlorothiazide (a diuretic)
EMLA	lidocaine (a local anesthetic)/prilocaine (an anesthetic)
Eryzole	erythromycin (a macrolide)/sulfisoxazole (a sulfonamide)
Etrafon	perphenazine (an antipsychotic)/amitriptyline (an antidepressant)
Extra Strength Maalox	magnesium hydroxide (an antacid)/simethicone (an antiflatulent)
Femhrt	norethindrone (a hormone)/estradiol (an estrogen)
Ferro-Sequels	ferrous fumarate (a hematinic)/docusate (a laxative)
Fioricet	butabarbital (a sedative-hypnotic)/acetaminophen (a non-narcotic analgesic)/caffeine (a CNS stimulant)
Fiorinal	butabarbital (a sedative-hypnotic)/aspirin (a non-narcotic analgesic)/caffeine (a CNS stimulant)
Gaviscon (oral suspension)	aluminum hydroxide (an antacid)/magnesium carbonate (an antacid)
Gaviscon (tablets)	aluminum hydroxide (an antacid)/magnesium trisilicate (an antacid)
Gelusil	aluminum hydroxide (an antacid)/magnesium hydroxide (a laxative)/simethicone (an antiflatulent)
Gentlax-S	senna (a laxative)/docusate (a laxative)
Glucovance	glyburide (an antidiabetic)/metformin (an antidiabetic)
Haley's M-O	magnesium (a laxative)/mineral oil (a lubricant laxative)
Helidac	bismuth (an antidiarrheal)/metronidazole (an anti-infective)/ tetracycline (an anti-infective)
Hyzaar	losartan (an angiotensin II receptor antagonist)/ hydrochlorothiazide (a diuretic)
Imodium Advanced	loperamide (an antidiarrheal)/simethicone (an antiflatulent)
Inderide	propranolol (a beta-blocker)/hydrochlorothiazide (a diuretic)
Inderide LA	propranolol (a beta-blocker)/hydrochlorothiazide (a diuretic)
Lexxel	enalapril (an ACE inhibitor)/felodipine (a calcium channel blocker)

Librax	chlordiazepoxide (an antianxiety agent)/clidinium (an anticholinergic)
Lidocaine with epinephrine	lidocaine (a local anesthetic)/epinephrine (a vasoconstrictor)
Limbitrol	chlordiazepoxide (an antianxiety agent)/ amitriptyline (an antidepressant)
Lomotil	diphenoxylate (an antidiarrheal)/atropine (an anticholinergic-antispasmodic)
Lopressor HCT	metoprolol (a beta-blocker)/hydrochlorothiazide (a diuretic)
Lortab	hydrocodone (a narcotic analgesic)/ acetaminophen (a non-narcotic analgesic)
Lortab Elixir	hydrocodone (a narcotic analgesic)/ acetaminophen (a non-narcotic analgesic)
Lortab/ASA	hydrocodone (a narcotic analgesic)/aspirin (a non-narcotic analgesic)
Lotensin HCT	benazepril (an ACE inhibitor)/hydrochlorothiazide (a diuretic)
Lotrel	amlodipine (a calcium channel blocker)/benazepril (an ACE inhibitor)
Lotrisone	clotrimazole (an antifungal)/betamethasone (and adrenocortical steroid)
Lunelle	medroxyprogesterone (a progestin)/estradiol (an estrogen)
Maalox	aluminum hydroxide (an antacid)/magnesium hydroxide (an antacid)
Maalox Plus	aluminum hydroxide (an antacid)/magnesium hydroxide (an antacid)/simethicone (an anti-flatulent)
Maxitrol	neomycin (an anti-infective)/polymyxin (an anti-infective)/dexamethasone (an adrenocortical steroid)
Maxzide	triamterene (a potassium-sparing diuretic)/ hydrochlorothiazide (a diuretic)
Metaglip	glipizide (an antidiabetic)/metformin(an antidiabetic)
Micardis HCT	telmisartan (an angiotensin II receptor antagonist)/ hydrochlorothiazide (a diuretic)
Minizide	prazosin (an antihypertensive)/polythiazide (a diuretic)
Moduretic	amiloride (a potassium-sparing diuretic)/ hydrochlorothiazide (a diuretic)
Mycitracin	neomycin (an aminoglycoside)/polymyxin B (an anti-infective)/ bacitracin (an anti-infective)
Myco II	nystatin (an antifungal)/triamcinolone (an adrenocortical steroid)

(continued)

Combination Product Name	Generic Components
Mycolog II	nystatin (an antifungal)/triamcinolone (an adreno-cortical steroid)
Myco-Triacet	nystatin (an antifungal)/triamcinolone (an adreno-cortical steroid)
Mylanta (oral suspension)	aluminum hydroxide (an antacid)/magnesium hydroxide (an antacid)/simethicone (an antiflatulent)
Mylanta (tablets)	calcium carbonate/magnesium hydroxide
Naphcon-A	naphazoline (a nasal decongestant/pheniramine (an antihistamine)
Neosporin GU Irrigant	neomycin (an aminoglycoside)/polymyxin B (an anti-infective)
Neosporin Ointment, Triple Antibiotic	neomycin (an aminoglycoside)/polymyxin B (an anti-infective)/bacitracin (an anti-infective)
Norco	hydrocodone (a narcotic analgesic)/acetaminophen (a non-narcotic analgesic)
Normozide	labetalol (a beta-blocker)/hydrochlorothiazide (a diuretic)
Pediazole	erythromycin (a macrolide)/sulfisoxazole (a sulfonamide)
Pepcid Complete	famotidine (an H_2 antagonist)/calcium chloride (an antacid)/magnesium hydroxide (an antacid)
Percocet	oxycodone (a narcotic analgesic)/acetaminophen (a non-narcotic analgesic)
Percodan	oxycodone (a narcotic analgesic)/aspirin (a non-narcotic analgesic)
Phenergan with Codeine	promethazine (an antihistamine)/codeine (a cough suppressant)
Phenergan VC	promethazine (an antihistamine)/phenylephrine (a vasopressor)
Phenergan VC with Codeine	promethazine (an antihistamine)/phenylephrine (a vasopressor)/codeine (a cough suppressant)
Polysporin	polymyxin B (an anti-infective)/bacitracin (an anti-infective)
Pravigard	aspirin (an antiplatelet)/pravastatin (an antihyperlipidemic)
Premphase	conjugated estrogens (an estrogen)/medroxyprogesterone (an androgen)
Prempro	conjugated estrogens (an estrogen)/medroxyprogesterone (an androgen)
Prinzide	lisinopril (an ACE inhibitor)/hydrochlorothiazide (a diuretic)

Rebetron	ribavirin (an antiviral)/interferon alpha-2b (an immunologic agent)
Rifamate	rifampin (an antitubercular)/isoniazid (an antitubercular)
Rifater	rifampin (an antitubercular)/isoniazid (an antitubercular)/pyrazinamide (an antitubercular)
Robitussin AC	guaifenesin (an antitussive)/codeine (a narcotic analgesic)
Robitussin DM	dextromethorphan (a cough suppressant)/guaifenesin (an antitussive)
Roxicet	oxycodone (a narcotic analgesic)/acetaminophen (a non-narcotic analgesic)
Senokot-S	senna (a laxative)/docusate (a laxative)
Septra	sulfamethoxazole (a sulfonamide)/trimethoprim (an anti-infective)
Silain-Gel	magnesium hydroxide (an antacid)/aluminum hydroxide (an antacid)/simethicone (an antiflatulent)
Stalevo	carbidopa-levodopa (an antiparkinson agent)/entacapone (an antiparkinson agent)
Suboxone	buprenorphine (a non-narcotic analgesic)/naloxone (a narcotic antagonist)
TAC	tetracaine (an anesthetic)/epinephrine (a vasoconstrictor)/cocaine (an anesthetic)
Tarka	trandolapril (an ACE inhibitor)/verapamil (a calcium channel blocker)
Teczem	enalapril (an ACE inhibitor)/diltiazem (a calcium channel blocker)
Tenoretic	atenolol (a beta-blocker)/chlorthalidone (a diuretic)
Teveten HCT	eprosartan (an angiotensin II receptor antagonist)/hydrochlorothiazide (a diuretic)
Thyrolar	liothyronine (a thyroid agent)/levothyroxine (a thyroid agent)
Timolide	timolol (a beta-blocker)/hydrochlorothiazide (a diuretic)
Tobradex	tobramycin (an aminoglycoside)/dexamethasone (an adrenocortical steroid)
Triavil	perphenazine (an antipsychotic)/amitriptyline (an antidepressant)
Trizivir	abacavir (an antiretroviral)lamivudine (an antiretroviral)/zidovudine (an antiretroviral)
Tylenol with Codeine	acetaminophen (a non-narcotic analgesic)/codeine (a narcotic analgesic)
Tylox	acetaminophen (a non-narcotic analgesic)/oxycodone (a narcotic analgesic)

(continued)

Combination Product Name	Generic Components
Ultracet	tramadol (a non-narcotic analgesic)/ acetaminophen (a non-narcotic analgesic)
Uniretic	moexipril (an ACE inhibitor)/hydrochlorothiazide (a diuretic)
Vaseretic	enalapril (an ACE inhibitor)/hydrochlorothiazide (a diuretic)
Vasocidin	sulfacetamide (an anti-infective)/prednisolone (an adrenocortical steroid)
Vicodin	hydrocodone (a narcotic analgesic)/ acetaminophen (a non-narcotic analgesic)
Vicodin ES	hydrocodone (a narcotic analgesic)/ acetaminophen (a non-narcotic analgesic)
Vicodin HP	hydrocodone(a narcotic analgesic)/acetaminophen (a non-narcotic analgesic)
Vicoprofen	hydrocodone (a narcotic analgesic)/ibuprofen (an NSAID)
Zestoretic	lisinopril (an ACE inhibitor)/hydrochlorothiazide (a diuretic)
Ziac	bisoprolol (a beta-blocker)/hydrochlorothiazide (a diuretic)
Zotrim	trimethoprim (an anti-infective)/sulfamethoxazole (a sulfonamide)/phenazopyridine (a spasmolytic)
Zydone	hydrocodone (a narcotic analgesic)/ acetaminophen (a non-narcotic analgesic)
Zyrtec D 12 hour tablets	cetirizine (an antihistamine)/pseudoephedrine (a nasal decongestant)

Appendix F

CONTROLLED DRUGS (UNITED STATES)

Schedule I: Medications having no legal medical use. These substances may be used for research purposes with proper registration (e.g., heroin, LSD).

Schedule II: Medications having a legitimate medical use but are characterized by a very high abuse potential and/or potential for severe physical and psychic dependency. Emergency telephone orders for limited quantities of these drugs are authorized, but the prescriber must provide a written, signed prescription order (e.g., morphine, amphetamines).

Schedule III: Medications having significant abuse potential (less than Schedule II). Telephone orders are permitted (e.g., opiates in combination with other substances such as acetaminophen).

Schedule IV: Medications having a low abuse potential. Telephone orders are permitted (e.g., benzodiazepines, propoxyphene).

Schedule V: Medications having the lowest abuse potential of the controlled substances. Some Schedule V products may be available without a prescription (e.g., certain cough preparations containing limited amounts of an opiate).

CULTURAL ASPECTS OF DRUG THERAPY

The term *ethnopharmacology* was first used to describe the study of medicinal plants used by indigenous cultures. More recently, it is being used as a reference to the action and effects of drugs in people from diverse racial, ethnic, and cultural backgrounds. Although there are insufficient data from investigations involving people from diverse backgrounds that would provide reliable information on ethnic-specific responses to all medications, there is growing evidence that modifications in dosages are needed for some members of racial and ethnic groups. There are wide variations in the perception of side effects by patients from diverse cultural backgrounds. These differences may be related to metabolic differences that result in higher or lower levels of the drug, individual differences in the amount of body fat, or cultural differences in the way individuals perceive the meaning of side effects and toxicity. Nurses and other health care providers need to be aware that variations can occur with side effects, adverse reactions, and toxicity so that patients from diverse cultural backgrounds can be monitored.

Some cultural differences in response to medications include the following:

African Americans: Generally, African Americans are less responsive to beta-blockers (e.g., propranolol [Inderal]) and angiotensin-converting enzyme (ACE) inhibitors (e.g., enalapril [Vasotec]).

Asian Americans: On average, Asian Americans have a lower percentage of body fat, so dosage adjustments must be made for fat-soluble vitamins and other drugs (e.g., vitamin K used to reverse the anticoagulant effect of warfarin).

Hispanic Americans: Hispanic Americans may require lower dosages and may experience a higher incidence of side effects with the tricyclic antidepressants (e.g., amitryptyline).

Native Americans: Alaskan Eskimos may suffer prolonged muscle paralysis with the use of succinylcholine when administered during surgery.

There has been a desire to exert more responsibility over one's health and, as a result, a resurgence of self-care practices. These practices are often influenced by folk remedies and the use of medicinal plants. In the United States, there are several major ethnic population subgroups (white, black, Hispanic, Asian, and Native Americans). Each of these ethnic groups has a wide range of practices that influence beliefs and interventions related to health and illness. At any given time, in any group, treatment may consist of the use of traditional herbal therapy, a combination of ritual and prayer with medicinal plants, customary dietary and environmental practices, or the use of Western medical practices.

African Americans

Many African Americans carry the traditional health beliefs of their African heritage. Health denotes harmony with nature of the body, mind, and spirit, whereas illness is seen as disharmony that results from natural causes or divine punishment. Common practices to the art of healing include treatments with herbals and rituals known empirically to restore health. Specific forms of healing include using home remedies, obtaining medical advice from a physician, and seeking spiritual healing.

Examples of healing practices include the use of hot baths and warm compresses for rheumatism, the use of herbal teas for respiratory illnesses, and the use of kitchen condiments in folk remedies. Lemon, vinegar, honey, saltpeter, alum, salt, baking soda, and Epsom salt are common kitchen ingredients used. Goldenrod, peppermint, sassafras, parsley, yarrow, and rabbit tobacco are a few of the herbals used.

Hispanic Americans

The use of folk healers, medicinal herbs, magic, and religious rituals and ceremonies are included in the rich and varied customs of Hispanic Americans. This ethnic group believes that God is responsible for allowing health or illness to occur. Wellness may be viewed as good luck, a reward for good behavior, or a blessing from God. Praying, using herbals and spices, wearing religious objects such as medals, and maintaining a balance in diet and physical activity are methods considered appropriate in preventing evil or poor health.

Hispanic ethnopharmacology is more complementary to Western medical practices. After the illness is identified, appropriate treatment may consist of home remedies (e.g., use of vegetables and herbs), use of over-the-counter patent medicines, and use of physician-prescribed medications.

Asian Americans

For Asian Americans, harmony with nature is essential for physical and spiritual well-being. Universal balance depends on harmony between the elemental forces: fire, water, wood, earth, and metal. Regulating these universal elements are two forces that maintain physical and spiritual harmony in the body: the *yin* and the *yang*. Practices shared by most Asian cultures include meditation, special nutritional programs, herbology, and martial arts.

Therapeutic options available to the traditional Chinese physicians include prescribing herbs, meditation, exercise, nutritional changes, or acupuncture.

Native Americans

The theme of total harmony with nature is fundamental to traditional Native American beliefs about health. It is dependent on maintaining a state of equilibrium among the physical body, the mind, and the environment. Health practices reflect this holistic approach. The method of healing is determined traditionally by the medicine man, who diagnoses the ailment and recommends the appropriate intervention.

Treatment may include heat, herbs, sweat baths, massage, exercise, diet changes, or other interventions performed in a curing ceremony.

European Americans

Europeans often use home treatments as the front-line interventions. Traditional remedies practiced are based on the magical or empirically validated experience of ancestors. These cures are often practiced in combination with religious rituals or spiritual ceremonies.

Household products, herbal teas, and patent medicines are familiar preparations used in home treatments (e.g., salt water gargle for sore throat).

Appendix H

DRUGS OF ABUSE

Name (Brand)	Class	Signs and Symptoms	Treatment
Acid (see LSD) Adam (see MDMA) Amphetamine (Adderall, Dexedrine)	Stimulant	Tachycardia, hypertension, diaphoresis, agitation, headache, seizures, dehydration, hypokalemia, lactic acidosis. Severe overdose: hyperthermia, dysrhythmia, shock, rhabdomyolysis, liver necrosis, acute renal failure.	Control agitation, reverse hyperthermia, support hemodynamic function. **Antidote:** No specific antidote.
Angel dust (see phencyclidine) Apache (see fentanyl) Barbiturates (Nembutal, Seconal)	Depressant	Hypotension, hypothermia, apnea, nystagmus, ataxia, hyporeflexia, somnolence, stupor, coma.	Airway management, decontamination, supportive care. **Antidote:** No specific antidote.
Barbs (see barbiturates) Benzodiazepines (Xanax, Valium, Librium, Halcion)	Depressant	Respiratory depression, hypothermia, hypotension, nystagmus, miosis, diplopia, bradycardia, nausea, vomiting, impaired speech and coordination, amnesia, ataxia, somnolence, confusion, depressed deep tendon reflexes.	**Antidote:** Flumazenil (Romazicon) is a specific antidote.
Black tar (see heroin) Horse (see heroin) Boomers (see LSD) Buttons (see mescaline) Cactus (see mescaline) Candy (see benzodiazepines) China girl (see fentanyl) China white (see heroin)			

(continued)

Name (Brand)	Class	Signs and Symptoms	Treatment
Cocaine	Stimulant	Hypertension, tachycardia, mild hyperthermia, mydriasis, pallor, diaphoresis, psychosis, paranoid delusions, mania, agitation, seizures.	Control agitation, seizures, hyperthermia, support hemodynamic function. **Antidote:** No specific antidote.
Codeine	Opioid	Miosis, respiratory depression, decreased mental status, hypotension, cardiac dysrhythmia, hypoxia, bronchoconstriction, constipation, decreased intestinal motility, ileus, lethargy, coma.	Airway management, hemodynamic support. **Antidote:** Naloxone, nalmefene.
Coke (see cocaine) **Crank** (see amphetamine) **Crank** (see heroin) **Crystal** (see amphetamine) **Crystal meth** (see methamphetamine) **Cubes** (see LSD) **Downers** (see benzodiazepines) **Ecstasy** (see MDMA)			
Fentanyl (Sublimaze)	Opioid	Miosis, respiratory depression, decreased mental status, hypotension, cardiac dysrhythmia, hypoxia, bronchoconstriction, constipation, decreased intestinal motility, ileus, lethargy, coma.	Airway management, hemodynamic support. **Antidote:** Naloxone, nalmefene.
Flunitrazepam (Rohypnol)	Depressant	Drowsiness, slurred speech, impaired judgment and motor skills, hypothermia, hypotension, bradycardia, diplopia, blurred vision, nystagmus, respiratory depression, nausea, constipation, depression, lethargy, headache, ataxia, coma, amnesia, incoordination, tremors, vertigo.	Supportive care, airway control. **Antidote:** Flumazenil (Romazicon).

Name (Brand)	Class	Signs and Symptoms	Treatment
Forget me pill (see flunitrazepam)			
GHB (gammahydroxybutyrate)	CNS depressant	Dose-related CNS depression, amnesia, hypotonia, drowsiness, dizziness, euphoria. Other effects: bradycardia, hypotension, hypersalivation, vomiting, hypothermia. Higher dosages: Cheyne-Stokes respiration, seizures, coma, death. Users become highly agitated, flailing.	Supportive care. Severe intoxication may require airway support, including intubation. **Antidote:** No specific antidote.
Gib (see GHB)			
Goodfellas (see fentanyl)			
Grass (see marijuana)			
Hashish (see marijuana)			
Heroin	Opioid	Miosis, coma, apnea, pulmonary edema, bradycardia, hypotension, pinpoint pupils, CNS depression, seizures.	Airway management. **Antidote:** Naloxone, nalmefene.
Ice (see amphetamine)			
Ketamine (Ketalar)	Anesthetic	Feeling of dissociation from one's self (sense of floating over one's body), visual hallucinations, lack of coordination, hypertension, tachycardia, palpitation, respiratory depression, apnea, confusion, negativism, hostility, delirium, reduced awareness.	Supportive care, esp. respiratory and cardiac function. **Antidote:** No specific antidote.
Keets (see ketamine)			
Kit-kat (see ketamine)			
Liquid ecstasy (see GHB)			
Liquid X (see GHB)			

(continued)

Name (Brand)	Class	Signs and Symptoms	Treatment
LSD	Halluci-nogen	Diaphoresis, mydriasis, dizziness, twitching, flushing, hyperreflexia, hypertension, psychosis, behavioral changes, emotional lability, euphoria or dysphoria, paranoia, vomiting, diarrhea, anorexia, restlessness, incoordination, tremors, ataxia.	Airway management, control activity associated with hallucinations, psychosis, panic reaction. **Antidote:** No specific antidote.
Ludes (see methaqualone)			
Magic mushroom (see psilocybin)			
Marijuana	Canna-binoid	Increased appetite, reduced motility, constipation, urinary retention, seizures, euphoria, somnolence, heightened awareness, relaxation, altered time perception, short-term memory loss, poor concentration, mood alterations, disorientation, decreased strength, ataxia, slurred speech, respiratory depression, coma.	Airway management, supportive care. **Antidote:** No specific antidote.
MDMA (Methylene dioxymethamphetamine)	Stimu-lant	Euphoria, intimacy, closeness to others, loss of appetite, tachycardia, jaw tension, bruxism, sweating.	**Antidote:** No specific antidote.
Mescaline	Halluci-nogen	Diaphoresis, mydriasis, dizziness, twitching, flushing, hyperreflexia, hypertension, psychosis, behavioral changes, emotional instability, euphoria or dysphoria, paranoia, vomiting, diarrhea, anorexia, restlessness, incoordination, tremors, ataxia.	Airway management, control activity associated with hallucinations, psychosis, panic reaction. **Antidote:** No specific antidote.
Meth (see methamphetamine)			

Name (Brand)	Class	Signs and Symptoms	Treatment
Methamphetamine (Desoxyn)	Stimulant	Hypertension, hyperthermia, hyperpyrexia, agitation, hyperactivity, fasciculation, seizures, coma, tachycardia, dysrhythmias, pale skin, diaphoresis, restlessness, talkativeness, insomnia, headache, coma, delusions, paranoia, aggressive behavior, visual, tactile, or auditory hallucinations.	Airway control, hyperthermia, seizures, dysrhythmias. **Antidote:** No specific antidote.
Methaqualone (Quaalude)	Depressant	Slurred speech, impaired judgment and motor skills, hypothermia, hypotension, bradycardia, diplopia, blurred vision, nystagmus, mydriasis, respiratory depression, depression, lethargy, headache, ataxia, coma, amnesia, incoordination, hypertonicity, myoclonus, tremors, vertigo.	Airway management, supportive care. **Antidote:** No specific antidote.
Methylphenidate (Ritalin)	Stimulant	Agitation, hypertension, tachycardia, hyperthermia, mydriasis, dry mouth, nausea, vomiting, anorexia, abdominal pain, agitation, hyperactivity, insomnia, euphoria, dizziness, paranoid ideation, social withdrawal, delirium, hallucinations, psychosis, tremors, seizures.	Control agitation, hyperthermia, seizures, support hemodynamic function. **Antidote:** No specific antidote.
Miss Emma (see morphine) **Mister blue** (see morphine)			

(continued)

Name (Brand)	Class	Signs and Symptoms	Treatment
Morphine (MS-Contin, Roxanol)	Opioid	Miosis, respiratory depression, decreased mental status, hypotension, cardiac dysrhythmia, hypoxia, bronchoconstriction, constipation, decreased intestinal motility, ileus, lethargy, coma.	Airway management, hemodynamic support. **Antidote:** Naloxone, nalmefene.
Oxy (see oxycodone)			
Oxycodone (OxyContin)	Opioid	Miosis, respiratory depression, decreased mental status, hypotension, cardiac dysrhythmia, hypoxia, bronchoconstriction, constipation, decreased intestinal motility, ileus, lethargy, coma.	Airway management, hemodynamic support. **Antidote:** Naloxone, nalmefene.
OxyContin (see oxycodone)			
Peace pill (see phencyclidine)			
Phencyclidine (PCP)	Hallucinogen	Nystagmus, hypertension, tachycardia, agitation, hallucinations, violent behavior, impaired judgment, delusions, psychosis.	Support blood pressure, manage airway, control agitation. **Antidote:** No specific antidote.
Phennies (see barbiturates)			
Pot (see marijuana)			
Propoxyphene (Darvon)	Depressant	Respiratory depression, seizures, cardiac toxicity, miosis, dysrhythmias, nausea, vomiting, anorexia, abdominal pain, constipation, drowsiness, coma, confusion, hallucinations.	Maintain airway, seizures, cardiac toxicity. **Antidote:** Naloxone.

Name (Brand)	Class	Signs and Symptoms	Treatment
Psilocybin	Hallucinogen	Diaphoresis, mydriasis, dizziness, twitching, flushing, hyperreflexia, hypertension, psychosis, behavioral changes, emotional lability, euphoria or dysphoria, paranoia, vomiting, diarrhea, anorexia, restlessness, incoordination, tremors, ataxia.	Manage airway, control activity associated with hallucinations, psychosis, panic reaction. **Antidote:** No specific antidote.
Purple passion (see psilocybin)			
Quay (see methaqualone)			
Reefer (see marijuana)			
Rock (see cocaine)			
Rocket fuel (see phencyclidine)			
Roofies (see flunitrazepam)			
Rope (see flunitrazepam)			
Rophies (see flunitrazepam)			
Salty water (see GHB)			
Schoolboy (see codeine)			
Scoop (see GHB)			
Snow (see cocaine)			
Special K (see ketamine)			
Speed (see amphetamine)			
STP (see MDMA)			
Super acid (see ketamine)			
Super K (see ketamine)			
Tranks (see benzodiazepines)			
Uppers (see amphetamine)			
White girl (see cocaine)			
Yellow jackets (see barbiturates)			
Yellow sunshine (see LSD)			

"CLUB DRUG" WEB SITES

www.drugfreeamerica.org	Partnership for a Drug-Free America
www.clubdrugs.org	Consumer-oriented site sponsored by the National Institute on Drug Abuse
www.health.org	Substance Abuse and Mental Health Services Administration
www.projectghb.org	Independent site devoted to risks and dangers of GHB use
www.nida.nih.gov	National Institute on Drug Abuse
www.dea.gov	Drug Enforcement Administration
www.whitehousedrugpolicy.org	Office of National Drug Control Policy

Appendix I

ENGLISH TO SPANISH DRUG PHRASES AND TERMS

TAKING THE MEDICATION HISTORY

* Are you allergic to any medications? (If yes:)
  ¿Es alérgico a algún medicamento? (sí:)
  (Ehs ah-lehr-hee-koh ah ahl-goon meh-dee-kah-mehn-toh) (see:)

  —Which medications are you allergic to?
  ¿A cuál medicamento es alérgico?
  (ah koo-ahl meh-dee-kah-mehn-toh ehs ah-lehr-hee-koh)

  —What happens when you develop an allergic reaction?
  ¿Qué le pasa cuando desarrolla una reacción alérgica?
  (Keh leh pah-sah koo-ahn-doh deh-sah-roh-yah oo-nah reh-ahk-see-ohn ah-lehr-hee-kah)

  —What did you do to relieve or stop the allergic reaction?
  ¿Qué hizo para aliviar o detener la reacción alérgica?
  (Keh ee-soh pah-rah ah-lee-bee-ahr oh deh-teh-nehr lah reh-ahk-see-ohn ah-lehr-hee-kah)

* Do you take any over-the-counter, prescription, or herbal medications? (If yes:)
  ¿Toma medicamentos sin receta, con receta, o naturistas (hierbas medici-nales)? (sí:)
  (Toh-mah meh-dee-kah-mehn-tohs seen reh-seh-tah, kohn reh-seh-tah, oh nah-too-rees-tahs [ee-ehr-bahs meh-dee-see-nah-lehs]) (see:)

  —Why do you take each medication?
  ¿Porqué toma cada medicamento?
  (Pohr-keh toh-mah kah-dah meh-dee-kah-mehn-toh)

  —What is the dosage for each medication?
  ¿Cuál es la dosis de cada medicamento?
  (Koo-ahl ehs lah doh-sees deh kah-dah meh-dee-kah-mehn-toh)

  —How often do you take each medication?
  ¿Con qué frequencia toma cada medicamento?
  (Kohn keh freh-koo-ehn-see-ah toh-mah kah-dah meh-dee-kah-mehn-toh)

Once a day?	¿Una vez por día; diariamente? (Oo-nah behs pohr dee-ah; dee-ah-ree-ah-mehn-teh)
Twice a day?	¿Dos veces por día? (dohs beh-sehs pohr dee-ah)
Three times a day?	¿Tres veces por día? (Trehs beh-sehs pohr dee-ah)
Four times a day?	¿Cuatro veces por día? (Koo-ah-troh beh-sehs pohr-dee-ah)
Every other day?	¿Cada tercer día? (Kah-dah tehr-sehr dee-ah)
Once a week?	¿Una vez por semana? (Oo-nah behs pohr seh-mah-nah)

- How does each medication make you feel?
  ¿Como le hace sentir cada medicamento?
  (Koh-moh leh ah-seh sehn-teer kah-dah meh-dee-kah-mehn-toh)

  —Does the medication make you feel better?
  ¿Le hace sentir mejor el medicamento?
  (Heh ah-seh sehn-teer meh-hohr ehl meh-dee-kah-mehn-toh)

  —Does the medication make you feel the same or unchanged?
  ¿Le hace sentir igual o sin cambio el medicamento?
  (Leh ah-seh sehn-teer ee-goo-ahl oh seen kam-bee-oh ehl meh-dee-kah-mehn-toh)

  —Does the medication make you feel worse? (If yes:)
  ¿Se siente peor con el medicamento? (si:)
  (Seh see-ehn teh peh-ohr kohn ehl meh-dee-kah-mehn-toh) (see:)

    What do you do to make yourself feel better?
    ¿Qué hace para sentirse mejor?
    (Keh ah-seh pah-rah sehn-teer-seh meh-hohr)

PREPARING FOR TREATMENT TO MEDICATION THERAPY
Medication Purpose
This medication will help relieve:

Este medicamento le ayudará a aliviar:

(Ehs-teh meh-dee-kah-mehn-toh leh ah-yoo-dah-rah ah ah-lee-bee-ahr)

English	Spanish	Pronunciation
abdominal gas	gases intestinales	(gah-sehs een-tehs-tee-nah-lehs)
abdominal pain	dolor intestinal; dolor en el abdomen	(doh-lohr een-tehs-tee-nahl; doh-lohr ehn ehl ahb-doh-mehn)
chest congestion	congestión del pecho	(kohn-hehs-tee-ohn dehl peh-choh)
chest pain	dolor del pecho	(doh-lohr dehl peh-choh)
constipation	constipación; estreñimiento	(Kohns-tee-pah-see-ohn; ehs-treh-nyee-mee-ehn-toh)
cough	tos	(tohs)
headache	dolor de cabeza	(doh-lohr-deh kah-beh-sah)
muscle aches and pains	achaques musculares y dolores	(ah-chah-kehs moos-koo-lah-rehs ee doh-loh-rehs)
pain	dolor	(doh-lohr)

This medication will prevent:

Este medicamento prevendrá:

(Ehs-teh meh-dee-kah-mehn-toh preh-behn-drah)

English	Spanish	Pronunciation
blood clots	coágulos de sangre	(koh-ah-goo-lohs deh sahn-greh)
constipation	constipación; estreñimiento	(Kohns-tee-pah-see-ohn; ehs-treh-nyee-mee-ehn-toh)
contraception	contracepción; embarazo	(kohn-trah-sehp-see-ohn; ehm-bah-rah-soh)
diarrhea	diarrea	(dee-ah-reh-ah)
infection	infección	(een-fehk-see-ohn)
seizures	convulciónes; ataque epiléptico	(kohn-bool-see-ohn-ehs; ah-tah-keh eh-pee-lehp-tee-koh)
shortness of breath	respiración corta; falta de aliento	(rehs-pee-rah-see-ohn kohr-tah; fahl-tah deh ah-lee-ehn-toh)
wheezing	el resollar; la respiración ruidosa, sibilante	(ehl reh-soh-yahr; lah rehs-pee-rah-see-ohn roo-ee-doh-sah, see-bee-lahn-teh)

This medication will increase your:
Este medicamento aumentará su:
(Ehs-teh meh-dee-kah-mehn-toh ah-oo-mehn-tah-rah soo:)

English	Spanish	Pronunciation
ability to fight infections	habilidad a combatir infecciones	(ah-bee-lee-dahd ah kohm-bah-teer een-fehk-see-oh-nehs)
appetite	apetito	(ah-peh-tee-toh)
blood iron levels	nivel de hierro en la sargre	(nee-behl deh ee-eh-roh ehn lah sahn-greh)
blood sugar	azúcar en la sangre	(ah-soo-kahr ehn lah sahn-greh)
heart rate	pulso; latido	(pool-soh; lah-tee-doh)
red blood cell count	cuenta de células rojas	(koo-ehn-tah deh seh-loo-lahs roh-hahs)
thyroid hormone levels	niveles de hormona tiroide	(nee-beh-lehs deh ohr-moh-nah tee-roh-ee-deh)
urine volume	volumen de orina	(boh-loo-mehn deh oh-ree-nah)

This medication will decrease your:
Este medicamento reducirá su:
(Ehs-teh meh-dee-kah-mehn-toh reh-doo-see-rah soo:)

English	Spanish	Pronunciation
anxiety	ansiedad	(ahn-see-eh-dahd)
blood cholesterol level	nivel de colesterol en la sangre	(nee-behl deh koh-lehs-teh-rohl ehn lah sahn-greh)
blood lipid level	nivel de lípido en la sangre	(nee-behl deh lee-pee-doh ehn lah sahn-greh)
blood pressure	presión arterial; de sangre	(preh-see-ohn ahr teh-ree-ahl; deh sahn-greh)
blood sugar level	nivel de azúcar en la sangre	(nee-behl deh ah-soo-kahr ehn lah sahn-greh)
heart rate	pulso; latido	(pool-soh; lah-tee-doh)
stomach acid	ácido en el estómago	(ah-see-doh ehn ehl ehs-toh-mah-goh)
thyroid hormone levels	niveles de hormona tiroide	(nee-beh-lehs deh ohr-moh-nah tee-roh-ee-deh)
weight.	peso	(peh-soh)

This medication will treat:
Este medicamento sirve para:
(Ehs-teh meh-dee-kah-mehn-toh seer-beh pah-rah)

English	Spanish	Pronunciation
cancer of your _____	cancer de su _____	(kahn-sehr deh soo)
depression	depresión	(deh-preh-see-ohn)
HIV infection	infección de VIH	(een-fehk-see-ohn deh beh ee ah-cheh)
inflammation	infamación	(een-flah-mah-see-ohn)
swelling	hinchazón	(een-chah-sohn)
the infection in your _____	la infección en su _____	(lah een-fehk-see-ohn ehn soo)
your abnormal heart rhythm	su ritmo anormal de corazón	(soo reet-moh ah-nohr-mahl deh koh-rah-sohn)
your allergy to _____	su alergia a _____	(soo eh-lehr-hee-ah ah)
your rash	su erupción; sarpullido	(soo eh-roop-see-ohn; sahr-poo-yee-doh)

ADMINISTERING MEDICATION

- Swallow this medication with water or juice.
  Tragüe este medicamento con agua o jugo
  (Trah-geh ehs-teh meh dee-kah-mehn-toh kohn ah-goo-ah oh hoo-goh)

- If you cannot swallow the medication whole, I can crush it and put it in food.
  Si no puede tragar el medicamento entero puedo aplastarlo (triturarlo) y ponerlo en el alimento.
  (See noh poo-eh-deh trah-gahr ehl meh-dee-kah-mehn-toh ehn-teh-roh poo-eh-doh ah-plahs-tahr-loh [tree-too-rahr-loh] ee poh-nehr-loh ehn ehl ah lee-mehn-toh)

- I need to mix this medication with water or juice before you drink it.
  Necesito mezclar este medicamento en agua o jugo antes de que lo tome.
  (Neh-seh-see-toh mehs-klahr ehs-teh meh-dee-kah-mehn-toh ehn ah-goo-ah oh hoo-goh ahn-tehs deh keh loh toh-meh)

- Do not chew this medication. Swallow it whole.
  No mastique este medicamento. Tragüelo entero.
  (Noh mahs-tee-keh ehs-teh meh-dee-kah-mehn-toh. Trah-geh-loh ehn-teh-roh)

- Gargle with this medication and then swallow it.
  Haga gargaras con este medicamento y luego tragüelo.
  (Ah-gah gahr-gah-rahs koh ehs-teh meh-dee-kah-mehn-toh ee loo-eh-goh trah-geh-loh)

- Place this medication under your tongue and let it dissolve.
  Ponga este medicamento bajo la lengua y deje que se disuelva
  (Pohn-gah ehs-teh meh-dee-kah-mehn-toh bah-hoh lah lehn-goo-ah ee deh-heh keh seh dee-soo-ehl-bah)

- I would like to give this injection in your:
  Quiero aplicar esta injección en su:
  (Kee-eh-roh ah-plee-kahr ehs-tah een-yehk-see-ohn ehn soo:)

    —abdomen
    abdomen
    (ahb-doh-mehn)

    —arm
    brazo
    (brah-soh)

—buttocks
nalga
(nahl-gah)

—hip
cadera
(kah-deh-rah)

—thigh.
muslo
(moos-loh)

- I will give you this medication through your intravenous line.
  Le daré este medicamento por el tubo de suero intravenoso.
  (Leh dah-reh ehs-teh meh-dee-kah-mehn-toh pohr ehl too-boh deh soo-eh-roh een-trah-beh-noh-soh)

- Let me know if you feel burning or pain at the intravenous site.
  Digame si siente ardor o dolor en el sitio del suero intravenoso.
  (Dee-gah-meh see see-ehn-teh ahr-dohr oh doh-lohr ehn ehl see-tee-oh dehl soo-eh-roh een-trah-beh-noh-soh)

- I need to insert this suppository into your rectum (or vagina).
  Necesito meter este supositorio en el recto (o vagina).
  (Neh-seh-see-toh meh-tehr ehs-teh soo-poh-see-toh-ree-oh ehn ehl rehk-toh [oh bah-hee-nah])

- I need to put this medication into each ear; left ear; right ear.
  Necesito poner este medicamento en cada oreja; oreja izquierda; oreja derecha.
  (Neh-seh-see-toh poh-nehr ehs-teh meh-dee-kah-mehn-toh ehn kah-dah oh-reh-hah; oh-reh-hah ees-kee-ehr-dah; -oh-reh-hah deh-reh-chah)

- I need to put this medication into each eye; left eye; right eye.
  Necesito poner este medicamento en cada ojo; ojo izquierdo; ojo derecho.
  (Neh-seh-see-toh poh-nehr ehs-teh meh-dee-kah-mehn-toh ehn kah-dah oh-hoh; oh-hoh ees-kee-ehr-doh; oh-hoh deh-reh-choh)

PREPARING FOR DISCHARGE

- The generic name for this medication is _____ .
  El nombre genérico (sin marca) de este medicamento es _____ .
  (Ehl nohm-breh heh-neh-ree-koh [seen mahr-kah] deh ehs-teh meh-dee-kah-mehn-toh ehs _____)

- The trade name for this medication is _____ .
  El nombre comercial de este medicamento es _____ .
  (Ehs nohm-breh koh-mehr-see-ahl deh ehs-teh meh-dee-kah-mehn-toh
  ehs _____)

- Take the medication exactly as prescribed.
  Tome el medicamento exactamente como se receta.
  (Toh-meh ehl meh-dee-kah-mehn-toh ehx-ahk-tah-mehn-teh koh-moh seh
  reh-seh-tah)

- You can safely break a scored tablet in half.
  Puede partir por la mitad la tableta que tiene una muesca (marca).
  (Poo-eh-deh pahr-teer pohr lah mee-tahd lah tah-bleh-tah keh tee-eh-neh
  oo-nah moo-ehs-kah [mahr-kah])

- Do not crush or chew enteric-coated, extended-release, or sustained-
  release tablets or capsules.
  No aplaste (triture) o mastique una tableta con capa entérica, de acción
  prolongada o de mantenimiento.
  (Noh ah-plahs-teh [tree-too-reh] oh mahs-tee-keh oo-nah tah-bleh-tah
  kohn-kah-pah ehn-teh-ree-kah, deh ahk-see-ohn proh-lohn-gah-dah oh deh
  mahn-teh-nee-mee-ehn-toh)

- If you miss a dose:
  Si pierde una dosis:
  (See pee-ehr-deh oo-nah doh-sees:)

      —take it as soon as you remember it.
      tómela tan pronto se acuerde.
      (toh-meh-lah tahn prohn-toh seh ah-koo-ehr-deh)

      —wait until the next dose.
      espere hasta la siguiente dosis.
      (ehs-peh-reh ahs-tah lah see-ghee-ehn-teh doh-sees)

      —do not double the next dose.
      No doble la siguiente dosis.
      (noh doh-bleh lah see-ghee-ehn-teh doh-sees)

      —contact your physician.
      llame a su médico.
      (yah-meh ah soo meh-dee-koh)

- Do not stop taking your medication without first speaking with your
  physician.
  No deje de tomar su medicamento sin hablar primero con su médico.
  (Noh deh-heh deh toh-mahr soo meh-dee-kah-ehn-toh seen ah-blahr pree-
  meh-roh kohn soo meh-dee-koh)

- Do not drink alcohol while taking this medication.
  No tome alcohol cuando tome este medicamento.
  (Noh toh-meh ahl-kohl koo-ahn-doh toh-meh ehs-teh meh-dee-kah-mehn-toh)

- Do not drive or operate machinery while taking this medication.
  No maneje o use maquinaria cuando toma este medicamento.
  (Noh mah-neh-heh oh oo-seh mah-kee-nah-ree-ah koo-ahn-doh toh-mah ehs-teh meh-dee-kah-mehn-toh)

- Notify your physician right away if you experience a dangerous side effect.
  Llame a su médico inmediatamente si tiene efectos secundarios peligrosos.
  (Llah-meh ah soo meh-dee-koh een-meh-dee-ah-tah-mehn-teh see tee-eh-neh eh-fehk-tohs seh-koon-dah-ree-ohs peh-lee-groh-sohs)

- Check with your physician before taking any over-the-counter medications.
  Cheque con su médico antes de tomar medicamentos sin receta.
  (Cheh-keh kohn soo meh-dee-koh ahn-tehs deh toh-mahr meh-dee-kah-mehn-tohs seen reh-seh-tah)

- Notify your physician if you are pregnant or are planning to become pregnant while taking this medication.
  Dígale a su médico si está embarazada o planea el embarazo cuando toma este medicamento.
  (Dee-gah-leh ah soo meh-dee-koh see ehs-tah ehm-bah-rah-sah-dah oh plah-neh-ah ehl ehm-bah-rah-soh koo-ahn-doh toh-mah ehs-teh meh-dee-kah-mehn-toh)

- Notify your physician if you are breast-feeding while taking this medication.
  Dígale a su médico si está amamantando (dando de pecho) cuando toma este medicamento.
  (Dee-gah-leh ah soo meh-dee-koh see ehs-tah ah-mah-mahn-tahn-doh [dahn-doh deh peh-choh] koo-ahn-doh toh-mah ehs-teh meh-dee-kah-mehn-toh)

- Refill your prescription right away, unless you don't need it anymore.
  Rellene su receta inmediatamente, a menos que no la necesite.
  (Reh-yeh-neh soo reh-seh-tah een-meh-dee-ah-tah-mehn-teh, ah meh-nohs keh noh lah neh-seh-see-teh)

PROPER MEDICATION STORAGE

- Discard expired medications because they may become dangerous or ineffective.
  Tire los medicamentos con fecha vencida (caducados) porque pueden ser peligrosos o infectivos.
  (Tee-reh lohs meh-dee-kah-mehn-tohs kohn feh-chah behn-see-dah [kah-doo-kah-dohs] pohr-keh poo-eh-dehn sehr peh-lee-groh-sohs oh een-eh-fehk-tee-bohs)

- Keep all medications out of the reach of children at all times.
  Guarde todos los medicamentos fuera del alcance de los niños todo el tiempo.
  (Goo-ahr-deh toh-dohs lohs meh-dee-kah-mehn-tohs foo-eh-rah dehl ahl-kahn-seh deh lohs nee-nyohs toh-doh ehl tee-ehm-poh)

- Store the medication:
  Almacene (guarde) el medicamento:
  (Ahl-mah-seh-neh [goo-ahr-deh] ehl meh-dee-kah-mehn-toh:)

      —in its original container.
      en su empaque original.
      (ehn-soo ehm-pah-keh oh-ree-hee-nahl)

      —in a cool, dry place.
      en un lugar fresco y seco.
      (ehn oon loo-gahr frehs-koh ee seh-koh)

      —away from heat.
      lejos del calor.
      (leh-hohs dehl kah-lohr)

      —at room temperature.
      a temperatura ambiente
      (ah tehm-peh-rah-too-rah ahm-bee-ehn-teh)

      —out of direct sunlight.
      fuera de la luz directa del sol.
      (foo-eh-rah deh lah loos dee-rehk-tah dehl sohl)

      —in the refrigerator.
      en el refrigerador.
      (ehn ehl reh-free-heh-rah-dohr)

Selected Drug Classes
Clasificación de Drogas Selectas (Medicamentos Selectos)
(Klah see-fee-kah-see-ohn deh droh-gahs seh-lehk-tahs
[Meh-dee-kah-mehn-tohs Seh-lehk-tohs])

English	Spanish	Pronunciation
Analgesic (narcotic, nonnarcotic)	Analgésico (narcótico, no narcótico)	(Ah-nahl-heh-see-koh [nahr-koh-tee-koh, noh nahr-koh-tee-koh])
Antacid	Antiácido	(Ahn-tee-ah-see-doh)
Antianginal	Antianginoso	(Ahn-tee-ahn-hee-noh-soh)
Antianxiety	Ansiolítico	(Ahn-see-oh-lee-tee-koh)
Antiarrhythmic	Antiarritmico	(Ahn-tee-ah-reet-mee-koh)
Antibiotic	Antibiótico	(Ahn-tee-bee-oh-tee-koh)
Anticoagulant	Anticoagulante	(Ahn-tee-koh-ah-goo-lahn-teh)
Anticonvulsant	Anticonvulsivo	(Ahn-tee-kohn-bool-see-boh)
Antidepressant	Antidepresivo	(Ahn-tee-deh-preh-see-boh)
Antidiarrheal	Antidiarréicos	(Ahn-tee-dee-ah-reh-ee-kohs)
Antifungal	Antimicótico	(Ahn-tee-mee-koh-tee-koh)
Antihistamine	Antihistamínico	(Ahn-tee-ees-tah-mee-nee-koh)
Antihyperlipemic	Antihiperlipémico	(Ahn-tee-ee-pehr-lee-peh-mee-koh)
Antihypertensive	Antihipertensivo	(Ahn-tee-ee-pehr-tehn-see-boh)
Anti-inflammatory	Antiinflamatorio; Contra la inflamación	(Ahn-tee-een-flah-mah-toh-ree-oh; kohn-trah lah een-flah-mah-see-ohn)
Antimigraine	Antimigrañoso	(Ahn-tee-mee-grah-nyoh-soh)
Antiparkinsonian	Contra el Parkinson	(Kohn-trah ehl Pahr-keen-sohn)
Antipsychotic	Medicamentos sicóticos	(Meh-dee-kah-mehn-tohs see-koh-tee-kohs)
Antipyretic	Antitérmicos	(Ahn-tee-tehr-mee-kohs)
Antiseptic	Antiséptico	(Ahn-tee-sehp-tee-koh)
Antispasmodic	Antiespasmódico	(Ahn-tee-ehs-pahs-moh-dee-koh)
Antithyroid	Antitiroideos	(Ahn-tee-tee-roh-ee-deh-ohs)
Antituberculosis	Antifímicos	(Ahn-tee-fee-mee-kohs)
Antitussive	Antitusígenos	(Ahn-tee-too-see-heh-nohs)
Antiviral	Antivirales	(Ahn-tee-bee-rah-lehs)

English	Spanish	Pronunciation
Appetite Suppressant	Antisupresivos del Apetito	(Ahn-tee-soo-preh-see-bohs dehl ah-peh-tee-toh)
Appetite stimulant	Estimulantes del apetito	(Ehs-tee-moo-lahn-tehs dehl ah-peh-tee-toh)
Bronchiodilator	Bronquiolíticos	(Brohn-kee-oh-lee-tee-kohs)
Cancer Chemotherapy	Quimioterapia de Cancer	(Kee-mee-oh teh-rah-pee-ah deh kahn-sehr)
Decongestant	Anticongestivo	(Ahn-tee-kohn-hehs-tee-hoh)
Digestant	Digestible	(Dee-hehs-tee-bleh)
Diuretic	Diurético	(Dee-oo-reh-tee-koh)
Emetic	Emético	(Eh-meh-tee-koh)
Fertility	Inductor de la Ovulación	(Een-doohk-tohr deh lah Oh-boo-lah-see-ohn)
Herbal	Medicamentos Naturales; Hierbas Medicinales	(Meh-dee-kah-mehn-tohs Nah-too-rah-lehs, Ee-ehr-bhas Meh-dee-see-nah-lehs)
Hypnotic	Hipnótico	(Eep-noh-tee-koh)
Insulin	Insulina	(Een-soo-lee-nah)
Laxative	Laxante	(Lahx-ahn-teh)
Mineral	Mineral	(Mee-neh-rahl)
Muscle Relaxant	Relajante Muscular	(Reh-lah-hahn-teh Moos-koo-lahr)
Oral Contraceptive	Anticonceptivos Orales	(Ahn-tee-kohn-sehp-tee-bohs Oh-rah-lehs)
Oral Hypoglycemic	Hipoglicémico Oral	(Ee-poh-glee-seh-mee-koh Oh-rahl)
Sedative	Sedantes	(Seh-dahn-tehs)
Steroid	Esteroide	(Ehs-teh-roh-ee-deh)
Thyroid Hormone	Tiroideos, Hormona Tiroide	(Tee-roh-ee-deh-ohs, Ohr-moh-nah Tee-roh-ee-deh)
Vaccine	Vacuna	(Bah-koo-nah)

Administration Routes
Modo de Uso
(Moh-doh deh Oo-soh)

English	Spanish	Pronunciation
By mouth	Oral	(Oh-rahl)
Intradermal	Intradermica	(Een-trah-dehr-mee-kah)
Intramuscular	Intramuscular	(Een-trah-moos-koo-lahr)

(continued)

English	Spanish	Pronunciation
Intravenous	Intravenosa	(Een-trah-beh-noh-sah)
Nasal	Nasal	(Nah-sahl)
Oral	Oral	(Oh-rahl)
Otic	Ótica	(Oh-tee-kah)
Patch	Parche	(Pahr-cheh)
Rectal	Rectal	(Rehk-tahl)
Subcutaneous	Subcutanea	(Soob-koo-tah-neh-ah)
Sublingual	Sublingual	(Soob-leen-goo-ahl)
Topical	Topical, Local	(Toh-pee-kahl, Loh-kahl)
Vaginal	Vaginal	(Bah-hee-nahl)

Drug Preparations
Presentación del Medicamento
(Preh-sehn-tah-see-ohn dehl Meh-dee-kah-mehn-toh)

English	Spanish	Pronunciation
Capsule	Cápsula	(Kahp-soo-lah)
Cream	Crema	(Kreh-mah)
Drops	Gotas	(Goh-tahs)
Elixir	Elixir, Jarabe	(Eh-leex-eer, Hah-rah-beh)
Fluid	Líquido	(Lee-kee-doh)
Gel	Gel, Jalea	(Hehl, Hah-leh-ah)
Inhaler	Inhalador*	(Een-ah-lah-dohr)
Injection	Inyección	(Een-yehk-see-ohn)
Liquid	Líquido	(Lee-kee-doh)
Lotion	Loción	(Loh-see-ohn)
Lozenge	Trocisco, pastilla	(Troh-sees-koh, Pahs-tee-yah)
Ointment	Ungüento	(Oon-goo-ehn-toh)
Pill	Píldora, Pastilla	(Peel-doh-rah, Pahs-tee-yah)
Powder	Polvo	(Pohl-boh)
Spray	Spray	(Sp-rah-ee)
Suppository	Supositorio	(Soo-poh-see-toh-ree-oh)
Syrup	Jarabe	(Hah-rah-beh)
Tablet	Tableta	(Tah-bleh-tah)

*The h is silent.

Administration Frequency
Frecuencia de la Administración
(Freh-koo-ehn-see-ah deh lah Ahd-mee-nees-trah-see-ohn)

English	Spanish	Pronunciation
Once a day	Una vez por día; diariamente	(Oo-nah behs pohr dee-ah; dee-ah-ree-ah-mehn-teh)
Twice a day	Dos veces por día	(Dohs beh-sehs pohr dee-ah)
Three times a day	Tres veces por día	(Trehs beh-sehs pohr dee-ah)
Four times a day	Cuatro veces por día	(Koo-ah-troh beh-sehs pohr dee-ah)
Every other day	Cada tercer día	(Kah-dah tehr-sehr dee-ah)
Once a week	Una vez por semana	(Oo-nah behs pohr seh-mah-nah)
Every 4 hours	Cada cuatro horas	(Kah-dah koo-ah-troh oh-rahs)
Every 6 hours	Cada seis horas	(Kah-dah seh-ees oh-rahs)
Every 8 hours	Cada ocho horas	(Kah-dah oh-choh oh-rahs)
Every 12 hours	Cada doce horas	(Kah-dah doh-seh oh-rahs)
In the morning	En la mañana	(Ehn lah mah-nyah-nah)
In the afternoon	En la tarde	(Ehn lah tahr-deh)
In the evening	En la noche	(Ehn lah noh-cheh)
Before bedtime	Antes de acostarse	(Ahn-tehs deh ah-kohs-tahr-seh)
Before meals	Antes de la comida; Antes del alimento	(Ahn-tehs deh lah koh-mee-dah; Ahn-tehs dehl ah-lee-mehn-toh)
With meals	Con los alimentos; Con la comida	(Kohn lohs ah-lee-mehn-tohs; Kohn lah koh-mee-dah)
After meals	Después de los alimentos, Después de la comida	(Dehs-poo-ehs deh lohs ah-lee-mehn-tohs; Dehs-poo-ehs deh lah koh-mee-dah)
Only when you need it	Solo cuando la necesite	(Soh-loh koo-ahn-doh lah neh-seh-see-teh)
When you have _____ (pain)	Cuando tiene _____ (dolor)	(Koo-ahn-doh tee-eh-neh _____) (doh-lohr)

50 Common Side Effects
Cincuenta Efectos Secundarios Comúnes
(Seen-koo-ehn-tah Eh-fehk-tohs Seh-koon-dah-ree-ohs Koh-moo-nehs)

English	Spanish	Pronunciation
Abdominal cramps	Retorcijón abdominal	(Reh-tohr-see-hohn ahb-doh-mee-nahl)
Abdominal pain	Dolor abdominal	(Doh-lohr ahb-doh-mee-nahl)
Abdominal swelling	Inflamación abdominal	(Een-flah-mah-see-ohn ahb-doh-mee-nahl)
Anxiety	Ansiedad	(Ahn-see-eh-dahd)
Blood in the stool	Sangre en el excremento	(Sahn-greh ehn ehl ehx-kreh-mehn-toh)
Blood in the urine	Sangre en la orina	(Sahn-greh ehn la oh-ree-nah)
Bone pain	Dolor de hueso*	(Doh-lohr deh oo-eh-soh)
Chest pain	Dolor de pecho	(Doh-lohr deh peh-choh)
Chest pounding	Palpitación; latidos fuertes en el pecho	(Pahl-pee-tah-see-ohn; lah-tee-dohs foo-ehr-tehs ehn ehl peh-choh)
Chills	Escalofrío	(Ehs-kah-loh-free-oh)
Confusion	Confusión	(Kohn-foo-see-ohn)
Constipation	Constipación, estreñimiento	(Kohns-tee-pah-see-ohn, ehs-treh-nyee-mee-ehn-toh)
Cough	Tos	(Tohs)
Mental depression	Depresión mental	(Deh-preh-see-ohn mehn-tahl)
Diarrhea	Diarrea	(Dee-ah-reh-ah)
Difficult urination	Dificultad al orinar	(Dee-fee-kool-tahd ahl oh-ree-nahr)
Difficulty breathing	Dificultad al respirar	(Dee-fee-kool-tahd ahl rehs-pee-rahr)
Difficulty sleeping	Dificultad al dormir	(Dee-fee-kool-tahd ahl dohr-meer)
Dizziness	Mareos; vahídos	(Mah-reh-ohs; bah-ee-dohs)
Dry mouth	Boca seca	(Boh-kah seh-kah)
Easy bruising	Fragilidad capilar; le salen moretones con facilidad	(Frah-hee-lee-dahd kah-pee-lahr; leh sah-lehn moh-reh-toh-nehs kohn fah-see-lee-dahd)
Faintness	Desvanecimiento; sintió un vahído	(Dehs-bah-neh-see-mee-ehn-toh; seen-tee-oh oon bah-ee-doh)
Fatigue	Fatiga, cansancio	(Fah-tee-gah, kahn-sahn-see-oh)

English	Spanish	Pronunciation
Fever	Fiebre	(Fee-eh-breh)
Frequent urination	Orina frecuente	(Oh-ree-nah freh-koo-ehn-teh)
Headache	Dolor de cabeza	(Doh-lohr deh kah-beh-sah)
Impotence	Impotencia	(Eem-poh-tehn-see-ah)
Increased appetite	Aumento en el apetito	(Ah-oo-mehn-toh ehn ehl ah-peh-tee-toh)
Increased gas	Flatulencia	(Flah-too-lehn-see-ah)
Increased perspiration	Aumento en el sudor	(Ah-oo-mehn-toh ehn ehl soo-dohr)
Indigestion	Indigestión	(Een-dee-hehs-tee-ohn)
Itching	Comezón	(Koh-meh-sohn)
Loss of appetite	Pérdida en el apetito	(Pehr-dee-dah ehn ehl ah-peh-tee-toh)
Menstrual changes	Cambios en la menstruación; Cambio en el ciclo menstrual	(Kahm-bee-ohs ehn la mehns-truh-ah-see-ohn; Kahm-bee-oh ehn ehl see-kloh mehns-truh-ahl)
Mood changes	Cambio en el humor; Cambio en la disposición	(Kahm-bee-oh ehn ehl oo-mohr, Kahm-bee-oh ehn lah dees-poh-see-see-ohn)
Muscle pain	Dolores musculares	(Doh-loh-rehs moos-koo-lah-rehs)
Muscle aches	Achaques musculares	(Ah-chah-kehs moos-koo-lah-rehs)
Muscle cramps	Calambre muscular	(Kah-lahm-breh moos-koo-lahr)
Nasal congestion	Congestión nasal	(Kohn-hehs-tee-ohn nah-sahl)
Nausea	Nausea	(Nah-oo-seh-ah)
Ringing in the ears	Zumbido en los oidos	(Soom-bee-doh ehn lohs oh-ee-dohs)
Skin rash	Erupción en la piel	(Eh-roop-see-ohn ehn lah pee-ehl)
Swelling on the hands, legs or feet	Hinchazón en las manos, piernas, o pies	(Een-chah-sohn ehn lahs mah-nohs, pee-ehr-nahs, oh pee-ehs)
Vaginal bleeding	Sangrado vaginal	(Sahn-grah-doh bah-hee-nahl)
Vision changes	Cambios en la visión; cambios en la vista	(Kahm-bee-ohs ehn lah bee-see-ohn; cahm-bee-ohs ehn lah bees-tah)
Vomiting	Vomitando	(Boh-mee-tahn-doh)

(continued)

English	Spanish	Pronunciation
Weakness	Debilidad	(Deh-bee-lee-dahd)
Weight gain	Aumento de peso	(Ah-oo-mehn-toh deh peh-soh)
Weight loss	Pérdida de peso	(Pehr-dee-day deh peh-soh)
Wheezing	Resollar; respiración sibilante	(Reh-soh-yahr; rehs-pee-rah-see-ohn see-bee-lahn-teh)

*The h is silent.

Appendix J

ENTERAL AND PARENTERAL NUTRITION

INDICATIONS: ENTERAL NUTRITION

Enteral nutrition (EN), also known as *tube feedings,* provides food and nutrients via the gastrointestinal (GI) tract, using special formulas, delivery techniques, and equipment. All EN routes consist of a tube through which liquid formula is infused.

Tube feedings are used in patients with major trauma or burns; those undergoing radiation or chemotherapy; and those with liver failure, severe renal impairment, or physical or neurologic impairment. They're also used preoperatively and postoperatively to promote anabolism. In addition, they're used to prevent cachexia and malnutrition.

ROUTES OF ENTERAL NUTRITION DELIVERY

NASOGASTRIC (NG):
INDICATIONS: This route is most common for short-term feeding in patients who can't or won't consume adequate nutrition by mouth. It requires at least a partially functioning GI tract. **ADVANTAGES:** NG tube placement doesn't require surgery, and the tube is fairly easily inserted. It allows full use of the digestive tract. It decreases the risk that hyperosmolar solutions may cause distention, nausea, and vomiting. **DISADVANTAGES:** This route is temporary, and the NG tube may be easily pulled out during routine nursing care. The patient is at risk for pulmonary aspiration of gastric contents, reflux esophagitis, and regurgitation.

NASODUODENAL (ND), NASOJEJUNAL (NJ):
INDICATIONS: These routes may be used in patients who can't or won't consume adequate nutrition by mouth. They require at least a partially functioning GI tract. **ADVANTAGES:** These tubes don't require surgical placement, are fairly easily inserted, and are preferred for patients at risk of aspiration. They're valuable for patients with gastroparesis. **DISADVANTAGES:** These routes are temporary. ND or NJ tubes may be pulled out during routine nursing care and may be dislodged by coughing or vomiting. Their small lumens increase the risk of clogging when drugs are given through them, and make them more susceptible to rupture when an infusion device is used. These tubes require x-rays for confirmation of placement and are frequently extubated.

GASTROSTOMY:
INDICATIONS: This route is used in patients with esophageal obstruction or impaired swallowing; those in whom the NG, ND, and NJ routes aren't feasible; and those who need long-term feeding. **ADVANTAGES:** Gastrostomy provides permanent feeding access. The tubing has a larger bore, allowing noncontinuous (bolus) feeding (300 to 400 ml over 30 to 60 min q

3 to 6 hr). It may be inserted endoscopically using local anesthetic (in a procedure called *percutaneous endoscopic gastrostomy* [PEG]). **DISADVANTAGES:** This route requires surgical placement, although the tubing may be inserted during other surgery or endoscopically (see **ADVANTAGES**). The tube may be inadvertently dislodged. Gastrostomy requires stoma care and increases the risk of aspiration, peritonitis, cellulitis, and leakage of gastric contents.

JEJUNOSTOMY:

INDICATIONS: This route is used for patients with stomach or duodenal obstruction or impaired gastric motility; those in whom the NG, ND, and NJ routes aren't feasible; and those who need long-term feeding. **ADVANTAGES:** Jejunostomy allows early postoperative feeding because small bowel function is least affected by surgery. It reduces the risk of aspiration, and its tubing is rarely pulled out inadvertently. **DISADVANTAGES:** This route requires surgical placement (laparotomy) and stoma care. It poses a risk of intraperitoneal leakage, and its tubing can be dislodged easily.

INTIATING ENTERAL NUTRITION

With continuous feeding, expect to begin feedings of isotonic (about 300 mOsm/L) or moderately hypertonic (up to 495 mOsm/L) formula at full strength, usually at a slow rate (30 to 50 ml/hr), and gradually increase it (25 ml/hr q 6 to 24 hr). Start formulas with an osmolality above 500 mOsm/L at half strength and gradually increase the rate and then the concentration. Tolerance increases when the rate and concentration aren't increased simultaneously.

SELECTION OF ENTERAL FORMULAS

Protein has many important physiologic roles and is the primary source of nitrogen in the body. It provides 4 kcal/g of protein. Sources of protein in enteral feedings include sodium caseinate, calcium caseinate, soy protein, and dipeptides.

Carbohydrate (CHO) provides energy for the body and heat to maintain the body temperature. It provides 3.4 kcal/g of carbohydrate. Sources of carbohydrate in enteral feedings include corn syrup, cornstarch, maltodextrin, lactose, sucrose, and glucose.

Fat provides a concentrated source of energy, referred to as *kilocalorie dense or protein sparing.* It provides 9 kcal/g of fat. Sources of fat in enteral feedings include corn oil, safflower oil, and medium chain triglycerides.

Electrolytes, vitamins, and trace elements are contained in formulas, but not in specialized products for patients with renal or hepatic insufficiency. All products containing protein, fat, carbohydrate, vitamins, electrolytes, and trace elements are nutritionally complete and designed to be used by patients for long periods.

COMPLICATIONS OF ENTERAL NUTRITION

MECHANICAL: These complications usually relate to some aspect of the feeding tube.

Aspiration pneumonia can result from delayed gastric emptying, gastroparesis, gastroesophageal reflux, or decreased gag reflex. To prevent or treat it, reduce the infusion rate, use lower fat formulas, feed beyond the pylorus, check residuals, use small-bore feeding tubes, elevate the head of the bed 30° to 45° during and for 30 to 60 minutes after each intermittent feeding, and regularly check tube placement.

Esophageal, mucosal, and pharyngeal irritation and otitis are caused by using a large-bore NG tube. To prevent these problems, use small-bore tubing whenever possible.

Irritation and leakage at the ostomy site can stem from digestive juice drainage from the site. To prevent them, provide frequent skin and stoma care.

Tube or lumen obstruction is caused by thickened formula residue and formation of formula-medication complexes. To prevent this, frequently irrigate the tube with clear water (also before and after giving formulas and medications) and avoid medication instillation if possible.

GASTROINTESTINAL: These complications usually relate to the formula, the delivery rate, or unsanitary handling of solutions or the delivery system.

Diarrhea may result from low-residue formulas, rapid delivery, hyperosmolar formulas, hypoalbuminemia, malabsorption, microbial contamination, or rapid GI transit time. To prevent it, use fiber-supplemented formulas, decrease the delivery rate, use dilute formula, and gradually increase its strength.

Cramping, gas, and abdominal distention are caused by nutrient malabsorption or rapid delivery of refrigerated formula. To prevent them, deliver formula by a continuous method, give formulas at room temperature, and decrease the delivery rate.

Nausea and vomiting can result from rapid delivery of formula and gastric retention. To prevent them, reduce the delivery rate, use dilute formulas, and select low-fat formulas.

Constipation is caused by inadequate fluid intake, reduced bulk, and inactivity. To prevent it, supplement the patient's fluid intake, use fiber-supplemented formula, and encourage ambulation.

METABOLIC: These complications require fluid and electrolyte monitoring. (See Monitoring of EN section.) Very young and very old patients have a greater risk of developing such complications as dehydration or overhydration.

MONITORING OF ENTERAL NUTRITION

Daily: Estimate the patient's nutrient intake. Measure the patient's fluid intake and output and body weight and carefully monitor the patient's general health status.

Weekly: Evaluate the levels of serum electrolytes (potassium, sodium,

magnesium, calcium, and phosphorus), blood glucose, blood urea nitrogen (BUN), creatinine, liver enzymes (such as SGOT [AST] and alkaline phosphatase), 24-hr urea and creatinine excretion, total iron-binding capacity (TIBC) or serum transferrin, triglycerides, and cholesterol.
Monthly: Check the serum albumin level.
Other: Assess the urine glucose and acetone levels (when the blood glucose exceeds 250 mg/dl). Check vital signs (temperature, respirations, pulse, and blood pressure) every 8 hours.

INDICATIONS: PARENTERAL NUTRITION

Parenteral nutrition (PN), also known as *total parenteral nutrition* (TPN) or *hyperalimentation* (HAL), provides required nutrients to patients by the IV route of administration. The goal of PN is to maintain or restore nutritional balance, which may be upset by disease, injury, or inability to consume nutrients by other means.

PN is used in patients with conditions that preclude use of the alimentary tract by the oral, gastrostomy, or jejunostomy routes. Such conditions include impaired protein absorption due to obstruction, inflammation, or antineoplastic therapy; bowel rest after GI surgery or ileus, fistulas, or anastomotic leaks; and conditions with increased metabolic requirements, such as burns, infection, and trauma. PN also is used to preserve tissue reserves (as in acute renal failure) and to provide adequate nutrition when tube-feeding methods can't.

COMPONENTS OF PARENTERAL NUTRITION

To meet IV nutritional requirements, PN needs six essential components for tissue synthesis and energy balance.
Protein takes the form of crystalline amino acids (CAA), which are primarily used for protein synthesis. Several products are designed to meet specific needs for patients with renal failure (such as NephrAmine), liver disease (such as HepatAmine), or stress and trauma (such as Aminosyn HBC) and for use in neonates and children (such as Aminosyn PF and TrophAmine). PN provides 4 kcal/g of protein.
Energy takes the form of dextrose, which is available in concentrations of 5% to 70%. Dextrose concentrations below 10% may be given peripherally; those above 10% must be given centrally. PN provides 3.4 kcal/g of dextrose.
IV fat emulsion comes in 10% or 20% concentrations and provides a concentrated source of energy (9 kcal/g of fat). It's also a source of essential fatty acids. It may be administered peripherally or centrally.
Electrolytes include calcium, magnesium, potassium, sodium, acetate, chloride, and phosphate. Electrolyte doses must be individualized, based on many factors, such as kidney function, liver function, and fluid status.
Vitamins are essential for maintaining metabolism and cellular function. They're widely used in PN.
Trace elements are needed in long-term PN. Trace elements include zinc, copper, chromium, manganese, selenium, molybdenum, and iodine.

Miscellaneous additives include insulin, albumin, heparin, and histamine$_2$ blockers, such as cimetidine, ranitidine, and famotidine. Other medications may be added on an individual basis, but admixture compatibility should be checked first.

ROUTES OF PARENTERAL NUTRITION DELIVERY

PN is administered by a peripheral or central vein.

Peripheral administration usually involves 2 to 3 L/day of 5% to 10% dextrose with 3% to 5% amino acid solution along with IV fat emulsion. Electrolytes, vitamins, and trace elements are added based on the patient's needs. Peripheral solutions provide about 2,000 kcal/day and 60 to 90 g protein/day. **ADVANTAGES:** Peripheral administration poses lower risks than central administration. **DISADVANTAGES:** Peripheral veins may not be suitable (especially in patients with long-term illness); may be more susceptible to phlebitis (because osmolality exceeds 600 mOsm/L); and may be viable for only 1 to 2 weeks. Also, large volumes of fluid are needed to meet nutritional requirements, which may be contraindicated in many patients.

Central administration usually uses hypertonic dextrose (in a concentration of 15% to 35%) and amino acid solution of 3% to 7% with IV fat emulsion. Electrolytes, vitamins, and trace elements are added based on patient needs. Central solutions provide 2,000 to 4,000 kcal/day. They must be given through a large central vein with high blood flow, allowing rapid dilution and avoiding phlebitis and thrombosis. Usually, a catheter is inserted percutaneously into the subclavian vein and then advanced to the superior vena cava. **ADVANTAGES:** Central administration allows more alternatives and flexibility in regimens and a greater ability to meet full nutritional requirements without the need for daily fat emulsion. It's useful in patients with fluid restrictions (because of increased solution concentration), in those with large nutritional requirements (such as from trauma or malignancy), and those for whom PN is indicated for more than 7 to 10 days. **DISADVANTAGES:** The insertion, use, and maintenance of a central line increase the risk of infection, catheter-induced trauma, and metabolic changes.

COMPLICATIONS OF PARENTERAL NUTRITION

MECHANICAL: Malfunction of the IV delivery system may include pump failure and problems with lines, tubing, administration sets, and catheters. Catheter placement may cause pneumothorax, catheter misdirection, arterial puncture, bleeding, and hematoma formation.

INFECTIOUS: Infections can occur because these patients are typically more susceptible to infection. Catheter sepsis can occur when no other site of infection is identified; it may cause fever, shaking chills, and glucose intolerance.

METABOLIC: These complications include hyperglycemia, elevated cholesterol and triglyceride levels, and abnormal liver function test results. They may also include altered potassium, sodium, phosphate, and magnesium levels and, therefore, require fluid and electrolyte monitoring.

NUTRITIONAL: Clinical effects may results from lack of adequate vitamins, trace elements, and essential fatty acids.

MONITORING OF PARENTERAL NUTRITION

Monitoring requirements may vary slightly among institutions.

Baseline: Document the CBC; blood platelet count; prothrombin time; body weight; body length and head circumference (in infants); levels of serum electrolytes, glucose, BUN, creatinine, uric acid, total protein, cholesterol, triglycerides, bilirubin, alkaline phosphatase, LDH, SGOT (AST), and albumin; and other test results as appropriate.

Daily: Measure the patient's body weight, vital signs (TPR), and nutritional intake (kcal, protein, fat). Check the levels of serum electrolytes (potassium, sodium, and chloride), glucose (serum, urine), acetone, and BUN. Evaluate osmolarity and the results of other tests as needed.

2 to 3 times/week: Record the CBC, acid-base status, results of coagulation studies (PT, PTT) and other tests, and levels of serum creatinine, calcium, magnesium, and phosphorus as needed.

Weekly: Evaluate the nitrogen balance; levels of total protein, albumin, prealbumin, transferrin, liver enzymes (SGOT [AST], SGPT [ALT]), alkaline phosphatase, LDH), bilirubin, hemoglobin, uric acid, cholesterol, and triglycerides; and results of other tests as needed.

Appendix K

EYE AND TOPICAL AGENTS

ANTIGLAUCOMA AGENTS

USES	ACTION
Antiglaucoma agents are used to reduce elevated intraocular pressure (IOP) in patients with open-angle glaucoma and ocular hypertension.	Some antiglaucoma agents decrease IOP by increasing the outflow of aqueous humor: *Miotics (direct acting)* are cholinergic agents or miotics. They stimulate ciliary muscles, leading to increased contraction of the iris sphincter muscle. *Miotics (indirect acting)* primarily inhibit cholinesterase, allowing acetylcholine to accumulate, which prolongs parasympathetic activity. *Sympathomimetics* increase the rate of fluid flow out of the eyes and decrease the rate of aqueous humor production. Other antiglaucoma agents decrease IOP by decreasing aqueous humor production: *Alpha₂ agonists* activate receptors in the ciliary body, inhibiting aqueous secretion and increasing uveoscleral aqueous outflow. *Beta-blockers* reduce the production of aqueous humor. *Carbonic anhydrase inhibitors* reduce fluid flow into the eyes by inhibiting the enzyme carbonic anhydrase. *Prostaglandins* increase the outflow of aqueous fluid by the uveoscleral route.

Name	Availability	Dosage Range	Side Effects
Miotics			
Carbachol (Isopto-Carbachol)	**S:** 0.75%, 1.5%, 2.25%, 3%	1 drop 2 times/day	Ciliary or accommodative spasm, blurred vision, reduced night vision, sweating, increased salivation, urinary frequency, nausea, diarrhea

(continued)

EYE AND TOPICAL AGENTS—cont'd

ANTIGLAUCOMA AGENTS—cont'd

Name	Availability	Dosage Range	Side Effects
Miotics—cont'd			
Echothiophate (Phospholine Iodide)	**S:** 0.03%, 0.06%, 0.125%, 0.25%	1 drop 2 times/day	Headaches, accommodative spasm, sweating, vomiting, nausea, diarrhea, tachycardia
Pilocarpine (Isopto Carpine)	**S:** 0.25%, 0.5%, 1%, 2%, 3%, 4%, 5%, 6%, 8%, 10%	1–2 drops 3–4 times/day	Same as carbachol
Physostigmine (Eserine)	**O:** 0.25%	Apply up to 3 times/day	Blurred vision, eye pain
Sympathomimetics			
Dipivefrin (Propine)	**S:** 0.1%	1 drop q12h	Ocular congestion, burning, stinging
Epinephrine (Epifrin, Epinal)	**S:** 0.5%, 1%, 2%	1 drop 1–2 times/day	Mydriasis, blurred vision, tachycardia, hypertension, tremors, headaches, anxiety
Alpha-Agonists			
Apraclonidine (Iopidine)	**S:** 0.5%	1–2 drops 3 times/day	Ocular allergic-like reactions, hypersensitivity reaction, change in visual activity, lethargy
Brimonidine (Alphagan)	**S:** 0.2%	1–2 drops 2–3 times/day	Ocular allergy, headaches, drowsiness, fatigue

Prostaglandins

Bimatoprost (Lumigan)	S: 0.03%	1 drop daily in evening	Ocular hyperemia, eyelash growth, pruritus
Latanoprost (Xalatan)	S: 0.005%	1 drop daily in evening	Burning, stinging, iris pigmentation
Travoprost (Travatan)	S: 0.004%	1 drop daily in evening	Ocular hyperemia, eye discomfort, foreign body sensation, pain, pruritus
Unoprostone (Rescula)	S: 0.15%	1 drop 2 times/day	Iris pigmentation

Beta-Blockers

Betaxolol (Betoptic)	Suspension: 0.25% S: 0.5%	1–2 drops 1–2 times/day	Transient irritation, burning, tearing, blurred vision
Carteolol (Ocupress)	S: 1%	1 drop 2 times/day	Mild, transient ocular stinging, burning, discomfort
Levobetaxolol (Betaxon)	S: 0.5%	1 drop 2 times/day	Transient irritation, burning, tearing, blurred vision
Levobunolol (Betagan)	S: 0.25%, 0.5%	1 drop 1–2 times/day	Local discomfort, conjunctivitis, brow ache, tearing, blurred vision, headache, anxiety
Metipranolol (OptiPranolol)	S: 0.3%	1 drop 2 times/day	Transient irritation, burning, stinging, blurred vision
Timolol (Timoptic)	S: 0.25%, 0.5% G: 0.25%, 0.5%	S: 1 drop 2 times/day G: 1 drop daily	Same as betaxolol

Carbonic Anhydrase Inhibitors

Acetazolamide (Diamox)	T: 125 mg, 250 mg C: 500 mg	0.25–1 g/day	Diarrhea, loss of appetite, metallic taste, nausea, tingling in hands and fingers
Brinzolamide (Azopt)	Suspension: 1%	1 drop 3 times/day	Blurred vision, bitter taste
Dorzolamide (Trusopt)	S: 2%	1 drop 2–3 times/day	Burning, stinging, blurred vision, bitter taste

C, Capsules; *G,* gel; *O,* ointment; *S,* solution; *T,* tablets.

EYE AND TOPICAL AGENTS—cont'd

MISCELLANEOUS OPHTHALMIC AGENTS

USES	ACTION
Miscellaneous ophthalmic agents are used to prevent and treat mild ophthalmic disorders, such as allergic conjunctivitis, keratitis, and dry eyes.	Miscellaneous ophthalmic agents act in various ways. For example, *hydroxypropyl methylcellulose* stabilizes and thickens precorneal tear film, protecting and lubricating the eyes. *Azelastine, emedastine,* and *levocabastine* antagonize histamine (H_1)-receptors, thus inhibiting histamine-stimulated responses in the conjunctiva, such as redness and itching. By stabilizing mast cells, *lodoxamide* prevents antigen-stimulated release of histamine, which inhibits Type 1 hypersensitivity reactions. A broad-spectrum anti-infective, *sulfacetamide* interferes with the synthesis of folic acid that bacteria require for growth. *Vidarabine* blocks deoxyribonucleic acid (DNA) polymerase, blocking viral DNA synthesis.

Name	Indications	Dosages	Side Effects
Azelastine (Optivar)	Relief of itching eyes caused by allergic conjunctivitis	1 drop 2 times/day	Transient eye burning or stinging, headache, bitter taste, eye pain, fatigue, flu-like symptoms, pharyngitis, rhinitis, blurred vision
Emedastine (Emadine)	Treatment of signs and symptoms of allergic conjunctivitis	1–2 drops 2 times/day	Headache, bad taste, blurred vision, eye burning or stinging, dry eyes, tearing
Epinastine (Elestat)	Treatment of allergic conjunctivitis	1 drop 4 times/day	Headache, taste disturbance, drowsiness, blurred vision, eye burning or stinging, dry eyes, foreign body sensation, rhinitis

Hydroxypropyl methylcellulose (Artificial Tears, Isopto Tears, Tears Naturale)	Relief of eye dryness and irritation caused by insufficient tear production	1–2 drops 3–4 times/day	Eye irritation, blurred vision, eyelash stickiness
Ketotifen (Zaditor)	Temporary relief of itching eyes caused by allergic conjunctivitis	1 drop every 8–12 hours	Conjunctival infection, headache, rhinitis, eye burning or stinging, ocular discharge, eye pain
Levocabastine (Livostin)	Treatment of signs and symptoms of seasonal allergic conjunctivitis	1 drop 4 times/day	Transient eye stinging, burning, or discomfort; headache; dry eyes; eyelid edema
Lodoxamide (Alomide)	Treatment of vernal keratoconjunctivitis and keratitis	1 drop 4 times/day	Transient eye stinging or burning, instillation discomfort, itching eyes, blurred vision, dry eyes, tearing, headache
Olopatadine (Patanol)	Treatment of signs and symptoms of allergic conjunctivitis	1–2 drops 2 times/day	Headache, drowsiness, eye burning or stinging, foreign body sensation, pharyngitis, rhinitis, pruritus

(continued)

EYE AND TOPICAL AGENTS—cont'd

MISCELLANEOUS OPHTHALMIC AGENTS—cont'd

Name	Indications	Dosages	Side Effects
Pemirolast (Alamast)	Prevention of itching eyes caused by allergic conjunctivitis	1–2 drops 3–4 times/day	Transient eye stinging or burning, instillation discomfort, itching eyes, blurred vision, tearing, headache
Sulfacetamide (Sulf-10)	Treatment of corneal ulcers, bacterial conjunctivitis, other superficial eye infections; prevention of infection after eye injury	1–3 drops every 2–3 hours; or 1.25- to 2.5-cm strip of ointment 4 times/day and at bedtime	Transient eye burning or stinging, headache, rash, itching eyes, eye swelling, photosensitivity
Vidarabine (Ara-A)	Treatment of keratitis or keratoconjunctivitis caused by herpes simplex virus, type 1 or 2	½" 5 times/day at 3-hour intervals; after re-epithelialization, ½" 2 times/day for 7 days	Eye burning or irritation, itching eyes, tearing, eye pain, photophobia

TOPICAL ANTI-INFLAMMATORY AGENTS

USES	ACTION
Topical anti-inflammatory agents relieve inflammation and pruritus caused by corticosteroid-responsive disorders, such as contact dermatitis, eczema, insect bite reactions, first- and second-degree localized burns, and sunburn.	Topical anti-inflammatory agents diffuse across cell membranes and form complexes with cytoplasm. These complexes stimulate the synthesis of inhibitory enzymes that are responsible for the agents' anti-inflammatory effects, which include inhibition of edema, erythema, pruritus, capillary dilation, and phagocyte activity. Topical corticosteroids can be classified based on potency: *Low potency agents* provide modest anti-inflammatory effects. They're safest for long-term application, facial and intertriginous application, use with occlusive dressings, and for infants and young children. *Medium potency agents* are active against moderate inflammatory conditions, such as chronic eczematous dermatoses. They may be used for facial and intertriginous application for a limited time only. *High potency agents* are effective in more severe inflammatory conditions, such as lichen simplex chronicus and psoriasis. They may be used for facial and intertriginous application for a short time only and can be used on skin thickened by chronic conditions. *Very high potency agents* offer an alternative to systemic therapy for local effects, such as with chronic lesions caused by psoriasis. Because they pose an increased risk of skin atrophy, they should be used only for short periods on small areas without occlusive dressings.

TOPICAL CORTICOSTEROIDS

Name	Availability	Potency	Side Effects
Alclometasone (Aclovate)	C, O: 0.05%	Low	Burning, stinging, irritation, itching, rash
Amcinonide (Cyclocort)	C, O, L: 0.1%	High	Same as above

(continued)

EYE AND TOPICAL AGENTS—cont'd

TOPICAL CORTICOSTEROIDS—cont'd

Name	Availability	Potency	Side Effects
Betamethasone dipropionate (Diprosone)	C, O, G, L: 0.05%	High	Same as above
Betamethasone valerate (Valisone)	C: 0.01%, 0.05%, 0.1% O: 0.1% L: 0.1%	High	Same as above
Clobetasol (Temovate)	C, O: 0.05%	High	Same as above
Desonide (Tridesilon)	C, O, L: 0.05%	Low	Same as above
Desoximetasone (Topicort)	C: 0.25%, 0.5% O: 0.25% G: 0.05%	High	Same as above
Dexamethasone (Decadron)	C: 0.1%	Medium	Same as above
Fluocinolone (Synalar)	C: 0.01%, 0.025%, 0.2% O: 0.025%	High	Same as above
Fluocinonide (Lidex)	C, O, G: 0.05%	High	Same as above
Fluticasone (Cutivate)	C: 0.05% O: 0.005%	Medium	Same as above
Halobetasol (Ultravate)	C, O: 0.05%	High	Same as above
Hydrocortisone (Cort-Dome, Hytone)	C, O: 0.5%, 1%, 2.5%	Medium	Same as above
Mometasone (Elocon)	C, O, L: 0.1%	Medium	Same as above
Prednicarbate (Dermatop)	C: 0.1%	—	Same as above
Triamcinolone (Aristocort, Kenalog)	C, O, L: 0.025%, 0.1%, 0.5%	Medium	Same as above

C, Cream; *G,* gel; *L,* lotion; *O,* ointment.

MISCELLANEOUS TOPICAL AGENTS

USES	ACTION
Miscellaneous topical agents are used to treat dermatologic disorders, such as acne, dermatitis, and infections. Some are also used to prevent certain dermatologic disorders and relieve localized pain.	Miscellaneous topical agents act in various ways. Some *anti-infectives*, such as *docosanol, mupiricin,* and *penciclovir,* prevent viral or bacterial replication; *silver sulfadiasine* acts on bacterial cell walls, producing bactericidal effects. *Becaplermin* is a platelet-derived growth factor that stimulates new tissue growth to heal open wounds. *Capsaicin* depletes and prevents the accumulation of substance P (a mediator of pain impulses) from peripheral sensory neurons to the central nervous system, relieving pain. *Pimecrolimus* is an anti-inflammatory agent that inhibits the release of cytokine, an enzyme that produces inflammatory reactions. *Tretinoin* decreases the cohesiveness of follicular epithelial cells and increases their turnover.

Name	Indications	Dosages	Side Effects
Azelaic acid (Azelex)	Treatment of mild to moderate acne vulgaris	Apply to affected area 2 times/day.	Pruritus, stinging, burning, tingling
Becaplermin (Regranex)	Treatment of lower leg diabetic neuropathic ulcers extending into subcutaneous tissue or beyond	Apply once daily. After 12 hours, rinse ulcer and recover with saline gauze.	Local rash near ulcer
Capsaicin (Zostrix)	Treatment of neuralgia, osteoarthritis, and rheumatoid arthritis	Apply directly to affected area 3–4 times/day.	Burning, stinging, erythema at application site
Collagenase (Santyl)	Debridement of necrotic tissue in chronic dermal ulcers and severe burns	Apply once daily, or more frequently if dressing becomes soiled.	Transient erythema

(continued)

EYE AND TOPICAL AGENTS—cont'd

MISCELLANEOUS TOPICAL AGENTS—cont'd

Name	Indications	Dosages	Side Effects
Docosanol (Abreva)	Treatment of cold sores or fever blisters caused by herpes simplex virus, type 1 or 2	Apply to lesions 5 times/day at onset of symptoms and until lesions are healed, up to a maximum of 10 days.	Headache, skin irritation
Eflornithine (Vaniqa)	Reduction of unwanted facial and chin hair	Apply to affected area 2 times/day at least 8 hours apart.	Anemia, leukopenia, thrombocytopenia, dizziness, alopecia, vomiting, diarrhea, hearing impairment
Imiquimod (Aldara)	Treatment of external genital and perianal warts (condylomata acuminata)	Apply 3 times/week before normal sleeping hours. Leave on skin for 6-10 hours, then remove. Continue for a maximum of 16 weeks.	Local skin reactions, erythema, itching, burning, excoriation, flaking, fungal infection
Mupirocin (Bactroban)	**Topical:** Treatment of impetigo and infected traumatic skin lesions **Nasal:** Reduction of spread of methicillin-resistant S. aureus	**Topical:** Apply 3 times/day. **Nasal:** Apply 2 times/day for 5 days.	**Topical:** Pain, burning, stinging, itching **Nasal:** Headache, rhinitis, upper respiratory congestion, pharyngitis, altered taste
Penciclovir (Denavir)	Treatment of recurrent herpes labialis (cold sores)	Apply every 2 hours while awake for 4 days.	Headache, mild erythema, altered taste, rash

Pimecrolimus (Elidel)	Treatment of mild to moderate atopic dermatitis (eczema)	Apply 2 times/day.	Upper respiratory tract infection, nasopharyngitis, burning, pyrexia, cough, nasal congestion, abdominal pain, sore throat, headache
Povidone iodine (Betadine)	External antiseptic action	Apply as needed.	Rash, pruritus, local edema
Sertaconazole (Ertaczo)	Treatment of superficial dermatophytic and candidal infections	Apply 2 times/day.	Headache, drowsiness, pruritus, erythema
Silver sulfadiazine (Silvadene)	Prevention and treatment of infection in second- and third-degree burns; protection against conversion from partial- to full-thickness wounds	Apply 1-2 times/day.	Burning feeling at application site, rash, itching, increased skin sensitivity to sunlight
Tretinoin (Retin-A)	Treatment of acne vulgaris	Apply once daily at bedtime.	Transient pigmentation changes, photosensitivity, local inflammatory reactions (peeling, dry skin, stinging, pruritus)

Appendix L

FDA PREGNANCY CATEGORIES

Alert: Medications should be used during pregnancy only if clearly needed.

A: Adequate and well-controlled studies have failed to show a risk to the fetus in the first trimester of pregnancy (also, no evidence of risk has been seen in later trimesters). Possibility of fetal harm appears remote.

B: Animal reproduction studies have failed to show a risk to the fetus and there are no adequate/well-controlled studies in pregnant women.

C: Animal reproduction studies have shown an adverse effect on the fetus and there are no adequate/well-controlled studies in humans. However, the benefits may warrant use of the drug in pregnant women despite potential risks.

D: There is positive evidence of human fetal risk based on data from investigational or marketing experience or from studies in humans, but the potential benefits may warrant use of the drug despite potential risks (e.g., use in life-threatening situations in which other medications cannot be used or are ineffective).

X: Animal or human studies have shown fetal abnormalities and/or there is evidence of human fetal risk based on adverse reaction data from investigational or marketing experience where the risks in using the medication clearly outweigh potential benefits.

Appendix M

NORMAL LABORATORY VALUES

HEMATOLOGY/COAGULATION

Test	Specimen	Normal Range
Activated partial thromboplastin time (APTT)	Whole blood	25–35 sec
Erythrocyte count (RBC count)	Whole blood	M: 4.3–5.7 million cells/mm^3 F: 3.8–5.1 million cells/mm^3
Hematocrit (HCT, Hct)	Whole blood	M: 39%–49% F: 35%–45%
Hemoglobin (Hb, Hgb)	Whole blood	M: 13.5–17.5 g/dl F: 12.0–16.0 g/dl
Leukocyte count (WBC count)	Whole blood	4.5–11.0 thousand cells/mm^3
Leukocyte differential count	Whole blood	
Basophils		0%–0.75%
Eosinophils		1%–3%
Lymphocytes		23%–33%
Monocytes		3%–7%
Neutrophils-bands		3%–5%
Neutrophils-segmented		54%–62%
Mean corpuscular hemoglobin (MCH)	Whole blood	26–34 pg/cell
Mean corpuscular hemoglobin concentration (MCHC)	Whole blood	31%–37% Hb/cell
Mean corpuscular volume (MCV)	Whole blood	80–100 fL
Partial thromboplastin time (PTT)	Whole blood	60–85 sec
Platelet count (thrombocyte count)	Whole blood	150–450 thousand/mm^3
Prothrombin time (PT)	Whole blood	11–13.5 sec
RBC count (see Erythrocyte count)		

SERUM/URINE VALUES

Test	Specimen	Normal Range
Alanine aminotransferase (ALT, SGPT)	Serum	0–55 units/L
Albumin	Serum	3.5–5 g/dl
Alkaline phosphatase	Serum	M: 53–128 units/L F: 42–98 units/L
Anion gap	Plasma or serum	5–14 mEq/L
Aspartate aminotransferase (AST, SGOT)	Serum	0–50 units/L
Bilirubin (conjugated direct)	Serum	0–0.4 mg/dl

Test	Specimen	Normal Range
Bilirubin (total)	Serum	0.2–1.2 mg/dl
Calcium (total)	Serum	8.4–10.2 mg/dl
Carbon dioxide (CO_2) total	Plasma or serum	20–34 mEq/L
Chloride	Plasma or serum	96–112 mEq/L
Cholesterol (total)	Plasma or serum	<200 mg/dl
C-Reactive protein	Serum	68–8,200 ng/ml
Creatine kinase (CK)	Serum	M: 38–174 units/L F: 26–140 units/L
Creatine kinase isoenzymes	Serum	Fraction of total: <0.04–0.06
Creatinine	Plasma or serum	M: 0.7–1.3 mg/dl F: 0.6–1.1 mg/dl
Creatinine clearance	Plasma or serum and urine	M: 90–139 ml/min/ 1.73 m^2 F: 80–125 ml/min/ 1.73 m^2
Free thyroxine index (FTI)	Serum	1.1–4.8
Glucose	Serum	Adults: 70–105 mg/dl >60 yrs: 80–115 mg/dl
Hemoglobin A_{1c}	Whole blood	5.6%–7.5% of total Hgb
Homovanillic acid (HVA)	Urine, 24 hr	1.4–8.8 mg/day
17-Hydroxycorticosteroids (17-OHCS)	Urine, 24 hr	M: 3–10 mg/day F: 2–8 mg/day
Iron	Serum	M: 65–175 mcg/dl F: 50–170 mcg/dl
Iron-binding capacity, total (TIBC)	Serum	250–450 mcg/dl
Lactate dehydrogenase (LDH)	Serum	0–250 units/L
Magnesium	Serum	1.3–2.3 mg/dl
Oxygen (Po_2)	Whole blood, arterial	83–100 mm Hg
Oxygen saturation	Whole blood, arterial	95%–98%
pH	Whole blood, arterial	7.35–7.45
Phosphorus, inorganic	Serum	2.7–4.5 mg/dl
Potassium	Serum	3.5–5.1 mEq/L
Protein (total)	Serum	6–8.5 g/dl
Sodium	Plasma or serum	136–146 mEq/L
Specific gravity	Urine	1.002–1.030
Thyrotropin (hTSH)	Plasma or serum	2–10 mcgU/ml
Thyroxine (T_4) total	Serum	5–12 mcg/dl
Triglycerides (TG)	Serum, after 12-hr fast	20–190 mg/dl
Triiodothyronine resin uptake test (T_3RU)	Serum	22%–37%
Urea nitrogen	Plasma or serum	7–25 mg/dl
Urea nitrogen/creatinine ratio	Serum	12/1–20/1
Uric acid	Serum	M: 3.5–7.2 mg/dl F: 2.6–6 mg/dl
Vanillylmandelic acid (VMA)	Urine, 24 hr	2–7 mg/day

Appendix N

ORAL, VAGINAL, AND TRANSDERMAL CONTRACEPTIVES

ACTION	CLASSIFICATION
Oral contraceptives decrease fertility primarily by inhibiting ovulation. In addition, they can promote thickening of the cervical mucus, thereby creating a physical barrier to the passage of sperm. Also, they can modify the endometrium, making it less favorable for implantation. Contraception can also be achieved through the use of vaginal and transdermal agents.	Oral contraceptives may contain an estrogen and a progestin (combination oral contraceptives) or may contain only a progestin (progestin-only oral contraceptives). Combination oral contraceptives have four subgroups: *Monophasic contraceptives* have daily estrogen and progestin dosages that remain constant. *Biphasic contraceptives* have a constant estrogen dosage, and a progestin dosage that increases during the second half of the cycle. *Triphasic contraceptives* have a progestin dosage that changes for each phase of the cycle. *Estrophasic contraceptives* have a constant progestin dosage, and an estrogen dosage that gradually increases through the monthly cycle.

ORAL CONTRACEPTIVES

Brand Names	Estrogen (mcg)	Progestin (mg)	Brand Names	Estrogen (mcg)	Progestin (mg)
Monophasic			Monophasic		
Genora 1/50	50 mestranol	1 norethindrone	**Modicon**	35 ethinyl estradiol	0.5 norethindrone
Nelova 1/50M	50 mestranol	1 norethindrone	**Nelova 0.5/35E**	35 ethinyl estradiol	0.5 norethindrone

(continued)

ORAL, VAGINAL, AND TRANSDERMAL CONTRACEPTIVES—cont'd

ORAL CONTRACEPTIVES—cont'd

Brand Names	Estrogen (mcg)	Progestin (mg)	Brand Names	Estrogen (mcg)	Progestin (mg)
Monophasic—cont'd			Monophasic—cont'd		
Norethin 1/50M	50 mestranol	1 norethindrone	Ovcon-35	35 ethinyl estradiol	0.4 norethindrone
Norinyl 1+ 50	50 mestranol	1 norethindrone	Ortho-Cyclen	35 ethinyl estradiol	0.25 norgestimate
Ortho-Novum 1/50	50 mestranol	1 norethindrone	Demulen 1/35	35 ethinyl estradiol	1 ethynodiol diacetate
Ovcon-50	50 ethinyl estradiol	1 norethindrone	Loestrin 21 1.5/30	30 ethinyl estradiol	1.5 norethindrone acetate
Demulen 1/50	50 ethinyl estradiol	1 ethynodiol diacetate	Loestrin Fe 1.5/30	30 ethinyl estradiol	1.5 norethindrone acetate
Ovral	50 ethinyl estradiol	0.5 norgestrel	Lo/Ovral	30 ethinyl estradiol	0.3 norgestrel
Genora 1/35	35 ethinyl estradiol	1 norethindrone	Desogen	30 ethinyl estradiol	0.15 desogestrel
Nelova 1/35E	35 ethinyl estradiol	1 norethindrone	Ortho-Cept	30 ethinyl estradiol	0.15 desogestrel
Norethin 1/35E	35 ethinyl estradiol	1 norethindrone	Levlen	30 ethinyl estradiol	0.15 levonorgestrel

Norinyl 1+35	35 ethinyl estradiol	1 norethindrone
Ortho-Novum 1/35	35 ethinyl estradiol	1 norethindrone
Brevicon	35 ethinyl estradiol	0.5 norethindrone
Genora 0.5/35	35 ethinyl estradiol	0.5 norethindrone
Ortho Evra	0.02 ethinyl estradiol	0.15 norelgestromin
NuvaRing	2.7 ethinyl estradiol	11.7 etonogestrel

Levora	30 ethinyl estradiol	0.15 levonorgestrel
Nordette	30 ethinyl estradiol	0.15 levonorgestrel
Loestrin 21 1/20	20 ethinyl estradiol	1 norethindrone acetate
Yasmin	30 ethinyl estradiol	3 drospirenone

Biphasic

	Phase 1	Phase 2
Jenest-28	0.5 mg norethindrone 35 mcg ethinyl estradiol	1 mg norethindrone 35 mcg ethinyl estradiol
Nelova 10/11	0.5 mg norethindrone 35 mcg ethinyl estradiol	1 mg norethindrone 35 mcg ethinyl estradiol
Ortho-Novum 10/11	0.5 mg norethindrone 35 mcg ethinyl estradiol	1 mg norethindrone 35 mcg ethinyl estradiol

(continued)

ORAL, VAGINAL, AND TRANSDERMAL CONTRACEPTIVES—cont'd

ORAL CONTRACEPTIVES—cont'd

	Phase 1	Phase 2	Phase 3
Triphasic			
Estrostep	1 mg norethindrone 20 mcg ethinyl estradiol	1 mg norethindrone 30 mcg ethinyl estradiol	1 mg norethindrone 35 mcg ethinyl estradiol
Tri-Norinyl	0.5 mg norethindrone 35 mcg ethinyl estradiol	1 mg norethindrone 35 mcg ethinyl estradiol	0.5 mg norethindrone 35 mcg ethinyl estradiol
Ortho-Novum 7/7/7	0.5 mg norethindrone 35 mcg ethinyl estradiol	0.75 mg norethindrone 35 mcg ethinyl estradiol	1 mg norethindrone 35 mcg ethinyl estradiol
Tri-Levlen Triphasil	0.05 mg levonorgestrel 30 mcg ethinyl estradiol	0.075 mg levonorgestrel 40 mcg ethinyl estradiol	0.125 mg levonorgestrel 30 mcg ethinyl estradiol
Ortho Tri-Cyclen	0.18 mg norgestimate 35 mcg ethinyl estradiol	0.215 mg norgestimate 35 mcg ethinyl estradiol	0.25 mg norgestimate 35 mcg ethinyl estradiol
Progestin Only			
Micronor Nor Q D	0.35 mg norethindrone		
Ovrette	0.075 mg norgestrel		

(continued)

NEW CONTRACEPTIVE OPTIONS

Name	Ingredients	Cycle duration
Oral Contraceptive		
Yasmin 28	30 mcg ethinyl estradiol 3 mg drospirenone	28-day cycle (21 days active; 7 days placebo)
Micrette, Kariva	20 mcg ethinyl estradiol 0.15 mg desogestrel 10 mcg placebo, ethinyl estradiol	28-day cycle (21 days active, 2 days placebo, 5 days ethinyl estradiol 10 mcg)
Ortho Tri-Cyclen Lo	25 mcg ethinyl estradiol 180 mcg norgestimate (7 days); 215 mcg (7 days), 250 mcg (7 days), 7 days placebo	28-day cycle (21 days active; 7 days placebo)
Nortrel 7/7/7	35 mcg ethinyl estradiol norethindrone 0.5 mg (7 days), 0.75 mg (7 days), 1 mg (7 days), 7 days placebo	28-day cycle (21 days active; 7 days placebo)
Extended Contraceptive Regimen		
Seasonale	30 mcg ethinyl estradiol 150 mcg levonorgestrel	91-day cycle (84 days active; 7 days placebo)
Intrauterine System		
Mirena	52 mg levonorgestrel; total releasing 20 mcg/ day	Device inserted into uterus once every 5 years
Vaginal Ring		
Nuva-Ring	15 mcg ethinyl estradiol 120 mcg/day etonogestrel	28-day cycle; self-inserted vaginal ring left in place for 21 days, then replaced after 7 days

(continued)

NEW CONTRACEPTIVE OPTIONS—cont'd

Name	Ingredients	Cycle duration
Transdermal Patch		
Ortho-Evra	20 mcg ethinyl estradiol 150 mcg norelgestromin released per day	28-day cycle; one new patch applied and kept in place for one week and then replaced weekly for 3 weeks with a new patch. During week 4 a transdermal patch isn't used.
Injectable		
Lunelle	5 mg ethinyl cypionate 25 mg medroxyprogesterone	28-day cycle administered IM once q28 days

Appendix O

OVARIAN STIMULANTS

Ovarian stimulants (medications that induce ovulation) are used to treat infertility (a decreased ability to reproduce), but not sterility (the inability to reproduce). Infertility may result from reproductive dysfunction of the male, female, or both.

Female infertility can be caused by disruption of any phase of the reproductive process. The most critical phases are follicular maturation, ovulation, ovum transport through the fallopian tubes, fertilization of the ovum, implantation, and growth and development of the conceptus. Female infertility can have a number of causes:

Anovulation and failure of follicular maturation can result from lack of adequate hormonal stimulation. As a result, ovarian follicles don't ripen, and ovulation doesn't occur.

Unfavorable cervical mucus may be scant, thick, or sticky. Normally, the cervical glands secrete large volumes of thin, watery mucus; if the mucus is unfavorable, sperm can't pass through to the uterus.

Hyperprolactinemia causes excessive prolactin secretion, which may lead to amenorrhea, galactorrhea, and infertility.

Luteal phase defect can occur in which progesterone secretion by the corpus luteum is insufficient to maintain endo-metrial integrity.

Endometriosis (abnormal implantation of endometrial tissue, such as in the uterine wall and ovaries) can prevent normal implantation of the ovum.

Androgen excess may decrease fertility, commonly by causing polycystic ovaries.

Male infertility may result from decreased density or motility of sperm or abnormal volume or quality of semen. The most obvious manifestation of male infertility is impotence (inability to achieve erection). Unlike female infertility, which usually stems from an identifiable endocrine disorder, most cases of male infertility have no identifiable endocrine cause.

(continued)

OVARIAN STIMULANTS—cont'd

Name	Category	Availability	Uses	Side Effects
Cetrorelix (Cetrotide)	GnRH antagonist	I: 0.25 mg, 3 mg	Inhibition of premature luteinizing hormone (LH) surges in women undergoing ovarian hyperstimulation	Ovarian hyperstimulation syndrome (OHSS): Abdominal pain, indigestion, bloating, decreased urine, nausea, vomiting, diarrhea, rapid weight gain, shortness of breath, swelling of the lower legs. Headaches, pain and redness at the injection site
Chorionic gonadotropin (APL, Pregnyl, Profasi, Profasi HP)	Gonadotropin	I: 5,000 units, 10,000 units, 20,000 units	In conjunction with clomiphene, human menotropins, or urofollitropin to stimulate ovulation	OHSS: Abdominal pain, indigestion, bloating, decreased urine, nausea, vomiting, diarrhea, rapid weight gain, shortness of breath, swelling of the lower legs. Ovarian enlargement, ovarian cyst formation
Clomiphene (Clomid, Milophene, Serophene)	Antiestrogen	T: 50 mg	Anovulation, oligo-ovulation with intact pituitary-ovarian response and endogenous estrogen	Ovarian cyst formation, ovarian enlargement, visual disturbances, premenstrual syndrome, hot flashes

Follitropin alpha (Gonal-F)	Gonadotropin	I: 37.5 international units follicle-stimulating hormone (FSH), 75 international units FSH, 150 international units FSH	In conjunction with human chorionic gonadotropin (hCG) to stimulate ovarian follicular development in patients with ovulatory dysfunction not due to primary ovarian failure (such as anovulation or oligo-ovulation)	OHSS: Abdominal pain, indigestion, bloating, decreased urine, nausea, vomiting, diarrhea, rapid weight gain, shortness of breath, swelling of the lower legs. Flu-like symptoms, upper respiratory tract infections, bleeding between menstrual periods, ovarian enlargement, ovarian cysts, acne, breast pain or tenderness
Follitropin beta (Follistem)	Gonadotropin	I: 75 international units FSH	Same as above	OHSS: Abdominal pain, indigestion, bloating, decreased urine, nausea, vomiting, diarrhea, rapid weight gain, shortness of breath, swelling of the lower legs. Flu-like symptoms, breast tenderness, dry skin, rash, dizziness, fever, headaches, unusual tiredness
Ganirelex (Antagon)	Gonadotropin-releasing hormone (GnRH) antagonist	I: 250 mcg/0.5 ml	Inhibition of premature LH surges in women undergoing ovarian hyperstimulation	Same as cetrorelix

(continued)

OVARIAN STIMULANTS—cont'd

Name	Category	Availability	Uses	Side Effects
Gonadorelin	GnRH agonist	**I:** 100 mcg, 500 mcg	Evaluation of hypothalamic-pituitary-gonadotropic function; evaluation of abnormal gonadotropin regulation as in precocious puberty or delayed puberty; treatment of primary hypothalmic amenorrhea	Swelling, pain, or itching at injection site with SubQ administration. Local or generalized skin rash with long-term SubQ administration. Headache, nausea, light-headedness, abdominal discomfort, hypersensitivity reactions (bronchospasm, tachycardia, flushing, urticaria), induration at injection site
Goserelin (Zoladex)	GnRH agonist	**Implant:** 3.6 mg	Endometriosis, adjunct to menotropins and hCG for ovulation induction	Hot flashes, amenorrhea, blurred vision, edema, headaches, nausea, vomiting, breast tenderness, weight gain
Leuprolide (Lupron)	GnRH agonist	5 mg/ml for SC injection	Endometriosis, adjunct to menotropins and hCG for ovulation induction	Same as goserelin
Menotropins (Humegon, Pergonal)	Gonadotropin	**FSH:** 75 units, 150 units **LH activity:** 75 units, 150 units	In conjunction with hCG for ovulation stimulation in patients with ovulatory dysfunction due to primary ovarian failure	Same as chorionic gonadotropin

| Nafarelin (Synarel) | GnRH agonist | **Nasal Spray:** 2 mg/ml | Same as leuprolide | Loss of bone mineral density, breast enlargement, bleeding between regular menstrual periods, acne, mood swings, seborrhea, hot flashes |
| Urofol-litropoin (Fertinex, Metrodin) | Gonadotropin | **FSH activity:** 75 units, 150 units | In conjunction with hCG for ovulation stimulation in patients with polycystic ovary syndrome who have an elevated LH/FSH ratio and have failed clomiphene therapy | Same as chorionic gonadotropin |

I, injection; *T,* tablets.

Appendix P

(POISON) ANTIDOTE CHART

Poison/Drug	Indications	Antidote	Dosage
acetamino-phen	Treatment of acetaminophen overdose to protect against hepatotoxicity.	*N*-acetylcysteine (Mucomyst)	Dilute to 5% solution with carbonated beverage, fruit juice, or water and administer orally. **Loading:** 140 mg/kg for one dose. **Maintenance:** 70 mg/kg for 17 doses, starting 4 hrs after loading dose and given q4h.
arsenic, gold, mercury, lead	Treatment of arsenic, gold, mercury if started within 1–2 hrs; treatment of acute lead poisoning of levels >70 mcg/dl (with calcium EDTA) (do **not** use for chronic mercury poisoning).	Dimercaprol (BAL in oil)	Deep IM injections. **Mild arsenic/gold:** 2.5 mg/kg 4×/day for 2 days, 2×/day for 1 day, then once daily for up to 10 days. **Severe arsenic/gold:** 3 mg/kg q4h for 2 days then 4×/day for 1 day, then 2×/day for up to 10 days. **Mercury:** 5 mg/kg, then 2.5 mg/kg 1–2×/day for 10 days. **Acute lead encephalopathy:** 4 mg/kg alone in first dose, then at 4-hr intervals with calcium EDTA (give at separate sites). **Less severe lead:** After first dose, 3 mg/kg. Continue for 2–7 days as needed.
arsenic, lead, mercury	Treatment of lead poisoning with levels of >45 mcg/dl. Treatment of arsenic and mercury poisoning.	Succimer, DMSA	10 mg/kg orally 3×/day for 5 days, then 10 mg/kg 2×/day for additional 14 days.

Poison/Drug	Indications	Antidote	Dosage
atropine, anticholinergic agents, antihistamines, plants containing anticholinergic agents	Reverse toxic effects on the central nervous system (CNS) caused by drugs and plants capable of producing anticholinergic poisoning in clinical or toxic dosages (including tricyclic antidepressants).	physostigmine (Antilirium)	**Children:** 0.02 mg/kg IM or slow IV injection (0.5 mg/min). May repeat at 5- to 10-min intervals until therapeutic response or maximum dose of 2 mg is attained. **Adults:** Slow IV push (1 mg/min): 0.5–2 mg; may repeat if life-threatening signs, including arrhythmias, convulsions, coma, occur.
benzodiazepines	Complete or partial reversal of sedative effects of benzodiazepines when general anesthesia has been induced and/or maintained with benzodiazepines, when sedation has been produced with benzodiazepines for diagnostic and therapeutic procedures, management of benzodiazepine overdosage.	flumazenil (Romazicon)	**IV: Adults, elderly:** Initially, 0.2 mg (2 ml) over 30 sec; may repeat after 30 sec with 0.3 mg (3 ml) over 30 sec if desired level of consciousness not achieved. Further doses of 0.5 mg (5 ml) over 30 sec may be administered at 60-sec intervals. **Maximum:** 3 mg (30 ml) total dose. **Alert:** If resedation occurs, repeat dose at 20-min intervals. **Maximum:** 1 mg (given as 0.5 mg/min) at any one time, 3 mg in any 1 hr.
cyanide, nitroprusside	Begin treatment at first sign of toxicity if exposure is known or strongly suspected.	amyl nitrite, sodium nitrite, sodium thiosulfate (Cyanide Antidote Kit)	First, crush amyl nitrite pearls in gauze and allow patient to inhale for 15 sec, then remove for 15 sec. Use a fresh pearl every 3 min. Continue until injection of 10 ml of 3% (300 mg) sodium nitrite in adults. Inject over 2–5 min. Pediatric dose based on Hgb level; if normal Hgb assumed, then 0.15–0.33 ml/kg sodium nitrite up to 10 ml may be used. After sodium

(continued)

(POISON) ANTIDOTE CHART—cont'd

Poison/Drug	Indications	Antidote	Dosage
cyanide, nitroprusside—cont'd			nitrite, immediately inject 50 ml of 25% sodium thiosulfate (12.5 g), slow IV, over 10 min. Use 7 g/m^2 maximum of 12.5 g, in children.
digoxin	Treatment of potentially life-threatening digoxin intoxication.	digoxin-immune Fab (Digibind)	Dose in number of vials = steady-state digoxin level in mg/ml × patient weight in kg divided by 100. 4–6 vials adequate to treat 90%–95% of patients with chronic digoxin toxicity. If ingested amount is unknown, give 10–20 vials (400–800 mg). Administer IV over 30 min through a 0.22-micron filter. A bolus injection can be given if cardiac arrest is imminent.
ethylene glycol	Ethylene glycol blood levels >20 mg/dl. Blood levels not readily available and suspected ingestion of toxic amounts. Any symptomatic patient with a history of ethylene glycol ingestion.	fomepizole (Antizol)	**Loading:** 15 mg/kg IV over 30 min followed by 10 mg/kg q12h for 4 doses, then 15 mg/kg q12h until ethylene glycol levels are <20 mg/dl.
hydrofluoric acid (HF), fluoride salts	Calcium gluconate 2.5% gel for dermal exposure to HF <20% concentration. Subcutaneous injections of calcium gluconate for dermal exposures of HF in >20% concentration or failure to respond to calcium gluconate gel. IV calcium	calcium gluconate	Massage 2.5% gel into exposed area for 15 min, repeating as necessary for pain. Infiltrate each cm^2 of exposed area with 0.5 ml 10% calcium gluconate SC, using a 30-gauge needle. Give 0.1–0.2 ml/kg IV 10% calcium gluconate slowly up to 10 ml. Repeat dose if necessary.

Poison/Drug	Indications	Antidote	Dosage
hydrofluoric acid (HF), fluoride salts—cont'd	gluconate 10% for serious systemic toxicity following dermal exposure, or ingestion of fluoride salts.		
iron	Acute iron intoxication. Chronic iron overload.	deferoxamine (Desferal)	**Acute iron intoxication:** *IM:* 1 g, then 0.5 g q4h × 2 doses, then 0.5 g q4–12h. May give IV infusion 10–15 mg/kg/hr. Do not exceed 6 g in 24 hrs. **Chronic iron overload:** *IM:* 0.5–1 g daily. *Subcutaneous:* 1–2 g/day (20–40 mg/kg/day) over 8–24 hrs. **Children:** Maximum of 6 g/24 hrs or 2 g/dose.
lead	Acute and chronic lead poisoning, lead encephalopathy.	calcium EDTA	**Adults:** 1 g in 250–500 ml NaCl or D_5W over >1 hr for 5 days, stop for 2 days, then repeat for 5 days if needed.
miscellaneous medications	Treatment of drug overdose.	ipecac	**Children <1 yr:** 5–10 ml, then ½–1 glass of water. **Children ≥1–12 yrs:** 15 ml followed by 1–2 glasses of water. **Adults:** 15–30 ml followed by 3–4 glasses of water. **Alert:** Repeat dose (15 ml) once in those >1 yr if vomiting does not occur within 20–30 min. Perform gastric lavage if vomiting does not occur within 30–45 min after second dose.

(continued)

Poison/Drug	Indications	Antidote	Dosage
miscellaneous medication poisoning	Treatment of drug poisoning.	charcoal, activated	**Adults:** 25–100 g (or 1 g/kg or approx. 10 times the amount of poison ingested) as a suspension (4–8 oz of water). Multiple doses may be used in severe poisoning to prevent desorption from the charcoal; also increases GI clearance and rate of elimination of drugs that undergo an enteral recirculation pattern.
opiates, alpha$_2$-agonists (e.g., clonidine)	Opiate overdose. Coma or respiratory depression of unknown origin.	naloxone (Narcan) nalmefene (Revex)	**Naloxone: Adults:** Give 0.4–2 mg IV bolus. Doses may be repeated q2–5min up to 10 mg if no response. **Children:** 0.01 mg/kg. May repeat with 0.1 mg/kg. **Alert:** AAP recommends initial dose of 0.1 mg/kg for infants and children up to 5 yrs and weighing <20 kg. **Children >5 yrs or ≥20 kg:** Recommended initial dose 2 mg. **Nalmefene:** 0.5–1 mg IV q2min as needed to a total of 2 mg.
organophosphate insecticides	Synergistic adjunct to atropine therapy. Reverses nicotinic effects such as profound muscle weakness, respiratory depression, and muscle twitching. Organophosphate poisoning. Anticholinesterase drug overdose.	pralidoxime (2-PAM) (Protopam)	**Children:** *IV:* 25–50 mg/kg up to 1 g in 250 ml NaCl over 30 min. **Adults:** *IV:* 1–2 g in 100 ml NaCl over 15–30 min. If pulmonary edema present, may give as a 5% solution slow IV push over not less than 5 min. Dosage may be repeated in 1 hr followed by q8h if indicated.

RECOMMENDED CHILD AND ADULT IMMUNIZATION SCHEDULES

Recommended Childhood and Adolescent Immunization Schedule—United States, 2003

Legend: range of recommended ages | catch-up vaccination | preadolescent assessment

Age ▶ Vaccine ▼	Birth	1 mo	2 mos	4 mos	6 mos	12 mos	15 mos	18 mos	24 mos	4–6 yrs	11–12 yrs	13–18 yrs
Hepatitis B[1]	HepB #1 only if mother HbsAg (−)	HepB #2			HepB #3						HepB series	
Diphtheria, Tetanus, Pertussis[2]			DTaP	DTaP	DTaP		DTaP			DTaP	Td	
Haemophilus influenzae type b[3]			Hib	Hib	Hib	Hib						
Inactivated Polio			IPV	IPV		IPV				IPV		
Measles, Mumps, Rubella[4]						MMR #1				MMR #2		MMR #2
Varicella[5]						Varicella					Varicella	
Pneumococcal[6]			PCV	PCV	PCV	PCV			PCV	PCV	PPV	
Hepatitis A[7]										Hepatitis A series		
Influenza[8]						Influenza (yearly)						

----- Vaccines below this line are for selected populations -----

This schedule indicates the recommended ages for routine administration of currently licensed childhood vaccines, as of December 1, 2002, for children through age 18 years. Any dose not given at the recommended age should be given at any subsequent visit when indicated and feasible. ▨ Indicates age groups that warrant special effort to administer those vaccines not previously given. Additional vaccines may be licensed and recommended during the year. Licensed combination vaccines may be used whenever any components of the combination are indicated and the vaccine's other components are not contraindicated. Providers should consult the manufacturers' package inserts for detailed recommendations.

1. Hepatitis B vaccine (HepB). All infants should receive the first dose of hepatitis B vaccine soon after birth and before hospital discharge; the first dose may also be given by age 2 mos if the infant's mother is HBsAg negative. Only monovalent HepB can be used for the birth dose. Monovalent or combination vaccine containing HepB may be used to complete the series. Four doses of vaccine may be administered when a birth dose is given. The second dose should be given at least 4 wks after the first dose, except for combination vaccines, which cannot be administered before age 6 wks. The third dose should be given at least 16 wks after the first dose and at least 8 wks after the second dose. The last dose in the vaccination series (third or fourth dose) should not be administered before age 6 mos.

Infants born to HBsAg-positive mothers should receive HepB and 0.5 mL Hepatitis B Immune Globulin (HBIG) within 12 hrs of birth at separate sites. The second dose is recommended at age 1–2 mos. The last dose in the vaccination series should not be administered before age 6 mos. These infants should be tested for HBsAg and anti-HBs at 9–15 mos of age.

Infants born to mothers whose HBsAg status is unknown should receive the first dose of the HepB series within 12 hrs of birth. Maternal blood should be drawn as soon as possible to determine the mother's HBsAg status; if the HBsAg test is positive, the infant should receive HBIG as soon as possible (no later than age 1 wk). The second dose is recommended at age 1–2 mos. The last dose in the vaccination series should not be administered before age 6 mos.

2. Diphtheria and tetanus toxoids and acellular pertussis vaccine (DTaP). The fourth dose of DTaP may be administered as early as age 12 mos, provided 6 mos have elapsed since the third dose and the child is unlikely to return at age 15–18 mos. **Tetanus and diphtheria toxoids (Td)** is recommended at age 11–12 yrs if at least 5 yrs have elapsed since the last dose of tetanus and diphtheria toxoid-containing vaccine. Subsequent routine Td boosters are recommended every 10 yrs.

3. Haemophilus influenzae type b (Hib) conjugate vaccine. Three Hib conjugate vaccines are licensed for infant use. If PRP-OMP (PedvaxHIB or ComVax [Merck]) is administered at ages 2 and 4 mos, a dose at age 6 mos is not required. DTaP/Hib combination products should not be used for primary immunization in infants at ages 2, 4, or 6 mos, but can be used as boosters after any Hib vaccine.

4. Measles, mumps, and rubella vaccine (MMR). The second dose of MMR is recommended routinely at age 4–6 yrs but may be administered during any visit, provided at least 4 wks have elapsed since the first dose and that both doses are administered beginning at or after age 12 mos. Those who have not previously received the second dose should complete the schedule by the 11- to 12-yr-old visit.

5. Varicella vaccine. Varicella vaccine is recommended at any visit at or after age 12 mos for susceptible children (i.e., those who lack a reliable history of chickenpox). Susceptible persons aged ≥13 yrs should receive two doses, given at least 4 wks apart.

6. Pneumococcal vaccine. The heptavalent **pneumococcal conjugate vaccine (PCV)** is recommended for all children age 2–23 mos. It is also recommended for certain children age 24–59 mos. **Pneumococcal polysaccharide vaccine (PPV)** is recommended in addition to PCV for certain high-risk groups. See *MMWR* 2000;49(RR-9);1–38.

7. Hepatitis A vaccine. Hepatitis A vaccine is recommended for children and adolescents in selected states and regions, and for certain high-risk groups; consult your local public health authority. Children and adolescents in these states/regions and high-risk groups who have not been immunized against hepatitis A can begin the hepatitis A vaccination series during any visit. The two doses in the series should be administered at least 6 mos apart. See *MMWR* 1999;48(RR-12);1–37.

8. Influenza vaccine. Influenza vaccine is recommended annually for children age ≥6 mos with certain risk factors (including but not limited to asthma, cardiac disease, sickle cell disease, HIV, diabetes, and household members of persons at high risk; see *MMWR* 2002;51(RR-3);1–31), and can be administered to all others wishing to obtain immunity. In addition, healthy children age 6–23 mos are encouraged to receive influenza vaccine if feasible because children in this age group are at substantially increased risk for influenza-related hospitalizations. Children aged ≤12 yrs should receive vaccine in a dosage appropriate for their age (0.25 mI if age 6–35 mos or 0.5 mI if aged ≥3 yrs). Children aged ≤8 yrs who are receiving influenza vaccine for the first time should receive two doses separated by at least 4 wks.

For additional information about vaccines, including precautions and contraindications for immunization and vaccine shortages, please visit the National Immunization Program Website at **www.cdc.gov/nip** or call the National Immunization Information Hotline at 800-232-2522 (English) or 800-232-0233 (Spanish).

Approved by the Advisory Committee on Immunization Practices (ACIP) (www.cdc.gov/nip/acip), the American Academy of Pediatrics (www.aap.org), and the American Academy of Family Physicians (www.aafp.org).

Recommended Adult Immunization Schedule, United States, 2002–2003

Legend:
- For all persons in this group
- Catch-up on childhood vaccinations
- For persons with medical/exposure indications

Vaccine▼ Age Group ▶	19–49 yrs	50–64 yrs	≥65 yrs
Tetanus, Diphtheria (Td)*	1 dose booster every 10 years[1]		
Influenza	1 dose annually for persons with medical or occupational indications, or household contacts of persons with indications[2]	1 annual dose	
Pneumococcal (polysaccharide)	1 dose for persons with medical or other indications. (1 dose revaccination for immunosuppressive conditions)[3,4]		1 dose for unvaccinated persons[3] / 1 dose for revaccination[4]
Hepatitis B*	3 doses (0, 1–2, 4–6 mos) for persons with medical, behavioral, occupational, or other indications[5]		
Hepatitis A	2 doses (0, 6–12 mos) for persons with medical, behavioral, occupational, or other indications[6]		
Measles, Mumps, Rubella (MMR)*	1 dose if measles, mumps, or rubella vaccination history is unreliable; 2 doses for persons with occupational or other indications[7]		
Varicella*	2 doses (0, 4–8 wks) for persons who are susceptible[8]		
Meningococcal (polysaccharide)	1 dose for persons with medical or other indications[9]		

This schedule indicates the recommended age groups for routine administration of currently licensed vaccines for persons ≥19 yrs. Licensed combination vaccines may be used whenever any components of the combination are indicated and the vaccine's other components are not contraindicated. Providers should consult the manufacturers' package inserts for detailed recommendations.

Report all clinically significant postvaccination reactions to the Vaccine Adverse Event Reporting System (VAERS). Reporting forms and instructions on filing a VAERS report are available by calling 800-822-7967 or from the VAERS website at **www.vaers.org**.

For additional information about the vaccines listed above and contraindications for immunization, visit the National Immunization Program Website at **www.cdc.gov/nip/** or call the National Immunization Hotline at 800-232-2522 (English) or 800-232-0233 (Spanish).

Approved by the Advisory Committee on Immunization Practices (ACIP), and accepted by the American College of Obstetricians and Gynecologists (ACOG) and the American Academy of Family Physicians (AAFP).

Footnotes for Recommended Adult Immunization Schedule, United States, 2002–2003

1. Tetanus and diphtheria (Td)—A primary series for adults is 3 doses: the first 2 doses given at least 4 wks apart and the 3rd dose, 6–12 mos after the second. Administer 1 dose if the person had received the primary series and the last vaccination was 10 yrs ago or longer. *MMWR* 1991;40(RR-10):1–21. The ACP Task Force on Adult Immunization supports a second option: a single Td booster at age 50 yrs for persons who have completed the full pediatric series, including the teenage/young adult booster. *Guide for Adult Immunization*, ed 3, ACP 1994:20.

2. Influenza vaccination—Medical indications: chronic disorders of the cardiovascular or pulmonary systems, including asthma; chronic metabolic diseases, including diabetes mellitus, renal dysfunction, hemoglobinopathies, immunosuppression (including immunosuppression caused by medications by human immunodeficiency virus [HIV]), requiring regular medical follow-up or hospitalization during the preceding year; women who will be in the second or third trimester of pregnancy during the influenza season. Occupational indications: health care workers. Other indications: residents of nursing homes and other long-term care facilities; persons who might transmit influenza to persons at high risk (in-home caregivers to persons with medical indications, household contacts and out-of-home caregivers of children birth to 23 mos of age, or children with asthma or children with high-risk conditions); and anyone who wishes to be vaccinated. *MMWR* 2002;51(RR-3):1–31.

3. Pneumococcal polysaccharide vaccination—Medical indications: chronic disorders of the pulmonary system (excluding asthma), cardiovascular diseases, diabetes mellitus, chronic liver diseases (including liver disease as a result of alcohol abuse [e.g., cirrhosis]), chronic renal failure or nephrotic syndrome, functional or anatomic asplenia (e.g., sickle cell disease or splenectomy), immunosuppressive conditions (e.g., congenital immunodeficiency, HIV infection, leukemia, lymphoma, multiple myeloma, Hodgkin's disease, generalized malignancy, organ or bone marrow transplantation), chemotherapy with alkylating agents, antimetabolites, or long-term systemic corticosteroids. Geographic/other indications: Alaskan Natives and certain American Indian populations. Other indications: residents of nursing homes and other long-term care facilities. *MMWR* 1997;47(RR-8):1–24.

4. Revaccination with pneumococcal polysaccharide vaccine—One-time revaccination after 5 yrs for persons with chronic renal failure or nephrotic syndrome, functional or anatomic asplenia (e.g., sickle cell disease or splenectomy), immunosuppressive conditions (e.g., congenital immunodeficiency, HIV infection, leukemia, lymphoma, multiple myeloma, Hodgkin's disease, generalized malignancy, organ or bone marrow transplantation), chemotherapy with alkylating agents, antimetabolites, or long-term systemic corticosteroids. For persons 65 years and older, one-time revaccination if they were vaccinated 5 yrs or more previously and were aged less than 65 yrs at the time of primary vaccination. *MMWR* 1997;47(RR-8):1–24.

5. Hepatitis B vaccination—Medical indications: hemodialysis patients, patients who receive clotting-factor concentrates. Occupational indications: health care workers and public safety workers who have exposure to blood in the workplace, persons in training in schools of medicine, dentistry, nursing, laboratory technology, and other allied health professions. Behavioral indications: injecting drug users, persons with more than one sex partner in the previous 6 mos, persons with a recently acquired sexually transmitted disease (STD), all clients in STD clinics, men who have sex with men. Other indications: household contacts and sex partners of persons with chronic HBV infection, clients and staff of institutions for the developmentally disabled, international travelers who will be in countries with high or intermediate prevalence of chronic HBV infection for more than 6 mos, inmates of correctional facilities. *MMWR* 1991;40(RR-13):1–25. (www.cdc.gov/travel/diseases/hbv.htm)

6. Hepatitis A vaccination—For the combined HepA-HepB vaccine use 3 doses at 0, 1, 6 mos. Medical indications: persons with clotting factor disorders or chronic liver disease. Behavioral indications: men who have sex with men, users of injecting and noninjecting illegal drugs. Occupational indications: persons working with HAV-infected primates or with HAV in a research laboratory setting. Other indications: persons traveling to or working in countries that have high or intermediate endemicity of hepatitis A. *MMWR* 1999;48(RR-12):1–37. (www.cdc.gov/travel/diseases/hav.htm)

7. Measles, Mumps, Rubella vaccination (MMR)—Measles component: Adults born in or before 1957 may be considered immune to measles. Adults born in or after 1957 should receive at least one dose of MMR unless they have a medical contraindication, documentation of at least one dose or other acceptable evidence of immunity. A second dose of MMR is recommended for adults who:
- Are recently exposed to measles in an outbreak setting
- Were previously vaccinated with killed measles vaccine
- Were vaccinated with an unknown vaccine between 1963 and 1967
- Are students in postsecondary educational institutions
- Work in health care facilities
- Plan to travel internationally

Mumps component: 1 dose of MMR should be adequate for protection. Rubella component: Give 1 dose of MMR to women whose rubella vaccination history is unreliable and counsel women to avoid becoming pregnant for 4 wks after vaccination. For women of childbearing age, regardless of birth year, routinely determine rubella immunity and

counsel women regarding congenital rubella syndrome. Do not vaccinate pregnant women or those planning to become pregnant in the next 4 wks. If pregnant and susceptible, vaccinate as early in postpartum period as possible. *MMWR* 1998;47(RR-8):1–57.

8. Varicella vaccination—Recommended for all persons who do not have reliable clinical history of varicella infection, or serologic evidence of varicella-zoster virus (VZV) infection; health care workers and family contacts of immunocompromised persons, those who live or work in environments where transmission is likely (e.g., teachers of young children, day care employees, residents and staff members in institutional settings), persons who live or work in environments where VZV transmission can occur (e.g., college students, inmates and staff members of correctional institutions, military personnel), adolescents and adults living in households with children, women who are not pregnant but who may become pregnant in the future, international travelers who are not immune to infection. Note: Greater than 90% of U.S.-born adults are immune to VZV. Do not vaccinate pregnant women or those planning to become pregnant in the next 4 wks. If pregnant and susceptible, vaccinate as early in postpartum period as possible. *MMWR* 1996;45(RR-11):1–36, *MMWR* 1999;48(RR-6):1–50.

9. Meningococcal vaccine (quadrivalent polysaccharide for serogroups A, C, Y, and W-135)—Consider vaccination for persons with medical indications: adults with terminal complement component deficiencies, with anatomic or functional asplenia. Other indications: travelers to countries in which disease is hyperendemic or epidemic ("meningitis belt" of sub-Saharan Africa, Mecca, Saudi Arabia for Hajj). Revaccination at 3–5 yrs may be indicated for persons at high risk for infection (e.g., persons residing in areas in which disease is epidemic). Counsel college freshmen, especially those who live in dormitories, regarding meningococcal disease and the vaccine so that they can make an educated decision about receiving the vaccine. *MMWR* 2000;49(RR-7):1–20.
Note: The AAFP recommends that colleges should take the lead on providing education on meningococcal infection and vaccination and offer it to those who are interested. Physicians need not initiate discussion of the meningococcal quadrivalent polysaccharide vaccine as part of routine medical care.

Recommended Immunizations for Adults with Medical Conditions, United States, 2002-2003

Legend:
- ▓ For all persons in this group
- ▓ Catch-up on childhood vaccinations
- ▓ For persons with medical/exposure indications
- ▓ Contraindicated

Medical Conditions ▼ / Vaccine ▲	Tetanus-Diphtheria (Td)*	Influenza	Pneumococcal (polysaccharide)	Hepatitis B*	Hepatitis A	Measles, Mumps, Rubella, (MMR)*	Varicella*
Pregnancy		A					
Diabetes, heart disease, chronic pulmonary disease, chronic liver disease, including chronic alcoholism		B	C		D		
Congenital immunodeficiency, leukemia, lymphoma, generalized malignancy, therapy with alkylating agents, antimetabolites, radiation or large amounts of corticosteroids			E				F
Renal failure/end stage renal disease, recipients of hemodialysis or clotting factor concentrates			E	G			

Asplenia including elective splenectomy and terminal complement deficiencies										E, H, I		
HIV infection										E, J		K

A. If pregnancy is at 2nd or 3rd trimester during influenza season.

B. Although chronic liver disease and alcoholism are not indicator conditions for influenza vaccination, give 1 dose annually if the patient is ³ 50 years, has other indications for influenza vaccine, or if the patient requests vaccination.

C. Asthma is an indicator condition for influenza but not for pneumococcal vaccination.

D. For all persons with chronic liver disease.

E. Revaccinate once after 5 years or more have elapsed since initial vaccination.

F. Persons with impaired humoral but not cellular immunity may be vaccinated. *MMWR* 1999;48(RR-06):1-5.

G. Hemodialysis patients: Use special formulation of vaccine (40 ug/mL) or two 1.0 mL 20 ug doses given at one site. Vaccinate early in the course of renal failure disease. Assess antibody titers to hep B surface antigen (anti-HBs) levels annually. Administer additional doses if anti-HBs levels decline to < 10 milliinternational units (mIU)/mL.

H. Also administer meningococcal vaccine.

I. Elective splenectomy: vaccinate at least 2 weeks before surgery.

J. Vaccinate as close to diagnosis as possible when CD4 cell counts are highest.

K. Withhold MMR or other measles containing vaccines from HIV-infected persons with evidence of severe immunosuppression. *MMWR* 1996;45:603-606. *MMWR* 1992;41(RR-17):1-19.

Appendix R

SIGNS AND SYMPTOMS
OF ELECTROLYTE IMBALANCE

HYPOGLYCEMIA (excessive insulin)

Tremulousness, cold/clammy skin, mental confusion, rapid/shallow respirations, unusual fatigue, hunger, drowsiness, anxiety, headache, muscular incoordination, paresthesia of tongue/mouth/lips, hallucination, increased pulse/blood pressure, tachycardia, seizures, coma.

HYPERGLYCEMIA (insufficient insulin)

Hot/flushed/dry skin, fruity breath odor, excessive urination (polyuria), excessive thirst (polydipsia), acute fatigue, air hunger, deep/labored respirations, mental changes, restlessness, nausea, polyphagia (excessive appetite).

HYPOKALEMIA (potassium level <3.5 mEq/L)

Weakness/paresthesia of extremities, muscle cramps, nausea, vomiting, diarrhea, hypoactive bowel sounds, absent bowel sounds (paralytic ileus), abdominal distention, weak/irregular pulse, postural hypotension, difficulty breathing, disorientation, irritability.

HYPERKALEMIA (potassium level >5.0 mEq/L)

Diarrhea, muscle weakness, heaviness of legs, paresthesia of tongue/hands/feet, slow/irregular pulse, decreased blood pressure, abdominal cramps, oliguria/anuria, respiratory difficulty, cardiac abnormalities.

HYPONATREMIA (sodium level <130 mEq/L)

Abdominal cramping, nausea, vomiting, diarrhea, cold/clammy skin, poor skin turgor, tremulousness, muscle weakness, leg cramps, increased pulse rate, irritability, apprehension, hypotension, headache.

HYPERNATREMIA (sodium level >150 mEq/L)

Hot/flushed/dry skin, dry mucous membranes, fever, extreme thirst, dry/rough/red tongue, edema, restlessness, postural hypotension, oliguria.

HYPOCALCEMIA (calcium level <8.4 mg/dl)

Circumoral/peripheral numbness and tingling, muscle twitching; Chvostek's sign (facial muscle spasm; test by tapping of facial nerve anterior to earlobe, just below zygomatic arch), muscle cramping, Trousseau's sign (carpopedal spasm), seizures, arrhythmias.

HYPERCALCEMIA   (calcium level >10.2 mg/dl)

Muscle hypotonicity, incoordination, anorexia, constipation, confusion, impaired memory, slurred speech, lethargy, acute psychotic behavior, deep bone pain, flank pain.

Appendix S

TECHNIQUES OF MEDICATION ADMINISTRATION

OPHTHALMIC
Eye Drops

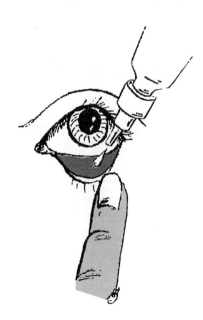

1. Wash hands.
2. Instruct patient to lie down or tilt head backward and look up.
3. Gently pull lower eyelid down until a pocket (pouch) is formed between eye and lower lid (conjunctival sac).
4. Hold dropper above pocket. Without touching tip of eye dropper to eyelid or conjunctival sac, place prescribed number of drops into the center pocket (placing drops directly onto eye may cause a sudden squeezing of eyelid, with subsequent loss of solution). Continue to hold the eyelid for a moment after the drops are applied (allows medication to distribute along entire conjunctival sac).
5. Instruct patient to close eyes gently so that medication will not be squeezed out of sac.
6. Apply gentle finger pressure to the lacrimal sac at the inner canthus (bridge of the nose, inside corner of the eye) for 1–2 min (promotes absorption, minimizes drainage into nose and throat, lessens risk of systemic absorption).

7. Remove excess solution around eye with a tissue.

8. Wash hands immediately to remove medication on hands. Never rinse eye dropper.

Eye Ointment

1. Wash hands.

2. Instruct patient to lie down or tilt head backward and look up.

3. Gently pull lower eyelid down until a pocket (pouch) is formed between eye and lower lid (conjunctival sac).

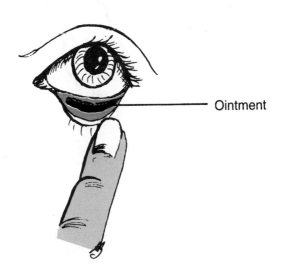

Ointment

4. Hold applicator tube above pocket. Without touching the applicator tip to eyelid or conjunctival sac, place prescribed amount of ointment (¼–½ inch) into the center pocket (placing ointment directly onto eye may cause discomfort).

5. Instruct patient to close eye for 1–2 min, rolling eyeball in all directions (increases contact area of drug to eye).

6. Inform patient of temporary blurring of vision. If possible, apply ointment just before bedtime.

7. Wash hands immediately to remove medication on hands. Never rinse tube applicator.

OTIC

1. Ear drops should be at body temperature (wrap hand around bottle to warm contents). Body temperature instillation prevents startling of patient.

2. Instruct patient to lie down with head turned so affected ear is upright (allows medication to drip into ear).

3. Instill prescribed number of drops toward the canal wall, not directly on eardrum.

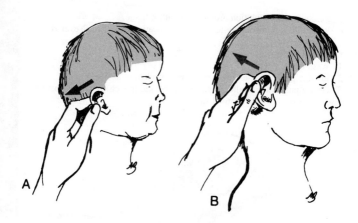

4. To promote correct placement of ear drops, pull the auricle down and posterior in children (A) and pull the auricle up and posterior in adults (B).

NASAL
Nose Drops and Sprays
1. Instruct patient to blow nose to clear nasal passages as much as possible.
2. Tilt head slightly forward if instilling nasal spray, slightly backward if instilling nasal drops.
3. Insert spray tip into 1 nostril, pointing toward inflamed nasal passages, away from nasal septum.
4. Spray or drop medication into 1 nostril while holding other nostril closed and concurrently inspire through nose to permit medication as high into nasal passages as possible.
5. Discard unused nasal solution after 3 mos.

INHALATION
Aerosol (Multidose Inhalers)
1. Shake container well before each use.
2. Exhale slowly and as completely as possible through the mouth.
3. Place mouthpiece fully into mouth, holding inhaler upright, and close lips fully around mouthpiece.
4. Inhale deeply and slowly through the mouth while depressing the top of the canister with the middle finger.
5. Hold breath as long as possible before exhaling slowly and gently.
6. When 2 puffs are prescribed, wait 2 min and shake container again before inhaling a second puff (allows for deeper bronchial penetration).
7. Rinse mouth with water immediately after inhalation (prevents mouth and throat dryness).

SUBLINGUAL
1. Administer while seated.
2. Dissolve sublingual tablet under tongue (do not chew or swallow tablet).
3. Do not swallow saliva until tablet is dissolved.

TOPICAL
1. Gently cleanse area prior to application.
2. Use occlusive dressings only as ordered.
3. Without touching applicator tip to skin, apply sparingly; gently rub into area thoroughly unless ordered otherwise.
4. When using aerosol, spray area for 3 sec from 15-cm distance; avoid inhalation.

TRANSDERMAL
1. Apply transdermal patch to clean, dry, hairless skin on upper arm or body (not below knee or elbow).
2. Rotate sites (prevents skin irritation).
3. Do not trim patch to adjust dose.

RECTAL
1. Instruct patient to lie in left lateral Sims position.
2. Moisten suppository with cold water or water-soluble lubricant.
3. Instruct patient to slowly exhale (relaxes anal sphincter) while inserting suppository well up into rectum.

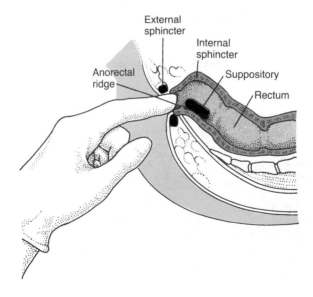

External sphincter

Internal sphincter

Anorectal ridge

Suppository

Rectum

4. Inform patient as to length of time (20–30 min) before desire for defecation occurs or <60 min for systemic absorption to occur, depending on purpose for suppository.

SUBCUTANEOUS

1. Use 25- to 27-gauge, ½- to ⅝-inch needle; 1–3 ml. Angle of insertion depends on body size: 90° if patient is obese. If patient is very thin, gather the skin at the area of needle insertion and administer also at a 90° angle. A 45° angle may be used in a patient with average weight.
2. Cleanse area to be injected with circular motion.
3. Avoid areas of bony prominence, major nerves, blood vessels.
4. Aspirate syringe before injecting (to avoid intra-arterial administration), except insulin, heparin.
5. Inject slowly; remove needle quickly.

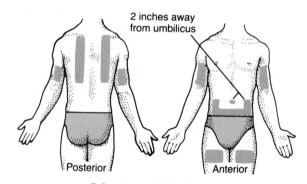

Subcutaneous injection sites

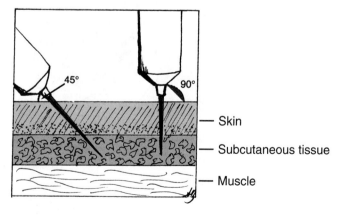

**IM
Injection Sites**

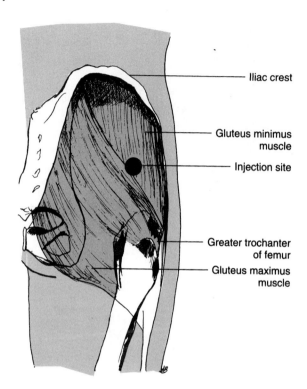

- Iliac crest
- Gluteus minimus muscle
- Injection site
- Greater trochanter of femur
- Gluteus maximus muscle

Dorsogluteal (upper outer quadrant)

1. Use this site if volume to be injected is 1–3 ml. Use 18- to 23-gauge, 1.25- to 3-inch needle. Needle should be long enough to reach the middle of the muscle.
2. Do not use this site in children <2 yrs or in those who are emaciated. Patient should be in prone position.
3. Using 90° angle, flatten the skin area using the middle and index fingers and inject between them.

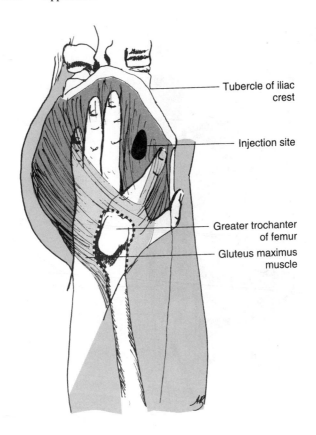

Tubercle of iliac crest

Injection site

Greater trochanter of femur

Gluteus maximus muscle

Ventrogluteal

1. Use this site if volume to be injected is 1–5 ml. Use 20- to 23-gauge, 1.25- to 2.5-inch needle. Needle should be long enough to reach the middle of the muscle.
2. Preferred site for adults, children >7 mos. Patient should be in supine lateral position.
3. Using 90° angle, flatten the skin area using the middle and index fingers and inject between them.

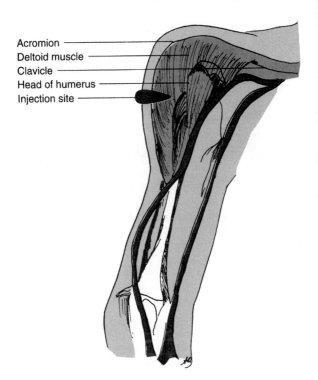

Acromion
Deltoid muscle
Clavicle
Head of humerus
Injection site

Deltoid

1. Use this site if volume to be injected is 0.5–1 ml. Use 23- to 25-gauge, ⅛- to ½-inch needle. Needle should be long enough to reach the middle of the muscle.
2. Patient may be in prone, sitting, supine, or standing position.
3. Using 90° angle or angled slightly toward acromion, flatten the skin area using the thumb and index finger and inject between them.

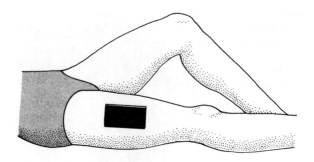

Anterolateral thigh

1. Anterolateral thigh is site of choice for infants and children <7 mos. Use 22- to 25-gauge, ⅝- to 1-inch needle.
2. Patient may be in supine or sitting position.
3. Using 90° angle, flatten the skin area using the thumb and index finger and inject between them.

Z-TRACK TECHNIQUE
1. Draw up medication with one needle, and use new needle for injection (minimizes skin staining).
2. Administer deep IM in upper outer quadrant of buttock only (dorsogluteal site).
3. Displace the skin lateral to the injection site before inserting the needle.
4. Withdraw the needle before releasing the skin.

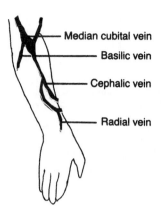

Median cubital vein

Basilic vein

Cephalic vein

Radial vein

IV

1. Medication may be given as direct IV, intermittent (piggyback), or continuous infusion.
2. Ensure that medication is compatible with solution being infused (see IV compatibility chart in this drug handbook).
3. Do not use if precipitate is present or discoloration occurs.
4. Check IV site frequently for correct infusion rate, evidence of infiltration, extravasation.

Intravenous medications are administered by the following:

1. Continuous infusing solution.
2. Piggyback (intermittent infusion).
3. Volume control setup (medication contained in a chamber between the IV solution bag and the patient).
4. Bolus dose (a single dose of medication given through an infusion line or heparin lock). Sometimes this is referred to as an IV push.

Adding medication to a newly prescribed IV bag:

1. Remove the plastic cover from the IV bag.
2. Cleanse rubber port with an alcohol swab.
3. Insert the needle into the center of the rubber port.
4. Inject the medication.
5. Withdraw the syringe from the port.
6. Gently rotate the container to mix the solution.
7. Label the IV including the date, time, medication, and dosage. It should be placed so it is easily read when hanging.
8. Spike the IV tubing and prime the tubing.

Hanging an IV piggyback (IVPB):

1. When using the piggyback method, lower the primary bag at least 6 inches below the piggyback bag.
2. Set the pump as a secondary infusion when entering the rate of infusion and volume to be infused.
3. Most piggyback medications contain 50–100 cc and usually infuse in 20–60 min, although larger-volume bags will take longer.

Administering IV medications through a volume control setup (Buretrol):

1. Insert the spike of the volume control set (Buretrol, Soluset, Pediatrol) into the primary solution container.
2. Open the upper clamp on the volume control set and allow sufficient fluid into volume control chamber.
3. Fill the volume control device with 30 cc of fluid by opening the clamp between the primary solution and the volume control device.

Administering an IV bolus dose:

1. If an existing IV is infusing, stop the infusion by pinching the tubing above the port.
2. Insert the needle into the port and aspirate to observe for a blood return.
3. If the IV is infusing properly with no signs of infiltration or inflammation, it should be patent.
4. Blood indicates that the intravenous line is in the vein.
5. Inject the medication at the prescribed rate.
6. Remove the needle and regulate the IV as prescribed.

PEDIATRIC MEDICATION INDEX

Generic names appear first, followed by brand names in parentheses.

GENERAL INDEX

D

NANDA Nursing Diagnoses

Activity intolerance
Activity intolerance, Risk for
Adjustment, Impaired
Airway clearance, Ineffective
Allergy response, Latex
Allergy response, Risk for latex
Anxiety
Anxiety, Death
Aspiration, Risk for
Attachment, Risk for impaired
   parent/infant/child
Autonomic dysreflexia
Autonomic dysreflexia, Risk for

Body image, Disturbed
Body temperature, Risk for imbalanced
Bowel incontinence
Breastfeeding, Effective
Breastfeeding, Ineffective
Breastfeeding, Interrupted
Breathing pattern, Ineffective

Cardiac output, Decreased
Caregiver role strain
Caregiver role strain, Risk for
Communication, Impaired verbal
Communication, Readiness for enhanced
Conflict, Decisional
Conflict, Parental role
Confusion, Acute
Confusion, Chronic
Constipation
Constipation, Perceived
Constipation, Risk for
Coping, Compromised family
Coping, Defensive
Coping, Disabled family
Coping, Ineffective
Coping, Ineffective community
Coping, Readiness for enhanced
Coping, Readiness for enhanced
   community
Coping, Readiness for enhanced family

Denial, Ineffective
Dentition, Impaired
Development, Risk for delayed
Diarrhea
Disuse syndrome, Risk for
Diversional activity, Deficient

Energy field, Disturbed
Environmental interpretation syndrome,
   Impaired

Failure to thrive, Adult
Falls, Risk for
Family processes: Alcoholism,
   Dysfunctional
Family processes, Interrupted
Family processes, Readiness for enhanced
Fatigue
Fear
Fluid balance, Readiness for enhanced
Fluid volume, Deficient
Fluid volume, Excess
Fluid volume, Risk for deficient
Fluid volume, Risk for imbalanced

Gas exchange, Impaired
Grieving, Anticipatory
Grieving, Dysfunctional
Growth, Risk for disproportionate
Growth and development, Delayed

Health maintenance, Ineffective
Health-seeking behaviors
Home maintenance, Impaired
Hopelessness
Hyperthermia
Hypothermia

Identity, Disturbed personal
Incontinence, Functional urinary
Incontinence, Reflex urinary
Incontinence, Stress urinary
Incontinence, Total urinary
Incontinence, Urge urinary
Incontinence, Risk for urge urinary
Infant behavior, Disorganized
Infant behavior, Readiness for enhanced
   organized
Infant behavior, Risk for disorganized
Infant feeding pattern, Ineffective
Infection, Risk for
Injury, Risk for
Injury, Risk for perioperative-positioning
Intracranial adaptive capacity, Decreased

Knowledge, Deficient
Knowledge, Readiness for enhanced

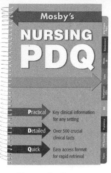
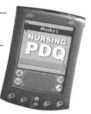